This book is to be returned on or before
the last date stamped below.

Volume I

Pediatric Otolaryngology

Edited by

CHARLES D. BLUESTONE, M.D.

Professor of Otolaryngology
University of Pittsburgh
School of Medicine
Director, Department of Otolaryngology
Children's Hospital of Pittsburgh

and

SYLVAN E. STOOL, M.D.

Professor of Otolaryngology and Pediatrics
University of Pittsburgh
School of Medicine
Director of Education, Department of Otolaryngology
Children's Hospital of Pittsburgh

SANDRA K. ARJONA, B.A.

Associate Editor

1983

W. B. SAUNDERS COMPANY
Philadelphia   London   Toronto   Mexico City   Rio de Janeiro   Sydney   Tokyo

W. B. Saunders Company: West Washington Square
Philadelphia, PA 19105

1 St. Anne's Road
Eastbourne, East Sussex BN21 3UN, England

1 Goldthorne Avenue
Toronto, Ontario M8Z 5T9, Canada

Apartado 26370—Cedro 512
Mexico 4, D.F., Mexico

Rua Coronel Cabrita, 8
Sao Cristovao Caixa Postal 21176
Rio de Janeiro, Brazil

9 Waltham Street
Artarmon, N.S.W. 2064, Australia

Ichibancho, Central Bldg., 22-1 Ichibancho
Chiyoda-Ku, Tokyo 102, Japan

Library of Congress Cataloging in Publication Data

Main entry under title:

Pediatric otolaryngology.

1. Pediatric otolaryngology.   I. Bluestone, Charles D.
II. Stool, Sylvan E.   III. Arjona, Sandra K. [DNLM:
1. Otorhinolaryngologic diseases—In infancy and childhood.
WV 100 P3703]

RF47.C4P38   618.92'09751   78-64698
ISBN 0–7216–1758–1 (set)
ISBN 0–7216–1761–1 (v. 1)
ISBN 0–7216–1762–X (v. 2)

Volume I ISBN   0–7216–1761–1
Volume II ISBN   0–7216–1762–X
SET ISBN   0–7216–1758–1

Pediatric Otolaryngology

Last digit is the print number: 9   8   7   6   5   4   3   2   1

CONTRIBUTORS

JOHN C. ADKINS, M.D.

Clinical Assistant Professor of Pediatric Surgery, University of Pittsburgh School of Medicine. Attending Surgeon, Children's Hospital of Pittsburgh, Pittsburgh, Pennsylvania.

Congenital Malformations of the Esophagus

WILLIAM A. ALONSO, M.D.

Associate Professor, Department of Surgery (Otolaryngology), University of South Florida College of Medicine, Tampa. Chairman, Department of Otolaryngology and Head and Neck Surgery, St. Joseph's Hospital, Tampa; Attending Otolaryngologist, Veterans Administration Hospital of Tampa and Tampa General Hospital, Tampa, Florida.

Injuries of the Lower Respiratory Tract

JOSEPH P. ATKINS, Jr., M.D.

Clinical Assistant Professor of Otorhinolaryngology, University of Pennsylvania School of Medicine, Philadelphia. Head, Division of Otolaryngology, Pennsylvania Hospital; Attending Physician, Graduate Hospital, Children's Hospital of Philadelphia, Veterans Hospital, Hospital of the University of Pennsylvania, Northeastern Hospital, and Albert Einstein Medical Center: Daroff Division, Philadelphia, Pennsylvania.

Embryology and Anatomy of the Neck

BYRON J. BAILEY, M.D.

Wiess Professor and Chairman, Department of Otolaryngology, The University of Texas Medical Branch, Galveston. Consultant, U.S. Public Health Service Hospital, Clear Lake City; Consultant, Brooke General Army Hospital, San Antonio, Texas.

Methods of Examination of the Larynx, Trachea, Bronchi, and Lungs

THOMAS J. BALKANY, M.D.

Clinical Assistant Professor, University of Colorado, Director, Pediatric Otolaryngology Clinic, Health Sciences Center, Denver. Chairman, Department of Otolaryngology, Porter Memorial Hospital and Swedish Medical Center, Denver, Colorado.

Injuries of the Neck

WALTER M. BELENKY, M.D.

Chief, Department of Pediatric Otolaryngology, Children's Hospital of Michigan, Detroit, Michigan.

Nasal Obstruction and Rhinorrhea

LaVONNE BERGSTROM, M.D.

Professor of Surgery, Division of Head and Neck Surgery, U.C.L.A. School of Medicine, Center for the Health Sciences, Los Angeles. Attending Physician, U.C.L.A. Center for the Health Sciences, and Wadsworth Veterans Hospital, Los Angeles; Courtesy Staff, Harbor/U.C.L.A. Medical Center, Los Angeles, and Olive View Hospital, Van Nuys, California.

Diseases of the External Ear; Diseases of the Labyrinthine Capsule

F. OWEN BLACK, M.D.

Chief, Division of Neuro-otology, Good Samaritan Medical Center, and Neurological Sciences Institute, Portland, Oregon.

Tinnitus in Children

CHARLES D. BLUESTONE, M.D.

Professor of Otolaryngology, University of Pittsburgh School of Medicine; Director, Department of Otolaryngology, Children's Hospital of Pittsburgh; Senior Staff, Eye and Ear Hospital, Pittsburgh, Pennsylvania.

Clinical Examination of the Ear; Otitis Media with Effusion, Atelectasis, and Eustachian Tube Dysfunction; Intratemporal Complications and Sequelae of Otitis Media; Intracranial Suppurative Complications of Otitis Media and Mastoiditis; Burns and Acquired Strictures of the Esophagus

SIDNEY N. BUSIS, M.D.

Clinical Professor of Otolaryngology, University of Pittsburgh School of Medicine. Senior Staff, Eye and Ear Hospital, Montefiore Hospital, and Children's Hospital of Pittsburgh; Chief of Otology, Montefiore Hospital, Pittsburgh, Pennsylvania.

Vertigo

THOMAS C. CALCATERRA, M.D.

Professor, Department of Surgery, Division of Head and Neck Surgery, U.C.L.A. School of Medicine, Los Angeles. Staff Physician, U.C.L.A. Medical Center, Los Angeles, California.

Orbital Swellings

VINCENT G. CARUSO, M.D.

Clinical Instructor in Otolaryngology, Columbia University, New York. Attending Surgeon, Southampton Hospital, Southampton, New York.

Embryology and Anatomy of the Mouth, Pharynx, and Esophagus

WERNER D. CHASIN, M.D.

Professor and Chairman of Otolaryngology, Tufts University School of Medicine, Boston. Otolaryngologist-in-Chief, Tufts–New England Medical Center; Visiting Surgeon, Boston City Hospital; Associate Surgeon, Massachusetts Eye and Ear Infirmary, Boston, Massachusetts.

Otalgia

M. MICHAEL COHEN, Jr., D.M.D., Ph.D.

Professor of Oral Pathology, Faculty of Dentistry, and Professor of Pediatrics, Faculty of Medicine, Dalhousie University, Halifax, Nova Scotia.

Craniofacial Anomalies and Syndromes

SEYMOUR R. COHEN, M.D.

Clinical Professor of Surgery, Department of Otolaryngology, University of Southern California School of Medicine, Los Angeles. Chief, Division of Otolaryngology, Children's Hospital; Chief, Section of Pediatric Otolaryngology, University of Southern California–Los Angeles County Medical Center, Los Angeles, California.

Difficulty with Swallowing

GEORGE H. CONNER, M.D.

Professor of Surgery and Chief, Division of Otolaryngology, Head and Neck Surgery, The Milton S. Hershey Medical Center of the Pennsylvania State University, Hershey, Pennsylvania.

Idiopathic Conditions of the Mouth and Pharynx

ROBIN T. COTTON, M.D., F.R.C.S.(C)

Professor, Department of Otolaryngology and Maxillofacial Surgery, University of Cincinnati College of Medicine. Director, Department of Otolaryngology and Maxillofacial Surgery, Children's Hospital Medical Center, Cincinnati, Ohio.

Stridor and Airway Obstruction; Congenital Malformations of the Larynx; Tumors of the Larynx, Trachea, and Bronchi; Velopharyngeal Insufficiency

WILLIAM N. CRAIG, Ph.D.

Superintendent, Western Pennsylvania School for the Deaf, Pittsburgh, Pennsylvania.

Education of the Deaf

WILLIAM S. CRYSDALE, M.D., F.R.C.S.(C)

Associate Professor, Department of Otolaryngology, University of Toronto. Staff Physician, Hospital for Sick Children and Wellesley Hospital; Attending Consultant, Ontario Crippled Children's Centre, Toronto, Canada.

Craniofacial Malformations and Syndromes

M. C. CULBERTSON, Jr., M.D.

Clinical Professor, Department of Otolaryngology, University of Texas Health Science Center, Southwestern Medical School, Dallas. Senior Otolaryngologist, Children's Medical Center of Dallas, Texas.

Epistaxis

RICHARD F. CURLEE, Ph.D.

Professor of Speech-Language Pathology, Department of Speech and Hearing Sciences, University of Arizona, Tucson, Arizona.

Disorders of Articulation, Voice, and Fluency

DOUGLAS D. DEDO, M.D.

Clinical Assistant Professor of Otolaryngology, University of Miami Medical School. Attending Physician, Jackson Memorial Hospital; Consultant, Veterans Administration Hospital, Miami; Active Staff, Good Samaritan Hospital and St. Mary's Hospital, West Palm Beach, and Palm Beach Gardens Hospital, North Palm Beach, Florida.

Neurogenic Diseases of the Larynx

HERBERT H. DEDO, M.D.

Professor and Vice-Chairman, Department of Otolaryngology, University of California Medical School, San Francisco. Attending Otolaryngologist, University of California Hospital, San Francisco, California.

Neurogenic Diseases of the Larynx

PHILIP J. DUBOIS, M.B., B.S., F.R.C.R., M.R.A.C.R.

Associate Professor of Radiology, Duke University Medical School, Durham. Staff Radiologist, Department of Radiology, Division of Neuroradiology, Duke University Medical Center, Durham, North Carolina.

Radiologic Aspects of Examination of the Ear

ROLAND D. EAVEY, M.D.

Assistant Professor of Otolaryngology, Harvard Medical School, Boston. Director, Pediatric Services and Emergency and Ambulatory Services, Massachusetts Eye and Ear Infirmary; Assistant in Pediatrics, Children's Service, Massachusetts General Hospital, Boston, Massachusetts.

Tracheotomy

ABRAHAM EVIATAR, M.D.

Professor of Otolaryngology, Albert Einstein College of Medicine of Yeshiva University, New York. Director of Otolaryngology, Hospital of the Albert Einstein College of Medicine; Attending Physician, Montefiore Hospital and Medical Center, Bronx Municipal Hospital Center, and North Central Bronx Hospital, New York, New York.

Neurovestibular Testing of Infants and Children

LYDIA EVIATAR, M.D.

Associate Professor of Pediatrics and Neurology, State University of New York at Stony Brook Health Sciences Center School of Medicine, Stony Brook, New York. Attending Physician, Department of Pediatrics, Division of Pediatric Neurology, Long Island Jewish/Hillside Medical Center, New Hyde Park, New York.

Neurovestibular Testing of Infants and Children

DAVID N. F. FAIRBANKS, M.D.

Clinical Professor of Otolaryngology, George Washington University School of Medicine and Health Sciences, Washington, D.C. Director, Division of Otolaryngology, George Washington University Hospital; Active Staff, Sibley Memorial Hospital, Washington, D.C.

Embryology and Anatomy of the Nose, Paranasal Sinuses, Face, and Orbit

PHILIP FIREMAN, M.D.

Professor of Pediatrics, University of Pittsburgh School of Medicine. Director, Allergy and Immunology, Children's Hospital of Pittsburgh, Pittsburgh, Pennsylvania.

Allergic Rhinitis

THOMAS J. FRIA, Ph.D.

Assistant Professor of Otolaryngology, University of Pittsburgh School of Medicine. Director, Audiology Division, Department of Otolaryngology, Children's Hospital of Pittsburgh, Pittsburgh, Pennsylvania.

Assessment of Hearing and Middle Ear Function in Children

JACOB FRIEDBERG, M.D., F.R.C.S.(C)

Assistant Professor, Department of Otolaryngology, University of Toronto. Consultant in Otolaryngology, Hospital for Sick Children, Mount Sinai Hospital, and Sunnybrook Medical Centre, Toronto, Ontario, Canada.

Hoarseness

ANTONIO G. GALVIS, M.D.

Associate Professor of Anesthesiology and Pediatrics, University of Pittsburgh School of Medicine. Director, Intensive Care Unit, Children's Hospital of Pittsburgh, Pittsburgh, Pennsylvania.

Intensive Care of Respiratory Disorders

GEORGE A. GATES, M.D.

Professor and Head, Department of Surgery, Division of Otorhinolaryngology, University of Texas Health Science Center at San Antonio, Texas.

Diseases of the Salivary Glands

EDWARD R. GRAVISS, M.D.

Associate Professor of Radiology and Pediatrics, St. Louis University School of Medicine, St. Louis. Staff Physician, Cardinal Glennon Memorial Hospital for Children, St. Louis, Missouri.

Methods of Examination of the Neck

KENNETH M. GRUNDFAST, M.D.

Associate Professor, Division of Otolaryngology, Department of Surgery, George Washington University School of Medicine, Washington, D.C. Chairman, Department of Otorhinolaryngology, Children's Hospital, National Medical Center, Washington, D.C.

Hearing Loss; Physiology of the Nose, Paranasal Sinuses, Face, and Orbit

DAVID J. HALL, D.D.S., M.Sc.O.

Clinical Assistant Professor, Department of Orthodontics, University of North Carolina School of Dentistry, Chapel Hill, North Carolina. Consultant Staff, Moore Memorial Hospital, Pinehurst, North Carolina.

Orthodontic Problems in Children

STEVEN D. HANDLER, M.D.

Assistant Professor, Department of Otorhinolaryngology and Human Communication, University of Pennsylvania School of Medicine, Philadelphia. Associate Director, Division of Otolaryngology and Human Communication, Children's Hospital of Philadelphia, Philadelphia, Pennsylvania.

Methods of Examination of the Mouth, Pharynx, and Esophagus

DONALD B. HAWKINS, M.D.

Associate Professor of Otolaryngology, University of Southern California School of Medicine, Los Angeles. Director of Pediatric Otolaryngology, Los Angeles County–University of Southern California Medical Center, Los Angeles, California.

Noninfectious Disorders of the Lower Respiratory Tract

GERALD B. HEALY, M.D.

Associate Professor of Otolaryngology, Harvard Medical School and Boston University School of Medicine; Instructor in Otolaryngology, Tufts University School of Medicine, Boston. Otolaryngologist-in-Chief, Children's Hospital Medical Center, Boston, Massachusetts.

Methods of Examination of the Nose, Paranasal Sinuses, Face, and Orbit

ARTHUR S. HENGERER, M.D.

Professor of Surgery, Chairman, Division of Otolaryngology, University of Rochester School of Medicine and Dentistry, Rochester. Staff Physician, Strong Memorial Hospital, The Genesee Hospital, Rochester General Hospital, Monroe Community Hospital, Rochester, New York.

Complications of Nasal and Sinus Infections

JAMES A. HOLLIDAY, M.D.

Clinical Assistant Professor in Surgery, Division of Otolaryngology, University of South Florida College of Medicine, Tampa. Attending Otolaryngologist, St. Joseph's Hospital, Tampa General Hospital, and Veterans Administration Hospital, Tampa, Florida.

Injuries of the Lower Respiratory Tract

BRUCE W. JAFEK, M.D.

Professor and Chairman, Department of Otolaryngology, Division of Head and Neck Surgery, University of Colorado School of Medicine, Denver. Chief of Service, University Hospital; Consultant, Denver Veterans Administration Medical Center and Fitzsimons Army Medical Center; Courtesy Staff, Rose Medical Center; Attending Staff, Denver General Hospital and Children's Hospital, Denver, Colorado, and Indian Health Service Hospital, Gallup, New Mexico.

Injuries of the Neck

JOHN K. JONES, M.D.

Clinical Assistant Professor, Department of Otorhinolaryngology and Communication Science, Baylor College of Medicine, Houston. Staff, Kelsey-Seybold Clinic, P.A., Houston, Texas.

Methods of Examination of the Larynx, Trachea, Bronchi, and Lungs

COLLIN S. KARMODY, M.D.

Senior Surgeon, New England Medical Center; Consultant in Otolaryngology, Boston City Hospital, Boston, Massachusetts.

Developmental Anomalies of the Neck

WILLIAM M. KEANE, M.D.

Clinical Assistant Professor of Otorhinolaryngology, University of Pennsylvania School of Medicine, Philadelphia. Associate Surgeon, Pennsylvania Hospital; Attending Staff, Hospital of the University of Pennsylvania, Graduate Hospital, Children's Hospital of Philadelphia, Northeastern Hospital, Albert Einstein Medical Center, Daroff Division, Philadelphia, Pennsylvania.

Embryology and Anatomy of the Neck

WILLIAM B. KIESEWETTER, M.D. (Deceased)

Former Professor of Pediatric Surgery, University of Pittsburgh. Former Surgeon-in-Chief, Children's Hospital of Pittsburgh, Pittsburgh, Pennsylvania.

Congenital Malformations of the Esophagus

JEROME O. KLEIN, M.D.

Professor of Pediatrics, Boston University School of Medicine, Boston. Director, Division of Pediatric Infectious Diseases, Boston City Hospital, Boston, Massachusetts.

Otitis Media with Effusion, Atelectasis, and Eustachian Tube Dysfunction; Intratemporal Complications and Sequelae of Otitis Media; Intracranial Suppurative Complications of Otitis Media and Mastoiditis

DAN F. KONKLE, Ph.D.

Associate Professor, Department of Otorhinolaryngology and Human Communication, University of Pennsylvania School of Medicine, Philadelphia. Director, Speech and Hearing Center, Children's Hospital of Philadelphia Pennsylvania

Hearing Aids for Children

SHARON G. KULIG, Ph.D.

Private Practice, Dallas, Texas.

Screening for Speech and Language Disorders

GERALD LEONARD, M.B., F.R.C.S., F.R.C.S.(I)

Assistant Professor of Surgery, and Director, Department of Otolaryngology and Head and Neck Surgery, University of Connecticut Health Center, Farmington, Connecticut.

Tinnitus in Children

MARTHA L. LEPOW, M.D.

Professor of Pediatrics, Albany Medical College, Albany. Attending Pediatrician, Albany Medical Center; Consulting Pediatrician, St. Peter's Hospital, Albany, New York.

Infections of the Lower Respiratory Tract

JESSICA K. LEWIS, M.D.

Clinical Assistant Professor of Pediatrics, Baylor College of Medicine, Houston. Staff Physician, Pediatric Intensive Care and Pediatric Pulmonology, Kelsey-Seybold Clinic, P.A., Houston, Texas.

Intensive Care of Respiratory Disorders

JOSE A. LIMA, M.D.

Assistant Professor of Otolaryngology, St. Louis University School of Medicine, St. Louis. Section Chief, Pediatric Otolaryngology. Cardinal Glennon Memorial Hospital for Children; Staff Physician, St. Louis University Medical Center Hospitals, Deaconess Hospital, St. Mary's Health Center, Compton Hill Medical Center, Bethesda General Hospital, and St. Louis City Hospital, St. Louis, Missouri.

Methods of Examination of the Neck

J. THOMAS LOVE, M.D.

Assistant Professor, University of Texas Medical School at Galveston. Staff Physician, St. Mary's Hospital and John Sealy Hospital, Galveston; County Memorial Hospital and Danforth Hospital, Texas City, Texas.

Embryology and Anatomy of the Larynx, Trachea, Bronchi, and Lungs

FRANK E. LUCENTE, M.D.

Associate Professor, Department of Otolaryngology, Mount Sinai School of Medicine, New York. Director, Department of Otolaryngology, City Hospital Center at Elmhurst; Associate Attending Physician, Mount Sinai Hospital, New York, New York.

Facial Pain and Headache

ROBERT H. MAISEL, M.D.

Associate Professor of Otolaryngology, University of Minnesota School of Medicine, Minneapolis. Chief of Otolaryngology, Hennepin County Medical Center, Minneapolis, Minnesota.

Injuries of the Mouth, Pharynx, and Esophagus

FRANK I. MARLOWE, M.D.

Professor of Surgery (Otolaryngology), Medical College of Pennsylvania, Philadelphia. Chief, Division of Otolaryngology, Presbyterian–University of Pennsylvania Medical Center. Consultant, Otolaryngology and Maxillofacial Surgery, Naval Regional Medical Center, Philadelphia, Pennsylvania.

Injuries of the Nose, Facial Bones, and Paranasal Sinuses

ROBERT HENRY MATHOG, M.D.

Professor and Chairman, Wayne State University School of Medicine, Detroit. Chief of Otolaryngology, Harper-Grace Hospitals and Detroit Receiving Hospital; Staff Physician, Children's Hospital of Michigan and Hutzel Hospital; Consulting Physician, Veterans Administration Medical Center (Allen Park), Detroit, Michigan.

Injuries of the Mouth, Pharynx, and Esophagus

JACK MATTHEWS, Ph.D., D.Sc.

Professor of Speech, University of Pittsburgh, Pittsburgh, Pennsylvania.

Disorders of Language

MARK MAY, M.D.

Clinical Associate Professor, Department of Otolaryngology and Head and Neck Surgery, University of Pittsburgh School of Medicine. Chief of Division of Ear, Nose, and Throat, Shadyside Hospital; Attending Physician, Eye and Ear Hospital, and Children's Hospital of Pittsburgh; Consultant, Presbyterian Hospital, Magee Women's Hospital, Montefiore Hospital, and Veterans Administration Hospital, Pittsburgh, Pennsylvania.

Facial Paralysis in Children; Neck Masses

BETTY JANE McWILLIAMS, Ph.D.

Professor, Speech Pathology; Director, Cleft Palate Center, University of Pittsburgh, Pittsburgh, Pennsylvania.

Multiple Speech Disorders (Cleft Palate and Cerebral Palsy Speech)

ARLEN D. MEYERS, M.D.

Associate Professor of Otolaryngology, University of Colorado Health Sciences Center, Denver. Chief of Otolaryngology, Denver. Children's Hospital and Attending Physician, Denver Veterans Administration Hospital, Denver, Colorado.

Aspiration

AAGE R. MØLLER, Ph.D.

Research Professor of Otolaryngology and Physiology, University of Pittsburgh School of Medicine, Pittsburgh, Pennsylvania.

Physiology of the Ear

ROBERT D. MUNDELL, Ph.D.

Professor and Chairman, Department of Anatomy and Histology, School of Dental Medicine, University of Pittsburgh. Consulting Staff, Children's Hospital of Pittsburgh, Pittsburgh, Pennsylvania.

Phylogenetic Aspects and Embryology of Craniofacial Growth

EUGENE N. MYERS, M.D.

Professor and Chairman, Department of Otolaryngology, University of Pittsburgh School of Medicine; Professor, Department of Diagnostic Services, University of Pittsburgh School of Dental Medicine. Chief, Department of Otolaryngology, Eye and Ear Hospital; Consultant in Otolaryngology, Veterans Administration Hospital, and Children's Hospital of Pittsburgh, Pittsburgh, Pennsylvania.

Tumors of the Neck

NIZAR S. NUWAYHID, M.D.

Clinical Assistant Professor of Otolaryngology, American University, Beirut, Lebanon.

Velopharyngeal Insufficiency

MICHAEL J. PAINTER, M.D.

Associate Professor of Neurology and Pediatrics, University of Pittsburgh. Chief, Division of Child Neurology, Children's Hospital of Pittsburgh, Pittsburgh, Pennsylvania.

Neurologic Disorders of the Mouth, Pharynx, and Esophagus

JACK L. PARADISE, M.D.

Professor of Pediatrics and Community Medicine, University of Pittsburgh School of Medicine. Medical Director, Ambulatory Care Center, Children's Hospital of Pittsburgh, Pittsburgh, Pennsylvania.

Primary Care of Infants and Children with Cleft Palate; Tonsillectomy and Adenoidectomy

SIMON C. PARISIER, M.D.

Professor of Clinical Otolaryngology, Mt. Sinai School of Medicine. Attending Otolaryngologist, Mt. Sinai Hospital, New York, New York.

Injuries of the Ear and Temporal Bone

JAMES L. PARKIN, M.D.

Professor and Chairman, Division of Otolaryngology—Head and Neck Surgery, University of Utah School of Medicine, Salt Lake City. Staff Physician, University Hospital, Salt Lake City; Consultant, Veterans Administration Hospital, Primary Children's Hospital, and Shriner's Crippled Children's Hospital, Salt Lake City, Utah.

Congenital Malformations of the Mouth and Pharynx

STEPHEN I. PELTON, M.D.

Assistant Professor of Pediatrics, Boston University School of Medicine. Assistant Director, Department of Pediatrics, Boston City Hospital, Boston, Massachusetts.

Cervical Adenopathy

WILLIAM P. POTSIC, M.D.

Assistant Professor of Otorhinolaryngology and Human Communication, University of Pennsylvania School of Medicine, Philadelphia. Director,

Division of Otorhinolaryngology and Human Communication; Children's Hospital of Philadelphia, Philadelphia, Pennsylvania.

Methods of Examination of the Mouth, Pharynx, and Esophagus

DANIEL D. RABUZZI, M.D.

Professor and Chairman, Department of Otolaryngology, New York Medical College and New York Eye and Ear Infirmary, Valhalla, New York.

Complications of Nasal and Sinus Infections

ROBERT RAPP, D.D.S., F.R.C.D.(C)

Professor and Chairman, Department of Pedodontics, School of Dental Medicine, University of Pittsburgh. Chief of Dentistry, Children's Hospital of Pittsburgh, Pittsburgh, Pennsylvania.

Dental and Gingival Disorders

TIMOTHY J. REICHERT, M.D.

Chief, Division of Otolaryngology, St. Luke's Hospital; Department of Otolaryngology, St. John's Mercy Medical Center, St. Louis, Missouri.

Physiology of the Mouth, Pharynx, and Esophagus; Foreign Bodies of the Larynx, Trachea, and Bronchi

JAMES S. REILLY, M.D.

Assistant Professor of Otolaryngology, University of Pittsburgh School of Medicine. Full-Time Staff Surgeon, Children's Hospital of Pittsburgh; Associate Staff Surgeon, Eye and Ear Hospital, Pittsburgh, Pennsylvania.

Stridor and Airway Obstruction; Congenital Malformations of the Larynx

KEITH H. RIDING, M.D., F.R.C.S.(C)

Clinical Assistant Professor of Otolaryngology, University of British Columbia, Vancouver. Director, ENT Department, Children's Hospital; Attending Otolaryngologist; Vancouver General Hospital, Vancouver, British Columbia, Canada.

Burns and Acquired Strictures of the Esophagus

STEWART R. ROOD, M.P.H., Ph.D.

Assistant Professor, Department of Otolaryngology, University of Pittsburgh School of Medicine. Adjunct Medical Staff, Eye and Ear Hospital, Pittsburgh, Pennsylvania.

Anatomy and Physiology of Speech

ROBERT J. RUBEN, M.D.

Professor and Chairman, Department of Otorhinolaryngology, Albert Einstein College of Medicine of Yeshiva University. Staff Physician, Montefiore Hospital and Medical Center, Hospital of the Albert Einstein College of Medicine, Bronx Municipal Hospital Center, and North Central Bronx Hospital, New York, New York.

Diseases of the Inner Ear and Sensorineural Deafness

ISAMU SANDO, M.D., D.M.S.

Professor of Otolaryngology and Pathology, Department of Otolaryngology, University of Pittsburgh School of Medicine, Pittsburgh, Pennsylvania.

Congenital Anomalies of the External and Middle Ear

EBERHARDT K. SAUERLAND, M.D.

Professor of Anatomy, Department of Anatomy, University of Texas Medical School at San Antonio. Staff Physician, Department of Radiology, Wilford Hall Medical Center, Lackland Air Force Base, San Antonio, Texas.

Embryology and Anatomy of the Mouth, Pharynx, and Esophagus

JOYCE A. SCHILD, M.D.

Professor in Otolaryngology—Head and Neck Surgery, University of Illinois College of Medicine, Chicago. Attending Physician, University of Illinois Hospital; Consultant Staff, Children's Memorial Hospital, Chicago, Illinois.

Congenital Malformations of the Trachea and Bronchi

MELVIN D. SCHLOSS, M.D., F.R.C.S.(C)

Associate Professor, Department of Otolaryngology, McGill University, Montreal. Director, Division of Otolaryngology, Montreal Children's Hospital, Montreal, Quebec, Canada.

Otorrhea

VICTOR L. SCHRAMM, Jr., M.D.

Associate Professor, Department of Otolaryngology, University of Pittsburgh School of Medicine. Chief, Department of Otolaryngology, Veterans Administration Hospital. Associate Physician, Department of Otolaryngology, Eye and Ear Hospital, Pittsburgh, Pennsylvania.

Tinnitus in Children; Tumors of the Nose, Paranasal Sinuses, and Nasopharynx; Neck Masses

DANIEL M. SCHWARTZ, Ph.D.

Associate Professor and Chairman of Audiology, Department of Otorhinolaryngology and Human Communication, University of Pennsylvania School of Medicine, Philadelphia. Director, Speech and Hearing Center, Hospital of the University of Pennsylvania, Philadelphia, Pennsylvania.

Hearing Aids for Children

· M. WILLIAM SCHWARTZ, M.D.

Associate Professor of Pediatrics, University of Pennsylvania School of Medicine, Philadelphia. Senior Physician, Section of General Pediatrics and Nephrology, Children's Hospital of Philadelphia, Pennsylvania.

Oropharyngeal Manifestations of Systemic Disease

ALLAN B. SEID, M.D.

Associate Clinical Professor of Surgery, Division of Otolaryngology and Head and Neck Surgery, University of California, San Diego. Attending

Physician, Children's Hospital and Health Center, Mercy Hospital, and University Hospital, San Diego, California.

Tumors of the Larynx, Trachea, and Bronchi

EDWARD M. SEWELL, M.D.

Professor of Pediatrics, Jefferson Medical College, Thomas Jefferson University, Philadelphia. Attending Physician, Thomas Jefferson University Hospital, Philadelphia, Pennsylvania.

Cough

ROBERT S. SHAPIRO, M.D., F.R.C.S.(C)

Associate Professor of Otolaryngology, McGill University, Montreal. Attending Otolaryngologist, Montreal Children's Hospital, Montreal, Quebec, Canada.

Foreigh Bodies of the Nose

RALPH L. SHELTON, Ph.D.

Professor of Speech Pathology, Department of Speech and Hearing Sciences, University of Arizona, Tucson, Arizona.

Disorders of Articulation, Voice, and Fluency

PAUL A. SHURIN, M.D.

Assistant Professor of Pediatrics, Case Western Reserve University School of Medicine, Cleveland. Associate Director, Pediatric Infectious Disease Service, Cleveland Metropolitan General Hospital, Cleveland, Ohio.

Inflammatory Diseases of the Nose and Paranasal Sinuses

WILLIAM K. SIEBER, M.D.

Clinical Professor of Surgery, University of Pittsburgh School of Medicine. Senior Staff, Surgery, Children's Hospital of Pittsburgh; Active Staff, Department of Surgery, Presbyterian Hospital, West Penn Hospital, and E. Suburban Hospital; Courtesy Staff, Mercy Hospital, Pittsburgh, Pennsylvania.

Functional Abnormalities of the Esophagus

KENNETH B. SKOLNICK, M.D.

Clinical Instructor, Department of Otolaryngology, University of Pittsburgh School of Medicine. Staff Physician, Ear and Eye Hospital, Sewickley Valley Hospital, Alliquippa Hospital, and Medical Center of Beaver County, Pennsylvania.

Tumors of the Neck

F. T. SPORCK, M.D.

Clinical Assistant Professor, Department of Otolaryngology, West Virginia University School of Medicine, Morgantown. Staff Physician, St. Francis Hospital and Charleston Area Medical Center, Charleston, West Virginia.

Congenital Malformations of the Nose and Paranasal Sinuses

P. M. SPRINKLE, M.D.

Professor and Chairman, Department of Otolaryngology, West Virginia University School of Medicine. Chief, Department of Otolaryngology, West Virginia University Medical Center, Morgantown, West Virginia.

Congenital Malformations of the Nose and Paranasal Sinuses

SYLVAN E. STOOL, M.D.

Professor of Otolaryngology and Pediatrics, University of Pittsburgh School of Medicine. Director of Education, Department of Otolaryngology, Children's Hospital of Pittsburgh, Pittsburgh, Pennsylvania.

Phylogenetic Aspects and Embryology of Craniofacial Growth; Postnatal Craniofacial Growth and Development; Craniofacial Anomalies and Syndromes; Foreign Bodies of the Pharynx and Esophagus; Tracheotomy

JOHN R. STRAM, M.D.

Assistant Clinical Professor of Otolaryngology, Boston University School of Medicine; Chairman, Committee on Otolaryngologic Pathology, American Academy of Ophthalmology and Otolaryngology, 1974–1979. Consultant, Veteran's Administration Hospital (Jamaica Plains), Boston, Massachusetts.

Tumors of the Ear and Temporal Bone

SUSUMU SUEHIRO, M.D.

Assistant Professor, Department of Otolaryngology, Kyoto University Faculty of Medicine, Kyoto, Japan. Chief, Department of Otolaryngology, Amagasaki Hospital, Amagasaki, Hyogo, Japan.

Congenital Anomalies of the External and Middle Ear

DAVID W. TEELE, M.D.

Associate Professor of Pediatrics, Boston University School of Medicine. Director, In-Patient Pediatrics, Boston City Hospital, Boston, Massachusetts.

Sore Throat in Childhood: Diagnosis and Management; Inflammatory Diseases of the Mouth and Pharynx

I. DAVID TODRES, M.D.

Associate Professor of Anesthesia (Pediatrics), Harvard Medical School, Boston. Director, Pediatric Intensive Care Unit, Massachusetts General Hospital, Boston, Massachusetts.

Respiratory Disorders of the Newborn

JAMES M. TOOMEY, M.D., D.M.D.

Attending Staff, Sturdy Memorial Hospital, Attleboro, and Morton Hospital, Taunton, Massachusetts.

Tumors of the Mouth and Pharynx

MYLES G. TURTZ, M.D.

Associate Professor of Otorhinolaryngology and Bronchoesophagology, Temple University School of Medicine; Visiting Professor, Hahnemann

Medical College, Philadelphia. Chief of Pediatric Ear, Nose, and Throat Service; Chairman, Board of Managers, St. Christopher's Hospital for Children, Philadelphia, Pennsylvania.

Foreign Bodies of the Pharynx and Esophagus

DONALD W. WARREN, D.D.S., Ph.D.

Kenan Professor and Chairman, Department of Dental Ecology, and Professor, Department of Surgery, University of North Carolina at Chapel Hill Schools of Dentistry and Medicine. Attending Physician, Hospital Dental Service, North Carolina Memorial Hospital, Chapel Hill, North Carolina.

Orthodontic Problems in Children

RICHARD C. WEBSTER, M.D.

Lecturer on Otolaryngology, Harvard Medical School, Boston. Chief of Plastic Service, Melrose-Wakefield Hospital, Melrose; Associate Surgeon in Plastic and Reconstructive Surgery and in Otolaryngology, Massachusetts Eye and Ear Infirmary, Boston, Massachusetts.

Cosmetic Problems Involving the Face; Cosmetic Problems Involving the Nose

LINTON A. WHITAKER, M.D.

Professor of Surgery (Plastic) and Director, Craniofacial Program, University of Pennsylvania School of Medicine, Philadelphia. Chief of Plastic Surgery, Children's Hospital of Philadelphia; Attending Surgeon, Hospital of the University of Pennsylvania, Philadelphia, Pennsylvania.

Principles and Methods of Management of Craniofacial Malformations

MATTHEW L. WONG, M.D.

Clinical Assistant Professor, Department of Otolaryngology, University of Washington, Seattle. Otologist, Providence Medical Center, Swedish Hospital Medical Center, Virginia Mason Hospital, and Children's Orthopedic Hospital and Medical Center, Seattle, Washington.

Embryology and Developmental Anatomy of the Ear

RAYMOND P. WOOD, II, M.D.

Associate Professor and Vice-Chairman, Department of Otolaryngology–Head and Neck Surgery, University of Colorado Health Sciences Center, Denver. Attending Otolaryngologist, University Hospital, Denver; Consultant in Otolaryngology, National Jewish Hospital and Asthma Center, Denver, Colorado.

Congenital Anomalies of the External and Middle Ear

ROBERT E. WOOD, Ph.D., M.D.

Associate Professor of Pediatrics, Case/Western Reserve University, Cleveland. Associate Pediatrician, Rainbow Babies' and Children's Hospital, Cleveland, Ohio.

Physiology of the Larynx, Airways, and Lungs

FOREWORD

Pediatric Otolaryngology has finally come of age. It is now firmly established and widely recognized as an important and legitimate subspecialty. Nearly two decades ago in a Foreword to the Symposium on Ear, Nose and Throat Problems in *Pediatric Clinics of North America* (1962) I stated:

Pediatric Otolaryngology has not as yet attained the status of a true subspecialty and the chances are that it may never do so. Nevertheless, each year finds certain otolaryngologists among us devoting increasing time and consideration to those problems peculiar to infancy and childhood. . . . Only a relatively few years ago the term "Pediatric Surgery" was unknown, as there had never been any question but that the general surgeon was capable and adequately equipped to care for all surgical ailments in infancy and childhood. It gradually became apparent, however, . . . that customary methods of treatment were often not successfully adaptable to the very young age-group, and mortality here was notoriously much higher than it should have been when compared to similar conditions in the adult. . . . Many other conditions were considered totally inoperable, simply because of the age barrier.

From our vantage point, the passage of time has more than justified a subspecialty devoted to the general surgery of infancy and childhood. Its establishment has improved methods of diagnosis and treatment and has led to the development of more appropriate and successful techniques for use in treating the very young, thereby considerably diminishing morbidity and mortality at this stage of life. I am very happy that my original fears proved unfounded, because Pediatric Otolaryngology later assumed a similar challenge and now vindicates its own existence by its rapid advances in this particular area of the broad field of ear, nose, and throat disease and has already taken its rightful place as a true subspecialty.

For several decades now, the programs of the annual and sectional meetings of the various specialty societies have contained more and more essays on otolaryngologic problems peculiar to infancy and childhood. When a student or resident, however, wished more information on a specific problem, he had to go back to the literature and survey those original papers. To be sure, for some time there had been many excellent textbooks on otolaryngology, but little space was devoted to the important area of congenital malformations or to special techniques so essential in treating the very young. Over the years it was felt that a compact source of the rapidly accumulating knowledge relating to specific pediatric conditions should be available to students, residents, and pediatricians who knew little about otolaryngology, as well as to otolaryngologists who dealt only very occasionally with pediatric problems.

In 1960 J. F. Birrell, Consultant Ear, Nose and Throat Surgeon at The Royal Hospital for Sick Children in Edinburgh, authored the first such volume, but it was primarily a compendium, considerably abridged, and unfortunately covered the conditions in little depth. However, it remained the only pediatric otolaryngologic textbook of its kind until 1972 when *Pediatric Otolaryngology* by Ferguson and Kendig was published.

When the publishers were contemplating a much-needed second edition of Dr. Edwin L. Kendig's very well-received volume entitled *Disorders of the Respiratory Tract in Children* (to which I had contributed several chapters on otolaryngologic problems), Mr. Robert B. Rowan, Vice-President of W. B. Saunders Publishing Company, suggested that the otolaryngologic material be very greatly expanded and become the basis of a separate volume entitled *Pediatric Otolaryngology* and be a companion to *Pulmonary Disorders* under the covering title *Disorders of the Respiratory Tract in Children*. The publishers felt that such a textbook should be edited by one who for over 25 years had been devoting full time to this special branch of otolaryngology. They graciously asked me to assume that very challenging responsibility.

My first hope and inclinations were to use for this purpose many of the papers I had presented before medical organizations. On rereading them, however, it was readily apparent that a new approach would be essential, because those papers were for the most part oriented to groups of highly trained specialists and would not be practical or appropriate for use by the average medical student, resident, or practitioner. Fortunately, many of my friends and colleagues responded to the call for assistance, and *Pediatric Otolaryngology* was finally published in 1972 and five years later translated in its entirety into Spanish for use in Latin America (*Otorinolaringología Pediátrica*). After 40 years at Children's Hospital Medical Center in Boston the inevitable time for my retirement came in 1974, so the publisher's request for the editing of a second edition of *Pediatric Otolaryngology* unfortunately had to be declined. Many modifications of our first, but heroic, attempt to create a source book for otolaryngology of the young were going to be indicated the second time around and extensive revisions would become necessary. I am happy that younger and better-trained editors have been recruited to accomplish this monumental task that produced the present two volumes. The new *Pediatric Otolaryngology* is larger in scope, more comprehensive, and more detailed than its predecessor, and it has been well updated for this rapidly changing and expanding field. Perhaps the original volume served its purpose by blazing the trail!

During the past 40 years there have been many amazing advances in otolaryngology. It is hard to believe that I was trained to perform tonsillectomies on patients sitting upright in a specialized chair, under insufflation ether anesthesia, with their heads held by anesthetists, who pumped bellows to force the ether vapor from the Richardson bottle that regulated its concentration. Lipiodol was used for bronchograms, performed with the child under ether anesthesia and lying on the x-ray table under a poorly shielded tube that buzzed and sparked when activated. A wet towel held over the mouth and nose was supposed to prevent sparks from igniting the ether vapor, and luck was apparently with us, as we had no accidents!

In my earlier days chemotherapeutic and antibiotic drugs were nonexistent and infections could be treated only symptomatically, except for streptococcal infections, which sometimes responded a bit to immune-transfusions, and pneumococcal infections, which were treated with type-specific sera. This meant, however, that a laborious typing of the organism had to be done first. Staphylococcal infections were untreatable and carried an extremely high mortality. The bulk of the otolaryngologist's practice in those days was the treatment of infections and their serious complications. Transfusions were done by the direct method from donor to recipient, and processed blood and bloodbanks were never even envisioned. Mastoidectomies were frequently performed on seriously ill patients with meningitis and/or septicemia as emergency procedures during the middle of the night as soon as the patient was admitted. The middle fossa dura was exposed, the jugular vein ligated, the lateral sinus opened, and any thrombus removed. Mortality was high. Osteomyelitis of the frontal bone and brain abscess frequently followed sinus infections due to swimming, and every fall epidemics of poliomyelitis kept the otolaryngologist busy with tracheotomies and respirators. Now that dreaded scourge has mercifully been eliminated and fortunately is only a nightmare of the past.

A new day has finally dawned, and undoubtedly the next decade will bring even greater progress than the past, marvellous though it has been. Pediatric otolaryngology, I am sure, will be on the frontier of that progress.

The evolution of pediatric otolaryngology as a true subspecialty in my own lifetime is a dream fulfilled. It is most exciting, and also very gratifying, to learn that there are now over a score of otolaryngologists who devote over 80 per cent of their professional time to this new subspecialty. This fact augurs well for the infant and young child of the future, as well as of today, and assures him of a much more normal and productive life of health and happiness and freedom from crippling disease, as more and more of the previously considered "untreatable" conditions are now being cured.

CHARLES F. FERGUSON
Senior Otolaryngologist Emeritus
Children's Hospital Medical Center
Boston, Massachusetts

PREFACE

Just as otolaryngology has grown into an important and broad specialty, so has increasing interest in its various subspecialties proportionately expanded. Diseases and disorders of the head and neck and of the air and food passages are the most common conditions encountered by health care professionals who care for children. Therefore, interest in pediatric otolaryngology has progressively increased during the past decade, which has resulted in an information explosion. As clinicians and teachers, we have been aware that there has been a need for a comprehensive text that would embody the principles of otolaryngology and pediatrics. We undertook the task of writing and editing this book in order to fill this perceived need. Since the areas covered by such a text cannot be adequately written by only one or two pediatric otolaryngologists, we have selected the most knowledgeable and experienced authors for the chapters, and since the field is so diverse, we have asked specialists not only in medicine, but in other disciplines as well, to contribute their expertise.

It is the hope of the editors and publishers that this textbook will provide as complete a coverage of the field of pediatric otolaryngology as possible, with an authoritative, discriminating, precise, and concise presentation of what is currently known about the diseases of the ear, nose, and throat in infants and children. The text is geared to medical students and to house staff officers in otolaryngology, pediatrics, and primary medicine, as well as to the practicing otolaryngologist, pediatrician, generalist, and other health professionals. It is not the intent of the editors that this book should compete with existing texts in pediatrics or otolaryngology, but rather that it should provide a single reference source oriented to pediatric otolaryngology. With this concept in mind, there has been no attempt to provide extensive details of surgical techniques that have been covered adequately in texts and atlases. The emphasis is on concepts of surgical management rather than on explicit descriptions of techniques. At the end of each chapter, there are, in addition to the bibliography, selected references, which are annotated. Included are the references that are considered to have the best descriptions of surgical procedures that are applicable to children.

We believe that the text is unique in that we have combined the problem-oriented approach with an authoritative, comprehensive presentation of what is currently known about disorders of the head and neck and air and food passages in childhood. This has been accomplished by including several chapters early in each section that present the differential diagnoses of the common presenting signs and symptoms. The reader can then turn to the comprehensive review of the condition in the appropriate chapter. The length of these chapters varies considerably, since we have attempted to emphasize the conditions that are most common in children. Otitis media and its related conditions have been extensively covered in this text, since this disease is the most common condition otolaryngologists and primary care physicians encounter in children.

It is the hope of the editors of this text that the health care of infants and children will be improved by those physicians who increase their knowledge by using this book as a reference.

CHARLES D. BLUESTONE
SYLVAN E. STOOL

ACKNOWLEDGMENTS

In a work of this scope, the editors and contributors receive help from many sources. It is difficult to adequately acknowledge each of these; however, first, we wish to acknowledge Sandra Arjona's dedication and commitment to the coordination and collation of the entire manuscript, from initial contact with the contributors down through all editorial phases. She has orchestrated this most all-encompassing, arduous, and mammoth task with efficiency, skill, and a great sense of humor.

Manuscripts and revisions were graciously prepared and submitted by the various contributing authors. Assistance with reading of galleys was cheerfully provided by Suzanne Stewart. Diana Mathis has copy-edited the entire text so that it would be cohesive in spite of the fact that there are a large number of contributors.

Artwork provides visual emphasis to the text. Jon Coulter created many excellent illustrations, while Robert Coulter provided valuable photographic support. We have been delighted with their contributions. Additional high-quality photography has been provided by Norman Rabinovitz and his staff at Children's Hospital of Pittsburgh.

A number of colleagues have been most helpful in reviewing chapters and providing advice—Jack L. Paradise, M.D., participated in the early planning for the book. In Pittsburgh, members of the Departments of Pediatrics, Infectious Disease, Neurosurgery, and Radiology have been most accommodating.

The book is in memoriam to William B. Kiesewetter, M.D. (1915–1981), who was both a teacher and a colleague during his tenure as Chief of Surgical Services at Children's Hospital of Pittsburgh, from 1955 to June, 1981. His contribution to this book is living proof of his expertise.

Brian Decker initiated our contact with the W. B. Saunders Company and gave impetus to the production; Shauna Garay followed him for a period; and finally, Mary Cowell, our current editor, has maintained interest and offered all possible assistance to complete the project.

In any effort as time-consuming as this, the authors' families must provide support—and ours have made this task easier by their understanding and encouragement throughout.

CHARLES D. BLUESTONE
SYLVAN E. STOOL

CONTENTS

VOLUME I

Chapter 17

INTRATEMPORAL COMPLICATIONS AND SEQUELAE OF
OTITIS MEDIA 513

Charles D. Bluestone, M.D., and Jerome O. Klein, M.D.

Section I

CRANIOFACIAL GROWTH, DEVELOPMENT, AND MALFORMATIONS

Chapter 1

PHYLOGENETIC ASPECTS AND EMBRYOLOGY

Sylvan E. Stool, M.D.
Robert D. Mundell, Ph.D.

It is appropriate that the first chapter of a text on pediatric otolaryngology should be devoted to the broad subject of the development of the craniofacial complex. This is the major region that is involved in diseases of the ear, nose, and throat and which serves as the entryway to the air and food passages. The more we know about the embryology, growth, and development of the face and about the various factors involved in normal variations and anomalies of this region, the better will be our understanding of the many otorhinolaryngologic disorders affecting infants and children.

The first region that the clinician and, indeed, the layman usually inspect on encountering another person is the face. Usually, an impression of the face and an evaluation of the facial type and facial expression are made instantly. Following this, the general body type and posture are noted, and the degree of interpersonal communication is ascertained. DeMyer (1975) states,

One glance at the patient's face may settle the diagnostic issue, an Augenblick, or eyeblink diagnosis, in which the clinician immediately knows what syndrome the patient has. I am neither describing nor advocating a hasty, careless snap judgment, I am merely pointing out that the clinician, utilizing the pattern recognition attributes of his own brain, sometimes can diagnose abnormal faces with the speed and certainty with which he distinguishes the faces of family and friends.

The clinician may decide, on the basis of certain facial features, that the patient has a recognizable syndrome that identifies him with a group of similar patients more than it does with his own family. The face and the cranial configuration, therefore, contribute immeasurably to the total or *gestalt* diagnosis.

One of the characteristics any observer can appreciate is the great variation in the appearance of the normal face. In addition, there are certain characteristics that we associate with facial types almost on an instinctive basis. These variations and expectations in facial types can be appreciated by examining Figure 1–1, which is a sketch of a group of Caucasian children from the same grammar school class. The variations in facial configuration are obvious: there are round, oval, and triangular faces. Individual characteristics of the eyes and nose also show tremendous variation. A diagnosis of an abnormality that is based on facial configuration may be very difficult to make unless the observer knows what hereditary background the individual represents, although there are some abnormalities, such as Down syndrome, that are expressed in similar facial features regardless of the child's origin. Thus, although we recognize great variations in facial type as being normal, we also instinctively recognize other features as being abnormal in a particular individual, based on our ability to assess facial patterns in the contexts of age, race, and hereditary background.

The human craniofacial complex is the result of at least 500 million years of progressive development. These structures, which developed in the anterior portion of an an-

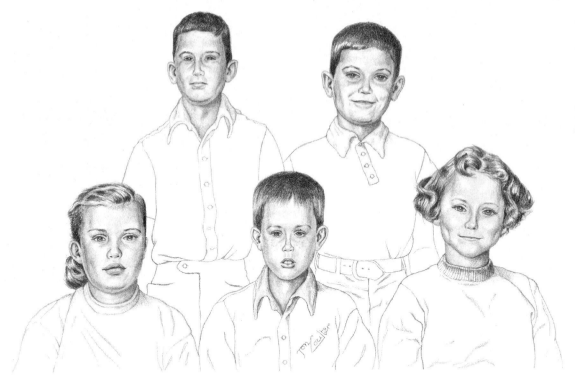

Figure 1–1 Children from a sixth grade class. Note the variation of facial types, even though all are the same age and race.

cestral organism, were designed to obtain and maintain initial contact with the environment. The pattern initially developed in the invertebrates was continued in the vertebrates, and, according to Krogman (1974), there can be no doubt that the craniofacial complex from its beginning was a multistructured, highly integrated, diversely systematized center for almost every life need of the organism. In the development of the craniofacial complex in the human embryo and fetus, the form and functions that have evolved over many millions of years take shape in fantastically rapid sequence. Those structures that required many millions of years of natural selection to evolve may form in minutes or hours in a human. This is especially true in the embryonic stages of development and is the reason why any interference with these processes in the early embryonic stages may have catastrophic consequences in the developing human. The embryogenesis of the craniofacial complex is indeed an amazing phenomenon; form and function must relate to one another with an almost unbelievable precision and at exactly the right moments in time. In order to appreciate the structures and physiology that the physician interested in

diseases of the ear, nose, and throat so frequently sees go awry, we begin this text with a very abbreviated review of the normal development of the human head.

Although this text is organized into sections on the basis of organ systems, and although each section has a discussion of the most important embryologic and developmental anatomy of that particular organ system, of necessity there is some duplication and lack of continuity in this method of presentation. Therefore, this section will be primarily concerned with the cranium, base of the skull, face, and eyes and will concentrate on the broad concepts involved in the development of these structures.

The subject of embryology is a complex one, running the gamut from descriptive chronology of events that transpire during prenatal life to details of genetic types and mutations and how they affect the individual proteins and nucleic acids that are part of the molecular biology of the embryo (Moore, 1977). A complete survey of even a portion of the aspects of subcellular structure is beyond the scope of this text; however, since many of the advances in embryology of interest to the physician involved with craniofacial anomalies will undoubtedly occur because of a better understanding of subcellular events, it is important to mention these, if only briefly. A general overview of the structure of the human face will be presented first, followed by a discussion of the cellular and subcellular mechanisms that lead to the facial configuration. This method of presentation parallels the way in which the clinician usually views patients with anomalies of this region.

PLAN OF THE HUMAN FACE

The assumption of the upright posture in man has been associated with a number of anatomic developments, as can be appreciated from an examination of Figure 1–2A and B (Enlow, 1975). With the enlargement of the brain, especially of the frontal region, and the concomitant rotation of the eyes to the midline, there has been a relative decrease in the intraorbital distance in man compared to that in lower mammals. This has resulted in a smaller region at the root of the nose and a shortening of the muzzle or snout. Thus, man has close-set eyes and a short, narrow nose that does not interfere with binocular vision.

The growth of the frontal lobes and other evolutionary changes have resulted in flexure of the cranial base, as illustrated in Figure 1–2C, making the face appear to hang from the base of the skull. Other less obvious changes have occurred, such as rotation of the olfactory bulbs and nerves, so that the nasal region in man has a vertical orientation and most of its important functional components are housed within the face. This placement of the face within the flexure of the cranial base may be of some clinical significance, as any condition that affects the cranial base may have some secondary effect on the airway and, ultimately, on the speech mechanisms, which are discussed in Chapter 82.

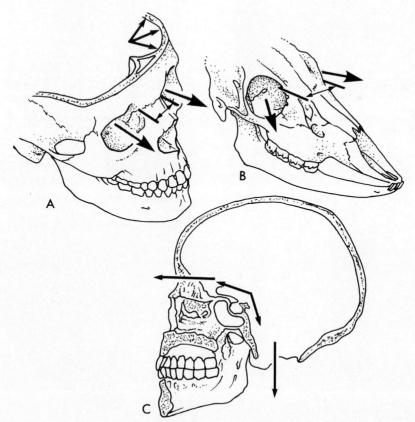

Figure 1–2 *A,* Plan of the human face demonstrating an enlargement of the frontal lobes in the human and rotation of the orbit, resulting in a narrow nasal root, in contrast to *B,* a lower animal. *C,* Flexure of the cranial base results in an alteration of facial orientation. (Modified from Enlow, 1975.)

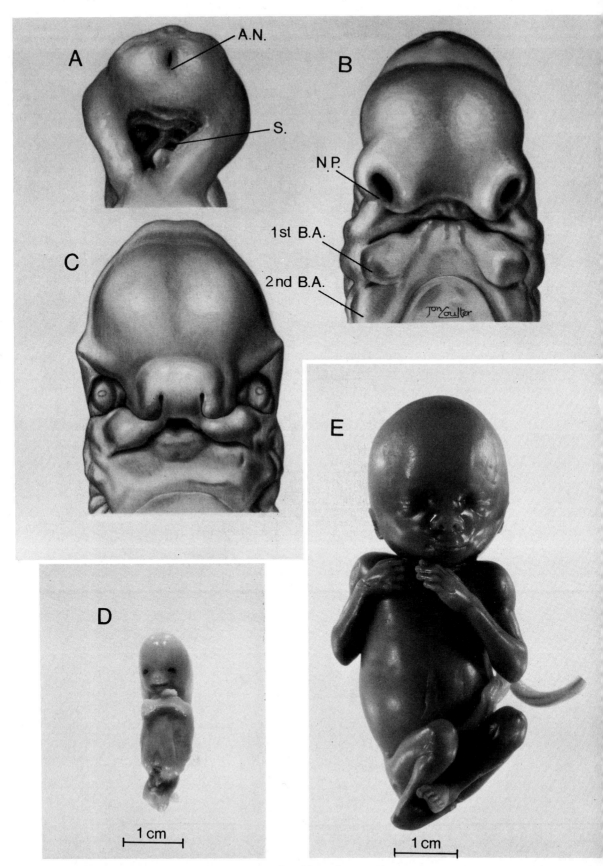

Figure 1–3 *See legend on the opposite page*

PRENATAL DEVELOPMENT OF THE FACE

The development of the face from midembryonic through midfetal life is illustrated in Figure 1–3. The embryo at about three to four weeks of age is illustrated in Figure 1–3A. At this stage, the embryo does not have a face, the head is composed of a brain covered with a membrane, and the anterior neuropore (AN) is still present. The eyes, which are represented by optic vesicles, are on the lateral aspects of the head, as is seen in fish, and the future mouth is represented by a stomadeum (S). It is only in the later part of this period of embryonic growth that nasal pits develop. At the embryonic age of five to six weeks, as is illustrated in Figure 1–3B, the general shape of the face has begun to develop. The frontonasal process is prominent, the nasal pits (NP) are forming laterally, and, with the increase in size of the first and second branchial arches (1st BA, 2nd BA), there is a suggestion of a mouth. In the subsequent weeks of embryonic life, as illustrated in Figure 1–3C, those structures that we associate with the human face — jaws, nose, eyes, ears, and mouth — will take on human configurations.

During this period of rapid growth and expansion, there is also tremendous *differential* growth. Thus, the development of a human baby is not merely the enlargement or rearrangement of a previous form, but, by differential growth, the development of a new configuration. This is a concept that has been difficult for students to comprehend, perhaps because of the tendency to illustrate different stages of embryonic development with drawings of equal size. These illustrating techniques have been used because minute structures are difficult to demonstrate without magnification, but it is important to try to view human embryologic development in perspective in order to appreciate both its similarities to phylogenetic development and its unique course in man.

The embryonic period ends at about eight weeks, when the embryo has achieved sufficient size and form so that facial characteristics can be recognized and photographed at actual size, as shown in Figure 1–3D. At this stage of late embryonic or early fetal development, the facial features are characterized by the appearance of hypertelorism; during subsequent growth, it will appear as though the eyes are moving closer together. This is not happening, however; the eyes continue to move farther apart, but the remainder of the face is growing at a much more rapid rate and thus it appears that the eyes are moving closer together; hypertelorism is actually decreasing as a result of differential development. These observations may be of importance in understanding some of the craniofacial syndromes in which hypertelorism is a prominent feature.

The continued rapid growth and change in configuration, not only of the face but also of the extremities and body during the next few months, are illustrated in Figure 1–3E. The fetus has facial features that are easily recognized and associated with the human. The ears, nasal alae, and lips are well-developed, and the head constitutes a large portion of the body mass — a relationship that will exist at birth and gradually change during extrauterine life.

The concept of differential growth is vital to the comprehension of both prenatal and postnatal development. Although this concept is difficult to grasp when the student must view development of structures of different ages magnified to the same size and when illustrations are in two dimensions, it is important to visualize the process in three dimensions *and* in the fourth dimension — time.

FORMATION OF THE CRANIOFACIAL COMPLEX

The structures and factors that form the craniofacial complex have been the subject of investigation by embryologists for many years, and their study has involved use of a number of sophisticated, time-consuming techniques (Stewart, 1976). Among the most interesting studies has been the research of

Figure 1–3 Prenatal facial development. *A*, An embryo of three to four weeks. *A.N.*, anterior neuropore; *S*, stomadeum. *B*, An embryo of five to six weeks: *N.P.*, nasal pit; *1st B.A.*, first branchial arch; *2nd B.A.*, second branchial arch. *C*, An embryo of seven to eight weeks. *D*, A fetus of eight to nine weeks. *E*, A fetus of three to four months. (Fetal specimens are from the Krause Collection, the Cleft Palate Center, University of Pittsburgh.)

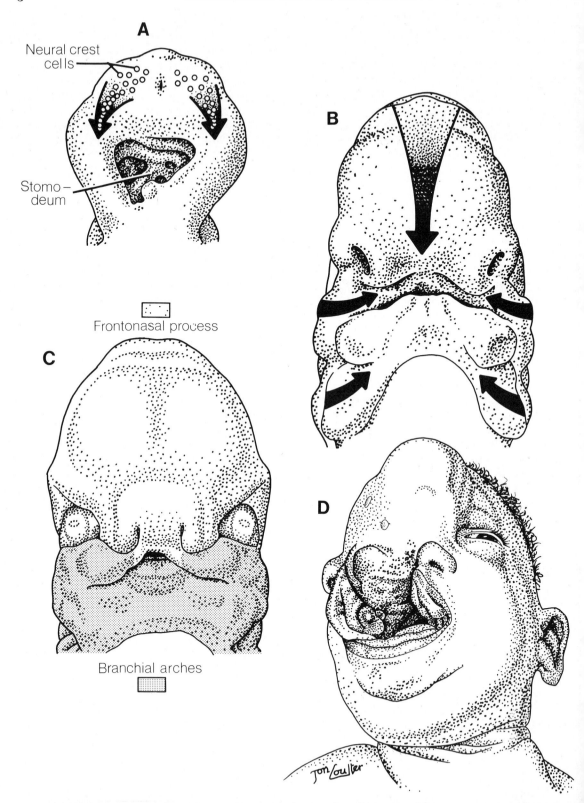

Figure 1–4   Formation of the craniofacial complex. *A*, An embryo of three to four weeks showing development and beginning migration of neural crest cells. *B*, Migration of neural crest cells to the forebrain and the branchial arches. *C*, Contributions to the face of the frontonasal process and branchial arches. *D*, Deformity caused by failure of neural crest cell migration.

Johnston (1975) into the development and migration of cells in the neural crest. These cells are initially composed of ectoderm found at the junction of the neural plate and surface ectoderm; Figure 1–4*A* shows the neural crest cells forming around the anterior neuropore. It has been shown that the face of the amphibian, as well as of mammals, develops as a consequence of massive cell migrations and the interactions of loosely organized embryonic tissue. In most of the body, this embryonic tissue is derived from mesoderm; however, in the craniofacial complex, neural crest cells give rise to a large variety of connective and nervous tissues of the skull, face, and branchial arches. This ectodermal tissue therefore constitutes the majority of the pluripotential tissue of the face. The sequence of events after the initial formation of the neural crest cells is illustrated in Figure 1–4*B*. The differentiation, proliferation, and migration of those cells are critical in the formation of the face.

Migration occurs at different rates. For instance, those cells forming the frontonasal process are derived from the forebrain fold, and their migration is relatively short as they pass into the nasal region. However, those cells that form the mesenchyme of the maxillary processes have a considerably longer distance to migrate, since they must move into the branchial arches where they surround the corelike mesodermal muscle plates (Krogman, 1974). In Figure 1–4*C*, the ultimate distribution of neural crest cells from the frontonasal process and from the branchial arches is illustrated. Since this mesenchymal tissue contributes the majority of the soft tissues and bone to the face, failure of proliferation or migration may be responsible for a number of abnormalities, such as orofacial clefts (Stark, 1977). An illustration of a severe facial abnormality secondary to failure of migration is illustrated in Figure 1–4*D*. Less severe clefts of the lip and palate or both may also develop. In some cases, such as with severe arhinencephalia, not only are mesodermal tissues involved but there are central nervous system abnormalities as well (DeMyer, 1975).

DIVISIONS OF THE HUMAN FACE

From the foregoing, it can be seen that the human face may be divided embryologically, as illustrated in Figure 1–4*C*. The median facial structures arise from the frontonasal processes, and the lateral structures arise from the branchial arches. This dual embryonic origin provides a basis for dividing the face into three *vertical* segments. The central segment, primarily the frontonasal process, includes the nose and central portion of the upper lip. The two lateral segments that arise from the branchial arches may be called the otomaxillomandibular segments. For convenience of description, the face can also be divided into three almost equal *horizontal* planes. The upper, or frontal horizontal segment derives solely from the frontonasal process. The middle, or maxillary, segment derives from the maxillary process of the first branchial arch, and the prolabium comes from the frontonasal process. The third horizontal segment, the lower, or mandibular, segment, comes from the mandibular process of the first branchial arch (DeMyer, 1975).

PRENATAL CRANIOFACIAL SKELETAL COMPONENTS

The craniofacial skeleton provides support and protection for the human's most vital functions. Conceptually, it is a region with two divisions: that which is involved with the central nervous system — the *neurocranium* — and that which is involved with respiration and mastication — the *visceral cranium*. It consists of four components: the cranial base, cranial vault, nasomaxillary complex, and the mandible. Although most of these structures are derived from the mesodermal germinal layer, a portion of the dental structures are of ectodermal origin.

The skeletal structures originate spontaneously from two types of bone. One type of bone is first formed in cartilage, and the other is derived from membrane. In general, the bones of the skull that represent the earliest phylogenetic structures are first formed as cartilage, which subsequently ossifies, and the more recently developed craniofacial structures are derived from membranous bone.

The components and structures of the fetal craniofacial complex are illustrated in Figures 1–5 through 1–8. Figure 1–5 is a parasagittal section through the cranial base and the facial structures. The cranial base is cartilaginous and provides a floor for the calvarium and a roof for the face. The nasal space and nasopharynx are part of the airway system. Although the airway is not functional

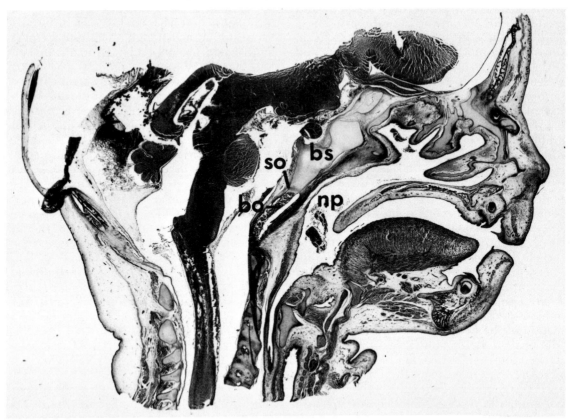

Figure 1–5 Photomicrograph of a parasagittal section of a 15 week old fetal head. *bo,* Basiocciput; *bs,* basisphenoid cartilage; *np,* nasopharynx; *so,* sphenooccipital synchondrosis. (From the Krause Collection, the Cleft Palate Center, University of Pittsburgh.)

in the fetus, alterations of the cranial base during fetal life may affect its subsequent development. Figure 1–6*A* and *B* shows the cartilaginous continuity of the cranial base and nasal septum as well as the arrangement of the fetal facial bones and teeth around the cartilaginous nasal capsule. The nasal septum is attached to the cranial base and the palate, and thus constitutes a large portion of the skeletal structure in the fetal midface. Although there is much difference of opinion on this subject, growth of craniofacial cartilage is considered by some to be of prime importance in facial development (Latham, 1976).

As previously mentioned, the craniofacial skeletal complex is composed of bones of different embryonic origins. Figure 1–7 shows the bones of cartilaginous origin (dark stipple) and those of membranous origin (light stipple); cartilage that is of branchial arch origin is indicated by solid black. In general, the base of the skull and the sphenoid, petrosal, and ethmoid bones are of cartilaginous

origin. The growth of the cartilage of the cranial base will be primarily at the cartilaginous synchondrosis until cartilage is replaced by bone; thereafter, growth is at the periosteal margins. Most of the cranial and facial bones are membranous, and growth takes place primarily at the margins of these bones. The major facial bones are formed from multiple ossification centers, which subsequently produce single bones in later fetal life. The importance of understanding the dual embryonic origin of the skeleton is that many diseases that affect the craniofacial complex may be manifest because of their influence on particular types of bone; for example, achondroplasia, which affects bones of cartilaginous origin, usually results in a characteristic alteration of facial configuration. The formation of membranous and enchondral bones and remodeling of bone are discussed and illustrated in Chapter 2.

The sequential development of the fetal skeleton has been studied extensively by radiographic methods (Kier, 1971). It is an-

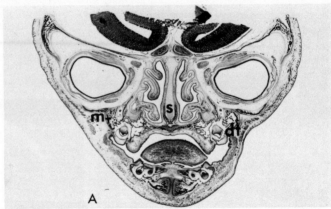

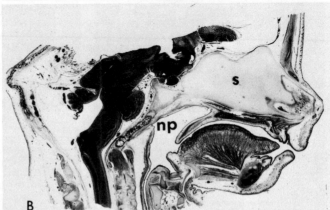

Figure 1–6 *A,* Coronal section of a 15 week old fetal head. *B,* Sagittal section of a 15 week old fetal head. *dt,* Deciduous tooth germ; *m,* maxillary bone center; *np,* nasopharynx; *s,* nasal septum.

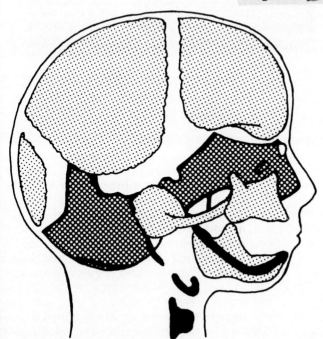

Figure 1–7 Schematic illustration of the components of the fetal craniofacial complex of membranous origin (light stipple) and cartilaginous origin (dark stipple). The cartilage of branchial arch origin is indicated in black. (Redrawn from Stewart, 1976.)

 Cartilaginous bone

 Membranous bone

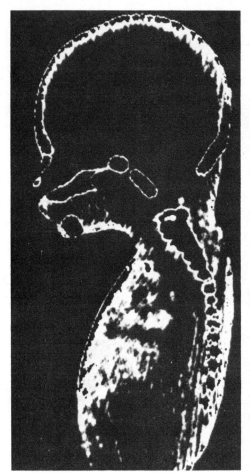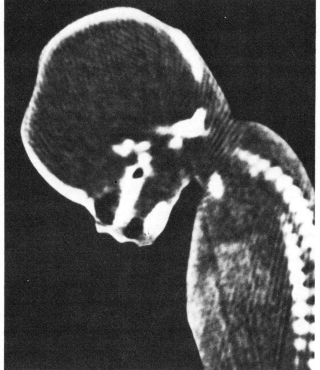

Figure 1–8   Computerized axial tomography of a fetus, about 16 weeks old, showing the extent of skeletal development.

ticipated, however, that newer developments such as computerized axial tomography (Fig. 1–8) will provide better visualization of the relationship of the various tissues and improve our understanding of craniofacial morphogenesis by use of nondestructive techniques (Maue-Dickson and Trefler, 1977; Prewitt, 1976).

DEVELOPMENT OF CRANIOFACIAL ARTERIES, MUSCLES, AND NERVES

Figure 1–9 illustrates the development of the cranium, arteries, nerves, and muscles during embryonic and early fetal life. The characteristics of these structures will be discussed in their respective sections, since their growth and development are interrelated.

Arteries

Figure 1–9A shows that the early arterial supply to the head consists primarily of the dorsal aorta and an arch with a small branch coming from it, which is the primitive internal carotid artery. The future musculature consists of mesenchymal tissue in the first and second branchial arches, which are just beginning to form. As the head begins to grow and the embryo starts to develop a face, the internal carotid artery increases in both size and length, and the aortic arches begin to develop. Each of the branchial arches contains not only an artery but also a nerve and a core of mesodermal tissue. Figure 1–9B shows an embryo of about six weeks when the first and second aortic arches and their arteries have formed. As the face continues to develop, these vessels will ultimately disappear. It must

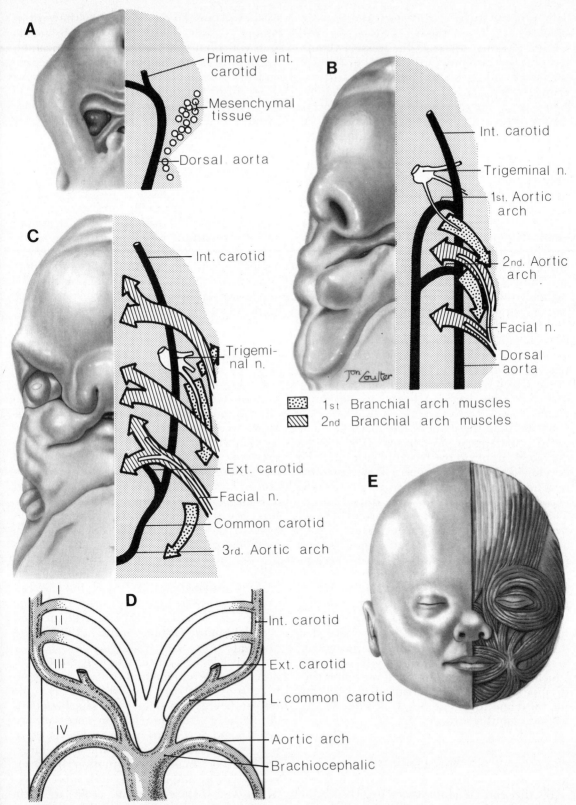

Figure 1–9 Development of the craniofacial arteries, muscles, and nerves. *A*, A three to four week old embryo. *B*, A five to six week old embryo. *C*, A seven to eight week old embryo. *D*, The fate of the aortic arches (shaded vessels persist). (After Avery, 1974.) *E*, Distribution of the facial musculature in the 15 week old fetus. (After Gasser, 1961.)

be appreciated that at this stage the fetus is still very small and these vessels are correspondingly tiny. In fact, the vessels themselves are responding to the needs of the tissue surrounding them, and with further growth their anastomosis will ultimately come from another source. The internal carotid artery at this stage has increased in size, and the facial muscles are beginning to develop in a laminar fashion. One group of muscles develops a lamina that grows posteriorly, and the other group of muscles comes from a lamina that extends anteriorly.

The nerves are beginning to develop as outgrowths of the central nervous system. Growth of the nerves induces bone to form around them, so that the nerves form first and induce the formation of their foramina as they grow. The fifth cranial nerve (trigeminal), which will ultimately supply sensation to the face, is really a combination of three nerves with ophthalmic, mandibular, and maxillary divisions and a division to the muscles of mastication. The seventh cranial nerve, which is the nerve supply to the second branchial arch, has also begun its development.

By the time the embryo has facial characteristics that appear more human (Fig. 1–9C), the blood supply to the face and cranium has developed the pattern that will persist into fetal and postnatal life. The third aortic arch is connected to the embryonic dorsal aorta. This arch becomes a common carotid artery, from which the external carotid artery develops to provide the major blood supply for the face. In general, these vessels have a recognizable pattern, but there is tremendous variation in their sites of origin and in the anastomosis between the internal and external carotid arteries. Figure 1–9D illustrates the formation of the arterial supply. Note the disappearance of the first and second aortic arches, the persistence of the third arch, which becomes the common carotid, and the disappearance of the dorsal aorta between the third and fourth arches, which on the left will become the aorta.

Muscles

By the end of embryonic life, the facial musculature has become rather well developed and has migrated extensively superiorly into the craniofacial region. Figure 1–9E shows the muscles contributed by the various lamina (Gasser, 1961). The first branchial arch contributes the muscles of mastication, which lie beneath the musculature of the second branchial arch and, in general, have a different orientation. These muscles include the temporalis, masseter, pterygoid, mylohyoid, anterior belly of the digastric, tensor veli palatini, and tensor tympani.

Nerves

The nerve supply to the muscles of the face (Gasser, 1961) follows the musculature because of the inductive influence of the mesoderm. These cranial nerves are mixed nerves, having autonomic, sensory and motor components. By the time the fetus has reached 37 mm crown–rump length, all of the peripheral branches of the facial nerve are identifiable.

SUBCELLULAR EMBRYOLOGY

Having looked at some of the broad, important details of morphogenesis and development of the prenatal cranium and face, it is appropriate — even in a text which is primarily clinically oriented — to discuss some aspects of molecular biology. In the past 20 years there has been a remarkable increase in our understanding of many evolutionary and developmental processes at a molecular level. It is anticipated that further definition at this level of development will provide us with methods of diagnosis, therapy, and perhaps prevention of many of the conditions discussed in this text. An immense body of literature is available on this subject, but the concepts expressed here are primarily from Ayala (1978), Roberts (1973), Williams and Wendel-Smith (1969), Burdi (1976), and Moore (1977).

The cell is the structural as well as the functional and developmental unit of the organism (Burdi, 1976). It is obvious that the human begins as a single cell, which contains all of the genetic information necessary for growth and development, and that every subsequent cell should contain the same information. The unanswered question, however, is exactly why and how cells and, subsequently tissues, differentiate in order to form organ systems. To understand this at our current state of knowledge, we must look at two features of cells. One is the mechanism by which the cells express the genetic code, and the other is the ability of the cell and of its environment to determine which parts of its genetic material will be expressed.

To elucidate the first feature, the current concept of molecular biology acknowledges that the nucleus of the cell is the repository of encoded information, which is stored in an extremely long, deoxyribonucleic acid (DNA) molecule. A sequence of amino acids is arranged along a strand of DNA and represents a linear code (or language). The gene is one segment of this molecule. In order for this information to reach the cytoplasm, a portion of the DNA uncoils, and a single strand of ribonucleic acid (RNA) picks up the message, which it takes through the nuclear wall to the cytoplasm. This RNA is called messenger RNA and the process is called transcription (the genetic code or "language" is transcribed). In a second process, called translation, the genetic program of the organism is "read" in the cytoplasm so that appropriate protein substances may be formed.

What is the clinical significance of this process? The characteristics and behavior of organisms depend ultimately on the sequence of amino acids in their proteins, and evolution consists largely of progressive substitution of one amino acid for another (Ayala, 1978). Figure 1–10 gives an example of what might happen if one of the molecules in DNA is modified so that the messenger RNA

formed has an error in its information code. This error will be perpetuated in subsequent generations of the cell, resulting in an entire line of cells producing a defective protein. If this accident occurred late in embryologic development and if the amino acid is not significant, the defect might not be noticed or it might merely contribute to one of the myriad of individual variations illustrated in Figure 1–1. If the defect is not fatal, it may still involve an important enzyme and be passed on to succeeding generations, where it could result in a whole-system abnormality, such as hemophilia. In general, the more genetic material involved in producing an abnormality, the more likely it is that there will be dire consequences for the organism. Most of the chromosomal abnormalities, such as Down syndrome and 13–15 translocation, are at least partially expressed as abnormalities of the craniofacial complex.

The second feature is the susceptibility of the cell's process of gene expression to outside control. Since each cell has a full genetic code but does not function the same as all other cells, there must be some mechanism for genetic control. Some substance must induce a gene to be expressed, or turned "on," and others must repress the gene, or turn it "off." This repression has been observed in some instances to be reversible and in others to be irreversible. In the instance of cellular differentiation, it is obvious that at any particular time in embryonic life a cell may come

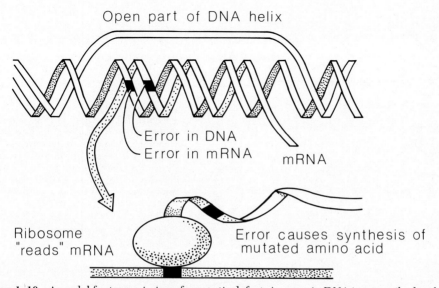

Figure 1–10 A model for transmission of a genetic defect. An error in DNA is transcribed to the messenger RNA and subsequently translated into an abnormal protein.

into contact with any number of substances that are produced by or contained in adjacent tissue. This contact results in interaction with, or induction of, the gene to form new gene products. This interaction is compatible with observations made over the years in descriptive embryology and may be seen in the induction of surface ectoderm to form a lens and of mesoderm to form an orbit in the presence of an optic stalk. Thus, an optic stalk induces the formation of the whole eye.

The phenomenon of induction introduces another level at which developmental deviations can occur (Fig. 1–11). In the normal course of events (Fig. 1–11*A*), the inducer acts on *A,* which in turn produces products *B* and *C.* The inducer is usually a small metabolite, an ion, or some reaction product resulting from the presence of such a low molecular weight substance. If, instead of the inducer, a teratogen (*T*) acts on the tissues, the inductive phenomenon shown in Figure 1–11*B* might occur: instead of *B* and *C, A* would produce *X* and *Y.* If this occurs early in embryologic life, it is likely that the effects would be devastating to that cell line. If this teratogen is present after *A* has induced *B,* however, it will not prevent the normal formation of *C.* Thus, in the induction phenomenon, timing is crucial and anything that interferes with an orderly sequence of events will result in some type of developmental abnormality. In order to appreciate this, one need only review the vari-

ous functions of cells: filling spaces in the developing embryo; producing a sticky substance to adhere to other cells, thus allowing fusion between parts; producing hormones — the list is long. In addition, if one considers the sequence of events necessary to form a cell line — differentiation, multiplication, and proliferation — it is obvious that there are many steps at which the intervention of a teratogen could act to prevent the proper functioning of cells and their products and in turn influence surrounding cells.

In the embryology of the craniofacial complex, cells that initially look alike and have similar genetic codes gradually assume different functional appearances or phenotypes. This differentiation then becomes the foundation for growth and development. Cytogenesis, or cytologic and biochemical differentiation, is followed by morphogenesis — change in shape and position of cell aggregates. Both cytogenesis and morphogenesis must occur in proper temporal sequence if normal craniofacial development is to occur. (For example, it would be of little functional value for salivary glands to secrete enzymes if there were no salivary duct system [Burdi, 1977].) By the time the embryo has reached the age of five weeks, when the craniofacial structures first become identifiable, most of these basic developmental events have occurred. During the next three weeks of embryologic life, these cells must

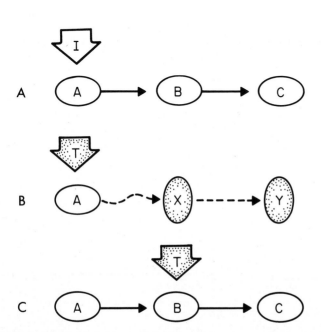

Figure 1–11 A model illustrating one concept of the influence of a teratogen on induction phenomena. *A,* Normal induction of A produces a normal cell sequence. *B,* Introduction of a teratogen at A when the cell line is developing results in faulty protein formation. *C,* Introduction of the same teratogen at B has no influence, as the cell line is not sensitive at this time.

proliferate and migrate to their proper locations so that by eight weeks the embryonic face is recognizably human.

During subsequent fetal and postnatal life, there will be a continuation of differential growth and development, including precocious growth of the nervous system, resulting in enlargement of the calvarium in the fetus and infant out of proportion to enlargement of the face and the remainder of the body. The concepts of this chapter furnish the basis for understanding normal postnatal growth and possible abnormalities of the craniofacial complex.

SELECTED REFERENCES

Ayala, F. 1978. The mechanisms of evolution. Scientific American, *239*:56–69.
A well-illustrated article that explains the current concepts of molecular biology as related to evolution. This entire issue is devoted to evolution.

Burdi, A. 1976. Biological forces which shape the human midface before birth. *In* McNamara, J. (Ed.) Craniofacial growth series, Monograph No. 6. Ann Arbor, MI, Center for Human Growth and Development, the University of Michigan.
A comprehensive article which relates molecular biology to embryonic and fetal growth.

Enlow, D. 1975. Handbook of Facial Growth. Philadelphia, W. B. Saunders Co.
This book is written primarily in atlas style and illustrates craniofacial growth from embryonic to adult life.

Moore, K. 1977. The Developing Human. Philadelphia, W. B. Saunders Co.
A clinically oriented embryology text that is well-illustrated.

Stewart, R. 1976. Genetic factors in craniofacial morphogenesis. *In* Stewart, R., and Prescott, G. (Eds.) Oral Facial Genetics. St. Louis, The C. V. Mosby Co.
This is a comprehensive text with extensive references which describes the genetic aspects of craniofacial abnormalities and gives other extensive descriptions of oral abnormalities.

REFERENCES

Avery, T. 1974. Developmental Anatomy, 7th ed. Philadelphia, W. B. Saunders Co.

Ayala, F. 1978. The mechanisms of evolution. Scientific American, *239*:56–69.

Burdi, A. R. 1977. Early development of the human basicranium: Morphogenic basicranium: Morphogenic controls, growth patterns and relations. *In* Bosma, J. F. (Ed.) NIH symposium on development of the basicranium. U.S. Government Printing Office, pp. 81–92. (Available from Superintendent of Documents as No. 017–047–00011–61).

Burdi, A. R. 1976. Biological forces which shape the human midface before birth. *In* McNamara, J. (Ed.) Craniofacial growth series, Monograph No. 6, Ann Arbor, MI, Center for Human Growth and Development, the University of Michigan.

DeMyer, W. 1975. Median facial malformations and their implications for brain malformations. *In* Bergsma, V. (Ed.) Morphogenesis and Malformation of Face and Brain. New York, Alan Rhise, Inc., pp. 155–181.

Enlow, D. 1975. Handbook of Facial Growth. Philadelphia, W. B. Saunders Co.

Gasser, R. 1961. The development of the facial nerve in man. Ann. Otol. Rhinol. Laryngol., *76*:37.

Johnston, M. 1975. The neural crest in abnormalities of the face and brain in birth defects. Original Article Series II, no. 7, pp. 1–18.

Kier, S. 1971. Fetal skull. *In,* Newton, T., and Potts, D., (Eds.) Radiology of the Skull and Brain, Vol. 1, Chap. 7. St. Louis, The C. V. Mosby Co.

Krogman, W. 1974. Craniofacial Growth and Development: An Appraisal. Yearbook of Physical Anthropology, *18*, pp. 31–64.

Latham, R. 1976. An appraisal of the early maxillary growth mechanism. *In* McNamara, J. (Ed.) Craniofacial growth series, Monograph No. 6, Ann Arbor, MI, Center for Human Growth and Development, the University of Michigan.

Maue-Dickson, W., and Trefler, M. 1977. Image quality in computerized and conventional tomography in the assessment of craniofacial anomalies. SPIE, *127*:353–361.

Moore, K. 1977. The Developing Human, 2nd ed. Philadelphia, W. B. Saunders Co.

Prewitt, J. 1976. Prospective medical advances in computerized tomography. *In,* Bosma, J. (Ed.) Development of the Basicranium. DHEW Publication No. (NIH) 789.

Roberts, J. A. 1973. An Introduction to Medical Genetics. London, Oxford University Press.

Stark, R. 1977. Embryology of Cleft Palate. *In* Converse, J. (Ed.) Reconstructive Plastic Surgery. Philadelphia, W. B. Saunders Co., pp. 1941–1949.

Stewart, R. 1976. Genetic factors in craniofacial morphogenesis. *In* Stewart, R., and Prescott, G. (Eds.) Oral Facial Genetics, St. Louis, The C. V. Mosby Co., pp. 46–66.

Williams, P., and Wendell-Smith, C. 1969. Basic Human Embryology, 2nd ed. Philadelphia, J. B. Lippincott Co.

Chapter 2

POSTNATAL CRANIOFACIAL GROWTH AND DEVELOPMENT

Sylvan E. Stool, M.D.

Growth implies an increase in dimension and mass, whereas development implies a progression to more adult characteristics. In this chapter, we shall start by describing the appearance of the soft tissues of the human head and then examine the underlying skeletal components in order to relate the development of these components to some of the basic principles and concepts of cartilage and bone growth. The infant face rarely projects an image of the adult configuration. Conversely, attempting to identify an adult by examination of his or her "baby pictures" is usually impossible. The face of the infant or child is not a miniature of an adult face but has definite proportions that are different from those of the adult. The changes that take place during maturation are part of a differential growth process. In general, newborns, regardless of their ethnic backgrounds, resemble each other more than each one does his or her parents. The different proportions of infant and adult faces have been studied extensively by artists and anthropologists and are appreciated almost instinctively by the layman (Hogarth, 1965; Ligett, 1974). These changes in the facial configuration and proportions are illustrated in Figure 2–1.

The infant has a very prominent forehead because of the early development of the neurocranium in relationship to the face. About 90 per cent of the child's facial height is achieved by five years of age, but 90 per cent of the facial width is present at two years. Thus, the young child's head appears round.

The *face* of the infant is diminutive compared with the calvarium. As seen in Figure 2–1, the proportion of facial mass to cranial mass, as viewed laterally, is 1 to 3. Subsequent growth in childhood alters this proportion so that the ratio becomes about 1 to 2½, while in the adolescent and adult the proportion becomes 1 to 2. If, however, this proportion does not change as described, the adult is frequently referred to as having a "baby face." In addition, because the soft tissue of the face includes fat, the external appearance does not necessarily reflect the underlying musculoskeletal structure of the face; thus the underlying proportions may change but the general outline of the adult face may still appear child-like. The infant face has a very "flat" configuration, which changes during adolescence when sharper angles develop as a result of orbital, chin, and nasal growth. The upper jaw of the infant is small but increases in size during childhood to present a wide, full appearance of the tissue overlying the maxilla. This is because of the growth of dental tissues (Fig. 2–6). The *chin* of the infant is almost nonexistent but is usually a very prominent adult structure as a result of mandibular and dental growth. The cheekbones become very prominent in the adult owing to loss of baby fat and rotation of the skeletal components. The *ears* of the infant appear to

18

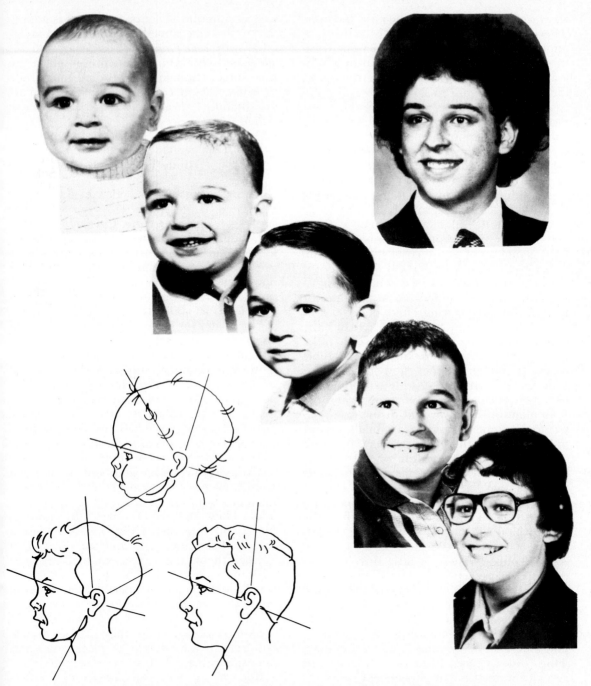

Figure 2–1 Postnatal growth of a Caucasian boy. The diagonal from above downward shows the boy at ages six months, two years, four years, eight years, and 12 years; the photograph in the upper right corner is the same child at 18 years. Drawings in the lower left show the changes in proportion of face mass to cranial mass. In the infant, it is 1 to 3; during childhood, it gradually changes to 1 face mass to 2½ cranial mass. From adolescence through adult life, it is 1 face mass to 2 cranial mass.

be very low-set because the head in general is more ovoid than elongated; the ears appear to "rise" with growth because of the increase in the vertical dimension of the face, particularly growth of the mandible and lower facial structures. The configuration of the ear remains the same throughout life, although its mass increases.

The most prominent facial features, the relationship of which has become characteristic of human faces, are the nose and eyes. The *nose* of the infant has a distinctive pug appearance. It is diminutive and remains so throughout most of childhood. During adolescence and later, especially in the male, there is an increase in length, breadth, and protrusion of the nose, which is related to the increase in airway requirements at this age and which is accompanied by a similar increase in the size of the internal airway. Humans are the only animals with a truly external nose, and this particularly human trait is subject to many variations, depending in part on ethnic background.

The *eyes* of the infant appear to be wide-set and have a very prominent inner canthal fold, giving an appearance of hypertelorism because of the lack of vertical dimension of the face. If the infant's face is bisected horizontally, the eyes are located in the inferior half of the face. During childhood the eyes appear to move upward, but in actuality the bottom half of the face grows more than the upper half so that the maxilla and mandible become more prominent, and in the older child the eyes are placed midway in the face. In adolescence, with further growth and development of the lower half of the face relative to the upper half, the eyes finally appear to be just above the dividing line. This adult configuration is the result of differential growth of facial components, and the same principle may be used to explain why in adults the eyes are less prominent than they appear to be in children: with growth of the superorbital rim during adolescence, less of the eye is exposed.

Until puberty there is little difference in the appearance between girls and boys. However, as female craniofacial growth ceases and male craniofacial growth continues throughout the second decade, the eyes, lips, nose, and chin achieve adult proportions, and the jaw and cheeks become more prominent. Thus, distinct facial features distinguish the sexes from the time of adolescence on.

GROWTH CONCEPTS

"Parallel evaluation of the cranium and of other parts of the skeleton is at the present time the basis for the clinical distinction of generalized skeletal disorders from cranial abnormalities" (Pierce, et al., 1977). Therefore, in order to understand the normal morphologic changes that occur with growth, as well as craniofacial abnormalities, it is important to describe some basic concepts of skeletal growth: *bone formation, remodeling,* and *displacement.* The information presented in the following section may be studied more fully in Williams and colleagues (1969), Sokoloff and Bland, (1975), Rubin (1964), and Enlow (1975).

Bone Formation

Humans possess an endoskeleton that is fabricated from specialized connective tissue — cartilage and bone. Cartilage is a special, tough, pliable tissue that has the capacity to form in regions that experience direct pressure; it does not always calcify and does not necessarily have a surface membrane. Its most important feature in the craniofacial complex is its ability to function as a precursor or model for bone. The characteristics of bone are hardness and rigidity and the possession of a surface membrane or periosteum. It is a complex substance that is viewed by the chemist as a compound of protein, polysaccharide, mineral, and cellular constituents. To the histologist, it is a tissue composed of osteogenic cells and intracellular matrix. To the gross anatomist, it is an organ with vascular and nerve supplies.

The cells of cartilage and bone are derived from fetal mesenchymal tissue, which has a fairly uniform and undifferentiated appearance. These cells differentiate into chondroblasts and osteoblasts. Osteoblasts secrete a matrix that mineralizes and surrounds and encases them; they mature into osteocytes. Multinucleated giant cells called osteoclasts, which are known to destroy mineralized bone, also develop. They do not act on uncalcified bone — a fact of some importance in certain dysplasias — but they play an important role in the process of destruction and deposition that results in bone formation.

Bone always forms in preexisting connective tissue. When this tissue is cartilage, the process is called endochondral ossification; when it is noncartilaginous, it is called intramembranous ossification. The sequence of events is illustrated in Figure 2–2.

Membranous bone in the skull forms as a layer of mesenchyme with points of condensation. These areas of condensation begin to ossify, and the process extends until the areas meet to form suture lines. The sutures are active growth sites owing to the depositional

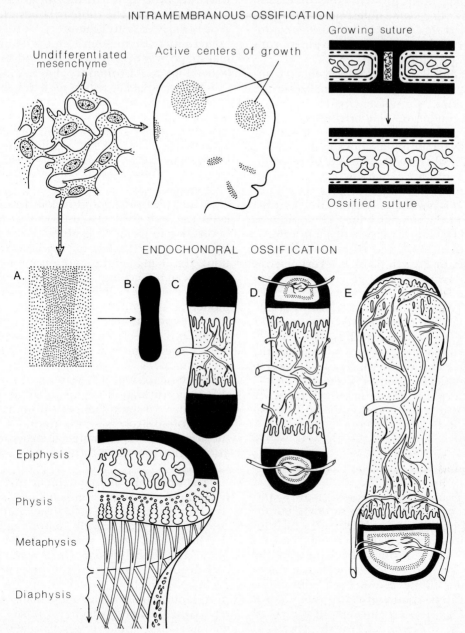

Figure 2–2   This figure illustrates the mechanism of formation of the two types of bone found in the head. Undifferentiated mesenchyme is the precursor of both. *Intramembranous ossification:* mesenchyme condenses to form centers of growth, which enlarge until they meet to form a suture. Growth proceeds at these sutures and remains active until the stimulus is removed and the suture ossifies. *Endochondral ossification:* A, Endochondral bone formation also begins with condensation. B, Cartilage *anlage* is formed. C, Vascular mesenchyme forms a primary marrow and a periosteal collar forms. D, Ossification centers develop at the extremities, resulting in the four segments illustrated in the lower left. E, Eventually the bone is completely ossified and the segmental differences disappear. The segments of a typical long bone are shown in the lower left. Epiphysis — a secondary ossification center, covered with cartilage. Physis — the cartilage growth plate. Metaphysis — the segment in which cartilage is transformed to bone by endochondral bone formation. Diaphysis — the shaft separating the growing ends. (Redrawn in part from Williams et al., 1969, and Rubin, 1964).

activity of osteoblasts, but at varying times, usually when brain growth slows or ceases, the sutures will become quiescent and eventually ossify. If this occurs prematurely, conditions such as craniosynostosis, with its consequent deformities, result.

Endochondral ossification is a more complex process that is easier to visualize in the tubular bones. The mesenchyme condenses and then undergoes chondrification. This forms a precise model for future bone surrounded by a limiting membrane. Formation of a periosteal collar is followed by development of a primitive marrow cavity and an ossification center, which forms at the end of the bone. It is possible to identify four distinct segments in the tubular bone. The epiphysis is covered by an articular cartilage in tubular bones and includes the ossification center. The physis, or growth plate, is a very narrow but highly active region that consists of four zones all related to chondrogenesis. The metaphysis is a zone where the transformation, or change of growing cartilage into bone, takes place. Growth in length is achieved primarily through the activities of cells in the metaphysis. This is also an important region in the remodeling process. Eventually, when growth ceases, the physis or growth plate will undergo ossification and disappear. The diaphysis is the shaft of the bone.

Remodeling and Displacement

In the craniofacial complex, growth and development depend on two separate but interrelated processes: displacement, which involves motion of segments of bone, and remodeling, which involves a change in the configuration of the bone while displacement is occurring. Bone grows by a continuous process of deposition and resorption. This is not a uniform process throughout the entire bone but is a differential growth process. If this were not so, the adult skeleton would be the same as the fetal configuration. The mechanism by which these two different but complementary functions are achieved is influenced by a number of factors, such as stress on the surface and various nutritional, hormonal, and genetic influences. The biodynamics have been studied for years and are still undergoing conceptual changes (Bassett, 1972).

In the simplest terms, bone grows because of osteoblastic activity and is resorbed by os-teoclastic activity; anything that interferes with this process will result in an abnormal configuration. In the tubular bones, this concept is fairly easy to visualize. In order for a bone to increase in length and retain its normal shape, it is necessary to add and substract bone. This is illustrated in Figure 2–3.

The craniofacial region is a much more complex area, and perhaps the process of bone growth in this region can best be visualized by describing the technique by which an artist working with clay might construct a bowl, using coils. A basic hollow form is constructed, to which clay is added superficially. The edges may be smoothed in order to achieve a pleasing configuration. In order to keep the wall thickness uniform, it may be necessary to remove (subtract) some clay from the inner surface of the bowl (resorption). If a change in the configuration is desirable, it can be accomplished by applying pressure on the inner surface (displacement) and modeling the outer surface. Although this simple explanation is of some help in understanding the mechanics of bone formation, it does not explain why these events occur in the human.

For the clinician, it is important to realize that bone formation begins in the fetus and undergoes constant changes throughout life. This twofold process is important not only in the formation of craniofacial structures but also in the growth of other bones and cartilage.

To amplify the first statement in this section, there are some abnormalities, such as dyschondroplasia, that affect the craniofacial complex but are clinically more familiar in the limbs and trunk than in the cranium. Some dyschondroplasias which result in cranial distortions, such as Crouzon syndrome, occur exclusively or principally in the chondrocranium, but with an abnormality such as Apert syndrome, which produces facial characteristics similar to the Crouzon abnormalities, the extremities will also be affected. A certain group of disorders are affected by alterations in the remodeling process. For instance, a craniometaphyseal abnormality involves alterations of the remodeling process, which are best understood by examination of the extremities. Some systemic diseases, such as hemolytic and iron deficiency anemias, may first be recognized in the cranium. Obviously, complete diagnosis of some cranial abnormalities necessitates evaluation of the remainder of the skeleton.

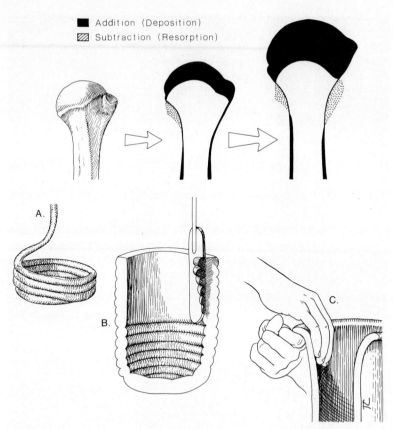

■ Addition (Deposition)
▨ Subtraction (Resorption)

Figure 2–3 The concept of remodeling is illustrated. In order to prevent distortion of growing bone, there is osteoclastic cut-back at the metaphysis. An example is this tubular bone, in which there is addition — deposition — at the epiphysis and subtraction — resorption — at the metaphysis.

The concepts involved in skeletal growth and development are illustrated using the analogy of the ancient coil technique of clay construction. *A,* The initial step is formation by deposition (addition); during this process there is concomitant removal, resorption (subtraction) resulting in differential growth. *B,* The final configuration is achieved by these two processes as well as an additional one, displacement *(C).*

Postnatal Skeletal Growth

The external features and some of the basic concepts of bone growth of the craniofacial complex have been discussed. We will now examine those changes that occur in the skeleton. Skeletal growth is more readily assessed and easier to document than soft tissue growth, as it is subject to radiographic examination and physical measurements (Dorst, 1971). These methods yield good estimates of skeletal proportions. Because of the availability of these tools, skeletal growth parameters have come to be widely used as indices for general growth evaluation. "Skeletal age" is one of the "biologic ages" used to ascertain the normality of growth and development. Usually this is evaluated not only with cephalometric radiography but also by examination of the extremities, most commonly the wrist.

Figure 2–4A shows the skulls of a newborn, child, and adult; Figure 2–4B is a three-quarter view of the same skulls. Figure 2–4C shows these same skulls with the infant and child enlarged to the same size as the adult so that the vertical dimensions are equal. This provides a graphic means of illustrating changes in proportion. There has been intense interest, especially among physicians, anthropologists, and dental scientists, in the factors responsible for the control of growth (Bassett, 1972). These will be discussed as they pertain to the various segments of the craniofacial complex: the calvarium, mandible, nasomaxillary complex, and cranial base.

Calvarium

The calvarium of the newborn is very prominent in comparison with that of the child and adult. Indeed, as can be seen in Figure 2–4C, the skull of an infant is almost round. Growth in this region is fairly easy to evaluate, as it seems to be passive and dependent on the size of the neural mass. As the bones grow, they become thicker because of deposits on both the endocranial and ectocranial surfaces. Ultimately, growth ceases, and irregular, interdigitated suture lines develop.

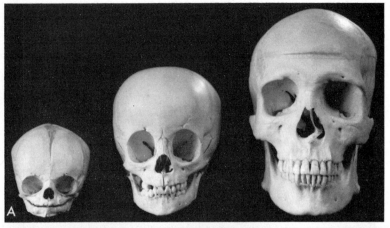

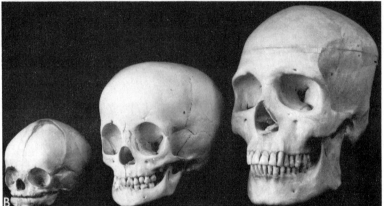

Figure 2–4 Skulls of a newborn, child, and adult illustrate skeletal changes during growth and development. *A*, Frontal view. *B*, Three-quarter view. *C*, The newborn and child skulls have been enlarged to the same size as the adult skull to demonstrate the changes in proportion with growth.

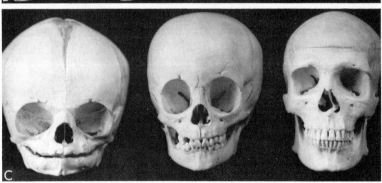

Mandible

The mandible in the newborn is very small compared with the rest of the craniofacial complex. Growth is multidirectional but primarily downward and forward. In the child, the stimulation of developing dentition contributes to the increase in size of the mandible seen at this stage of life; it is necessary for mandibular growth to keep pace with maxillary growth so that dental occlusion will be accurate. The most marked changes in man-

dibular shape take place between childhood and adolescence and may be appreciated by examining Figure 2–4B. The ramus of the jaw increases in height and width, a change which is felt to be due to the increase in size of the pharynx, as the mandible serves to protect its lateral wall. The mandibular condyle is covered with cartilage to protect it from the great pressures to which it is subject as the condyle grows generally upward and backward with a resulting downward and forward thrust to the chin.

Nasomaxillary Complex

Development of the nasomaxillary complex has been the subject of extensive investigation (McNamara, 1976). Although long ago it was observed that growth of these structures occurs downward and forward, the mechanism of such growth has been the subject of debate. The problem has been that it is difficult to design studies in which the variables are effectively controlled (Enlow, 1973).

In addition, this is a very complex anatomic region that is difficult to visualize from one perspective. Growth in this region occurs in both the horizontal and vertical planes, and different segments grow at varying rates. This can be appreciated by examining Figure 2–5, which shows the change in configuration and relationship of the orbits and the nasal apertures with age. Figure 2–5A is a photograph of a newborn; Figure 2–5B, a child; and Figure 2–5C, an adult skull; all have

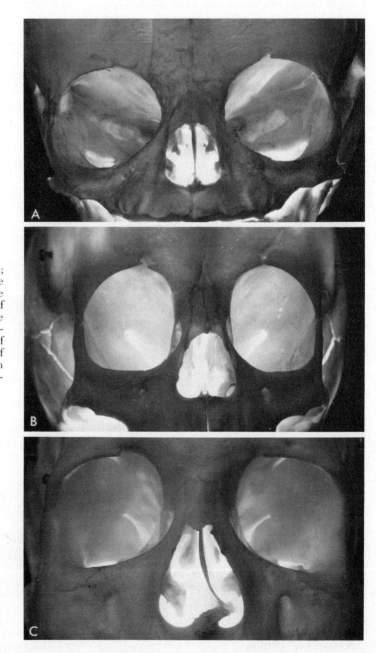

Figure 2–5 Skulls of A, a newborn; B, a child; and C, an adult, which have been transilluminated to emphasize the change in the relationship of the floor of the orbit to the floor of the nose. In the newborn and child, there is little separation; however, in the adult, because of downward growth and displacement of the floor of the nose and upward growth of the floor of the orbit the distance increases.

been transilluminated so that the changes in density of the bone and the outline of the nasal apertures are more apparent.

The remodeling changes in the orbit are very complex because so many bones are involved, each of which undergoes different amounts of growth and displacement. One of the most marked changes is the difference in the relationship of the floor of the nose to the floor of the orbit. In the newborn they are almost level, and in the child there is some separation; however, in the adult there is a marked change due to the downward displacement of the whole maxilla. This change is more complex as the floor of the orbit grows up and the floor of the nose grows down. The change in the bony septum with age is rather dramatic. In the newborn the septum appears straight, and in the adult skull shown, there is marked septal deviations, a common finding. It is interesting that the breadth of the nasal bridge does not increase noticeably from early childhood to adulthood, although the shape of the nasal aperture changes from almost circular to pear shaped — a characteristic that shows marked racial variation. The horizontal plane of the growth of the nasomaxillary complex is related to growth of the anterior cranial fossa until five or six years of age. During the time in which this region is growing, the bones are also being displaced forward. After five or six years of age, growth in the palate is primarily posterior.

The biomechanical force for displacement of the nasomaxillary complex is the subject of much controversy. According to Scott (1953), it is due to the expansion of the nasal septum, whereas Latham (1970) believes that it is due to traction on the septopremaxillary ligaments. Moss (1968) has proposed "the functional matrix" to describe development of the nasomaxillary complex, and Enlow (1973) thinks that this concept is of great significance, as it proposes that the genetic determinants of skeletal growth do not reside within the actual bony part itself. That is, the pacemakers of the displacement and the bony remodeling processes occur in the surrounding soft tissue parts. It is important to understand that the functional matrix concept describes essentially what happens during displacement and remodeling but is not intended to explain how this growth happens or what the regulating processes actually are at the tissue and cellular levels. Much is yet to be learned with regard to the "local growth control mechanism" (Enlow, 1973).

A factor influencing the configuration of the face, especially of the nasomaxillary complex, is dentition. There is little evidence in the newborn's jaws of the dental structures that will develop. However, inspection of Figure 2–6, which shows the maxilla and mandible of a child, reveals a pallisade of multi-tiered primary and permanent teeth in many stages of development (Enlow, 1975). The growth and development of teeth and related dental architecture have been studied extensively, and methods of evaluation and modalities of treatment of these structures are discussed in Chapters 45 and 46.

Basicranium

The basicranium is a particularly fascinating region that has been the subject of much investigation (Bosma, 1976). It is phylogenetically the oldest skeletal component and anatomically may be considered the keystone of craniofacial growth. The basicranium is derived from separate cartilage masses which house the oto-olfactory anlage and surrounding membranous bone. It is through this region that the majority of cranial nerves pass.

It is very difficult to visualize the basicranium from the anterior perspective. Figure

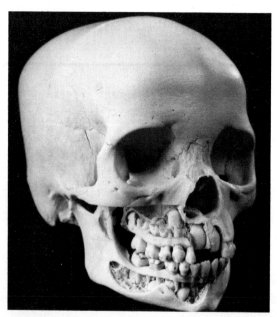

Figure 2–6 Skull of a child that demonstrates mixed dentition. The multitiered battery of teeth is partially responsible for the increase in the vertical and horizontal dimensions of the jaws with increasing age.

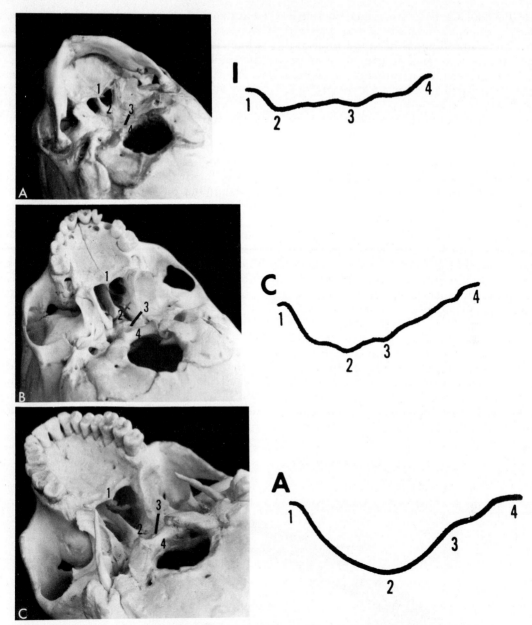

Figure 2–7 A, Tangential views of the inferior aspect of the skulls of an infant (I). B, child (C), C, adult (A). All illustrate the change in configuration of the nasopharynx. The anatomical landmarks indicated are: 1, posterior nasal spine; 2, junction of vomer with the base of the skull; 3, spheno-occipital synchondrosis; and 4, edge of the foramen magnum. The change in size and configuration of the posterior choanae and the nasal airway with age can be appreciated.

2–7, which is a tangential view of the inferior aspect of the skull, reveals that the nasomaxillary complex covers the anterior portion, beneath the anterior cranial fossa. The posterior portion of the cranial base, which provides the roof of the nasopharynx, is most important. In Figure 2–7 the shape of this region has been traced on three skulls from different age groups. In the infant (I) this line is relatively flat, but with growth and development it assumes a more curved appearance in the child (C). This is due not only to increased depth, which results from remodeling of the palate, but also to the flexure of the basicranium. These changes provide an enlarged nasal airway to meet the requirements for gas exchange and speech resonance in the adult (A). The spheno-occipital synchondrosis has been presumed to represent the primary growth site of the basicranium. This assumption has been the subject of much controversy, and at present it is believed that there are a number of centers within the cranial base that are responsible for growth.

The relationship of the cranial base to craniofacial development has been described by Burdi (1976) (Fig. 2–8). As previously stated, the cranial base is the keystone in craniofacial development. As such, it is influenced by a number of forces. During fetal life and early childhood, neural influences predominate because of the rapid development of the brain. With the postnatal development of the airway, the nasal influences play a more important role, and, because of speech and nutritional requirements, pharyngeal influences develop. The cranial base in turn will, via a biofeedback mechanism, influence development of the pharynx, palate, and face. Thus, there is a reciprocal relationship in which morphogenic changes in one area can influence development of a surrounding area. This is indeed a complex mechanism by which the control of facial development has evolved. It is important, however, to realize

that many of the normal and abnormal facial characteristics have their origin in this region, which is phylogenetically the oldest part of the skull.

For the clinician who is interested in ear, nose, and throat disorders, this is an important region for several reasons. Many of the dysplasias will affect this region, and since vital structures pass through its foramina, their function may be affected. The size of the nasopharyngeal airway is in part determined by the configuration of the cranial base, and this has an effect on respiration and middle ear function because of the dynamics of airflow. The ear can also be affected because the osseous eustachian tube passes through the cranial base, and the muscles that control the cartilaginous portion of the tube take their origin from the cranial base.

FUNCTIONS OF THE HUMAN CRANIOFACIAL COMPLEX

In these first two chapters, we have discussed prenatal and postnatal development and have alluded to some of the many functions of the craniofacial complex: respiration,

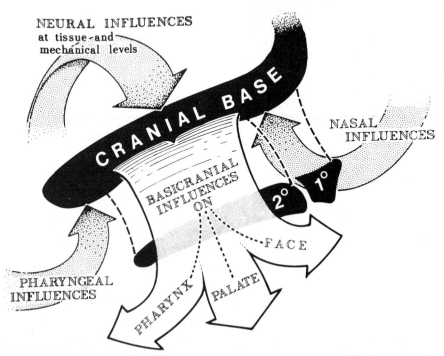

Figure 2–8 A conceptual summary of developmental forces involved in shaping the basicranium (stippled arrows) and the subsequent biofeedback influences from the cranial base (large, light arrow) onto the pharynx, face, primary palate (1 °), and secondary palate (2 °). (Reprinted with permission from Burdi, A.R. Development of the Basicranium. DHEW Publication (NIH) No. 76–989.)

olfaction, speech, digestion, hearing, balance, vision, and neural integration. The tissue components of this complex can be classified as skeletal tissue, soft tissue, and functional spaces (nasopharyngeal and oropharyngeal). Space permits only a brief discussion of these functions, but since the musculature is intimately related to skeletal development, it will be discussed in more detail.

Eye. One of the most salient elements of human evolution has been the development of vision as a dominant sense. It was this sense that enabled primitive humans to survive as a species and to develop our present state of technology. The development of binocular vision enabled humans to evolve a system of eye–hand coordination that their increased cerebral function can utilize.

Ear. The ear has dual functions of hearing and balance. The balance mechanism is of earlier phylogenetic development and is represented by paired organs that are connected to the brain. Hearing is a person's most important contact with his or her environment, for without adequate hearing, speech and communication will not develop.

Nose. The sense of smell, which is of such importance in the lower animals, is one of the less important basic functions in man. However, the conditioning of inhaled air and the provision of a nasal airway are two important functions of the nose in respiration.

Mouth. The facial part of the digestive tract — the mouth — has a vital function, and, although it may be temporarily bypassed by artificial means, the ultimate growth and development of the organism will be affected if the anatomy of this area is altered.

Speech, which utilizes both the air and food passages, is a relatively recent phylogenetic function. For the human, however, speech is one of the major achievements and represents the most important means of communication and expression. The neuromuscular functions of the craniofacial complex are concerned with both the aesthetic and the expressive functions of the face. The human face covers a highly complicated skeletal framework with extremely flexible and expressive soft tissue. It is capable of an amazing number of motions and has the ability to convey emotion. Since the face is not covered, even slight facial deformities may be difficult to conceal and can seriously affect the appearance, and thus the interpersonal relationships, of a child. This was expressed beautifully by Charles Bell in 1821.

The human countenance performs many functions — in it we have combined the organs of mastication, of breathing, of natural voice and speech, and of expression. These motions are performed directly by the will; here also are seen signs of emotions, over which we have but a very limited or imperfect control; the face serves for the lowest animal enjoyment, and partakes of the highest and most refined emotions.

The distribution of the facial musculature is illustrated in Figure 2–9, which demonstrates the relationship of the vaious facial muscle masses. Facial movements that occur during fetal life were described by Hooker (1939) and have been discussed in detail by Humphrey (1970).

At birth the infant's musculature is primarily involved with the functions of suckling and swallowing. The airway is maintained, and there are primitive facial reflexes which provide some expression. Experiments have shown that there are responses to taste such as sweet and sour (Steiner, 1973). Early postnatal facial expressions are largely imitations, but most of the facial muscles are used for mandibular stabilization and airway functions. During subsequent postnatal growth and development, there will be tremendous changes in the facial neuromusculature. According to Enlow (1975), more attention has been given to the study of growth of the craniofacial skeleton than to the neuromusculature. One of the reasons for this is that it is much more difficult to study the neuromusculature of the face than it is to study bony structures of the face; consequently, we know less about the facial and jaw muscles and are less certain of what we do know than we are about the knowledge of bones and teeth.

During the early periods of embryonic growth, an intimate functional relationship exists between the muscles and the bones to which they are attached. Obviously, when the bones grow the muscles also must change their size and shape. As a consequence, the muscles occupy different positions, and there is constant adjustment in the attachments of muscles to the skeleton. For instance, changes in the vertical dimensions of the skull will result in a reorientation of the angles at the musculo-osseous junctions.

The influence of the facial musculature on skeletal growth will depend on the region involved. Since the most powerful of the facial muscles are involved with mastication, the influence of musculature on the dentition

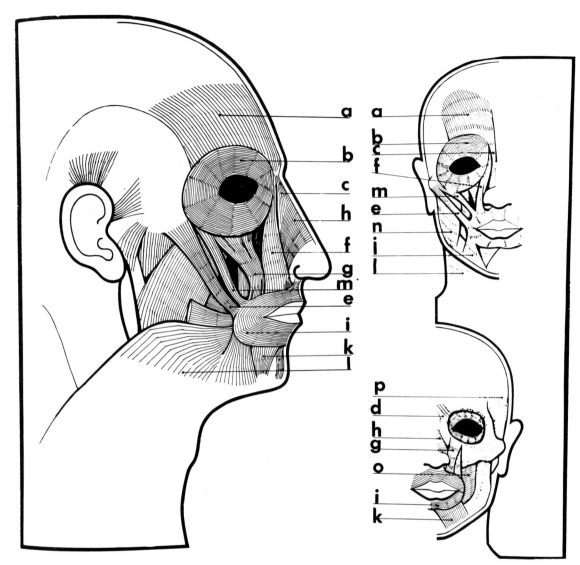

Figure 2-9   The distribution of the facial muscles and the complexity of this musculature are illustrated in this figure. The muscles originate in laminal form and segment into specific muscles, as described by Gasser (1967), a, frontalis; b, orbicularis oculi; c, procerus; d, corrugator; e, zygomaticus major; f, levator labii superioris et alae nasi; g, levator labii; h, compressor naris; i, orbicularis oris; j, depressor anguli oris; k, depressor labii inferioris; l, platysma; m, zygomaticus minor; n, masseter nonexpressive; o, buccinator nonexpressive; p, temporal nonexpressive.

and especially on the mandible will be considerable. Muscles of the airway and food passages compete for influence with the tongue, one of the most powerful muscles of the head.

As a final comment on postnatal craniofacial growth and development, just as the embryo begins as an undifferentiated cell mass, the newborn appears as an undifferentiated craniofacial complex. Because of differential growth, highly developed individual characteristics will appear as the newborn matures. In the skeleton, osteoblastic and osteoclastic activity lead to bone deposition, resorption, and displacement. The stimuli for alterations in skeletal development are both genetic and environmental, and it is a balance of these two factors that is responsible for the ultimate craniofacial configuration. The functions of the craniofacial complex, the most characteristic of which in humans are binocular vision (so important in eye–hand coordination), speech, and an infinite variety of facial expressions, have evolved over millions of years. It is understandable that we should desire to know more about this very important area of development, but it is also obvious why study of the craniofacial complex involves deep concentration and unusual effort to yield results.

SELECTED REFERENCES

Dorst, J. P. 1971. Changes of the skull during childhood. *In,* Newton, T. H., and Potts, D. G. (Eds.) Radiology of the Skull and Brain, Vol. 1. St. Louis, The C. V. Mosby Co.
   This is a concise description of skeletal growth during childhood; it also discusses some cranial abnormalities.

Enlow, D. A. 1975. Handbook of Craniofacial Growth. Philadelphia, W. B. Saunders Co.
   This is a well-organized text that illustrates the various growth concepts and also includes an extensive bibliography.

Rubin, P. 1964. Dynamic Classification of Bone Dysplasias. Chicago, Yearbook Medical Publishers, Inc.
   This book describes some of the anomalies of the craniofacial complex and also discusses the growth mechanisms by which they occur.

REFERENCES

Bassett, A. H. 1972. The biophysical approach to craniofacial morphogenesis. Acta Morphol. Neerl. Scand., *10*:71–86.

Bell, C. 1833. The nervous system of the human body. Papers delivered to the Royal Society on the Subject of the Nerves. Stereotyped by Duff Green, for the Register and Library of Medical and Chirurgical Science.

Bosma, J. (Ed.) 1976. Symposium on the Development of the Basicranium. Bethesda, MD., U.S. Dept. of Health, Education and Welfare. DHEW Pub. No. (NIH) 76–989.

Burdi, A. R. 1976. Biological forces which shape the human midface before birth. *In* McNamara, J. (Ed.) Factors Affecting the Growth of the Midface. Ann Arbor, MI, Center for Human Growth and Development, University of Michigan.

Burdi, A. R. 1976. Early development of the human basicranium: Its morphogenic controls, growth patterns and relations. *In* Bosma, J. (Ed.) Symposium on the Development of the Basicranium. Bethesda, MD., U.S. Dept. of Health, Education and Welfare, DHEW Pub. No. (NIH) 76–989.

Dorst, J.P. 1971. Changes of the skull during childhood. *In,* Newton, T. H., and Potts, D. G. (Eds.) Radiology of the Skull and Brain, Vol. 1. St. Louis, The C. V. Mosby Co.

Enlow, D. H. 1973. Growth and the problem of the local antral mechanism. Am. J. Anat., *178*:2.

Enlow, D. H. 1975. Handbook of Craniofacial Growth. Philadelphia, W. B. Saunders Co.

Gasser, R. F. 1967. The development of the facial muscles in man. Am. J. Anat., *120*:357–375.

Hogarth, B. 1965. Drawing the Human Head, 9th ed. New York, Watson-Guptill Publications.

Hooker, D. 1939. Fetal behavior. Association for Research in Nervous and Mental Disease XIX. Interrelationship of Mind and Body, pp. 237–243, Baltimore, The Williams and Wilkins Co.

Humphrey, T. 1970. Reflex activity in the oral and facial area of the human fetus. *In* Bosma, J. (Ed.) Second Symposium on Oral Sensation and Perception. Springfield, IL, Charles C Thomas Pub.

Latham, R. A. 1970. Maxillary development and growth: The septomaxillary ligament. J. Anat., *107*:471.

Ligett, J. 1974. The Human Face. London, Constable & Co., Ltd.

McNamara, J. 1976. Factors Affecting the Growth of the Midface. Craniofacial Growth Series, Monograph No. 6. Ann Arbor, MI, Center for Human Growth and Development. University of Michigan.

Moss, M. L. 1968. The primacy of functional matrices in one facial growth. Dent. Pract. Dent. Rec., *19*:65–73.

Pierce, R., et al. 1977. The Cranium of the Newborn Infant. Bethesda, MD, U.S. Dept. of Health, Education and Welfare, DHEW Pub. No. (NIH) 76–788.

Rubin P. 1964. The Dynamic Classification of Bone Dysplasias. Chicago, Yearbook Medical Publishers, Inc.

Scott, J.A. 1953. The cartilage of the nasal septum. Br. Dent. J., *95*:37.

Sokoloff, L., and Bland, J. 1975. The Musculoskeletal System. Baltimore, The Williams and Wilkins Co.

Steiner, J. 1973. The gustofacial response: Observations on normal and anencephalic infants. *In* Bosma, J. (Ed.) Oral Sensation and Perception. Bethesda, MD, U.S. Dept. of Health, Education and Welfare, DHEW Pub. No. (NIH) 73–546.

Williams, P. L., et al. 1969. Basic Human Embryology, 2nd ed. Philadelphia, J. B. Lippincott Co.

Chapter 3

CRANIOFACIAL ANOMALIES AND SYNDROMES

M. Michael Cohen, Jr., D.M.D., Ph.D.
Sylvan E. Stool, M.D.

INTRODUCTION

The first two chapters of this text have discussed normal prenatal and postnatal growth and development and have mentioned how alterations in these processes may result in abnormalities. In this chapter we will discuss some of the current concepts regarding genesis of the abnormalities that are seen by the physician who is interested in ear, nose, and throat disorders in children. This vast and complex field encompasses the concepts of a number of disciplines, such as embryology, chemistry, molecular biology, and genetics, and information is increasing at such a rapid rate that it is not possible for any text to remain current. However, several general principles have now been well established that will enable the physician to develop an orderly approach to the evaluation of the abnormal child. Even though there are great variations among individuals with abnormal characteristics, those individuals with syndrome complexes by definition will resemble each other more than each will resemble the normal members of his or her family.

SYNDROMES

The word "syndrome" is of Greek derivation and means "running together." Minimally, a syndrome is viewed as several abnormalities in the same individual. One of

the misconceptions about this term is the logic that many use when they see a unique patient. They do not acknowledge that a single patient can represent a syndrome. This is the equivalent of saying that if you see a unicorn, you cannot acknowledge that the animal exists until you see a herd of unicorns. Thus, it is important to discuss how a syndrome is delineated.

THE PROCESS OF SYNDROME DELINEATION

Because craniofacial anomalies are associated with a great many syndromes, the physician who treats children may see a wide variety of anomalies, many of which are not readily recognized as being associated with any one syndrome. In a large study of newborn infants with multiple anomalies of all kinds (syndromes), only 40 per cent had known, recognized syndromes (Marden et al., 1964). The other 60 per cent had provisionally unique-pattern syndromes that needed to be further delineated. A major task in medicine is to delineate the unknown-genesis syndromes as rapidly as possible because such delineation fosters good patient care. As an unknown-genesis syndrome becomes delineated, its phenotypic spectrum, its natural history, and its risk of recurrence become known, allowing for better patient care and family counseling. The process of syndrome delineation also aids in

Table 3-1 SYNDROME DELINEATION

Type
A   Unknown-genesis syndrome
    A-1   Provisionally unique-pattern syndrome
    A-2   Recurrent-pattern syndrome

B   Known-genesis syndrome
    B-1   Pedigree syndrome
    B-2   Chromosomal syndrome
    B-3   Biochemical-defect syndrome
    B-4   Environmentally induced syndrome

the study of pathogenesis by sorting anomalies into meaningful biologic categories (Cohen, in press).

The process of syndrome delineation can be divided into stages (Cohen, 1977) (Table 3–1). In an *unknown-genesis syndrome* (Type A) the cause is simply not known.

In a *provisionally unique-pattern syndrome* (Type A–1), two or more abnormalities are observed in the same patient in such a way that the clinician does not recognize the overall pattern of defects from his own experience, nor from searching the literature, nor from consultation with the most learned colleagues in the field. The patient shown in Figures 3–1 and 3–2 has a provisionally unique-pattern syndrome. This baby has craniosynostosis involving the sagittal suture, as well as prominent veins, strabismus,

micrognathia, an umbilical hernia, complete anterior dislocation of the tibia, and deformed feet. It is most likely that these abnormalities have a common cause (even though we do not yet know what that is) rather than being caused by different factors acting independently. The probability that such abnormalities occur in the same patient by chance becomes less likely the more abnormalities the patient has and the rarer these abnormalities are individually in the general population. Obviously if a second example comes to light, the condition is no longer unique. A provisionally unique-pattern syndrome is a one-of-a-kind syndrome to a particular observer at a particular point in time (Cohen, 1977).

The next stage in syndrome delineation is the *recurrent-pattern syndrome* (Type A–2). A recurrent-pattern syndrome can be defined as a similar or identical set of abnormalities in two or more unrelated patients. A recurrent-pattern syndrome is illustrated in Figures 3–3 through 3–5. These two patients from different families share in common a wide bifrontal diameter, ocular hypertelorism, large ears, micrognathia, finger contractures at the proximal interphalangeal joints, deeply set fingernails, umbilical hernias, excessive growth, and a variety of other abnormalities. The presence of the same abnormalities in two or more patients

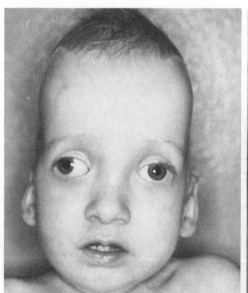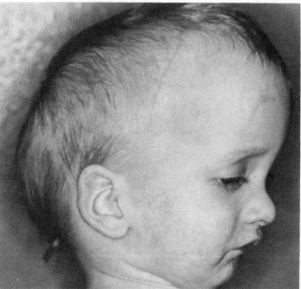

Figure 3–1 Provisionally unique-pattern syndrome. Craniosynostosis involving the sagittal suture, prominent veins, strabismus, and micrognathia. (From Cohen, M. M., Jr. 1977. Genetic perspectives on craniosynostosis and syndromes with craniosynostosis. J. Neurosurg., 47:886.)

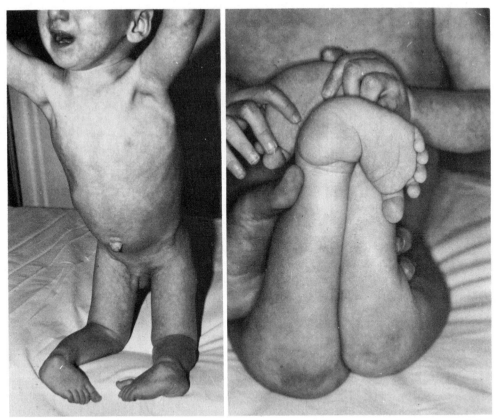

Figure 3–2 Provisionally unique-pattern syndrome. Umbilical hernia, complete anterior dislocation of the tibia allowing the knees to be flexed in reverse with the feet against the chest, metatarsus adductus. (From Cohen, M. M., Jr. 1977. Genetic perspectives on craniosynostosis and syndromes with craniosynostosis. J. Neurosurg., *47*:886.)

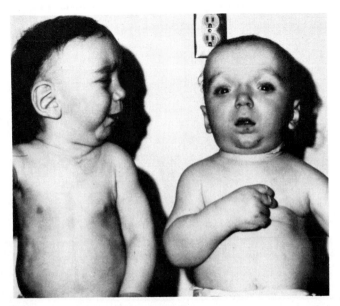

Figure 3–3 Recurrent-pattern syndrome in two patients. Note wide bifrontal diameter, ocular hypertelorism, large ears, long philtrum, and micrognathia. (From Weaver, D. D. et al. 1974. A new overgrowth syndrome with accelerated skeletal maturation, unusual facies, and camptodactyly. J. Pediatr., *84*:547.)

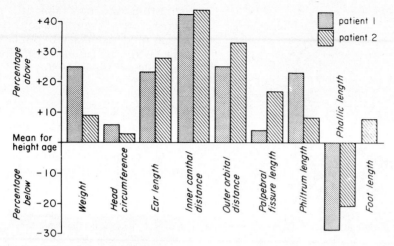

Figure 3–4   Recurrent-pattern syndrome in two patients. Note similarity of measurement patterns. (From Weaver, D. D. et al. 1974. A new overgrowth syndrome with accelerated skeletal maturation, unusual facies, and camptodactyly. J. Pediatr., *84:*547.)

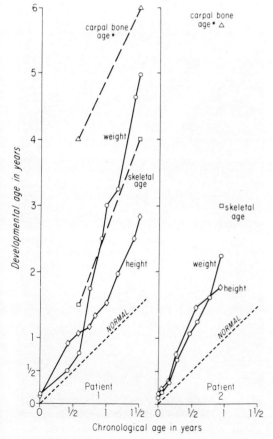

Figure 3–5   Recurrent-pattern syndrome in two patients. Note similarity in accelerated osseous maturation pattern. (From Weaver, D. D. et al. 1974. A new overgrowth syndrome with accelerated skeletal maturation, unusual facies, and camptodactyly. J. Pediatr., *84:*547.)

suggests (but does not prove) that the pathogenesis in both cases may be the same. At the recurrent-pattern stage of syndrome delineation, the etiology is still not known. In general, the validity of a recurrent-pattern syndrome increases the more abnormalities there are in the condition and the more patients that are known to have the syndrome (Cohen, 1977).

A *known-genesis syndrome* (Type B) can be defined as two or more abnormalities causally related on the basis of (1) occurrence in the same family or, less conclusively, the same mode of inheritance in different families; (2) a chromosomal defect; (3) a specific defect in an enzyme or structural protein; or (4) a teratogen or environmental factor (Cohen, 1977). These four types of known-genesis syndromes have been respectively termed pedigree, chromosomal, biochemical-defect, and environmentally induced syndromes.

A *pedigree syndrome* (Type B–1) is of known-genesis on the basis of pedigree evidence alone; the basic defect itself remains undefined, although the condition is known to represent a monogenic disorder. A good example is the autosomal recessive Meckel syndrome (Fig. 3–6) characterized by features such as occipital encephalocele, polydactyly, polycystic kidneys, and other anomalies (Cohen, 1980).

A *chromosomal syndrome* (Type B–2) is cytogenetically defined and may be typified by the trisomy 13 syndrome (Fig. 3–7). This

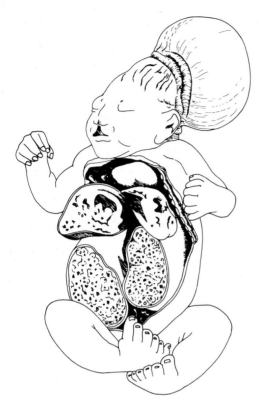

Figure 3–6 Known-genesis syndrome of the pedigree type. Autosomal recessively inherited Meckel syndrome. Note encephalocele, cleft lip, polydactyly, polycystic kidneys, and cysts of liver. (From Cohen, M. M., Jr. 1980. The Patient with Multiple Anomalies. New York, Raven Press.)

condition is characterized by holoprosencephaly, microphthalmia, posterior scalp defects, forehead hemangiomas, orofacial clefting, polydactyly, hyperconvex fingernails, cardiac defects, and many other abnormalities (Cohen, 1980).

In a *biochemical-defect syndrome* (Type B–3), specific enzymatic defects are known in recessive syndromes. The term is also meant to include specific defects in structural proteins when these become known in some of the dominant disorders. The Lesch-Nyhan syndrome (Fig. 3–8), characterized by hypoxanthine-guanine-phosphoribosyl-transferase deficiency, is an X-linked recessive biochemical defect syndrome (Cohen, 1980).

An *environmentally induced syndrome* (Type B–4) is defined in terms of the causative teratogen or environmental factor. Infants born to mothers who are chronic alcoholics during their pregnancies have an increased risk of having growth deficiency of prenatal onset

persisting into postnatal life, microcephaly, mental deficiency, narrow palpebral fissures, mild maxillary hypoplasia, short nose (Fig. 3–9), cardiac malformations, and other anomalies (Cohen, 1980).

COMMENTS ON THE SYNDROME DELINEATION PROCESS

The process of syndrome delineation is summarized in Figure 3–10. Generally, a

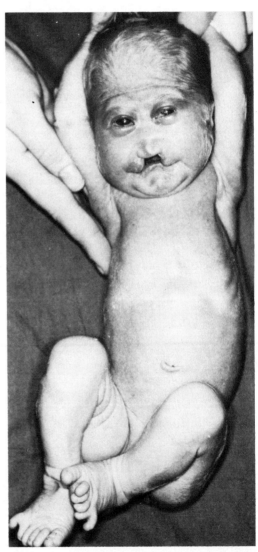

Figure 3–7 Known-genesis syndrome of the chromosomal type. Trisomy 13 syndrome. Patient has holoprosencephaly, ocular hypotelorism, absent nasal bones, premaxillary agenesis, and extra digits. (From Conen, P. E. et al. 1966. The "D" syndrome. Report of four trisomic and one D/D translocation case. Am. J. Dis. Child, *111*:236–247.)

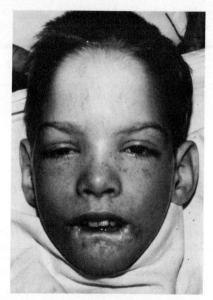

Figure 3–8. Biochemical-defect syndrome of the enzymatic type. Lesch-Nyhan syndrome with enzymatic defect in purine metabolism that leads to self-mutilation of lips. (From Cohen, M. M., Jr. 1980. The Patient with Multiple Anomalies. New York, Raven Press.)

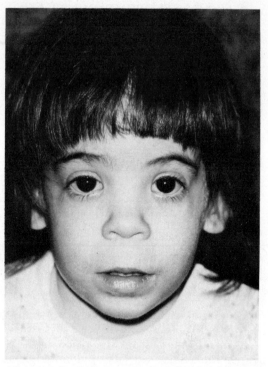

Figure 3–9 Known-genesis syndrome of the environmentally induced type. Fetal alcohol syndrome. Note microcephaly, narrow palpebral fissures, mild maxillary hypoplasia, and short nose. (From Clarren, S. K., and Smith, D. W. 1978. The fetal alcohol syndrome. N. Engl. J. Med., 289:1063.)

syndrome can be placed into one of the categories discussed previously. Occasionally, a syndrome may be delineated in a one-step delineation, thus bypassing several of the stages mentioned earlier. For example, if a new chromosomal abnormality is discovered during the laboratory investigation of a patient clinically defined as having a provisionally unique-pattern syndrome, the patient represents a known-genesis syndrome of the chromosomal type in a one-step delineation. However, the variability of the clinical expression must await the discovery of more patients with that syndrome. In other instances, such as a large dominant pedigree with many affected individuals, a known-genesis syndrome of the pedigree type and much of its phenotypic variability can be determined in one step (Cohen, 1980).

THE PACE OF SYNDROME DELINEATION

Syndrome delineation is proceeding at a very rapid rate. In 1971, for example, 72 syndromes were known in which orofacial clefting was one feature. By 1978, however, 154 syndromes with orofacial clefting were

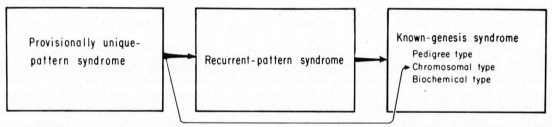

Figure 3–10 A diagrammatic summary of the process of syndrome delineation. (From Cohen, M. M., Jr. 1980. The Patient with Multiple Anomalies. New York, Raven Press.)

Table 3–2   SYNDROME DELINEATION
INVOLVING CLEFTS FROM 1971 TO 1978

Etiology	Gorlin et al., 1971	Cohen, 1978
Monogenic	39	79
Autosomal dominant	(17)	(35)
Autosomal recessive	(18)	(39)
X-linked	(4)	(5)
Environmentally induced	0	6
Chromosomal	15	29
Unknown genesis	18	40
Total	72	154

The criteria for inclusion or exclusion of a syndrome with orofacial clefting differ slightly in these two compilations. Thus, a small proportion of the increase from 1971 to 1978 is attributable to this factor rather than to syndrome delineation *per se.*
Adapted from Gorlin, R. J., et al. 1971. Facial clefting and its syndromes. Birth Defects, 7(7):3, and Cohen, M. M., Jr. 1978. Syndromes with cleft lip and cleft palate. Cleft Palate J., 15:306–328.

recognized — an increase of more than 100 per cent (Table 3–2). Thus, the discovery of new syndromes is taking place at a very rapid rate. Since various epidemiologic surveys have shown that other anomalies may accompany as many as 13 to 50 per cent of all cases of cleft palate, the delineation of many more new syndromes from this group can be anticipated.

SIGNIFICANCE OF SYNDROME DELINEATION

The significance of syndrome delineation cannot be overestimated. If the phenotypic spectrum is known, the clinician can search for suspected defects that may not be apparent immediately but that may produce clinical problems at a later date, such as a hemivertebra in the Goldenhar syndrome. If a certain complication may occur in a given syndrome, such as a Wilms tumor in the Beckwith-Wiedemann syndrome, the clinician is forewarned to monitor the patient with intravenous pyelograms. Finally, if the recurrence risk is known, the parents can be counseled properly about future pregnancies. This is especially important if the risk is high and the disorder is severely handicapping or disfiguring, has mental deficiency as one component, or entails a dramatically shortened life span. For example, cleft palate or the Robin complex is a common

feature of the Stickler syndrome, an autosomal dominant disorder with a 50 per cent recurrence risk when one parent is affected. In this condition, retinal detachment occurs in 20 per cent of reported cases and blindness occurs in 15 per cent. Genetic counseling is of great importance because the risk of developing serious ocular problems is high. This relatively common condition also illustrates the importance of syndrome delineation because the entity was unrecognized before 1965, although surely it existed before that time. Thus, syndrome delineation fosters good patient care; the overall treatment program gains rationality. In contrast, with a provisionally unique-pattern syndrome, the treatment program and overall management frequently leave something to be desired (Cohen, 1980).

BIOLOGIC TYPES OF SYNDROMES AND SYNDROME MODELS

Syndromes can be analyzed at different levels of organization. In the broadest possible context, there are perhaps four general classes of syndromes: the dysmetabolic syndrome, the dyshistogenetic syndrome, the malformation syndrome, and the deformation syndrome. They represent disturbances in metabolism, tissues, organs, and regions, respectively. The four types of syndromes and their relationships are illustrated by the inverted triangle shown in Figure 3–11. It will be observed that the syndromes are stratified. For example, a malformation syndrome has dyshistogenetic and dysmetabolic levels underlying it. However, the syndrome expresses itself at the organ formation level (Cohen, 1980).

The four different syndrome models and their characteristics are summarized in Table 3–3 and will be discussed in detail in the following section. The term syndrome model is used to convey the notion that not necessarily every finding in a given syndrome can be accounted for. In fact, the power of any model is that it is an abstract conception and, as such, it can ignore some of the realities in the same manner as the law of gravity ignores friction. "Science," says the noted philosopher Morris Cohen, "must abstract some phenomena and neglect others because not all things that exist

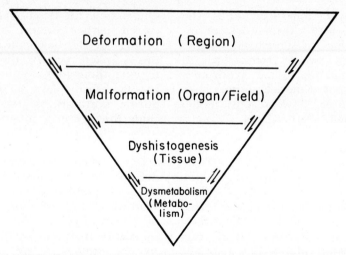

Figure 3–11 Stratification of syndromes into dysmetabolic, dyshistogenetic, malformational, and deformational syndromes that represent expression at the metabolic, tissue, organ, and regional levels, respectively. (From Cohen, M. M., Jr. 1980. The Patient with Multiple Anomalies. New York, Raven Press.)

Table 3–3 BIOLOGIC TYPES OF SYNDROMES

Type	Level of Disturbance	Features
Dysmetabolic syndrome	Metabolism	Child frequently normal at birth with generalized progressive disturbances after birth Clinical features relatively uniform compared with other types of syndromes Not associated with congenital malformations Biochemically defined or potentially so Commonly recessive mode of inheritance
Dyshistogenetic syndrome	Tissues	Simple dyshistogenetic syndrome Characterized by involvement of only one germ layer Inheritance may be dominant or recessive Hamartoneoplastic syndrome Characterized by hamartomas, hyperplasia, and a propensity for neoplasia May involve one, two, or all three germ layers Inheritance is commonly dominant
Malformation syndrome	Organs	Two or more malformations or malformation complexes in the same patient Characterized by embryonic pleiotropy in which the pattern of malformations or malformation complexes are developmentally unrelated at the embryologic level Lack of biochemical definition; highest state of definition is a known-genesis syndrome of the chromosomal or pedigree type
Deformation syndrome	Regions	Characterized by alterations in the shape or structure of previously normal parts Most important cause is lack of fetal movement whether the cause be a mechanical, functional, or malformational disturbance Commonly affects musculoskeletal system

together are relevant together." Thus, the models provide us with a framework for analyzing various types of syndromes by giving us convenient points from which to move in our thinking. Some syndromes closely fit the proposed models; others have overlapping features between one model and another (Cohen, 1980).

Dysmetabolic Syndromes

Dysmetabolic syndromes are characterized by inborn errors of metabolism. Metabolism is carried out as a stepwise series of reactions, each step being catalyzed by a specific enzyme. The pathway may be blocked at any step, either completely or partially, by impaired activity of the required enzyme resulting from a mutation in the gene that codes for the normal enzyme. Enzymatic blocks have various consequences: a precursor substance may accumulate just proximal to the block, and the excess precursor itself may be harmful; alternative minor pathways may open, resulting in overproduction of toxic metabolites; the deficient product itself may be a substrate for a subsequent reaction that cannot proceed normally; or a feedback inhibition type of control mechanism may be impaired (Cohen, 1980).

The clinical manifestations of dysmetabolic syndromes depend upon the particular metabolic pathway involved, the availability of alternative pathways, the solubility of metabolites, the particular organ systems involved, and a variety of other factors. A typical example of a dysmetabolic syndrome is the Hurler syndrome — an autosomal recessive disorder characterized by α-L-iduronidase deficiency, which inhibits degradation of α-L-iduronide-containing mucopolysaccharides. Accumulation of undegraded or partially degraded acid mucopolysaccharides interferes with the normal function of affected cells and leads to the characteristic clinical symptoms, which are progressive: a coarse facial appearance, thick lips, and a large tongue are evident by two years of age. Other progressive features include growth deficiency, mental retardation, cloudy corneas, hepatosplenomegaly, cardiomegaly, and excessive urinary excretion of dermatan sulfate and heparin sulfate. Another example of a dysmetabolic

syndrome is the Lesch-Nyhan syndrome discussed earlier under known-genesis syndromes of the biochemical defect type. In this X-linked recessive disorder, the enzyme hypoxanthine-guanine-phosphoribosyl-transferase, which plays a role in regulating purine synthesis, is missing. Features include uric aciduria, mental retardation, and self-mutilation of the lips and fingers (Fig. 3–8).

Dysmetabolic syndromes have enzymatic defects and are primarily recessively inherited. Some dominantly inherited dysmetabolic syndromes may be caused by basic defects in structural proteins in some instances and by regulator mutations that result in excessive or reduced enzyme reduction rates in other instances (Cohen, 1980).

In small molecular weight dysmetabolic syndromes, a patient is usually normal at birth, since intrauterine compensation has taken place by placental or maternal metabolism. In large molecular weight dysmetabolic syndromes, abnormalities may be present during fetal life or at birth. Generalized progressive disturbances may appear after birth in some instances or considerably later in some instances, or only under special circumstances in still other instances (Cohen, 1980).

Pure dysmetabolic syndromes are not associated with congenital malformations such as cleft lip, ventricular septal defect, or syndactyly. There are a few exceptions to this general rule of thumb. First, it is possible for a malformation to occur coincidentally in a dysmetabolic syndrome. However, the frequency would not be expected to be any more common than the frequency of isolated malformations in the general population. Second, it has been observed that albinism (a dysmetabolic disorder in which melanin is not produced) is associated with a defect in decussation of the optic nerve fibers. Finally, pseudovaginal perineoscrotal hypospadias accompanies the 5-α-reductase deficiency (Cohen, 1980).

Dyshistogenesis and Dyshistogenetic Syndromes

The term dyshistogenesis is used here to mean a developmental disturbance of tissue structure. There are two classes of dyshistogenetic syndromes: simple dyshistogenetic syndromes and hamartoneoplastic syndromes (Cohen, 1980).

In simple dyshistogenetic syndromes, only one germ layer is involved, and either dominant or recessive inheritance may be encountered. The Marfan syndrome is a good example. Its features include tall stature with a disproportionately long lower segment, long fingers and toes, detachment of the lens from the zonular fibers in the eye, and aortic aneurysms. All of these features trace their origin to a basic defect in connective tissue (derived from the mesodermal germ layer) even though the exact nature of the defect is unknown. The Marfan syndrome is inherited as an autosomal dominant trait (Cohen, 1980).

In hamartoneoplastic syndromes one, two, or all three germ layers are involved. The major distinguishing features consist of hamartomas and a marked propensity for neoplasia. Autosomal dominant inheritance is characteristically observed, although a few such conditions occur only sporadically (Cohen, 1980).

Hamartomas are tumor-like, non-neoplastic admixtures of tissues indigenous to the part with an excess of one or more of these. Hamartomas are either present at birth or appear later during postnatal maturation of the tissue. Hemangiomas are excellent examples of hamartomas. They may occur singly or multiply and, in contrast to malformations such as cleft lip, hamartomas are located variably throughout the body with the consequences of the abnormality depending upon the location. For example, a large hemangioma of the face has an obvious psychologic impact, while the same lesion on a limb may result in hemihypertrophy. If such a lesion occurs in the gastrointestinal tract, bleeding may occur that results in anemia (Cohen, 1980).

The impact of a hamartoma on the patient depends upon (1) the type, (2) the location, (3) the size, and (4) the number of lesions. On this basis, hamartomas may be classified as major or minor. A small hemangioma and an intradermal nevus are examples of minor hamartomas. Minor hamartomas differ from minor malformations in being much more common in the general population; for example, the average caucasian person has 20 melanotic nevi. Hemangiomas are common and frequently

occur internally (e.g., hemangiomas of the liver) as well as on the skin (Cohen, 1980).

Both hamartomas and neoplasms are nonspecific. Each may occur as an isolated abnormality or may be a component part of various syndromes. For instance, a hemangioma may occur alone or together with multiple enchondromas in the Maffucci syndrome. An angiomyolipoma may occur alone or as part of tuberous sclerosis, and a Wilms tumor may occur alone, with hemihypertrophy, or as part of trisomy 18 syndrome (Cohen, 1980).

Hamartomatous tissue varies in its predisposition to neoplasia. The lesions of neurofibromatosis are prone to neurofibrosarcomatous degeneration. On the other hand, malignant transformation of angiomyolipomas of the kidney in tuberous sclerosis is uncommon, and neoplasia in the angiomatous lesions of the Klippel-Trénaunay-Weber syndrome is virtually unknown (Cohen, 1980).

Hamartoneoplastic syndromes can be divided into unilaminar, bilaminar, or trilaminar types depending upon which germ layers are involved. A good example of a hamartoneoplastic syndrome is the dominantly inherited Gardner syndrome characterized by osteomas, odontomas, colonic polyposis, fibromas, and sometimes lipomas and leiomyomas.

Malformations and Malformation Syndromes

A *malformation* may be defined as a primary structural defect resulting from a localized error of morphogenesis (Anonymous, 1975). Malformations are defects of organ structure that arise during the formation or developmental placement of an organ. Approximately 3 per cent of all newborns have significant malformations, and approximately 1 per cent have multiple malformations or malformation syndromes.

There are three general classes of malformations — incomplete morphogenesis, redundant morphogenesis, and aberrant morphogenesis. The most common class is incomplete morphogenesis, which has a number of different subtypes (Cohen, 1980).

In *incomplete morphogenesis,* embryogenesis

proceeds normally until the time of developmental arrest. Of the many different types of incomplete morphogenesis, only three will be considered here. In *aplasia*, there is total failure of development. If, for instance, the optic vesicle fails to contact the surface ectoderm, the lens fails to form. In *hypoplasia*, there is partial failure of development. Micrognathia is an example of such underdevelopment. *Failure of fusion* is a third type of incomplete morphogenesis. If the palatine processes fail to contact each other during embryogenesis, for example, a cleft palate results (Cohen, 1980).

Redundant morphogenesis is much less common. In this class of malformations, the redundant organ passes through the same stage of morphogenesis at the same time as does its normal counterpart. A good example of redundant morphogenesis is an ear tag in the presence of a perfectly normal ear. Such a tag may be interpreted as having developed from a supernumerary auricular hillock (Cohen, 1980).

Aberrant morphogenesis is rare and has no counterpart in normal morphogenesis. A good example is a mediastinal thyroid gland. During normal morphogenesis, the

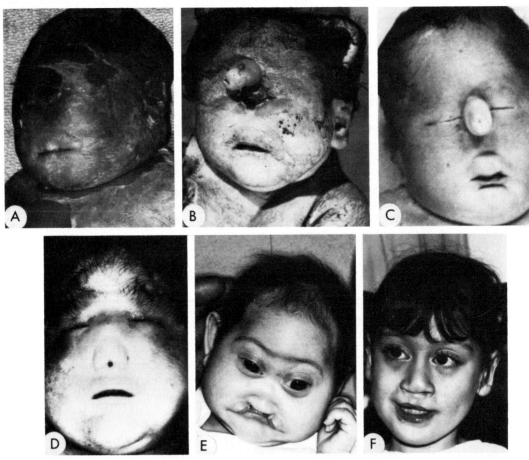

Figure 3–12 Spectrum of dysmorphic facies associated with variable degrees of holoprosencephaly. *A*, Cyclopia without proboscis formation; note single central eye. *B*, Cyclopia with proboscis. *C*, Ethmocephaly. Ocular hypotelorism with proboscis formation. *D*, Cebocephaly; ocular hypotelorism with single nostril nose. *E*, Premaxillary agenesis, flat nose, and ocular hypotelorism. *F*, Ocular hypotelorism and surgically repaired cleft lip. (*A* and *F* from Cohen, M. M., Jr. 1976b. Etiologic heterogeneity in holoprosencephaly and facial dysmorphia with comments on the facial bones and cranial base. *In* Bosma, J. F. (Ed.) Development of the Basicranium. Bethesda, MD, U.S. Dept. of Health, Education and Welfare. (NIH) 76–989, p. 384. *B*, *C*, and *D* from Cohen, M. M., Jr., et al. 1971. The holoprosencephalic disorders: Clinical, pathogenetic, and etiologic considerations. Birth Defects, 7(7):125. *E* from DeMyer, W. E., and Zeman, W. 1963. Alobar holoprosencephaly (arhinencephaly) with median cleft lip and palate. Confin. Neurol., 23:1.)

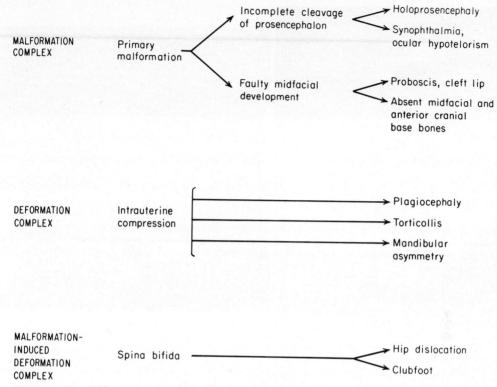

Figure 3–13 Malformation complex with holoprosencephaly as an example (top). Deformation complex with intrauterine compression as an example (middle). Malformation-induced deformation complex with spina bifida as an example (bottom). (From Cohen, M. M., Jr. 1980. The Patient with Multiple Anomalies. New York, Raven Press.)

thyroid gland is never found in the mediastinum (Cohen, 1980).

Malformations may be relatively simple or complex. The later the defect is initiated, the simpler the malformation. Examples of simple malformations include microphthalmia, cleft lip, and choanal atresia. Malformation complexes are initiated earlier during organogenesis and have more far-reaching consequences. A *malformation complex* may be defined as a malformation together with its subsequently derived structural changes. The primary defect sets off a morphologic chain of secondary and tertiary events, resulting in what appear to be multiple malformations. All such malformations, however, are developmentally interrelated. Holoprosencephaly and facial dysmorphia represent an example of a malformation complex (Fig. 3–12). In holoprosencephaly the embryonic forebrain fails to cleave sagittally into cerebral hemispheres, transversely into telencephalon and diencephalon, and horizontally into olfactory and optic bulbs. Holoprosencephaly varies in its degree of severity. At the mild end of the spectrum is simple absence of the olfactory tracts and bulbs. Holoprosencephaly is associated with facial dysmorphia, which also varies from mild to severe (Fig. 3–12). A single eye or closely set eyes, proboscis formation, a single-nostril nose, a flattened nose, and a median cleft lip may be observed variably or in combination. All of the malformations encountered trace their origins developmentally to a single primary defect in morphogenesis (Fig. 3–13 top).

Malformations may be minimally or maximally expressed. For example, bifid uvula is a minimal expression of cleft palate. Malformation complexes may also be minimally or maximally expressed.

Major malformations are of surgical, medical, or cosmetic importance and may lead to secondary functional disturbances. Examples of major malformations include cleft lip, congenital heart defects, and omphalocele. *Minor malformations* are generally not

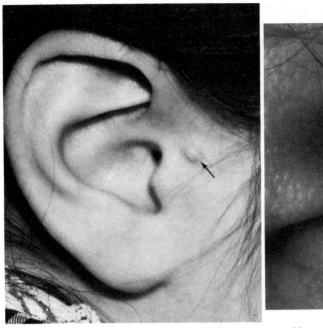 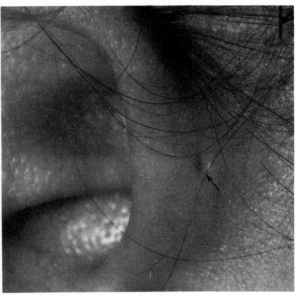

Figure 3–14 Ear tag as an example of a minor malformation (left). Ear pit as an example of a minor malformation (right). (From Cohen, M. M., Jr., 1980. The Patient with Multiple Anomalies. New York, Raven Press.)

of surgical or medical significance, although in some instances they may be of cosmetic concern, such as webbed neck, ptosis of the eyelids, or prominent epicanthic folds. Rarely, they may cause complications such as an infected branchial arch fistula (Marden et al., 1964). Some minor anomalies are pictured in Figure 3–14. A representative but by no means exhaustive list of minor malformations of the head and neck is presented in Table 3–4.

The occurrence of single minor malformations is common in the general population, being found in 15 per cent of all newborns. The occurrence of two is less common, and the presence of three or more minor anomalies is distinctly unusual, occurring in approximately 1 per cent of all newborns. Of great interest is the occurrence of a major malformation in 90 per cent of all newborns with three or more minor malformations (Marden et al., 1964). The implication is clear that any newborn with three or more minor malformations should be carefully evaluated for possible hidden major malformations such as cardiac, renal, or vertebral defects.

Minor malformations occur with high frequency in many malformation syndromes. For example, in the Down syndrome, 79 per cent of all malformations detectable by clinical examination are minor malformations; in trisomy 18 syndrome, 38 per cent of the malformations are minor; in trisomy 13, 50 per cent of the malformations are minor; and in the Turner syndrome, 73 per cent of detectable malformations are minor. Thus, minor malformations serve as diagnostic aids for many malformation syndromes.

Finally, 42 per cent of patients with idiopathic mental retardation have three or more malformations of which 80 per cent are minor (Smith and Bostian, 1964). Thus, minor malformations may be considered aids in the predicting of mental deficiency associated with other abnormalities.

The significance of minor malformations is summarized in Table 3–5. Of all minor anomalies, 71 per cent occur in the head and neck region and the hand — easily accessible areas for the pediatric otolaryngologist to evaluate (Fig. 3–15).

All malformations, whether major or minor, and all malformation complexes are nonspecific. Each may occur as an isolated abnormality; each may also occur as a component part of various syndromes. Cleft palate, for example, may occur alone or as part of the autosomal dominant Stickler syndrome, characterized by high myopia, retinal detachment, and various abnormalities of bones and joints. A minor malformation such as epicanthic folds may occur alone or as part of the Down syndrome. Holoprosencephaly and facial dysmorphia may occur alone or as part of the trisomy 13 syndrome (Cohen, 1980).

Because malformations occur with various frequencies in different syndromes, they are facultative rather than obligatory; that is, they may or may not be present in a given

Table 3–5 SIGNIFICANCE OF MINOR ANOMALIES

Fact	Implication
In newborns with three or more minor anomalies, 90 per cent have a major anomaly	Search for major anomaly
Minor anomalies are present in many multiple congenital anomaly syndromes	Aid in diagnosis
42 per cent of idiopathic mental retardation cases have three or more anomalies of which 80 per cent are minor anomalies	Aid in prognosis

Table 3–4 MINOR MALFORMATIONS

Head
Aberrant scalp hair patterning
Flat occiput
Bony occipital spur
Third fontanel

Eyes
Epicanthic folds
Epicanthus inversus
Upward-slanting palpebral fissures
Downward-slanting palpebral fissures
Short palpebral fissures
Dystopia canthorum
Minor hypertelorism
Minor hypotelorism
Minor ptosis
Coloboma (eyelid, iris)

Ears
Primitive shape
Lack of helical fold
Asymmetric size
Posterior rotation
Small ears
Protuberant ears
Absent tragus
Double lobule
Auricular tag
Auricular pit
Narrow external auditory meatus

Nose
Small nares
Notched alae

Oral Regions
Borderline small mandible
Incomplete form of cleft lip
Bifid uvula
Aberrant frenulum
Enamel hypoplasia
Malformed teeth
Malocclusion

Neck
Mild webbed neck
Branchial cleft fistula

Adapted from Marden, P. M., et al. 1964. Congenital anomalies in the newborn infant, including minor variations. J. Pediatr., 64:358.

example of a condition in which they are known to be features. For example, two common features of the Beckwith-Wiedemann syndrome are macroglossia and omphalocele, yet cases are known in which both malformations are absent. Pathognomonic abnormalities for various syndromes are rare.

Since malformations are both nonspecific and facultative for various disorders, syndrome diagnosis is made from the overall pattern of abnormalities. It cannot be stressed strongly enough that diagnosis is never made on the basis of specific abnormalities but on the basis of the overall pattern. The more abnormalities there are in a given syndrome, the easier the condition is to diagnose because even if some of the features are not expressed, the overall pattern is still discernible. Conversely, the fewer abnormalities there are in a given syndrome, the more difficult the condition is to diagnose if some of the features are not expressed. In general, diagnosis of any syndrome with some of its features not expressed is more of a problem in a sporadic case than in a familial instance. For example, if an eight year old child has ocular hypertelorism and bifid ribs but no other abnormalities, the diagnosis of the basal cell nevus syndrome is extremely probable if the child comes from a family in which one or more members are known to have the syndrome. It is highly likely that such a child will go on to develop other features of the syndrome, such as jaw cysts, bridging of the sella turcica, and basal cell carcinomas. On the other hand, the diagnosis is extremely uncertain if a child with the same anomalies comes from a perfectly normal family (Cohen, 1980).

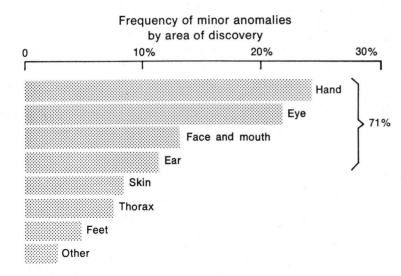

Figure 3–15 Frequency of minor anomalies by region. Of all minor anomalies, 71 per cent occur in the head and neck region and the hand. (Modified from Smith, D. W., and Bostian, K. E. 1964. Congenital anomalies associated with idiopathic mental retardation. J. Pediatr., 65:189.)

A *malformation syndrome* may be defined as two or more malformations or malformation complexes in the same individual. A true malformation syndrome is characterized by *embryonic pleiotropy* in which a pattern of developmentally unrelated malformations or malformation complexes occurs. The difference between a malformation syndrome and a malformation complex is diagrammed in Figure 3–16. We have already discussed holoprosencephaly and facial dysmorphia as an isolated malformation complex. In the trisomy 13 syndrome — a true malformation syndrome — holoprosencephaly and facial dysmorphia occur together with congenital heart defects, polydactyly, and other anomalies (Fig. 3–7). These malformations are unrelated at the embryonic level, although at a more basic level they have a common cause — an extra chromosome No. 13.

Another example of a true malformation syndrome exhibiting embryonic pleiotropy is the previously discussed Meckel syndrome (Fig. 3–6). Suppose the patient has an encephalocele, polycystic kidneys, polydactyly, a ventricular septal defect, and cleft palate. It will be observed that the embryonic timing of each of these malformations is different (Fig. 3–17). This is true for many malformation syndromes. The only statement that can be made about embryonic

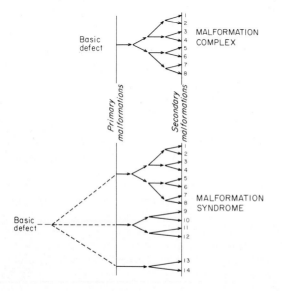

Figure 3–16 Diagram comparing malformation complex (top) with true malformation syndrome (bottom). Isolated holoprosencephaly is an example of a malformation complex. When holoprosencephaly occurs with polydactyly, congenital heart defects, and other anomalies as in trisomy 13 syndrome, the condition is a malformation syndrome. (From Cohen, M. M., Jr. 1980. The Patient with Multiple Anomalies. New York, Raven Press.)

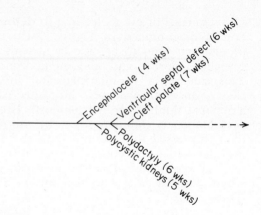

Figure 3–17 Embryonic timing of various malformations in a patient with the Meckel syndrome. (From Cohen, M. M., Jr. 1980. The Patient with Multiple Anomalies. New York, Raven Press.)

timing is that something happened *prior to* the earliest induced malformation. In the case of the Meckel syndrome, the earliest induced malformation occurred at four weeks of development. However, we cannot pinpoint the syndrome as being induced *at* four weeks because the other four malformations were induced *later* during development. Furthermore, since the Meckel syndrome has autosomal recessive inheritance, the abnormality was present *earlier* than four weeks of development — specifically at the zygotic stage of development since two mutant genes in the homozygous state were present at that time (Cohen, 1980).

Malformation syndromes lack biochemical definition. The highest stage in malformation syndrome delineation is a known-genesis syndrome of the pedigree or chromosomal type. Pedigree syndromes may involve mutant embryonic proteins that are switched off before birth, thus masking the basic defect. Many other malformation syndromes remain unknown-genesis syndromes of the provisionally unique or recurrent-pattern type (Cohen, 1980).

Deformations and Deformation Syndromes

A *deformation* is an alteration in the shape or structure of a previously normal part (Anonymous, 1975). Deformations arise most frequently during fetal life. Since the most common cause is intrauterine molding, the musculoskeletal system is usually affected. The most important factor contributing to deformations is lack of fetal movement, whatever the cause. Important deformations include clubfoot, congenital hip dislocation, congenital postural scoliosis, plagiocephaly in the absence of craniosynostosis, and some cases of sternomastoid torticollis. An example of a mandibular deformation is illustrated in Figure 3–18. Approximately 2 per cent of all newborns have deformations (Dunn, 1976).

Figure 3–18 Mandibular deformation resulting from sharply lateroflexed position of the head *in utero* with the shoulder pressed against the mandible for a long period of time. (Courtesy of Mead Johnson and Company.)

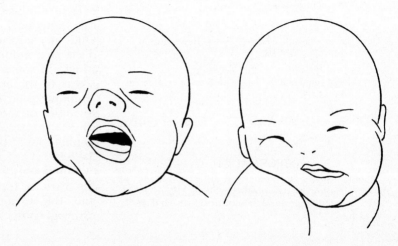

A sequence of events leading to deformation is diagrammed in Figure 3–19. First pregnancies tend to be associated with unstretched uterine and abdominal muscles. This can result in uteroplacental insufficiency which, in turn, can lead to decreased amnionic fluid (oligohydramnios). Breech presentation is common since the uterus is too compressed to allow the fetus to rotate into the cephalic position. Uterine restraints on fetal movement allow the mild but persistent extrinsic forces to deform the fetus (Dunn, 1976).

The characteristic features of deformations and malformations are contrasted in Table 3–6. Malformations tend to arise during the organogenetic period of embryonic life. Deformations, on the other hand, tend to arise during the fetal period after organogenesis is already completed. Thus, deformations affect intact regions. A clubfoot is not an organ defect but a regional defect, since the limbs have already formed. Furthermore, deformations tend not to have structural defects, in contrast to malformations which do. With clubfoot, for example, five digits and the proper number of phalanges and metatarsals are present. This is not true of malformations such as ectrodactyly (missing digits) or polydactyly (extra digits). Some degree of perinatal mortality accompanies every statistical survey of malformations because of the high incidence of central nervous system and cardiovascular anomalies. In contrast, the perinatal mortal-

Table 3–6 COMPARISON OF MALFORMATIONS AND DEFORMATIONS

	Malformation	Deformation
Time of Occurrence	Embryonic Period	Fetal Period
Level of Disturbance	Organ	Region
Structural Changes	Present	Absent
Perinatal Mortality	Present	Absent
Spontaneous Correction	Absent	Present
Correction by Posture	Absent	Present

ity tends to be extremely low in surveys of deformations. Finally, spontaneous correction in some instances or, more commonly, correction by posturing is possible for many deformations. Tibial torsion present in newborns, for example, undergoes spontaneous correction in most cases. Postural correction is feasible in many cases of scoliosis, congenital hip dislocation, and clubfoot. In contrast, spontaneous correction of malformations is rare (except for septal defects of the heart) and correction by posturing is not possible.

Since the deformations discussed thus far have a common mechanical origin, more than one deformation might be expected to occur in some patients. In a study of approximately 4500 newborns, Dunn (1976) indicated that one third of all patients with deformations had multiple deformations or deformation complexes. A *deformation complex* may be defined as two or more deformations in the same patient that have a common cause. For example, plagiocephaly, torticollis, and mandibular asymmetry in the same patient may all be caused by intrauterine compression. A deformation complex is contrasted with a malformation complex in Figure 3–13 (top, middle).

Deformations may result from mechanical, functional, or malformational causes. One mechanical cause of deformations is decreased amnionic fluid (oligohydramnios) which, in some instances, may be caused by a tear in the amnion. The resultant lack of amnionic fluid can lead to the multiple deformities of the Potter syndrome, which include compressed facies and abnormal positioning and bowing of the limbs (Fig. 3–20A).

Functional causes of deformation include the various forms of congenital hypotonia and the various neuromuscular types of arthrogryposis. Congenital hypotonia may

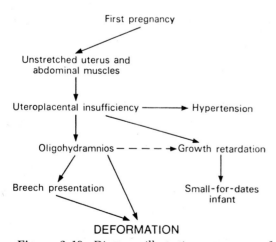

DEFORMATION

Figure 3–19 Diagram illustrating sequence of events leading to deformation. (From Dunn, P. M. 1976. Congenital postural deformities. Brit. Med. Bull., 32:71.)

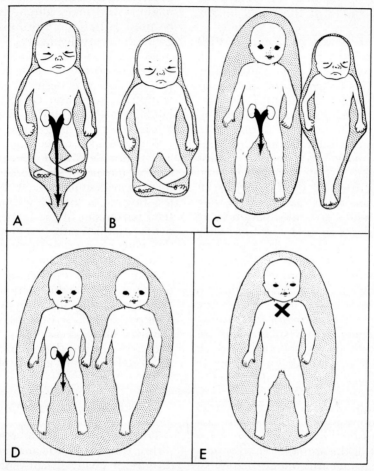

Figure 3–20 Decreased amnionic fluid (oligohydramnios) has different causes and, except under unusual circumstances, leads to facial and limb deformities of the Potter syndrome. Normally, small amounts of amnionic fluid cross the amnion as a transudate, but most of the amnionic fluid results from fetal urination. *A*, Amnionic tear with chronic leakage of fluid leading to oligohydramnios, Potter facies, and limb positioning defects. Both kidneys are present and urination is normal. All the features in this fetus are deformations. Therefore, this is a pure deformation syndrome. *B*, Patient has bilateral renal agenesis. Lack of fetal urination results in compression, producing the features of the Potter syndrome. This is a malformation-induced deformation syndrome. *C*, Monozygotic twins with separate amnions. Fetus on left has kidneys, and enough fetal urine is contributed to the amnionic fluid to protect the fetus from the deformities of the Potter syndrome. Fetus on right has sirenomelia, a more extensive caudal axis defect in which both kidneys and genitalia are absent. Since there is no urinary contribution to the amnionic fluid, compression results in the facial and upper limb deformities of the Potter syndrome. *D*, Monozygotic twins sharing a common amnionic sac. Note that although fetus on right has sirenomelia, Potter deformities are not present because fetus on left provides enough urine in the amnionic fluid to protect cotwin from deformities of the Potter syndrome. *E*, Patient has bilateral renal agenesis and therefore does not contribute fetal urine to amnionic fluid. Fetus does not have Potter syndrome because fetus has neurologic swallowing deficit. Thus, amnionic fluid crossing the amnion does not pass through the fetus but remains external to it and protects it from extrinsic deforming forces. (From Cohen, M. M., Jr. 1980. The Patient with Multiple Anomalies. New York, Raven Press.)

be accompanied by micrognathia, microglossia, prominent lateral palatine ridges, abnormal flexion creases, pes planovalgus, and other deformities. The arthrogryposes are characterized by congenital immobility of the limbs and fixation of the joints in certain positions.

In a study of newborns, Dunn (1976) found that approximately 8 per cent of all malformations were associated with deformations. When this occurred, the malformations primarily involved the central nervous system and the urinary tract, and most frequently the deformations were secondary to the malformations. Both central nervous system and urinary tract malformations cause deformations by interfering with fetal movements. Figure 3–13 (bottom) gives an example of a *malformation-induced deformation complex*. Spina bifida, a malformation, may lead to hip dislocation and clubfoot since the malformation produces partial paralysis of the legs. The resultant muscular imbalance is an intrinsic deforming force that limits the ability to kick and hence to change the position of the fetus to alter the direction along which extrinsic deforming forces may be acting. Hip dysplasia, hip dislocation, and clubfoot may be explained on this basis, as may hypoplastic lower limbs (a growth disturbance caused by deficient innervation).

Amnionic fluid protects the fetus from extrinsic deforming forces. Some of the amnionic fluid crosses the amnion as a transudate, but most of the amnionic fluid is produced by fetal urine. Any malformation of the urinary tract that significantly reduces the output of fetal urine results in a decrease in amnionic fluid, thus producing the deformities of the Potter syndrome. Earlier we indicated that a mechanical tear in the amnion could result in the Potter syndrome (Fig. 3–20*A*). However, malformations such as bilateral renal agenesis (Fig. 3–20*B*), severe hypoplastic kidneys, severe polycystic kidneys, or urethral atresia can also cause oligohydramnios and its consequences. A more severe caudal axis malformation complex such as sirenomelia, in which kidneys and genitalia are both missing, also produces oligohydramnios and the deformed face and hands of the Potter syndrome (Fig. 3–20*C*).

We have already defined deformation, deformation complex, and malformation-induced deformation complex. The term *deformation syndrome* should be reserved for conditions in which all the abnormalities are deformities. There is no basic distinction between a deformation complex and a deformation syndrome, although the latter can be used to indicate more extensive or more generalized involvement.

As with hamartomas and malformations, deformations too are nonspecific. For example, clubfoot may occur as an isolated deformation. It may also be secondary to spina bifida. Finally, it may be a component part of one of the arthrogryposes.

A distinction can be made between major and minor deformations on the basis of the clinical impact of the deformity. Minor deformations include absent flexion creases on the fingers or hands secondary to lack of fetal movement of the involved joints. Cutaneous dimples and prominent lateral palatine ridges are other examples of minor deformities (Cohen, 1980).

Although the distinction between deformations and malformations based upon fetal and embryonic periods is useful, rigid adherence to these time periods can be misleading since occasionally a deformation may arise during the embryonic period and many deformations arise after birth.

Comments on Syndrome Models

To reiterate, syndrome models provide us with a framework for analyzing various syndromes by giving us convenient points from which to move in our thinking. As we indicated earlier, some syndromes closely fit the models proposed, and others have overlapping features that express themselves at more than one level. Figure 3–21 shows the four types of syndromes and how they are stratified. The representative syndromes at the margins of the inverted triangle all express themselves at two different levels. As we have already noted, bilateral renal agenesis results in oligohydramnios, producing the Potter syndrome. Here, we have a malformation-induced deformation syndrome. The basal cell nevus syndrome has dyshistogenetic features such as basal cell carcinomas and medulloblastoma. True malformations, such as ocular hypertelorism, bifid ribs, and cervical spina bifida occulta, are also present. In one form of the

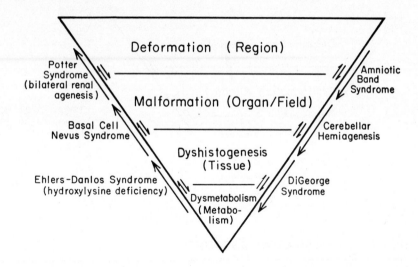

Figure 3–21 Examples of compound syndromes that express themselves at more than one level. (From Cohen, M. M., Jr. 1980. The Patient with Multiple Anomalies. New York, Raven Press.)

Ehlers-Danlos syndrome, hydroxylysine deficiency results in dyshistogenetic skin changes (Cohen, 1980).

Figure 3–22 shows a patient with the Zellweger syndrome who has a tower-like skull, an enlarged liver, and is severely hypotonic. Figure 3–23 shows that the Zellweger syndrome expresses itself at all four levels. The patient has a progressive downhill course with an early demise, typical of individuals with dysmetabolic syndromes. The brain exhibits neuronal malmigration, which is dyshistogenetic. Patent ductus arteriosus and patent foramen ovale are frequently present, and they represent malformations. Finally, clubfoot and flexion contractures of the fingers represent deformations (Cohen, 1980).

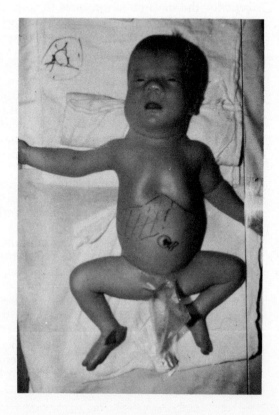

Figure 3–22 Patient with the Zellweger syndrome. Severe hypotonia, enlarged liver, and tower-like skull. (From Cohen, M. M., Jr. 1980. The Patient with Multiple Anomalies. New York, Raven Press.)

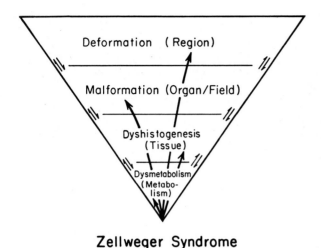

Zellweger Syndrome

Figure 3–23 Diagram of the Zellweger syndrome showing clinical expression at all four levels. See text. (From Cohen, M. M., Jr. 1980. The Patient with Multiple Anomalies. New York, Raven Press.)

AN APPROACH TO SYNDROME DIAGNOSIS AND PATIENT MANAGEMENT

As previously stated, because a great many syndromes have craniofacial anomalies as one of their components, the clinician who is interested in ear, nose, and throat disorders may become involved in the evaluation of the child. Since there are so many syndromes it is difficult to remember them except for the most common ones. A logical approach to any patient who exhibits anomalies is to narrow the possibilities systematically by first using the least expensive and invasive techniques and by consulting texts devoted exclusively to the subject of syndromology (Gorlin et al., 1976). If a syndrome can be found in a syndromology textbook, the clinician will immediately become aware of the phenotypic spectrum of abnormalities known in the disorder and will therefore know the appropriate tests to perform.

A history and physical examination should be performed in all cases. The history should include pedigree, maternal and paternal ages at the time of conception, the presence or absence of parental consanguinity, the number of abortions, and possible maternal exposure to environmental teratogens. Physical examination should include not only a description of the obvious anomalies but also a search for the more obscure ones. Otoscopic and audiometric evaluation may be of special importance because of the cryptic nature of this system and the fact that early identification of hearing loss may be amenable to therapy.

Since the syndromes of known genesis and many of the recurrent-pattern syndromes can be found in syndromology textbooks, they can be properly identified, and a rational workup of such patients may be planned from the description of the syndrome. This cannot be done for provisionally unique-pattern syndromes nor for some of the less well-known recurrent-pattern syndromes. With the aid of the child's history and physical examination, the clinician should strive to classify unknown-genesis syndromes as dysmetabolic, dyshistogenetic, malformational, or deformational. Such classification allows the physician to evaluate the patient rationally. One of the first steps in evaluating an unusual appearing child is to decide whether the manifestations were present prenatally or postnatally. If the patient has no malformations of the embryonic type, was normal at birth, and shows progressive deterioration with time, the patient has a dysmetabolic syndrome. It is unlikely, although not impossible, that the unknown metabolic defect will be discovered in the patient in question. Nevertheless, consultation in an academic medical center should be sought in selected cases since it is sometimes possible to define a new dysmetabolic disorder. Even if the patient represents a sporadic instance in the family, the highest recurrence risk for future affected offspring is 25 per cent since all known dysmetabolic syndromes are recessive.

If the unknown-genesis syndrome is dyshistogenetic, is it simple or hamartoneoplastic? If it is the latter type, the patient should be monitored frequently for the possibility of neoplasms.

If the unknown-genesis syndrome is malformational, it is not rational to perform amino acid screening and similar tests, since pure malformation syndromes are not known to be dysmetabolic. Certainly, a chromosomal study is indicated.

Many patients with multiple malformations may have growth deficiency of prenatal onset in which the infant is small for gestational age. If this type of growth deficiency is regarded as a malformation, that is, as hypoplasia of the whole individual, it is not surprising that other malformations, especially those of incomplete morphogenesis, frequently accompany the growth deficiency. Organ formation and developmental placement are susceptible to malformation if hypoplasia occurs during the period of rapid differentiation and growth. Endocrine studies and various other tests for humorally mediated growth deficiency are contraindicated in pure malformation syndromes. Such growth deficiency usually persists into postnatal life and has no known treatment.

In the patient with multiple malformations of unknown genesis, it is important to sort out malformation complexes from true malformation syndromes whenever this is possible. Malformation complexes tend to have a multifactorial recurrence risk, whereas true malformation syndromes are more likely to be monogenic or chromosomal.

The finding of multiple deformations of unknown genesis defines a deformation syndrome. When growth deficiency accompanies multiple deformations, it is usually caused by intrauterine compression or uteroplacental insufficiency. Endocrine studies and various tests for humorally mediated growth deficiency are contraindicated. Catch-up growth is expected following birth once the fetus is no longer compressed within the uterus.

There are, of course, many syndromes of unknown genesis that may express their phenotypes at more than one level. When malformations and deformations occur together in the same syndrome of unknown genesis, the clinician should strive to explain the deformations in terms of the malformations when this is possible. Some unknown-genesis syndromes with phenotypic expression at more than one level are occasionally refractory to the type of analysis proposed here.

As an aid to the physician's understanding of congenital anomalies and syndromes, each section of this text has a review of the embryology and development of the organ system discussed, as well as a detailed review of the congenital anomalies usually associated with that particular region. It is possible in many instances that if the most obvious abnormality is recognized and reviewed, insight may be gained into the biologic type and possible associated manifestations of the specific abnormality.

SELECTED REFERENCES

Cohen, M. M., Jr. 1977. On the nature of syndrome delineation. Acta Genet. Med. Gemellol. (Roma), 26:103.
  A comprehensive article about the process of syndrome delineation.
Gorlin, R. J., Pindborg, J. J., and Cohen, M. M., Jr. 1976. Syndromes of the Head and Neck, 2nd ed. New York, McGraw-Hill.
  An encyclopedic text that catalogs over 700 syndromes that have various head and neck components.

Cohen, M. M., Jr. 1980. The Patient with Multiple Anomalies. New York, Raven Press.
  A new text that offers a systematic understanding of syndromology.

REFERENCES

Anonymous. 1975. Classification and nomenclature of morphological defects. Lancet, 1:513.
Clarren, S. K., and Smith, D. W. 1978. The fetal alcohol syndrome. N. Engl. J. Med., 289:1063.
Cohen, M. M., Jr. 1976a. Dysmorphic syndromes with craniofacial manifestations. In Oral Facial Genetics. St. Louis, C. V. Mosby Co., p. 500.
Cohen, M. M., Jr. 1976b. Etiologic heterogeneity in holoprosencephaly and facial dysmorphia with comments on the facial bones and cranial base. In Bosma, J. F., (Ed). Development of the Basicranium. U. S. Dept. of Health, Education and Welfare, (NIH) 76–989, Bethesda, MD, p. 384.
Cohen, M. M., Jr. 1977. On the nature of syndrome delineation. Acta Genet. Med. Gemellol, (Roma), 26:103.
Cohen, M. M., Jr. 1978. Syndromes with cleft lip and cleft palate. Cleft Palate J.. 15:306–328.
Cohen, M. M., Jr. 1980. The Patient with Multiple Anomalies, New York, Raven Press.
Conen, P. E., Phillips, K. G., and Manntuer, L. S. 1962. Multiple developmental anomalies and trisomy of a 13–15 group chromosome ("D" syndrome). Can. Med. Assoc. J., 87:709.
DeMyer, W. E., and Zeman, W. 1963. Alobar holopro-

sencephaly (arhinencephaly) with median cleft lip and palate. Confin. neurol., *23*:1.

Dunn, P. M. 1976. Congenital postural deformities. Brit. Med. Bull., *32*:71.

Gorlin, R. J., Cervenka, J., and Pruzansky, S. 1971. Facial clefting and its syndromes. Birth Defects, 7(7):3.

Gorlin, R. J., Pindborg, J. J., and Cohen, M. M., Jr. 1976. Syndromes of the Head and Neck, 2nd ed. New York, McGraw-Hill.

Marden, P. M., Smith, D. W., and McDonald, M. J. 1964. Congenital anomalies in the newborn infant, including minor variations. J. Pediatr, *64*:358.

Smith, D. W., and Bostian, K. E. 1964. Congenital anomalies associated with idiopathic mental retardation. J. Pediatr., *65*:189.

Weaver, D. D., Graham, C. B., Thomas, I. T., et al. 1974. A new overgrowth syndrome with accelerated skeletal maturation, unusual facies, and camptodactyly. J. Pediatr., *84*:547.

Chapter 4

MALFORMATIONS AND SYNDROMES

William S. Crysdale, M.D.

Normal growth and development and the pathogenesis of congenital anomalies have been discussed in the preceding chapters. These chapters, along with the works of Smith (1976), Cohen et al. (1976), and Konigsmark and Gorlin (1976) may be utilized to understand the many facets of congenital anomalies involving the craniofacial complex. In this chapter, the specific concerns of the otolaryngologist will be discussed. He or she is an integral member of the team that cares for these children and is most concerned with management of hearing and airway problems. This material primarily reflects the methods utilized at the clinics of the Hospital for Sick Children in Toronto. There will obviously be different approaches in other institutions when dealing with such complex medical and surgical problems.

Congenital abnormalities stem from errors in morphogenesis and genetic factors. An anomaly is an isolated local structural defect or malformation that results in a structural change, such as an isolated cleft of the bony or secondary palate. A syndrome comprises several defects in a recognizable pattern and is not a consequence of a single local error of morphogenesis (for example, Crouzon syndrome). Thus, each craniofacial syndrome has certain clinical features (albeit of varied frequency and degree), and the condition has a recognized natural history and an established mode of inheritance or risk of occurrence. Syndrome labels are confusing because they are described by different types of terms: eponyms, anatomic terms, enzyme deficiencies, or chromosome abnormalities, for instance. As medical knowledge expands, the descriptions of syndromes may become obsolete, changed, or eliminated. In the meantime, we use various catalogues to describe the incidence and association of congenital defects in anomalies and syndromes (Smith, 1976; Gorlin et al., 1976; Konigsmark and Gorlin, 1976). This chapter discusses the aspects of interest to the otolaryngologist of the normal growth and development and the pathogenesis of congenital anomalies that have been described in the preceding chapters.

THE TEAM APPROACH

Children with craniofacial abnormalities are best managed by a team of specialists (Munro, 1975). The head of the team should accept the responsibility for coordinating the patient's needs from birth to adulthood. Good communication within the team is essential and can be achieved only by group review of the patients and delineation of their needs in open discussion. Team review of patients is time-consuming and hence relatively inefficient, but the byproducts of good intrateam communication and the increased appreciation of other team members' problems, concerns, and special skills are worth the effort. At The Hospital for Sick Children, Toronto, we have two such teams: the maxillofacial team, for treating children with isolated oral clefts, and the craniofacial team, for treating children with other (usually more severe) craniofacial anomalies.

The maxillofacial team, headed by a plastic surgeon, routinely includes a dentist, orthodontist, otolaryngologist, pediatrician, social worker, and speech pathologist (Fig. 4–1). They meet once a week to review all current

55

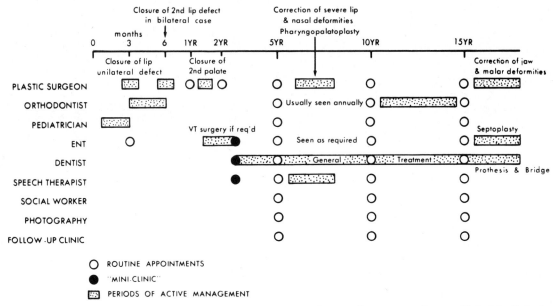

Figure 4-1 Diagrammatic summary of routine specialist involvement in the maxillofacial clinic through which children with cleft lip and palate deformities are followed.

cases, usually five or six patients. Other specialists are consulted as the need arises. All patients with isolated orofacial clefts are reviewed by the team at 5, 10, and 15 years of age, and most are also reviewed between 2 and 3 years of age by a subteam composed of a dentist, otolaryngologist, and speech pathologist. Needless to say, new patients are seen individually by an otolaryngologist and undergo audiologic assessment within a few months of birth.

The craniofacial team, headed by a craniofacial surgeon, has members from 15 other disciplines — anesthesiology, audiology, dentistry, facial anthropology, genetics, medical art, neuro-ophthalmology, neuroradiology, neurosurgery, orthodontics, otolaryngology, psychiatry, psychology, social work, and speech pathology. During the past six years, this team has evaluated 300 children and adults (Munro, 1977).

In our center, the otolaryngologist on the teams mentioned previously is involved in the assessment and management of hearing loss, airway obstruction, speech disorders, chronic infections, and disorders of olfaction.

HEARING LOSS

The importance of early detection and expeditious management of significant hearing

loss cannot be overemphasized. Even mild hearing losses, if not detected early, can significantly retard the acquisition of language skills (Holm and Kumze, 1969). Untreated hearing losses of moderate or greater degree have a measurable — even devastating — effect on speech and intellectual development.

All infants with craniofacial anomalies have a high risk of having a hearing loss and require diligent otologic and audiologic follow-up until their audiologic status has been established (Downs and Silver, 1972). Unfortunately, detection of hearing loss is delayed in a large percentage of children with craniofacial anomalies but without any obvious structural aural defects. This occurs as many persons, lay and medical alike, hold the erroneous belief that because of their odd appearance, such children are mentally retarded (Crysdale, 1978), and thus the delayed acquisition of communication skills is attributed to mental deficiency and not to a possible hearing loss (Fig. 4–2).

Hearing loss in children with craniofacial anomalies may be congenital or acquired. The loss is congenital if there is present at birth significant malformation of the structures of the external, middle, or inner ear. Acquired hearing loss is a consequence of any postnatal process, perhaps a consequence of the malformation that interferes with auditory function.

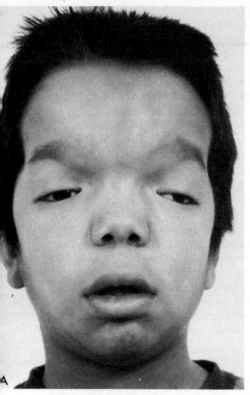

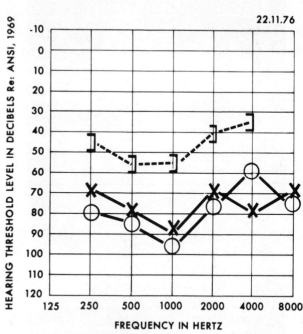

Figure 4–2 A, Poor language development in this North American Indian boy with isolated primary hypertelorism was attributed to mental retardation. B, The mixed congenital hearing loss was finally detected at 10 years of age. Psychologic reassessment now suggests above normal intelligence (Crysdale, 1978).

Congenital Hearing Loss

Congenital hearing loss, usually conductive, is an intrinsic component of many craniofacial syndromes. Deafness associated with an aural anomaly may be due to a primary defect of the temporal bone or secondary defects in bone contiguous to the temporal bone (Caldarelli, 1977). In most craniofacial anomalies, sensorineural hearing loss is thought to be coincidental only.

Atresia of the external auditory meatus, with various degrees of obliteration of the middle ear cleft, is usually associated with microtia. The latter anomaly is frequently seen in Treacher-Collins syndrome (mandibulofacial dysostosis) and hemifacial microsomia (Figs. 4–3 and 4–4). Bilateral atresia of the external auditory meatus with microtia was seen in one patient who had Crouzon disease. Microtia, being visible, is "helpful" to the patient, as it usually stimulates the physician to determine the patient's level of auditory function. In patients who have a craniofa-

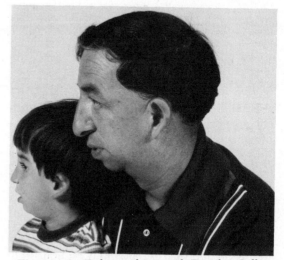

Figure 4–3 Father and son with Treacher-Collins syndrome at 42 and 4 years of age, respectively. Note retrognathia in both individuals. Audiometry in father documents substantial conductive hearing loss. His tympanic membranes are small and oblique, but the middle ear is air-containing. The boy's hearing is normal, although middle ear ventilating tubes have been inserted for the management of serous otitis media.

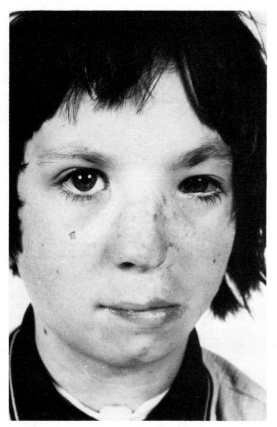

Figure 4–4 Left hemifacial microsomia in an 11 year old boy. Bony ankylosis of the left temporomandibular joint severely limits the jaw movement. Left-sided microtia with 60 dB conductive hearing loss is present. Airway control prior to mandibular surgery was established by inserting a rigid bronchoscope through the opening to the left of the upper incisors after unsuccessful attempts at nasal intubation.

cial syndrome with bilateral microtia and atresia, the middle ear cleft is almost invariably obliterated, and reconstructive middle ear surgery is not possible. However, these patients manage quite well when provided with an appropriate hearing aid, as their intelligence has been found to be normal except when the condition is part of Apert syndrome (acrocephalosyndactyly). We do not recommend reconstructive middle ear surgery for patients with unilateral microtia and atresia, but CROS (Contralateral Routing of Signal) hearing aids may be helpful in auditory rehabilitation.

If a child's ears have a normal appearance, a congenital conductive hearing loss — an invisible deformity — may not be detected until it has adversely affected the development of speech and language. In the absence of microtia, a conductive hearing loss may be a consequence of ossicular deformity or ankylosis or fixation of the stapes. In many of these patients, the tympanic membrane is small and oblique and has abnormal landmarks, an otoscopic finding that should make the physician suspect the presence of a hearing loss. Middle ear surgery may improve the hearing for these children.

Studies of a temporal bone from a patient with Apert syndrome showed the stapedial vestibular joint region to be abnormal with incomplete development of the annular ligament and fixation of the stapes by undifferentiated cartilage in two areas (Lindsay et al., 1975). In another patient with this syndrome, the stapes was found to be fixed when it was inspected at tympanotomy; a gush of perilymphatic fluid occurred from the oval window when the stapes was removed (Bergstrom et al., 1972).

Some patients with hypertelorism have a congenital sensorineural hearing loss; this combination may represent a variant of Waardenburg syndrome.

Acquired Hearing Loss

Acquired hearing loss is usually conductive and is most often the consequence of eustachian tube dysfunction. The degree of middle ear pathology is in proportion to the duration and severity of this eustachian tube dysfunction. Thus, one may observe patients with middle ear effusions or various degrees of middle ear atelectasis or even attic cholesteatoma. Perforations of the pars tensa and extensive tympanosclerosis may be a consequence of middle ear infection or therapeutic procedures such as tympanostomy tube insertion.

Eustachian tube insufficiency is most frequently seen in patients with a cleft secondary palate. It is present also in patients with a craniosynostosis in whom the nasopharynx is distorted, obstructed, or both as a result of aberrant growth of the midface and skull base. It has been suggested that in patients with Apert syndrome the ciliated epithelium in the eustachian tube is abnormal, retarding clearance of middle ear secretions (Selder, 1973).

Successful management of middle ear effusions in patients with palatal clefts usually requires the insertion of tympanostomy tubes, as middle ear effusions in these patients rarely respond to conservative measures. In our center, palatal clefts are repaired at 18 months of age, and the decision to insert tympanostomy tubes is usually deferred for a further three months; then, if the middle ear effusion has not resolved, the tubes are inserted (Crysdale, 1976). Care should be taken when performing myringotomy on patients with craniosynostosis; we found unilateral dehiscence of the jugular bulb in three of our patients (Witzel et al., unpublished observations).

Other pathology related to eustachian tube dysfunction, such as atelectasis of the middle ear and attic cholesteatoma, is observed in older patients; the management of these problems is discussed in another chapter. In our experience, tympanoplastic procedures in children with a history suggestive of eustachian tube dysfunction are unsuccessful in the majority of cases and should be deferred until late adolescence. Extensive tympanosclerosis may cause significant conductive hearing loss; if bilateral, amplification may be required, as surgery is rarely beneficial.

AIRWAY OBSTRUCTION

The otolaryngologist is responsible for managing problems that may compromise the airway from the anterior nares to the segmental bronchi. In children with craniofacial abnormalities, the causes of obstruction may be legion, and the effects of the obstruction may be dependent on the age of the child. Neonates may experience life-threatening nasal or oropharyngeal obstruction; older children may have obstructive apneic episodes during sleep or troublesome nasal obstruction from day to day, and some children undergoing maxillofacial or craniofacial surgery may also experience difficulty in airway maintenance.

Neonatal Nasal Airway Obstruction

Neonates are obligate nose-breathers for the first two to three months of life (Stool and Houlihan, 1977) and therefore experience respiratory distress, even asphyxia, if the nasal airway obstruction is unrelieved. Newborn infants whose nasal passages are blocked exhibit "paradoxical cyanosis": they become cyanotic when quiet with their mouths closed but lose their cyanosis when crying and hence using the oral airway.

Characteristically, paradoxical cyanosis occurs in infants with bilateral choanal atresia and in neonates with midfacial hypoplasia (such as those with Crouzon or Apert syndrome) (Fig. 4–5). It has also been observed in patients with frontal nasal dysplasia, who have a defect of the cribriform plate and a nasal encephalocele. Neonatal nasal airway obstruction can usually be relieved by taping an oral airway in place. Conscientious nursing care is necessary for these children. When the infant learns to use his oral airway (by two to three months of age), the danger of asphyxia is past.

Neonatal Oropharyngeal Obstruction

Neonatal respiratory distress may be a consequence of glossoptosis, which will occur when the relationship of mandible to hyoid is altered (as in infants with retrognathia or micrognathia) so that the tongue falls back and obstructs the oropharynx (Farnsworth and Pacik, 1971) (Fig. 4–6). This obstructing posture of the tongue seems to occur more readily, hence causing more problems clinically, when associated with cleft palate. Cor pulmonale has been detected as early as 5 weeks of age in an infant with Pierre Robin syndrome who was experiencing airway distress (Cogswell and Easton, 1974); certainly, asphyxia will occur in severe cases.

Our experience is that this type of airway obstruction can usually be relieved by nursing the infant carefully in the prone position for the first few months of life. Creating a tongue–lip adhesion and suturing the tongue in front of this (Hawkins and Simpson, 1974) is rarely helpful; nasopharyngeal intubation (Stern et al., 1972) or tracheotomy is the treatment of choice in refractory cases. Before tracheotomy, the airway obstruction is relieved by inserting a rigid bronchoscope — a challenging task for a pediatric endoscopist to accomplish in a hypoxic but struggling retrognathic infant. The rigid bronchoscope (3 or 3.5 mm in diameter) must be inserted without the aid of a laryngoscope and in the absence of anesthesia; it is passed through the glottis from the lateral retromolar position, and the tracheotomy proceeds in an orderly fashion with the bronchoscope in place. By 6 months of age, mandibular growth has usually been sufficient to decrease glossoptosis to an insignificant level, and decannulation is possible. If the palate is cleft in these infants,

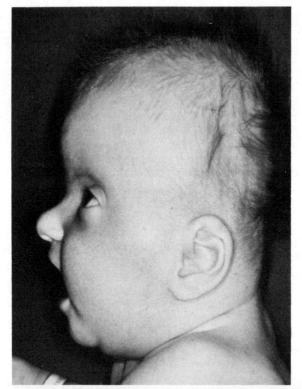

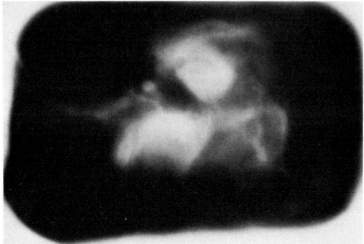

Figure 4–5   Top, Apert syndrome or acrocephalosyndactyly. These children frequently have airway obstruction due to the midfacial anomaly. Bottom, Frontal tomography of the petrous area demonstrates the obliquity of the external meatus and the medial upward rotation of the petrous apex.

some physicians prefer to maintain the tracheotomy until this defect has been repaired.

Obstructive Apneic Episodes

Obstructive apneic episodes during sleep, in some cases associated with the development of cor pulmonale, have been documented in children with normal craniofacial con-

figurations but in whom adenoidal hypertrophy is causing chronic nasopharyngeal obstruction (Mangat et al., 1977). Children with craniofacial anomalies that affect the configuration of the upper airway will also experience similar obstruction during sleep.

Children with craniofacial anomalies in which there is severe posterior displacement of the midfacial structures (as in Apert and Crouzon syndromes) have very narrow na-

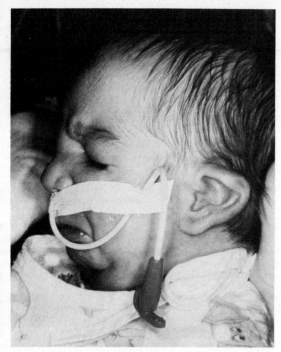

Figure 4–6 This boy was born with a cleft of the secondary palate and experienced increasing respiratory distress secondary to glossoptosis (Pierre Robin syndrome). Tracheotomy at 5 weeks of age eliminated the respiratory obstruction and was maintained for five months.

sopharyngeal airways and will suffer apneic episodes during sleep. In fact, the development of cor pulmonale in a three year old child with Crouzon disease and clinical improvement after adenotonsillectomy has been reported (Don and Siggers, 1971). We have observed substantial reduction in obstructive apneic episodes during sleep, with near disappearance of the associated stridor, after adenotonsillectomy in two children two years of age.

Noisy, stridorous breathing during sleep, with occasional obstructive apneic episodes, increased in severity over several months in a five year old child with retrognathia. This night-time airway obstruction was almost eliminated by removing the palatine tonsils, which were large and pedunculated. Presumably, tonsillar hypertrophy in this child with glossoptosis caused significant oropharyngeal obstruction when the pharyngeal musculature was relaxed, as is normal during deep rapid eye movement (REM) sleep.

Life-threatening obstructive apneic episodes will occur if palatopharyngoplasty is performed in a child who has glossoptosis.

Cor pulmonale developed in two of three children with Pierre Robin syndrome who had undergone palatopharyngoplasty to overcome velopharyngeal incompetence (VPI), and one of these children died of respiratory obstruction at eight years of age (Jackson et al., 1976). A three year old patient who had Treacher-Collins syndrome experienced moderately severe obstructive apneic episodes during sleep after successful palatopharyngoplasty. To have some periods of uninterrupted sleep, she formed the habit of sleeping prone in the knee–chest position. Eventually, the child became hypersomniac, and tracheotomy was necessary four months after the successful palatopharyngoplasty to eliminate the obstructive episodes. The girl now sleeps well with a tracheotomy tube in place at night but wears a small Silastic stent during the daytime that plugs the tracheocutaneous fistula and permits speech. Children with a history that suggests airway obstruction and who have retrognathia or micrognathia are poor candidates for pharyngeal flap surgery, as they may experience significant upper airway obstruction during sleep postoperatively.

Less troublesome night-time obstruction may develop in adolescents in whom palatopharyngoplasty has been "too successful." These patients with repaired palatal clefts and persistent VPI have normal mandibular configurations. Following palatopharyngoplasty, they develop almost total nasal obstruction and speech that is noticeably hyponasal. Characteristically, they sleep poorly, with frequent nightmares. One girl reported waking frequently and "gasping for air." Dilatation of the small lateral ports with Tucker bougies gave only transient relief, and surgical revision of the pharyngeal flap was necessary.

Chronic Nasal Obstruction

Individuals with craniofacial anomalies commonly are open-mouthed. However, mouth-breathing is not always indicative of nasal airway obstruction; it may be a consequence of malocclusion or retrognathia. If it is due to nasal obstruction, the latter may be secondary to causes (allergic rhinitis, adenoidal hypertrophy) unrelated to the anomaly. In most of these patients, however, nasal obstruction is consequent upon distortion of the midfacial anatomy.

As clefts of the primary and secondary palate are a common anomaly, nasal obstruction is most frequently observed in that group of patients. Reduction in the caliber of the nasal airway may be a consequence of several factors unique to these children: distortion of nasal soft tissue, nasal mucosa edema, and deviation of the nasal septum. In children who have a unilateral cleft of the primary palate, slumping and collapse of the ipsilateral lower lateral cartilage may cause obstruction. Significant nasal mucosal edema may be a consequence of an ipsilateral oronasal fistula, heterotopic dental eruption in the floor of the nose, or sinusitis. If the cleft is unilateral, the nasal septum is deviated: the anterior aspect of the nasal septum is visible in the contralateral nostril; posteriorly, however, the septum angulates sharply to the cleft side, to articulate with the tilted, malpositioned vertical plate of the vomer bone (Fig. 4–7).

In the absence of anterior nasal obstruction due to alar collapse, successful septoplasty with improvement of the airway will be achieved by removing the septal obstruction and reducing mucosal edema. The former is accomplished by relatively conservative excision of the caudal aspect of the quadrilateral

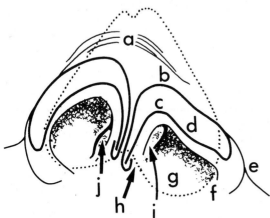

Figure 4–7 Diagrammatic illustration of nasal deformity in the patient with unilateral cleft of primary palate. (a) Nasal tip deviated to normal side. (b) Ipsilateral upper lateral cartilage flatter. (c) Dome of lower lateral cartilage lower, retroposed, and less well-developed. The angle between medial and lateral crurae is less acute. (d) Lateral crus of lower lateral cartilage flatter, and alar base (f) displaced downwards in association with flat, underdeveloped maxilla (e). (g) Nasal floor wider. (h) Columella and cartilaginous septum deviated to normal side. (i) Posterior cartilaginous deviation usually will cause ipsilateral nasal obstruction while anteriorly, the caudal strut of the quadrilateral cartilage is visible in the normal side (j).

cartilage, maintaining dorsal and caudal struts, combined with radical removal of the nasal crest of the maxilla and the thickened, tilted vomer bone. Management of mucosal edema with turbinate hypertrophy is difficult. Elimination of sinusitis and closure of the oronasal fistula is helpful, as may be outfracturing of the ipsilateral turbinate; turbinate bulk can be reduced by cauterization, cryosurgery, or laser application. We reserve aggressive management of nasal obstruction until early adolescence, when the patients are embarking upon more active orthodontic management, as persistent mouth-breathing then will have a deleterious effect on the teeth.

Airway Obstruction and Craniofacial Surgery

During surgical correction of craniofacial anomalies under general anesthesia, the airway is protected and controlled by the use of an endotracheal tube (nasal or oral) or tracheotomy tube. In many cases, this operative protection must be maintained postoperatively to prevent aspiration of blood from the oropharynx or if airway obstruction by swollen soft tissues is anticipated.

Elective tracheotomy is necessary for operative and postoperative airway management in two groups of patients: (1) those with poor or inaccessible nasal airways who will have interdental wiring in the postoperative period and (2) those in whom intubation for anesthesia is extremely difficult or impossible. Thus, children with Crouzon or Apert syndrome (all of whom have poor nasal airways) who will have interdental wiring postoperatively will require tracheotomy for the major craniofacial surgery to correct the midfacial deformity. Most children undergoing mandibular osteotomy will be managed postoperatively with nasoendotracheal tubes, whereas those who have already undergone palatopharyngoplasty may require tracheotomy prior to the osteotomy. However, it is possible to nasally intubate a teenager with a preexisting palatopharyngoplasty flap if the lateral ports are relatively commodious. In children who have severe retrognathia or ankylosis of the temporomandibular joint (Fig. 4–4) and who require tracheotomy, blind nasal intubation may be possible (Sklar and King, 1976) or, alternatively, a rigid bronchoscope can usually be inserted without using a laryngoscope. If severe retrognathia is accompanied by cervical spondylosis, tracheotomy can be performed without airway control but under light anesthesia induced intravenously and supplemented with local infiltration of an anesthetic agent.

Discussion between the anesthetist and the otolaryngologist is essential, to plan pre-, intra-, and postoperative airway management. From 1972 to 1976, 21 of our patients underwent elective tracheotomy before a major craniofacial surgery. The only major complication was surgical emphysema, which developed in one child when the posterior wall of the trachea was lacerated during introduction of the tracheotomy tube. Intraoperative aspiration of blood is minimized by the routine use of cuffed tracheotomy tubes. In children under 6 years of age, we use a cuffed armored endotracheal tube, which is sutured in place; 24 hours after surgery, this tube is replaced by a metal, noncuffed tra-

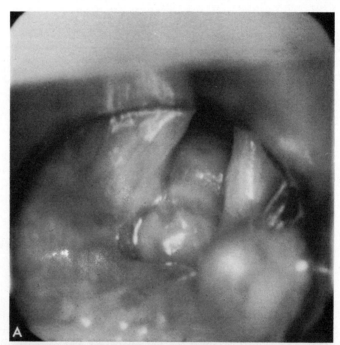

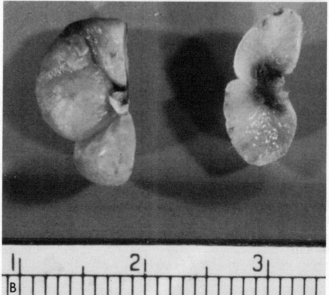

Figure 4–8 *A,* Larynx at time of microlaryngoscopy in 16 year old girl who had nasoendotracheal intubation for seven days following bilateral mandibular osteotomies four months previously. A mature epithelialized polyp is attached by a narrow stalk to the arytenoid process of the left vocal cord. *B,* Surgical specimen.

cheotomy tube. Decannulation usually occurs within one week. Children in whom a tracheotomy has been created because intubation would be difficult or impossible and who will require further surgery within six months should be fitted after decannulation with a solid Silastic plug, to maintain the tracheocutaneous fistula.

After mandibular osteotomy, nasotracheal intubation is maintained until soft tissue swelling subsides. Most children have been extubated uneventfully within five days postoperatively, but two of our 63 adolescent patients who underwent mandibular osteotomy from 1972 to 1976 required semi-urgent tracheotomy to relieve upper airway obstruction that developed at the time of extubation three and ten days after surgery. In both, subglottic stenosis responded to endoscopy, and decannulation was achieved within six months. Also during this five year period, persistent laryngeal granulomas developed in three adolescent girls who had been nasoendotracheally intubated for six days after mandibular osteotomies (Fig. 4–8A). Their symptoms were surprisingly minor — mildly husky speech, transient aphonia, and slight dyspnea with exercise. The granulomata were readily removed by microlaryngoscopy (Fig. 4–8B).

SPEECH DISORDERS

Hypernasality

Hypernasality is most often observed in children who have velopharyngeal insufficiency (VPI) after cleft palate repair. It may also be apparent (and it is important that the otolaryngologist stress this to other team members) as "deaf speech" in a child who does not have VPI but who has a craniofacial anomaly and a hearing loss exceeding 30 dB (Yules, 1970). Hypernasal speech can be reduced to an acceptable degree with speech therapy in most youngsters. Persistent VPI has been eliminated in some children by injecting Teflon beneath the mucous membrane of the nasopharynx (Smith and McCabe, 1977), but palatopharyngoplasty is the treatment of choice in most centers. It is usually done at five years of age when speech therapy has been unsuccessful. Cineradiography and nasopharyngoscopy with a flexible tube are helpful adjuncts in determining the degree of VPI.

Hyponasality

Hyponasality indicates lack of nasal resonance and is invariably due to nasal airway obstruction. It occurs in patients with severe posterior displacement of the midface or persistent congenital choanal atresia or with iatrogenic velopharyngeal atresia consequent upon too successful palatopharyngoplasty. Ironically, in these last patients, their original speech disorder was hypernasality. Removal of nasal airway obstruction diminishes and may eliminate hyponasality.

Hoarseness

Nodules of the vocal cords are present in approximately 20 per cent of children who have VPI; they are thought to be a result of increased laryngeal activity to compensate for loss of vocal power. The nodules and the hoarseness disappear after elimination of the VPI and the evolution of normal speech patterns. Hoarseness — even transient aphonia in some cases — develops after nasotracheal intubation in a minority of patients.

INFECTIONS OF THE UPPER RESPIRATORY TRACT

Purulent otitis media seems to occur more often in children who have craniofacial anomalies. Persistent, painless otorrhea without pyrexia or other evidence of coalescent mastoiditis probably indicates dysfunction of the eustachian tube. The condition may be unresponsive to even rigorous conservative measures, including daily aural toilet under microscopy, instillation of topical medications, and the parenteral administration of aminoglycoside antibiotics. Frequently, at this juncture the therapy is abandoned; then, two to three months later, the ear is found to be dry. In such cases, presumably, cessation of the otorrhea marks the resumption of some degree of eustachian tube function.

In patients with unremitting, recurrent, acute otitis media, adenoidectomy may be advised, even in children who have a repaired cleft of the secondary palate. Velopharyngeal insufficiency will occur postoperatively, and the parents must be advised that palatopharyngoplasty will be required later to eliminate the hypernasality that will be present after adenoidectomy. Adenoidectomy is also indicated before palatopharyngoplasty if there is excessive adenoid tissue obstructing the nasal airway.

Sinusitis is more common than usual in cleft palate patients (Jaffee and DeBlanc, 1971). In our five year study, unilateral maxillary sinusitis developed in a few adolescents after nasal intubation for four or five days following mandibular osteotomy. Presumably, the nasoendotracheal tube obstructed the ostium of the sinus, preventing normal drainage and providing ideal conditions for opportunistic infection.

Purulent, foul-smelling rhinorrhea indicates the presence of infected foreign material in the nasal airway or paranasal sinuses. The foreign material may be autogenous. Infected bone sequestra and teeth, driven into the sinus during LeFort osteotomy, have been removed from antra via an anterior approach through the canine fossa; preoperative tomography and intraoperative use of an image intensifier were most helpful to localize and remove these foreign bodies. Foreign material may also be exogenous in origin. It may be food that has been forced into the anterior aspect of the nasal cavity through an oronasal fistula or into the posterior choana past an incompetent palate. In one of our patients, a foul-smelling gauze pack was removed from the back of the nose six months after palatopharyngoplasty.

Tonsillitis does not seem to occur with increased frequency in this group of patients. Tonsillectomy can be done safely if recurrent infections are a problem; in many cleft palate patients, articulation is markedly improved afterwards.

DISORDERS OF OLFACTION

We have not attempted evaluation of the sense of smell in patients with craniofacial anomalies, but some adolescents have commented spontaneously after major corrective surgery that their sense of smell has improved. Presumably, partial or total anosmia is not uncommon in patients with congenital obstruction of the nasal airway.

REFERENCES

Bergstrom, L., Neblett, L. M., and Hemenway, W. G. 1972. Otologic manifestations of acrocephalosyndactyly. Arch. Otolaryngol., 96:117–123.

Caldarelli, D. E. 1977. Congenital middle ear anomalies associated with craniofacial and skeletal syndromes. In Jaffe, B. F. (Ed.) Hearing Loss in Children. A Comprehensive Text. Baltimore, University Park Press, pp. 310–340.

Cogswell, J. J., and Easton, D. M. 1974. Cor pulmonale in the Pierre Robin syndrome. Arch. Dis. Child., 49:905–908.

Crysdale, W. S. 1978. Abnormal facial appearance and delayed diagnosis of congenital hearing loss. J. Otolaryngol., 7:349–352.

Crysdale, W. S. 1976. Rational management of middle ear effusions in the cleft palate patient. J. Otolaryngol., 5:463–467.

Don, N., and Siggers, D. C. 1971. Cor pulmonale in Crouzon's disease. Arch. Dis. Child., 46:394–396.

Downs, M. P., and Silver, H. K. 1972. The A.B.C.D.'s to H.E.A.R.; early identification in nursery, office and clinic of the infant who is deaf. Clin. Pediatr., 11:563–566.

Farnsworth, P. B., and Pacik, P. T. 1971. Glossoptotic hypoxia and micrognathia — the Pierre Robin syndrome reviewed. Early recognition and prompt surgical treatment is important for survival. Clin. Pediatr., 10:600–606.

Gorlin, R. J., Pindborg, J. J., and Cohen, M. M., Jr. (Eds.) 1976. Syndromes of the Head and Neck, 2nd ed. New York, McGraw-Hill.

Hawkins, D. B., and Simpson, J. V. 1974. Micrognathia and glossoptosis in the newborn. Clin. Pediatr., 13:1066–1073.

Holme, V. A., and Kumze, L. H. 1969. Effect of chronic otitis media on language and speech development. Pediatrics, 43:833–839.

Jackson, P., Whitaker, L. A., and Randall, P. 1976. Airway hazards associated with pharyngeal flaps in patients who have the Pierre Robin syndrome. Plast. Reconstr. Surg., 58:184–186.

Jaffe, B. F., and DeBlanc, C. B. 1971. Sinusitis in children with cleft lip and palate. Arch. Otolaryngol., 93:479–482.

Konigsmark, B. W., and Gorlin, R. J. 1976. Genetic and Metabolic Deafness. Philadelphia, W. B. Saunders Co.

Lindsay, J. R., Black, F. O., and Donelly, W. H., Jr. 1975. Acrocephalosyndactyly (Apert's syndrome): temporal bone findings. Ann. Otol. Rhinol. Laryngol., 84:174–178.

Mangat, D., Orr, W. C., and Smith, R. O. 1977. Sleep apnea, hypersomnolence, and upper airway obstruction secondary to adenotonsillar enlargement. Arch. Otolaryngol., 103:383–386.

Munro, I. R. 1975. Orbito-cranio-facial surgery: the team approach. Plast. Reconstr. Surg., 55:170–176.

Munro, I. R. 1977. Craniofacial surgery: a change of face. Can. Med. Assoc. J., 117:210–211.

Robson, M. C., Stankiewicz, J. A., and Mendelsohn, J. S. 1977. Cor pulmonale secondary to cleft palate repair. Case report. Plast. Reconstr. Surg., 59:754–757.

Selder, A. 1973. Hearing disorders in children with otocraniofacial syndromes. In Proceedings of the Conference: Orofacial Anomalies. Clinical and Research Implications, April 15–17, 1972. Phoenix, Ariz., American Speech and Hearing Assoc., ASHA Report #8, 95–110.

Sklar, G. S., and King, B. D. 1976. Endotracheal intubation and Treacher-Collins syndrome. Anesthesiology, 44:247–249.

Smith, D. W. 1976. Recognizable Patterns of Human

Malformation. Genetic, Embryologic and Clinical Aspects, 2nd ed. Philadelphia, W. B. Saunders Co.

Smith, J. K., and McCabe, B. F. 1977. Teflon injection in the nasopharynx to improve velopharyngeal closure. Ann. Otol. Rhinol. Laryngol., *86*:559–563.

Stern, L. M., Fonkalsrud, E. W., Hassakis, P., et al. 1972. Management of Pierre Robin syndrome in infancy by prolonged nasoesophageal intubation. Am. J. Dis. Child., *124*:78–80.

Stool, S. E., and Houlihan, R. 1977. Otolaryngologic management of craniofacial anomalies. Otolaryngol. Clin. North Am., *10*:41–44.

Witzel, M. A., Crysdale, W. S., and Munro, I. R. Speech and hearing problems in 38 patients with Apert's, Crouzon's and Pfeiffer's syndrome. Unpublished observations, the Hospital for Sick Children, Toronto.

Yules, R. B. 1970. Hearing in cleft palate patients. Arch. Otolaryngol., *91*:319–323.

Chapter 5

PRINCIPLES AND METHODS OF MANAGEMENT

Linton A. Whitaker, M.D.

BACKGROUND

In 1949 Sir Harold Gillies, a pioneer in plastic surgery in England, did what was probably the first craniofacial procedure (Gillies and Harrison, 1950). This was a Le-Fort III osteotomy along the classic craniofacial disjunction lines as originally described by Rene LeFort. Because of the difficulties Gillies encountered, he was not anxious to repeat the procedure. Between 1949 and 1965, there were scattered attempts at correction of major craniofacial anomalies, with Dr. Paul Tessier of Paris laying the groundwork in the late 1950s for what is currently the field of craniofacial surgery. Many of his ideas apparently evolved from observations in trauma patients, and it was during these operative procedures, in conjunction with neurosurgeons, that the concept of an intracranial approach to correction of facial deformity was conceived.

About 1965 Dr. Tessier did his first intracranial approach for correction of a major facial deformity, representing probably the earliest procedure done by a deliberate, planned method. While others contributed to the early development of craniofacial surgery, Dr Tessier has been the prime force in the development of this field. There are now a number of major centers in North America and around the world where this type of surgical procedure is done frequently. Most of the surgical teams have been developed from existing cleft palate teams by adding neurosurgical and ophthalmological elements and utilizing more sophisticated radiographic techniques. Involvement of the intensive care unit in the correction of the craniofacial anomalies has also become important.

THE SPECTRUM OF CORRECTABLE ANOMALIES

Craniofacial surgery, by definition of those working in the field, means surgery concentrated about the orbits and has indeed been called orbitocranial surgery (Whitaker et al., 1976). To qualify as a craniofacial operation, at least one orbit must be entirely stripped of soft tissue except for the attachments at the nasolacrimal apparatus and the point of entry of the optic nerve. The most common structural deformities that can be corrected by a craniofacial technique are acrocephalosyndactyly and craniofacial dysostosis (Apert and Crouzon syndromes), orbital hypertelorism, mandibulofacial dysostosis, hemifacial microsomia, and certain instances of craniofacial trauma and tumors of the midface and orbit. While these deformities primarily involve the middle and upper thirds of the face, the lower third is often an integral part of the abnormality, as when dealing with deformities of the external ears. Maldevelopment of portions of these interrelated areas often results in distorted growth of adjacent structures, resulting in a complex deformity of bony and soft tissue (Goodman and Gorlin, 1977).

Mandibulofacial dysostosis, or Treacher-Collins syndrome, generally represents the simplest form of deformity correctable by craniofacial surgical techniques. It is characterized by zygomatic hypoplasia of a subtle to extreme degree, often with absent areas of bone in the zygomas, antimongoloid slant of the eyes, nasal deformity, and low-set ears; sometimes with other ear abnormalities; and frequently with mandibular and palatal abnormalities. The basis for correction of the deformity is addition of bone in areas of bony deficiency, with simultaneous correction of the antimongoloid slant of the eyes and correction of the ears. Mandibular osteotomies may also be necessary for correction of such deformities. Hemifacial microsomia is structurally similar to a unilateral form of mandibulofacial dysostosis, manifesting zygomatic and mandibular hypoplasia and ear abnormalities that may be particularly prominent (Franceschetti, 1968).

Craniofacial dysostosis, or Crouzon syndrome, can be identical in appearance to acrocephalosyndactyly and usually involves craniostenosis with forehead and skull abnormalities as well as orbits that are too shallow for the ocular globes, producing exorbitism. Minimal grades of orbital hypertelorism may be associated with the exorbitism in the craniofacial dysostoses, and typically midface hypoplasia with retromaxillism is present. Correction of these deformities involves a more complicated procedure that includes advancing the areas of bony deficiency and holding the advanced bone in place with bone grafts (Block, 1957; Dingman, 1956; Lewin, 1952; Tessier, 1971c and d).

Orbital hypertelorism and similar craniofacial defects represent perhaps the most complicated of the deformities correctable by craniofacial techniques. The orbits in these patients are too far apart, not having achieved adequate rotation toward the midline *in utero*. The inadequate rotation can be a result of several intrauterine events, including encephalocoeles at the frontonasal area, paramedian facial clefts, or other as yet unknown reasons (Currarino and Silverman, 1960; Gonzales-Ulloa, 1964; Tessier, 1971a, 1972, 1976; Trautman, Converse, and Smith, 1962).

In certain instances the residua of craniofacial trauma, particularly of secondary reconstructions with displacement of the orbit or structures about the upper face, can be corrected using craniofacial techniques (Whitaker and Schaffer, 1977; Jones, Whitaker, and Murtagh, 1977).

PLANNING RECONSTRUCTION

The major craniofacial abnormalities can be considered as a group for the purposes of operative planning. Since the abnormalities are predominantly structural, with few functional and physiologic problems, the goal of surgical correction is normal facial structure and function. Standards of normal that have been widely described in the plastic surgery, physical anthropology, and dental literature are used for evaluating craniofacial procedures and problems. Such norms are the basis for determining what is abnormal and for defining the goal of the surgery (Broadbent and Mathews, 1957; Cameron, 1931; Duke-Elder and Wybar, 1961; Gonzales-Ulloa, 1962, 1964; Whitaker, La-Rossa, and Randall, 1975).

Physical examination of the craniofacial structure as a whole must be considered, utilizing concepts of symmetry and facial form. Operations on soft tissue, the nose, and the ears are based on the principles of symmetry in facial form. The hairline in the frontal region should be more or less horizontal, and the eyebrows should be in the same plane. The medial and lateral canthi normally are on the same horizontal line, approximately parallel to the eyebrows. Slight variations from this can exist, but in general there should be a straight line from the lateral canthi through the medial canthi. The upper edge of the ear is normally at approximately the lower edge of the eyebrow on each side.

Bony shifts represent the foundation of craniofacial surgery, and measurements between bones are the foundation for such shifts. The interpupillary distance is measured between the midpoints of the pupils. Although the measurement is often inaccurate because of strabismus, it is a useful preliminary guide; the normal range is 58 to 71 mm in the adult. The medial intercanthal distance is obtained by using calipers to measure between the medial-most extents of the palpebral fissures; this distance is the final determinant of the success of the correction. However, the measurement that is used as the basis for planning orbital shifts is the bony interorbital distance. It is determined by using standard 2-

meter films (to reduce magnification errors) and making measurements directly on radiographs. Cephalograms also may be utilized for this. The normal medial intercanthal distance is 5 to 8 mm more than the bony interorbital distance.

Measurement of orbital volume is still difficult; perhaps the most accurate way of evaluating volume at present is to use the Luedde exophthalmometer to directly measure the distance from the lateral orbital margin to the apex of the cornea. This distance normally is from 10 to 14 mm. The difference between the measured and expected value is the distance an orbit of insufficient volume must be advanced to produce an orbit of normal depth and volume.

By measuring the medial intercanthal distance and obtaining a direct exophthalmometer reading on the patient, determinations can be made as to how far medially or forward to shift the orbits. In addition, measuring levels of the orbital rims, pupils, and canthi aids in determining how far superiorly or inferiorly to move an orbit. By such determinations, precise planning can be made for movement of orbits in any direction.

Bitemporal distance may be considered also, as if it is too wide, it must be narrowed, and if too narrow, expanded. The same is true for the zygomas. Prominence of the zygomatic bones is essential to normal facial appearance, and as they are often hypoplastic in the syndromes referred for corrective surgery and may be completely absent, they must be considered in reconstruction of the face. The zygomatic arches are the key to reconstruction of defects in mandibulofacial dysostosis. They average 1.5 cm at the widest, 0.5 cm anterior-to-posterior in the adult, and the distance from the external auditory canal to the zygomaticomaxillary sutures averages 6 cm in the adult. The exact length can be determined in each individual by direct measurement from the tragus to the lateral side of the nose. Bone grafts to correct defects must approximate these dimensions.

Photographs are essential in planning the craniofacial operative procedures, as they give a fixed point of reference for soft tissue and bony shifts. Life-sized black and white photographs in full face and profile views are utilized, with plans for orbital and jaw shifts as well as ear and nose changes based on such photographs. They are used in conjunction with direct patient measurements, radiograph measurements, and dental study models in planning the corrective surgery.

Dental study models determine the jaw shifts that are necessary to correct the malocclusion that usually occurs in these syndromes. The lips must be taken into consideration with such jaw shifts, and changes in the form of the lips must be made if necessary to accommodate shifts of either the mandible or maxilla.

Standard 2-meter radiographs in the posterior-anterior and lateral views or cephalometrograms are essential for measurements of the bony distances of the face. They are particularly necessary in determining the cribriform plate level, which is important in deciding whether or not to operate intracranially to correct hypertelorism. Tomograms may be useful in defining abnormalities within the orbits or in the cranial base: computed tomography (CT) is a precise tool for determining structures within the orbit and cranium. Computer analysis of craniofacial structures is in its infancy, but it potentially has the capacity for predicting exactly what movements of orbits or other structures about the face will be necessary for establishing normal relations. Standardized radiographs are essential for long-term follow-up and for determining whether growth or relapse has occurred.

Multispecialty evaluation of the patient's condition and potential for rehabilitation are essential in craniofacial surgery (Munro, 1975); thus, the team concept is extremely important. In particular, neurosurgeons must work in conjunction with plastic surgeons in all operative procedures performed on patients with intracranial problems. In our institution, airway problems are handled by the otolaryngology service, and all patients having surgery to correct orbit deformities are seen by ophthalmologists (strabismus following craniofacial surgery is frequent, although most of the time it is self-limiting). Input from the anesthesiology group is essential because of the frequent difficulties that occur with airway maintenance and the prolonged time that the patient is anesthetized. In our institution, the anesthesiologists regularly attend the planning sessions for craniofacial surgery. The need for specialized radiographs means that an unusual amount of input is necessary from the radiology department.

Dental help, particularly from orthodontics and pedodontics, is necessary both for planning and in providing methods of fixation following surgical reconstructive procedures about the jaws. Physical anthropology has been useful in helping to determine the normal values for facial measurements and the proper goals for surgical procedures. The nursing services and intensive care units are alerted to provide the special care required by these patients, who have massive facial swelling and often large bandages following surgery.

SURGICAL METHODS

Preliminary Surgical Preparation. Preparations for a major, prolonged operative procedure must be made (Davies and Munro, 1975; Munro, 1975). All patients in whom the oral or nasal cavities or any of the sinuses is entered receive preoperative antibiotics in the highest appropriate dose for their body weight and age. The antibiotic is started 12 hours before surgery and is given at 4-hour intervals during the operative procedure.

Decadron in doses of 1.5 mg/kg of body weight to a maximum of 20 mg, starting 24 hours before surgery and continuing 2 days after surgery, has been given in the past, but we have now stopped using this drug, since there is no evidence that it affects the outcome of intracranial procedures in any beneficial way.

Because of the prolonged nature of the procedure, and because frequently a large volume of blood is lost, the following preparations are made by the anesthesia group:

1. Standard intravenous lines
2. Central venous pressure line
3. Arterial lines
4. Indwelling urinary catheter
5. Rectal thermometer probe
6. Electrocardiograph leads connected to a visual display screen
7. Endotracheal anesthesia tube
8. Preparation for hypotensive anesthesia
9. Cerebrospinal fluid drainage catheter, which is left open to drip during the operative procedure in intracranial cases.

The Exposure. The unique feature of, and, in fact, the foundation of craniofacial surgery is the coronal incision. This incision is carried from the superior tragal notch on one side to the superior tragal notch on the opposite side, going directly across the vertex of the skull. The scalp flap and forehead tissue are then turned down and a subperiosteal dissection of the entire upper facial skeleton is carried out (Fig. 5–1). Un-

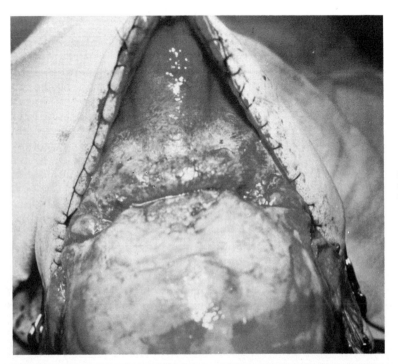

Figure 5–1 Coronal incision showing subperiosteal dissection to base of nose and exposing upper portions of both orbits.

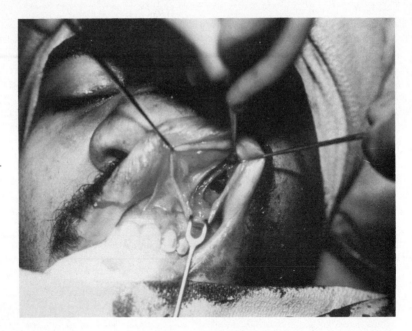

Figure 5–2 Buccal sulcus incision for exposure of lower face.

usually good visualization of the upper face is thus provided and the orbits and nasal bones can be exposed, except for a small segment of tissue that remains in the infraorbital areas bilaterally. To complete exposure of the orbits, a conjunctival incision is done in most instances that allows visualization of the area from the nasolacrimal apparatus medially to the juncture of the inferior and lateral orbital walls. Also, visualization of the orbital floor is provided by this means. Only when a considerable amount of bone grafting has to be done on the anterior zygoma is an external eyelid incision used. If scars are present, particularly after trauma, they may be used for access. External nasal incisions are sometimes made in instances of hypertelorism; other than in these two exceptions, all incisions are kept in the hairline and in the conjunctival area so that visible scars are kept to a minimum.

The lower face, below the level of the zygomas, is approached by means of buccal sulcus incisions, in combination with conjunctival or eyelid incisions (Fig. 5–2). By means of the buccal sulcus incision, the entire maxilla and lower portion of the zygoma including the zygomatic arch can be cleared. Such incisions are used for midface osteotomies such as in a LeFort I, II, or III osteotomy. When possible, entry into the oral cavity is avoided because of concern about contaminating the wound, although infections have been rather rare.

By means of these combined approaches, all soft tissue is stripped from the face from the level of the forehead to the level of the maxilla, leaving the orbital contents attached only at the optic foramen and the nasolacrimal apparatus. The soft tissue orbits are, therefore, circumferentially mobilized and the nose is detached of all soft tissue in most instances to a level below the nasal bones (Tessier, 1971*d*).

Extracranial Corrections. In its simplest form, craniofacial surgery involves adding bone to areas of deficiency. This occurs primarily in instances of mandibulofacial dysostosis, hemifacial microsomia, and posttraumatic problems, as well as in a host of other, rare problems.

Bone grafts are harvested from standard donor site areas, most often the ribs. Up to four ribs can be taken without concern by skipping one rib in the middle and taking two on either side of the strut. In general, a 4 to 5 cm inframammary incision is made and the ribs are dissected out subperiosteally in 8 to 15 cm segments depending upon the size of the patient. Rib regrowth can then be expected and the same ribs reharvested at a later date (Longacre and deStefano, 1957; Pagnell, 1960).

As an alternative, especially when cancellous bone is specifically desired or when larger amounts of bone are needed, iliac bone can be used, but its use is attended with the disadvantage of greater and more prolonged donor site discomfort. The scarring is also generally more obvious. Cancellous bone, however, is useful in areas of marginal vascularity where a more certain take of the bone graft is desirable, so that in certain instances the disadvantages are outweighed by better results.

The bone grafts are tailored to the appropriate size and shape and wired into place. In mandibulofacial dysostosis, two or three layers of split ribs are usually needed across the body of the zygoma and one or two layers are needed along the lateral orbit of each side of the face. In hemifacial microsomia, the reconstruction is similar but usually unilateral (Figs. 5–3 and 5–4) (Converse et al., 1973a and b; Converse et al., 1974a and b; Longacre, Stevens, and Holmstrand, 1963; Obwegeser, 1974).

Osteotomies with en bloc movements of segments of bone are sometimes done extracranially. In particular, subcranial LeFort III osteotomies or movements of segments of hypoplastic zygomas are instances in which this technique is used. The segments of bone to be moved are cut loose using power tools and osteotomes and moved into position. Bone grafts are placed behind them to fill the gap and to hold the segment in its new position. Wires are used to fix the bones in place when necessary, although interlocking segments of bone held by tension

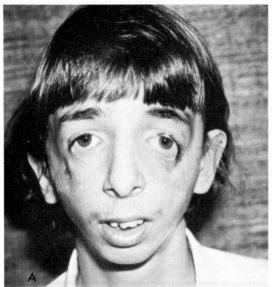
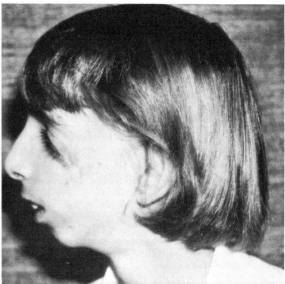
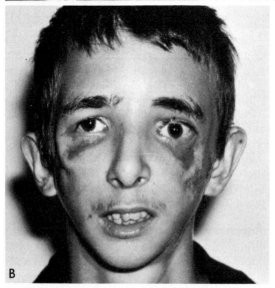

Figure 5–3 A, Preoperative full face and profile views of patient with Treacher Collins syndrome, showing pseudocolobomas, extreme zygomatic hypoplasia, and hypoplasia of the chin. B, Postoperative view showing correction of colobomas, zygomatic hypoplasia, and chin deficiency. The zygomatic hypoplasia was corrected with onlay grafts and the chin deformity with a combination of sliding genioplasty and onlay grafts.

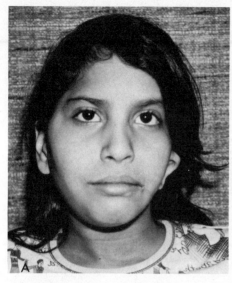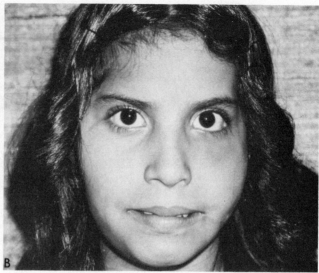

Figure 5–4 *A*, Preoperative view of patient with left hemifacial microsomia. *B*, Postoperative view of same patient, following onlay grafts to zygoma, dermal graft, and lateral canthopexy on the left. From Whitaker, L. A. 1978. Evaluation and treatment of upper facial asymmetry. *In* Whitaker, L. A., and Randall, P. (Eds.) Symposium on reconstruction of jaw deformity. St. Louis, The C. V. Mosby Co.

are preferred if possible (Murray and Swanson, 1968).

Following corrections, the wounds are generally closed with single layer sutures.

Limited Intracranial Approaches with En Bloc Movements. These approaches involve doing limited intracranial dissection, typically with burr holes to protect the frontal or temporal lobes of the brain. This is most applicable in an extended LeFort III osteotomy, or in moving the lateral wall of the orbit, or in certain instances of LeFort II osteotomies. The burr holes are made in the frontal and temporal regions in the LeFort III procedure so that the extended LeFort III can be carried up to the supraorbital area with the frontal lobes protected by the burr holes, using packing to move the frontal lobe of the brain and to move the temporal lobe backward (Fig. 5–5*A* through *D*).

In all instances in which the jaws are moved, some form of fixation is necessary. Generally, this means intermaxillary fixation, often with cast-capped splints or with orthodontic bands. This must be carefully planned with the orthodontists preoperatively (Freihofer, 1973; Hogemann and Willmar, 1974; Jabaley and Edgerton, 1969; Longacre, 1968; Obwegeser, 1969; Tessier, 1971*b*, *c*, and *e*).

Intracranial Procedures. Full-scale intracranial approaches are required in the most complex craniofacial procedures. These involve complete shifts of one or both orbits or of any of the bones about the skull. The orbits may be cut loose posteriorly near the apex and shifted in any direction desired to correct the structural deformities (Fig. 5–6). It is only by means of such an intracranial approach that techniques can be used to protect the frontal lobe of the brain.

The neurosurgeon does a unilateral or bilateral craniotomy after stripping of the soft tissue has been completed. The frontal lobes of the brain and, where necessary, the temporal lobes are retracted after the craniotomy is done, and the osteotomies of the orbits are next accomplished. Protecting both the brain and the orbital contents and using power instruments, the orbits are cut loose and moved in the direction desired. In the correction of orbital hypertelorism, a segment of bone is removed from the region of the glabella and the nose, both orbits are cut loose, and are moved medially. For downward displacement of an orbit, it is cut and moved into the position desired. Inferior orbital movement can be accomplished if an orbit is, as occasionally occurs with craniostenosis, positioned too high. Orbits may be advanced by cutting them near the apex, moving them into a

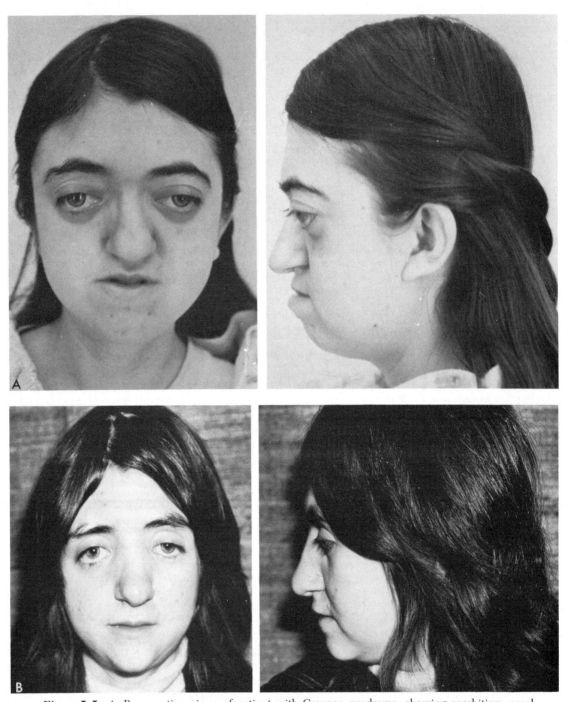

Figure 5–5 *A,* Preoperative views of patient with Crouzon syndrome, showing exorbitism, nasal deformity, and zygomaticomaxillary hypoplasia.
B, Postoperative views showing deformities corrected following Le Fort III midface advancement.

Illustration continued on the opposite page

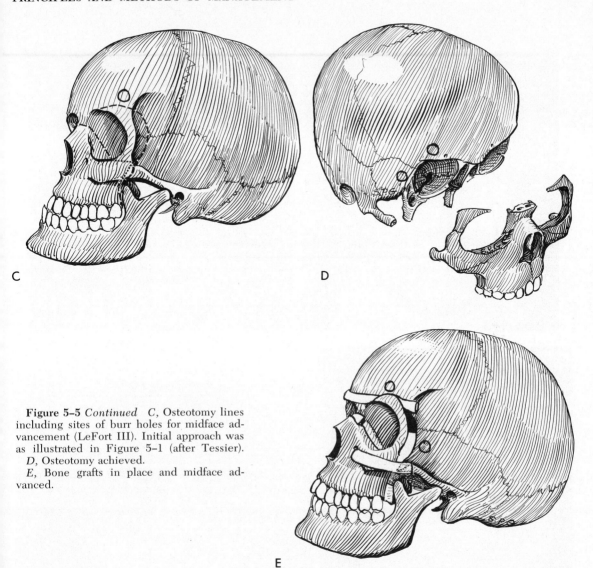

C

D

E

Figure 5–5 *Continued C*, Osteotomy lines including sites of burr holes for midface advancement (LeFort III). Initial approach was as illustrated in Figure 5–1 (after Tessier).
  D, Osteotomy achieved.
  E, Bone grafts in place and midface advanced.

forward position, and holding them there with bone grafts. This is particularly applicable in the correction of exorbitism (Converse, Wood-Smith, and McCarthy, 1975; Converse et al., 1970; Converse and Wood-Smith, 1971; Edgerton, Udvarhely, and Knox, 1970; Longacre, 1968; Tessier, 1972, 1974).

After orbital movements, gaps should be filled with bone grafts — typically split rib — and the segments wired in place. Interlocking bone segments, where possible, are preferred.

Shifts of areas of skull to correct deformities of any area but particularly about the frontal or temporal region may be made by cutting the bones loose, repositioning them, and molding or shaping them as necessary by burring, cutting, or by refashioning with bone grafts (Munro, 1976).

Preventive Surgery. Surgery on children of less than 1 year old is an exciting new clinical area in the correction of craniofacial deformities. It is particularly applicable in structural deformities of the upper face and utilizes the developing brain and globes as molding influences on reconstructed structures. The brain nearly triples in volume during the first year of life, and the ocular globes follow a similar pattern of growth. After 3 months of age, it is technically simpler to do the soft tissue dissection required in a craniofacial exposure and the bones are much more pliable and easily cut.

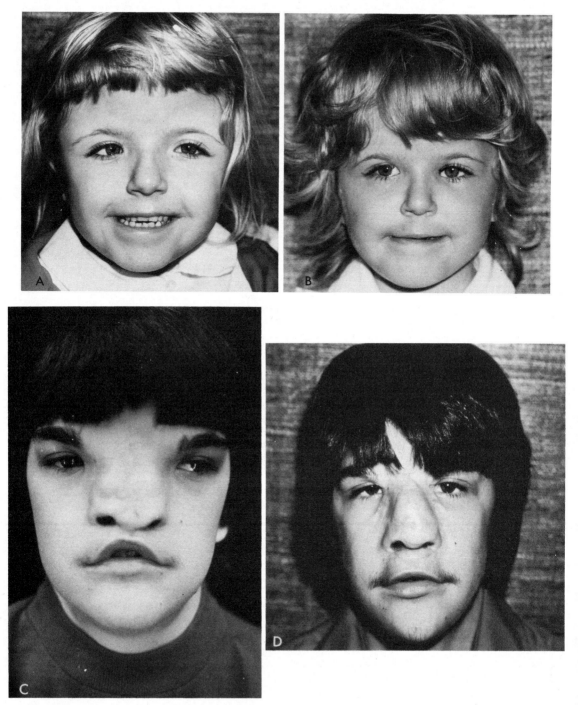

Figure 5–6　*A,* Patient with craniofacial dysostosis, forehead deformity, and orbital hypertelorism.
　B, Postoperative view showing correction of orbital hypertelorism and reshaping of forehead intracranially.
　C, Preoperative view of patient with orbital hypertelorism, nasal deformity and extremely short upper lip.
　D, Postoperative view showing correction of orbital hypertelorism, correction of nasal deformity, and lengthening of lip.

Illustration continued on the opposite page

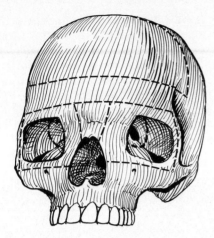

E

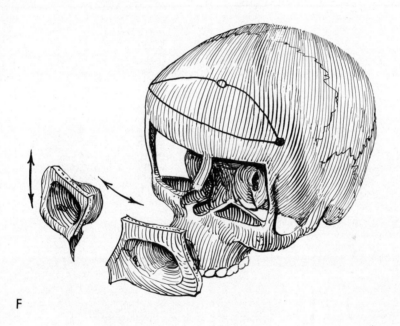

F

Figure 5–6 *Continued*   *E*, Basic osteotomy sites for orbital shifts used with variations in the two patients. Full craniotomy was necessary for brain protection.

F, Orbits mobilized.

G, Orbits in place with bone grafts.

(*A* and *B* from Whitaker, L. A., Broennle, M. A., Kerr, L. P., et al. 1980. Improvements in craniofacial reconstruction: Methods evolved in 235 consecutive patients. Plast. Reconstr. Surg., 65:561.)

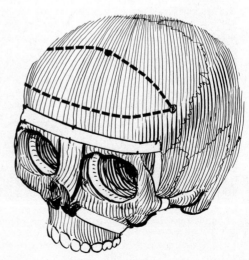

G

At the same time, the neurosurgeon does a craniectomy for craniostenosis; in children with deformities about the upper face, the orbits can be partially advanced into new positions, or less severe cases of hypertelorism can be corrected. Following that correction, and after placement of structures into more normal relation with one another, growth progresses normally under the influence of the developing brain and ocular globes (Fig. 5–7). In addition to the technical and psychologic advantages of early correction, distant bone graft donor sites are not necessary, since bone obtained from a craniectomy can be used for grafting (Edgerton et al., 1974a and b; Freihofer, 1974; Ingraham, Alexander, and Matson, 1948; Longacre, deStefano, and Holmstrand,

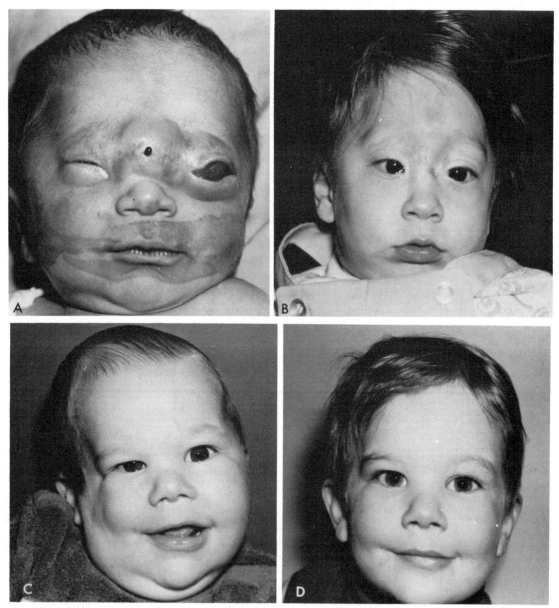

Figure 5–7 *A,* Preoperative view of patient with encephalocele and orbital hypertelorism. *B,* Postoperative view of same patient. *C,* Preoperative view of patient with isolated craniostenosis. *D,* Postoperative view of same patient. (*A* and *B* from Whitaker, L. A., Broennle, M. A., Kerr, L. P., et al. 1980. Improvements in craniofacial reconstruction: Methods evolved in 235 consecutive patients. Plast. Reconstr. Surg., *65:*561. *C* and *D* from Whitaker, L. A., Schut, L., and Kerr, L. P. 1977. Early surgery for isolated craniofacial dysostosis. Plast. Reconstr. Surg., *60:*575.)

1961; Whitaker and Randall, 1974; Whitaker, Schut, and Randall, 1976; Whitaker, Schut, and Kerr, 1977).

RESULTS

Ancillary Procedures. By means of alterations in the major bony and soft tissues of the face the basic architecture of the face is changed. Additional procedures are usually required to attain the best corrections of facial deformities: medial canthopexies with orbital hypertelorism; lateral canthopexies with hypertelorism, mandibulofacial dysostosis, and craniofacial dysostosis; and corrections of nasolacrimal apparatus problems. Various forms of osteoplasty may be necessary. Nasolacrimal apparatus drainage problems are frequent in orbital hypertelorism, in which an inadequate drainage system often exists. Often canthoplasties are advisable in addition to canthopexies in instances of webbing at the medial canthi following correction of orbital hypertelorism. Eyebrows may have to be repositioned. Nasal soft tissue changes may be necessary, particularly in patients with clefts going through the nose and the interorbital area. These are done in tandem with bony changes about the orbit. Plastic procedures on the lip and ear and changes in the lower jaw may be essential to completing the reconstruction. Mandibular and maxillary osteotomies may be required, particularly in patients with mandibulofacial dysostosis and in hemifacial microsomia or other types of facial asymmetry.

Problems and Complications. The involved and major nature of this surgery makes it hazardous: the mortality rate world wide has been around 1.5 per cent. Death is generally related to intracranial problems associated with the length of the surgery, brain damage during surgery, or intracranial infections. Blindness has been reported, but is rare and has generally occurred as a result of shifts of the orbits for orbital hypertelorism.

Infection has been the most frequent serious problem occurring in this surgery, with an approximate 7 per cent infection rate documented in one large series (Whitaker et al., 1976). There is a slightly higher incidence of infection associated with intracranial procedures in which the oral cavity is entered, but in general the infection rate has been rather uniform for intra- and extracranial procedures. By means of the routines outlined earlier, the infection rate has been diminished considerably in our series. Generally temporary, although sometimes permanent, damage to the cranial nerves has been reported, particularly to the sixth nerve and to a frontal branch of the seventh nerve. Areas of hypesthesia with fifth nerve deficit are frequent following the surgery but are usually transient.

Canthal drift following medial repositioning or upward or downward repositioning of the lateral canthus is a significant problem that has not been satisfactorily solved. Strabismus is another problem that occurs in the orbital region, following stripping of the orbits. In most instances, this is self-correcting, but a small number of patients will require strabismus surgery. Velopharyngeal incompetence following midface advancement has been reported but is seemingly rare.

Structural losses, or bony resorption, are difficult to measure accurately. There is undoubtedly a small amount of this in every case, but the precise amount is difficult to determine. It is felt that en bloc movements have less tendency to resorb or relapse while onlay grafts result in unpredictable amounts of resorption.

Although the facial structures may be repositioned to reflect normal or near-normal relations to each other, the most difficult structural problem remaining is still the soft tissue deformity in overall facial form and function. With the less severe deformities, a normal facial appearance can often be achieved, but with increasingly severe deformities the residua of correction, especially the soft tissue problems, continue to be difficult to deal with.

Growth has seemed to progress normally in faces following upper face surgery. Lower face surgery at an early age is less certain, and major procedures should probably be delayed until more definite understanding of lower face growth is achieved. It is to be remembered that the recovery period is long, and that postoperatively the face is bandaged and the patients frequently have tracheotomies so that communication is difficult. This situation is extremely well tolerated, particularly in younger children. The facial bandages are removed 3 to 4 days postoperatively, but postoperative swelling is present for weeks, and patients are advised to wait at least 6 weeks before attempting to return to anything like normal activities. One year is necessary for all changes to "settle in" and for the final result to be observed (Converse, Wood-Smith, and McCarthy, 1975; Converse et al., 1974*b*; Salyer et al., 1975; Whitaker, Schut, and Randall, 1976).

REFERENCES

Block, F. C. 1957. Developmental anomalies of the skull affecting the eye. Arch. Ophthalmol., 57:593.

Broadbent, T. R., and Mathews, V. L. 1957. Artistic relationships in surface anatomy of the face: Application to reconstructive surgery. Plast. Reconstr. Surg., 20:1.

Cameron, J. 1931. Interorbital width, new cranial dimension. Am. J. Phys. Anthropol., 15:509.

Converse, J. M., Coccaro, P. J., Becker, M., and Wood-Smith, D. 1973*a*. On hemifacial microsomia. Plast. Reconstr. Surg., 51:268.

Converse, J. M., Horowitz, S. L., Coccaro, P. J., and Wood-Smith, D. 1973*b*. Corrective treatment of skeletal asymmetry in hemifacial microsomia. Plast. Reconstr. Surg., 52:221.

Converse, J. M., McCarthy, J. G., and Wood-Smith, D. 1975. Orbital hypertelorism: Pathogenesis, associated faciocerebral anomalies and surgical correction. Plast. Reconstr. Surg., 56:389.

Converse, J. M., Ransohoff, J., Mathews, E. S., Smith, B., and Molenaar, A. 1970. Ocular hypertelorism and pseudohypertelorism. Plast. Reconstr. Surg., 45:1.

Converse, J. M., and Wood-Smith, D. 1971. An atlas and classification of midfacial and craniofacial osteotomies. Transactions of the Fifth International Congress of Plastic and Reconstructive Surgery. Melbourne, Butterworth's, p. 931.

Converse, J. M., Wood-Smith, D., and McCarthy, J. G. 1975. Report on a series of 50 craniofacial operations. Plast. Reconstr. Surg., 55:283.

Converse, J.M., Wood-Smith, D., McCarthy, J.G., and Coccaro, P.J. 1974*a*. Craniofacial surgery. Clin. Plast. Surg., 1(3):499.

Converse, J. M., Wood-Smith, D., McCarthy, J. G., Coccaro, P. J., and Becker, M. H. 1974*b*. Bilateral facial microsomia. Plast. Reconstr. Surg., 54:413.

Currarino, G., and Silverman, F. N. 1960. Orbital hypertelorism, arhinencephaly and trigonocephaly. Radiology, 74:206.

Davies, D. W., and Munro, I. R. 1975. The anesthetic management and intra-operative care of patients undergoing major facial osteotomies. Plast. Reconstr. Surg., 55:50.

Dingman, R. D. 1956. A syndrome of craniofacial dysostosis. Report of 2 cases. Plast. Reconstr. Surg., 18:113.

Duke-Elder, S., and Wybar, K. C. 1961. The Anatomy of the Visual System. (Vol. 2, System of Ophthalmology Series). St. Louis, C.V. Mosby Co.

Edgerton, M. T., Jane, J. A., and Berry, F. 1974*a*. Craniofacial osteotomies and reconstructions in infants and young children. Plast. Reconstr. Surg., 54:13.

Edgerton, M. T., Jane, J. A., Berry, F. A., and Fuher, J. C. 1974*b*. Feasibility of craniofacial osteotomies in infants and young children. Scand. J. Plast. Reconstr. Surg., 8:164.

Edgerton, M. T., Udvarhely, G. B., and Knox, D. L. 1970. The surgical correction of ocular hypertelorism. Ann. Surg., 172:3.

Franceschetti, A. 1968. Craniofacial dysostoses. In Symposium on Surgical Medical Management of "Congenital Anomalies of the Eye." Trans. New Orleans Acad. Ophthalmol. St. Louis, C. V. Mosby Co., p. 77.

Freihofer, H. P. 1973. Results after midface osteotomies. J. Maxillofac. Surg., 1:30.

Freihofer, H. P. 1974. Kieferorthopadische operationen im jugendalter—ja oder nein? Vortrag Dtsch Ges Kiefer–u Gesichtschir (Hamburg).

Gillies, H. D., and Harrison, S. H. 1950. Operative correction by osteotomy of recessed malar maxillary compound in a case of oxycephaly. Br. J. Plast. Surg., 3:123.

Gonzales-Ulloa, M. 1962. Quantitative principles in cosmetic surgery of the face (profileplasty). Plast. Reconstr. Surg., 29:186.

Gonzales-Ulloa, M. 1964. Quantum method for the appreciation of the morphology of the face. Plast. Reconstr. Surg., 34:241.

Goodman, R. M., and Gorlin, R. J. 1977. Atlas of the Face in Genetic Disorders, 2nd ed. St. Louis, C. V. Mosby Co.

Hogemann, K. E., and Willmar, K. 1974. On LeFort III osteotomy for Crouzon's disease in children. Scand. J. Plast. Reconstr. Surg., 8:169.

Ingraham, F. D., Alexander, E., Jr., and Matson, D.D. 1948. Clinical studies in craniosynostosis; analysis of 50 cases and description of a method of surgical treatment. Surgery, 24:518.

Jabaley, M. E., and Edgerton, M. T. 1969. Surgical correction of congenital midface retrusion in the presence of mandibular protrusion. Plast. Reconstr. Surg., 44:1.

Jones, W. D., III, Whitaker, L. A., and Murtagh, F. 1977. Applications of reconstructive craniofacial techniques to acute upper facial trauma. J. Trauma, 17:339.

Lewin, M. L. 1952. Facial deformity in acrocephaly and its surgical correction. Arch. Ophthalmol., 47:321.

Longacre, J. J. 1968. The early reconstruction of congenital hypoplasia of the facial skeleton and skull: Surgical management of facial deformation secondary to craniosynostosis. In Longacre, J. J. (Ed.): Craniofacial Anomalies: Pathogenesis and Repair. Philadelphia, J. B. Lippincott Co., p. 151.

Longacre, J. J., and deStefano, G. A. 1957. Reconstruction of extensive defects of the skull with split rib grafts. Plast. Reconstr. Surg., 19:186.

Longacre, J. J., DeStefano, A., and Holmstrand, K. E. 1961. The early versus the late reconstruction of congenital hypoplasia of the facial skeleton and skull. Plast. Reconstr. Surg., 27:489.

Longacre, J. J., Stevens, G. A., and Holmstrand, K. E. 1963. The surgical management of first and second branchial arch syndrome. Plast. Reconstr. Surg., 31:507.

Munro, I. R. 1975. Orbito-cranio-facial surgery: The team approach. Plast. Reconstr. Surg., 55:170.

Munro, I. R. 1976. Cranial vault reshaping. Presented at the Second International Conference on the Diagnosis and Treatment of Craniofacial Anomalies, New York, May 1976.

Murray, J. E., and Swanson, L. T. 1968. Midface oste-otomy and advancement for craniostenosis. Plast. Reconstr. Surg., *41*:299.

Obwegeser, H. 1969. Surgical correction of small or retrodisplaced maxillae. Plast. Reconstr. Surg., *43*:351.

Obwegeser, H. L. 1974. Correction of skeletal anomalies of otomandibular dysostosis. J. Maxillofac. Surg., *2*:73.

Pagnell, A. 1960. The use and behavior of bone grafts to the deformed facial skeleton. Transactions of the Second International Congress of Plastic Surgery. Edinburgh, E and S Livingstone, Ltd.

Salyer, K. E., Munro, I. R., Whitaker, L. A., et al.: Difficulties and problems to be solved in the approach to craniofacial malformations. Birth Defects: The National Foundation. Original Article Series XI: 315–399.

Tessier, P. 1971a. Orbitocranial surgery. Trans. Fifth Intl. Congress Plast. Reconstr. Surg., Melbourne, Butterworth's, p. 903.

Tessier, P. 1971b. Relationship of craniostenoses to craniofacial dysostoses, and to faciostenoses. Plast. Reconstr. Surg., *48*:224.

Tessier, P. 1971c. The definitive plastic surgical treatment of the severe facial deformities of craniofacial dysostosis. Plast. Reconstr. Surg., *48*:419.

Tessier, P. 1971d. The scope and principles—dangers and limitations—and the need for special training—in orbitocranial surgery. Trans. Fifth Intl. Congress Plast. Reconstr. Surg., Melbourne, Butterworth's, p. 903.

Tessier, P. 1971e. Total osteotomy of the middle third of the face for faciostenosis or for sequelae of Le-Fort III fractures. Plast. Reconstr. Surg., *48*:533.

Tessier, P. 1972. Orbital hypertelorism. 1. Successive surgical attempts, material and methods, causes and mechanisms. Scand. J. Plast. Reconstr. Surg., *6*:135.

Tessier, P. 1974. Experiences in the treatment of orbital hypertelorism. Plast. Reconstr. Surg., *53*:1.

Tessier, P. 1976. Anatomical classification of facial, craniofacial and laterofacial clefts. J. Maxillofac. Surg., *4*:69.

Trautman, R. C., Converse, J. M., and Smith, B. 1962. Plastic and Reconstructive Surgery of the Eye and Adnexa. Washington, Butterworth's.

Whitaker, L. A., and Randall, P. 1974. The developing field of craniofacial surgery. Pediatrics, *54*:571.

Whitaker, L. A., LaRossa, D., and Randall, P. 1975. Structural goals in craniofacial surgery. Cleft Palate J., *12*:23.

Whitaker, L. A., Munro, I. R., Jackson, I. T., and Salyer, K. E. 1976. Problems in craniofacial surgery. J. Maxillofac. Surg., *4*:131.

Whitaker, L. A., Schut, L., and Randall, P. 1976. Craniofacial surgery: Present and future. Ann. Surg., *184*:558.

Whitaker, L. A., and Schaffer, D. 1977. Severe traumatic oculo-orbital displacement: Diagnosis and treatment. Plast. Reconstr. Surg., *59*:352.

Whitaker, L. A., Schut, L., and Kerr, L. P. 1977. Early surgery for isolated craniofacial dysostosis. Plast. Reconstr. Surg., *60*:575.

Section II

THE EAR AND RELATED STRUCTURES

Chapter 6

EMBRYOLOGY AND DEVELOPMENTAL ANATOMY OF THE EAR

Matthew L. Wong, M.D.

Disease of the ear — inner, middle and outer — is an important part of pediatric otolaryngology. To understand ear disease, knowledge of the embryology and anatomy of the ear is essential. The anatomy of the ear is divided into three distinct parts: the external ear, the middle ear, and the inner ear. Each part has its own distinct embryological development.

EXTERNAL EAR

The external ear is divided into two parts: the auricle, or pinna, and the external auditory canal, or external acoustic meatus.

Auricle

In the fourth fetal week, the auricle develops around the first branchial groove as tissue growths of the first (mandibular) and second (hyoid) branchial arches (Fig. 6–1*A*). These tissue growths are called hillocks, and there are six of them. The first three are from the first branchial arch, and the second three are from the second branchial arch. The hillocks fuse to form the auricle. Eventually, the first hillock gives rise to the tragus; the second forms the crus of the helix; the third develops into the major part of the helix; the fourth becomes the anthelix; the fifth produces the antitragus; and

the sixth forms the lobule and lower part of the helix (Fig. 6–1*B*).

The middle part of the first branchial groove gives rise to the cavum conchae. The upper part develops into the cymba, and the lower part into the intertragal notch.

The auricle changes position. When first formed, it is more ventromedial, but with the growth of the mandible and face during the second fetal month, it is displaced dorsolaterally. By the 20th fetal week, the auricle has attained the adult configuration; but although the newborn auricle has the adult configuration, it is only about two thirds of the adult size (Fig. 6–1*C*). The auricle increases to almost adult size by 4 to 5 years of age and reaches its final size at about 9 years. Otoplasty for protruberant auricles can, therefore, be performed by the fifth year without fear of auricular development retardation.

The neonate auricular cartilage is more immature, softer, and more pliable than that of the adult. Histologically, there are relatively more chondrocytes and the cartilage matrix is more immature. By young childhood, the cartilage is rapidly maturing; by age 8 to 9 years it has the adult consistency.

The fully developed auricle is a cartilaginous structure covered by skin and subcutaneous tissue. The lateral aspect has little subcutaneous tissue, and the skin is tightly bound. The medial aspect is less tightly bound and has more subcutaneous tissue.

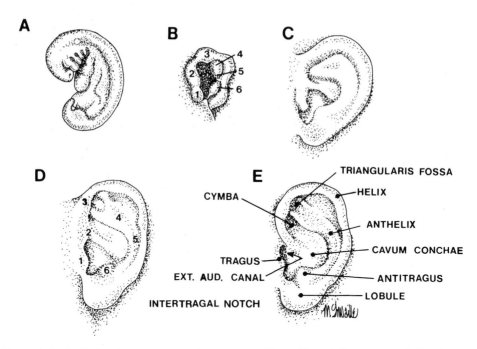

Figure 6-1 Auricular development and anatomy. *A*, Fetus (5 mm): Branchial arch development is evident.

B, First and second branchial arches in 11-mm fetus: six hillocks are present; hillocks 1,2, and 3 are from first (mandibular) arch; hillocks 4, 5, and 6 are from the second (hyoid) arch.

C, Newborn auricle: adult configuration but smaller.

D, Auricle, fully developed, showing hillock's relationship to anatomy.

E, Auricle fully developed showing anatomical parts. (Adapted from Anson, B., and Donaldson, J. 1973. Surgical Anatomy of the Temporal Bone and Ear. 2nd ed. Philadelphia, W. B. Saunders Co., p. 31.)

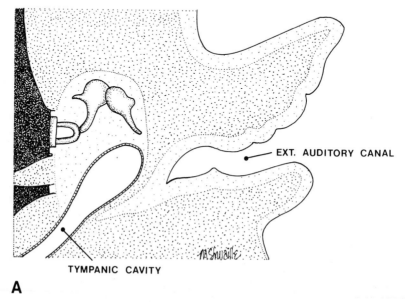

Figure 6-2 Development of external auditory canal.

A, Primitive external auditory canal of a 3-month-old fetus: External auditory canal develops from first branchial groove. Tympanic cavity is from tubotympanic recess of first and second pharyngeal pouches. Primitive tympanic membrane is present.

Illustration continued on the opposite page

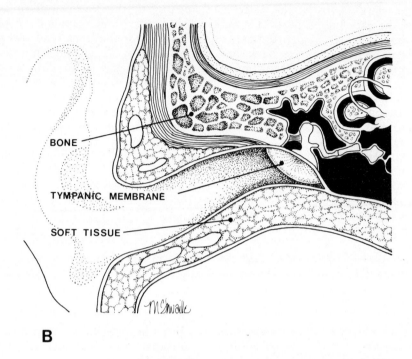

B

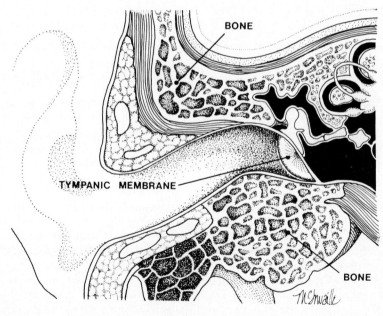

C

Figure 6–2 *Continued   B,* Newborn: Tympanic membrane is almost horizontal. Bone of squamosa forms the superior bony canal wall. Inferior bony canal is fibrous (lamina fibrosa) and has not ossified; cartilaginous (outer third) of canal is unchanged.

C, Adult: Bony (inner two-thirds) canal wall is completely ossified; cartilaginous (outer third) canal is unchanged. Tympanic membrane is more vertical.

The auricular cartilage consists of a series of ridges and depressions. The largest and deepest of the depressions is the concha, which leads to the external auditory meatus. In front of the concha is a prominence called the tragus, which projects backward over the meatus. A less marked elevation is the antitragus, which lies behind the tragus and is separated from it by the intertragal notch. The margin of the auricle is the helix. It surrounds another curved ridge called the anthelix; the two ridges are separated by a depression, or groove, called the scapha. The anthelix has two superior crura that enclose a space called the triangular fossa. The lobule is the inferior-most part of the auricle and is devoid of cartilage, consisting only of fibrous tissue and fat (Fig. 6–1D and E).

The medial aspect of the auricle is the reverse relief of the lateral surface. The concha, triangular fossa, and scapha are seen as eminences, while the anthelix appears as a fossa.

The auricle attaches to the head by: skin, a cartilage extension to the external auditory canal, ligaments, and three small auricular muscles. These muscles are vestigial and are the anterior, superior, and posterior auricular muscles (Anson, 1973).

External Auditory Canal

The external auditory canal is derived from the first branchial groove (between the first and second branchial arches). It consists of two parts: a cartilaginous outer one-third and an osseous inner two-thirds. All other branchial grooves normally disappear, although they occasionally persist to form a cyst or sinus.

At the fourth to fifth fetal week, the ectoderm of the first branchial groove is in contact with the endoderm of the first pharyngeal pouch for a short time, and a primitive tympanic membrane is found. Then the mesoderm grows between the two and contact is lost. The primary meatus is formed at the eighth week by the cavum conchae at the bottom of the first branchial groove deepening to form a narrow, funnel-shaped tube, called the *primary external auditory canal*. This represents the outer one third of the ear canal, is persistent, and is later surrounded by cartilage (Fig. 6–2A).

In the eighth fetal week, a solid cord of epithelial cells called the meatal plate extends from the primary external auditory meatus to the lower wall of the tympanic membrane. This solid meatal plate remains closed until the 21st fetal week, when it is hollowed by the disintegration of its central cells, forming a canal. This new ectodermal tube will become the inner two-thirds of the external auditory canal, and membranous bone will develop around it to form the bony external auditory canal. External auditory canal atresia can develop in two ways. Early in fetal life (2 to 3 months) malformation of the first and second branchial arches can occur, with associated mastoid, middle ear, and auricular deformity. Later (21 weeks of fetal life), the cause is lack of resorption of mesenchymal tissue, so that middle ear, mastoid, and auricular development are normal.

At birth the posterior portion and roof of the bony external auditory canal are formed by the eardrum and the squamosa. The anterior portion and floor of the bony canal consist of a fibrous plate (lamina fibrosa). Thus the anterior portion and floor of the newborn bony ear canal has no bone (Fig. 6–2B). Bone soon forms in the remaining unossified portion of the fibrous plate so that the anterior and inferior walls of the bony canal become osseous by the second postfetal year.

In the neonate, the ear canal is short and straight, collapsed, and impacted with vernix caseosa (Balkany et al., 1978). It becomes longer and extends medially, forward, and inferiorly in a slightly curved course; adult size is attained by the ninth year (Fig. 6–2C).

The skin within the cartilaginous canal has sebaceous and ceruminous glands and hair follicles. The skin overlying the bony canal is tight and has no subcutaneous tissue except the periosteum.

The boundaries of the fully formed external auditory canal are (1) anteriorly, the mandibular fossa and parotid gland, (2) posteriorly, the mastoid, (3) superiorly, the epitympanic recess medially and the cranial cavity laterally, and (4) inferiorly, the parotid gland (Pearson and Jacobson, 1970).

Blood Supply and Nerve Supply

The arterial supply is the superficial temporal and posterior auricular arteries. The venous drainage is via the posterior auricular and posterior facial veins. The auricle's nerve supply is from five sources: the mandibular division of the trigeminal nerve, the greater auricular (C3), lesser occipital (C2,3), facial, and vagus nerves. The ear canal is innervated by the trigeminal, vagus, and facial nerves.

MIDDLE EAR

Developmentally, the middle ear consists of the tympanic cavity and associated ossicles, muscles, and tendons; the eustachian (auditory) tubes; epitympanum; and the mastoid antrum and other air cells. The development of the tympanic membrane and tympanic ring is discussed in this middle ear section, but they actually derive from both external and middle ear tissues. The tympanic cavity and its associated structures are adult size at birth (as is the inner ear), except for the mastoid and other air cells, which continue to enlarge until 9 years of age. The mesoderm of the first and second branchial arches give rise to the ossicles, muscles, tendons, and related connective tissues.

Tympanic Membrane and Ring

The development of the tympanic membrane and its bony tympanic ring begins early and is nearly complete by the fourth fetal month. A primitive tympanic membrane is formed by the fourth to fifth week and separates the first branchial groove from the first pharyngeal pouch. The mesodermal tissue grows between the two layers of the primitive tympanic membrane by the eighth week (Fig. 6–3A). This tissue hollows out to form the bony external auditory canal by the 21st fetal week, and a new, thin tympanic membrane is formed.

The three layers of the eardrum are the outer epithelial layer, which forms from the ectoderm of the first branchial groove; the middle fibrous layer, which forms from the mesoderm between the first branchial groove and the tubotympanic recess; and the inner mucosal layer, which forms from the endoderm of the first and second pharyngeal pouches.

The tympanic ring is formed in the ninth fetal week from four ossification centers as membranous bone. After the fusion of these centers, growth proceeds. By the 15th fetal week, the tympanic ring is almost fully developed and ossification follows. The ring is incomplete at the upper cranial end, called the tympanic incisure, or notch of Rivinus. The tympanic membrane inserts into a sulcus in the annulus and directly into the petrous bone in the tympanic incisure. The fixation of the tympanic ring begins around the 34th fetal week and is complete at birth.

At birth, the tympanic membrane is nearly horizontal; the pars flaccida is thicker and more vascular than the adult tympanic membrane; the tympanic membrane is dull and opaque; the lateral process of the malleus is the most prominent structure; and light reflex is inconsistent (Balkany et al., 1978) (Fig. 6–3B). The tympanic membrane converts to the more vertical position with the development of the external auditory canal. The tympanic membrane is surrounded by a bony tympanic ring, which is incomplete at the superior end at the notch of Rivinus (tympanic incisure).

The mature eardrum consists of two parts: the pars flaccida superiorly and the pars tensa inferiorly. The pars flaccida is a V-shaped flaccid area that overlies the epitympanum and notch of Rivinus. The pars tensa is an almost circular, tense area that overlies the mesotympanum. Histologically, the pars tensa of the tympanic membrane is of three layers: the outer layer is of squamous epithelium; the middle layer consists of outer radial fibers and inner nonradial fibers — circular, parabolic, and transverse; the medial layer is the mucosal layer. The pars flaccida consists only of the lateral cutaneous and medial mucosal layers (Fig. 6–3C).

The manubrium of the malleus is attached to the eardrum and pulls it medially to form its characteristic conical shape. The point of maximum concavity is called the umbo. The annulus is a fibrocartilaginous ring of tissue that attaches to the tympanic ring except superiorly where it attaches to the squamosa. The nerve supply is the same as that of the external auditory canal laterally. The medial innervation of the eardrum is the tympanic branch of the ninth cranial nerve. The deep auricular branch of the internal maxillary artery supplies the lateral surface of the eardrum, while the medial surface is supplied by the posterior auricu-

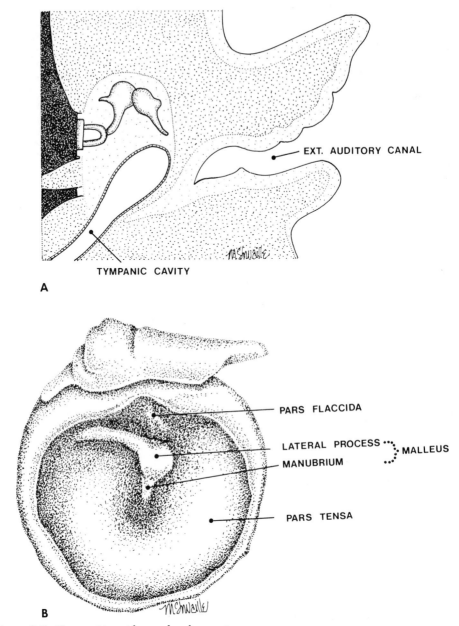

EXT. AUDITORY CANAL

TYMPANIC CAVITY

A

PARS FLACCIDA

LATERAL PROCESS

MANUBRIUM

MALLEUS

PARS TENSA

B

Figure 6–3   Tympanic membrane development.
A, Primitive tympanic membrane of 3-month-old fetus: Malleus has not attached to tympanic membrane.
B, Newborn: Tympanic membrane is almost horizontal. Lateral process of malleus is most prominent. Pars flaccida is thicker and more vascular.

Illustration continued on the opposite page

lar artery via its stylomastoid branch and the internal maxillary artery via its anterior tympanic branch.

Eustachian (Auditory) Tube

The eustachian tube develops from the tubotympanic recess by the third fetal week and serves to equalize the air pressure on both sides of the tympanic membrane (Fig. 6–4*A*). This tube extends downward, forward, and medially, terminating on the lateral wall of the nasopharynx. It is 17 to 18 mm long at birth and elongates to 35 mm in adult life (Donaldson and Miller, 1973). At birth, the tube is horizontal; it is gradually depressed medially with skull growth,

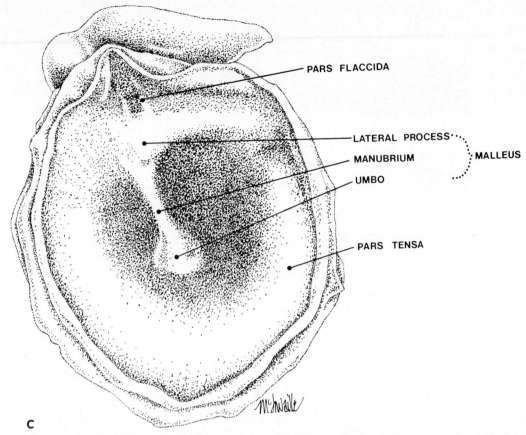

C

Figure 6–3 *Continued   C,* Adult: Tympanic membrane is more vertical. Lateral process of malleus is less prominent. Manubrium of malleus is more vertical. Pars flaccida appears less vascular.

so that in the adult it lies at an incline of 45 degrees (Figs. 6–4*B* and *C*).

The adult eustachian tube is divided into an anteromedial cartilaginous portion (24 mm) and a posterolateral bony portion (11 mm). The narrowest part is called the isthmus and is the junction of the bony and cartilaginous portions. The eustachian tube lies below the tensor tympani muscle and its canal. The muscle opening the eustachian tube is the tensor veli palatini, innervated by the trigeminal nerve. The eustachian tube function of the levator veli palatini muscle, which is innervated by the vagus nerve, is still not certain. The lymphoid tissue located at the pharyngeal opening is called the tonsil of Gerlach (Lim, 1974).

The respiratory epithelium of the nose and nasopharynx is continuous into the eustachian tube and to a variable degree onto the walls of the middle ear space. The ciliary "stream" is from the middle ear toward the nasopharynx. Abundant goblet cells and

seromucinous glands provide a mucous blanket, so that the ciliary beat toward the nasopharynx can be effective.

Changes with age take place continuously during childhood but are most marked at age 7 years. At this age the muscle mass of the tensor palatini is greater than before and the tubal cartilage is much larger. These two changes probably account for the better eustachian tube ventilating function that so often becomes evident by age 8 to 10 years. Also, the seromucinous glands so numerous in early years become less evident at age 7 (Holborow, 1970). (See Chap. 16.)

Tympanic Cavity and Epitympanic Recess (Epitympanum)

The development of the middle ear starts at the third fetal week with the expansion of the endodermally lined first and second pharyngeal pouches, called the tubotympan-

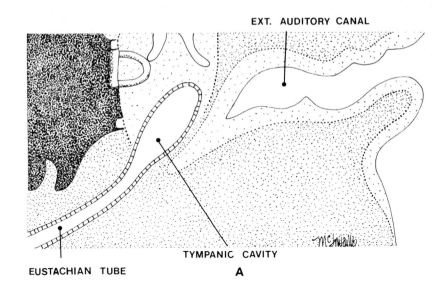

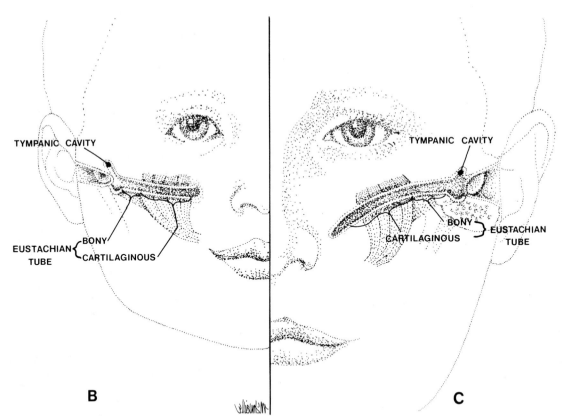

Figure 6–4   Eustachian tube development.

A, Fetus, 3 months old.

B, Infant: tube is 17 mm in length, straighter and more horizontal. Medial two-thirds is cartilaginous; lateral third is bony.

C, Fully developed: tube is 37 mm in length, slightly curved, with more vertical incline medially and anteriorly. Medial two-thirds is cartilaginous; lateral third is bony.

ic recess. This develops into the eustachian tube and tympanic cavity. Through slow lengthwise growth, the tympanic cavity extends backward and is nearly complete by the 30th fetal week.

The epitympanum forms from an extension of the tympanic cavity. It starts to develop at the 18th fetal week and is nearly complete by the 34th fetal week.

At the 23rd fetal week, ossification starts around the tympanic cavity, first at the medial and lateral parts of the tegmen tympanum. This process is complete at the end of the fetal period.

The fully developed tympanic cavity is an air space lined by respiratory epithelium. The mucosa near the eustachian tube has columnar cells and mucus-secreting cells, while the mucosa farther away from the eustachian tube has flat, cuboidal epithelium. With chronic infection, there is proliferation of the goblet cells and seromucinous glands in the middle ear, especially those around the eustachian tube orifice (Holborow, 1970).

The roof of the tympanic cavity is called the tegmen tympani and separates the middle ear from the middle cranial fossa. The floor of the tympanic cavity consists of the fundus tympani posteriorly (a thin sheet of bone that forms the floor of the jugular fossa) and anteriorly the posterior wall of the ascending part of the carotid canal. Posteriorly, the border of the tympanic cavity is the mastoid, stapedius muscle, and pyramidal prominence. The medial wall of the tympanic cavity consists of: the promontory (a round, hollow prominence resulting from the first turn of the cochlea); the fenestra vestibuli, or oval window, just above and behind the promontory; the prominence of the facial canal; the fenestra cochlea or round window; and the sinus tympani. The lateral wall of the tympanic cavity is the tympanic membrane and the scutum, a part of the squamosa (Fig. 6–5).

The epitympanum lies above the level of the tympanic membrane and contains the greater part of the incus and the upper half of the malleus. Its boundaries are medially, the lateral semicircular canal and eighth cranial nerve; superiorly, the tegmen; anteriorly, the zygomatic arch; laterally, the scutum of the squamosa; inferiorly, the fossa incudis; and, posteriorly, the aditus ad antrum (the connection with the antrum).

Contents of Tympanic Cavity

Muscles

There are two muscles in the middle ear. The first is the tensor tympani, derived from the first branchial arch. The tensor tympani is described as bipinnate muscle. The most medial group of fibers arise from the sphenoid bone and superior tubal cartilage. The lateral group of fibers arise as a continuation of the most inferoposterior fibers of the tensor veli palatini, which lack bony attachment, but rather extend lateral to the tube and into the semicanal to join the tendon of the medial fibers. This tendon bears many interspersed muscle fibers for almost its full course to the tympanum and just anterior to the cochleariform process (Rood and Doyle, 1978). It inserts near the root of the manubrium of the malleus. It has its own canal, above the eustachian tube, and is formed from the middle of the 8th to the 11th fetal week. Its action is to tighten and draw the tympanic membrane medially when an extremely loud sound is heard (startle reflex). Its nerve supply is the trigeminal nerve. The second muscle is the stapedius muscle, derived from the second branchial arch. It originates from the pyramidal eminence and inserts into the neck of the stapes. Its action is to tilt the anterior end of the base of the stapes laterally on the stimulus of a loud noise. Its nerve supply is the seventh cranial nerve.

Development of Ossicles

There are three ossicles in the middle ear. The malleus, incus, and stapes develop from the mesenchymal tissue (cartilage) at the dorsolateral end of the first two branchial arches. The first branchial cartilage is called Meckel's cartilage and gives rise to the head and neck of the malleus and body and short process of the incus. The second branchial cartilage is called Reichert's cartilage and gives rise to the long process of the incus, the manubrium of the malleus, and all of the stapes except the medial aspect of the footplate (Fig. 6–6).

Malleus. The malleus has a dual origin. The head and neck are from the first branchial arch, and the manubrium is from the second arch. Development starts at the fourth to fifth fetal week. By the eighth

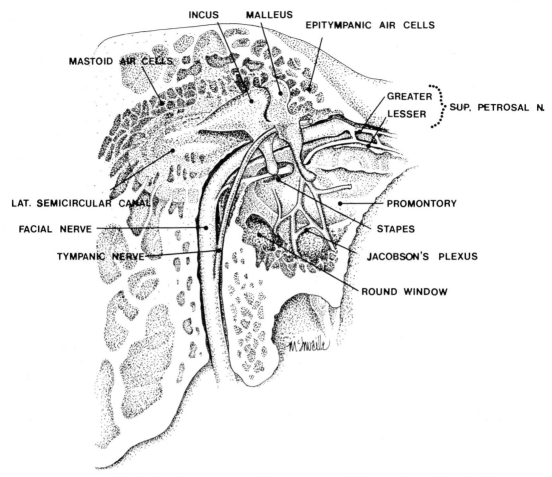

Figure 6–5 Fully developed anatomy of middle ear and mastoid. Note relationships of facial nerve, tympanic nerve, ossicles, lateral semicircular canal, mastoid air cells, and epitympanum.

week, the malleus has a cartilage form similar to its form in the adult. The cartilaginous malleus develops to full adult size by the 15th fetal week; then ossification begins.

The malleus is the lateral-most ossicle. Fully formed, it has a round head and a constricted neck, which lie in the epitympanum. The manubrium extends downward, medially, and backward from the neck and is embedded in the upper half of the tympanic membrane. The anterior process projects from the neck and is connected by the anterior ligament to the petrotympanic fissure. The lateral process projects toward the tympanic membrane from the root of the manubrium, and malleolar folds are attached to it.

Incus. The incus also has a dual origin. The body and short process are from the first branchial arch, while the long process

is from the second. The incus reaches adult size by the 15th fetal week as a cartilage and then begins ossifying.

The incus is the second (intermediate) bone, is shaped like an anvil, and has a body and short and long processes. The short process projects backward from the body toward the fossa incudis, where it is attached to the wall by the posterior ligament. The long process extends downward; its lower end bends medially and terminates in a knob, the lenticular process. The incus articulates with the head of the stapes at the incudostapedial joint, an enarthrodial joint. The body of the incus joins with the head of the malleus at the incudomalleal joint, a diarthrodial joint.

Stapes. The stapes has a dual origin as well: all of the stapes except the medial part of the footplate is from the second branchial arch. The medial, or vestibular, portion of the footplate (lamina stapedis) is from the otic capsule.

The blastemic mass of the stapes is first recognized at four and a half weeks fetally. This is the first ossicle that is recognizable. This blastema divides into the stapes and the interhyal and laterohyal cartilages. Initially, the stapes is a round solid mass. During the 5th to 6th fetal week, the stapedial mass grows around the stapedial artery (artery of the second branchial arch), forming a ring-shaped stapes with the stapedial artery in the center (Fig. 6–7A). As the stapes differentiates and assumes its stirrup shape, the stapedial artery regresses (Bolz

and Lim, 1972) (Fig. 6–7B). By the middle of the fourth fetal month, the stapes is almost adult shape and configuration. By the sixth fetal month, the stapes assumes the adult shape and configuration but is cartilaginous (Figs. 6–7C and D).

The laterohyal cartilage fuses to the otic capsule and takes part in the formation of the facial canal's anterior wall and the bone of the stapedius pyramid. The interhyal cartilage becomes the stapedius muscle and its tendon.

The stapes is the third and innermost of the ossicles. Fully developed, it is stirrup-shaped and has a small head and neck. From the neck are two diverging limbs,

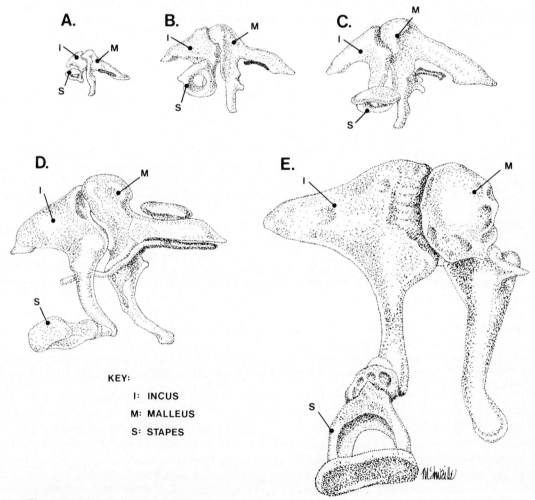

KEY:

I: INCUS

M: MALLEUS

S: STAPES

Figure 6–6 Ossicular development.

A, Fetus of 2 months: cartilaginous ossicles recognizable. B, Fetus of 3 months. C, Fetus of 4 months: attaining adult configuration, but cartilaginous. D, Fetus of 6 months: adult configuration and size; ossification begins. E, Adult ossicles. (Adapted from Anson, B. 1973. Developmental anatomy of the ear. In Paparella, M. and Shumrick, D. (Eds.): Otolaryngology, Vol I. Philadelphia, W. B. Saunders Co., p. 20.)

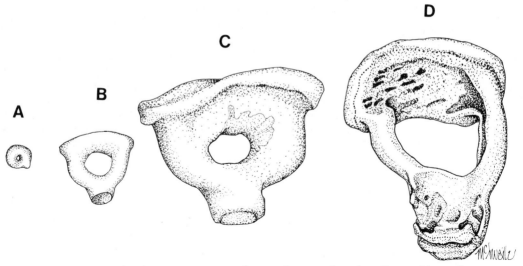

Figure 6–7   Stapes development. *A*, Fetus of 2 months: ring shaped. *B*, Fetus of 3 months: stirrup shaped. *C*, Fetus of 4.5 months: almost adult shaped and cartilaginous. *D*, Fetus of 6 months: adult size and configuration; ossification begins. (Adapted from Anson, B., and Donaldson, J. 1973. Surgical Anatomy of the Temporal Bone and Ear. 2nd ed. Philadelphia, W. B. Saunders Co., pp. 56–57.)

called crura, which extend to the oval base, the footplate. The footplate is attached to the oval window by the annular ligaments in a syndesmotic joint. The stapedius muscle and tendon attach to the neck of the stapes.

Ossification of the Ossicles

Ossification of the ossicles is similar to that of the otic capsule, with formation of outer periosteal, endochondral, and inner periosteal bone. This process starts at the 16th fetal week and is nearly complete by the 32nd fetal week. Erosion of the malleus and incus continues in postfetal life with secondary and tertiary bone formation in the adult.

The stapes ossifies later, beginning at the 18th fetal week. Remodeling does not occur after birth, so the fetal bone remains throughout life.

Mucosal Pouches and Folds

There are four mucosal pouches that appear between the 12th and 28th fetal weeks. They are the saccus anterior, the saccus medius, the saccus superior, and the saccus posterior. The saccus medius forms the epitympanic recess and divides into three saccules — anterior, medial, and posterior. It is the posterior saccule that pneumatizes that

part of the mastoid that develops into the petrous portion of the temporal bone. The saccus superior develops into the posterior pouch of Tröltsch and inferior incudal space and later pneumatizes the mastoid portion of the temporal bone. The saccus posterior extends along the floor of the middle ear to form the round window niche, sinus tympani, and a large part of the oval window niche. The saccus anterior forms the anterior pouch of Tröltsch.

During the development of the tympanic cavity, the cavity is filled with mucoid tissue. Between the third and seventh fetal months this tissue is slowly absorbed. Mucosal folds are formed where the pouches were in contact with each other.

There are five malleal folds and four incudal folds. The significant ones will be described. The anterior malleal fold is from the neck of the malleus to the anterosuperior margin of the tympanic sulcus. The posterior malleal fold is from the neck of the malleus to the posterosuperior margin of the tympanic sulcus. The lateral malleal fold is from the malleal neck to the malleal neck in an arch form and attaches to Shrapnell's membrane, enclosing Prussak's space. The anterior pouch of Tröltsch lies between the anterior malleal fold and that portion of the tympanic membrane anterior to the handle of the malleus. The posterior pouch of Tröltsch lies between the posterior malleal fold and the portion of the tympanic membrane posterior to the handle of the malleus (Proctor, 1964).

Tympanic Antrum, Mastoid Air Cells, and Related Air Spaces

The tympanic antrum appears in the 22nd fetal week as a lateral extension of the epitympanum. The antrum lumen is well developed by the 34th fetal week, and its pneumatization is completed in the first year of postfetal life.

The other related air spaces are first found in the tympanic floor, the tympanic ostium of the auditory (eustachian) tube, the antral lumen and along the tegmen and the medial wall of the middle ear. Development of these related air cells is so extensive that in the adult nearly all parts of the temporal bone show air cells. Most of these air cells complete their development postfetally.

Air cell formation in the petrous pyramid starts as early as the 28th fetal week, and most are developed during the first 2 years of life. Pneumatization of the mastoid air cells starts as early as the 33rd fetal week, but most are formed after birth. The process continues and reaches a near-adult state between 5 and 10 years postfetally. The majority of the mastoid air cells originate from the antrum, but some communicate directly with the middle ear.

The fully developed antrum is the proximal-most mastoid air cell and often the largest. It is connected with the epitympanum by the aditus ad antrum and is an important landmark. Except in rare congenital malformations, it is always present, just posterior to the attic and just behind and medial to the posterosuperior meatal wall. Leading into the antrum are the rest of the mastoid air cells (Palva and Palva, 1966).

The entire, fully developed temporal bone is filled with air cells, including the zygoma, the jugular wall, the petrous apex, and around and through the semicircular canals. These air cells usually originate from the antrum but can start from the tympanic cavity proper. The exact pattern and degree of pneumatization vary greatly, but tend to be symmetrical unless hindered by otitis media, especially in infancy and early childhood (Flisberg and Zsigmoind, 1965).

There are several important landmarks in the developed mastoid air cells. Trautmann's triangle is a triangular area of the posterior fossa plate behind the antrum. It is bound posteroinferiorly by the sigmoid sinus, anterosuperiorly by the bony labyrinth, and superiorly by the superior petrosal sinus. The solid angle is the angle formed by the three semicircular canals and Citelli's angle is the sinodural angle. The tegmen, or roof of the attic and antrum, lies in a horizontal plane and is delineated externally by the linea temporalis, a line extending posteriorly from the root of the zygoma. This thin plate of bone separates the middle fossa from the tympanic cavity and mastoid air cells.

Temporal Bone

The temporal bone forms part of the side and base of the skull. It constitutes two thirds of the floor of the middle cranial fossa and one third of the floor of the posterior fossa. There are four parts to the temporal bone: petrous, squamous, tympanic, and mastoid. At birth only three have formed: petrous, squamous, and tympanic. The squamous part starts to develop at the eighth fetal week, and the tympanic part starts to develop at the ninth to tenth fetal week. The periotic capsule constitutes the petrous portion and results from the condensation of mesenchymal tissue around the membranous labyrinth (fourth fetal week). This tissue changes to cartilage during the seventh fetal week and starts to ossify by the sixth fetal month. The squamous, tympanic, and mastoid bones are formed by membranous bony development, while the petrous part is first formed in cartilage (endochondral). All bones except the petrous portion continue to develop postfetally.

Most of the mastoid part of the temporal bone develops after birth by growing over and lateral to the mastoid antrum. At the end of the first year, the mastoid forms a distinct process and is well developed by the third year of life. Its final configuration is not attained until years later.

Lateral Surface

At birth and in infancy, there is no external osseous meatus, except for its superior

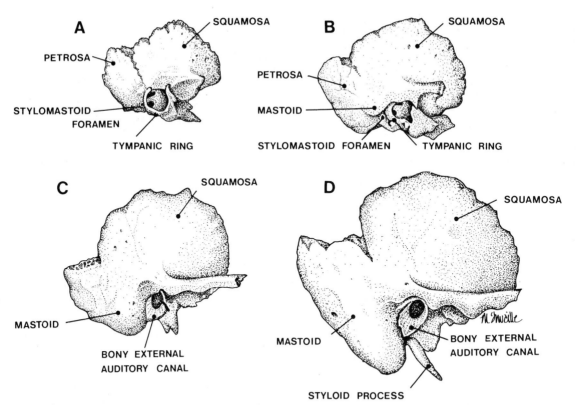

Figure 6–8 Lateral temporal bone development.

A, Newborn: Petrous, squamous, and tympanic portions are present; mastoid portion is not developed. Stylomastoid foramen (exit of facial nerve) is just behind tympanic ring.

B, Infant, 1.5 years old: Mastoid development is underway. Stylomastoid foramen can still be exposed and not covered by mastoid process. Tympanic ring is ossifying.

C, Child, 5 years: Mastoid process is well developed and covers stylomastoid foramen. Tympanic ring has completely ossified and entire bony external auditory canal is osseous.

D, Adult: normal anatomy.

portion, and no mastoid process (Fig. 6–8*A*). The facial nerve emerges from the stylomastoid foramen just behind the tympanic membrane and is at risk with the usual postauricular incision. The bone over the infant's antrum is cribriform; consequently, otitis media can easily extend subperiosteally. It is not until the second year that the mastoid process begins to appear and the osseous meatus develops more fully (Fig. 6–8*B*). At 5 years of age, mastoid process development is well advanced and the stylomastoid foramen is covered (Fig. 6–8*C*).

Lateral surface anatomy is important to surgery. The superoposterior aspect of the external auditory canal is usually marked by a small spine, the suprameatal spine of Henle. Medially to the spine is the antrum. The fossa mastoidea or cribriform area is 1 cm posterior to the spine of Henle and is a shallow depression on the mastoid cortex. It is perforated by numerous emissary vessels, especially in infancy. In infancy and young childhood a subperiosteal abscess may result from extension of otitis media and mastoiditis through this cribriform area, with production of an inflamed mass in the mastoid area and displacement of the auricle downward, outward, and forward (Shambaugh, 1967). The temporal line marks the inferior margin of the insertion of the temporalis muscle and is used as an approximate guide to the level of the middle fossa. In the bony auditory canal are two sutures: the tympanosquamous superiorly, and the tympanomastoid posteriorly (Fig. 6–8*D*).

Middle Fossa Surface

The middle fossa is the roof of the tympanic and mastoid cavities. The area is a trapezoid in a transverse plane. The middle meningeal artery and its foramen, the foramen spinosum, lie anteriorly and laterally. About 8 mm medial to the middle meningeal artery at its foramen is the greater superficial petrosal nerve. Within its canal, the greater superficial petrosal nerve runs posteriorly to join the geniculate ganglion. Posteriorly, a ridge called the arcuate eminence houses the superior semicircular canal. Along the medial ridge of the middle fossa bone is the superior petrosal sinus (Parisier, 1977).

The apex of the petrous bone houses many important structures. Laterally is the foramen spinosum. Anteriorly and medially is the foramen ovale (the opening for the mandibular division of the trigeminal nerve). Just posterior to this is the trigeminal (Gasserian) ganglion within its depression, Meckel's cave. Dorello's canal is between the petrous tip and the sphenoid bone and is the groove for the sixth cranial nerve. Most medial is the foramen lacerum, containing the internal carotid artery (Gacek, 1975).

Posterior Fossa Surface

The posterior fossa lies in a sagittal (vertical) plane and runs posteriorly and laterally at a 45-degree angle. The anterior part is more medial than the posterior part. The internal auditory meatus and the endolymphatic sac lie in the posterior fossa.

The anterior-most structure is the internal auditory meatus. Fully developed, its diameter is about 8 mm; the anterior lip is more medial than its posterior lip. There are four nerves in this meatus: anterosuperiorly the facial nerve; anteroinferiorly the cochlear nerve; superoposteriorly the superior vestibular nerve; and posteroinferiorly the inferior vestibular nerve. A vertical crest of bone, called Bill's bar, separates the superior half of the canal vertically. The horizontal, or falciform, crista separates the canal into a superior and inferior half.

The subarcuate artery is 5 to 6 mm directly posterior to the internal auditory meatus. At an angle of 30 degrees posteroinferiorly and a distance of 10 to 11 mm from the internal auditory meatus is the operculum of the endolymphatic sac. Just inferior to that is the jugular notch.

The cochlear canaliculus (periotic duct) exits the temporal bone near the jugular notch. The posterior-most portion of the posterior fossa is the sigmoid sinus. Anteroinferiorly is the inferior petrosal sinus, which empties into the sigmoid sinus (Geurkink, 1977).

Miscellaneous Middle Ear Structures

Meninges and Venous Sinuses

The meninges cover the middle and posterior fossae. The middle fossa dura is more easily elevated and less easily torn. The posterior fossa lacks arachnoid prolongations; therefore, a cerebral spinal fluid leak here is more difficult to heal than one in the middle fossa, which has arachnoid prolongations.

Blood flow in the veins of the head relies on gravity; the veins are without valves. Venous sinuses are splits in the dura; the largest of them is the lateral (transverse) sinus, which begins at the occipital protuberance, extends forward horizontally and then descends medially in a deep groove to become the sigmoid sinus, which ends in the jugular bulb. The right lateral sinus is larger than the left because the large, superior longitudinal sinus flows into the right lateral sinus and the smaller, straight sinus flows into the left. The superior petrosal sinus carries blood from the cavernous sinus to the lateral sinus and lies in the attachment of the tentorium to the petrous ridge. The inferior petrosal sinus contains blood from the cavernous sinus and runs along the inferior portion of the posterior fossa to empty into the sigmoid sinus at the jugular bulb. This accounts for bleeding from the jugular bulb area even with tamponade of the sigmoid sinus and the internal jugular vein in glomus jugulare tumor excision (Shambaugh, 1967).

Facial Nerve

Facial nerve development is intimately connected with temporal bone development as it is the nerve of the second branchial arch. In the third fetal week, the acousticofacial ganglion is formed in the region lateral to the rhombencephalon, in a close relationship with the auditory vesicle. Then the facial ganglion separates from the original acousticofacial ganglion. (The acoustic ganglion retains its close relationship to the developing auditory vesicle; see the section of this chapter that discusses the inner ear, especially the acoustic ganglion.) The facial nerve comes into view. Nerve fibers grow from the neural tube into the mesenchyme of the second branchial arch. The chorda tympani nerve arises from the peripheral nerve fibers of the geniculate (formerly facial) ganglion. The chorda tympani nerve joins the developing facial nerve for a short distance, and by the fifth fetal week unites

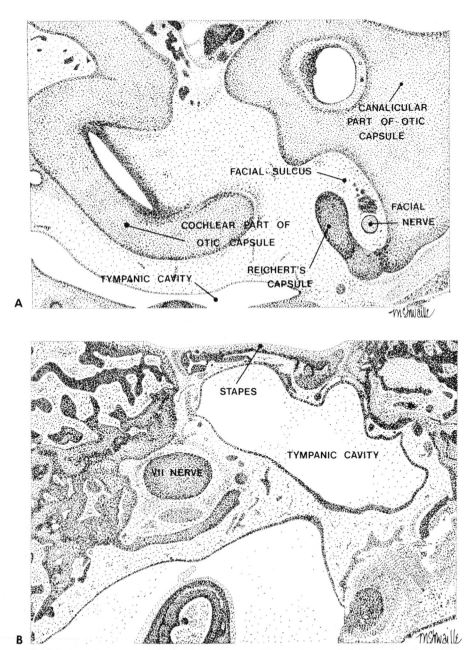

Figure 6–9   Facial nerve and canal development. A, Fetus of 2.5 months: Facial nerve develops early and parallels the development of the middle and inner ears, being complete by the time of ossification of the middle and inner ears (6 months).

B, Term newborn: fully developed facial nerve.

Illustration continued on the opposite page

with the third branch of the trigeminal nerve (Gasser, 1967).

The primordial form of the facial canal begins as a shallow sulcus on the lateral surface of the otic capsule by the 10th fetal week. At this stage, its outer wall is contributed by the second branchial arch and contains the triad of structures that make up its mature content — facial nerve, stapedius muscle, and blood vessels (Fig. 6–9*A*).

Closure of the sulcus to form the facial nerve canal is well underway by the sixth fetal month and almost complete by the seventh fetal month. By the eighth fetal month, bone of the otic capsule approaches a petrous texture and vessels have taken their positions surrounding the nerve. At birth, facial nerve development is complete (Figs. 6–9*B* and *C*).

The most common anomaly of the facial nerve in the temporal bone is dehiscence, with an incidence of up to 63 per cent in the horizontal and 6 per cent in the vertical part (Baxter, 1971). The stapedius muscle is absent in 1 per cent of people (Donaldson and Anson, 1974).

The fully developed facial nerve originates from the facial nucleus and leaves the brain stem at the inferior border of the pons in the recess between the olive and the inferior cerebellar peduncle. It enters the porus of the internal acoustic meatus ac-companied by the nervus intermedius and enters its bony canal, the facial or fallopian canal. The nerve continues laterally, close to the middle fossa, to the geniculate ganglion. In the newborn, the geniculate ganglion is not covered by bone but lies against the middle fossa dura. In the adult, it is usually covered by a thin bony plate except for the hiatus of the facial canal, which allows for the emergence of the greater and lesser superficial petrosal nerves onto the surface of the petrous apex. At the geniculate ganglion, the facial nerve bends posteriorly to begin its tympanic course along the medial wall of the middle ear. The tympanic portion of the facial nerve lies in its bony canal just above the oval window niche and slopes backward and downward at a 30-degree angle. Dehiscences of this canal are noted in up to 63 per cent of bone-studies (Baxter, 1971).

At the pyramidal eminence for the stapedius muscle, the facial nerve makes its second turn, the pyramidal turn, to begin its vertical or mastoid course. At the beginning of its vertical portion, the nerve lies just lateral and inferior to the horizontal semicircular canal. As it descends, the facial nerve moves inferiorly and slightly laterally; it is surrounded here by perifacial air cells. The tympanomastoid suture acts as a landmark, as the nerve lies medial or sometimes poste-

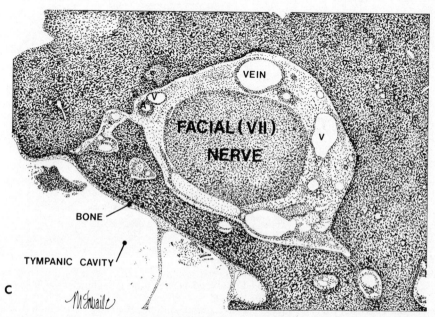

Figure 6–9 *Continued*   C, Adult.

rior, but never anterior, to the plane of this canal suture. The nerve exits at the stylomastoid foramen at the anterior end of the diagastric groove. At birth, due to the lack of development of the mastoid process, the facial nerve exits very close to the tympanic ring and can be transected by the usual adult postauricular incision. With mastoid process development, the exit of the facial nerve is carried more inferiorly (Shambaugh, 1967).

The chorda tympani nerve leaves the facial nerve at its mastoid (vertical) portion, but can leave as high as the midtympanic portion or as low as a site outside the temporal bone. The chorda tympani proceeds in its own canal to the posterior iter, from which it exits and passes lateral to the long process of the incus and medial to the handle of the malleus toward the anterior iter. Here it enters the anterior petrotympanic fissure (canal of Huguier) to leave the ear (Donaldson and Anson, 1974; Anson et al., 1963).

Important Landmarks of Tympanic Cavity: Prussak's space or the superior recess of the

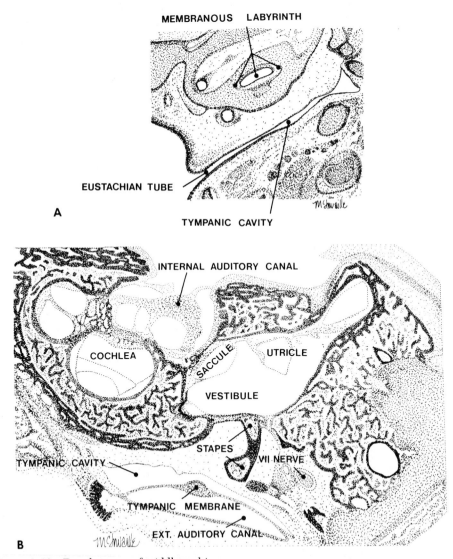

Figure 6–10 Development of middle and inner ear.

A, Fetus, 3 months: Early development of labyrinth; eustachian tube and tympanic cavity are developing, ossicular formation is not recognizable.

B, Fetus, 6 months: Inner ear and middle ear have attained full development; ossification commences.

Illustration continued on the opposite page

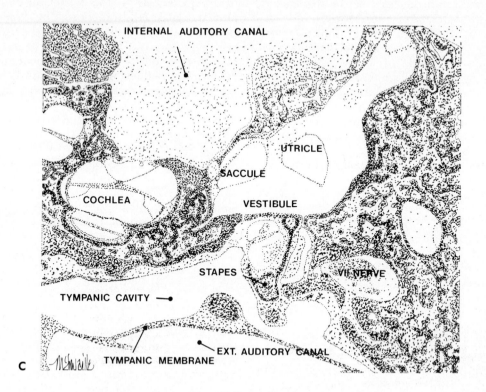

C

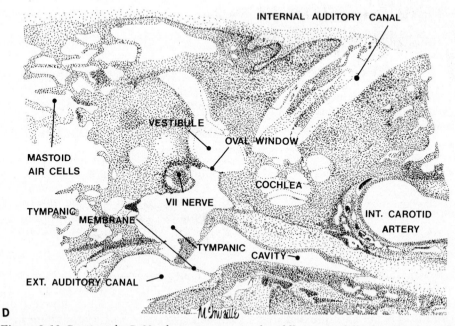

D

Figure 6–10 *Continued* *C,* Newborn: inner ear and middle ear are fully developed; ossification is almost complete except for minimal postfetal changes in the malleus and incus and outer periosteal layer of the bony labyrinth.

D, Adult.

tympanic membrane is situated between the pars flaccida and the neck of the malleus. It is bound anteriorly, posteriorly, and superiorly by the lateral malleal fold; inferiorly by the lateral process of the malleus; medially by the neck of the malleus; and laterally by Shrapnell's membrane.

The *canal of Huguier* (anterior petrotympanic fissure) exits the temporal bone from the anterior mesotympanum; the chorda tympani nerve leaves the temporal bone through this canal.

The *sinus tympani* is the area where cholesteatoma may remain hidden. Its boundaries are medially, the bony labyrinth; laterally, the pyramidal eminence; superiorly, the ponticulus and lateral semicircular canal; posteriorly, the posterior semicircular canal; and inferiorly, the subiculum and jugular wall (Wigard and Trilbich, 1973).

The *ponticulus* is the ridge of bone between the oval window niche and the sinus tympani, and forms the superior border of the sinus tympani.

The *subiculum* is the ridge of bone between the round window niche and the sinus tympani, and forms the inferior border of the sinus tympani.

The *facial recess* is another area where cholesteatoma can be difficult to remove. It is bound medially by the facial nerve, laterally by the bony annulus and chorda tympani, and superiorly by the short process of the incus.

The *cochleariform process* is the curved end of the bony semicanal in which the tensor tympani muscle runs, and is in the anterior medial wall of the tympanic cavity. It is where the tensor tympani muscle turns laterally from its canal to attach to the malleus. In revision radical mastoidectomies, this is one of the few safe landmarks to locate.

Vascular and Nerve Supplies of the Middle Ear and Mastoid

The middle ear and mastoid air cells receive their arterial supply from the external and internal carotid arteries. The external carotid contribution is via the internal maxillary, posterior auricular, and ascending pharyngeal arteries. The internal maxillary artery gives rise to the anterior tympanic branch and the superior tympanic and superficial petrosal branches (via the middle meningeal artery). The posterior auricular artery gives rise to the posterior tympanic and stylomastoid branches. The ascending pharyngeal artery gives rise to the inferior tympanic branch. The internal carotid artery contribution is via the caroticotympanic artery, which anastomoses with branches of the stylomastoid, internal maxillary, and ascending pharyngeal arteries. The mastoid is also supplied by the occipital artery through its meningeal branch and the internal carotid artery via the subarcuate vessels.

The middle ear is innervated by the auriculotemporal nerve of the mandibular division of the trigeminal nerve, Jacobsen's portion of the ninth cranial nerve, and the auricular portion of the vagus nerve (Fig. 6–10).

INNER EAR

The inner ear consists of the membranous labyrinth housed in a bony labyrinth in the petrous portion of the temporal bone. At birth, both of these structures are of adult size and configuration except for minimal subsequent changes of the periosteal layer of the bony labyrinth and postfetal continued growth of the endolymphatic sac and duct.

Membranous Labyrinth

Formation

Auditory Vesicle. At the third fetal week, the primordium of the membranous labyrinth appears on either side of the rhombencephalon as a thickening of ectoderm called the auditory placode. During the fourth fetal week, the placode rapidly invaginates, forming initially the auditory (otic) pit and finally the auditory vesicle (otocyst).

The auditory vesicle develops and is divided into two pouches by three folds. The ventral (cochlear) pouch forms the saccule and cochlear duct. The dorsal (vestibular) pouch gives rise to the endolymphatic duct, utricle, and semicircular canal (Pearson and Jacobson, 1970). These two pouches are evident by the fifth fetal week and grow rapidly (Figs. 6–11*A* and *B*). The membranous labyrinth develops rapidly and, at two and a

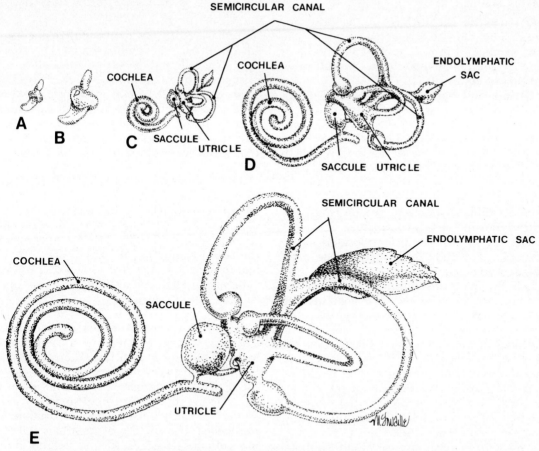

Figure 6–11   Development of membranous labyrinth.

A, Fetus, 5 weeks: development of ventral (cochlear) and dorsal (vestibular) pouches.

B, Fetus, 6 weeks: rapid growth.

C, Fetus, 2.5 months: Adult structures easily recognizable. Cochlea has attained its 2.5 turns; semicircular canals, utricle, saccule, and endolymphatic sac and duct are well developed.

D, Fetus, 6 months: Membranous labyrinth development is complete except endolymphatic sac and duct continue to grow postfetally.

E, Adult: fully developed labyrinth. (Adapted from Anson, B. 1973. Developmental Anatomy of the Ear. *In* Paparella, M., and Shumrick, M. (Eds.): Otolaryngology, Vol. 1. Philadelphia, W. B. Saunders Co., p. 35.)

half months, adult structures are easily recognizable (Fig. 6–11*C*). By the sixth fetal month, the membranous labyrinth is completely developed, except that the endolymphatic sac and the duct continue to grow postfetally (Figs. 6–11*D* and *E*).

Structures

The membranous labyrinth is filled with endolymph, is bathed by the perilymph, and lies in the bony labyrinth. It includes the utricle, saccule, semicircular canals, and endolymphatic sac and duct.

Endolymphatic Duct and Sac. The growth of the endolymphatic duct and sac starts at the sixth fetal week from the dorsal pouch of the auditory vesicle. The duct remains straight for the first half of fetal life, but later the duct and sac acquire a curved course. In the mature state, the endolymphatic sac turns downward at a 30- to 60-degree angle. The fully developed endolymphatic duct lies in the vestibular aqueduct, except for the proximal (utricular) extremity, which is within the perilymphatic labyrinth. It is connected to both the saccule and utricle by the utricular and saccular ducts. At the utricular duct is the endolymphatic valve of Bast. The endolymphatic sac lies partly within the vestibular aqueduct and partly on the surface of the posterior fossa. The sac itself is often rugose. The duct averages 4 mm in length and the sac is 7 to 16 mm long and 5 to 10 mm wide (Arenberg et al., 1977).

Utricle and Saccule. The utricle develops from the dorsal (vestibular) pouch of the auditory vesicle, and the saccule is from the ventral (cochlear) pouch of the auditory vesicle. They begin to develop at the sixth fetal week. By the eighth fetal week, the utricle and saccule show the characteristics of their adult forms. By the eleventh fetal week, the development of the neuroepithelial cells and supporting cells is complete.

The utricle and saccule are located in the vestibule. The fully developed utricle is an oblong, flattened sac with a rounded end which occupies the elliptical recess in the posterosuperior portion of the vestibule. On its posterior wall are the openings of the semicircular canals and on its anterior wall is the utriculosaccular duct. The saccule is smaller and is a spherical organ, located in the anteroinferior portion of the vestibule. It connects with the cochlea via the ductus reuniens, with the utricle via the utriculosaccular duct, and with the endolymphatic duct via the utricular duct.

The sensory receptors and their supporting structures form the maculae of the utricle and saccule. The macula of the utricle is a spade-shaped area located anteriorly and laterally within the utricle while the macula of the saccule is located on the medial wall of the saccule. The macula of the saccule lies in the vertical plane, perpendicular to the utricular macula.

Both maculae are structurally similar. The primary receptor cells are the hair cells, which are of two types: Type I has an expanded base (goblet-shaped) and is surrounded by afferent nerve endings; Type II is tubular and supplied by smaller nerve endings. The upper surface of each cell has a cuticular region in which nonmotile stereocilia are embedded and a cuticular-free region with a kinocilium. The stereocilia project into an otolithic membrane, which contains crystals of calcium carbonate. The hair cells are supported by columnar supporting cells.

Semicircular Canal. Development of the semicircular ducts begins at the sixth fetal week; the first to develop is the superior, the second the posterior, and the third the lateral canal. At the seventh fetal week, the crista ampullaris with its neuroepithelial cells is formed in each semicircular canal. The neuroepithelial cells and the supporting cells of the cristae are completely formed by the 11th fetal week. By the 19th fetal week, the superior semicircular canal has reached maximum growth, followed soon by the posterior semicircular canal. The lateral semicircular canal reaches its maximum growth by the 22nd fetal week.

The membranous labyrinth of the fully formed semicircular canal is tubular. At one end of each canal is the ampulla; the other end is nonampullated. These ducts all open into the utricle, but there are only five openings as the two nonampullated ends of the superior and posterior canals are joined as the crus commune. All three ampullated ends open directly into the utricle.

At the ampulla of each canal is an expanded area, called the crista ampullaris, that contains a transverse ridge of sensorineural epithelium and supporting structures. Microscopically, the cristae are very similar to the maculae of the utricle and saccule. Type I and Type II hair cells are found. The outer surface of each hair cell has a cuticular area which contains 50 stereocilia. The surface of each hair cell also has cuticular-free region and a kinocilium. The cilia of these cells insert into a gelatinous cupula.

Cochlear Duct. At the sixth fetal week, the cochlear duct forms from the tubular outpouching of the ventral portion of the auditory vesicle. At the seventh fetal week, one turn of the cochlear duct is formed. By the eighth fetal week, the entire two and a half turns have been formed.

The organ of Corti starts to differentiate at the eighth fetal week, initially forming two ridges of high columnar cells. The inner ridge becomes the spiral limbus. The outer ridge differentiates into the organ of Corti; by the 22nd fetal week, it has differentiated into inner and outer hair cells, pillar cells and Hensen's cells. The supporting cells develop in relation to the hair cells.

At the eighth fetal week, the stria vascularis starts to develop and is well developed by the 20th fetal week.

The cochlear duct contains the sensory receptors of hearing. It follows the bony cochlea through its two and a half turns. The duct extends from the cochlear recess of the vestibule to end in a blind pouch, the cupular cecum, at the apex of the cochlea. At its basal end, a small ductus reuniens communicates with the saccule (Pearson and Jacobson, 1970).

In a transverse section, the fully formed cochlear duct is triangular. The floor is the basilar membrane, which inserts laterally along the spiral ligament. Overlying the spiral ligament and forming the lateral wall of the cochlear duct is the stria vascularis. At the upper limit of the stria, a thin bicellular vestibular membrane called Reissner's membrane extends from the spiral ligament to the limbus overlying the osseous spiral lamina (Duvall and Rhodes, 1967). The basilar and Reissner's membranes divide the cochlear labyrinth into three canals. The enclosed central canal is the endolymph-filled cochlear duct or scala media (Johnson, 1971). Adjacent to Reissner's membrane is the scala vestibuli, and adjacent to the basilar membrane is the scala tympani. Both scalae vestibuli and tympani are perilymph-filled, and their fluid is in communication through the helicotrema.

Organ of Corti.   The organ of Corti contains the hearing sensory receptors and their supporting structures and is located on the basilar membrane of the cochlear duct. The tunnel of Corti is formed by the two pillar cells between the outer and inner hair cells. There is a single row of inner hair cells just medial to the tunnel of Corti and three rows of outer hair cells lateral to the tunnel. Near the apex, a fourth and even fifth row of outer hair cells can usually be seen. The basilar membrane is divided into two parts: the zona arcuata, from the osseous spiral lamina to the outer pillars; and the zona pectinata, from the lateral pillars to the spiral ligament.

The inner hair cells are more flask-shaped, while the outer hair cells are more tubular in shape. The upper surface of each hair cell is formed by a cuticular plate; in this plate are embedded stereocilia. On the outer hair cell, the stereocilia are arranged in three rows, forming a "W" pattern. Two rows of 50 stereocilia are found on the inner hair cells. Each inner hair cell rests in a cuplike phalangeal cell. The outer hair cells rest similarly on supporting Deiter's cells. The cells of Hensen are located beyond the most laterally placed phalangeal process, and they extend from the lateral border of the organ of Corti to the cells of Claudius (Fig. 6–12).

Beneath each hair cell are two types of nerve endings. The primary endings are terminal endings of the afferent eighth cranial nerve. They extend as unmyelinated fibers through the tunnel of Corti and enter the osseous spiral lamina via the habenula perforata. At this point, these nerve fibers acquire a myelin sheath and proceed through Rosenthal's canal to the modiolus to join the main body of the afferent eighth cranial nerve. The second type is the efferent nerve endings that connect with each hair cell and which originate from the olivocochlear bundle in the brain stem (Bredberg et al., 1965).

Bony Labyrinth

Formation

The formation of the otic capsule and of the enclosed perilymphatic spaces occurs in three stages. The first is the condensation of the mesenchymal tissue around the membranous labyrinth and its subsequent conversion into a cartilaginous capsule. The second is the hollowing out of the perilymphatic spaces in the inner ear. The third stage is the ossification of the cartilaginous capsule to form a bony capsule.

Formation of Cartilaginous Periotic Capsule and Ossification.   Condensation of the mesenchyme starts around the auditory vesicle during the fourth fetal week. Precartilage differentiation develops at the sixth fetal week. This is soon followed by precartilage differentiation to the first true cartilage in the seventh fetal week. However, precartilage is retained in areas immediately adjacent to the membranous labyrinth. The perichondrium of the otic capsule appears in the 12th fetal week.

Ossification of the otic capsule starts in the 15th fetal week and proceeds from 14 centers of ossification. At the 23rd fetal week, all centers have fused to form a complete bony capsule. In the adult, the bony labyrinth consists of three layers: the outer periosteal bone, the middle layer of endochondral bone and the inner periosteal bone. While the periosteal bones ossify with a bony union if fractured, the endochondral bones heal with a fibrous union, so late-onset meningitis can occur after temporal bone fractures (Bast, 1930).

Development of Perilymphatic Spaces. The development of the vestibule starts at the eighth fetal week. The development of the

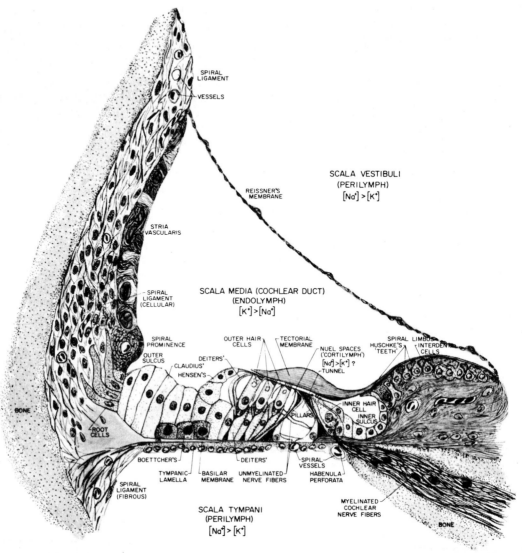

Figure 6–12   Diagram of transverse midmodiolar view of cochlear duct. (From Hawkins, J. E. 1966. Hearing: anatomy and acoustics. *In* Best, C. H., and Taylor, W. B. (Eds.): Physiological Basis of Medical Practice, 8th ed. Baltimore, Williams & Wilkins Co., Chapter 17.)

scalae vestibuli and tympani soon follows at the eighth to ninth fetal week. The first area starts under the round window as the beginning of the scala tympani. The scala vestibuli starts slightly later near the oval window as an outpouching of the vestibule. The development of the scalae is closely associated with the development of the cochlear duct and the scalae attain the adult size by the 16th fetal week. The development of the perilymph spaces around the semicircular canals starts later than the development of the vestibule (Fig. 6–13).

There are four outpouchings of the perilymphatic spaces: an unnamed one along the endolymphatic duct (proximal or utricular extremity of the duct); the perilymphatic or periotic duct; the fissula ante fenetram; and the fossula post fenestram. The unnamed perilymphatic space is short, so that only part of the endolymphatic duct is closed by perilymphatic space. The periotic duct development parallels the development of the scalae tympani and vestibuli and forms a gap in the developing cartilaginous periotic capsule in the region between the cochlear duct and the subarachnoid space. It usually runs parallel to the internal auditory canal and is 12 to 13 mm in length (Rask-Anderson et al., 1977). The fissula ante fenestram is an irregular projection of perilymphatic connective tissue through a slitlike space in the lateral wall of the otic capsule just anterior to the oval window. This starts at the ninth fetal week. The fossula post fenestram is a similar evagination of vestibular periotic tissue into the lateral wall of the otic capsule, posterior to the oval window.

Structures

The bony labyrinth encloses the membranous labyrinth and consists of the vestibule, the three semicircular canals, and the cochlea.

Vestibule. The vestibule is an oval cavity with the following boundaries: medially, the fundus of the internal auditory canal; laterally, the oval window; anteriorly, the communication with the cochlear; and posteriorly, the communication with the semicircular canals. The vestibular aqueduct extends from the posteroinferior surface of the vestibule to the posterior fossa via a narrow canal. This contains the endolymphatic duct and sac. The vestibule contains the utricle and saccule.

Semicircular Canal. Located above and posterior to the vestibule are the three semicircular canals. Each canal approximates a circle. They terminate as enlarged osseous ampullae. The superior canal arches laterally in a vertical plane (transverse to the axis of the petrous temporal bone) and produces the arcuate eminence on the middle fossa surface. Its lateral end is ampullated. The medial, nonampullated end joins the nonampullated end of the posterior canal to form the crus commune. The posterior semicircular canal lies vertically and arches parallel to the long axis of the petrous temporal bone. Its lower end is ampullated and has a separate opening into the vestibule. Its upper end forms the crus commune with the superior semicircular canal. The lateral canal arches laterally in an approximately horizontal plane. This canal has an ampullated lateral end; both ends have separate openings into the vestibule.

Cochlea. The cochlea looks like a snail shell placed on its side. Its base is at the fundus

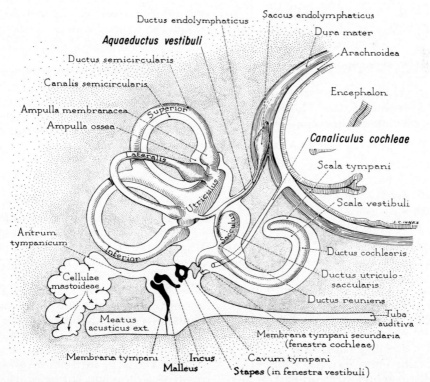

Figure 6–13 Vestibular and cochlear aqueduct in relation to the labyrinthine systems for endolymph and perilymph: dark grey, perilymph; light grey, endolymph. (From Anson, B., Warpeha, R., and Rensink, M. 1968. Ann Otol Rhinol Laryngol, 77:583–607, 1968.)

of the internal auditory meatus, and its apex is directed anterolaterally. It is a tapering canal, coiled approximately two and a half turns around the modiolus (a horizontal central core). Projecting sideways from the modiolus, the osseous spiral laminae subdivide the cochlear canal into the scala vestibuli above, and scala tympani below. The scalae communicate with each other near the apex of the modiolus by an aperture called the helicotrema. The helicotrema is bound by a bony process called the hamulus of the spiral lamina. Both the modiolus and the osseous spiral lamina contain numerous canals for nerve fiber passage. The cochlear aqueduct extends from the basal turn of the cochlea through the petrous temporal bone to open at the anterior margin of the jugular foramen in the posterior fossa.

Other Otic Capsule Structures

The walls of the internal auditory canal form around the eighth cranial nerve and the accompanying internal and auditory artery and vein. The canal is initially a cartilaginous channel and later becomes a bony channel.

The subarcuate fossa is the channel for smaller blood vessels (offshoots of the internal auditory artery and vein) to go into the temporal bone. It is formed in the fetus by erosive vascular buds. The capacity of the fossa is reduced after the fifth fetal month and is small in the adult. It is a small opening into the bone of the posterior fossa, situated above and behind the opening of the internal auditory canal. The arteries that enter the fossa are sometimes large enough to be a factor in surgery involving the cerebellopontine angle (Mazzoni, 1970).

The vestibular aqueduct forms around the endolymphatic duct and sac. It is initially cartilaginous and later becomes osseous.

Acoustic (Eighth Cranial Nerve) Ganglion

In the third fetal week, the acousticofacial ganglion is formed in the region lateral to the rhombencephalon, in close proximity to the auditory vesicle. The ganglion divides into a dorsal part, which becomes the geniculate ganglion of the seventh cranial nerve, and a ventral part, which becomes the statoacoustic ganglion of the eighth cranial nerve. (For a discussion of the embryology of the seventh cranial nerve ganglion, see the part of this chapter which discusses the facial nerve.)

The acoustic nerve ganglion further divides into a superior and an inferior portion. The superior portion (pars superior) becomes the superior division of the vestibular nerve and supplies the macula of the utricle and cristae of the lateral and superior semicircular canals. The inferior portion (pars inferior) divides into an upper portion, which forms the inferior division of the vestibular nerve and supplies the macula of the saccule and the crista of the posterior semicircular canal, and a lower portion which becomes the spiral ganglion of the cochlear nerve and supplies the hair cells of the organ of Corti.

The nerve cells in the ganglion of the cochlear and vestibular nerves remain bipolar throughout life. The central processes terminate in the brain stem and their peripheral processes in the sensory areas of the developing labyrinth.

The efferent fibers of the cochlear nerve are thought to arise in the brain stem and to end in the inner ear. They are thought to be parasympathetic neurons which serve a vasomotor function and suppress the normal responses.

The fully developed cochlear nerve supplies the cochlea with both afferent and efferent fibers. The vestibular division of the eighth cranial nerve is divided into superior and inferior vestibular nerves. The superior vestibular nerve supplies the superior and horizontal semicircular canals and the utricle. The inferior vestibular nerves goes to the saccule and posterior semicircular canal.

Arterial Supply. Labyrinthine blood supply is established early in conjunction with the development of the labyrinth. In the fourth month of fetal life, internal auditory blood vessels can be traced into the internal acoustic meatus and their branches followed, as they course through the area of the developing modiolus to the osseous spiral lamina. Blood vessels are well developed in the cochlea at the onset of ossification (15th fetal week).

The arterial supply of the inner ear comes from the internal auditory artery (a branch of the anterior inferior cerebellar artery). The internal auditory artery divides into two branches, the common cochlear and the anterior vestibular arteries. The anterior vestibular artery supplies the superior portion of the utricle and saccule and the superior and horizontal semicircular canals. The common cochlear artery further divides into two branches: the main cochlear artery and the cochlear-vestibular artery. The main cochlear artery supplies all of the cochlea except the last third of the basal turn. The cochlear-vestibular artery supplies this one-third of the cochlear basal turn via its cochlear ramus and the inferior portion of the utricle and saccule and the posterior semicircular canal via its posterior vestibular branch (Mazzoni and Hansen, 1970).

The blood supply to the organ of Corti and other structures of the cochlear duct is provided by vessels within the stria vascularis and by the spiral vessels underlying the basilar membrane. The arterial supply enters the cochlea through the modiolus along with the eighth cranial nerve fibers. The arterioles divide at the osseous spiral lamina, with one group proceeding under the basilar membrane. The second group travels within the periosteal lining, across the wall of the scala vestibuli, to the spiral ligament and stria vascularis (Johnson, 1972; Lawrence, 1971).

SELECTED REFERENCES

Anson, B. J., and Donaldson, J. 1973. Surgical Anatomy of the Temporal Bone and Ear, 2nd ed. Philadelphia, W. B. Saunders Co.

This is the classic textbook and reference source for the embryology and anatomy of the ear and temporal bone. The illustrations are superb. Each otolaryngologist should have a copy for his personal use.

Pearson, A., and Jacobson, A. 1970. Development of the Ear. Amer. Acad. Ophthal. and Otol., Section on Instructions—Home Study Courses, Univ. of Oregon Medical School Printing Department.

The embryology of the ear is a difficult topic to learn. This is a comprehensive yet simple manual on a complex topic. The question and answer section at the end of each unit helps to develop and retain knowledge.

REFERENCES

Arenberg, I., Rask-Anderson, H., Wilbrand, H., et al. 1977. Surgical anatomy of the endolymphatic sac. Arch. Otolaryngol., *103*:1–11.

Anson, B. J. 1973. Developmental anatomy of the ear. *In* Paparella, M. M., and Shumrick, D. A. (Eds.): Otolaryngology, Vol. I. Philadelphia, W. B. Saunders Co., pp. 3–74.

Anson, B. J., and Donaldson, J. 1973. Surgical Anatomy of the Temporal Bone and Ear, 2nd ed. Philadelphia, W. B. Saunders Co.

Anson, B. J., Harper, D., and Warpeha, R. 1963. Surgical anatomy of facial canal and facial nerve. Ann. Otol. Rhinol. Laryngol., *72*:713–734.

Anson, B., Warpeha, R., and Rensink, M. 1968. Ann. Otol. Rhinol. Laryngol., *77*:583–607.

Balkany, T., Berman, S., Simmons, M. E., et al. 1978. Middle ear effusions in neonate. Laryngoscope, *88*:398–405.

Bast, T. H. 1930. Ossification of Capsule in Human Fetus. Carnegie Contribution to Embryology, *21*:53–82.

Baxter, A. 1971. Dehiscence of the fallopian canal. J. Laryngol. Otol., *85*:587–594.

Bolz, E., and Lim, D. 1972. Morphology of stapedovestibular joint. Acta, Otolaryngol., *73*:10–17.

Bredberg, C., Engstrom, H., and Ades, H. 1965. Cellular pattern and nerve supply of human organ of Corti. Arch. Otolaryngol., *82*:462–469.

Donaldson, J., and Miller, J. 1973 Anatomy of ear. *In* Paparella, M. M., and Shumrick, D. A. (Eds.): Otolaryngology, Vol. 1, Philadelphia, W. B. Saunders Co., pp. 75–110.

Donaldson, J. A., and Anson, B. J., 1974. Surgical anatomy of the facial nerve. Otolaryngol. Clin. North Am., *7*(2):289–308.

Duvall, A., and Rhodes, V. 1967 Reissner's membrane. Arch. Otolaryngol., *86*:143–151.

Flisberg, K., and Zsigmoind, W. 1965. Size of mastoid air cells. Acta Otolaryngol., *60*:23–29.

Gacek, R. 1975. Diagnosis and management of primary tumor of the petrous apex. Ann. Otol. Rhinol. Laryngol., *84*:Suppl. 18.

Gasser, R. 1967. Development of facial nerve in man. Ann. Otol. Rhinol. Laryngol., *76*:37–56.

Geurkink, N. 1977. Surgical anatomy of temporal bone posterior to internal auditory canal — an operative approach. Laryngoscope, *87*:975–986.

Hawkins, J. E. 1966. Hearing: Anatomy and acoustics. *In* Best, C. H., and Taylor, W. B. (Eds.): Physiological Basis of Medical Practice, 8th ed. Baltimore, Williams & Wilkins Co., Chap. 17.

Holborow, C. 1970. Eustachian tube function. Arch. Otolaryngol., *92*:624–626.

Johnson, L. 1971. Reissner's membrane in human cochleas. Ann. Otol. Rhinol. Laryngol., *80*:425–439.

Johnson, L. 1972. Cochlear blood vessel pattern in human fetus and post-natal vascular involution. Ann. Otol. Rhinol. Laryngol., *81*:22–40.

Lawrence, M. 1971. Blood flow through basilar membrane capillaries. Acta Otolaryngol., *71*:106–114.

Lim, D. 1974. Functional morphology of the lining membrane of the middle ear and eustachian tube. Ann. Otol. Rhinol. Laryngol., *83*:Suppl. 11:5–26.

Mazzoni, A. 1970. Subarcuate artery in man. Laryngoscope, *80*:69–79.

Mazzoni, A., and Hansen, C. 1970. Surgical anatomy of arteries of internal auditory canal. Arch. Otolaryngol., *91*:128–135.

Palva, I., and Palva, A. 1966. Size of human mastoid air cells system. Acta Otolaryngol. *62*:237–251.

Parisier, S. 1977. Middle cranial fossa approach to internal auditory canal — an anatomical study stressing critical distances between surgical landmarks. Laryngoscope, *87*:Suppl. 4.

Pearson, A., and Jacobson, A. 1970. Development of the Ear. Amer. Acad. Ophthal. and Otol., Section on Instructions—Home Study Courses, University of Oregon Medical School. Printing Department.

Proctor, B. 1964. Development of middle ear spaces and their surgical significance. J. Laryngol. Otol., *78*:631–648.

Rask-Anderson, H., Stahle, J., Wilbrand, H. 1977. Human cochlear aqueduct and its accessory canals. Ann. Otol. Rhinol. Laryngol., *86*:Supp, 42.

Rood, S. R., and Doyle, W. J. 1978. Morphology of tensor veli palatini, tensor tympani, and dilatator tubae muscles. Ann. Otol. Rhinol. Laryngol., *87*:202–209.

Shambaugh, G. 1967. Surgery of the Ear, 2nd ed. Philadelphia, W. B. Saunders Co.

Wigard, M., and Trilbich, K. 1973. Surgical anatomy of sinus epitympani. Ann. Otol. Rhinol. Laryngol., *82*:378–383.

Chapter 7

PHYSIOLOGY OF THE EAR

Aage R. Møller, Ph. D.

INTRODUCTION

When considering the function of the ear, it is appropriate to divide the auditory system into (1) the sound conducting apparatus, (2) the auditory part of the inner ear, and (3) the auditory nervous system.

The sound conducting apparatus comprises *the outer ear, the ear canal, and the middle ear,* the last being the most interesting from a clinical point of view. The auditory part of the inner ear includes the cochlea. The *sensory cells* (hair cells) that are located along the *basilar membrane* in the organ of Corti transform the mechanical vibration of the basilar membrane into neural activity. The auditory nervous system consists of the *ascending auditory pathway,* including a number of *brain nuclei,* and the *primary auditory cortex.* There is also a *descending auditory pathway* that conveys information from higher to lower levels of the auditory nervous system.

GENERAL FUNCTION OF THE EAR

Sound that is transmitted through the ear canal sets the tympanic membrane into vibration. These vibrations are transmitted to the cochlea via the three ossicles: malleus, incus, and stapes. The stapes perform piston-like movements whereby the fluid in the cochlea is set into vibration. These vibrations, in turn, set the basilar membrane, a partition separating the cochlea into two canals, into wave-like motion. By means of the hair cells located along it, the basilar membrane, in motion, controls the discharge pattern in the nerve fibers of the auditory portion of the eighth cranial nerve (auditory nerve). The informa-

tion carried by the auditory nerve is transformed extensively by the nuclei of the ascending auditory pathway before it reaches the primary auditory cortex, located in the temporal lobe.

Before we go into a detailed description of the function of the individual parts of the ear, such basic psychoacoustic features as range of hearing, perception of loudness, and ability to discriminate frequency and intensity will be considered briefly. For a more detailed description of sound perception, the reader is referred to textbooks such as Stevens (1951) Stevens and Davis (1938), and Tobias (1970).

PSYCHOACOUSTICS

The Sensitivity of the Ear

The threshold of hearing is shown in Figure 7–1, where the minimum audible pressure (MAP) is given as a function of frequency for pure tones applied to one ear through an earphone. The curve shows median values of a number of normal-hearing subjects.*

It is seen that the threshold has its lowest value between 0.5 and 5 kHz. Above 10 kHz it increases rapidly, whereas toward lower frequencies it increases gradually. The high frequency limit for hearing of 20 kHz usually given in young people with normal ears may thus be regarded as well defined, whereas the low frequency limit, usually given at 16 or 10 Hz, should be regarded as

---

*The sound pressure is expressed in dB relative to 20 μPa, the commonly used reference level. Decibel is a logarithmic measure of the physical sound pressure.

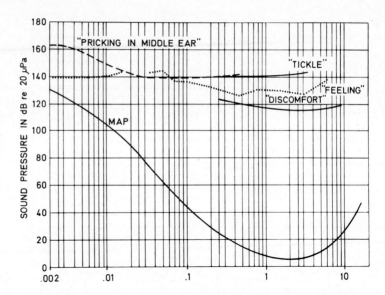

Figure 7–1 Threshold of monaural hearing (MAP = minimum audible pressure) as a function of frequency together with the sound level at which sound gives rise to sensations other than hearing. (Modified from Licklider, J. C. R. 1951. Basic correlates of the auditory stimulus. *In* Stevens, S. S. (ed.). Handbook of Experimental Psychology. New York, John Wiley and Sons.)

rather arbitrary. Figure 7–1 also illustrates the intensity above which a sound gives rise to sensations other than hearing and even to pain. These intensity values are usually regarded as the upper limit of hearing.

In a free sound field in which sound reaches both ears, the threshold is lower than the threshold for monaural listening shown in Figure 7–1. Figure 7–2 compares the monaural thresholds (1) with the free field thresholds (MAF = Minimum Auditory Field). It shows the threshold for sound coming from a source directly in front of the head (0° azimuth) (2) and for sound coming from all directions (random incidence) (3). The difference in threshold for the three listening situations illustrated in Figure 7–2 can be

explained to some extent by the diffractive effect of the head and the resonance of the ear canal (p. 116).

Loudness

Our subjective sensation of loudness does not follow the increase in the physical sound intensity. Moreover, it increases at a different rate for different frequencies. Figure 7–3 shows *equal loudness curves,* that is, curves that give the sound pressure of a sound that is subjectively equally as loud as a 1000 Hz tone 10 to 20 to 30 . . . dB above threshold. These curves are sometimes referred to as phon curves.

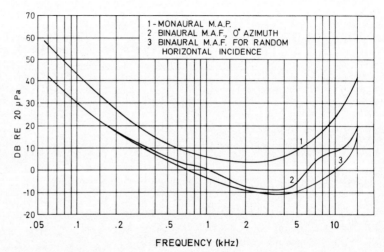

Figure 7–2 Threshold of hearing in a free sound field (MAF = minimum audible field) for sounds coming from a source directly in front of the head (0° azimuth) (2), and MAF from random incidence (3). The monaural hearing threshold (MAP) is seen for comparison (1). (Modified from Sivian, L. J., and White, S. D. 1933. On minimum audible sound fields. J. Acoust. Soc. Am. 4:288–321.)

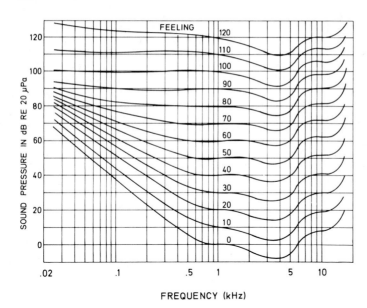

Figure 7–3 Equal loudness curves (phon curves). (From Fletcher, H., and Munson, W. A. 1933. Loudness, its definition, measurement and calculation. J. Acoust Soc. Am., 5:82–108.)

The sensation of loudness also depends on the duration of the tone when the tone is shorter than about 100 msec. This means that the auditory system integrates energy over a time span of about 100 msec. Figure 7–4 shows how much the intensity of a tone (frequency Hz) must be increased in order for this tone to sound equally as loud as a tone of a duration longer than 500 msec. It is seen that a 10 msec tone must have a sound pressure that is about 10 dB higher than a 500 msec tone to sound equally as loud as the 500 msec tone. The curve in Figure 7–4 is representative of sound intensities between 40 dB and 80 dB. At threshold the integration time is larger (about 200 msec). Thus, tones that are shorter than 200 msec have a higher threshold than tones that are longer.

In the frequency range around 1000 Hz, the subjective perception of loudness of a pure tone increases as an exponential function with a mean exponent of 0.6. There is a great individual spread. As an approximation it can be said that a tone sounds twice as loud every time the sound pressure is increased with 10 dB.

Pitch

Just as is the case for the perception of loudness, the subjective perception of pitch of a tone does not follow the physical frequency of the tone, as seen in Figure 7–5.

Complex Sounds

The previously depicted experimental results were obtained using simple sounds such

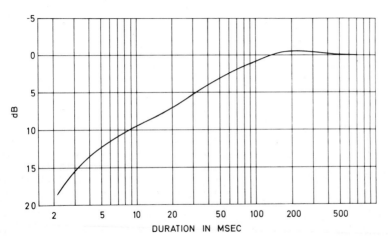

Figure 7–4 Loudness level of a tone as a function of its duration. The amount (in dB) that a sound must be increased in order for the tone to sound equally loud as tone of a duration longer than 500 msec.

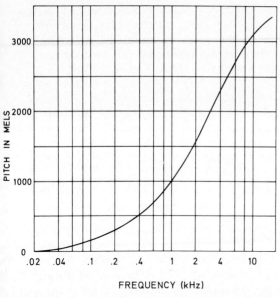

Figure 7–5 Perception of pitch (in mel, measure of subjective perception of pitch) as a function of the physical frequency of a tone. (From Stevens, S. S., and Volkman, J. 1940. The relation of pitch to frequency. Am. J. Psychol., 53:329–353.)

as pure tones. The discrepancy between physical measures and perception is even more apparent when it comes to such complex sounds as speech that contain energy over a large frequency range and that have spectrum and intensity varying rapidly in time. A simple physical measurement of a sound's intensity or frequency thus does not provide direct information about how it is perceived.

Sensitivity to Changes

The ear has a great ability to perceive small changes in frequency and intensity of a sound. Figure 7–6 shows the difference limen for frequency, that is, the smallest change in the frequency of a pure tone that can be detected. Roughly, we can detect that two tones are different if their frequency differs 1 Hz as long as these tones have frequencies of 1000 Hz or less. For tones above 1000 Hz, our frequency discrimination is approximately 0.1 per cent of the frequency.

Discrimination of changes in the intensity of a sound, which varies somewhat depending on intensity, is roughly 1 dB in the physiologic range of intensities.

Directional Hearing

In a free sound field we can determine the direction to a sound source with an accuracy of about 2 degrees when that source is directly in front of us (around 0 degrees azimuth). This ability is best for transient sounds or low-frequency tones. When the source is not located directly in front of the head, we are able to notice a difference in the arrival time of the sound at the two ears. This difference depends on the angle of the head in relation to the sound source and thus on the different distances that the sound will have to travel to reach the respective ears. We can detect very small time differences between arrival of sound in the two ears. When the sounds are continuous pure tones, it can be said that a phase difference is being discriminated. This discriminative ability exists only for frequen-

Figure 7–6 Difference limen (DL) for frequency, i.e., the smallest change in frequency that can be detected by a trained observer. (Modified from Nordmark, J. 1968. Mechanisms of frequency discrimination. J. Acoust. Soc. Am. 44:1533–1540.)

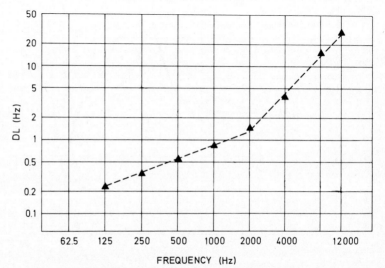

cies below approximately 1500 Hz. Directional hearing of high-frequency sounds is based on the diffraction of the head in a free field (see next section). A sound pressure difference between the two ears then arises that is a function of the head's angle to the sound source.

SOUND CONDUCTION TO THE COCHLEA

Effect of Head and Ear Canal

In a free sound field, the head and the outer ear cause the sound pressure at the entrance of the ear canal to become different, usually higher, than it is at the same location in space when the person is absent. The magnitude of the increase in sound pressure depends on the frequency of the sound, the greatest increase taking place in the frequency range between 2 and 3 kHz as is illustrated in Figure 7–7 (heavy line). As mentioned before, the degree of the sound pressure at the entrance of the ear canal also depends on the direction to the sound source relative to the head. The pinna has a significant influence on the sound pressure at the entrance of the ear canal with respect to sounds of high frequency.

The ear canal acts as a resonator, and consequently the sound pressure near the tympanic membrane is higher in a certain frequency range than it is at the entrance of

the ear canal (Fig. 7–8, thin line). At the resonance frequency (near 4 kHz), this difference reaches a peak of about 10 dB. The total effect of the head and the resonance in the ear canal is seen in Figure 7–8. This graph shows how much larger the sound pressure near the tympanic membrane is compared with the sound pressure at the same place but with the person absent. The curves in Figures 7–9 and 7–10 concern sound coming from a source directly in front of the head (0 degrees azimuth).

Middle Ear

Anatomy

Figure 7–9 shows a schematic drawing of the middle ear. The tympanic membrane is a cone-shaped membrane. The manubrium of the malleus is imbedded in the tympanic membrane from about its central part almost to its periphery. The connection between the malleus and the incus is a relatively stiff joint, whereas the connection between the incus and the stapes is loose for movements perpendicular to the piston-like movements of the stapes. There are two small muscles in the middle ear: the tensor tympani and stapedius muscles. These muscles are innervated by the trigeminal and facial nerves, respectively, and they contract as an acoustic reflex at sound levels well above threshold. In humans only the stapedius muscle seems to respond to sound.

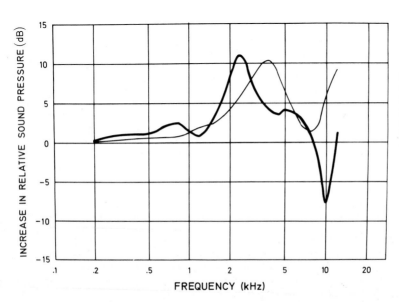

Figure 7–7 The heavy line shows the difference between the sound pressure between that in a free sound field when the observer is not there and the sound pressure at the entrance of the ear canal. The thin line shows the difference between the sound pressure at the entrance of the ear canal and that at the tympanic membrane. (The results concern sounds coming from a source directly in front of the head.) (Data from Shaw, E. A. C. 1974. Transformation of sound pressure level from the free field to the eardrum in the horizontal plane. J. Acoust. Soc. Am. 56:1848–1861.)

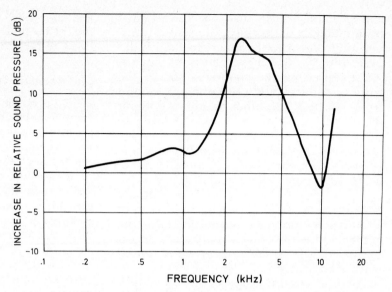

Figure 7–8 Total effect of the outer ear and the resonance of the ear canal. The curve shows the difference between the sound·pressure at the tympanic membrane and that in a free sound field when the observer is not there. (Data from Shaw, E. A. C. 1974. Transformation of sound pressure level from the free field to the eardrum in the horizontal plane. J. Acoust. Soc. Am. 56:1848–1861.)

Function of the Middle Ear

Acoustically, the middle ear acts as a lever that increases the efficiency of transmission of sound to the cochlear fluid. If sound were to be transmitted directly to one of the windows of the fluid-filled cochlea, 99.9 per cent of its energy would be reflected, and consequently only 0.1 per cent would be transmitted further.

The middle ear improves the sound transmission to the oval window of the cochlea by reducing this reflection. The function of the middle ear can also be said to be that of an impedance transformer that changes the high impedance of the cochlear fluid into a low impedance resembling that of air (impedance = resistance, high impedance = low mobility).

The increase in transmission that takes place in the middle ear is mainly a result of hydraulic lever action. This is brought about by the interaction of the tympanic membrane and the stapes footplate, having different areas as they do, and to some extent even by the mechanical lever action of the ossicles. The tympanic membrane and the stapes footplate provide a lever ratio of about 17 in humans, whereas the ossicles have a ratio of only 1.3. If the reflection is totally eliminated

Figure 7–9 Schematic drawing of the middle ear as viewed from inside the head. (From Møller, A. R. 1981. Fundamentals of Auditory Physiology. New York. Academic Press.)

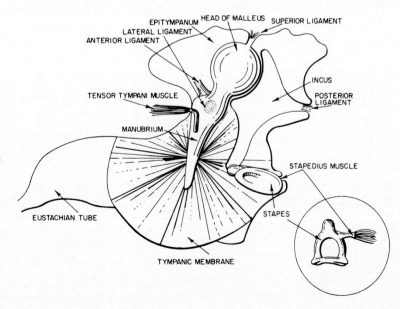

and all sound energy that reaches the ear is transmitted to the cochlea, the sound transmission from air to the inner ear fluid is improved by 30 dB at most. This is in comparison to directing the sound to one of the cochlear windows and preventing any sound from reaching the other window. Without the middle ear, sound would be likely to reach both the round and the oval windows because of the small distance between the windows with the same magnitude and in nearly the same phase. Such a course of events would not be effective in setting the fluid in motion. The efficient improvement of sound transmission to the cochlea by the middle ear is thus much more than 30 dB compared with a situation in which sound reaches both windows.

The transmission properties of the middle ear are frequency-dependent because of the inertia that results from the mass of the ossicles and because of the elasticity of the tympanic membrane and ligaments. Moreover, the efficient acoustic area of the tympanic membrane is somewhat frequency-dependent. The inertia resists the movements of the ossicles at high frequencies, and the stiffness resists movements at low frequencies. Transmission is thus best in the middle frequency range.

The transmission properties of the middle ear have been studied in animal experiments and in human cadaver ears using numerous methods. Figure 7–10 shows how the transmission of sound via the middle ear in a cat differs from transmission of sound applied directly to one of the windows. The lower graph shows how the middle ear improves transmission in the frequency range around 1 kHz, where it is about 30 dB, and somewhat

less above and below. The transmission taking place in the human middle ear is not likely to be very different.

The Acoustic Impedance of the Ear

The acoustic impedance of the ear is the tympanic membrane's "resistance" to being set into motion by sound. Since the tympanic membrane forms a more or less rigid connection with the ossicular chain, the mobility of that chain as well as the mobility of the cochlear fluid as a whole has an effect on the acoustic impedance of the ear. Because the middle ear contains mass, elasticity, and friction, the impedance must be expressed by two values, one for the real component and one for the imaginary. The impedance can also be expressed in terms of an absolute value and a phase angle (Figure 7–11). The absolute value of the impedance is the length of the vector (Z). The inverse of the impedance is called admittance and it is a measure of the system's mobility. The real component represents the friction and the imaginary one represents the inertia and stiffness. In a simple system containing one mass element suspended by a spring and one friction element (Fig. 7–11A), the real component is the resistance exerted by the friction element, whereas the imaginary component is the impedance of the mass and stiffness of the spring (Fig. 7–11B). The impedance of the mass increases proportionally with frequency, whereas that of the stiffness decreases proportionally with frequency. The sum of the impedance of the mass and the stiffness provides a value for the imaginary part of the impedance. Since the impedances of these two elements have opposite signs, the imag-

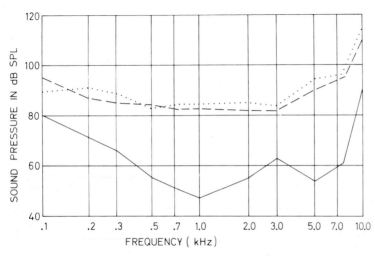

Figure 7–10 Sound pressure required to obtain a certain motion of the cochlear fluid when sound reaches the tympanic membrane and the middle ear is intact (solid line) compared with the case when sound reaches one cochlear window at a time (dashed line = oval window, dotted line = round window, SPL = sound pressure level, dB relative 20 μPa — micropascal). (Based on data from an experiment in a cat by Wever, E. G., and Lawrence, M. 1954. Physiological Acoustics. Princeton, Princeton University Press.)

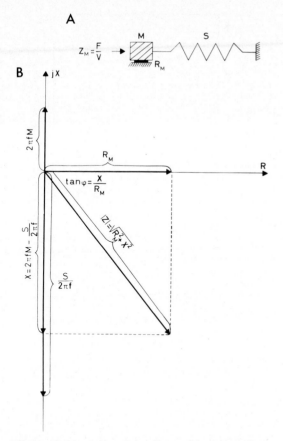

A

$$Z_M = \frac{F}{V}$$

B

Figure 7–11 A, Simple mechanical system with one mass (M), one stiffness (S), and one fricton (R_M). Z_M is the mechanical impedance, F is force, and V is velocity. B, Vector diagram of the impedance of the system illustrated in A. X is the imaginary part of the impedance ($j = \sqrt{-1}$), R_M is the real part, $\pi = 3.14$, f is the frequency, θ is the phase angle, tan is tangent, and $/Z/$ is the absolute value of the impedance. (From Møller, A. R. 1964. The acoustic impedance in experimental studies on the middle ear. Internat. Audiol. 3:123–135.)

inary component of the impedance of a mass and a spring becomes zero at the frequency where the two have the same absolute numerical value. This frequency is synonymous with the resonance frequency.

Measurements of the Ear's Acoustic Impedance. Measurements of the acoustic impedance of the ear can give valuable information concerning the function of the different components of the middle ear. Of particular value in audiologic diagnosis are measurements of changes in the ear's acoustic impedance as a result of changes in the air pressure in the ear canal or as a result of a contraction of the stapedius muscle.

Effect of Changes in Air Pressure. When

the air pressure on the two sides of the tympanic membrane, that is, in the middle ear cavity and in the ear canal, is not equal, the transmission of sound by the middle ear is impaired, more so for low frequencies than for high ones. Measurements of the ear's acoustic impedance in animals reveal that it is mainly the stiffness that is increased but that characteristic changes also occur in the resistive element. As illustrated in Figure 7–12A, the imaginary part of the impedance increases when the air pressure in the middle ear cavity of a cat is increased in relation to the pressure in the ear canal in an almost symmetrical way around zero (symmetrical in the sense of equal pressure on both sides of the tympanic membrane). This indicates that over-pressure and under-pressure in the middle ear cavity increases the stiffness of the middle ear in a similar way. The real component of the impedance (friction) (dashed line, Fig. 7–12A), behaves differently. A negative pressure in the middle ear cavity reduces this component almost to zero. Other experiments have shown that the resistive component of the ear's acoustic impedance originates mainly in the cochlea (Møller, 1965a). Thus, these results seem to indicate that under-pressure in the middle ear cavity (corresponding to an over-pressure in the ear canal) may cause a partial, functional decoupling of the cochlea from the middle ear. That such may be the case is further supported by the finding that an under-pressure in the middle ear cavity results in a larger decrease in transmission than does the same degree of over-pressure. This is illustrated in Figure 7–12B, where the absolute value of the change in impedance is plotted together with the change in transmission. These results are also from an experiment in a cat. If the middle ear did in fact function in the same way as a simple mechanical system consisting of one element of mass and one of elasticity (as that illustrated in Figure 7–11), the change in the admittance could be expected to be equal to the change in transmission. It is seen that such is approximately the case for over-pressure in the middle ear cavity but that for under-pressure the transmission change is larger than the admittance change. This supports the previous hypothesis that an under-pressure causes a decoupling of the cochlea from the middle ear.

Typanometry, which has been found to be

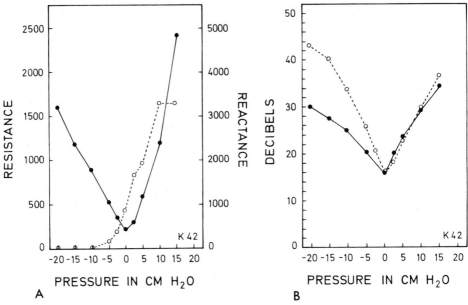

Figure 7–12 *A*, Acoustic impedance (reactance = solid line and resistance = dashed line) of the ear of a cat as a function of the air pressure in the middle ear cavity. *B*, Absolute values of the acoustic admittance at the tympanic membrane (solid lines) and of the change in transmission of sound from the tympanic membrane to the cochlear fluid in the same experiment as illustrated in *A*. (From Møller, A. R. 1965a. An experimental study of the acoustic impedance of the middle ear and its transmission properties. Acta Otolaryngol. *60*:129–149.)

of great value in the clinical diagnosis of various middle ear diseases, measures the change in acoustic impedance as a function of changes in air pressure in the ear canal. In a normal ear, such a recording, called a tympanogram, resembles the solid line in Figure 7–12*B*, but in the middle ear impairments, such as fluid in the middle ear cavity or otosclerosis, the tympanogram assumes a different and often disease-specific shape.

Effect of Contraction of the Middle Ear Muscles. When either of the two muscles, the tensor tympani or the stapedius, contracts, the mobility of the middle ear and consequently the transmission of sound through it are generally reduced.

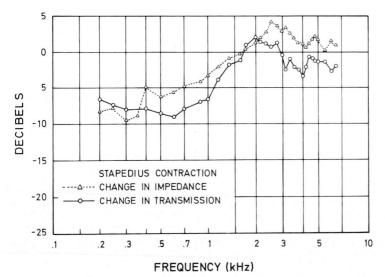

Figure 7–13 Change in the acoustic admittance at the tympanic membrane of a cat (dashed line) and the change in transmission (solid line) as a function of frequency as a result of contraction of the stapedius muscle. (From Møller, A. R. 1965a. An experimental study of the acoustic impedance of the middle ear and its transmission properties. Acta Otolaryngol. *60*:129–149.)

Figure 7–13 compares the change in acoustic admittance and the change in transmission of sound through the middle ear as a result of contraction of the stapedius muscle in a cat. It is seen that these changes are largest at low frequencies, which indicates that the contraction of the stapedius muscle adds stiffness to the middle ear. Since the transmission change is somewhat larger than the change in admittance, the middle ear probably cannot be regarded as functioning exactly like the simple mass-stiffness system earlier described and illustrated in Figure 7–11.

Changes in impedance as well as in transmission are larger when the two middle ear muscles contract together than when only one of them contracts. Although not precisely additive, the effects of the simultaneous contraction of the two muscles on impedance and transmission are synergistic (Møller, 1965b).

Contraction of the two muscles not only changes the acoustic properties of the middle ear but also causes a displacement of the ossicles. A contraction of the tensor tympani muscle causes the tympanic membrane to be displaced inwardly toward the tympanic cavity. This can be measured in terms of the change in the air pressure in the sealed ear canal. A contraction of the stapedius muscle in response to sound causes the stapes to be displaced perpendicular to its piston-like movement, and the displacement of the tympanic membrane as a result of the contraction of this muscle is small. When the two muscles contract simultaneously, the displacement is smaller than it is when the tensor tympani muscle alone contracts (Møller, 1965b). Thus, a contraction of the stapedius muscle counteracts the displacement of the tympanic membrane brought about by the tensor tympani contraction. The stapedius muscle acts antagonistically to the tensor tympani in this respect.

The physiology of the acoustic middle ear reflex will be treated later in this chapter.

INNER EAR

The Cochlea as a Frequency Analyzer

The inner ear consists of the vestibular apparatus (responsible for equilibrium) and the auditory cochlea. In this chapter only the function of the cochlea will be considered.

When the fluid of the inner ear is set into motion by the piston-like movements of the stapes footplate, the basilar membrane is also set into motion, whereby the sensory cells along the membrane are stimulated. In numerous experiments, the basilar membrane has been shown to have frequency selectivity in such a way that a low-frequency tone gives rise to a larger vibration in the apical end of the membrane, whereas higher frequency tones give rise to maximal amplitude near the base of the cochlea. It is thus possible to place a frequency scale with regard to maximal vibration along the basilar membrane, with low frequencies at the apical end and high frequencies at the base. It is assumed that this frequency selectivity is brought about by the particular type of basilar membrane wave motion in which a sound results. This wave motion has the character of a "traveling wave" that travels from the base toward the apex. For a pure tone, the distance it travels is a function of the frequency. A low-frequency tone travels a long distance and then suddenly decreases rapidly in amplitude, whereas a high-frequency tone travels a shorter distance before its amplitude decreases. The higher the frequency is, the shorter is the distance that the wave travels.

This description of the basilar membrane motion is based largely on von Bèkèsy's observations, made around 1940, and on his theoretical treatment of the cochlea's hydrodynamic properties (von Bèkèsy, 1960). He showed in experiments in human cadaver ears that each point along the basilar membrane has a maximal amplitude at a certain frequency and that the amplitude decreases as the frequency is increased or decreased (Fig. 7–14). The technical difficulties in performing measurements of the vibration of the basilar membrane become obvious when it is remembered that they were not repeated until 1967 when Johnstone and Boyle did so in anesthetized guinea pigs using the Mössbauer effect. This method made it possible to measure the vibration amplitude in the physiologic range of intensities. Von Bèkèsy, for whom only a light microscopy method was available, had to use an intensity of about 145 dB, rendering the situation highly unphysiologic. In 1971, Rhode performed an extensive study in the anesthetized squirrel monkey using the Mössbauer effect. Other methods such as the capacitive probe have come into use more recently. Some of the data obtained after 1967 indicate that the basilar membrane is more frequency selective than it seemed to be according to von Bèkèsy's data, whereas other recent data

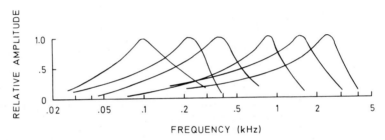

Figure 7-14 Frequency selectivity of the basilar membrane as it appears from the studies by von Békèsy. Each curve represents the relative vibration amplitude at various points along the basilar membrane in a human cadaver ear. (From von Békèsy, G. 1942. Über die Schwingungen der Schneckentrennowand beim Präparat und Ohrenmodel. Akust. Z. 7:173–186.)

show a low degree of frequency selectivity. Another discrepancy is that one investigation found that the basilar membrane vibrates in a nonlinear fashion in such a way that its selectivity decreases with sound intensity (Fig. 7–15). It is puzzling that other investigators have found a totally linear vibration of the basilar membrane. Indeed, the motion pattern of the basilar membrane seems to be more complex than previously believed. So far, it can by no means be considered to be known in detail.

It is assumed that the frequency selectivity of the basilar membrane, demonstrated using pure tones as in the experiments just discussed, also separates a complex sound whose energy covers a large frequency range into relatively narrow bands of frequencies. This occurs in such a way that certain hair cells (or small groups of hair cells) are stimulated mainly with frequencies within a certain frequency range. This frequency selectivity of the basilar membrane has been assumed to form the basis for the ear's ability to discriminate frequency. This series of assumptions is part of the so-called place theory of frequency discrimination.

Finally, it should be emphasized that most studies performed thus far have measured the vibration amplitude of the basilar membrane at one single point. It is, however, the distribution of vibration amplitude along the membrane that is of importance for the perception and discrimination of complex sounds. Only a few studies have been aimed at examining this distribution; therefore, our

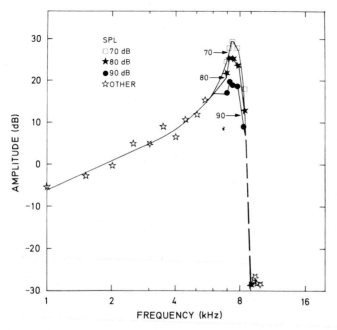

Figure 7-15 Relative vibration amplitude of a point along the basilar membrane of a squirrel monkey measured using the Mössbauer effect at three different sound intensities. The three curves are shifted vertically in such a way that they would coincide if the system was linear. (From Rhode, W. S. 1971. Observations of the vibration of the basilar membrane in squirrel monkeys using the Mössbauer technique. J. Acoust. Soc. Am. 49:1218–1231.)

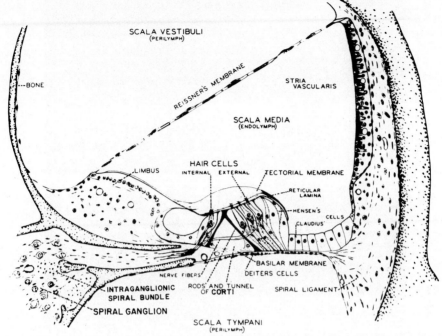

SCALA VESTIBULI
(PERILYMPH)

REISSNER'S MEMBRANE

STRIA
VASCULARIS

---BONE

SCALA MEDIA
(ENDOLYMPH)

HAIR CELLS
INTERNAL EXTERNAL

TECTORIAL MEMBRANE

LIMBUS

RETICULAR
LAMINA

HENSEN'S
CELLS

CLAUDIUS'

BASILAR MEMBRANE
DEITERS CELLS

NERVE FIBERS

INTRAGANGLIONIC
SPIRAL BUNDLE

RODS AND TUNNEL
OF CORTI

SPIRAL LIGAMENT

SPIRAL GANGLION

SCALA TYMPANI
(PERILYMPH)

Figure 7–16   Cross-section of the cochlea. (From Davis, H., et al. 1953. Acoustic Trauma in the Guinea Pig. J. Acoust. Soc. Am., 23:1180.)

knowledge of this matter is limited. It is not possible to estimate the distribution of vibration amplitude along the basilar membrane on the basis of knowledge about the vibration of a single point as a function of frequency.

Sensory Transduction in the Cochlea

The sensory cells in the cochlea are usually known as hair cells and are modified epithelial cells located in the organ of Corti along the basilar membrane. Similar cells may be found earlier in phylogenic development in the lateral line and the vestibular apparatus of the fish. Much of our knowledge about the function of hair cells has been gained in studies of the hair cells in the lateral line of fish because these cells are larger and more easily accessible for experimentation than those of the cochlea. On the basis of such studies, it has been concluded that the hair cells are excited when the hairs are deflected in one direction only. The hair cells in the mammalian cochlea have no kinocilium but they also are generally assumed to be sensitive to deflection of the hairs in one direction only (Flock, 1971).

The hair cells in the mammalian cochlea are organized into one row of inner hair cells,

and three to five rows of outer hair cells. Figure 7–16 shows a cross-section of the cochlea, and Figure 7–17 shows a scanning electron microscopic picture of the basilar membrane in a monkey.

The fibers of the auditory nerve terminate on the hair cells with synapse-like endings. The deflection of the hairs controls the firing in the individual fibers of the auditory part of the eighth nerve through a synaptic (chemical) transmission. The principle for the neural transduction is not known in detail, but it is believed that the all-or-none discharges of the afferent fibers are set up in the first node of Ranvier of a nerve fiber (Flock, 1971).

In addition, there are afferent and efferent endings on the hair cells themselves. These efferent synapses are the terminations of the fibers of the olivocochlear bundle (Rasmussen's bundle) that originate in the superior olive region of the brain stem. Electrical stimulation of the efferent fibers has been shown to decrease the sensitivity of the hair cells, but the normal function of this efferent system is not known. The recent finding that the hairs contain actin opens the possibility that their mechanical properties may be under some

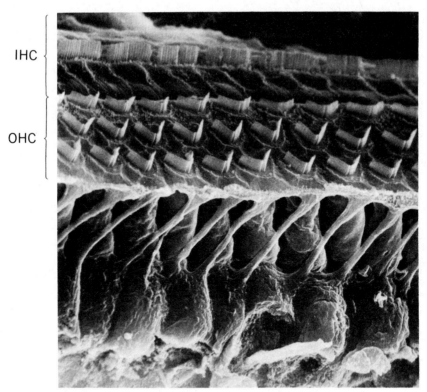

Figure 7-18 Schematic diagram of the innervation pattern of the organ of Corti. OHC = outer hair cells, IHC = inner hair cells, SG = spiral ganglion. Full thick lines: afferent fibers to outer hair cells. cells. (Courtesy of Prof. Hans Engström, Uppsala.)

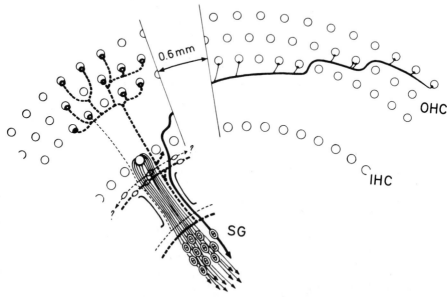

Figure 7-18 Schematic diagram of the innervation pattern of the organ of Corti. OHC = outer hair cells, IHC = inner hair cells, SG = spiral ganglion. Full thick lines: afferent fibers to outer hair cells. Full thin lines: afferent fibers to the inner hair cells. Interrupted thick lines: efferent nerve fibers from the contralateral olivocochlear bundle. Thin interrupted lines: efferent nerve fibers from the homolateral olivocochlear bundle. (From Spoendlin, H. 1970. Structural basis of peripheral frequency analysis. *In* Plomp, R., and Smoorenburg, G. F. (eds.) Frequency Analysis and Periodicity Detection in Hearing. Leiden, A. W. Sijthoff, pp. 2–36.)

form of neural or chemical control (Flock and Cheung, 1977).

The inner hair cells receive about 95 per cent of the afferent nerve fibers, the remaining 5 per cent being distributed to the outer hair cells (Fig. 7–18) (Spoendlin, 1970). The 400 to 600 efferent fibers terminate on those hair cells that have the efferent type of synaptic endings (dashed lines in Fig. 7–18). The functional importance of the separation of hair cells into inner and outer is not known, but recent electrophysiologic work indicates that some interaction may take place between inner and outer hair cells (Zwislocki, 1974).

Cochlear Electrophysiology

A number of electrical potentials can be recorded from the cochlea and its surroundings. These can be divided into those potentials that do not respond to sound stimulation and those that do. To the former belongs the endolymphatic potential, EP, illustrated in Figure 7–19. This potential is positive in the scala media (with 50 to 80 mV) relative to the scala tympani and scala vestibuli, both of which have potentials very close to the potentials of the surrounding tissue. The organ of Corti has a negative potential (about 30 mV) relative to that of the surrounding tissue.

Of all the sound-evoked potentials, the cochlear microphonic potential (CM) is by far the most studied. It is an electrical potential the wave form of which resembles the stimulus sound in the same way as does the electri-

cal output of a microphone. It can be recorded near the round window as well as in the cochlea. It is most likely generated by the hair cells, but its precise relationship and role in the neural transduction in the hair cells is not known. The CM recorded at the round window originates from hair cells at the basal part of the cochlea (probably outer hair cells) (Dallos, 1973). When recorded with differential electrodes in the cochlea, the CM shows a frequency selectivity resembling that of the basilar membrane (Dallos, 1973).

A somewhat less consistent potential is the summating potential (SP). This potential follows the envelope of a sound and may be positive or negative when recorded near the round window. Recorded in the cochlea, its value and polarity depend upon the recording location. It is not known how and where it is generated, but it has been speculated that it has a definite role in neural transduction. Recorded with microelectrodes near the hair cells, it is sharply tuned in a similar way as the basilar membrane. The response changes with frequency in accordance with the tuning of the particular point on the basilar membrane from which the recording is made.

The action potential (AP) is a whole nerve potential. It reflects the synchronous firing of a large number of fibers of the auditory nerve. Therefore, it is most pronounced in response to sharp transient sounds, such as clicks, that give rise to a synchronized firing of many fibers. It can be recorded from the round window, inside the cochlea, or in the internal auditory meatus (Fig. 7–20). Since the action potential reflects the neural excita-

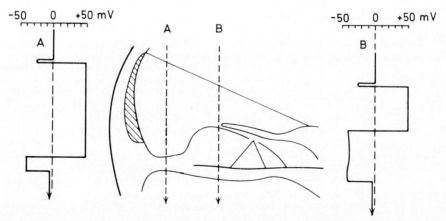

Figure 7–19 Electrical potentials in the cochlea. In the middle, a stylized organ of Corti of the cochlea with two electrode paths (A and B) indicated by dashed lines. The recorded potentials are seen in the graphs on each side. (From von Békésy, G. 1960. Experiments in Hearing. New York, McGraw-Hill.)

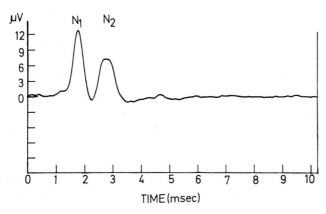

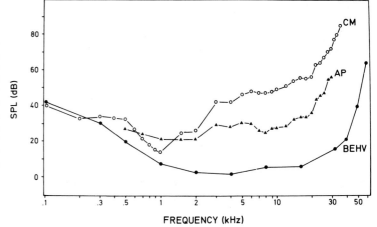

Figure 7–20 Typical action potential (AP) recorded from the round window of a rat in response to a click sound. Negative polarity is seen as upwards deflections. The two negative peaks are usually named N_1 and N_2.

Figure 7–21 Threshold of the action potentials (AP) compared with behavioral threshold (BHV) and the sound pressure necessary to produce a certain amplitude of the cochlear microphonics (CM). (The results are from experiments by Dallos, P., Harris, D., Özdamar, O., et al. 1978. Behavioral compound action potentials and single unit threshold: Relationship in normal and abnormal ears. J. Acoust. Soc. Am. 64:151–157.)

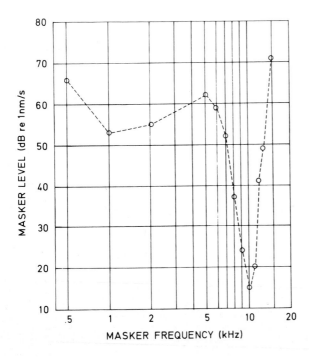

Figure 7–22 Tuning of the masking of the AP. Masker stapes velocity (dB re 1nm/sec), necessary to decrease the amplitude of N_1 by one third, is shown as a function of masker frequency. The probe tone was 10 kHz at 15 dB above AP threshold. (Modified from Dallos, P., and Cheatham, M A. 1976. Compound action potential (AP) tuning curves. J. Acoust. Soc. Am. 59:591–597.)

tion, the AP response to tone bursts or bandpass-filtered clicks is assumed to originate from special areas of the basilar membrane. The threshold of the AP response is almost parallel but not identical to the behavioral threshold curve. Figure 7–21 shows results from animal experiments in which both the behavioral threshold and the AP threshold were determined. Similar relationships have been seen in animals in whom parts of the hair cell population have been damaged by an ototoxic drug (kanamycin) (Dallos et al., 1978). Recording of the AP therefore gives information as to which parts of an impaired cochlea are intact. Such recordings are used clinically under the name electrocochleography (ECoG). The gap between the AP threshold and the behavioral threshold is probably due to the fact that the responses of the eighth nerve (AP) represent an integration of the stimulus over a much shorter period than does the behavioral threshold. The AP is assumed to be established on the basis of the first few msec of the stimulus, whereas the behavioral threshold is based on the summation of acoustic energy over 100 to 200 msec. Figure 7–22 illustrates the frequency tuning obtained by masking the AP in response to a weak tone burst by another tone. The curve shows how intense this masking tone must be in order to reduce the amplitude of the AP to two thirds of its original value.

AUDITORY NERVOUS SYSTEM

Ascending Auditory Pathway

The information about the vibrations of the basilar membrane as sensed by the hair cells is communicated to the auditory cortex via the ascending auditory pathway. On the way to the cortex, the information passes a number of brain nuclei. In these relay stations, incoming nerve fibers terminate on nerve cells, which in turn send axons to the next nucleus. Each nerve cell receives input from many axons, and numerous connections exist between the cells within one nucleus. Within the nuclei, an extensive interplay occurs between inhibition and excitation in such a way that incoming information may be either inhibitory or excitatory. Recurrent inhibition probably takes place in the nuclei. The ascending auditory pathway is more complex than just a string of relay stations on a straight line from the ear to the cortex. A simplified scheme of its organization is seen in Figure 7–23. It should be noted that the number of nerve fibers connecting the brain nuclei increases toward the cortex. The auditory nerve has about 20,000 to 30,000 fibers, and the connection between the medial geniculate and the primary auditory cortex includes about 250,000 fibers. Most fibers are observed to cross the midline at the level of the superior olive, but some fibers continue ipsilaterally to

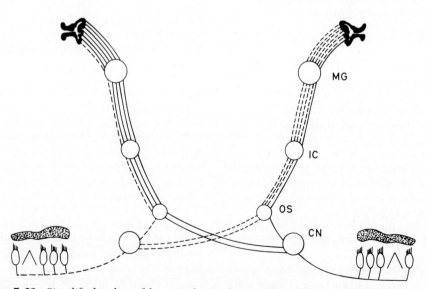

Figure 7–23 Simplified outline of the ascending auditory pathway illustrating the divergence and the partial crossing of fibers. CN = cochlear nucleus, OS = olive superior, IC = inferior colliculus, and MG = medial geniculate. (From Møller, A. R. 1981. Fundamentals of Auditory Physiology. New York, Academic Press.)

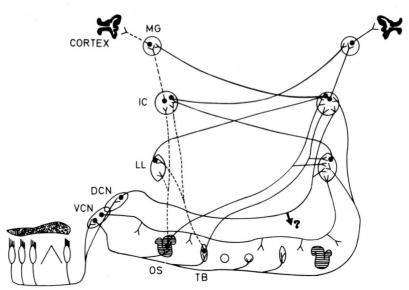

Figure 7–24 More detailed but still greatly simplified scheme of the ascending auditory pathway. VCN = ventral cochlear nucleus, DCN = dorsal cochlear nucleus, OS = olive superior, TB = trapezoid body; LL = lateral lemniscus, IC = inferior colliculus, MG = medial geniculate. (From Møller, A. R. 1981. Fundamentals of Auditory Physiology. New York, Academic Press.)

the inferior colliculus. It is assumed that the connections between the two sides at the level of the superior olive have to do with directional hearing and that the connections between the two sides at the level of the inferior colliculus (Fig. 7–24) also play a role in directional hearing.

Coding of Auditory Information in the Ascending Auditory Pathway

In neurophysiologic studies of the transformation of information in the various brain nuclei, recordings of the discharge pattern from single neurons with microelectrodes have constituted the method used extensively, indeed almost exclusively. The following discussion of the coding process will therefore be based on results from such recordings.

Frequency Tuning. When pure tones are used as stimuli, the most prominent feature of the responses of single fibers of the auditory nerve and of the cells in the various relay stations is frequency selectivity, or tuning. This means that a particular fiber or cell is responsive only within a certain range of frequencies and intensities upon stimulation with a pure tone. This range is called the fiber's response area. The border of this response area, that is, the threshold sound intensity as a function of frequency, is called

the fiber's frequency tuning curve (FTC). The frequency at which the threshold is lowest is called the fiber's characteristic frequency, or CF (Kiang et al., 1965; Evans, 1975).

Fibers of the auditory nerve usually discharge at a low rate; they show spontaneous discharges without any known stimulation. Upon stimulation with a pure tone whose intensity and frequency are within their response area, they will increase their discharge rate. The pattern as a whole is characterized by an irregular discharge rate. Fibers in the auditory nerve have different CFs, which is assumed to be a result of the fact that they terminate on hair cells having different positions along the basilar membrane. It is generally assumed that this frequency tuning of primary auditory fibers is at least partly a result of the mechanical tuning of the basilar membrane. The same is the case for most cells in the ascending auditory pathway, particularly at lower levels such as the cochlear nucleus.

Figure 7–25 shows typical tuning curves from primary auditory nerve fibers and from cochlear nucleus cells. Much attention has been devoted to the finding that the tuning curves of single auditory nerve fibers reveal a greater frequency selectivity than what would be expected from measurements of the displacement of the basilar membrane. In par-

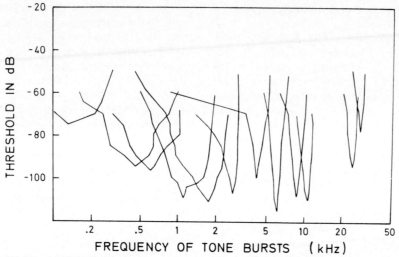

Figure 7–25 Typical frequency tuning curves of primary auditory nerve fibers in a cat. (Modified from Kiang, N. Y. S., Watanabe, T., Tomas, E. C., and Clark, L. F. 1965. Discharge patterns of single fibers in the cat's auditory nerve. Research Monograph No. 35. Cambridge, Mass., MIT Press.)

ticular, the low-frequency skirt of the tuning curves seems to be steeper than that of the basilar membrane's mechanical tuning curve. This discrepancy has given rise to the postulation that some additional frequency filtering must take place, perhaps in association with the neural transduction process (Evans, 1975). No anatomic evidence for such a filter has been put forth so far. Quantitative comparison between mechanical and neural tuning should be made with caution, however. Only if the system (neural transduction and basilar membrane vibration) can be regarded to function as a linear system is such comparison valid. In addition to their excitatory response area, most fibers of the cochlear nerve

have regions where the discharge rate resulting from stimulation with a tone within the response area can be slowed down. This inhibition, or suppression as it is more correctly designated, is seen in a region above the response area and sometimes in a region below the response area as well (Fig. 7–26). The origin of this suppression is not known, but some experimental results indicate that it may be the cochlea itself. Cells in the nuclei of the ascending auditory pathway have areas of suppression similar to those of the primary auditory fibers. There are some doubts as to whether the spontaneous activity of the eighth nerve fibers can be inhibited. In the cells of the cochlear nucleus, both sound-

Figure 7–26 Frequency tuning curve (filled circles) of a primary auditory nerve fiber together with area of inhibition, i.e., frequency and intensity ranges where the impulse frequency of the fiber in response to a tone (CTCF) is slowed down. (From Nomoto, M., Suga, N., and Katsuki, Y. 1964. Discharge pattern and inhibition of primary nerve fibers in the monkey. J. Neurophys., 27:768–787.)

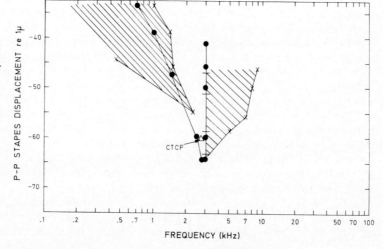

evoked activity and spontaneous activity can usually be inhibited.

Periodicity Coding. The temporal theory of frequency discrimination assumes that the periodicity of a sound is coded in the discharge pattern of single auditory nerve fibers and that this periodicity is decoded into formation about frequency somewhere in the auditory nervous system. According to the temporal theory, the frequency selectivity of the basilar membrane plays only a minor role in frequency discrimination.

The discharge rate of primary nerve fibers is modulated with the frequency of a low-frequency periodic sound such as a low-frequency tone. Complex sounds also seem to be coded in the discharge pattern in such a way that the probability of firing varies according to the estimated motion of the basilar membrane (Rose et al., 1971; Fig. 7–26). This phenomenon may be referred to as time-locking.

Place Hypothesis Versus Temporal Hypothesis in Frequency Discrimination. The characteristics just described of the frequency selectivity of single neurons are assumed to support the place theory of pitch perception. This theory assumes that the frequency (or spectral composition) of a sound is signalled to the higher nervous center in the form of the specific distribution of the discharge rate in the different nerve fibers terminating along the basilar membrane (p. 123). Although data on the function of the basilar membrane are now abundant, the sufficiency of the spectral resolving power of this membrane for explaining the psychoacoustic frequency resolution of the ears is still not certain. For one matter, it has been shown in numerous studies that the discharge rate of single auditory nerve fibers reaches a plateau only 20 to 30 dB above threshold. This finding seems to be an obstacle in explaining frequency discrimination solely on the basis of the place hypothesis.

When von Békésy's results were the only information available, it was generally assumed that some form of neural sharpening of the basilar membrane tuning took place between the membrane and the discharges of the eighth nerve fibers. It was assumed that such a sharpening would be similar to the lateral inhibition seen in connection with vision and touch. To date, it has not been possible to find evidence for such a neural sharpening in the cochlea, but recent studies, as mentioned earlier, indicate that some form

of interaction takes place between inner and outer hair cells and that this interaction may sharpen the frequency selectivity (Zwislocki, 1974). Other hypotheses claim that when the basilar membrane moves in directions other than merely up and down, the hair cells are stimulated and that such motions may represent a greater degree of frequency selectivity (Duifhuis, 1976).

Pursuit of the temporal hypothesis of frequency discrimination has generally been considered fruitless owing to the fact that it has not been possible to find evidence of a neural decoding of temporal information. However, it is perfectly clear from numerous neurophysiologic experiments that the temporal patterns of not only simple periodic sounds but also complex sounds are coded in the discharges of single auditory nerve fibers (cf. Rose et al., 1971). Only in one special case has it been possible to find neurons, that is, those in the ascending auditory pathway (n. cochlearis), that can transform a time code of a sound into a frequency code. Recent studies using noise stimuli and statistical signal analysis of the recorded discharge pattern support the notion that the temporal information is important. The fact that neurophysiologic experiments show that the auditory system can detect very small binaural time differences via directional hearing indicates that the nervous system has elements that are able to decode time information, or the interval between two sounds.

In conclusion, it is not yet known whether the ear's spectral resolving power and frequency discrimination can be explained on the basis of the place theory, on the basis of the temporal theory, or on the basis of some combination of the two that holds true for the type of sound being analyzed.

Transformation of Complex Sounds in the Ascending Auditory Pathway. If we were concerned only with the responses to pure tones, we might assume the transformation of information in the ascending auditory pathway to be relatively simple. We can observe that frequency tuning is a prominent feature of the responses of most cells in the ascending pathway to pure tones at threshold.

When more complex sounds are used and the responses at intensities above threshold are considered, we are faced with a substantially more complex processing of information. Indeed, it appears that the brain nuclei perform an extremely complex processing of information. A histogram of the discharges in

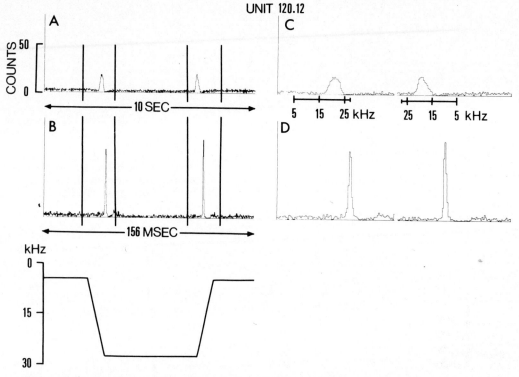

Figure 7–27 Histogram of the responses of a cell in the cochlear nucleus to a tone, the frequency of which was varied up and down according to the scheme seen below. The upper histogram (A and C) represents the responses when the tone was varied slowly (10 sec for a full sweep) while the lower histogram (B and D) represents the responses to a fast variation. The histograms on the right are enlarged parts of the histograms on the left. (From Møller, A. R. 1974. Coding of amplitude and frequency modulated sounds in the cochlear nucleus. Acustica *31*:292–299.)

response to a tone whose frequency is varied over its response area gives a measure of the unit's frequency selectivity. The frequency selectivity as it appears in such histograms greatly depends on the rate of change in the frequency of the tone. Figure 7–27 shows typical histograms for discharges recorded from a single cell in the cochlear nucleus in response to a tone whose frequency was varied at different rates according to the scheme seen in the figure. When the frequency of the tone was varied slowly (upper graph), the histograms of the responses are seen to indicate that the unit responds in a rather broad frequency range. Changing the frequency at a fast rate causes more nerve discharges to be evoked within a narrower range of frequencies. Natural sounds commonly undergo rapid changes in frequency, for which reason the resulting change in response pattern should be regarded as important for the transformation of information from such sounds in the auditory nervous system. Some units in the cochlear nucleus respond to fre-

quency changes in an extremely pronounced manner. Some units do not show any apparent frequency selectivity when stimulated with sounds that are slowly varied in frequency but do develop distinct response areas when stimulated with rapidly varying sounds. Such units thus respond to frequencies within a narrow range.

It is a rather common finding that units in the cochlear nucleus do not respond to broad-frequency bands of noise. As soon as the band width is increased beyond a certain value, the response of most units in fact decreases. This is assumed to be the result of an interaction between the excitatory areas and the inhibitory areas surrounding them. When the center frequency of broad-band noises is changed rapidly, the resulting responses will also be within a narrow range of frequencies (Fig. 7–28).

It is obvious, then, that changes in frequency are enhanced in the responses of single units in the cochlear nucleus. Such behavior cannot be predicted on the basis of the re-

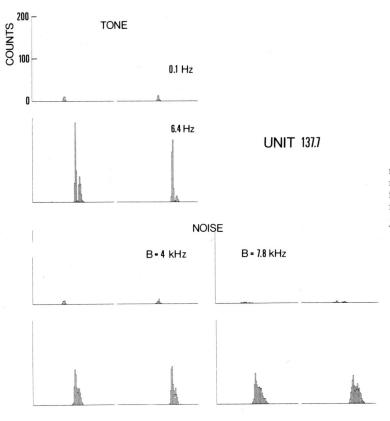

UNIT 137.7

Figure 7–28 Histogram of the responses of a cell in the cochlear nucleus to bands of noise, the center frequency of which is varied at different rates. (From Møller, A. R. 1982. Auditory Physiology. New York, Academic Press.)

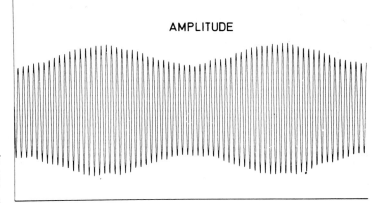

AMPLITUDE

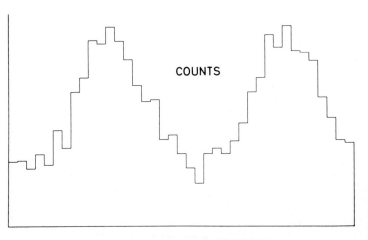

COUNTS

Figure 7–29 Cycle histogram of the responses of a unit in the cochlear nucleus to an amplitude modulated tone. The tone is illustrated above. (From Møller, A. R. 1972a. Coding of amplitude modulated sounds in the cochlear nucleus of the rat. In Møller, A. R. (ed.): Basic Mechanisms in Hearing. New York, Academic Press, pp. 539–619.)

sponses to steady tones or noise. A somewhat different type of enhancement in the responses of cochlear nucleus units is seen when slight changes, or modulations, are made in the amplitude of the stimulus tone. A period histogram of the responses to a sinusoidal, amplitude-modulated tone is seen in Figure 7–29. This histogram, which is synchronized or time-locked to the modulation, shows the probability of discharge during two cycles of an amplitude-modulated tone.

It is seen that a small (about 2 dB) modulation of the tone results in more than a 50 per cent modulation of the histogram. The degree to which small changes in amplitude are reproduced in the discharge pattern depends upon the modulation frequency as illustrated in Figure 7–30. The graph in the middle shows the relative modulation of the histogram as a function of the modulation frequency. The greatest modulation is observed

to occur at a modulation frequency of 200 Hz. This value varies somewhat from cell to cell, but the maximal reproduction is usually found between 50 and 300 Hz. The discharge rate of most neurons in the cochlear nucleus reaches a plateau, or saturates, only 20 to 30 dB above threshold, but these cells almost always respond to small changes in amplitude over a higher range of intensity (60 to 80 dB). This means that even an intensity range in which the average discharge rate has reached a saturation level, small rapid changes in the intensity of the sound bring about substantial changes in the probability of firing.

The findings described in the previous sections greatly emphasize that changes in a stimulus sound activate the neurons in the auditory nervous system in a specific way. At the same time, it must be remembered that the stimuli used have been rather simple, and only limited kinds of changes have been tested. Consequently, it is not possible to

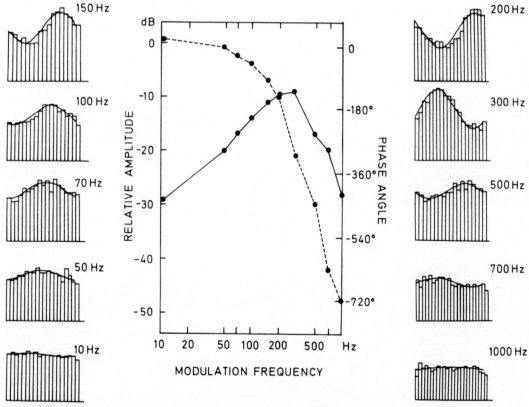

Figure 7–30 Cycle histograms of the responses of a unit in the cochlear nucleus to amplitude modulated tones of different frequencies (given by legend numbers). The middle graph gives the relative modulation of these cycle histograms as a function of modulation frequency. The phase lag between the modulation of the stimulus tone and the modulation of the histograms is also given. (From Møller, A. R. 1972b. Coding of amplitude and frequency modulated sounds in the cochlear nucleus of the rat. Acta Physiol. Scand. 86:223–238.)

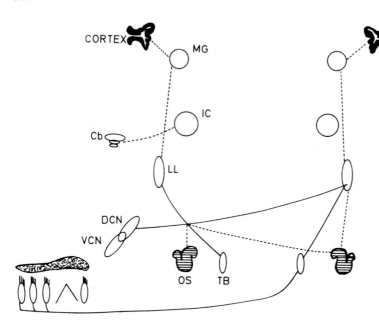

Figure 7–31 Simplified outline of the descending auditory pathway. The dashed lines show poorly verified connections. DCN = dorsal cochlear nucleus, VCN = ventral cochlear nucleus, OS = olive superior, TB = trapezoid body, LL = lateral lemniscus, IC = inferior colliculus, Cb = cerebellum, and MG = medial geniculate. (Modified from Whitfield, I. C. 1967. The Auditory Pathway. London, Edward Arnold, Ltd.)

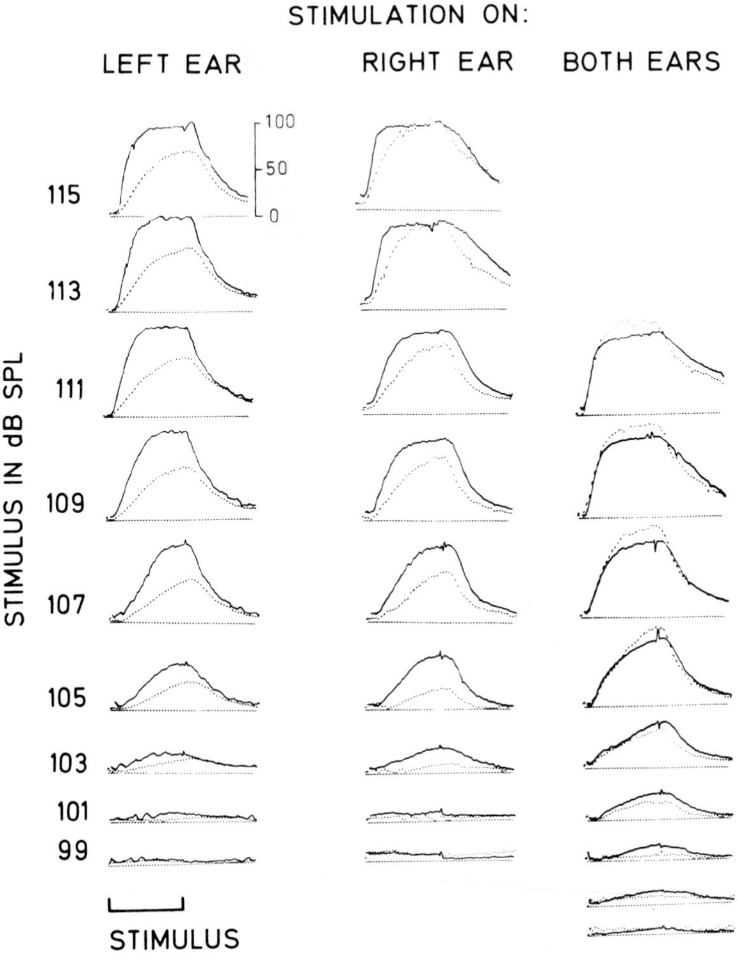

Figure 7–32 Typical responses of the acoustic middle ear reflex in a person with normal hearing recorded in both ears simultaneously. The left and middle columns represent stimulation of only one ear at a time. Solid lines represent the response in the ipsilateral ear and dashed lines are the responses in the contralateral ear. The right column shows responses recorded when both ears were stimulated simultaneously. The stimulus was 500 msec bursts of 1450 Hz tone. (From Møller, A. R. 1962. The acoustic reflex in man. J. Acoust. Soc. Am. *34*:1524–1534, Part II.)

STIMULATION ON:

LEFT EAR　　　　RIGHT EAR　　　BOTH EARS

STIMULUS IN dB SPL

115
113
111
109
107
105
103
101
99

STIMULUS

apply these results directly to such complex sounds as speech sounds.

With regard to the coding of complex sounds at higher levels of the ascending auditory pathway, our knowledge is very limited. There is no reason to assume that it should be less intricate than that seen in the cochlear nucleus.

Descending Pathway

There are extensive connections from higher auditory centers to lower ones, as outlined in Figure 7–31. The anatomy and, even more so, the physiology of these pathways are not known in any detail at all. Only the most peripheral of these pathways has been studied systematically using electrophysiologic methods. This pathway is the olivocochlear bundle, where electric stimulation of the fibers has been shown to decrease the sensitivity of the sound-evoked responses in the eighth nerve. Sectioning of the olivocochlear bundle has been shown to increase the sensitivity of the middle ear reflex in the rabbit. Nevertheless, the functional importance of the olivocochlear bundle is by and large unknown.

THE ACOUSTIC MIDDLE EAR REFLEX

The acoustic middle ear reflex involves only the stapedius muscle in humans, whereas in many animals, the tensor tympani muscle is activated regularly as well. The response of the middle ear reflex can be recorded conveniently in terms of changes in the ear's acoustic impedance (p. 118). The reflex is bilateral, that is, it is evoked in both ears when only one ear is stimulated. The threshold for the contralateral response is about 80 to 85 dB above the threshold of hearing. The ipsilateral reflex has a somewhat lower threshold (2 to 14 dB). When the reflex is elicited in both ears at the same time, the threshold is about 3dB lower than the thresholds for the ipsilateral reflex. Some people can contract their stapedius muscles voluntarily. Figure 7–32 shows typical responses of the middle ear reflex recorded in both ears simultaneously upon stimulation of either the left or the right ear. Also shown are the responses obtained when both ears are stimulated (right column). The response

appears in humans with a latency that decreases from about 150 msec for stimuli near threshold to about 35 msec for high-intensity stimuli. The reflex response has a buildup time that decreases with intensity from approximately 200 to 400 msec (until half the amplitude of the response is reached) at a low stimulus intensity to about 125 msec at a high stimulus intensity. The amplitude of the response grows monotonically with the stimulus intensity over an approximate range of 20 dB, as seen in Figure 7–32. Figure 7–33 illustrates the relative change in the ear's acoustic impedance as a function of the stimulus intensity.

Individual differences in the shape of these stimulus-response curves are rather great. Moreover, different stimulus frequencies give the stimulus-response curves different shapes (Fig. 7–33). The curves showing bilateral responses and those showing ipsilateral responses are in general parallel, whereas those showing contralateral responses have a different course and a generally smaller slope and do not reach such high values of impedance change. The difference between the impedance change of the ipsilateral and contralateral reflex is of clinical importance since it is usually the contralateral response that is studied.

The reflex arc of the stapedius reflex is illustrated schematically in Figure 7–34. The ascending part of the reflex arc is the ascending auditory pathway as far up as the superior olive nucleus. From this nucleus, connections go to the facial motor nucleus, which is the origin of the facial nerve (seventh cranial nerve) that innervates the stapedius muscle. There are also direct connections from the ventral cochlear nucleus to the ipsilateral facial motor neuron. The contralateral reflex is mediated by connections from the ipsilateral superior olive nucleus to the contralateral facial motor neuron.

Under normal circumstances, the reflex increases the dynamic range of the ear by reducing the transmission of sound through the middle ear. Because the reflex is relatively slow, fast changes in sound intensity may be transmitted to the cochlea under its influence. The ear's ability to handle changes in intensity is thereby preserved above the point at which the inner ear usually ceases to function adequately when presented with steady sounds.

Contractions of the stapedius muscle are elicited not solely as an acoustic reflex. Ex-

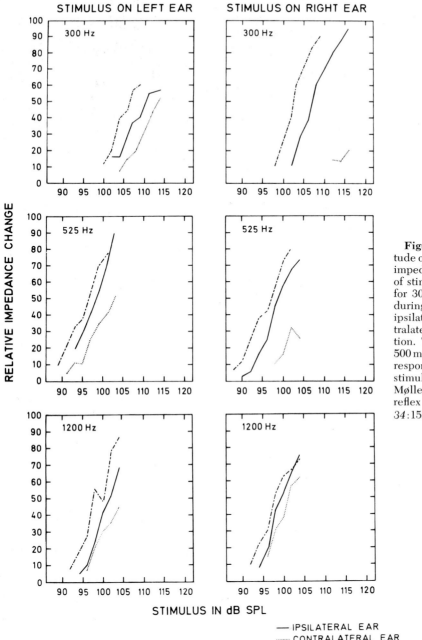

Figure 7–33 Relative amplitude of the changes in the acoustic impedance depicted as a function of stimulus intensity (in dB SPL) for 300, 500, and 1200 Hz tones during bilateral (dashed and dots), ipsilateral (solid lines), and contralateral (dotted lines) stimulation. The stimulus duration was 500 msec, and the amplitude of the responses was measured when the stimulus was terminated. (From Møller, A. R. 1962. The acoustic reflex in man. J. Acoust. Soc. Am. 34:1524–1534.)

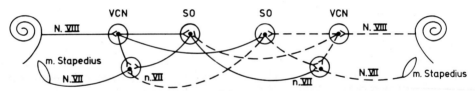

Figure 7–34 Components of the pathway of the acoustic stapedius reflex. VCN = ventral cochlear nucleus, SO = superior olive, n. VII = facial motor neuron, N. VII = facial nerve, N. VIII = auditory nerve. (From Møller, A. R. 1982. Auditory Physiology. New York, Academic Press.)

Figure 7-35 Recordings of the electrical activity (EMG) in the stapedius muscle in connection with vocalization in a patient during ear surgery. (From Borg, E., and Zakrisson, J. E. 1975. The activity of the stapedius muscle in man during vocalization. Acta Otolaryngol. 79: 325-333.)

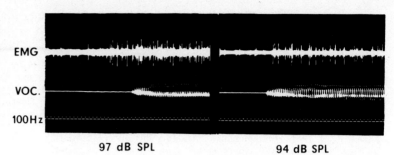

EMG

VOC.

100 Hz

97 dB SPL   94 dB SPL

perimental evidence shows that electrical potentials (EMG) can be recorded from the stapedius muscle in connection with vocalization at sound levels that could not possibly elicit the muscle contraction acoustically. In some cases, EMG potentials even appear immediately prior to vocalization (Fig. 7-35).

CONCLUSION

It is important to emphasize again that most of the findings on the function of the ear reported in this chapter are based on very simple sounds. We thus have to confess that we do not know very much about how the auditory system functions in response to complex sounds under natural conditions. Most of the methods used to test hearing clinically can be greatly improved as soon as we gain this knowledge. With regard to children, it is particularly important to remember that the auditory system can function in a seemingly normal manner for the simple signals we usually use in audiometric tests such as pure tone audiometry or brain stem auditory evoked potentials (BSEP), whereas it may function incompletely or not at all for such natural sounds as speech. It is of course of great importance to have this in mind when the hearing of a speech-retarded child is being tested.

REFERENCES

Borg, E., and Zakrisson, J. E. 1975. The activity of the stapedius muscle in man during vocalization. Acta Otolaryngol. 79:325-333.

This chapter was prepared with support from the Swedish Medical Research Council (contract 12 X 90 and B78-04P-05183-01). Pamela Boston corrected the language, Rigmor Joelsson typed the various versions of the manuscript, and Gunilla Jönsson prepared the illustrations.

Dallos, P., and Cheatham, M. A. 1976. Compound action potential (AP) tuning curves. J. Acoust. Soc. Am. 59:591-597.

Dallos, P. 1973. The Auditory Periphery. New York, Academic Press.

Dallos, P., Harris, D., Özdamar, Ö., et al. 1978. Behavioral compound action potentials and single unit threshold: Relationship in normal and abnormal ears. J. Acoust. Soc. Am. 64:151-157.

Davis, H., et al. 1953. Acoustic trauma in the guinea pig. J. Acoust. Soc. Am. 25:1180.

Duifhuis, H. 1976. Cochlear linearity and second filter: Possible mechanisms and applications. J. Acoust. Soc. Am. 59:408-423.

Evans, E. F. 1975. Cochlear nerve and cochlear nucleus. In Handbook of Sensory Physiology. New York, Springer Verlag, Chap. 1, pp. 1-108.

Fletcher, H., and Munson, W. A. 1933. Loudness, its definition, measurement and calculation. J. Acoust. Soc. Am. 5:82-108.

Flock, Å. 1971. Sensory transduction in hair cells. In Handbook of Sensory Physiology, Vol I. Chap. 14, pp. 396-441. Berlin, Springer-Verlag.

Flock, Å., and Cheung, H. C. 1977. Actin filaments in sensory hairs of inner ear receptor cells. J. Cell Biol. 75:339-343.

Johnstone, B. M., and Boyle, A. J. F. 1967. Basilar membrane vibration examined with the Mössbauer technique. Science N.Y. 158:389-390.

Keidel, W. D., and Neff, W. D. 1974. Handbook of Sensory Physiology, Vol. 5, Part 1. Auditory System: Anatomy and Physiology. Berlin, Springer-Verlag.

Kiang, N. Y. S., Watanabe, T., Tomas, E. C., et al. 1965. Discharge patterns of single fibers in the cat's auditory nerve. Research Monograph No 35. Cambridge, Mass., The MIT Press.

Licklider, J. C. R. 1951. Basic correlates of the auditory stimulus. In Stevens, S. S. (Ed.) Handbook of Experimental Psychology. New York, John Wiley and Sons.

Møller, A. R. 1962. The acoustic reflex in man. J. Acoust. Soc. Am. 34:1524-1534, Part II.

Møller, A. R. 1964. The acoustic impedance in experimental studies on the middle ear. Internat. Audiol. 3:123-135.

Møller, A. R. 1965a. An experimental study of the acoustic impedance of the middle ear and its transmission properties. Acta Otolaryngol. 60:129-149.

Møller, A. R. 1965b. Effects of tympanic muscle activity on movement of the eardrum, acoustic impedance and cochlear microphonics. Acta Otolaryngol. 58:525-534.

Møller, A. R. 1972a. Coding of amplitude modulated sounds in the cochlear nucleus of the rat. In Møller, A. R. (Ed.) Basic Mechanisms in Hearing. New York, Academic Press, pp. 593-619.

Møller, A. R. 1972b. Coding of amplitude and frequency modulated sounds in the cochlear nucleus of the rat. Acta Physiol. Scand. 86:223–238.

Møller, A. R. 1974. Coding of amplitude and frequency modulated sounds in the cochlear nucleus. Acustica, 31:292–299.

Møller, A. R. 1975. Noise as a health hazard. Ambio 4:6–13.

Møller, A. R. 1982. Auditory Physiology. New York, Academic Press.

Møller, A. R. 1981. Fundamentals of Auditory Physiology. New York. Academic Press.

Nomoto, M., Suga, N., and Katsuki, Y. 1964. Discharge pattern and inhibition of primary nerve fibers in the monkey. J. Neurophysiol. 27:768–787.

Nordmark, J. 1968. Mechanisms of frequency discrimination. J. Acoust. Soc. Am. 44:1533–1540.

Özdamar, O., Dallos, P., Ryan, A., et al. 1978. Comparison of auditory thresholds determined behaviorally and electrocochleographically in normal and kanamycin-treated gerbils. J. Acoust. Soc. Am.

Rhode, W. S. 1971. Observations of the vibration of the basilar membrane in squirrel monkeys using the Mössbauer technique. J. Acoust. Soc. Am. 49:1218–1231.

Rose, J. E., Hind, J. E., Anderson, D. J., et al. 1971. Some effects of stimulus intensity on response of auditory nerve fibers in squirrel monkey. J. Neurophysiol. 34:685–699.

Shaw, E. A. C. 1974. Transformation of sound pressure level from the free field to the eardrum in the horizontal plane. J. Acoust. Soc. Am. 56:1848–1861.

Spoendlin, H. 1970. Structural basis of peripheral frequency analysis. In Plomp, R., and Smoorenburg, G. F. (Eds.) Frequency Analysis and Periodicity Detection in Hearing. Leiden, A. W. Sijthoff, pp. 2–36.

Sivian, L. J., and White, S. D. 1933. On minimum audible sound fields. J. Acoust. Soc. Am. 4:288–321.

Stevens, S. S. 1951. Handbook of Experimental Psychology. New York, John Wiley & Sons.

Stevens, S. S., and Davis, H. 1938. Hearing. New York, John Wiley & Sons.

Stevens, S. S., and Volkman, J. 1940. The relation of pitch to frequency. Am. J. Psychol. 53:329–353.

Tobias, J. V. 1970. Foundations of Modern Auditory Theory I & II. New York, Academic Press.

Wever, E. G., and Lawrence, M. 1954. Physiological Acoustics. Princeton, Princeton University Press.

Whitfield, I. C. 1967. The auditory pathway. London, Edward Arnold, Ltd.

von Békèsy, G. 1942. Über die Schwingungen der Schneckentrennwand beim Präparat und Ohrenmodell. Akust. Z. 7:1973–186.

von Békèsy, G. 1960. Experiments in Hearing. New York, McGraw-Hill.

Zwislocki, J. J. 1974. A possible neuro-mechanical sound analysis in the cochlea. Acoustica 31:354–359.

METHODS OF EXAMINATION: CLINICAL EXAMINATION

Charles D. Bluestone, M.D.

Of the various methods currently used in the diagnosis of ear disease in children, the medical history and a physical examination that includes pneumatic otoscopy are usually sufficient to establish a reasonably accurate clinical diagnosis when inflammation is present. Although less common than the inflammatory diseases, congenital, traumatic, and neoplastic problems are also of significant importance.

SIGNS AND SYMPTOMS

There are eight prominent signs and symptoms primarily associated with diseases of the ear and temporal bone. *Otalgia* is most commonly associated with inflammation of the external and middle ear but may also be of nonaural origin, as from the temporomandibular joint, the teeth, or the pharynx. In young infants, pulling at the ear or general irritability, especially when it is associated with fever, may be the only sign of ear pain (Chap. 9A). Purulent *otorrhea* is a sign of otitis externa, otitis media with perforation of the tympanic membrane, or both. Bloody discharge may be associated with acute or chronic inflammation, trauma, or neoplasm. A clear drainage may be indicative of a perforation of the drum with a serous middle ear effusion or cerebrospinal fluid otorrhea draining through a defect in the external auditory canal or through the tympanic membrane from the middle ear (Chap. 9B).

Hearing loss is a symptom that may be the result of disease of either the external or middle ear (conductive hearing loss) or the result of a pathologic condition in the inner ear, retrocochlea, or the central auditory pathways (sensorineural hearing loss) (Chap. 10). *Swelling* about the ear is most commonly the result of inflammation (for example, external otitis, perichondritis, or mastoiditis), trauma (as a hematoma), or, on rare occasions, neoplasm. *Vertigo* is not a common complaint in children but is present more often than was formerly thought. The most common cause is eustachian tube–middle ear–mastoid disease, but vertigo may be due also to labyrinthitis; perilymphatic fistula between the inner and middle ear resulting from a congenital defect, trauma, or cholesteatoma; vestibular neuronitis; benign paroxysmal positional vertigo; Meniere disease; or disease of the central nervous system. Older children may describe a feeling of spinning or turning, while younger children may not be able to verbalize concerning the symptom but manifest the dysequilibrium by falling, stumbling, or "clumsiness." Unidirectional horizontal jerk *nystagmus,* usually associated with vertigo, is vestibular in origin (Chap. 11). *Tinnitus* is another symptom children infrequently describe but which is commonly present, especially in patients with eustachian tube–middle ear disease or conductive or sensorineural hearing loss (Chap. 12). *Facial paralysis* is an infrequent but frightening condition both for the child and for his or her parents. When it is due to disease within the temporal bone in children, it most commonly occurs as a complication of acute or chronic otitis media but also may be idiopathic (Bell palsy), the result of temporal bone fracture or neoplasm, or, on rare occasions, herpes zoster oticus (Chap. 13). Other signs and symptoms of conditions that may be associated with ear disease may also be present, such as symptoms of upper respiratory allergy associated with otitis media (Chap. 16).

PHYSICAL EXAMINATION

Aside from the history, the most useful method for diagnosing ear disease is a physical examination that includes pneumatic otoscopy. Adequate examination of the entire child, with special attention to the head and neck, can lead to the identification of a condition that may predispose to or be associated with ear disease. The appearance of the child's face and the character of his or her speech may be important clues to the possibility of an abnormal middle ear. Many of the craniofacial anomalies, such as mandibulofacial dysostosis (Treacher-Collins syndrome) and trisomy 21 (Down syndrome), are associated with an increased incidence of ear disease. Mouth breathing and hyponasality may indicate intranasal or postnasal obstruction, while hypernasality is a sign of velopharyngeal insufficiency. Examination of the oropharyngeal cavity may uncover an overt cleft palate or a submucous cleft (Fig. 8A–1), both of which conditions predispose the in-

fant to otitis media with effusion (Stool and Randall, 1967; Paradise et al., 1969). A bifid uvula is also associated with an increased incidence of middle ear disease (Taylor, 1972). An examination of the child's head and neck may also reveal posterior nasal or pharyngeal inflammation and discharge. Other pathologic conditions of the nose, such as polyposis, severe deviation of the nasal septum, or a nasopharyngeal tumor, may also be associated with otitis media.

Examination of the ear itself is the most critical part of the clinician's assessment of the patient, but it must be examined systematically. The auricle, periauricular area, and external auditory meatus should be examined first; all too frequently these areas are overlooked in the physician's haste to make a diagnosis by otoscopic examination, but the presence or absence of signs of infection in these areas may aid later in the differential diagnosis or evaluation of complications of ear disease. For instance, eczematoid external otitis may result from acute otitis media with discharge, or inflammation of the postauricular area may be indicative of a periosteitis or subperiosteal abscess that has extended from the mastoid air cells. Palpation of these areas will determine if tenderness is present; exquisite pain upon palpation of the tragus would indicate the presence of acute diffuse external otitis.

After the examination of the external ear and canal, then the clinician may proceed to the most important part of the physical assessment, the otoscopic examination.

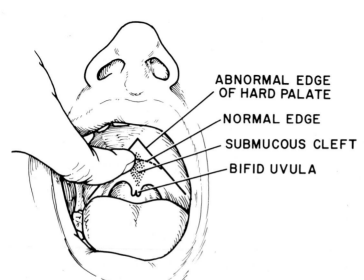

ABNORMAL EDGE
OF HARD PALATE

NORMAL EDGE

SUBMUCOUS CLEFT

BIFID UVULA

Figure 8A–1 Bifid uvula, widening, and attenuation of the median raphe of the soft palate and V-shaped midline notch, rather than a smooth curve, are diagnostic of a submucous cleft palate.

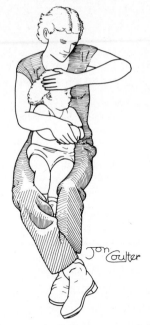

Figure 8A–2 Method of restraining child for examination of the ear.

OTOSCOPIC EXAMINATION

The position of the patient for otoscopy depends upon the patient's age, ability to cooperate, the clinical setting, and the preference of the examiner. Otoscopic evaluation of the neonate is best performed on an examining table, and a parent or assistant is necessary to restrain the baby since undue movement usually prevents an adequate evaluation. Some clinicians prefer to place the neonate prone on the table, while others prefer the patient to be supine. This method is also desirable for older infants who are uncooperative. However, infants and young children who are just apprehensive and not struggling actively can be evaluated adequately while sitting on the parent's lap; when necessary, the child may be restrained firmly on an adult's lap if the parent holds the child's wrists over his or her abdomen with one hand and holds the patient's head against the adult's chest with the other hand. If necessary, the child's legs can be held between the adult's thighs (Fig. 8A–2). Some young infants can be examined by placing the child's head on the parent's lap (Fig. 8A–3). Cooperative children can usually be evaluated successfully sitting in a chair or on the edge of an examination table. As shown in Figure 8A–4, the otoscope should be held with the hand or finger placed firmly against the child's head or face so that the otoscope will move with the head rather than causing trauma (pain) to the ear canal if the child moves suddenly.

Before adequate visualization of the external canal and tympanic membrane can be obtained, all obstructing cerumen must be removed from the canal. This can usually be accomplished with the aid of an otoscope with a surgical head and a wire loop or a blunt cerumen curet (Fig. 8A–5) or by irrigating the ear canal gently with warm water. A dental irrigation device (Water Pik) may be used for this purpose (Fig. 8A–6). Impacted cerumen can be softened by the instillation of a mixture of glycerine and peroxide (in equal parts) followed by irrigation of the canal at a later time. When it is necessary to make an immediate diagnosis, the cerumen should be removed under direct vision using an otoscope or otomicroscope without traumatizing the canal walls, since any bleeding will obscure the tympanic membrane. After the external canal has been cleaned thoroughly, it should be inspected for signs of inflammation. In the newborn, the external canal is filled with vernix caseosa, which disappears shortly after birth.

For proper assessment of the tympanic membrane and its mobility, a pneumatic otoscope in which the diagnostic head has an

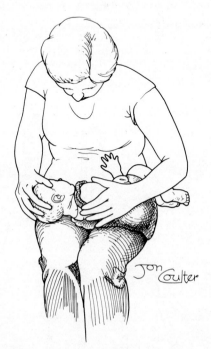

Figure 8A–3 Method for positioning baby for otoscopic examination.

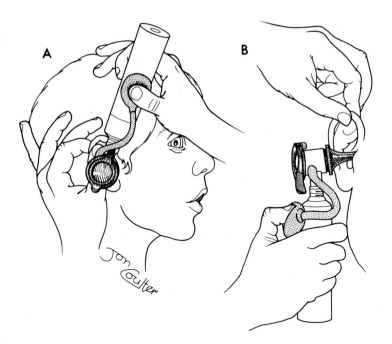

Figure 8A–4 Methods of positioning otoscope to enhance visualization and to minimize the chance that head movement will result in trauma to the ear canal. Both of the otoscopist's hands can be used (*A*), or, when the child is cooperative, a finger touching the child's cheek is sufficient (*B*).

adequate seal should be used. Currently, the quality of the otoscopic examination is limited by deficiencies in the designs of commercially available otoscopes. The speculum employed should have the largest lumen that comfortably can fit in the child's cartilaginous external auditory meatus. If the speculum is too small, adequate visualization may be impaired and the speculum may touch the bony canal, which can be painful. In most models, an airtight seal is usually not possible because of a leak of air within the otoscope head or between the stiff ear speculum and the exter-

nal auditory canal, although leaks at the latter location can be stopped by cutting off a small section of rubber tubing and slipping it over the tip of the ear speculum (Fig. 8A–7). Many otolaryngologists prefer to use a Bruenings or Siegle otoscope with the magnifying lens. Both of these instruments allow for excellent assessment of drum mobility since they have an almost airtight seal. A head mirror and lamp or a headlight (Fig. 8A–8) is necessary to provide light for the examination.

Inspection of the tympanic membrane should include evaluation of its position,

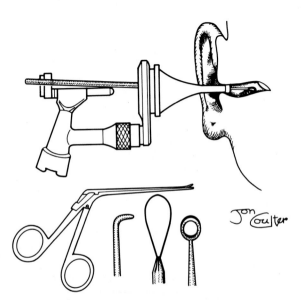

Figure 8A–5 Method for removing cerumen from the external ear canal employing the surgical head attached to the otoscope and instruments that can be used.

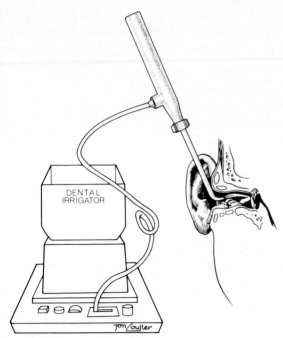

Figure 8A–6 Irrigation of the external canal with a dental irrigator to remove cerumen.

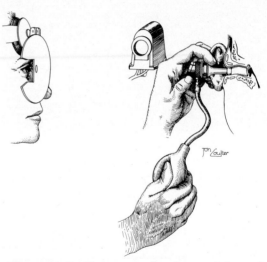

Figure 8A–8 Observation of eardrum mobility with the Bruenings otoscope with magnifying lens. The light source is from a lamp reflected off of a head mirror.

color, degree of translucency, and mobility. Assessment of the light reflex is of limited value in the evaluation of the tympanic membrane–middle ear since it may or may

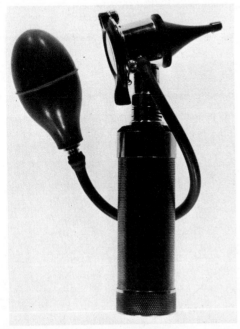

Figure 8A–7 Pneumatic otoscope with rubber tip on the end of the ear speculum to give a better seal in the external auditory canal.

not be absent when pathology is present. Figure 8A–9 shows the positions assumed by the tympanic membrane in various disease states. The normal eardrum should be in the neutral position, with the short process of the malleus visible but not prominent through the membrane. Mild retraction of the tympanic membrane usually indicates the presence of negative middle ear pressure, in which case the short process of the malleus and posterior mallear fold are prominent and the manubrium of the malleus appears to be foreshortened. Severe retraction (atelectasis) of the tympanic membrane is characterized by a very prominent posterior mallear fold and short process of the malleus and a severely foreshortened manubrium. In such an ear, a horizontal line may be visible below the umbo of the malleus; this represents the tympanic membrane resting on the promontory of the cochlea. However, the tympanic membrane may be severely retracted in the absence of high negative middle ear pressure as measured by pneumatic otoscopy or tympanometry or both; this retraction is presumably due to high negative pressure or inflammation within the middle ear with subsequent fixation of the ossicles, ligaments, and possibly the tensor tympani muscle. Fullness of the tympanic membrane is apparent initially in the posterosuperior portion of the pars tensa and the pars flaccida since these two areas are the most highly compliant parts of the tympanic membrane (Khanna and Tonndorf, 1972). The short process of the malleus usually is obscured. The fullness may be due

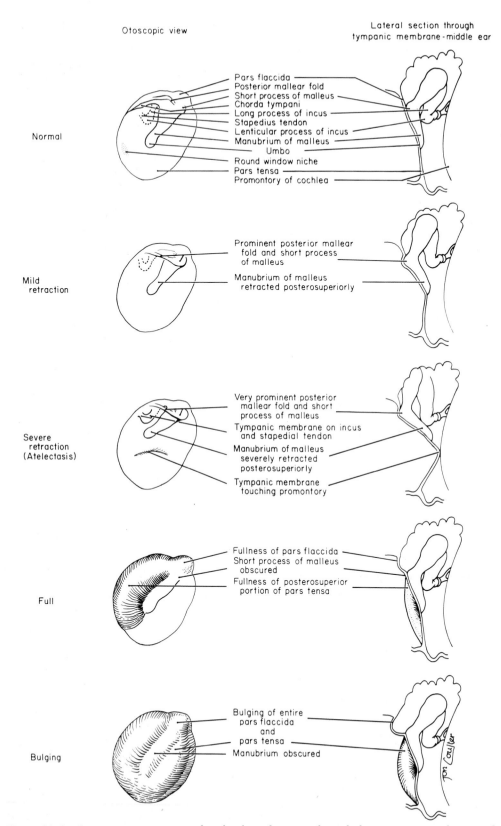

Otoscopic view

Lateral section through
tympanic membrane - middle ear

Normal
- Pars flaccida
- Posterior mallear fold
- Short process of malleus
- Chorda tympani
- Long process of incus
- Stapedius tendon
- Lenticular process of incus
- Manubrium of malleus
- Umbo
- Round window niche
- Pars tensa
- Promontory of cochlea

Mild
retraction
- Prominent posterior mallear fold and short process of malleus
- Manubrium of malleus retracted posterosuperiorly

Severe
retraction
(Atelectasis)
- Very prominent posterior mallear fold and short process of malleus
- Tympanic membrane on incus and stapedial tendon
- Manubrium of malleus severely retracted posterosuperiorly
- Tympanic membrane touching promontory

Full
- Fullness of pars flaccida
- Short process of malleus obscured
- Fullness of posterosuperior portion of pars tensa

Bulging
- Bulging of entire pars flaccida and pars tensa
- Manubrium obscured

Figure 8A–9 Otoscopic view compared with a lateral section through the tympanic membrane and middle ear to demonstrate the various positions of the drum with their respective anatomic landmarks (see text).

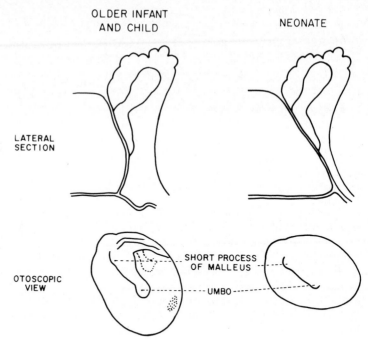

OLDER INFANT
AND CHILD

NEONATE

LATERAL
SECTION

OTOSCOPIC
VIEW

SHORT PROCESS
OF MALLEUS

UMBO

Figure 8A–10 Comparison of the tympanic membrane of an older infant or a child with that of a neonate. The lateral section shows the greater angulation of the neonate's external canal with regard to the tympanic membrane. The appearance of the eardrums and canals on otoscopy is depicted in the lower drawings; the neonate appears to have a smaller tympanic membrane because of angulation of the eardrum.

to increased air pressure or effusion or both within the middle ear. When bulging of the entire tympanic membrane occurs, the malleus is usually obscured.

The tympanic membrane of the neonate is in a different position from that of the older infant and child; if this is not kept in mind, the examiner may perceive the eardrum to be smaller and retracted, since in the neonate the tympanic membrane appears to be as wide as it is in older children but not as high. Figure 8A–10 shows that this perception is due to the more horizontal position of the neonatal eardrum, which frequently makes it difficult for the examiner to distinguish the pars flaccida of the tympanic membrane from the deep superior external canal wall skin. In addition, visualization of the inferior portion of the newborn's drum may be obscured by the redundant skin of the inferior canal wall since in the neonate the external canal consists of soft tissue and cartilage with the only bone being the tympanic ring, whereas the inner two thirds of the external canal skin in the child is firmly attached to the underlying tympanic bone. Adequate visualization of the inferior portion of the neonate's eardrum can be achieved if the examiner pulls the pinna inferiorly to distend the redundant skin of the ear canal before inserting the ear speculum deeply into the canal.

The normal tympanic membrane has a ground-glass appearance; a blue or yellow color usually indicates a middle ear effusion seen through a translucent tympanic membrane. A red tympanic membrane alone may not be indicative of a pathologic condition since the blood vessels of the drum head may be engorged as the result of the patient's crying, sneezing, or blowing his or her nose. It is critical to distinguish between translucency and opacification of the eardrum in order to identify a middle ear effusion. The normal tympanic membrane should be translucent, the observer being able to look through the drum and visualize the middle ear landmarks (the incudostapedial joint, promontory, round window niche, and frequently the chorda tympani nerve) (Fig. 8A–11). If a middle ear effusion is present medial to a translucent drum, an air-fluid level or bubbles of air admixed with the liquid may be visible (Fig. 8A–12). An air-fluid level or bubbles can be differentiated from scarring of the tympanic membrane by altering the position of the head while observing the drum with the otoscope (if fluid is present, the air-fluid level will shift in relation to gravity) or by seeing movement of the fluid during pneumatic otoscopy. The line frequently seen when a severely retracted membrane touches the cochlear promontory will

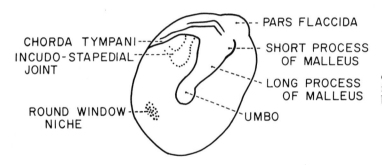

Figure 8A–11 Diagrammatic view of the tympanic membrane depicting important landmarks that usually can be visualized with the otoscope.

disappear (the drum will pull away from the promontory) if sufficient negative pressure can be applied with the pneumatic otoscope. Inability to visualize the middle ear structures indicates opacification of the drum, which is usually the result of thickening of the tympanic membrane, the presence of an effusion, or both. However, the normal tympanic membrane of the neonate is opaque, the only landmarks visible being the short process and umbo of the malleus. Obviously, it is necessary to have a bright light in order to evaluate opacity of the tympanic membrane. For this reason, otoscope batteries should be replaced frequently so that the ability of the examiner to "look through" the tympanic membrane

RETRACTED

AIR/FLUID LEVEL

BUBBLES IN FLUID

Figure 8A–12 Three examples of otoscopic findings (right ear).

will not be impaired. The electric otoscope is better than the battery type.

Abnormalities of the tympanic membrane and middle ear are reflected in the pattern of tympanic membrane mobility when first positive and then negative pressure is applied to the external auditory canal with the pneumatic otoscope. The technique of pneumatic otoscopy was originally described by Siegle in 1864, but unfortunately it has not been universally employed by clinicians during the past century. As shown in Figure 8A–13, this is achieved by first applying slight positive pressure on the rubber bulb (positive pressure) and then, after momentarily breaking the seal, releasing the bulb (negative pressure). The presence of effusion, high negative pressure, or both within the middle ear can markedly dampen the movements of the eardrum. When the middle ear pressure is ambient, the normal tympanic membrane moves inward with slight positive pressure in the ear canal and outward toward the examiner with slight negative pressure. The motion observed is proportionate to the applied pressure and is best visualized in the posterosuperior quadrant of the tympanic membrane (Fig. 8A–14). If a dimeric membrane or atrophic scar secondary to an old perforation is present, mobility of the tympanic membrane can also be assessed more readily by observing the movement of the flaccid area.

Figure 8A–15 shows the relationship between mobility of the tympanic membrane as measured by pneumatic otoscopy and the middle ear contents and pressure. In Figure 8A–15, Frame 1 shows the normal tympanic membrane when the middle ear contains only air at ambient pressure. A hypermobile eardrum (Frame 2) is seen most frequently in children whose membranes are atrophic or flaccid. The mobility of the tympanic membrane is greater than normal (the drum is said to be highly compliant) if the drum

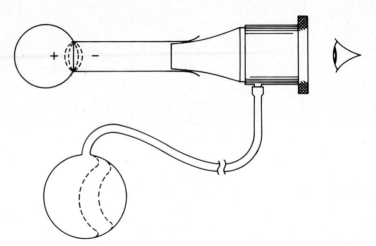

Figure 8A–13 Pressure applied to the rubber bulb attached to the pneumatic otoscope will deflect the normal tympanic membrane inward with applied positive pressure and outward with applied negative pressure if the middle ear air pressure is ambient. The movement of the eardrum is proportionate to the degree of pressure exerted on the bulb until the tympanic membrane has reached its limit of compliance.

moves when even slight positive or negative external canal pressure is applied, and if the drum moves equally well to both applied positive and negative pressures, the middle ear pressure is approximately ambient. However, if the tympanic membrane is hypermobile to applied negative pressure but is immobile when positive pressure is applied, the tympanic membrane is flaccid and negative pressure is present within the middle ear. Highly compliant tympanic membranes have been associated with abnormal function of the eustachian tube (Elner et al., 1971); it is speculated that wide fluctuations in middle ear pressure lead to loss of drum stiffness. A middle ear effusion is rarely present when the tympanic membrane is hypermobile, even though high negative middle ear pressure is present. A thickened tympanic membrane (secondary to inflammation or scarring or both) or a partly effusion-filled middle ear (in

which the middle ear air pressure is ambient) shows decreased mobility to applied pressures, both positive and negative (Frame 3).

Normal middle ear pressure is reflected by the neutral position of the tympanic membrane as well as by its response to both positive and negative pressures in each of the previous examples (Frames 1 to 3). In other cases, the eardrum may be retracted, usually because negative middle ear pressure is present (Frames 4 to 6). The compliant membrane is maximally retracted by even moderate negative middle ear pressure and hence cannot visibly be deflected inward farther with applied positive pressure in the ear canal. Negative pressure produced by releasing the rubber bulb of the otoscope will, however, cause a return of the eardrum toward the neutral position if a negative pressure equivalent to that in the middle ear can be created by releasing the rubber bulb, a condition that

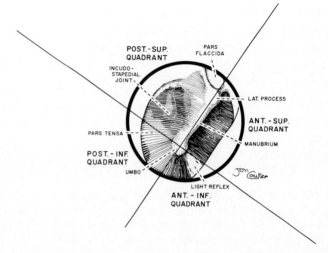

Figure 8A–14   The four quadrants of the pars tensa of a right tympanic membrane.

	TYMPANIC MEMBRANE POSITION*	OTOSCOPY	EXTERNAL CANAL PRESSURE† POSITIVE		NEGATIVE		MIDDLE EAR CONTENT	PRESSURE
			LOW	HIGH	LOW	HIGH		
1.	NEUTRAL	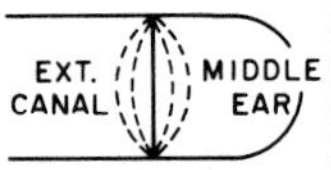 EXT. CANAL / MIDDLE EAR	1+	2+	1+	2+	AIR	AMBIENT
2.	NEUTRAL	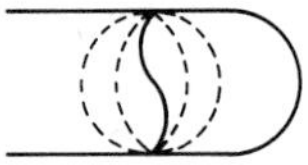	2+	3+	2+	3+	AIR	AMBIENT
3.	NEUTRAL	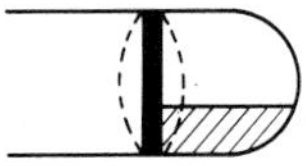	0	1+	0	1+	AIR OR AIR AND EFFUSION	AMBIENT
4.	RETRACTED	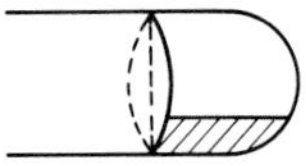	0	0	1+	2+	AIR OR AIR AND EFFUSION	LOW NEGATIVE
5.	RETRACTED	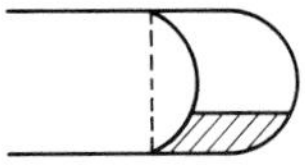	0	0	0	1+	AIR OR EFFUSION AND AIR	HIGH NEGATIVE
6.	RETRACTED	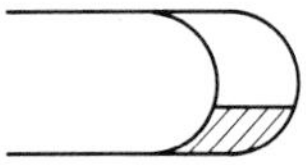	0	0	0	0	AIR OR EFFUSION OR BOTH	VERY HIGH NEGATIVE OR INDETERMINATE
7.	FULL	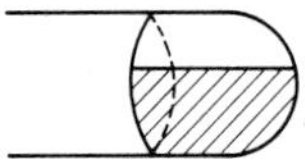	0	1+	0	0	AIR AND EFFUSION	POSITIVE OR INDETERMINATE
8.	BULGING	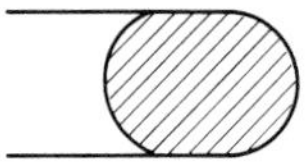	0	0	0	0	EFFUSION	POSITIVE OR INDETERMINATE

* POSITION AT REST (SOLID LINE) AND WITH APPLIED PRESSURE (DOTTED LINE)

† DEGREE OF TYMPANIC MEMBRANE MOVEMENT AS VISUALIZED THROUGH THE OTOSCOPE; 0 = NONE, 1+ = SLIGHT, 2+ = MODERATE, 3+ = EXCESSIVE

Figure 8A–15 Pneumatic otoscopic findings related to middle ear contents and pressure (see text).

occurs when air, with or without an effusion, is present in the middle ear (Frame 4). When the middle ear pressure is even lower, there may be only slight outward mobility of the tympanic membrane (Frame 5) because of the limited negative pressure that can be exerted through the otoscopes that are currently available. When assessing the mobility of the tympanic membrane in which a negative pressure is present within the middle ear, return of the tympanic membrane to the resting retracted position after the application of applied negative external canal pressure should not be confused with movement to applied positive pressure. This "rebound"

of the eardrum after applied negative pressure may lead the examiner to conclude erroneously that the tympanic membrane is mobile to both positive and negative pressure and that, therefore, the middle ear pressure is ambient. If the eardrum is severely retracted with extremely high negative middle ear pressure or in the presence of a middle ear effusion or both, the examiner is not able to produce significant outward movement (Frame 6).

The tympanic membrane that exhibits fullness (Frame 7) will move to applied positive pressure but not to applied negative pressure if the pressure within the middle ear is positive and air, with or without an effusion, is present. In such an instance, the tympanic membrane is stretched laterally to the point of maximal compliance and will not visibly move outward any farther to the applied negative pressure but will move inward to applied positive pressure as long as some air is present within the middle ear-mastoid air cell system. A full tympanic membrane and positive middle ear pressure without a middle ear effusion are frequently seen in neonates and in young infants who are crying during the otoscopic examination; in older infants and children, the same situation may be encountered after the patient has sneezed, blown his nose, or swallowed when his nose was obstructed. However, in the initial stage of acute otitis media with effusion, the tympanic membrane may be full, with the characteristic findings of pneumatic otoscopy described before, since air is usually present within the middle ear. When the middle ear–mastoid air cell system is filled with an effusion and little or no air is present, the mobility of the bulging tympanic membrane (Frame 8) is severely decreased or absent to both applied positive and negative pressure. In the neonate and young infant, in whom the skin of the ear canal is more floppy than in the older child, the skin may distend and pull into the lumen to applied positive and negative pressure, respectively; this can be mistaken for movement of an immobile tympanic membrane since the junction of the canal wall and drum is somewhat indistinct. For this reason, the anatomic characteristics of the tympanic membrane at different stages of development must be kept in mind.

ACCURACY, VALIDATION TECHNIQUES, AND INTEREXAMINER RELIABILITY OF OTOSCOPY

Otoscopy is subjective, and thus usually is an imprecise method of assessing the condition of the tympanic membrane and middle ear. Most clinicians do not use a pneumatic otoscope, and few have been trained adequately to make a correct diagnosis. The primary reason for this lack of proper education is the method of teaching employed. Since otoscopy is a monocular assessment of the tympanic membrane, the teacher cannot verify that the student actually visualized the anatomic features that led to the diagnosis. A

new otoscope with a teaching side arm observer head has been developed, but one of the most effective means of education currently available is the correlation of the otoscopic findings with those of the otomicroscope that has an observer tube for the student. In this manner, the instructor can point out the critical landmarks and can demonstrate tympanic mobility using the Bruenings otoscope.

Assessment techniques can also be improved by correlating otoscopy findings with a tympanogram taken immediately after the otoscopic examination (Bluestone and Cantekin, 1979). Lack of agreement between the otoscopic findings and tympanometry usually results in a second otoscopic examination since tympanometry is in general very accurate in distinguishing between normal and abnormal tympanic membranes and middle ears (specifically, in the identification of middle ear effusions). The presence or absen e of negative pressure within the middle ear as measured by pneumatic otoscopy can be verified only by similar results as measured on the tympanogram. Validation of the presence or absence of effusion as observed by otoscopy is best achieved by performing a tympanocentesis or myringotomy immediately after the examination. When surgical opening of the tympanic membrane is indicated, preliminary otoscopy by several examiners is a very effective way of teaching many students at once to evaluate the state of the middle ear.

In almost all studies of otitis media reported on in the past, the disease has been identified by otoscopy; however, no information has been offered to enable the reader to evaluate the ability of the otoscopist to make the diagnosis correctly. In an attempt to classify tympanometric patterns, Paradise and colleagues (1976) validated the diagnosis of the otoscopist by performing a myringotomy shortly after the otoscopic examination. This method of validation of otoscopic findings was also used in previous studies of infants with cleft palates in which two otoscopists were involved (Paradise et al., 1969; Paradise and Bluestone, 1974). However, other studies of otitis media have not reported validation of the diagnostic criteria, and when attempts have been made to determine interexaminer reliability in these studies, the results have been so poor as to infer that the data reported are not accurate. Jordan (1972) reported the inconsistency of the descriptions of the appearance of the tympanic membrane by

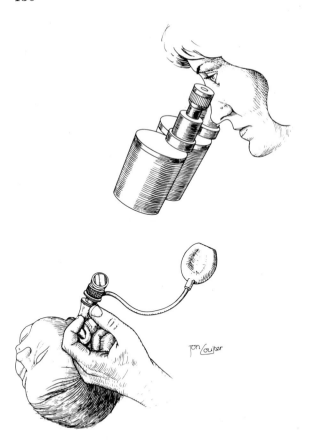

Figure 8A–16 Precise assessment of tympanic membrane mobility employing the otomicroscope and a Bruenings otoscope with a nonmagnifying lens.

the three otologists who participated in the Second Pittsburgh Study of Hearing Sensitivity and Ear Disease in Public School Children. In assessing normality or abnormality of the tympanic membrane, the examiners agreed in only 60 per cent of the observations in 10 children.

In the design of a study in which otoscopic examination is used in the identification of otitis media with effusion and related conditions, the diagnostic abilities of all otoscopists included in the study must be validated, and interexaminer reliability must be established. If the primary ear disease being studied is otitis media with effusion, then each otoscopist should have a high degree of accuracy in identifying otitis media with effusion. This can be achieved by performing otoscopy on a group of children immediately prior to tympanocentesis or myringotomy (Cantekin et al., 1980). The sensitivity (the total number of otoscopic diagnoses of otitis media with effusion present in ears with otitis media with effusion divided by the total myringotomy findings when otitis media with effusion is present) and specificity (total number of otoscopic diagnoses of otitis media with effusion

absent in ears without otitis media with effusion divided by the total myringotomy findings when otitis media with effusion is absent) should be as high as possible. Interexaminer reliability can be tested by having all the otoscopists involved in the study independently make an otoscopic diagnosis prior to the tympanocentesis or myringotomy.

OTOMICROSCOPY

Many otolaryngologists use the otomicroscope to improve the accuracy of diagnosis of otitis media and related conditions. For the assessment of tympanic membrane mobility, the microscope, when used with the Bruenings otoscope and nonmagnifying lens (Fig. 8A–16), is superior to conventional otoscopes; this is because the microscope provides binocular vision (and therefore depth perception), a better light source, and greater magnification. Under most conditions, otomicroscopic examination is impractical and generally is not necessary, but when a diagnosis by otoscopy is in doubt, then the otomicroscope is an invaluable diagnostic aid and frequently is essential in arriving at the correct diagnosis — for instance, in differentiating a deep retraction pocket in the posterosuperior quadrant of the tympanic membrane from a cholesteatoma. In addition to the advantages offered by the otomicroscope for certain diagnostic problems, it is superior to the conventional otoscopes for minor surgical procedures, such as tympanocentesis, since it allows for a more precise visualization of the field.

Even though several studies reported in the past have used the otomicroscopic examination as a validator for the presence or absence of middle ear disease (otitis media with effusion), no study has reported on the sensitivity and specificity of the microscopic examination for detecting middle ear effusion. It is purported to be superior to the standard otoscopic examination, but whether or not it is superior to tympanometry with otoscopy has not yet been shown. However, the otomicroscope with an observer tube attachment is superior to the currently available otoscope as a teaching device.

Whenever the otoscopic examination is unsatisfactory due to inability to adequately visualize the tympanic membrane (e.g., narrow external canal, uncooperative child), then an examination under general anesthesia is indicated employing the otomicroscope.

REFERENCES

Bluestone, C. D., and Cantekin, E. I. 1979. Design factors in the characterization and identification of otitis media and certain related conditions. Ann. Otol. Rhinol. Laryngol., 88(60):13–27.

Cantekin, E. I., Bluestone, C. D., Fria, T. J., et al. 1980. Identification of otitis media with effusion. Ann. Otol. Rhinol. Laryngol., 89(68):190–195.

Elner, A., Ingelstedt, S., and Ivarsson, A. 1971. The elastic properties of the tympanic membrane system. Acta Otolaryngol., 72:397.

Jordan, R. E. 1972. Epidemiology of otitis media. In Glorig, A., and Gerwin, K. S. (Eds.) Otitis Media. Proceedings of the National Conference, Gallier Hearing and Speech Center, Dallas, Texas. Springfield, IL., Charles C Thomas.

Khanna, S. M., and Tonndorf, J. 1972. Tympanic membrane vibrations in cats studied by time-averaged holography. J. Acoust. Soc. Am., 51:1904.

Paradise, J. L., Bluestone, C. D., and Felder, H. 1969. The universality of otitis media in fifty infants with cleft palate. Pediatrics, 44:3542.

Paradise, J. L., and Bluestone, C. D. 1974. Early treatment of universal otitis media of infants with cleft palate. Pediatrics, 53:48.

Paradise, J. L., Smith, C. G., and Bluestone, C. D. 1976. Tympanometric detection of middle ear effusion in infants and young children. Pediatrics, 58:198–210.

Siegle (Deutsch Klinik 1864), quoted by Politzer, A. 1909. Disease of the Ear, 5th ed. London, Baillière Tindall, p. 107.

Stool, S. E., and Randall, P. 1967. Unexpected ear disease in infants with cleft palate. Cleft Palate J., 4:99–103.

Taylor, G. D. 1972. The bifid uvula. Laryngoscope, 82:771–778.

Chapter 8B

THE ASSESSMENT OF HEARING AND MIDDLE EAR FUNCTION IN CHILDREN

Thomas J. Fria, Ph.D.

From the time of birth, a child exists in a world of sensory experiences. The reception and perception of these experiences provides the conceptual framework for communication and other interactive links to one's environment. Consequently, a decrement in sensory experience endangers the normal development of cognitive skills vital to the child's successful interaction with his or her environment. If a child has an undetected or unremediated sensory impairment in the months crucial to learning, a developmental lag results; this lag may prove irreversible, and the child may never realize his or her potential capabilities.

Hearing loss is one form of sensory impairment of particular concern in this text. The long-term effects of hearing loss cannot be dismissed as trivial even when the impairment appears to be mild or transient. As a result, we are obligated to identify children with impaired hearing, to assess the nature and extent of the impairment, and to manage the child's present and future environmental interactions in the context of the impairment. The present chapter will focus on those procedures used to assess hearing in children. The philosophies and techniques for the habilitation or rehabilitation of children with impaired hearing are presented in Chapters 88 and 89.

The methods for assessing hearing in chil-

dren can be considered as either behavioral or nonbehavioral. Obviously, techniques that require a behavioral response from the child would fall into the former category, and the latter category would be composed of those techniques requiring other than behavioral responses. Behavioral methods of assessment include behavioral observation audiometry (BOA), "play" audiometry, and conventional audiometry. Modifications of BOA that incorporate conditioning principles can also be considered behavioral assessment techniques.

Electroacoustic impedance measurements, auditory electric responses, and cardiac, respiratory, and galvanic skin responses to sound represent nonbehavioral assessment procedures that do not require a behavioral response. These techniques are further removed from the perceptual event called "hearing" than are the behavioral procedures, but they are nonetheless helpful assessment tools from which the integrity of the child's auditory system may be inferred.

The preceding paragraphs are meant to imply that regardless of the assessment technique employed, the examiner must interpret the behavioral or nonbehavioral responses obtained and judge whether a given child's hearing is normal or impaired. However, the precision of this judgment will depend on the particular assessment technique employed and its inherent limitations. For this reason, a judgment of impaired or unimpaired hearing, based on a single technique, should be regarded with caution, and often a combination of several techniques is necessary to arrive at a valid assessment.

In addition, the age of the child will significantly influence the precision with which assessment information may be obtained, since the nature of the auditory response is inherently gross and nonvolitional in the neonate and is refined and voluntary in the young child. The common misconception that some children are too young to evaluate is not true, but respect should be maintained for the imprecision of assessment information obtained in a young child and the intrinsic limitations of the assessment technique most suitable for a child of that age. With this in mind, it is hoped that the reader will have a more objective perspective of the discussion that follows.

BEHAVIORAL METHODS OF ASSESSMENT

As mentioned earlier, there are several techniques that fall into the general category of behavioral methods of hearing assessment. Since age has a significant impact on the nature and application of behavioral techniques, several age definitions are necessary: The "neonate" is the baby from birth to two months of age, the "infant" is defined here as the child from two months to two years of age, and the "young child" is two to five years of age. In each age group, a different assortment of behavioral responses to sound will be observed; consequently, an assessment technique must be used that requires responses commensurate with those in the child's repertoire. In other words, the age of the child has a significant influence on the choice of a particular assessment technique.

Age-Related Auditory Responses

The Neonate

A detailed discussion of the development of auditory integrity in the early months of life is beyond the scope of this chapter, but the interested reader will find Eisenberg's (1976) comprehensive text quite informative. Neonatal reactions to sudden, intense sound are predominantly reflexive and include the Moro reflex, the aural palpebral reflex, and the arousal and cessation responses.

The *Moro reflex* is a generalized motor response that classically consists of an upward and outward movement of the limbs and a backward thrust of the head. All components of this response are not readily observable in every child, and ordinarily the baby will simply "jump" when the stimulus is presented. For this reason, the reaction is commonly known as the startle reflex. Northern and Downs (1974) suggest that the startle reflex is clearly observable in normal neonates and infants up to 24 months of age when a stimulus of 80 to 85 decibels sound pressure level (dBSPL) is presented.

Another commonly observed neonatal response to sound is the *aural palpebral reflex.* This response consists of a contraction of the orbicularis oculi muscles and at times a full closure of the eyes. This latter feature has promoted the alternate term of "eyeblink" reflex to describe the response. However, full eye closure should not be considered a criterion for the aural palpebral reflex. Wedenberg (1963, 1972) reported that normal neonates produced this reflex to stimulus intensities of 105 to 115 dBSPL. Fröding (1960) found the response to be quite sensitive to impairment with a low false positive predictive error for impairment.

The *arousal* and *cessation reflexes* involve clear contrasts in the neonate's prestimulus and poststimulus activity. In the arousal reflex, the sleeping or drowsy neonate will awaken or arouse to the stimulus, and in the cessation reflex a decrease or inhibition of activity in the restless or crying baby is observed. Wedenberg (1963) found that normal neonates aroused to a 70 to 75 dBSPL stimulus. Downs (1967) reported that the cessation reflex was effectively elicited by a 90 dBSPL narrow-band stimulus.

It may be seen that neonatal reactions to sound are primarily reflexive and require rather intense stimulation. It follows that assessment of the neonate on the basis of these responses is a qualitative endeavor that can only identify the presence of impairment. There are additional considerations that can influence the interpretation of the neonatal response. The prestimulus activity of the baby is important, as pointed out by Bench (1970). The child's auditory system may be intact, but a response may not be observable if the child's prestimulus activity level is either very high or very low. Consequently, the examiner must give careful consideration to the child's readiness to respond.

Habituation is another important consideration. With repeated stimulation, the neonate's reactions will diminish considerably or will disappear altogether. This factor must be considered when forming assessment judgments.

The Infant

From two to 24 months of age, the infant's response to sound changes noticeably from that of the neonate. The two month old infant appears less interested than does the neonate in intense sounds that are percussive and unfamiliar (Gessell and Armatruda, 1948), and by three months of age the human voice is an effective stimulus. Moro reflexes begin to decrease in frequency by four months of age (Darley, 1961; Miller et al., 1963). Northern and Downs (1974) suggest that the neonatal reflexes persist into early infancy but require less stimulus intensity.

An infant reaction to sound used in many assessment paradigms is the "localization" response, which emerges at about four months of age (Ewing and Ewing, 1944; Murphy, 1961; Kendall, 1964). At this age, the response consists of rudimentary attempts to locate the sound source. The response is more fully developed by six to nine months of age (Darley, 1961; Northern and Downs, 1974) and consists of a full head and eye turn in the direction of the sound source.

Shepherd (1978) suggests that a form of the cessation response can be observed in infants, and he calls this the "distraction" response. In this response, the infant may cease play activity and at times actively may seek the sound source. The stimulus appears to distract the infant from the prestimulus activity.

Depending on the assessment technique employed, localization and distraction responses have been used to obtain response thresholds in infants as young as five months that approximate adult normal hearing levels (Thompson and Weber, 1974; Wilson et al., 1976).

At about 10 months of age, the infant begins to develop a differential response to speech stimuli. At this age, the child responds to his or her name, and by 12 months of age simple verbal commands are effective. By 18 to 24 months of age, the child can point to a parent or to a familiar object. In other words, as the child's receptive vocabulary develops, speech signals can be used to assess the integrity of the auditory system. While awareness of a speech stimulus can be demonstrated in both neonates and young infants, the human voice can be used most effectively to elicit behavioral responses in older infants (Northern and Downs, 1974; Wilson, 1978).

From the preceding discussion, one can appreciate the more refined nature of the infant's responses to sound in comparison to those of the neonate. The responses typical of the infant require less intense and more familiar stimuli and can provide a more quantitative assessment of the child's hearing than can responses typical of neonates.

The Young Child

The precursors of the adult voluntary response to sound are apparent in the two to three year old child, and by five years of age a child gives responses to auditory stimuli that are quite similar to those of the adult. In other words, the child is capable of producing a voluntary behavioral response to stimuli and at stimulus intensity levels that approximate adult threshold values. With the appropriate assessment technique, frequency-specific air and bone conduction thresholds are obtainable along with an indication of the reception of speech signals.

Although the young child is capable of refined voluntary responses, assessment procedures must be modified from those used with the adult in order to gain the cooperation of the child and thereby increase test reliability. "Play" audiometry techniques are particularly useful for assessing the young child, but only the exceptional two year old child will cooperate for the test. By 3 to 3½ years, however, such techniques are usually successful in obtaining voluntary behavioral responses to sound.

These age-related auditory responses demonstrate that responsivity develops from the reflex level in the neonate to the refined voluntary level in the young child. It should be noted that the responses described are those of normal children in whom there is a close correspondence between mental and chronologic age. In the developmentally delayed or mentally retarded child, such correspondence does not exist, and one must expect responses more appropriate to the age at which the child is functioning. Northern and

Downs (1974) suggest that this phenomenon can be used to one's advantage since the responses a child exhibits can give a gross estimation of developmental status.

The fact that behavioral assessment of hearing in infants and children must be conducted with techniques that require responses commensurate to the child's repertoire should now be apparent. Representative behavioral techniques include behavior observation audiometry, visual reinforcement audiometry, tangible reinforcement audiometry, play audiometry, and conventional audiometry.

Behavioral Observation Audiometry

Behavioral observation audiometry (BOA) is a term first used by Lloyd and Young (1969) to describe procedures for identifying neonates with impaired hearing. Many audiologists use this technique for neonates and infants less than 12 months of age. Several investigators (Murphy, 1961; Northern and Downs, 1974; Thompson and Weber, 1974) have reported norms for BOA in infants up to 24 months of age.

Very basically, BOA is any procedure in which the examiner presents a stimulus sound and observes the associated behavioral response of the child. True BOA procedures do not incorporate conditioning procedures and merely require the observation of the child's unconditioned responses. BOA is a viable screening procedure in the physician's office, or it can be used as a more diagnostic assessment tool in major audiology centers devoted to pediatric testing.

In the office setting, the baby typically is seated on the mother's lap, and the physician or examiner presents the stimulus to either of the baby's ears and observes the associated behavioral response. The age-related auditory responses, discussed in the previous section, are used as criteria for possible impairment. Simple noisemakers, such as rattles, squeak toys, Oriental bells, and crinkled onion-skin paper are common stimulus devices in the office setting. These devices produce sounds composed of a broad range of frequencies of indeterminant relative intensities, and consequently their use provides only a gross qualitative estimate of the normality of hearing. The chance for false positive judgments of impairment is usually small, since the child who fails to respond is at high risk for significant hearing impairment. Such a child must be referred for more extensive testing at a center devoted to pediatric hearing assessment.

False negative judgments of impairment, however, could be more serious, since a child with a significant high-frequency hearing loss may respond to a broad-frequency noise-maker in an apparently normal fashion. Concomitant persistence of parental or grandparental concern about the hearing of such children should alert the physician to the need for referral for more extensive tests. A comprehensive discussion of the use of noise-makers is presented by Northern and Downs (1974), and the reader intending to use these devices will profit from their suggestions.

In audiology centers concerned with assessing hearing in children, BOA is conducted in a manner different from the way it is performed in the office setting. The test environment is carefully controlled, and only calibrated stimuli are used. To avoid the unwanted influence of background sounds, the child is tested in a sound-treated test booth designed to attenuate ambient noise. To permit stimulation from either side, the child is situated (usually on the mother's lap) between two loudspeakers. Stimuli are presented through the loudspeakers from an adjoining control room with calibrated pure tone and speech audiometric equipment. The examiner is usually an experienced audiologist who observes the child through a window between the control room and the test booth. In some centers, two examiners conduct the test: one presents the stimuli from the control room, and the other, located in the test booth, observes the child's responses.

BOA in an audiology center is aimed at determining response thresholds for various stimuli, that is, the minimum intensity necessary to elicit a response on at least 50 per cent of the trials at that intensity. Pure tones, noise, and speech signals are commonly employed. When pure tones through loudspeakers are used, the tones are "warbled," which means they are electronically modulated in either frequency or amplitude to avoid standing waves in the test booth that would make stimulus intensity calibration impossible. These warbled tones have characteristic center frequencies; 500, 1000, 2000, and 4000 Hertz (Hz) are commonly used. Narrow bands of noise, with energy concentrated around the same frequencies, are used in

Table 8B–1   AUDITORY BEHAVIORAL INDEX FOR INFANTS*

Age	Noisemakers (Approx. SPL)	Warbled Pure Tones (Re: Audiometric Zero)	Speech (Re: Audiometric Zero)	Expected Response	Startle to Speech (Re: Audiometric Zero)
0–6 wk.	50–70 dB	78 dB (SD = 6 dB)	40–60 dB	Eye-widening, eye-blink, stirring or arousal from sleep, startle	65 dB
6 wk.–4 mo.	50–60 dB	70 dB (SD = 10 dB)	47 dB (SD = 2 dB)	Eye-widening, eye-shift, eye-blink, quieting, beginning rudimentary head turn by 4 mo.	65 dB
4–7 mo.	40–50 dB	51 dB (SD = 9 dB)	21 dB (SD = 8 dB)	Head-turn on lateral plane toward sound; listening attitude	65 dB
7–9 mo.	30–40 dB	45 dB (SD = 15 dB)	15 dB (SD = 7 dB)	Direct localization of sounds to side, indirectly below ear level	65 dB
9–13 mo.	25–35 dB	38 dB (SD = 8 dB)	8 dB (SD = 7 dB)	Direct localization of sounds to side, directly below ear level, indirectly above ear level	65 dB
13–16 mo.	25–30 dB	32 dB (SD = 10 dB)	5 dB (SD = 5 dB)	Direct localization of sound on side, above and below	65 dB
16–21 mo.	25 dB	25 dB (SD = 10 dB)	5 dB (SD = 1 db)	Direct localization of sound on side, above and below	65 dB
21–24 mo.	25 dB	26 dB (SD = 10 dB)	3 dB (SD = 2 dB)	Direct localization of sound on side, above and below	65 dB

*With permission from Northern, J. L., and Downs, M. P. 1974. Hearing in Children. Baltimore, Williams and Wilkins.

some centers as alternatives to warbled pure tone signals. Speech stimuli are also used and usually consist of the examiner's live voice, a recording of the parent's voice, or other recorded speech materials.

The Auditory Behavior Index for Infants, suggested by Northern and Downs (1974), is shown in Table 8–1 and serves as an example of BOA response norms that can be used to interpret the responses of a given child. Table 8B–1 shows the nature of the responses that can be expected for a child of a given age and the average stimulus levels necessary to produce the response for noisemakers, warbled pure tones, and speech signals. Noisemaker data are included in this table, but specific noisemakers were selected by the authors, and an analysis of the frequency and

intensity characteristics of the sounds produced by the selected devices was conducted.

As the data in Table 8–1 illustrate, the stimulus level necessary to produce a response decreases as age of the child increases. This is apparent for all three stimulus types shown. It is interesting also to note that only speech thresholds approximate normal adult levels and only for the child 12 months or older. Consequently, the responses obtained with BOA are interpreted as either age-appropriate or age-inappropriate with impairment inferred in the latter case, particularly for children less than 12 months of age.

Murphy (1961) and Thompson and Weber (1974) also published norms that can be used to interpret BOA results. Murphy (1961) found that normal infants required less stimulus intensity to elicit a response than was suggested by Northern and Downs (1974). Thompson and Weber (1974) found that normal infants responded to a wide range of stimulus intensities. These discrepancies have motivated many centers to generate their own norms for BOA. Wilson (1978) suggests that the response variability and unpredictable observer bias inherent in BOA preclude its use as an assessment tool and that it should serve only as an initial screening procedure to determine levels for further testing.

BOA, then, is a term used to describe a technique whereby a child's behavioral response to a variety of stimulus sounds is observed. The procedure is most commonly used to evaluate neonates and infants less than 12 months of age. The nature of the stimulus, the child's prestimulus activity, response habituation, and the unpredictable bias of the observer are factors that can endanger the reliability of the procedure as an assessment tool. For children less than 12 months of age, BOA should be considered as a subjective screening procedure that serves best to detect significant auditory impairment.

Modification of BOA procedures, incorporating conditioning principles, has been investigated as an alternative approach to assessing the auditory response of infants. As a result, visual reinforcement audiometry (Suzuki and Ogiba, 1960, 1961; Suzuki et al., 1972; Liden and Kankkunnen, 1969; Warren, 1972; Wilson et al., 1976) and tangible reinforcement audiometry (Lloyd et al., 1968; Fulton et al., 1975; Wilson and Decker, unpublished) have been used widely as clinical assessment tools.

Visual Reinforcement Audiometry

This assessment technique also involves the presentation of a stimulus sound and the observation of the child's associated behavioral response. The response, however, is rewarded with a visual reinforcer such as a blinking light, an illuminated picture or toy, or an animated toy that is located above the loudspeaker through which the stimulus is presented. This approach serves to strengthen the child's response to the sound, to decrease the effects of response habituation, and to increase the examiner's control of the child's responses.

In 1960, Suzuki and Ogiba suggested this technique to condition the "orientation" or localization reflex in young infants, and many clinics refer to the test as conditioning orientation reflex audiometry or CORA. As Wilson (1978) points out, however, the technique can be used for children who do not exhibit an unconditional orientation reflex, and consequently the general term visual reinforcement audiometry (VRA) is probably more appropriate.

VRA is most successful for assessing infants from 12 to 24 months of age, but several authors (Haug et al., 1967; Wilson et al., 1976; Moore et al., 1977) have demonstrated its effectiveness for infants as young as five months.

In the early VRA approaches, a simple visual reinforcer, such as a blinking light or illuminated toy, was used to reward localization responses. However, Moore and colleagues (1975) showed that a complex visual reinforcer (an animated toy) elicited a greater number of responses in normal 12 to 18 month old infants than did a simple blinking light reward. An animated toy has also been shown to be effective in rewarding responses in infants five to 12 months of age but not in infants less than four months of age (Moore et al., 1977).

Wilson (1978) cited the work of Wilson and coworkers (1976) and Thompson and Weber (1974) to demonstrate that VRA with an animated toy reward yielded thresholds that were significantly lower than those obtained with conventional BOA. In addition, the range of stimulus intensities required to elicit a response was significantly less with the VRA procedure, and the actual thresholds were not far removed from normal adult values.

Consequently, VRA is a particularly viable procedure for assessing auditory localization responses in infants as young as five months, and the technique is especially useful in providing hearing thresholds for 12 to 24 month old infants. This assessment tool appears to be reliable, to produce responses in normal infants to a narrow range of stimulus intensities, and to reflect response thresholds in normal infants that approximate adult values.

Tangible Reinforcement Audiometry

This technique uses tangible reinforcement, such as candy, sugar-coated cereal, or other edibles, to reward the child for pressing a bar when the stimulus is heard. A special apparatus is used that dispenses the reward when the bar is pressed. The appropriate term to describe this approach is "tangible reinforcement operant conditioning audiometry" (TROCA), and it is described by Lloyd and coworkers (1968) as a technique applicable for use with severely retarded children. Subsequent studies (Fulton et al., 1975; Wilson, 1978) have reported the utility of TROCA in obtaining auditory thresholds in infants. Fulton and colleagues (1975) used earphones in their study and obtained thresholds at the standard audiometric test frequencies, but they were able to do so only in infants 12 months of age or older. These same investigators found that an average of 11.4 test sessions was required for earphone testing.

In 1977, Wilson and Decker (Wilson, 1978) used both TROCA and VROCA (the same technique using visual reinforcement instead of a tangible reward) to assess 7 to 20 month old infants with warbled tone stimuli presented through loudspeakers. These investigators found that an average of four test sessions was required to establish thresholds. Of the infants less than 12 months of age, 64 per cent were successfully tested, while 84 per cent of the 13 to 20 month old children were successfully evaluated.

Owing to the special equipment required and the inordinate amount of time necessary for accurate threshold determination, TROCA has not been used widely in clinical settings as a primary assessment procedure. Yet the technique is quite promising as a tool for the assessment of difficult-to-test children such as the severely mentally retarded.

Play Audiometry

The behavioral assessment techniques discussed thus far are applied best to children less than three years of age. At two years of age a child can yield voluntary responses to sound that are premature prototypes of the adult response. Conventional audiometric techniques can be used, but they must be modified to be more interesting for the young child. This is accomplished by structuring the test situation in such a manner that the child can appropriately respond to stimuli by participating in a form of "play" activity. For this reason, the technique is often called "play" audiometry. It can be used for assess-

ing hearing levels for both speech and pure tone stimuli. Hearing levels for speech signals are determined by placing a small group of pictures or objects in front of the child and having the child identify the appropriate object or picture that is named through the loudspeaker or earphone by the examiner. The need for pictures or objects usually ends by four years of age, at which time the child can usually repeat the words presented by the examiner.

Play audiometry can provide air and bone conduction threshold information, but this requires a considerable amount of flexibility and creativity on the part of the examiner. A play activity must be used that (1) interests the child and (2) permits the child to respond appropriately while "playing." A common approach is to use a series of colored discs of different sizes that are stacked on a peg. The child is instructed to hold a disc up to his or her ear, and when the "bell" comes on to stack the disc on the peg. With a short practice session, the child can be taught to respond appropriately as stimulus frequency and intensity are varied. This technique is ideal for the two to five year old child but can also be helpful for evaluating chronologically older children who are mentally retarded or emotionally disturbed (Barr, 1955; Darley, 1961). Of course, there is nothing sacred about the colored discs on a peg, and a variety of other activities can be and have been used successfully, but the general principle underlying the technique is the same.

Conventional Audiometry

The use of conventional audiometric techniques is traditionally reserved for the child five years and older. Yet there are a surprising number of 3½ and four year olds who can be tested with conventional means. These techniques include pure tone and speech audiometry to determine air and bone conduction thresholds for tones, speech reception thresholds, and speech discrimination ability. The word list used for testing speech discrimination ability in the adult is typically beyond the capabilities of the young child, and pediatric lists, such as Haskins' PBK series (Haskins, 1949) are more suitable. In addition, the child who has difficulty repeating words can be evaluated with picture identification tests that are designed to assess word intelligibility. The Word Intelligibility with Pictures Identification (WIPI) test (Ross and Lerman, 1970) is a good example of such a test.

The Audiogram and Hearing Loss

The audiogram is a graphic representation of a child's hearing thresholds for air and bone conducted pure tone stimuli at octave frequencies from 250 Hz to 8000 Hz.* The octave stimulus frequencies are represented on the audiogram abscissa, and stimulus intensities, in decibels referenced to hearing level (dBHL, re:ANSI, 1969), are shown on the ordinate. At each stimulus frequency, coded symbols are used to denote threshold. An example of the audiogram form and coded symbols suggested by the American Speech and Hearing Association (ASHA, 1974) is shown in Figures 8B–1*A* and *B*, respectively.

A child's air conduction thresholds at the tested stimulus frequencies are connected with a solid line, and in some centers bone conduction thresholds are linked with a dashed line. Ordinarily the thresholds for both ears are plotted on the same graph, but some clinicians prefer to use a separate graph for each ear. For clarity, when a single graph is used, the right ear threshold symbols are written in red and those of the left ear in blue.

The audiogram most often represents the threshold obtained with either play or conventional audiometry through earphones. Thresholds obtained with warbled pure tones or narrow band noise through loudspeakers can be plotted using a "W" to denote thresholds for the former and "NBN" for the latter.

The audiogram indicates whether hearing is normal or impaired and, if impaired, the nature and degree of the hearing loss. Several guidelines can be used to retrieve this information from the audiogram. The decision as to whether certain results indicate normal or impaired hearing has been the subject of considerable disagreement among various clinicians and investigators, particularly in the context of hearing loss in children. Several authors (Lierle, 1959; Silverman, 1960; Goodman, 1965) have suggested

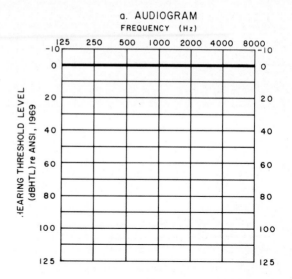

Figure 8B–1 The audiogram (*a*) and the symbols (*b*) used to denote hearing thresholds suggested by the American Speech and Hearing Association (1974).

that impairment begins when the average air conduction threshold at 500, 1000, and 2000 Hz exceeds 25 dBHL (ANSI, 1969). Northern and Downs (1974), on the other hand, suggest that significant impairment begins when the average threshold exceeds 15 dBHL, and such children may benefit from trial amplification with a hearing aid. As a compromise, one may consider 20 dBHL as the limit of normal hearing, with impairment beginning when air conducted sound thresholds exceed this level. As we shall see, however, this compromise may overlook significant conductive hearing loss.

Consequently, when the air and bone conduction thresholds of a given child are equal

---

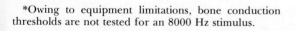

*Owing to equipment limitations, bone conduction thresholds are not tested for an 8000 Hz stimulus.

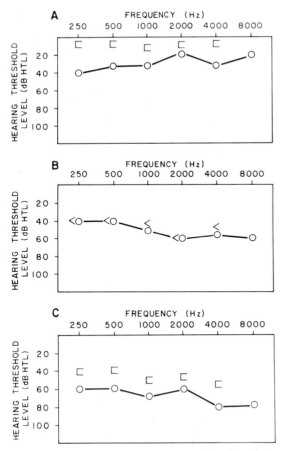

Figure 8B–2 Sample audiograms showing three different types of hearing loss in the right ear: *A*, conductive hearing loss; *B*, sensorineural hearing loss; and *C*, mixed hearing loss.

The nature of the hearing loss is sensorineural when the audiogram shows both air and bone conduction thresholds to be elevated but within 10 dB of each other (Fig. 8B–2B). When both air and bone conduction thresholds are elevated but are separated by more than 10 dB, the hearing loss is mixed in nature, as shown in Figure 8B–2C.

Aside from indicating the nature of the hearing impairment, if any, the audiogram also suggests the degree of impairment based on the average decibel threshold elevation for air conduction scores at 500, 1000, and 2000 Hz. Calculating the percentage of hearing impairment (Lierle, 1959) is one method of quantifying the degree of hearing loss indicated on the audiogram. In this method, each decibel of average hearing loss exceeding 26 dBHL (ANSI, 1969) is multiplied by 1.5 per cent, and an average loss of 93 dB HL represents 100 per cent impairment. This approach is useful in calculating compensation schemes for adults with occupation-related hearing losses, but it is not practical for describing hearing loss in children.

A preferable way to denote the degree of hearing loss in a child is to rate the loss as mild, moderate, moderately severe, severe, or profound. The average hearing thresholds (ANSI, 1969) associated with these ratings are 21 to 40 dB (mild), 41 to 55 dB (moderate), 56 to 70 dB (moderately severe), 71 to 90 dB (severe), and 91 dB or greater (profound). These levels are based on those suggested by Goodman (1965) with the mild hearing loss category adjusted to include a 20 dBHL lower limit of normal hearing.

Hence, the audiogram can describe the nature and degree of hearing impairment. This information can be used to infer the probable handicap a child with a particular hearing loss might realize. In this context, a description of the loss as either unilateral or bilateral is relevant. A bilateral impairment has more serious implications than a unilateral loss. However, Schwartz and Konkle (Chapter 88) present an interesting discussion of the impact of unilateral versus bilateral impairment.

The probable effects of bilateral hearing impairment on a child's function will depend on the degree of impairment, whether the impairment is conductive or sensorineural, and, if sensorineural, whether the loss is congenital or acquired. Downs (1974) outlined the interplay of these factors, and her suggestions are shown in Table 8B–2.

(or within 10 dB of each other) and 20 dBHL or better, hearing is within normal limits. When the audiogram reflects impaired hearing, the relative threshold of air and bone conduction will indicate the nature of the hearing loss — conductive, sensorineural, or mixed.

The audiogram of a child with a conductive hearing loss shows normal bone conduction thresholds and elevated air conduction thresholds (Fig. 8B–2A). The exception to this general guideline would be a case in which air conduction thresholds were within the 20 dB normal limit but the bone conduction thresholds were at least 15 dB better. In other words, the bone conduction scores could be −5 or 0 dBHL, and the air conduction scores would be 15 or 20 dBHL. This, too, would be considered a conductive impairment owing to the significant air-bone "gap" of 15 dB or more.

Table 8B–2 PROBABLE HANDICAPPED CONDITIONS ASSOCIATED
WITH HEARING LOSS*

Conductive Hearing Loss

Condition	Degree of Loss at Present	Probable Effect on Function
Evidence of past ear disease 1. Perforation 2. Scarring	5–20 dB	1. Subtle auditory dysfunction 2. Infantile speech 3. Articulation problems 4. Language retardation
Serous otitis	10–30 dB	1. Inattention 2. Speech and language retardation if persistent
Chronic otitis	15–55 dB	1. Inattention 2. Speech and language retardation if persistent
Middle ear anomaly	30–65 dB	1. Marked articulation problems 2. Serious language retardation

Sensorineural Hearing Loss

Condition	Degree of Loss	Probable Effect on Function	
Congenital loss	25–40 dB	Mild speech and language retardation	
	40–65 dB	Moderate to severe speech and language retardation	If habilitation is not started very early
	70–85 dB	Severe speech and language retardation	
	85 dB +	No speech or language	
Acquired loss	25–100 dB	If acquired after 2 years of age, speech and language need not be retarded if rehabilitation begins promptly. Speech deterioration if loss is profound.	

*From Downs, 1974, personal communication.

Behavioral Assessment Techniques — Summary

The material presented thus far has shown that a variety of age-dependent behavioral techniques are available for the audiologic assessment of neonates, infants, and young children. Ordinarily, the techniques for neonates and infants up to about four months of age provide only qualitative information about the auditory function of the child in question (hearing is either normal or impaired). At about four months of age, quantitative threshold information is obtainable with some behavioral techniques, particularly those involving conditioning procedures. By three years of age, most children can be assessed with "play" audiometric techniques, and from this age a pure tone audiogram is obtainable, which can indicate the nature and degree of impairment and the probable effect the loss might have on the child's function.

The various assessment techniques monitor a continuum of auditory responsivity from gross auditory reflexes to refined voluntary responses. Certain techniques are better suited for evaluating behavior at opposite ends of this continuum, while other techniques (for example, VRA and TROCA) can assess responsivity throughout the continuum. By knowing where on the continuum the child falls, the appropriate test can be employed, and the judgment as to whether the hearing is normal or impaired can be made on the basis of the appropriateness of the child's responses.

NONBEHAVIORAL ASSESSMENT TECHNIQUES

Nonbehavioral techniques to assess hearing include acoustic impedance measurements, auditory electric response recordings, cardiac audiometry, and respiration audiometry. Acoustic impedance measurements should be a routine part of the assessment of any child, with the possible exception of infants less than seven months old, in whom Paradise and colleagues (1976) suggest results can be misleading. The remaining nonbehavioral techniques are ordinarily used when the results of behavioral tests are ambiguous or unobtainable.

Nonbehavioral techniques are relatively independent of the child's behavioral response and rely instead on changes in the child's physiologic status in response to sound. These techniques are often referred to as "objective" tests, but they should not be considered to be completely objective since the interpretation of the results is often the subjective decision of the examiner. Nonbehavioral assessment techniques are comparatively objective when contrasted with the far more subjective behavioral procedures.

Acoustic Impedance Measurements

The major contribution of acoustic impedance measurements is that by measuring the degree of impedance a sound encounters at the tympanic membrane, certain inferences can be made about the status of the middle ear mechanism as a whole. This technique is particularly useful for assessing hearing in children when audiometric data may be inadequate to identify conductive impairment or when such data are poorly correlated with maladies that affect the middle ear (as in some cases of otitis media with effusion).

A mechanical means for measuring acoustic impedance was first described by Metz (1946), but in the United States it was not until much later that Zwislocki (1963) in-

troduced a measurement device that was the subject of several clinical investigations (Feldman, 1963; 1967; Nilges et al., 1969; Zwislocki and Feldman, 1970). The Scandinavians can be credited with advancing the clinical applications of acoustic impedance measurements originally introduced by Metz (1946). Terkildsen and Scott-Nielsen (1960) introduced the electroacoustic impedance bridge, which is the electronic version of Metz's original device and considerably more amenable to clinical use than Zwislocki's mechanical version. In 1970, papers by Alberti and Kristensen (1970) and Jerger (1970) marked the beginning of an extensive research effort in this country directed at making acoustic impedance measurements clinically useful.

A detailed discussion of the physical principles of acoustic impedance is beyond the scope of this chapter; however, such a discussion can be found in Northern and Grimes (1978). The basic principles of acoustic impedance measurement with an electroacoustic impedance bridge will be presented here.

Quite simply, the electroacoustic impedance bridge uses a miniature microphone and related circuitry to monitor the impedance an input sound encounters at the tympanic membrane. The input sound is a low-frequency (220 Hz) pure tone, usually called the probe tone.* The microphone circuit detects increased probe tone intensity (in the ear canal) when the encountered impedance is high and decreased intensity when the impedance encountered is low. The reason is that the intensity of a sound in a cavity (such as the ear canal) is inversely proportional to the size of the cavity. When impedance at the tympanic membrane is high, much of the probe tone energy is reflected, the cavity appears small to the microphone circuit, and the measured probe tone intensity is high. The reverse is true when the encountered impedance is low: Minimal probe tone energy is reflected, the cavity appears large, and the measured probe tone intensity is low.

Certain pathologic conditions of the middle ear will affect the acoustic impedance an input sound encounters at the tympanic membrane. Conditions that increase the stiff-

---

*Higher probe tone frequencies (e.g., 660 Hz or 800 Hz) are used by some investigators (Liden et al., 1970; Feldman, 1976). Interpretation of these measurements is somewhat different. For simplicity, this chapter will only discuss measurements obtained with a 220 Hz probe tone.

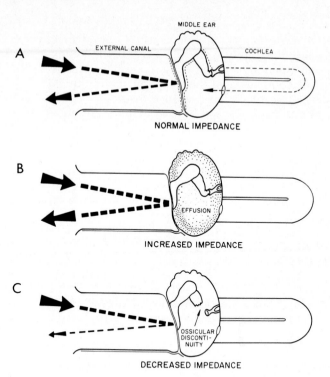

Figure 8B–3 A simplified diagram demonstrating that middle ear conditions influence impedance and, consequently, the transmission/reflection of an input sound. In the normal ear (A), more input sound energy is transmitted than is reflected. The increased impedance caused by a middle ear effusion (B) results in a decrease in transmitted energy and an increase in the amount reflected. An ossicular discontinuity (C) results in decreased impedance and an increase in transmitted energy with a much smaller proportion of reflected energy (even less than observed in the normal ear).

ness characteristics of the middle ear, such as ossicular fixation or some forms of otitis media, can significantly increase acoustic impedance. Ossicular discontinuity or other conditions that reduce the stiffness characteristics of the system can reduce the degree of measured acoustic impedance. Consequently, the measurement of significantly increased or reduced acoustic impedance can permit inferences to be made about middle ear status, and associations with specific pathologic conditions are possible (Fig. 8B–3).

Figure 8B–4 presents a simplified diagram of the electroacoustic impedance bridge and the manner in which the device is coupled to the ear for clinical measurements. A "probe" tip is sealed into the ear canal with a small rubber cuff. The probe tip has three small apertures. One aperture serves as an avenue for delivering the probe tone into the sealed ear canal, and the second aperture leads from the ear canal to a miniature microphone and related circuitry. The third aperture is connected to an air pump and manometer and provides a means for varying air pressure in the sealed ear canal.

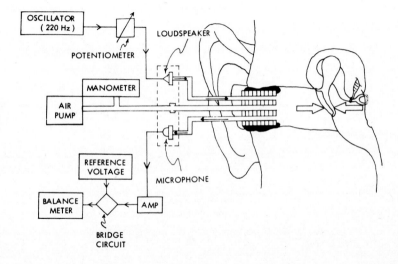

Figure 8B–4 A component diagram of the electroacoustic impedance bridge.

Acoustic impedance measurements involve three tests: tympanometry, static compliance, and the acoustic middle ear muscle reflex. Tympanometry and static compliance assess the compliance of the tympanic membrane in relation to the air pressure in the ear canal. Compliance is used here to denote the sound transmission characteristics of the tympanic membrane and by inference the encountered impedance. High tympanic membrane compliance denotes minimal acoustic impedance, and low compliance infers high acoustic impedance.

Tympanometry measures compliance across a range of varying air pressures and is sometimes called a "dynamic" compliance measure. Static compliance measurements are called "static" because compliance is compared under two fixed air pressure conditions. The acoustic middle ear muscle reflex is the third impedance test and involves stimulating the ear with an intense sound and detecting the associated change in impedance due to the contraction of the middle ear muscles.

Tympanometry

Tympanometry assesses the change in tympanic membrane compliance as air pressure is varied in the ear canal. The results are plotted on a chart, called a tympanogram, which graphically displays compliance as a function of air pressure. Compliance is represented on the ordinate in arbitrary units, and air pressure on the abscissa in millimeters of water pressure (mm H_2O).

Tympanometry is performed by first introducing 200 mm H_2O pressure into the sealed ear canal and then varying the pressure, usually from positive to negative, to -400 or -600 mm H_2O pressure. The associated change in compliance is transferred to the tympanogram either by hand or automatically with an X-Y plotter connected to the output of the impedance bridge's balance meter circuit.

The interaction of the impedance bridge and the ear in generating a tympanogram can be understood with the assistance of Figure 8B–5. With 200 mm H_2O pressure in the ear

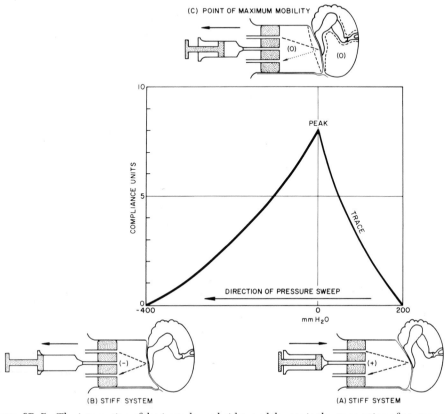

Figure 8B–5 The interaction of the impedance bridge and the ear in the generation of a tympanogram (see text).

canal, the tympanic membrane is effectively clamped, and compliance is minimal (Fig. 8B–5). In this situation, the bridge microphone circuit measures high probe tone intensity, and correspondingly the tympanogram trace is located at the bottom of the ordinate, at 200 mm H_2O pressure on the abscissa.

As pressure is released, the tympanogram begins to rise, indicating increased compliance and decreased probe tone intensity in the canal. As pressure is released further, the tympanogram will continue to rise until, at a certain air pressure value, it reverses direction and begins to fall (Fig. 8B–5). This reversal indicates that compliance is now decreasing and the measured probe tone intensity is increasing.

Consequently, tympanic membrane compliance is maximal at the point where the tympanogram reverses direction, and this also indicates where the probe tone intensity, measured in the canal, is lowest. This reversal point is often called the "peak" of the tympanogram or the point of maximal compliance (Fig. 8B–5C).

The tympanogram can be interpreted on the basis of three features: (1) the height of the peak, (2) the horizontal position of the peak in relation to atmospheric pressure, and (3) the rate of change in the curve height at the peak — the peak gradient (Brooks, 1969).

The height of the tympanogram peak reflects the degree of tympanic membrane compliance and the relative mobility of at least a portion of the membrane. The peak is normally located between half and full vertical scale on the tympanogram. A peak height of less than half scale is generally associated with middle ear conditions that reduce compliance or mobility. A peak height exceeding full vertical scale deflection is generally associated with conditions that increase compliance or mobility.

The horizontal location of the tympanogram peak in relation to atmospheric pressure gives an indirect approximation of the air pressure in the middle ear space. This is based on the principle that tympanic membrane compliance is maximal when the air pressure on both sides of the membrane is the same (Terkildsen and Thomsen, 1959). A number of investigators (Flisberg et al., 1963; Ingelstedt et al., 1967; Peterson and Liden, 1970; Elner et al., 1971; Renvall et al., 1975) have demonstrated that the tympanometri-

cally determined and actual middle ear pressures can differ and that the air pressure suggested by the tympanogram is influenced by tympanic membrane mobility and the volume of the middle ear space. Although the tympanometrically determined pressure may not be precisely that of the middle ear space, the horizontal position of the peak gives a general indication of pressure conditions in the middle ear, and it is consequently helpful in interpreting the tympanogram.

Figure 8B–6 demonstrates how shifts in the horizontal position of the tympanogram peak reflects pressure conditions in the middle ear. Positive and negative pressures produce corresponding shifts in the horizontal peak position, and in fact the absence of a peak can reflect extreme negative pressure in the middle ear space.

The normal range of middle ear pressure on the tympanogram has been the subject of some debate, and several values have been reported (Brooks, 1969; Jerger, 1970; Holmquist and Miller, 1972; Renvall et al., 1973; Paradise et al., 1976). In young children, there is support (Paradise et al., 1976; Schwartz et al., 1978) for a range of -150 to 50 mm H_2O pressure, inclusive, as normal. Deviations from this range can be rated as either abnormally negative or positive middle ear pressure. In children it should be realized that middle ear pressure tends to fluctuate from day to day (Cooper et al., 1974; Lewis et al., 1975; Schwartz et al., 1978), and a determination of abnormal pressure should be made on the basis of the persistence of the condition with time.

It follows that the height and horizontal position of the tympanogram peak, respectively, indicate tympanic membrane mobility and air pressure in the middle ear space. The gradient of the peak is also worthy of consideration. Recall that this feature represents the rate of change in curve height in the region of the peak. Typically, the gradient is rated as either "sharp" or "gradual." A gradual peak gradient implies a slower rate of change in curve height, which in turn implies a subtle degree of tympanic membrane "sluggishness" or a general dampening of the system's responsiveness to changes in external conditions. Gradient of the curve is a particularly pertinent feature in the tympanograms of children, since it has been found to be related to the presence of otitis media with effusion (Paradise et al., 1976).

Figure 8B–7 illustrates some commonly

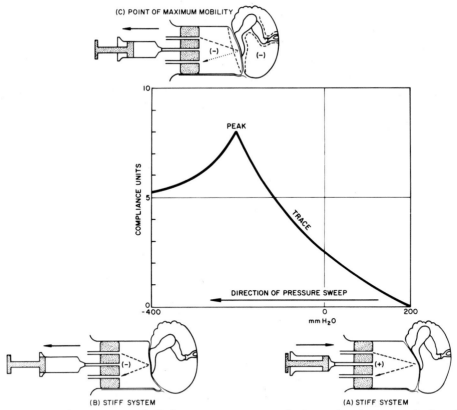

Figure 8B–6 The manner in which the tympanogram can reflect negative air pressure in the middle ear. Compliance is low when positive pressure (A) or negative pressure (B) is applied. The peak of the trace is indicative of middle ear pressure (C).

encountered types of tympanograms, with their associated middle ear pressures, tympanic membrane compliances, and presumptive conditions of the middle ear. This figure demonstrates how, in a very general way, the status of the middle ear can be inferred from the tympanogram. To make such an inference, one must consider pressure and mobility of the tympanic membrane and, in certain instances, peak gradient of the tympanogram curve.

Figure 8B–7 is intended to present general principles for the interpretation of tympanograms on the basis of pressure mobility and peak gradient. The reader must realize that the implied one-to-one relationship between tympanogram shape and specific middle ear conditions is an oversimplification. The conditions are "presumed" to be associated with given tympanograms, or, in other words, they are the "probable" associated conditions. There will be exceptions to the apparently simple relationships shown in Figure 8B–7, and tympanograms must be interpreted in

the context of other clinical information. For example, otoscopic examination and acoustic middle ear muscle reflex tests are important to the interpretation of tympanometric findings.

Several authors (Jerger, 1970; Liden et al., 1970; Paradise et al., 1976; Feldman, 1978) have suggested grouping various tympanograms into specific categories or types to facilitate their interpretation. The tympanogram categorizations of Jerger (1970) and Paradise and colleagues (1976) are of particular interest; the former has received widespread clinical use, and the latter is relevant to the pediatric population.

Jerger's (1970) classification has been used widely in the clinical setting, but it is based on only two of the three tympanogram features — peak height and horizontal position. The tympanogram types suggested by Jerger (1970) tend to oversimplify interpretation and are not validated, but since they are used in many centers, they will be given brief mention here (Fig. 8B–8).

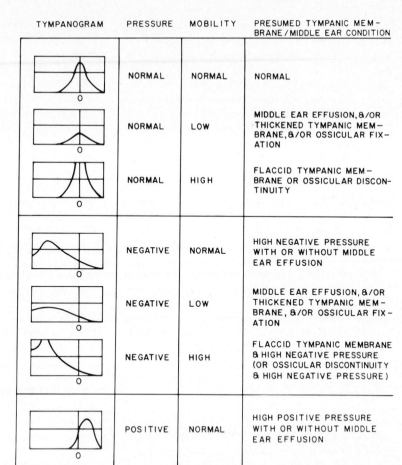

Figure 8B–7 Tympanogram types and property variants related to clinical findings.

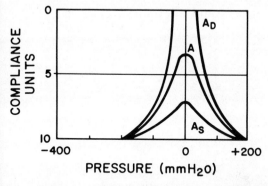

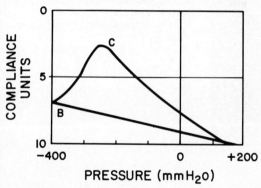

Figure 8B–8 Tympanogram classification according to Jerger (1970): A, A$_D$, A$_S$ (top graph) and B and C (bottom graph).

In Jerger's tympanogram types A, A$_S$, and A$_D$ the peaks are all placed horizontally to approximate atmospheric pressure ($\pm$ 100 mm H$_2$O), but the peak heights differ. The type A tympanogram has a peak height between half and full scale on the ordinate, and it is associated with a normal middle ear system. Type A$_S$ has a shallow peak, less than half scale on the ordinate, and is associated with conditions such as ossicular fixation and a thickened tympanic membrane in which the middle ear system demonstrates decreased mobility. The type A$_D$ tympanogram has a peak that exceeds full scale on the ordinate and is associated with a highly compliant system such as that found in ossicular disruption.

Jerger (1970) also described type B and C tympanograms. Type B is the tympanogram with no peak and is associated with otitis media with effusion, tympanic membrane perforation, or impacted cerumen. Type C tympanograms show a horizontal peak position at a pressure more negative than -100 mm H$_2$O and are generally associated with eustachian tube dysfunction.

It is of particular interest in children to identify those tympanogram types that are associated with the presence of otitis media with effusion. Several investigators (Jerger et al., 1974b; Paradise et al., 1976; Orchik et al., 1978) have confirmed the association of the so-called type B tympanogram with effusion,

but with one exception (Paradise et al., 1976), these authors concluded that other tympanogram types are poor predictors of the presence of otitis media.

Paradise and coworkers (1976) found that the probability of otitis media with effusion being present was, in tympanograms of other than type B (which they called type EFF), related to the gradient of the tympanogram peak and to a lesser extent to the height of the peak. These authors divided tympanogram shapes into seven types on the basis of the horizontal position, height, and gradient of the peak. These types represented regions on the tympanogram as shown in Figure 8B–9. The regions included normal (NL), high negative pressure (HN), high positive pressure (HP), transitional (TR), and effusion (EFF). The percentages shown in Figure 8B–9 denote the probability that ears with that tympanogram type contained effusions. The authors studied 141 children between the ages of seven months and six years; and the data are based on these examinations. The figure also shows a percentage dichotomy for the HN and TR regions. Tympanograms falling in these regions were found to reflect a higher probability of effusion if the peak gradient was gradual (g) rather than sharp (s).

Paradise and associates (1976) consequently found that tympanogram shapes or variants could be grouped into seven types —

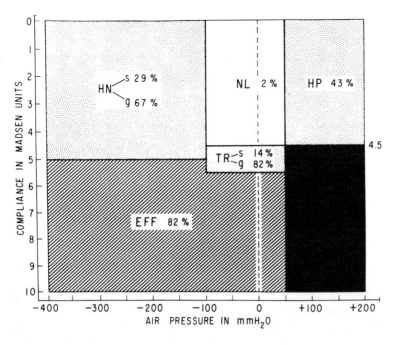

Figure 8B–9 Tympanogram classification suggested by Paradise and colleagues (1976). Percentages denote the associated incidence of effusion.

NL, HN-s, HN-g, HP, TR-s, TR-g, and EEF — and that these types were useful in detecting effusion in the children they studied.

Tympanometry, then, is a graphic representation of tympanic membrane compliance when air pressure is varied in the ear canal. The tympanogram provides an estimate of middle ear pressure and tympanic membrane mobility. The tympanogram peak height, horizontal position, and gradient can be used to infer the status of the middle ear. Tympanometry, however, is only one of three acoustic impedance measurements, and clinical judgments should not be made without a consideration of static compliance measurements and the results of the acoustic middle ear muscle reflex test. In addition, the results of the entire battery of acoustic impedance tests must be viewed in the context of other clinical findings.

Static Compliance Measurements

Static compliance measurements compare tympanic membrane compliance under two air pressure conditions: (1) with 200 mm H_2O pressure in the ear canal and (2) with a pressure in the canal that corresponds to the horizontal position of the tympanogram peak. The compliance (in cubic centimeters of equivalent volume) under the first condition is subtracted from that under the second condition, and the result is an estimate of the compliance of the middle ear system.

Extremely stiff middle ear systems generally yield very low static compliance values, and extremely compliant systems yield very high values. Between these extremes, however, the static compliance values of normal and abnormal systems tend to overlap. The extent of this overlap has essentially precluded using static compliance measurements as clinically important indicators of pathologic conditions.

When the tympanogram shows negative middle ear pressure and reduced mobility with little or no evidence of a peak, the static compliance value with 200 mm H_2O in the ear canal can be important. In these situations, a low compliance value (less than 0.4 cc) can suggest the presence of excessive cerumen or that the probe tip is resting against the canal wall. A high compliance value (greater than 1.5 cc) is suggestive of an opening in the tympanic membrane; this could be due to a perforation or the presence of a patent tympanostomy tube.

Consequently, the static compliance value with 200 mm H_2O in the ear canal can be used to confirm the reliability of the tympanogram and to detect a tympanic membrane perforation or patent tympanostomy tube. The application of this compliance value has been termed the physical volume test (PVT) by Northern and Grimes (1978) and is reported as such by some clinicians.

Acoustic Middle Ear Muscle Reflex

Acoustic impedance instrumentation can be used also to detect the contraction of the middle ear muscles, the stapedius and tensor tympani, to intensify sound stimulation. This contraction is called the acoustic middle ear muscle reflex or simply the acoustic reflex.

The anatomy of the acoustic reflex arc is described in Chapter 7. The afferent portion of the arc, up to and including the superior olivary complex, is shared with the hearing mechanism. The efferent fibers of the acoustic reflex arc arise from brain stem neuronal connections between the olivary complex and the facial nerve nucleus for the stapedius muscle and the trigeminal nerve nucleus for the tensor tympani muscle (Jepsen, 1963).

The acoustic impedance bridge indicates the status of the acoustic reflex in two ways: first, the reflex results in a stiffening of the ossicular chain and a concomitant increase in impedance; second, because the reflex is bilateral to a unilateral stimulus (the muscles of both sides contract when one ear is stimulated), an earphone can be placed on one ear to deliver an intense stimulus, and the probe tip of the impedance bridge inserted in the opposite ear can detect the impedance change caused by the reflex.

When the impedance bridge is used to detect an acoustic reflex elicited by stimulating the opposite ear, the response is commonly called the contralateral or crossed acoustic reflex. Many acoustic impedance bridges marketed today have probe tips designed both to stimulate and to detect the acoustic reflex in the same ear; the reflex is elicited and its effect on impedance is detected in the same ear. Under these conditions, the response is called the ipsilateral or uncrossed acoustic reflex.

For clinical purposes, three acoustic reflex

parameters are commonly considered. These include the reflex threshold intensity, its response amplitude decay in time, and the differential response to different types of sound stimuli. These features enable the examiner to make qualitative judgments about hearing, such as the type of impairment and the probable site of a lesion, as well as quantitative judgments, such as an estimation of the degree of hearing loss and hearing aid effectiveness.

The threshold of the acoustic reflex is operationally defined as the minimal stimulus intensity required to produce an observable change in monitored impedance. This minimal intensity, or acoustic reflex threshold, is typically specified as a certain number of decibels (dB) referenced to either "sensation level" or "hearing level." Sensation level (SL) refers to the individual's behavioral hearing threshold for a given stimulus, and hearing level (HL) refers to normal hearing for a group of young adults, i.e., 0 dB on the audiogram. For example, a reflex threshold of 85 dBHL for a 1000 Hz pure tone can also be expressed as 85 dBSL if the individual's hearing threshold for that stimulus is 0 dBHL. If the individual's hearing threshold for the same 1000 Hz pure tone is 30 dBHL, then the reflex threshold of 85 dBHL can also be expressed as 55 dBSL. These relationships between sensation level and hearing level are important to an understanding of the acoustic reflex parameters.

In adults with normal hearing, the contralateral acoustic reflex threshold for pure tones of different frequencies is approximately 85 dB poorer than behavioral hearing thresholds, i.e., 85 dBSL. The range of effective stimulus intensities is 70 to 95 dBSL (Metz, 1952; Jepsen, 1963; Alberti and Kristensen, 1970; Jerger, 1970). Approximately 20 dB less intensity is required to elicit a reflex with a broad-band noise stimulus (Metz, 1952; Jepsen, 1963; Skinner et al., 1978). Ipsilateral reflex thresholds are approximately 10 dB better than contralateral thresholds (Møller, 1962; Fria et al., 1975).

Age is an important factor relating to the presence of the acoustic reflex and its threshold. Only a small percentage of neonates exhibit an acoustic reflex when an impedance bridge with a 220 Hz probe tone frequency is used to detect the response (Kieth, 1971; McCandless and Allred, 1978). McCandless and Allred (1978) found that significantly more neonates (89 per cent) yielded acoustic

reflexes if a bridge with a 660 Hz probe tone frequency was employed. In one population of 1600 ears of school-age children (Liden and Renvall, 1978), 13 per cent had absent acoustic reflexes.

When the acoustic reflex is present in infants and young children, its threshold is slightly higher than that found in adults (Jepsen, 1963; Robertson et al., 1968). Average thresholds in neonates and infants approximate 95 dBHL (Kieth, 1971; McCandless and Allred, 1978). In school-age children the threshold is on the average 92 dBHL (Liden and Renvall, 1978). The adult with normal hearing, on the other hand, has an average threshold of about 85 dBHL (Metz, 1952; Jepsen, 1963; Jerger, 1970).

Various types of hearing impairment can influence the acoustic reflex. As Jerger and colleagues (1978) point out, the influence on the acoustic reflex of sensorineural impairment of cochlear origin is complex, but generally less difference exists between hearing and reflex thresholds (Metz, 1952). The reflex can occur at about the same absolute level as found in normal ears, but because of the elevated hearing threshold, ears with a sensorineural impairment apparently require less stimulus intensity above the hearing threshold to elicit the responses. Jerger and associates (1972) reported that the likelihood of eliciting the acoustic reflex was significantly reduced when the degree of sensorineural hearing loss exceeded 80 dBHL.

The influence of middle ear impairment and attendant conductive hearing loss on the reflex is not as straightforward, as a result of the mode of reflex stimulation. Recall that ipsilateral acoustic reflex tests stimulate and detect the response in the same ear through the impedance bridge probe tip assembly. In an impaired middle ear, the impedance is already abnormally altered, and further changes in impedance due to middle ear muscle contraction may not be observable; to be detectable, these changes may require elevated stimulus intensity levels.

It follows that ipsilateral acoustic reflex testing in an impaired middle ear will most probably yield no response; if the response is present, the threshold of the response will tend to be elevated.

The influence of middle ear impairment on the contralateral acoustic reflex may be somewhat harder to understand. The contralateral reflex will probably be absent if the middle ear having the probe tip assembly is impaired or if the impaired middle ear having the stimulus earphone has a moderate to moderately severe conductive hearing loss (Jerger et al., 1974c). The reason for the first situation was given in the previous paragraph. In the second situation, the conductive hearing loss necessitates reflex stimulus levels that may be beyond the instrument's output capabilities. For these reasons, the contralateral acoustic reflex is generally absent in cases of bilateral middle ear impairment. When the impairment is unilateral, the contralateral reflex will probably be absent for both ears, if the impaired ear has a moderate to moderately severe conductive hearing loss.

Lesions beyond the cochlea (at the eighth cranial nerve or brain stem level) can result in either an absent or elevated reflex or a reflex response amplitude that rapidly decays in time to a continuous stimulus (Anderson et al., 1970; Greisen and Rasmussen, 1970; Jerger et al., 1974a; Bosatra et al., 1975; Sheehy and Inzer, 1976; Jerger and Jerger, 1977). Anderson and colleagues (1970) first demonstrated that the acoustic reflex in eighth cranial nerve tumor cases tends to have a response amplitude that decays to half strength or less in less than 10 seconds of continuous pure tone stimulation.

Jerger and associates (1974a) and Sheehy and Inzer (1976) reported reflex findings in a larger series of such tumor cases and substantiated the clinical significance of reflex decay. However, these investigators found the reflex to be absent in most of the cases reviewed. In these studies, an abnormal reflex (absent or decaying) correctly identified 80 to 86 per cent of such retrocochlear impairments. Greisen and Rasmussen (1970) and Jerger and Jerger (1977) have demonstrated how the comparison of ipsilateral and contralateral reflexes can be used to identify eighth nerve and brain stem level impairments.

It should be apparent that the presence or absence of the acoustic reflex, its threshold, and degree of response amplitude decay can suggest a variety of underlying pathologic conditions. Consequently, the acoustic reflex alone cannot pinpoint a specific pathologic condition. Reflex findings must be viewed in the context of the tympanometric and behavioral audiometric results in order to infer the nature of hearing impairment and the possible location of the underlying lesion.

An absent acoustic reflex or a significantly elevated acoustic reflex threshold is highly suggestive of an impairment at some level of the auditory system. If the tympanogram is also abnormal, the level of impairment is likely to be the middle ear. An absent or elevated reflex with a normal tympanogram usually suggests a sensorineural impairment of either cochlear or retrocochlear origin, depending on the degree of associated sensorineural hearing loss. The probability of retrocochlear involvement is increased when the reflex is absent or elevated, and the tympanometrically normal ear has a sensorineural hearing loss of less than 80 dBHL. When the associated sensorineural hearing loss is 80 dBHL or more, an absent or elevated reflex can suggest either severe cochlear damage or a retrocochlear lesion. If the reflex occurs at essentially normal levels (70 to 100 dBHL) and does not decay in a tympanometrically normal ear with less than 80 dBHL sensorineural hearing loss, a probable location of the lesion is the cochlea.

Certain children are unable or unwilling to yield reliable behavioral hearing test results. In these cases, the reflex and tympanogram can provide evidence that corroborates impressions of the child's suspected impairment. If both the reflex and the tympanogram are normal, the likelihood of a sensorineural hearing loss exceeding 80 dBHL is low. A child with absent reflexes and a normal tympanogram in both ears, however, may well have a severe sensorineural hearing loss. Consequently, when less than reliable behavioral hearing tests suggest an impairment, measurement of the reflex and recording a tympanogram can add credence to associated clinical impressions.

Niemeyer and Sesterhenn (1974) first suggested that the difference between acoustic reflex thresholds for pure tones and broadband noise could be used to estimate the degree of hearing loss. Recall that ordinarily the reflex threshold for broad-band noise is approximately 20 dB better than that for pure tones. Niemeyer and Sesterhenn (1974) observed that this difference was reduced in ears with sensorineural hearing losses and that the reduction was systematically related to the degree of the sensorineural loss. Consequently, these authors concluded that the degree of loss could be predicted from the tone-noise difference in reflex thresholds.

The use of the acoustic reflex as a predictor of degree of hearing loss has been further investigated by several authors (Jerger et al., 1974d; Johnsen et al., 1976; Schwartz and

Sanders, 1976; Kieth, 1976; Margolis and Fox, 1977; Van Wagoner and Goodwine, 1977; Jerger et al., 1978). Generally, these investigations have shown that the tone-noise reflex threshold difference is best used to differentiate normal from impaired hearing but cannot accurately estimate the degree of associated hearing loss. An estimation of the degree of hearing loss is most effectively provided on the basis of the acoustic reflex threshold for broad-band noise, which tends to increase along with increased sensori-neural impairment (Johnsen et al., 1976; Jerger et al., 1978).

A number of investigators (McCandless and Miller, 1972; Tonnison, 1975; Denenberg and Altshuler, 1976; Rappaport and Tait, 1976; Snow and McCandless, 1976; Bragg, 1977; Rainville, 1977) have evaluated the utility of the acoustic reflex in choosing an appropriate hearing aid. In this context, the reflex is most useful in pediatric and geriatric populations when behavioral indices of hearing ability are unavailable.

In these cases, the acoustic reflex can provide information about the most effective hearing aid volume setting to avoid exceeding an individual's loudness discomfort level with a particular hearing aid. A more extensive discussion of this acoustic reflex application is given in Chapter 84. Because of the many variables involved and the lack of definitive experimental evidence, the use of the acoustic reflex in fitting hearing aids in children should be approached with caution.

The qualitative and quantitative uses of acoustic reflex data should be apparent at this point. The reflex, when interpreted in the context of tympanometry and behavioral hearing test results, can suggest the nature of impairment and the location of an underlying lesion. The response also shows promise as a tool for estimating or predicting the degree of hearing loss and for determining the suitability of a particular hearing aid for a given child. Certain clinical applications of the acoustic reflex are still in the experimental stage, but as further evidence is accumulated, a clearer picture of the response's utility will result.

Emphasis has been placed here on interpreting the three acoustic impedance measurements — tympanometry, static compliance, and the acoustic reflex — as a whole. This approach provides the best opportunity for accurate diagnostic assessment. There have been numerous attempts, however, to separate certain impedance measurements as screening tools, particularly for the detection of middle ear disease in children.

Several published investigations have evaluated the screening effectiveness of tympanometry and the acoustic reflex (Brooks, 1973; Renvall et al., 1973; Ferrer, 1974; Harker and Van Wagoner, 1974; Lewis et al., 1974; McCandless and Thomas, 1974; Orchik and Herdman, 1974; Cooper et al., 1974; Brooks, 1976; McCurdy et al., 1976; Roberts, 1976; Brooks, 1977). Brooks (1978) supported the utility of the acoustic reflex alone as a screening tool for detection of middle ear disease in children. These investigators commonly agree that impedance measurements are easy to perform, noninvasive, reliable, and highly sensitive to the presence of middle ear disease. These factors would favor the use of tympanometry and the acoustic reflex as screening measurements for the detection of disease. However, definitive data supporting the validity of using impedance measurements for screening are still lacking. Although the measurements are sensitive to disease when it is present, they are considerably less accurate in sorting out children without disease, and the percentage of false positive errors obtained is uncomfortably high (Paradise and Smith, 1978; Fria et al., unpublished). The resulting over-referral rate argues against the cost-effectiveness of mass screening for middle ear disease with acoustic impedance measurements. An excellent review of the state of the art and suggested guidelines for impedance screening for middle ear disease in children was presented at a symposium on this topic, the proceedings of which were published by Harford and colleagues in 1978.

Auditory Electric Responses

A variety of terms have been used to refer to this nonbehavioral assessment technique, including electric response audiometry (ERA), electroencephalographic (EEG) audiometry, and auditory evoked potentials (AEPs). However, the measured events are more appropriately called auditory electric responses. The technique is not routinely used for audiologic assessment; it is ordinarily used to evaluate children in whom behavioral hearing test information is either unobtainable or unreliable.

It would be possible to devote an entire chapter to auditory electric responses alone. In fact, the interested reader will find chapters by Gardi and Mendel (1977), Glatke (1978), McCandless (1978), Mendel (1977a, 1977b), and Skinner (1978) quite thorough in their treatment of the topic. The monograph entitled "Principles of Electric Response Audiometry" by Hallowell Davis (1976) is an additional excellent reference. The present chapter will not attempt to cover the entire area in as much depth but instead will offer a brief description of component auditory electric responses and how they are measured. A more extensive discussion will be given for those responses that are particularly valuable for evaluating hearing in children. Finally, a pragmatic approach will be taken that identifies those children to whom the procedure is most applicable.

There are several component auditory electric responses, and each component response occurs in a different time frame following stimulus onset. These components and their related time frames include (1) the "first" components — 0 to 2 msec, (2) the "fast" components — 0 to 10 msec, (3) the "middle" components — 0 to 50 msec, (4) the "slow" components — 0 to 300 msec; and (5) the "late" components — 0 to 800 msec.

Each of these components reflects electrical activity from different anatomic levels in the auditory system; the earlier components are from peripheral and brain stem levels, and the latter components are from midbrain and cortical levels.

Figure 8B–10 shows a diagram of the equipment used for evoked potential tests. Three miniature electrodes are used to record these responses. An "active" electrode is placed either in close proximity or in a favorable orientation to the neural generators responsible for the response component of interest. The "reference" electrode is placed on a site that is presumably "quiet" with respect to the component being measured. The third, or "ground," electrode is placed on an indifferent site — usually the forehead or contralateral neck or mastoid process. The actual placement of active, reference, and ground electrodes will vary with the component of interest.

The activity from the recording electrodes is then amplified, filtered, and analyzed by a special "averaging" computer. In essence the computer serves to "average out" background EEG and myogenic activity, thereby enhancing the response associated with multiple stimulus presentations. The computer analysis is "triggered" at the onset of each stimulus and continues for the time frame corresponding to the response component being measured.

Excessive muscle activity, as well as electrical artifacts from the surrounding environment, or line current inadequacies, can obliterate an otherwise observable electric response. Consequently, the child must be relaxed or preferably asleep. In addition, the test environment must be conducive to accurate recordings; the environment must be void of nearby sources of electrical artifacts,

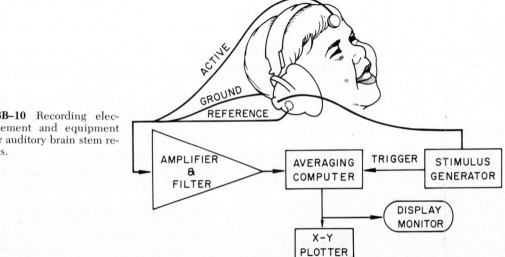

Figure 8B–10 Recording electrode placement and equipment diagram for auditory brain stem response tests.

such as transformers or fluorescent light ballasts, and adequate line current grounding is essential. These contaminating variables can seriously influence the interpretation of recordings.

In general, auditory electric responses provide perhaps the best data for nonbehavioral assessment of hearing and the auditory system's responsivity in children. However, all response components are not equally useful: The validity of the slow (0 to 300 msec) and late (0 to 800 msec) components for evaluating infants and children is still open to question (Mendel, 1977b), although these components can provide useful clinical information in an older child who is awake, cooperative, and alert (however, such a child is not often referred for such testing). Usually the child who is a candidate for auditory electric response testing is either too young, or unable, or unwilling to cooperate for conventional hearing tests.

With regard to the slow component, the inherent degree of intersubject and intrasubject variability, and of the variability due to the age and attentive state of the child can lead to significant clinical error (Barnet and Goodwin, 1965; Rapin and Bergman, 1969; Goodhill et al., 1970). In addition, if drugs are used to induce sleep in the child, the reliability of the slow components is adversely influenced (Davis, 1973; Skinner and Shimota, 1975). According to Davis (1976), the middle components show promise as tools for evaluating infants and children, but the clinical acceptance of these components has not been widespread. An in-depth discussion of the middle components is given by Mendel (1977b).

The first (0 to 2 msec) and fast (0 to 10 msec) components are rapidly gaining acceptance as clinical tools for assessing children. The common names for these components are electrocochleography (ECOCHG) and the auditory brainstem response (ABR), respectively.

Electrocochleography (ECOCHG)

These first components reflect cochlear and eighth cranial nerve activity; the latter is also known as the whole-nerve action potential or simply the eighth nerve action potential. The eighth nerve action potential is the response of interest in the procedure.

ECOCHG requires that the active electrode be placed in close proximity to the neural generator of the response (the eighth cranial nerve). For this reason, the most effective active electrode placement is through the tympanic membrane and onto the promontory in the middle ear (Aran, 1971; Eggermont et al., 1974). Because this electrode placement requires a surgical procedure and a general anesthetic in children, other less invasive electrode placements have been tried. The ear canal appears to be a reasonable compromise location for the active electrode in ECOCHG (Yoshie et al., 1967; Coats and Dickey, 1970; Salomon and Elberling, 1971; Cullen et al., 1972; Elberling, 1974). The compromise involved, however, is that the response is an order of magnitude smaller at this location, and consequently response sensitivity and reliability are open to question.

ECOCHG with a promontory electrode has been demonstrated to be useful in estimating the validity of the behavioral audiogram (Eggermont et al., 1974) and in the detection of eighth cranial nerve impairments (Brackmann and Selters, 1976; Odenthal and Eggermont, 1976).

The major limitation of ECOCHG as a tool for evaluating infants and children is the required surgical procedure for placing the active electrode and the related administration of a general anesthesia. The availability of the ABR, which is noninvasive and requires at most a sedative to induce sleep, has prompted many clinicians to choose the ABR in lieu of ECOCHG for evaluating infants and children. In addition, the ABR reflects activity not only of eighth cranial nerve fibers but also of central auditory centers as well. The reader interested in the principles and clinical application of ECOCHG should refer to Eggermont and associates (1974) and Ruben and colleagues (1976).

The Auditory Brain Stem Response (ABR)

The ABR consists of five to seven vertex-positive* waves, labeled I to VII, occurring in the first 10 msec following stimulus onset (Fig. 8B–11). The response was first reported by Sohmer and Feinmesser (1967), but the

---

*"Vertex-positive" refers to the condition in which the active electrode, on the vertex of the skull, is connected to the positive input of the preamplifier. The waves can also be referred to as "vertex-negative" if the active electrode is connected to the negative input of the preamplifier. The former situation, however, is becoming an accepted convention.

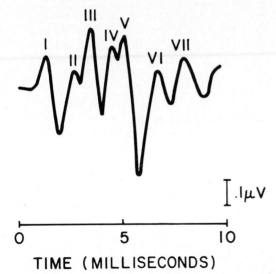

TIME (MILLISECONDS)

Figure 8B–11 The auditory brain stem response (ABR) for a young adult with normal hearing. Component waves are labeled I through VII.

landmark papers in this area were published by Jewett and his colleagues (Jewett, 1970; Jewett et al., 1970; Jewett and Williston, 1971; Jewett and Romano, 1972).

Waves I through III of the ABR presumably reflect activity of the eighth cranial nerve fibers (wave I) and auditory centers in the pons (waves II and III). Waves IV and V appear to represent activity of auditory centers in the mid to rostral pons and the caudal midbrain, respectively, while the neural generators for waves VI and VII are less certain but perhaps include thalamic auditory centers (Jewett, 1970; Lev and Sohmer, 1972; Buchwald and Huang, 1975; Starr and Hamilton, 1975).

The electrode configuration for the ABR includes the active electrode on the vertex of the skull or the midforehead at the hairline and the reference and ground electrodes respectively on the ipsilateral and contralateral mastoid processes or earlobes. The responses to 2000 to 4000 clicks, filtered clicks, or brief, pure tone bursts are typically averaged for each stimulus intensity employed. The stimuli are presented at a rapid rate (10 to 30 per second), and a complete run at a given stimulus intensity requires approximately 1.5 minutes; the entire procedure for both ears at several stimulus intensities averages 1.25 hours.

The deleterious effects of excessive muscle activity were mentioned earlier, and this factor is particularly pertinent to the obtaining of accurate ABR recordings. For this reason, a child must be completely relaxed, preferably asleep, for the procedure. Natural sleep can often be facilitated by feeding babies up to about six months of age immediately prior to the test. Often children seven years or older can lie quietly for the procedure. However, infants and children between these age extremes require sedation. In our experience, an intramuscular injection of meperidine (1.5 mg per kg) and secobarbital (3 mg per kg) is effective to induce sleep for the duration of the test.

Investigations subsequent to the early descriptions of the ABR have shown the response to possess excellent consistency between and within subjects and to be unchanged in awake and sleeping subjects. Of the five to seven waves comprising the ABR, waves I, III, and V can be obtained consistently, whereas waves II and IV appear inconsistently between and within subjects. The latency (the time of occurrence following stimulus onset) of the various waves increases, and wave amplitudes decrease with reductions in stimulus intensity; at stimulus intensities close to behavioral hearing threshold, only wave V can be discerned (Fig. 8B–12). These and other ABR properties have emerged from the extensive research efforts of a number of investigators (Lev and Sohmer, 1971; Sohmer and Feinmesser, 1973; Martin and Coats, 1973; Amadeo and Shagass, 1973; Hecox and Galambos, 1974; Hecox, 1975; Thornton, 1975; Buchwald and Huang, 1975; Blegvad, 1975; Ornitz and Walter, 1975; Salamy et al., 1975; Salamy and McKean, 1976; Starr and Achor, 1975; Starr, 1976; Starr and Hamilton, 1976; Starr et al., 1977; Hyde et al., 1976; Schulman-Galambos and Galambos, 1975, 1979; Kendall and Lawes, 1978; Rowe, 1978).

Hecox and Galambos (1974) reported differences in the ABRs of infants and adults. These investigators found prolonged wave V latencies in newborns and gradually shorter latencies in infants that approached adult values between 16 and 32 months of age. Salamy and McKean (1976) made similar observations, but they found that waves I and V matured at different rates. Wave I was essentially mature by six weeks of age, whereas two reductions in wave V latency were observed — one at six weeks and another between six and 12 months of age. These data suggest that the ABR may provide a maturational index of auditory system devel-

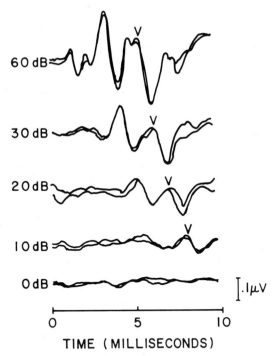

Figure 8B–12 The auditory brain stem response (ABR) to decreasing stimulus intensity. Each trace represents the averaged response to 1500 stimuli of the same intensity, and for successive traces stimulus intensity has been reduced by 10 dB. Note the reduction in amplitude and increase in response time (latency) of wave V with decreased stimulus intensity.

opment in neonates and infants. Apparently "immature" responses have been observed in developmentally delayed infants (Fria, unpublished) and in infants and children with autistic traits (Ornitz and Walter, 1975; Fria, 1978; Sohmer and Student, 1978). However, as Gardi and Mendel (1977) point out, behavioral correlates to these apparent maturational changes have not been documented.

The inherent properties of the ABR have provided a favorable milieu for the clinical application of the response. Both audiometric and otoneurologic applications are in common use today. In the pediatric population, the application has been primarily audiometric (but see Fria and Bartling, 1978; and Grundfast et al., 1978).

For the audiometric approach, a search is conducted for the minimum stimulus intensity yielding an observable ABR, and different stimulus types — clicks, filtered clicks, and brief tone bursts — are used to estimate responsivity in a frequency range comparable to that assessed by behavioral audiometry. In this context, response thresholds determined

with the ABR are correlated best with behavioral hearing thresholds in the higher frequencies (1000 to 4000 Hz), and the conventional ABR is unable to assess responsivity to lower stimulus frequencies (Davis, 1976). Modified ABR techniques, however, may provide a means for assessing the response to lower stimulus frequencies.

Davis and Hirsh (1979) described a slow negative wave (which was originally reported by Susuki et al., 1977), occurring at 10 msec in response to a low-frequency filtered click, that promises to be useful. Don and Eggermont (1978) applied a technique originally used for ECOCHG to generate a frequency-specific ABR audiogram. A major limitation of this "derived" ABR technique is that up to four hours may be required to assess a child completely. If these time factors can be overcome, the derived ABR should significantly augment audiometric applications of the ABR in general.

Galambos (1978) and Schulman-Galambos and Galambos (1979) suggested using the ABR to screen selected newborn populations for significant peripheral auditory impairment. This approach is based on preliminary evidence (Hecox and Galambos, 1974; Schulman-Galambos and Galambos, 1975; Starr et al., 1977) that the ABR can be recorded successfully in premature and term infants with stimulus intensities as low as 20 to 30 dBHL. Galambos (1978) emphasizes that this ABR technique will be most effective if applied to infant "graduates" of the intensive care nursery, those infants falling into a high-risk register for hearing loss, and those babies who fail neonatal behavioral hearing screening. Efforts are in progress (Despland and Galambos, 1980; Fria, unpublished; Riechert and Davis, unpublished) to specify further the reliability and validity of using the ABR for these purposes.

While one must be cognizant of the frequency specificity limitations of the ABR used for audiometric purposes, it is also important to realize that the technique does not assess the perceptual event called "hearing." The ABR reflects auditory neuronal electric responses that are adequately correlated to behavioral hearing thresholds, but a normal ABR only suggests that the auditory system, up to the midbrain level, is responsive to the stimulus employed, and it does not guarantee normal "hearing." Conversely, failure to elicit the ABR indicates an impairment of the system's synchronous response, but it does not insure that a child is totally "deaf" or that he or she has profoundly impaired "hearing." Consequently, ABR interpretation for audiometric purposes must be qualified by other clinical assessment data, either available at the time or resulting from follow-up evaluations.

The otoneurologic applications of the ABR use the response to infer the level of the auditory system — middle ear, cochlea, eighth cranial nerve, or brain stem — at which an impairment exists. The latency of the ABR waves is the primary consideration in these applications. For middle ear and cochlear impairments, wave latency as a function of stimulus intensity is important. Wave latencies at a fixed stimulus intensity provide the basis for detecting eighth cranial nerve and brain stem impairments.

In cases of middle ear impairment, the entire series of ABR waves is delayed in time by an amount commensurate with the degree of attendant conductive hearing loss (Hecox and Galambos, 1974; Yamada et al., 1975; Fria and Sabo, 1979). Typically, wave V latency as a function of decreasing stimulus intensity is used to detect such impairment, but recent evidence (Mendelson et al., 1979) suggests that wave I latency provides a better index of middle ear impairment.

The ABR in cases of cochlear impairment generally yields a steeper latency-intensity function. In other words, wave V latency is essentially normal at a high stimulus intensity, but it becomes excessively prolonged as stimulus intensity is decreased (Picton et al., 1977). Again, the convention has been to use wave V as the index of impairment, but wave I can also be used here since it normally precedes wave V by a constant 4 msec (Stockard and Rossiter, 1977). Consequently, the characteristic ABR finding in cochlear impairment includes a normal wave I-to-V latency difference in addition to the steep latency-intensity function. Stockard and Rossiter (1977) and Selters and Brachmann (1977) observed prolonged wave V latency to a high stimulus intensity in cochlear-impaired patients with severe, high-frequency sensorineural hearing losses, but the wave I-to-V latency difference was apparently normal.

The ABR has also proved to be effective in detecting eighth cranial nerve impairment (Selters and Brackmann, 1977; Terkildsen et al., 1977; Coats and Martin, 1977; Clemis and McGee, 1979; Thomsen et al., 1978) and brain stem impairment (Starr and Achor, 1975; Stockard and Rossiter, 1977; Stockard et al., 1977). In general, such impairments show an increased latency difference between waves I and V beyond the normal 4 msec. This increased I-to-V latency difference can be divided into two categories depending on where the delay begins: (1) beginning between waves I and III for defects at the lower pontine level and (2) beginning between waves III and V for defects at the rostral pons or caudal midbrain level. Eighth nerve tumor cases would tend to fall in the first category, as would certain brain stem defects occurring at this anatomic level. Brain stem lesions occurring at higher levels would tend to fall into the second category. Stockard and colleagues (1977) found that multifocal brain stem demyelinating processes predominantly showed ABR latency abnormalities; on closer examination, there existed a progressively increasing delay in the first six waves of the ABR.

Recently, Stockard (1978) has reviewed the utility of certain ABR amplitude measurements: Wave V amplitude that is reduced in comparison to that of wave I can be suggestive of impairment.

The ABR, then, is a series of positive waves occurring in the first 10 msec following stimulus onset that apparently reflect activity in successively higher levels of the auditory tract up to and perhaps including lower midbrain centers. Within limits, the response can be used audiometrically to estimate hearing acuity, and it also has utility for inferring at which level of the auditory system impairment might exist. The consistent nature of the ABR in newborns as well as in older children, and in sleeping as well as in awake subjects, makes the test a particularly useful tool for evaluating hearing in pediatric populations.

Candidate Pediatric Populations

As indicated earlier, testing auditory electric responses is not a routine procedure for assessing hearing in infants and children; however, it can be helpful in evaluating selected pediatric populations. In addition, ECOCHG and preferably ABR are the electric response components best suited for these populations.

In general, auditory electric responses are helpful in evaluating those infants and children for whom behavioral hearing test results are either unreliable or unobtainable or for whom the anatomic level of impairment is questioned. Clinical experience with the ABR in 240 infants and children (Fria and Bartling, 1978) has shown that the following pediatric populations are likely candidates for the technique:

1. Infants at risk for auditory impairment
   a. infants with meningitis
   b. infants with low birth weights or seizures
   c. infants with respiratory distress syndrome
   d. infants with recurrent acute otitis media or persistent otitis media with effusion, or both
   e. infants with other high-risk factors, including affected family members, craniofacial anomalies, hyperbilirubinemia, and evident intrauterine bacterial infection
2. Children with significant mental retardation, emotional disturbances or both
3. Children with suspected eighth cranial nerve or brain stem impairments
4. Children presenting with sudden-onset, fluctuating, or progressive sensorineural hearing loss

The utility of the ABR continues to be investigated for certain pediatric populations not listed here. As further experience is gained in using the ABR, there will no doubt be other pediatric populations added to the list.

Autonomic Response Audiometry

Certain nonbehavioral techniques utilize autonomic responses to sound to estimate hearing in infants and children. These approaches involve the presentation of an acoustic stimulus and the detection of an associated change in respiration rate or pattern (respiration audiometry), heart rate (cardiac audiometry), or skin resistance (electrodermal audiometry).

The data available at present suggest that cardiac and electrodermal responses show less promise as audiometric tools than do respiratory responses. While the cardiac response to sound has been studied by a number of investigators (Bartoshuk, 1962a, 1962b, 1964; Graham and Clifton, 1966; Schulman, 1970, 1974; Schulman and Kreiter, 1971; Eisenberg et al., 1974; Gerber

et al., 1976, 1977), no standard clinical approach to using the response audiometrically has been clearly documented. The cardiac response appears to be all-or-none and to be composed qualitatively of an accelerated heart rate in newborns and a deceleration later in infancy; however, Gerber and colleagues (1976) found that the nature of the cardiac response to sound was to some extent peculiar to the individual infant.

The most common electrodermal audiometric procedure involves pairing an acoustic stimulus with a mild shock. The shock produces an unconditioned change in skin resistance that is detected with recording electrodes placed on the palm or fingertips. With successive trials, an attempt is made to condition the skin response to the acoustic stimulus alone. When such conditioning is accomplished, stimulus parameters are varied in order to estimate hearing capabilities (Hardy and Pauls, 1952; Doerfler and McClure, 1954).

The required administration of a mild shock has proved to be a significant problem for electrodermal audiometry even in adult assessment, where the technique appears to work. In children, adequate results require a particularly cooperative child who can be easily conditioned and who is not troubled by the shock administration.

Hardy and Bordley (1951), Kodman and colleagues (1959), Moss and associates (1961), and Tizard (1968) found the technique to be particularly difficult to use with uncooperative or disturbed children. At present, electrodermal audiometry is not a popular procedure for assessing the hearing of infants and children.

Recent data (Kankkunnen and Liden, 1977) suggest that respiration audiometry has promise as a tool for estimating hearing thresholds in infants. The technique involves the detection of respiration rate and pattern changes secondary to acoustic stimulation. The method for detecting these changes has varied with the studies; some investigators have used a temperature-sensitive thermistor device placed 1 cm from the nasal opening, while others have employed a direct-pressure bellows strapped to the child's thorax. More recently, investigators have monitored respiration changes with thorax electrodes.

The audiometric utility of respiration measurement in adults remains uncertain. Certain studies (Rousey et al., 1964; Poole et al., 1966; Teel et al., 1967) support the reliability of respiration audiometry in adults, but at least one study (Hayes and Jerger, 1978) found the technique to have significant limitations when applied to adults with normal hearing.

Roseneau (1962) studied respiration responses in sleeping infants and young children with normal hearing, impaired hearing, experimentally induced hearing loss, and total deafness. Responses were not obtained from the deaf children. Other children in the study did yield responses, but there appeared to be uncomfortably large discrepancies between hearing threshold and the threshold for respiratory changes. Wagner (1963) suggested modifying Roseneau's (1962) technique to overcome apparent methodologic difficulties.

Bradford and colleagues (1968), Bradford (1975), and Kankkunnen and Liden (1977) had better success in assessing the hearing of newborns and infants with respiration audiometry. Kankkunnen and Liden (1977) used air- and bone-conducted pure tone stimuli to obtain "usable" respiration responses in 92 per cent of 218 high-risk infants and children. In this study, the technique yielded the highest percentage of usable responses in infants less than 12 months of age, and subsequent behavioral hearing tests on 13 selected infants confirmed the reliability of hearing thresholds predicted with respiration responses. Bradford and coworkers (1968) and Bradford (1975) also found good agreement between hearing thresholds predicted with respiration responses and those obtained with behavioral hearing tests in newborns and preschool-age children.

Although the procedural and subject-related variables related to respiration audiometry require additional attention, preliminary data would suggest that the technique can provide a useful estimation of hearing in infants. An in-depth discussion of respiration audiometry and related variables can be found in Gilchrist (1978).

OTHER ASSESSMENT TECHNIQUES

At least two other assessment techniques deserve mention here. The first involves the testing of speech-sound discrimination in infants, and the second involves the assessment of central auditory processing.

Eilers and colleagues (1977) developed a visual reinforcement procedure for testing speech-sound discrimination in infants. These authors called the technique visually reinforced infant speech discrimination (VRISD). VRISD procedures are essentially the same as those described earlier in this chapter for VRA, but here the infant is visually rewarded (with an animated toy) for localizing to a unique speech syllable presented among a series of other syllables. This and subsequent research (Eilers et al., 1977) found that a majority of infants 6 to 14 months of age can be tested successfully with the technique. Moore and Wilson (1978) suggest that VRISD may be useful in assessing infants suspected to be developmentally delayed, and the technique may provide an additional means for evaluating hearing aid performance in moderately to moderately severe hearing-impaired infants. The full clinical scope of this innovative assessment technique will surely emerge in the near future.

A number of approaches have been taken to assess central auditory processing in children. The perplexing pediatric problems of developmental delay and learning disabilities have motivated investigators to search for viable means to assess hearing in such children, many of whom have "normal" hearing on the basis of more conventional testing. Based on the pioneering principles and techniques described by Bocca and Calearo (1963), extensive research has been aimed at developing methodology for assessing pediatric populations. A current sample of this research is presented by Kieth (1977). It is difficult to lend enthusiastic credence to central auditory assessment results in children, since normative data for children less than 11 years of age are still being collected. However, certain centers devoted to pediatric testing have central auditory test batteries based on locally generated norms. When available, the information obtained with these techniques may be helpful in fully understanding a child's auditory interaction with his or her environment.

THE ROLE OF THE AUDIOLOGIST

This chapter has described the various techniques available for assessing hearing in infants. The reader should now have a basic understanding of the techniques for such assessment and an awareness of sources where more extensive treatment of a particular technique can be found. Throughout this chapter, it has been emphasized that no one method of assessment is definitive and that accurate assessment involves the consideration of information provided by several tests of hearing used in combination. Although certain techniques can be used in isolation as screening tools in certain situations (for example, BOA in the office situation), comprehensive assessment is based on the results of a combination of these tests.

The audiologist plays a multifaceted role in the assessment process. He or she must devise and implement an assessment strategy composed of procedures that are applicable to the child in question and must interpret the results in the context of the impairment suspected. The audiologist must also convey assessment results to the referral source and must provide suggestions that are meaningful for the management of the child. In concert with the referral source, the audiologist can also play an important role in interpreting the results to concerned family members and in counseling the family with regard to the impact an impairment may have on the child's future interaction with the environment from a social and educational point of view.

The audiologist can serve as a valuable resource for the implementation of habilitative or rehabilitative plans for a hearing-impaired child. Schwartz and Konkle (Chap. 88) present the manner in which the audiologist assists in determining the amplification needs of the hearing-impaired child. In addition, the audiologist is usually aware of the public and special school programs in the community that will play an active role in the child's education. The audiologist maintains contact with such programs so that the long-term follow-up of a particular child is maintained.

In conclusion, the audiologist should be an active team member in the general pediatric assessment of any child, regardless of age. At his or her disposal are the knowledge, experience, and techniques required to make a meaningful assessment of hearing in infants and children. Owing to the importance of adequate hearing in infancy and childhood, we as health care professionals are obligated to give the assessment of hearing the high priority it deserves.

SELECTED REFERENCES

Davis, H. 1976. Principles of electric response audiometry. Ann. Otol. Rhinol. Laryngol., Suppl. 28, 85(3):1–96, 1976.
  This article presents the background, classification, and clinical application of various auditory electric response components. It is particularly informative regarding subject and stimulus parameters relating to electric response audiometry.

Fria, T. J. 1980. The auditory brain stem response. Background and clinical applications. Monographs in Contemporary Audiology. Maico Hearing Instruments. Minneapolis. Minn., 2(2):1–44.
  A comprehensive review of the literature pertaining to the auditory brain stem response.

Gerber, S. E. 1977. Audiometry in Infancy. New York, Grune and Stratton.
  This reference contains a particularly thorough treatment of nonbehavioral assessment techniques.

Northern, J. L., and Downs, M. P. 1974. Hearing in Children. Baltimore, Williams and Wilkins.
  This book provides a good discussion of all aspects of hearing in children, including various assessment techniques and habilitative and rehabilitative considerations. Thorough discussions of newborn screening and behavioral observation audiometry are included.

Shepherd, D. C. 1978. Pediatric audiology. In Rose, D. E. (Ed.) Audiological Assessment. Englewood Cliffs, NJ, Prentice-Hall, pp. 261–300.
  This chapter presents a well-organized and thorough discussion of pediatric hearing testing. Behavioral hearing tests are covered best; electrophysiologic methods are presented with less thoroughness.

REFERENCES

Alberti, P. W., and Kristensen, R. 1970. The clinical application of impedance audiometry Laryngoscope, 80:735–746.

Amadeo, M., and Shagass, C. 1973. Brief latency click-evoked potentials during waking and sleeping in man. Psychophysiology, 10:244–250.

American National Standard Institute, 1969. Standard specifications for Audiometers, ANSI–S3.6–1969 (R 1973). American National Standards Institute, Inc., New York.

Anderson, H., Barr, B., and Wedenberg, E. 1970. Early diagnosis of VIIIth nerve tumors by acoustic reflex tests. Acta Otolaryngol., 263:232–237.

Aran, J. M. 1976. The electro-cochleogram: Recent results in children and in some pathological cases. Arch. Klin. Ohren. Nasen. Kehlkopf., 198:128–141.

ASHA, 1974. Committee on Audiometric Evaluation, Guidelines for audiometric symbols. ASHA, 16:260–264.

Barnet, A. B., and Goodwin, R. S. 1965. Averaged evoked electroencephalographic responses to clicks in the human newborn. EEG Clin. Neurophysiol., 18:441–450.

Barr, B. 1955. Pure-tone audiometry for pre-school children. Acta Otolaryngol., Suppl. 121, 1955.

Bartoskuk, A. K. 1962a. Response decrement with repeated elicitation of human neonatal cardiac acceleration to sound. J. Comp. Physiol. Psychol., 55:9–13.

Bartoshuk, A. K. 1962b. Human neonatal cardiac acceleration to sound; habituation and dishabituation. Percept. Mot. Skill, 15:15–27.

Bartoshuk, A. K. 1964. Human neonatal cardiac response to sound. A power function. Psychonomic Sci., 1:151–152.

Bench, J. 1970. The law of initial value: A neglected source of variance in infant audiometry. Int. Audiol., 9:314–322.

Blegvad, B. 1975. Binaural summation of surface recorded electrocochleographic responses, normal hearing subjects. Scand. Audiol., 4:233–238.

Bocca, E., and Calearo, C. 1963. Central hearing processes. In Jerger, J. (Ed.) Modern Developments in Audiology. New York, Academic Press, pp. 337–370.

Bosatra, A., Russolo, M., and Poli, P. 1975. Modifications of the stapedius muscle reflex under spontaneous and experimental brain-stem impairment. Acta Otolaryngol., 80:61–66.

Brackmann, D. E., and Selters, W. A. 1976. Electrocochleography in Meniere's disease and acoustic neuromas. In Ruben, R. J., Elberling, C. and Salomon, G. (Eds.) Electrocochleography. Baltimore, University Park Press, pp. 315–330.

Bradford, L. J. 1975. Respiration audiometry. In Bradford, L. J. (Ed.) Physiological Measures of the Audio-Vestibular System. New York, Grune and Stratton.

Bradford, L. J., Rousey, C. L., and Bradford, M. A. 1968. Respiration audiometry with the preschool child. Topeka, Kansas, The Menninger Foundation.

Bragg, V. C. 1979. Toward a more objective hearing aid fitting procedure. Hearing Instruments, September, 6–9.

Brooks, D. N. 1969. The use of the electroacoustic impedance bridge in the assessment of middle ear function. Int. Audiol., 8:563–569.

Brooks, D. N. 1973. Hearing screening: A comparative study of an impedance method and pure tone screening. Scand. Audiol., 2:67–72.

Brooks, D. N. 1976. School screening for middle ear effusions. Ann. Otol. Rhinol. Laryngol., 25(85):223–228.

Brooks, D. N. 1977. Mass screening with acoustic impedance. Proceedings of the Third International Symposium on Impedance Audiometry. New York, American Electromedics, May.

Brooks, D. N. 1978. Impedance screening for school children — State of the art. In Harford, E. R., Bess, F. H., Bluestone, C. D., and Klein, J. E. (Eds.) Impedance Screening for Middle Ear Disease in Children. New York, Grune and Stratton, pp. 173–180.

Buchwald, J. S., and Huang, C. M. 1975. Far field acoustic response: Origins in the cat. Science, 189:382–384.

Clemis, J. D., and McGee, T. 1979. Brainstem electric response audiometry in the differential diagnosis of acoustic tumors. Laryngoscope, 89(1):31–42.

Coats, A. C., and Dickey, J. R. 1970. Non-surgical recording of human auditory nerve action potentials from the tympanic membrane. Ann. Otol. Rhinol. Laryngol., 29:844.

Coats, A. C., and Martin, J. L. 1977. Nerve action potentials and brain stem evoked responses: Effects of audiogram shape and lesion location. Arch. Otolaryngol., 103:605–622.

Cooper, J. C., Gates, G., Owen, J., et al. 1974. An abbreviated impedance bridge technique for school screening. J. Speech Hear. Disord., 40:260–269.

Cullen, J. K., Ellis, M. S., Berlin, C. I., et al. 1972. Human acoustic nerve action potential recordings from the tympanic membrane without anesthesia. Acta Otolaryngol., 74:15–22.

Darley, F. L. 1961. Identification audiometry. J. Speech Hear. Disord., Suppl. 9.

Davis, H. 1973. Sedation of young children for evoked response audiometry (ERA). Summary of a symposium. Audiology, 12:55–57.

Davis, H. 1976. Principles of electric response audiometry. Ann. Otol. Rhinol. Laryngol., Suppl. 28, 85(3):1–96.

Davis, H., and Hirsh, S. K. 1979. A slow brain stem response for low-frequency audiometry. Audiology, 18:445–461.

Denenberg, L. J., and Altshuler, M. W. 1976. The clinical relationship between acoustic reflexes and loudness perception. J. Am. Audiol. Soc., 2(3):79–82.

Despland, P. A., and Galambos, R. 1980. The auditory brainstem response (ABR) as a useful diagnostic tool in the intensive care nursery. Pediatr. Res., 14:154–158.

Doerfler, L. G., and McClure, C. T. 1954. The measurement of hearing loss in adults by measurement of galvanic skin response. J. Speech Hear. Disord., 19:184–189.

Don, M., and Eggermont, J. J. 1978. Analysis of the click-evoked brainstem potentials in man using high-pass noise masking. J. Acoust. Soc. Am., 64(4):1084–1092.

Downs, M. P. 1967. Testing hearing in infancy and early childhood. In Freeman, M., and Ward, P. H. (Eds.) Deafness in Childhood. Nashville, Vanderbilt University Press.

Downs, M. P. 1974. Personal communication.

Eggermont, J. J., Odenthal, D. W., Schmidt, P. H., et al. 1974. Electrocochleography. Basic principles and clinical application. Acta Otolaryngol., Suppl. 316, 1–84.

Eilers, R. E., Wilson, W. R., and Moore, J. M. 1977. Developmental changes in speech discrimination in infancy. J. Speech Hear. Res., 20:766–780.

Eisenberg, R. B. 1976. Auditory Competence in Early Life. Baltimore, University Park Press.

Eisenberg, R. B., Marmarou, A., and Giovachino, P. 1974. Infant heart rate changes to a synthetic speech sound. J. Aud. Res., 14:21–28.

Elberling, C. 1974. Action potentials along the cochlear partition recorded from the ear canal in man. Scand. Audiol., 3:13.

Elner, A., Ingelstedt, S., and Ivarsson, A. 1971. Indirect determination of middle ear pressure. Acta Otolaryngol., 72:255.

Ewing, I. R., and Ewing, A. W. G. 1944. The ascertainment of deafness in infancy and early childhood. J. Laryngol. Otol., 59:309–333.

Feldman, A. S. 1963. Impedance measurements at the eardrum as an aid to diagnosis. J. Speech Hear. Disord., 6:315–327.

Feldman, A. S. 1967. A report of further studies of the acoustic reflex. J. Speech Hear. Res., 10:616–622.

Feldman, A. S. 1976. Tympanometry; application and interpretation. Ann. Otol. Rhinol. Laryngol., Suppl. 25, 85(2).

Feldman, A. S. 1978. Acoustic impedance-admittance battery. In Katz, J. (Ed.) Handbook of Clinical Audiology. 2nd ed. Baltimore, Williams and Wilkins.

Ferrer, H. 1974. Use of impedance audiometry in school screening. Public Health, *88*:153–163.

Flisberg, K., Ingelstedt, S., and Ortegren, U. 1963. On middle ear pressure. Acta Otolaryngol., Suppl. 182.

Fria, T. J. 1978. Brainstem auditory electric responses in autistic children. Presented at the XIV International Congress of Audiology, Acapulco, Mexico, November.

Fria, T. J., and Bartling, V. 1978. Brainstem auditory electric responses in selected pediatric populations. Presented at the National Convention of the American Speech and Hearing Association, San Francisco, November.

Fria, T. J., and Sabo, D. L. 1979. Brainstem auditory evoked potentials in children with otitis media with effusion. Presented at the Second International Symposium on Recent Advances in Otitis Media with Effusion, May 9–11.

Fria, T. J., Leblanc, J., Kristensen, R., et al. 1975. Ipsilateral acoustic reflex stimulation in normal and sensorineural impaired ears: A preliminary report. Can. J. Otolaryngol., *4*:695–703.

Fria, T. J., Sabo, D., and Beery, Q. C. 1979. The acoustic reflex in the identification of otitis media with effusion, unpublished.

Fröding, C. A. 1960. Acoustic investigation of newborn infants. Acta Otolaryngol., *52*:31–40.

Fulton, R. T., Gorzycki, P. A., and Hull, W. L. 1975. Hearing assessment with young children. J. Speech Hear. Disord., *40*:397–404.

Galambos, R. 1978. Use of auditory brainstem response in infant hearing screening testing. *In* Gerber, S. E., and Mencher, G. T. (Eds.) Early Diagnosis of Hearing Loss. New York, Grune and Stratton, pp. 243–258.

Gardi, J. N., and Mendel, M. 1977. Evoked brainstem potentials. *In* Gerber, S. E. (Ed.) Audiometry in Infancy. New York, Grune and Stratton, pp. 205–246.

Gerber, S. E., Mulac, A., and Swain, B. J. 1976. Idiosyncratic cardiovascular response of human neonates to acoustic stimuli. J. Am. Audiol. Soc., *1*:185–191.

Gerber, S. E., Mulac, A., and Lamb, M. E. 1977. The cardiovascular response to acoustic stimuli. Audiology, *16*:1–10.

Gessell, A., and Armatruda, C. 1948. Developmental Diagnosis. New York, Harper and Row.

Gilchrist, D. B. 1978. Respiratory measures. *In* Gerber, S. (Ed.) Audiometry in Infancy. New York, Grune and Stratton, pp. 117–133.

Glatke, T. J. 1978. Electrocochleography. *In* Katz, J. (Ed.) Handbook of Clinical Audiology, Baltimore, Williams and Wilkins, pp. 328–343.

Goodhill, V., Lowell, E. L., and Lowell, M. O. 1970. Computerized objective auditory testing in infancy. Final report of project DHEW H-181.

Goodman, A. 1965. Reference zero levels for pure-tone audiometers. ASHA, *7*:262–263.

Graham, F. K., and Clifton, R. K. 1966. Heart rate change as a component of the orientating response. Psychol. Bull., *65*:305–320.

Greisen, O., and Rasmussen, P. 1970. Stapedius muscle reflexes and otoneurological examinations in brain stem tumors. Acta Otolaryngol., *70*:366–370.

Grundfast, K., Fria, T. J., Bartling, V., and Stool, S. 1978. Clinical applications of brainstem auditory electric response testing at a children's hospital. Trans. Penn. Acad. Ophthalmol. Otolaryngol., *31*:205–210.

Hardy, W., and Bordley, J. 1951. Special techniques in

testing the hearing of children. J. Speech Hear. Disord., *16*:122–131.

Hardy, W. G., and Pauls, M. D. 1952. The test situation of PGSR audiometry. J. Speech. Hear. Disord., *17*:13–24.

Harford, E. R., Bess, F. H., Bluestone, C. D., et al. 1978. Impedance Screening for Middle Ear Disease in Children. New York, Grune and Stratton.

Harker, L. A., and Van Wagoner, R. 1974. Application of impedance audiometry as a screening instrument. Acta Otolaryngol., *77*:198–201.

Haskins, H. 1949. A phonetically balanced test of speech discrimination for children. Master's thesis, Northwestern University.

Haug, C. O., Boccaro, P., and Guilford, F. 1967. A puretone audiogram on the infant: The PIWI technique, Arch. Otolaryngol., *99*:30–33.

Hayes, D., and Jerger, J. 1978. Response detection in respiration audiometry. Arch. Otolaryngol., *104*:183–185.

Hecox, K. 1975. Electrophysiological correlates of human auditory development. *In* Cohen, L. B., and Salapatek, P. L. (Eds.) Infant Perception from Sensation to Cognition, Vol. 2. Perception of Space, Speech and Sound, New York, Academic Press.

Hecox, K., and Galambos, R. 1974. Brainstem auditory evoked responses in human infants and adults. Arch. Otolaryngol., *99*:30–33.

Holmquist, J., and Miller, J. 1972. Eustachian tube evaluation using the impedance bridge. Mayo Foundation Impedance Symposium. Mayo Clinic, Rochester, MN, 297–307, June.

Hyde, M. L., Stephans, S. D. G., and Thornton, A. R. D. 1976. Stimulus repetition rate and the early brainstem responses. Br. J. Audiol., *10*:41–50.

Ingelstedt, S., Ivarsson, A., and Jonsson, B. 1967. Mechanics of the human middle ear. Acta Otolaryngol., Suppl., 228.

Jepsen, O. 1963. Middle ear muscle reflexes in man. *In* Jerger, J. (Ed.) Modern Developments in Audiology. New York, Academic Press, pp. 193–239.

Jerger J. 1970. Clinical experience with impedance audiometry. Arch. Otolaryngol., *92*:311–324.

Jerger, J., Jerger, S., and Mauldin, L. 1972. Studies in impedance audiometry. I. Normal and sensorineural ears. Arch. Otolaryngol., *96*:513.

Jerger, J., Harford, E., Clemis, J., et al. 1974a. The acoustic reflex in eighth nerve disorders. Arch. Otolaryngol., *99*:409–413.

Jerger, S., Jerger, J., and Mauldin, L. 1974b. Studies in impedance audiometry. II. Children less than six years old. Arch Otolaryngol., *99*:1.

Jerger, J., Anthony, L., Jerger, S., et al. 1974c. Studies in impedance audiometry. III. Middle ear disorders. Arch. Otolaryngol., *99*:165–171.

Jerger, J., Burney, P., Mauldin, L., et al. 1974d. Predicting hearing loss from the acoustic reflex. J. Speech Hear. Disord., *18*:11–22.

Jerger, J., Hayes, D., Anthony, L., et al. 1978. Factors influencing prediction of hearing level from the acoustic reflex. Monographs in Contemporary Audiology, *1*:1–20. Minneapolis, Maico Hearing Instruments, Inc.

Jerger, S., and Jerger, J. 1977. Diagnostic value of crossed vs. uncrossed acoustic reflexes: Eighth nerve and brainstem disorders. Arch. Otolayngol., *103*:445–453.

Jewett, D. L. 1970. Volume-conducted potentials in response to auditory stimuli as detected by averaging in the cat. EEG Clin. Neurophysiol., *28*:609–618.

Jewett, D. L., and Romano, M. N. 1972. Neonatal development of auditory system potentials averaged from the scalp of the rat and cat. Brain Res., *36*:101–115.

Jewett, D. L., and Williston, J. S. 1971. Auditory evoked far fields averaged from the scalp of humans. Brain *94*:681–696.

Jewett, D. L., Romano, M. N., and Williston, J. S. 1970. Human auditory evoked potentials: Possible brainstem components detected on the scalp. Science, *167*:1517–1518.

Johnsen, N. J., Osterhammel, D., Terkildsen, K., et al. 1976. The white noise middle ear muscle reflex thresholds in patients with sensorineural hearing impairment. Scand. Audiol., *5*:313–335.

Kankkunnen, A., and Liden, G. 1977. Respiration audiometry. Scand. Audiol., *6*:81–86.

Kendall, D. C. 1964. Pediatrics and disorders in communication. III. The audiological examination of young children. Volta Rev., *66*:734–744.

Kendall, J. P., and Lawes, I. N. 1978. The clinical reliability of brainstem auditory evoked responses. Br. J. Audiol., *12*:23–30.

Kieth, R. W. 1971. Impedance audiometry with neonates. Presented at the Annual Convention of the American Speech and Hearing Association, November.

Kieth, R. W. 1976. An evaluation of predicting hearing loss from the acoustic reflex. Presented at the Annual Convention of the American Speech and Hearing Association. Houston, Texas, November.

Kieth, R. W. 1977. Central Auditory Dysfunction. New York, Grune and Stratton.

Kodman, F., Fein, A., and Mixon, A. 1959. Psychogalvanic skin response audiometry with severe mentally retarded children. Am. J. Ment. Defic., *64*:131–136.

Lev, A., and Sohmer, H. 1971. Sources of averaged neural responses recorded in animal and human subjects during cochlear audiometry. Arch. Klin. Exp. Ohren Nasen Kehlkopf, *201*:79–90.

Lewis, A. N., Barry, M., and Stuart, J. 1974. Screening procedures for the identification of hearing and ear disorders in Australian aboriginal children. J. Laryngol. Otol., *88*:335–347.

Lewis, N., Dugdale, A., Canty, A., and Jerger, J. 1975. Open ended tympanometric screening: A new concept. Arch. Otolaryngol., *101*:722–725.

Liden, G., and Kankkunnen, A. 1969. Visual reinforcement audiometry. Acta. Oto-laryngol. (Stockh.), *67*:281–292.

Liden, G., and Renvall, U. 1978. Impedance audiometry for screening middle ear disease in school children. *In* Harford, E. R., Bess, F. H., Bluestone, C. D., et al. (Eds.): Impedance Screening for Middle Ear Disease in Children. New York, Grune and Stratton, pp. 197–206.

Liden, G., Peterson, J., and Bjorkman, G. 1970. Tympanometry. Arch. Otolaryngol., *92*:248–257.

Lierle, D. M. 1959. Report of the Committee on Conservation of Hearing. Guide for the evaluation of hearing impairment. Trans. Am. Acad. Ophthalmol. Otolaryngol., *63*:238.

Lloyd, L. L., Spradlin, J. E., and Reed, M. J. 1968. An operant audiometric procedure for difficult-to-test patients. J. Speech Hear. Disord., *33*:236–245.

Lloyd, L. L., and Young, C. E. 1969. Pure tone audiometry. *In* Fulton, R., and Lloyd, L. (Eds.) Audiometry for the Retarded with Implications for the Difficult to Test. Baltimore, Williams and Wilkins.

Margolis, R. H., and Fox, C. M. 1977. A comparison of three methods for predicing hearing loss from acoustic reflex thresholds. J. Speech Hear. Res., *20*:241–253.

Martin, J. L., and Coats A. C. 1973. Short latency auditory evoked responses recorded from human nasopharynx. Brain Res., *60*:496–502.

McCandless, G. A. 1978. Neuroelectric measures of auditory function. *In* Rose, D. E. (Ed.) Audiological Assessment, 2nd ed. Englewood Cliffs, Prentice Hall, pp. 420–443.

McCandless, G. A., and Miller, D. 1972. Loudness discomfort and hearing aids. Natl. Hear. Aid J., *7*:28–32.

McCandless, G. A., and Thomas, G. K. 1974. Impedance audiometry as a screening procedure for middle ear disease. Trans. Am. Acad. Ophthalmol. Otolaryngol., *78*:98–102.

McCandless, G. A., and Allred, P. L. 1978. Tympanometry and emergence of the acoustic reflex in infants. *In* Harford, E. R., Bess, F. H., Bluestone, C. D., et al. (Eds.) Impedance Screening for Middle Ear Disease in Children. New York, Grune and Stratton, pp. 57–68.

McCurdy, J. A., Goldstein, J. L., and Gorski, D. 1976. Auditory screening of preschool children with impedance audiometry — a comparison with pure tone audiometry. Clin. Pediatr. (Phila), *15*:436–441.

Mendel, M. 1977a. Evoked cochlear potentials. *In* Gerber, S. E. (Ed.) Audiometry in Infancy. New York, Grune and Stratton, pp. 183–204.

Mendel, M. 1977b. Electroencephalic tests of hearing. *In* Gerber, S. E. (Ed.) Audiometry in Infancy. New York, Grune and Stratton, pp. 151–182.

Mendelson, T., Salamy, A., Lenoir, M., et al. 1979. Brainstem evoked potential findings in children with otitis media. Arch. Otolaryngol., *105*:17–20.

Metz, O. 1946. The acoustic impedance measured on normal and pathological ears. Acta Otolaryngol., Suppl. 63.

Metz, O. 1952. Threshold of reflex contractions of muscles of the middle ear and recruitment of loudness. Arch. Otolaryngol., *55*:536–543.

Miller, J. K., DeSchweinitz, L., and Goetzinger, C. P. 1963. How infants 3, 4 and 5 months of age respond to sound. J. of Except. Child., *30*:149–154.

Møller, A. R. 1962. The sensitivity of contraction of the tympanic muscles in man. Ann. Otol. Rhinol. Laryngol., *71*:86–95.

Moore, J. M., and Wilson, W. R. 1978. Visual reinforcement audiometry (VRA) with infants. *In* Gerber, S. E., and Mencher, G. T. (Eds.) Early Diagnosis of Hearing Loss. New York, Grune and Stratton, pp. 177–210.

Moore, J. M., Thompson, G., and Thompson, M. 1975. Auditory localization of infants as a function of reinforcement conditions. J. Speech Hear. Dis., *40*:29–34.

Moore, J. M., Wilson, W. R., and Thompson, G. 1977. Visual reinforcement of head-turn responses in infants under 12 months of age. J. Speech Hear. Dis., *42*:328–334.

Moss, J. W., Moss, M., and Tizard, J. 1961. Electrodermal response audiometry with mentally defective children. J. Speech Hear. Res., *4*:41–47.

Murphy, K. P. 1961. Development of hearing in babies. Hearing Instruments, November 9–11.

Niemeyer, W., and Sesterhenn, G. 1974. Calculating the hearing threshold from the stapedius reflex threshold for different sound stimuli. Audiology, *13*:421–427.

Nilges, T. C., Northern, J., and Burke, K. 1969. Zwislocki acoustic impedance bridge: Clinical correlations. Arch. Otolaryngol., *89*:69–86.

Northern, J. L., and Downs, M. P. 1974. Hearing in Children. Baltimore, Williams and Wilkins.

Northern, J. L., and Grimes, A. M. 1978. Introduction to acoustic impedance. In Katz, J. (Ed.) Handbook of Clinical Audiology. Baltimore, Williams and Wilkins, pp. 344–355.

Odenthal, D. W., and Eggermont, J. J. 1976. Electrocochleography study in Meniere's disease and pontine angle neuronoma. In Ruben, R. J., Elberling, C., and Solomon, G. (Eds.) Electrocochleography. Baltimore, University Park Press, pp. 331–352.

Orchik, D. J., and Herdman, S. 1974. Impedance audiometry as a screening device with school age children. J. Aud. Res., 14:283–286.

Orchik, D. J., Dunn, J. W., and McNutt, L. 1978. Tympanometry as a predictor of middle ear effusion. Arch. Otolaryngol., 104:4–6.

Ornitz, E. M., and Walter, D. O. 1975. The effect of sound pressure waveform on human brainstem auditory evoked responses. Brain Res., 92:490–498.

Paradise, J. L., Smith, C. G., and Bluestone, C. D. 1976. Tympanometric detection of middle ear effusion in infants and young children. Pediatrics, 58:198–210.

Paradise, J. L., and Smith, C. G. 1978. Impedance screening for preschool children — State of the art. In Harford, E. R., Bess, F. H., Bluestone, C. D. et al. (Eds.) Impedance Screening for Middle Ear Disease in Children. New York, Grune and Stratton, pp. 113–124.

Peterson, J., and Liden, G. 1970. Tympanometry in human temporal bones. Acta Otolaryngol., 92:258.

Picton, T. W., Woods, D. L., Baribeau-Braun, J., et al. 1977. Evoked potential audiometry. J. Otolaryngol., 6(2):90–119.

Poole, R., Goetzinger, C. P., and Rousey, C. A. 1966. A study of the effects of auditory stimuli on respiration. Acta Otolaryngol., 61:143–152.

Rainville, M. 1977. Hearing aid fitting using stapedial reflex measurement. Proceedings of Third International Symposium on Impedance Audiometry, Acton, Maine, American Electromedics Corp., 49–50.

Rapin, I., and Bergman, M. 1969. Auditory evoked responses in uncertain diagnosis. Arch. Otolaryngol., 90:307–314.

Rappaport, B. E., and Tait, C. A. 1976. Acoustic reflex threshold measurement in hearing aid selection. Arch. Otolaryngol., 102:129–132.

Renvall, U., Liden, G., Jungert, S., et al. 1973. Impedance audiometry as a screening method in school children. Scand. Audiol., 2:133–137.

Renvall, U., Liden, G., and Bjorkman, G. 1975. Experimental tympanometry in human temporal bones. Scand. Audiol., 4:135–144.

Roberts, M. E. 1976. Comparative study of pure tone, impedance, and otoscopic hearing screening methods. Arch. Otolaryngol., 102:690–694.

Robertson, E. O., Peterson, J. L., and Lamb, L. E. 1968. Relative impedance measurements in young children. Arch. Otolaryngol., 88:162–168.

Roseneau, H. 1962. Die Schlafbeschallung: Eine Methode der Horprufung beim Kleinstkind. Zeit. Laryngol. Rhinol. Otol. Ihre Grezg., 41:194–208.

Ross, M., and Lerman, J. 1970. A picture identification task for hearing impaired children. J. Speech Hear. Res., 13:44–53.

Rousey, C. L., Snyder, C., and Rousey, C. A. 1964. Changes in respiration as a function of auditory stimuli. J. Aud. Res., 4:107–114.

Rowe, M. J. 1978. Normal variability of the brain-stem auditory evoked response in young and old adult subjects. EEG Clin. Neurophysiol., 44:459–470.

Ruben, R. J., Elberling, C., and Solomon, G. 1976. Electrocochleography. Baltimore, University Park Press.

Salamy, A., and McKean, C. M. 1976. Postnatal development of human brainstem potentials during the first year of life. EEG Clin. Neurophysiol., 40:418–426.

Salamy, A., McKean, C. M., and Buda, F. B. 1975. Maturational changes in auditory transmission as reflected in human brainstem potentials. Brain Res., 96:361–366.

Salomon, G., and Elberling, G. 1971. Cochlear nerve potentials recorded from the ear canal in man. Acta Otolaryngol., 71:319.

Schulman, C. A. 1970. Heart rate response habituation in high-risk premature infants. Psychophysiology, 6:690–694.

Schulman, C. A. 1974. Heart rate audiometry. Part II. The relationship between heart rate change threshold and audiometric threshold in hearing-impaired children. Neuropaediatrie, 5:19–27.

Schulman, C. A., and Kreiter, R. 1971. The contribution of heart-rate audiometry in the identification of hearing impairment. Presented at the Annual Meeting of the California Speech and Hearing Association, Los Angeles.

Schulman-Galambos, C., and Galambos, R. 1975. Brainstem auditory evoked responses in premature infants. J. Speech Hear. Res., 18:456–465.

Schulman-Galambos, C., and Galambos, R. 1979. Brainstem evoked response audiometry in newborn hearing screening. Arch. Otolaryngol., 105:86–90.

Schwartz, D. M., and Sanders, J. 1976. Critical bandwidth and sensitivity prediction in the acoustic stapedial reflex. J. Speech Hear. Disord., 41:244–255.

Schwartz, D. M., Schwartz, R. H., Rosenblatt, M., et al. 1978. Variability in tympanometric pattern in children below five years of age. In Harford, E. R., Bess, F. H., Bluestone, C. D., et al. (Eds.) Impedance Screening for Middle Ear Disease in Children. New York, Grune and Stratton, pp. 145–152.

Selters, W. E., and Brackmann, D. E. 1977. Acoustic tumor detection with brainstem electric response audiometry. Arch. Otolaryngol., 103:181.

Sheehy, J. L., and Inzer, B. E. 1976. Acoustic reflex test in neuro-otologic diagnosis. Arch. Otolaryngol., 102:647–653.

Shepherd, D. C. 1978. Pediatric audiology. In Rose, D. E. (Ed.) Audiological Assessment, Englewood Cliffs, N.J., Prentice-Hall, pp. 261–300.

Silverman, S. R. 1960. Hard of hearing children. In Davis, H., and Silverman, S. R. (Eds.) Hearing and Deafness. Chap. 17. New York, Holt, Rinehart and Winston.

Skinner, P. H. 1978. Electroencephalic response audiometry. In Katz, J. (Ed.) Handbook of Clinical Audiology, Baltimore, Williams and Wilkins, pp. 311–327.

Skinner, B. K., Norris, T. W., and Jirsha, R. E. 1978. Contralateral ipsilateral acoustic reflex thresholds in preschool children. In Harford, E. R., Bess, F. H., Bluestone, C. D., et al. (Eds.) Impedance Screening for Middle Ear Disease in Children. New York, Grune and Stratton, pp. 161–170.

Skinner, P. H., and Shimota, J. 1975. A comparison of the effects of sedatives on the auditory evoked cortical response. J. Am. Audiol. Soc., *1*:71–78.

Snow, T., and McCandless, G. 1976. The use of impedance measures in hearing aid selection. Natl. Hear. Aid J., 7:32–33.

Sohmer, H., and Feinmesser, M. 1967. Cochlear action potentials recorded from the external ear in man. Ann. Otol. Rhinol. Laryngol., 76:427–435.

Sohmer, H., and Feinmesser, M. 1973. Routine use of electrocochleography (cochlear audiometry)· in human subjects. Audiology, *12*:167–173.

Sohmer, H., and Student, M. 1978. Auditory nerve and brain-stem evoked responses in normal, autistic, minimal brain dysfunction and psychomotor retarded children. EEG Clin. Neurophysiol., 44:380–388.

Starr, A. 1976. Auditory brainstem responses in brain death. Brain, 99:543–554.

Starr, A., and Achor, L. J. 1975. Auditory brainstem responses in neurological disease. Arch. Neurol., 32:761–768.

Starr, A., and Hamilton, A. 1976. Brain regions generating auditory brainstem responses: Correlating between site of pathology and response abnormalities. Neurology, 25:385.

Starr, A., Amlie, R., Martin, W. H., et al. 1977. Development of auditory function in newborn infants revealed by auditory brainstem potentials. Pediatrics, 6:831–839.

Stockard, J. J. 1978. Pathologic and non-pathologic factors influencing brainstem auditory evoked response. Presented at the Fourth Annual Auditory Evoked Response Workshop and Symposium, San Diego, November.

Stockard, J. J., and Rossiter, U. S. 1977. Clinical and pathologic correlates of brain stem auditory response abnormalities. Neurology, 27(4):316–325.

Stockard, J. J., Stockard, J. E., and Sharbrough, F. W. 1977. Detection and localization of occult lesions with brainstem auditory responses. Mayo Clin. Proc., 52:761–769.

Suzuki, T., and Ogiba, Y. 1960. A technique of pure tone audiometry for children under three years of age: Conditioned orientation reflex (COR) audiometry. Rev. Laryngol., 81:33–45.

Suzuki, T., and Ogiba, Y. 1961. Conditioned orientation reflex audiometry. Arch. Otolaryngol., 74:192–198.

Suzuki, T., Ogiba, Y., and Takei, T. 1972. Basic properties of conditioned orientation reflex audiometry. Minerva Otolaryngol., 22:181–186.

Suzuki, T., Hirai, Y., and Horiuchi, K. 1977. Auditory brain stem responses to pure tone stimuli. Scand. Audiol., 6:51–56.

Teel, J., Winston, M. A., Aspinall, K., et al., 1967. Thresholds of hearing by respiration using a polygraph. Arch. Otolaryngol., 86:172–174.

Terkildsen, K., and Thomsen, K. A. 1959. The influence of pressure variations on the impedance of the human ear drum. J. Laryngol. Otol., 73:409–418.

Terkildsen, K., and Scott-Nielsen, S. 1960. An electroacoustic impedance measuring bridge for clinical use. Arch. Otolaryngol., 72:339–346.

Terkildsen, K., Huis in't Veld, F., and Osterhammel, P. 1977. Auditory brain stem responses in the diagnosis of cerebellopontine angle tumors. Scand. Audiol., 3:123.

Thompson, G., and Weber, B. A. 1974. Responses of infants and young children to behavioral observation audiometry (BOA). J. Speech Hear. Disord., 39:140–147.

Thomsen, J., Terkildsen, K., and Osterhammel, P. 1978. Auditory brain stem responses in patients with acoustic neuromas. Scand. Audiol., 7:179–183.

Thomsen, K. A. 1958. Investigations of the tubal function and measurement of the middle ear pressure in pressure chamber. Acta Otolaryngol., Suppl. 140.

Thornton, A. R. D. 1975. Statistical properties of surface recorded electrocochleographic responses. Scand. Audiol., 4:91–102.

Tizard, B. 1968. Habituation of EEG and skin potentials changes in normal and severely subnormal children. Am. J. Ment. Defic., 73:34–40.

Tonnison, W. 1975. Measuring in the ear gain of hearing aids by the acoustic reflex method. J. Speech Hear. Res., 18:5–16.

Van Wagoner, R. S., and Goodwine, S. 1977. Clinical impressions of acoustic reflex measures in an adult population. Arch. Otolaryngol., 103:582–584.

Wagner, H. 1963. Zur Methodik der Schlafbeschallung. Zeit. Laryngol. Rhinol. Otol. Ihre Grezg., 42:139–146.

Warren, V. G. 1972. A comparative study of the auditory responses of normal and "at risk" infants from twelve to twenty-four months of age using COR audiometry. Doctoral dissertation, University of Southern California, Los Angeles.

Wedenberg, E. 1963. Objective audiometry tests on non-cooperative children. Acta Otolaryngologica, Suppl. 175.

Wedenberg, E. 1972. Auditory tests on newborn infants. *In* Cunningham, G. (Ed.) Conference on Newborn Hearing Screening, pp. 126–131, Washington, A. G. Bell Assoc.

Wilson, W. R. 1978. Behavioral assessment of auditory function in infants. *In* Minifie, F. D., and Lloyd, L. L. (Eds.) Communicative and Cognitive Abilities — Early Behavioral Assessment. Baltimore, University Park Press.

Wilson, W. R., Moore, J. M., and Thompson, G. 1976. Sound field auditory thresholds of infants utilizing visual reinforcement audiometry (VRA). Presented at the annual convention of the American Speech and Hearing Association, Houston, Texas, November.

Yamada, O., Yagi, T., Yamane, H., and Suzuki, J. I. 1975. Clinical evaluation of the auditory evoked brainstem response. Auris Nasus Larynx, 2:92–105.

Yoshie, N., Ohasi, T., and Suzuki, T. 1967. Non-surgical recording of auditory nerve action potentials in man. Laryngoscope, 77:76–85.

Zwislocki, J. 1963. An acoustic method for clinical examination of the ear. J. Speech Hear. Res., 6:303–314.

Zwislocki, J., and Feldman, A. S. 1970. Acoustic impedance of pathological ears. ASHA, Monogr. 15.

METHODS OF EXAMINATION: RADIOLOGIC ASPECTS

Philip J. Dubois, M.B.B.S., F.R.C.R., M.R.A.C.R.

INTRODUCTION

Since the advent of specialized projections for displaying the internal auditory canal (Stenvers, 1917; Towne, 1926) and mastoids (Schüller, 1918), radiology has had an established role in the evaluation of patients with otologic disease. Enthusiasm for preoperative radiology has varied greatly from country to country and from center to center within the same country.

New impetus was given to the use of preoperative radiology by the development of polydirectional tomography in the 1950s. Pioneering work by Brunner and others (1961) in Sweden and by Valvassori (1963) in the United States established a clearly defined role for tomography in the evaluation of certain patients, for example, those with congenital otologic anomalies. Use of this method in evaluating other problems such as inflammatory ear disease is still controversial, and again there is regional variation in the degree of utilization of these techniques.

The recent introduction of computed cranial tomography (CT) (Hounsfield, 1973) has opened new horizons in neuro-otologic radiology. Still in its infancy, this technique already can demonstrate the intracranial extension of otologic, pharyngeal, and sinus disease with more sensitivity and much less invasiveness than pneumoencephalography, cerebral angiography, or positive contrast cisternography.

In this chapter, a brief description of the radiologic examinations most often performed in pediatric otologic practice is presented. Since it is essential to minimize the radiation received by patients in this age group, it behooves the clinician to request only those radiologic examinations that address the clinical problem effectively and to order radiologic series in a logical sequence when more than one radiologic examination is required.

CONVENTIONAL RADIOGRAPHY

Skull Series

The full neurologic skull series includes two lateral projections, base or submentovertex projections, and Caldwell, posteroanterior, and Towne projections. Usually this series is inadequate for a detailed analysis of pathologic conditions of the temporal bone but is useful in the evaulation of lesions extending beyond the regions examined in specialized temporal bone projections (Fig. 8C–1). Fractures of the calvarium extending to the middle ear, cranial dysplasias, nasopharyngeal masses, and signs of raised intracranial pressure may thus be revealed by radiologic examination beyond the temporal bones.

Specialized Projections

In centers where polydirectional tomography is available, conventional specialized projections can usually be limited to two or three views. However, since many clinicians are unable to obtain adequate tomography in the locales in which they practice, the convention-

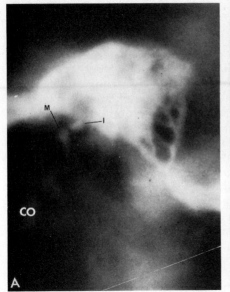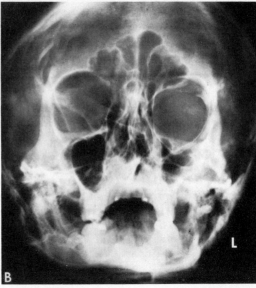

Figure 8C–1 *A*, Lateral projection tomogram through the left tympanic cavity showing inferior displacement of the ossicle (M, I), destruction of the tympanic ring anteriorly, and dislocation of the mandibular condyle (CO) by a soft tissue mass. *B*, Modified Caldwell projection from the full neurologic skull series of radiographs. The "bare orbit" characteristic of the dysplasia of neurofibromatosis is caused by defective ossification of the greater wing of the left sphenoid. This finding, as well as extensive destruction of the middle fossa floor seen on the submentovertex projection, demonstrated the full extent of a plexiform neurofibroma invading the temporal bone from the orbit and infratemporal fossa in this eight year old girl. (L = left.)

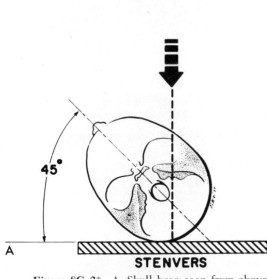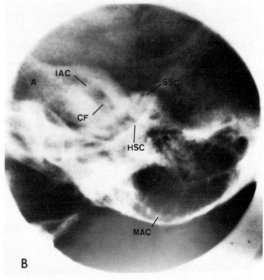

Figure 8C–2* *A*, Skull base seen from above. The Stenver projection is a "face-on" view of the posterior surface of the temporal bone. Thus, in this diagram the side farthest from the cassette is being examined. The sagittal plane is at a 45 degree angle to the cassette. *B*, The resulting radiograph of a Stenver projection. The internal auditory canal is foreshortened, the crista falciformis is easily identified, the superior and lateral semicircular canals are viewed tangentially and, therefore, are projected as linear lucencies, the petrous apex is well defined, and the mastoid air cells are somewhat overpenetrated.

Key to figures: A, mastoid antrum; AP, petrous apex; AT, auditory tube; C, cochlea; CA, carotid canal; CC, crus commune; CF, crista falciformis; CO, mandibular condyle; EAC, external auditory canal; ET, epitympanum; GF, glaserian (squamotympanic) fissure; HSC, horizontal semicircular canal; I, incus; IAC, internal auditory canal; KS, Körner's septum; M, malleus; MAC, mastoid air cells; MT, mesotympanum; OV, foramen ovale; OS, ossicles; OW, oval window; P, porus acusticus; POF, petro-occipital fissure; PSC, posterior semicircular canal; RS, recess for stapedius muscle; S, scutum; SD, sinodural angle; SS, sigmoid sinus; SSC, superior semicircular canal; V, vestibule; VA, vestibular aqueduct; VII, facial nerve canal; XII, hypoglossal canal.

*In the diagrams of Figures 8C–2 to 8C–4, the radiographic cassette containing film is represented by a rectangle with diagonal shading and the incident x-ray beam by a broken line at right angles to the cassette with an arrow indicating the direction of incident radiation.

al radiographic projections of the temporal bone must be utilized. Of the numerous projections described, all commonly used views fall into three categories.

Stenver Projection. (Fig. 8C–2) This is a "face on" view of the posterior surface of the petrous temporal bone and therefore provides an excellent demonstration of the petrous apex. The internal auditory canal is foreshortened so that differences in vertical diameters between the right and left sides can easily be detected in patients with suspected acoustic neurinomas. The bony labyrinth is well demonstrated. The mastoid is usually overpenetrated when this view is correctly exposed for examination of the petrous apex.

Lateral and Lateral Oblique Projections. (Fig. 8C–3) Since both mastoids are superimposed in true lateral skull radiographs, caudal angulation of the x-ray tube is used to examine one side at a time (Schüller projection). A second angulation achieved by tilting the patient's head is used in the Law and Owen projections. The former provides excellent visualization of the mastoid air cells, while the Owen projection is designed to demonstrate the ossicles within the epitympanum and mesotympanum, and the scutum (bony bridge) formed by the junction of the lateral epitympanic wall and the roof of the external auditory canal. Plain film detection of small cholesteatomas is based on the destruction of these structures early in the

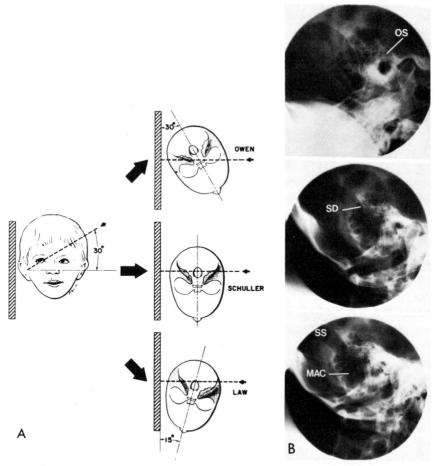

Figure 8C–3 Lateral type projections. *A,* Diagram illustrating, on the left, the primary caudal angulation of 30 degrees used to project the mastoid closest to the cassette away from the image of the contralateral mastoid. (In the Law projection, this angle is reduced to 15 degrees.) On the right, the secondary angulations for three commonly used projections are shown as being achieved by rotation of the patient's head. Sophisticated skull units achieve the same projections by a second angulation of the x-ray tube without moving the patient. *B,* The resultant radiographs. In this patient, the ossicles and sinodural angle are best demonstrated in Owen's projection.

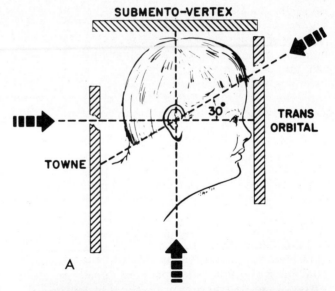

SUBMENTO-VERTEX

TRANS ORBITAL

30°

TOWNE

A

Figure 8C–4 Towne, base and posteroanterior projections. *A*, Diagram indicating the cassette position, incident beam, centering, and positioning for Towne, base (submentovertex), and posteroanterior (transorbital) projections of the temporal bones. *B*, Transorbital projection radiograph. The internal auditory canals, vestibules, and lateral and superior semicircular canals are usually well displayed. *C*, Towne projection radiograph. *D*, Submentovertex projection radiograph. TC = tympanic cavity.

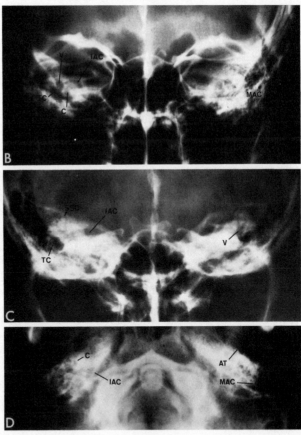

course of the disease. The Mayer projection is an "exaggerated" Owen projection — angulations of both the tube and the patient's head are increased to 45 degrees. In all these projections, the extent of mastoid pneumatization, position of the sinodural angle, pres-

ence of inflammatory mucosal thickening or fluid, destruction of bony septa by tumor, infection, or cholesteatoma, and course of fractures may be detected.

Towne, Base, and Posteroanterior Projections. (Fig. 8C–4) In each of these projections, the incident radiation beam is in the sagittal plane and the x-ray beam is tightly collimated to the temporal bone region, using either a small circular field to display individual sides or a narrow rectangular field to examine both sides simultaneously. In either case, the radiographic detail is markedly superior to that seen on the same projection with a large field, such as that used in the standard skull series. All these projections are useful in comparing the petrous apices, internal auditory canals, tympanic cavities, ossicles, and mastoids contralaterally. In addition, the foramina of the skull base, bony eustachian tube, and lateral pharyngeal walls are identified on the base projection.

Two modifications of the posteroanterior projection are occasionally useful. In the Guillen projection the patient's head is turned 15 to 20 degrees toward the side being examined so that the medial wall of the tympanic cavity and the oval window are projected in profile through the orbit. In the Chausse III projection, the head is turned 15 to 20 degrees away from the affected side so that the lateral attic wall is projected just lateral to the lateral orbital margin. These projections are seldom performed in pediatric practice.

Whenever the temporal bones are examined, it is usual to obtain the posteroanterior, Towne, and submentovertex projections. These are supplemented by one or more of the lateral or lateral oblique projections if inflammatory ear disease is suspected. If evaluation for suspected acoustic neurinoma or petrous apical pathologic conditions is required, the lateral views are usually omitted and the Stenver projection is used. When polytomography is available, one can limit plain film examination to Schüller or Law projections in mastoid disease or to Stenver projections for intrapetrous pathologic conditions.

TOMOGRAPHY

The use of tomography with thin (approximately 1 mm) body sections and polydirectional tube motion is now firmly established as part of the radiologic assessment of otologic disorders. The Philips polytome, CGR Stratomatic, and Siemens Optiplanimat, using hypocycloid, trispiral, and pentaspiral tube motion, respectively, are the currently available units capable of such polydirectional tomography. All require exposure times of 5 to 6 seconds for each section obtained, and an average examination requires approximately 8 to 12 sections per projection. Because of these long exposure times, it is our routine practice to use general anesthesia to secure immobility in all patients under three years of age and neuroleptanesthesia for most children under 12 years.

Shorter exposures may suffice if linear tomography is used, but the longitudinal "parasite" (false) shadows inherent in this method render the definition, particularly in lateral projections, vastly inferior to that obtained by polydirectional tomography. In centers where only linear tomography is available, adequate studies can often be obtained provided a stable tomographic unit capable of 60 degree tube travel is used by a trained technician supervised by a radiologist familiar with the procedure. Collimation to the smallest possible field size is mandatory for good detail, and a plesiosectional cassette (Lapayowkar et al., 1972) will help to reduce the number of exposures necessary.

Regardless of the tomographic method used, a definitive examination should be made with the smallest number of exposures possible since the radiation dose is high in these examinations (Chin et al., 1970).

The posteroanterior projection, which reduces the lens dose by 20 to 30 times (Berger et al., 1974) should be used when possible; otherwise, lead shielding of the eyes is mandatory. We aim to complete each examination in no more than two projections to minimize the radiation dose, patient discomfort, and time of examination. It is essential that the specific clinical problem that the tomograms are intended to resolve be conveyed to the radiologist supervising the examination so that the correct projection, levels of sections, and intervals between sections may be achieved on the first examination.

Although the otologist has a detailed knowledge of the surgical anatomy of the temporal bone, he or she may initially find difficulty in utilizing this knowledge in tomographic interpretations. Soft tissue landmarks are not reliably depicted, familiar bone structures may be invisible, and anatomically insignificant structures become prominent in tomograms. False (parasite) shadows may be confusing, and the projections used are not usually comparable to conventional anatomic sections. Therefore, some simple principles and pitfalls in interpretations should be ap-

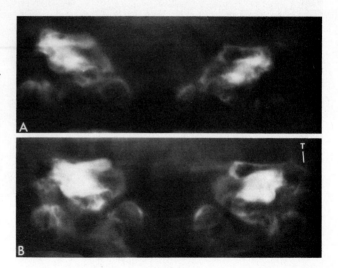

Figure 8C–5 Tomographic "invisibility" of thin bony structures when their orientation is not exactly at right angles to the plane of tomographic cut is demonstrated. *A*, Frontal projection tomogram at the level of the vestibule, standard anteroposterior projection. The tegmen tympani is not visible. *B*, With the head extended 15 degrees, a tomographic cut slightly more posterior shows the tegmen (T) clearly, since it is now oriented perpendicular to the plane of the tomographic section.

preciated, and "tomographic anatomy" should be relearned.

General physical principles and applications of tomography have been comprehensively reviewed by Littleton (1976). A tomographic section is created because adjacent structures are blurred much more than those in the plane of section. Nevertheless, very high or low densities in adjacent structures cannot be completely removed, and parasite shadows will result, obscuring detail in the plane of interest. In addition, there is always some blurring of structures in the plane of the tomographic cut, so that one does not see the same well-defined bony outlines as are obtained with conventional radiographs. Finally, a thin, bony plate such as the tegmen tympani will be depicted only when it lies in a plane perpendicular, or near perpendicular, to the plane of the tomographic section. When the patient is positioned so that the structure is more than 15 to 20 degrees from the perpendicular, it becomes tomographically "invisible" (Fig. 8C–5). In the same way, a fracture line will be demonstrated only when it is oriented near perpendicular to the plane of the tomographic section. Thus, searching for a longitudinal petrous fracture in coronal sections will often be futile, and sagittal, horizontal, or transverse axial projections will be necessary to exclude such a fracture.

Excellent texts are available that correlate anatomic with tomographic sections in all standard projections (Rabischong et al., 1976; Valvassori and Buckingham, 1975), and one of these should be available to any physician engaged in polydirectional tomography of the temporal bone. Since two tomographic projections, frontal and lateral, suffice for assessment of most pediatric patients, salient anatomic features of these are outlined here.

Coronal Sections (Frontal, Posteroanterior, or Anteroposterior Projection)

It is convenient to consider two levels that contain most of the structures of interest: the cochlear and vestibular planes. In the cochlear plane (Fig. 8C–6), no more than 1½ turns of the cochlea are identified since the section cuts obliquely across the cochlea. Immediately adjacent to its superolateral aspect, the facial nerve canal is usually identified as a slit or as paired round lucencies, depending on whether the section is at or behind the level of the geniculate ganglion. The mesotympanum and epitympanum contain the malleus and incus, which usually form a combined ossicular shadow because of their small size but which, fortuitously, may be represented separately in adjacent sections. The junction of the lateral epitympanic wall and roof of the external auditory canal normally forms a sharp ridge, the scutum. Erosion of the scutum is an early indication of cholesteatoma. The tympanic membrane is usually invisible, but when pathologically thickened it may be seen projecting at approximately 45 degrees inferomedially from the scutum to the floor of the external auditory canal. A thin, bony plate separates the hypotympanum from the carotid canal.

A section through the oval window may be

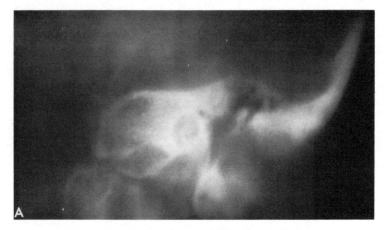

Figure 8C–6 *A,* Coronal tomographic section through the cochlea. *B,* Line drawing of *A.*

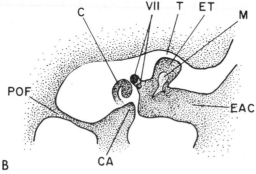

Figure 8C–7 *A,* Coronal tomographic section through the vestibule at the level of the oval window. In this section the incus is not displayed, although it is commonly seen at this level. The stapes is not readily demonstrated in normal pediatric patients. *B,* Line drawing of *A.*

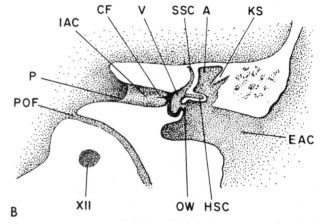

identified, the "vestibular plane," 2 to 3 mm posterior to the cochlear plane. When comparing the size and configuration of the internal auditory canals, the oval window provides a good landmark by which to check that identical levels of sectioning are being compared. In this plane (Fig. 8C–7) one may identify the crista falciformis, vestibule, oval window niche, and the ampullated ends of the horizontal and superior semicircular canals.

The tegmen separates the combined lucency of the epitympanum, aditus, and antrum from the middle cranial fossa. Körner's septum, the fused petrosquamous suture, is variably prominent and can usually be identified in normal subjects in this plane or in

more posterior sections through the antrum proper. Inferior to the tympanic cavity, the jugular foramen, jugular tubercle, hypoglossal canal, and petro-occipital fissure can be identified in the vestibular plane or in more posterior adjacent sections.

Parasagittal Sections (Lateral Projections)

In interpreting a series of lateral tomograms, it is helpful to search for recognizable landmarks at three key levels — the ossicles, the labyrinth, and the internal auditory canal. In the plane of the ossicles (Fig. 8C–8), one can usually identify the vertical portion of the facial nerve canal, the stapedial recess, the stylomastoid foramen, and the horizontal

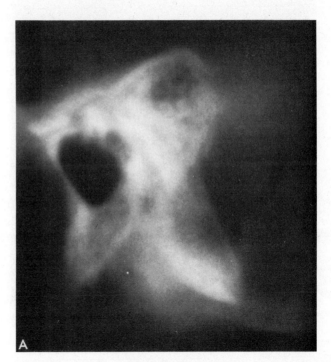

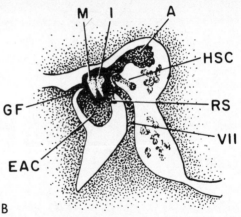

Figure 8C–8 *A,* Lateral (parasagittal) tomographic section through the plane of the ossicles. *B,* Line drawing of *A.*

semicircular canal. The ossicles appear as a tooth-like density, the head of the malleus and body of the incus forming the crown and the long processes forming the roots. Surrounding the ossicles is a figure eight–shaped lucency formed by the epitympanum above and the combined lucency of the external auditory canal and the mesotympanum below. The anterior tympanic spine forms the waist of the figure eight anteriorly, and the glaserian (squamotympanic) fissure is immediately anterosuperior. In this or adjacent sections, the aditus ad antrum can be seen as a more or less continuous lucency extending posteriorly from the epitympanum, separated from the middle fossa by the thin tegmen.

More medial sagittal sections through the labyrinth (Fig. 8C–9) enable identification of the individual semicircular canals, vestibule, round window, and cochlea. However, anomalies of the inner ear are better studied in base or transverse axial projections. The straight segment of the vestibular aqueduct is identified in sections at or adjacent to the level of the crus commune.

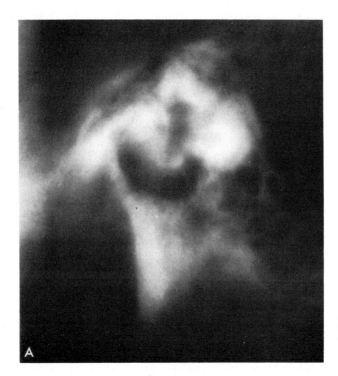

Figure 8C–9   *A*, Lateral (sagittal) tomographic section through the labyrinth at the level of the crus commune. *B*, Line drawing of *A*. VA = vestibular aqueduct.

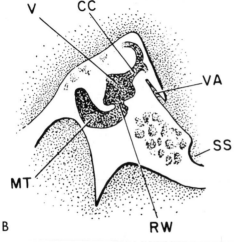

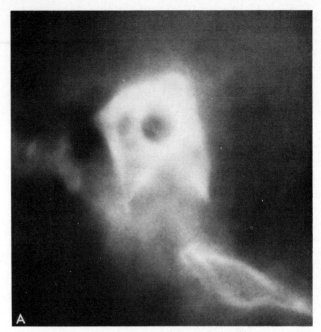

Figure 8C–10 *A*, Lateral (sagittal) tomographic section through the internal auditory canal. *B*, Line drawing of *A*.

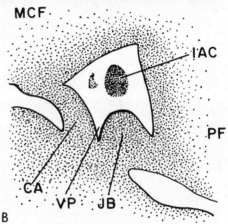

Sagittal sections medial to the labyrinth exhibit a much simpler anatomic configuration (Fig. 8C–10). A well-defined triangular bony ridge, the vaginal process or carotid crest, separates the carotid canal anteriorly from the jugular foramen posteriorly. The internal auditory canal is easily identified and may be surrounded by a variable number of petrous apical air cells.

COMPUTERIZED CRANIAL TOMOGRAPHY (CT)

In essence, this method produces on a cathode ray tube or television screen cross-sectional images of the brain, usually 13 or 8 mm thick. The final image, available for photography, is reconstructed by computer from a series of radiographic projections taken at different angles in the plane of interest using a narrow x-ray beam and sensitive scintillation detectors (Ter-Pogossian, 1977). Contrast resolution so far exceeds that of conventional radiography and tomography that differences between cerebrospinal fluid, gray matter, and white matter can be resolved. Pathologic processes such as tumor, abscess, edema, or hemorrhage are detected by distortion of normal intracranial anatomic landmarks (ventricles, subarachnoid spaces, and vascular structures) as well as by their differences in "density" (attenuation values) from that of normal structures. Intra-

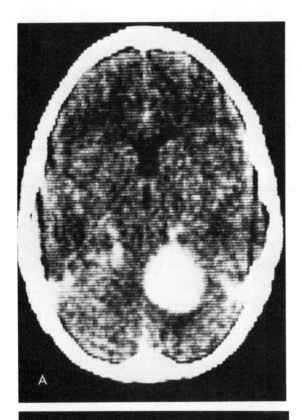

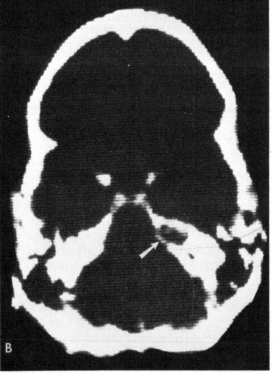

Figure 8C–11 *A,* Large (4 cm) acoustic neurilem-moma demonstrated by computed tomography in an eight year old boy with no stigmata of neurofibromatosis. *B,* In this case, bony erosion of the internal auditory canal was extensive enough to be demonstrable by CT (arrow).

venous contrast enhancement (Ambrose et al., 1973) and more recently, contrast enhancement of the subarachnoid spaces (Rosenbaum et al., 1978) have increased the sensitivity and specificity of the method.

Although the role of CT in pediatric otolaryngology has not yet been fully explored, it has become the most useful primary radiologic method in the evaluation of intracranial extension of mastoid inflammatory disease and aggressive tumors of the skull base, sinuses, or orbit. In detection of acoustic neurilemmomas greater than 1.5 cm in diameter, it is the most useful single radiographic investigative tool available (Fig. 8C–11). Despite superior contrast resolution, however, spatial resolution — the ability to portray fine detail — is inherently inferior to conventional radiography and tomography because of the section thickness and the process of electronic reconstruction. Thus, bony changes in the skull base and temporal bones are better portrayed by tomography, and pharyngeal and laryngeal lesions are better demonstrated by fluoroscopic contrast studies. It is likely that technologic advances will produce CT images of intrapetrous and extracranial lesions superior to those obtained by conventional radiologic methods, but at this time comparable thin-section images are not routinely available.

POSTERIOR FOSSA MYELOGRAPHY, PNEUMOENCEPHALOGRAPHY, AND ARTERIOGRAPHY

Tumors of the cerebellopontine angle are rare in children except in the presence of neurofibromatosis. These tumors, as well as the much more common intra-axial tumors (pontine and cerebellar) are usually investigated by CT, possibly followed by vertebral angiography. If differentiation between an intra-axial and extra-axial mass cannot be made by these studies, pneumoencephalography, after insuring that the intracranial pressure is not raised, is occasionally used. Other indications for pneumoencephalography are few since the advent of CT, which is less invasive. Posterior fossa myelography (iophendylate cisternography) should be strictly limited in its use to the detection of suspected small, predominantly intracanalicular acoustic neurilemmomas below the threshold of detection by CT (Dubois et al., 1977). There

would appear to be no other indication for introducing iophendylate into the posterior fossa of a child, since there is some risk of spilling the agent into the middle fossa, from which it cannot be retrieved. Residual droplets are present for life, may cause arachnoiditis or severe headache, and degrade subsequent CT images that may be crucial to effective care of the patient.

SELECTED REFERENCES

Compere, W. E., and Valvassori, G. E. Radiographic Atlas of the Temporal Bone. American Academy of Ophthalmology and Otolaryngology, home study course.
  This is probably the most useful single reference work for the practicing otologist interpreting radiographs.

Etter, L. E. 1972. Roentgenography and Roentgenology of the Temporal Bone, Middle Ear and Mastoid. 2nd Ed. Springfield, IL., Charles C Thomas.
  An old and valued text devoted entirely to conventional radiology of the temporal bone with a section on linear tomography by M. S. Lapayowkar. Normal anatomy, radiographic positionings, and pathologic illustrative cases are included.

Patter, G. D. (Ed.) 1974. Radiology of the Ear. Radiol. Clin. North Am., *12*(3).
  This comprehensive symposium contains excellent chapters on normal tomographic anatomy, congenital anomalies, inflammatory ear disease, trauma, and neoplasms of the temporal bone. A section on radiology of the ear in children by Fitz and Harwood-Nash is particularly recommended.

REFERENCES

Ambrose, J., Gooding, M. R., and Richardson, A. E. 1973. Sodium iothalamate as an aid to diagnosis of intracranial lesions by computerized transverse axial scanning. Lancet, *11*:669.

Berger, P., Gildersleever, S., and Poznanski, A. 1974. The feasibility of the PA projection for tomography of the petrous bone. Am. J. Roentgenol., *122*:67.

Brunner, S., Petersen, O., and Stoksted, P. 1962. Laminography of the temporal bone. Am. J. Roentgenol., *68*:281.

Chin, F. K., Anderson, W. B., and Gilbertson, J. D. 1970. Radiation dose to critical organs during petrous tomography. Radiology, *94*:623.

Compere, W. E., and Valvassori, G. E. Radiographic Atlas of the Temporal Bone. American Academy of Ophthalmology and Otolaryngology, home study course.

Dubois, P. J., Drayer, B. P., Bank, W. O., et al. 1977. An evaluation of current diagnostic radiologic modalities in the investigation of acoustic neurilemmomas. Radiology, *126*:173.

Etter, L. E. 1972. Roentgenography and Roentgenology of the Temporal Bone, Middle Ear and Mastoid. 2nd ed. Springfield, IL, Charles C Thomas.

Hounsfield, G. N. 1973. Computerized transverse axial scanning (tomography) Part 1. Description of system. Br. J. Radiol., *46*:1016.

Lapayowkar, M. S., Carter, B. L., and McGann, M. D. 1972. Plesiosectional tomography technique: Illustration of normal and pathologic roentgen anatomy. Section XII. *In* Etter, L. E. Roentgenography and Roentgenology of the Temporal Bone, Middle Ear and Mastoid Process, 2nd ed. Springfield, IL, Charles C Thomas.

Littleton, J. T. 1976. Tomography — physical principles and clinical applications. *In* Golden's Diagnostic Radiology, Sec. 17. Baltimore, Williams and Wilkins Co.

Potter, G. D. (Ed.) 1974. Radiology of the Ear. Radiol. Clin. North Am., *12*(3).

Rabischong, P., Vignaud, J., Paleirac, R., et al. 1976. Tomographie et Anatomie de L'Oreille. Amsterdam, Arts Graphiques.

Rosenbaum, A. E., Drayer, B. P., Dubois, P. J., et al. 1978. Visualization of small extracanalicular neu-rilemmomas by metrizamide cisternographic enhancement. Arch. Otolaryngol., *104*(5):239–243.

Schüller, A. 1918. Roentgen diagnosis of diseases of the head. (Translated by F. F. Stocking). St. Louis, The C. V. Mosby Co.

Stenvers, H. W. 1917. Roentgenology of the os petrosum. Arch. Radiol. Electrother., *22*:4.

Ter-Pogossian, M. M. 1977. Computerized cranial tomography: Physics and equipment. Semin. Roentgenol., *12*:13.

Towne, E. D. 1926. Erosion of petrous bone by acoustic nerve tumor. Arch. Otolaryngol., *5*:515.

Valvassori, G. E. 1963. Laminagraphy of the ear, normal roentgenographic anatomy. Am. J. Roentgenol., *89*:1155.

Valvassori, G. E., and Buckingham, R. A. 1975. Tomography and cross sections of the ear. Philadelphia, W. B. Saunders Co.

THE NEUROVESTIBULAR TESTING OF INFANTS AND CHILDREN

Lydia Eviatar, M.D.
Abraham Eviatar, M.D.

Vestibular dysfunction in children may present in a variety of ways, from the subtle lag in acquisition of head and postural control seen in infants with delayed maturation of vestibular function (such as premature babies) to the acute episodes of vertigo and loss of posture control encountered in diseases of the labyrinth. Because of the close interaction of the vestibular system with the visual, auditory, proprioceptive, cerebellar, and motor pathways in the maintenance of postural control and equilibrium in space, it is often difficult to single out which of the systems is directly responsible for a noted deficit. It is by a process of elimination that a correct diagnosis can be established. This implies that neurologic testing of sensory channels such as vision, hearing, and proprioception as well as of cerebellar motor pathways will be required. Both the neurologic examination and vestibular testing are adapted to the patient's age and level of maturation of the central nervous system.

BASIS OF THE EXAMINATION

A good history of the presenting complaints from the patient or parents and a detailed description of associated symptoms and signs are essential. It is important to review motor developmental milestones, his-

tory of drug intake (especially ototoxic drugs), and prior illnesses that may have affected the eighth nerve (Table 8D–1).

The method of examining children presented in this chapter has been tested in more than 500 children, and normative data were obtained and published (Eviatar and Eviatar, 1979a). The method evolved from information from embryologists, anatomists, neurophysiologists, and clinical investigators.

Table 8D–1   REVIEW OF HISTORY OF NEUROVESTIBULAR EXAMINATION

 I. Pregnancy
   1. Intrauterine infections: Toxoplasmosis, Rubella, Cytomegalic inclusion disease, Herpes (T.O.R.C.H.)
   2. Rh incompatibility
   3. Ingestion of ototoxic drugs
   4. Toxemia of pregnancy or gestational diabetes
 II. Neonatal period
   1. Neonatal asphyxia
   2. Neonatal jaundice
   3. Respiratory distress syndrome
   4. Central nervous system infection, sepsis, ingestion of ototoxic drugs
 III. Developmental milestones
   1. Sitting, standing, walking, speech
 IV. History of otitis, central nervous system infections, ingestion of ototoxic drugs, vertigo, head trauma
 V. Hereditary diseases affecting hearing or balance (degenerative or metabolic)

EMBRYOLOGIC DEVELOPMENT OF THE NEUROVESTIBULAR SYSTEM

A review of the basic information available on the development of the labyrinth and its gradual contribution to various postural and oculomotor reflexes is pertinent to a discussion of neurovestibular examination. From studies in embryos, it is known that brain stem reflexes controlling eyeball movements begin to operate at about the 15th week of gestation and become well established by the 24th week (Gesell and Amatruda, 1945; Hooker, 1952; Bergstrom, 1969).

Organized regional reflex responses to movements of the head and neck also emerge at about the 28th week (Gesell and Amatruda, 1945). The vestibular receptors in the inner ear become fully active by the 32nd week of gestation, at which time a well-developed Moro reflex can be elicited. This reflex persists until the child is between three and five months old (Schulte et al., 1969). Centripetal activity from the maturing ampullary cristae is detectable as a feeble Moro reflex as early as the eighth to ninth week of fetal life (Gesell and Amatruda, 1945; Humphrey, 1969; Cratty, 1970). At the 16th week of intrauterine life, myelin lamellae begin to appear for the first time in relation to the vestibular nerve fibers and in some of the intersegmental tract systems of the cervical spinal cord (Hamilton and Mossman, 1972). Thus, vestibular pathways are the first to myelinate, whereas the pyramidal tract is fully myelinated only by two years of age.

DEVELOPMENT OF THE VESTIBULAR SYSTEM AND ITS FUNCTIONS

The vestibular part of the inner ear consists of the three semicircular canals, the utricle, and the saccule. They are concerned with orientation in three-dimensional space, equilibrium, and modification of muscle tone.

The vestibular receptors of the semicircular canals are the cristae ampullares. The receptors of the utricle and saccule are the maculae. Angular acceleration causes movement of endolymphatic fluid of the semicircular canals and deflection of hair cells in the sensory epithelium of the cristae. This aspect of labyrinthine function is referred to as kinetic equilibrium. The utricular macula responds to changes in gravitational forces and

to linear acceleration and conveys information concerning the position of the head in space (static equilibrium) (Carpenter, 1974).

It is as yet unclear what the exact role of the saccular macula is. The macula and cristae are innervated by peripheral nerve endings originating in the bipolar cells of the vestibular ganglia. The central processes of the bipolar cells are primary vestibular fibers forming a vestibular nerve root, which enters the cerebellopontine angle where the root fibers pass dorsally between the inferior cerebellar peduncle and the spinal trigeminal tract. While entering the vestibular nuclear complex, which lies on the floor of the fourth ventricle, the fibers bifurcate into short ascending and long descending fibers. A small number of fibers will pass directly to the ipsilateral cerebellar cortex of the nodulus, uvula, and flocculus as mossy fibers. The peripheral processes of the ganglion cells, which innervate the cristae in the semicircular canals, project primarily to the superior vestibular nucleus and rostral parts of the medial vestibular nucleus (Stein and Carpenter, 1967). Cells of the inferior vestibular ganglion, which innervate the saccular macula, give rise to central fibers that descend and terminate mainly in the dorsolateral portions of the inferior vestibular nucleus. Secondary vestibular fibers arise from the vestibular nuclei and project to the cerebellum, to the nuclei of the oculomotor nerves, and to all spinal levels. From the vestibular nuclei arise ascending fibers, crossed and uncrossed, which run in the medial longitudinal fasciculus (MLF) and project to the nuclei of the extraocular muscles (abducens, trochlear, and oculomotor). These secondary vestibular fibers in the MLF play an important role in conjugate eye movements. Selective stimulation of the nerve endings from the ampulla of each semicircular canal produces specific deviation of both eyes, which is considered to be a primary vestibular response. Lesions of the MLF rostral to the abducens nuclei produce a disturbance of conjugate horizontal eye movements known as anterior internuclear ophthalmoplegia. Lesions or sectioning of the MLF rostral to the abducens nuclei abolish oculomotor responses, but nystagmus still results from labyrinthine stimulation, suggesting that impulses essential for nystagmus probably pass via the reticular formation. At the brainstem level, the descending secondary vestibular fibers in the MLF fibers are the medial vestibulospinal (crossed) and lateral vestibulospinal (uncrossed) tracts. Almost all the fibers reaching the spinal level are ipsilateral. Most fibers end at the cervical level, although some descend to the thoracic level. They terminate in the medial part of the anterior horn. The medial vestibulospinal tract plays an important role in the interaction of neck and vestibulo-ocular reflexes. The lateral vestibulospinal tract extends to the level of the sacral cord. In animal experiments, excitation by electric stimulation of the vestibulospinal fibers or the lateral nucleus produces excitation of extensor motor neurons and inhibition of flexor motor neurons (Baloh and Honrubia, 1979). Their influence is exerted primarily on axial and proximal extensor muscles by assisting local myotatic reflexes and producing enough extra force to support the body against gravity and to maintain an upright posture. A small number of primary vestibular fibers end in the reticular formation. The main influence on the reticulospinal outflow is mediated by way of secondary vestibular neurons. Muscular tone is highly dependent on myotatic reflexes (deep tendon reflexes), which in turn are under the influence of the combined excitatory and inhibitory influence of multiple supraspinal neural centers.

After transection of the midbrain, the inhibitory influence on cortex and basal ganglia is removed and the animal exhibits decerebrate rigidity manifested by increased tone in the extensor antigravity muscles. A significant decrease in tone will result if a bilateral labyrinthectomy is performed. Unilateral destruction of the labyrinth or of the lateral vestibular nucleus will result in an ipsilateral decrease in tone. Changes of position of the head in a decerebrate animal produce remarkable changes in posture and tone called tonic neck reflexes. Similar postural changes resulting from changes of position of the head will be seen in newborns until four months of age and are broadly designated as tonic neck reflexes.

When transection is performed at the midbrain level rostral to the red nucleus in an animal with intact labyrinths, righting responses of the head and body can be elicited. Similar responses are present in infants from six months on and persist with some modifications throughout life.

An understanding of the anatomy and function of vestibular pathways is necessary to recognize the various symptoms and signs of labyrinthine dysfunction. Vestibular irritation or disease causes the individual to experience vertigo, which is the illusion that he or his surroundings are moving. It may cause postural deviation, unsteadiness in the upright position, oculomotor deviation, or nystagmus. The presence of nystagmus is a good objective sign that the vestibular system is malfunctioning.

Nystagmus consists of rhythmic, involuntary oscillations of the eyes, characterized by alternating slow and rapid ocular excursions. Although the slow excursion represents the primary response to stimulation and the rapid phase is the reflex realignment, it is customary to name the nystagmus after the direction of the rapid phase.

The majority of laboratory tests for vestibular dysfunction rely on the evaluation of nystagmus evoked by stimulation of nerve endings in the semicircular canals by rotation or caloric irrigation. The vestibular impulses will then be transmitted to the vestibular nuclei and from there through the ascending secondary vestibular nerve fibers to the nuclei of the extraocular muscles in the brain stem.

The evaluation of postural responses of the head and extremities as a result of changes of position in space and changes in the center of gravity will test the integrity of the descending secondary vestibular fibers, the medial and lateral vestibulospinal tracts.

The central connections of the vestibular pathways are extensive and not well known. In addition to their close connections with the cerebellum and the reticular activating system of the brain stem, they also connect with the thalamus, specifically the ventroposterolateral nucleus (VPL), which projects to the precentral and postcentral gyrus. The cortical representation of the vestibular system is in the posterosuperior aspect of the temporal lobe, dorsal to Heschl's gyrus and at the intraparietal sulcus. Electrical stimulation of these areas can produce an illusion of rotation (de Morsier, 1938; Penfield and Kristiansen, 1951; Penfield and Jasper, 1954). Excitatory foci in these areas can produce focal seizures with vertigo as the presenting symptom.

METHODS OF EXAMINATION

The neurovestibular examination consists of the following procedures. (1) A neurodevelopmental evaluation adapted to the patient's age and level of central nervous system maturity.

(2) A comprehensive ear, nose, and throat examination to rule out the presence of infection, trauma, tumor, congenital anomalies, or fistula. Anomalies of the external ear and preauricular pits and branchial cleft fistulae are looked for. The use of the pneumatic otoscope in the diagnosis of middle ear disease and perilymphatic fistula (Hennebert sign) is helpful. In the presence of an intact tympanic membrane, negative pressure can be applied with a pneumatic otoscope and will presumably cause utriculofugal flow in the horizontal canal of the affected ear. A positive response is a slow ocular deviation (toward or away from the affected ear) followed by a few (three to four) nystagmic beats, even when pressure is sustained.

(3) A hearing test adapted to the patient's age and level of responsiveness should be performed. Infants can be tested by observing their behavioral responses to an infant auditory screener or with the help of a crib-o-gram. Orienting responses to sound in a free field will appear by four or five months of age. Play audiometry can be initiated after age two years. When responses to free-field screening are questionable, brain stem and cortical evoked responses will provide additional information.

(4) On radiographic examination, a transorbital view of the skull will demonstrate the inner ears and the internal auditory canals. Such an examination is helpful in screening for congenital anomalies, tumors in the acoustic meatus, and sometimes for cerebellopontine angle tumors. If a lesion is suspected, a complete mastoid series, tomograms or laminograms, and computerized axial tomography (with or without metrizamide) might be necessary to make a diagnosis. Rarely, a contrast study (a pantopaque myelogram or pneumoencephalogram) is required to evaluate the situation adequately.

(5) Laboratory tests, including a complete blood count with sickle cell preparation and baseline metabolic studies, such as fasting blood sugar and a two hour postprandial blood sugar, determinations of blood urea nitrogen, calcium, electrolytes, and T3 and T4 level, will help rule out some of the major blood dyscrasias and metabolic dysfunctions that may cause dizziness.

Neurologic Examination

Tables 8D–2 and 8D–3 present the basic procedures used in neurologic examinations of children of all ages. In infants under two years of age, information is obtained through observation, play, and evaluation of postural

Table 8D–2   NEUROLOGIC EXAMINATION OF CHILDREN FROM BIRTH TO 4 YEARS OLD

Cranial Nerves (No. to be tested)	Function (Test)
III, IV, VI	Following objects 2–4 weeks — wandering gaze 4–6 weeks — from midline to 90° to either side From 6 weeks — sideways from 180° up and down Nystagmus: Is it positional or spontaneous?
II	Funduscopy, visual fields
V	Corneal reflex and mastication
VII	Facial expression
VIII	Hearing test appropriate to patient's age Vestibular: Doll's eyes phenomenon (newborn), rotary nystagmus, verticular acceleration
IX, X	Palatal motions, gag reflex
XII	Tongue movements (rooting in the infant) Muscle tone, muscle power, deep tendon reflexes Posture: Head and body control (supine, prone, sitting, and standing) Developmental reflexes: Primitive reflexes (birth to 4 months), righting reflexes (6 months on) Fine motor coordination: Finger-light pursuit, building with blocks, copying figures

Table 8D–3 NEUROLOGIC EXAMINATION OF CHILDREN 4 YEARS OLD TO ADULT

I. Traditional examinations in Table 8D–2
II. Additional coordination and balance tests
    1. Finger-nose
    2. Heel-shin
    3. Tandem gait (blindfolded)
    4. Romberg
    5. Reinforced Romberg
    6. Stepping test
    7. Past-pointing test
III. Diadochokinesia
IV. Kinesthesia
    1. Expanded sensory examination
    2. Equilibrium reactions
    3. Electronystagmography

responses. Since many of the classic neurologic tests cannot be performed on children this young, additional tests of fine motor and gross motor coordination are not added until the child is older than two years. By age four, the general neurologic examination is comparable to the one performed in adults.

Assessment of postural responses in infants includes the evaluation of head control when in the prone position, when pulled from the supine position, while sitting, and while standing. Neck and trunk postures in response to various changes in position are noted. Tonic neck reflexes are normally present in the infant up to four months of age and gradually disappear thereafter (Paine and Oppe, 1966); in premature infants, they may last longer. In the infant, muscle tone and power can be assessed mostly through play. The presence of hypotonia or tremor may suggest cerebellar disease. Rigidity, posturing, or choreiform movements may suggest disease of the basal ganglia. The various preparatory stages of locomotion and finally gait are evaluated according to the norms expected for each age. All twelve cranial nerves can be evaluated even in the young child, as can fundi and visual fields (Paine and Oppe, 1966). Particularly important to evaluate are extraocular motions. Newborn infants may focus for a few seconds on the examiner's face but will not follow objects. After 14 days of age, the infant may follow objects or faces from the midline to 90 degrees laterally. By 6 weeks of age, he will follow objects throughout the horizontal and vertical fields of vision. Ocular alignment can thus be evaluated as well as the presence of nystagmus and its characteristics.

Congenital nystagmus is usually pendular on straight gaze and may convert to oscillatory when gaze is directed to the fast component. It is almost always dependent on fixation, disappearing or decreasing with loss of fixation or during convergence. Occasionally a reverse nystagmus, in the opposite direction, may be recorded with eyes closed. The optokinetic response may also be inverted. A latent congenital nystagmus may appear only during monocular vision (when one eye is covered) and is commonly associated with congenital ocular defects such as comitant squint and alternating hyperphoria (Baloh and Honrubia, 1979). Other types of nystagmus may be diagnosed later in life. A comprehensive discussion of the various types of nystagmus can be found elsewhere (Cogan, 1972).

Coordination tests used in evaluating infants are different from those used in older children: in the young infant, the finger-nose test is substituted by finger-light pursuit and the finger-apposition or alternate motion tests by building with blocks, picking up raisins, and scribbling.

Proprioception is difficult to evaluate in infants and may be inferred from tests that involve foot and hand placing or supporting and stepping as well as from manipulation of objects. The sensory examination of young infants is also rather crude.

By age four years, a complete, detailed neurologic evaluation can be performed (Table 8D–3), including more specific vestibular tests such as the sharpened Romberg test described by Fregly (1974). The patient is tested with feet aligned in the tandem heel-to-toe position with eyes closed and arms folded. A normal person can maintain this position for about 30 seconds. With unilateral or bilateral vestibular impairment, the patient can rarely sustain this position and may fall, mostly toward the affected side. Unilateral labyrinthine dysfunction or labyrinthectomy will cause transient hypotonia and loss of righting reflexes on the side of the lesion. With time, other supraspinal reflexes will compensate for the loss of tonic labyrinthine signals. However, difficulties in maintaining balance may persist in the blindfolded individual. With bilateral loss of labyrinthine function, righting reflexes are deficient and the blindfolded patient is unable to maintain the upright position or ambulate in the dark.

Stepping tests may also be helpful in the diagnosis of labyrinthine dysfunction. A variation of Fukuda's test (1959) is used in our laboratory. The patient is asked to mark time in place at the intersection of two perpendicular lines for 60 seconds with arms extended and eyes closed. A deviation over 45 degrees may signify vestibular disease, just as may falling or the past-pointing test. This test is usually performed with the patient seated, arms extended, his index finger touching that of the examiner. With eyes closed, the patient is asked to raise his extended arm and index finger and attempt to return it to the original position, touching the examiner's finger. In the presence of vestibular disease, there is consistent pointing past the examiner's finger toward the side of the lesion.

A detailed sensory examination, including stereognosis, proprioception, two-point discrimination, and determination of position and vibration sense, are performed on children older than four years.

DEVELOPMENTAL REFLEXES

We divide children into four groups according to their ages and levels of maturation of the central nervous system.

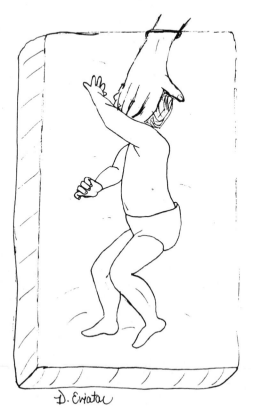

Figure 8D–1 Neck righting.

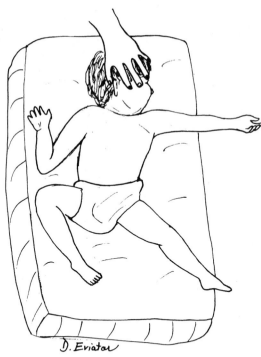

Figure 8D–2 Asymmetric tonic neck reflex.

Group 1: Birth to Four Months

In this group, tonic neck reflexes predominate. They are demonstrated by passive or active motions of the head relative to fixed positions of the body, which elicit movement of the endolymphatic fluid in the semicircular canals and stimulate the sensory nerve endings in the cristae ampullares. At the same time, proprioceptive stimuli arise from the cervical vertebrae and muscles. Appropriate tonic neck responses will depend on the integrity of the vestibular and proprioceptive afferents and of the efferent motor pathways. Although one cannot separate proprioceptive from labyrinthine stimuli, a well-coordinated reflex indicates a normal overall integrated response.

Neck Righting.   Active or passive rotation of the head from the midline to one side in an infant lying supine produces a rotation of the whole body in the direction of the head turn (Fig. 8D–1).

Asymmetric Tonic Neck Reflex (ATN, Fig. 8D–2).   This reflex is obtained with the baby lying supine with the head in the midline position. Active or passive rotation of the head to one side while the infant's chest is restrained will produce flexion of the extremities on the side of the occiput and exten-

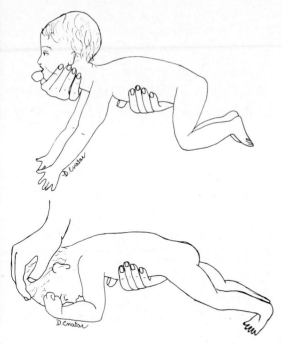

Figure 8D–3   Symmetric tonic neck reflex.

sion of the extremities on the side of the face.

Symmetric Tonic Neck Reflex (STN, Fig. 8D–3). There are two stages to this reflex. In the first stage, the baby is held in the horizontal prone position with the baby's chest on the examiner's arm or with the baby's chest on the examiner's lap. Dorsiflexion of the head will produce extension of the upper extremities and flexion of the lower extremities (Fig. 8D–3*A*). In the second stage, abrupt ventroflexion of the head will produce flexion of the upper extremities and extension of the lower extremities (Fig. 8D–3*B*).

Moro Reflex (Fig. 8D–4). For testing this reflex, the baby lies in the supine position with his head ventroflexed and supported by the examiner's hand. An abrupt backward deflexion of the head about 30 degrees in relation to the trunk will produce an extension and abduction of the arms followed by an embrace.

Absent tonic neck reflexes, including an absent Moro reflex, may occur in the severely asphyxiated hypotonic child with severe central nervous system depression and in those with severe myopathic disorders. Complete absence of labyrinthine function may also produce hypotonia, poor head control, and depressed tonic neck reflexes.

Specific vestibular reflexes are the response to vertical acceleration (introduced by the authors) and Doll's eye phenomenon.

Vertical Acceleration (Fig. 8D–5). The baby is held in the supine position on the examiner's extended forearms. The head and trunk must be aligned and parallel to the ground. A rapid downward acceleration is the stimulus produced to the baby's horizontal body by the examiner, who bends rapidly on his knees to a crouched position. A normal response consists of abduction and extension of the arms, with fanning of the hands. The response is similar to the Moro reflex. The difference is the absent dorsiflexion of the head, which eliminates proprioceptive input from the cervical vertebrae. Since the stimulus is vertical acceleration, it most likely stimulates the macula of the utricle as opposed to the cristae of the semicircular canals which are stimulated with the Moro reflex.

Doll's Eye Phenomenon (Fig. 8D–6). The baby is held vertically under the armpits with his head bent forward 30 degrees over the chest and is rotated for 360 degrees around an axis passing through the examiner's head. Ten rotations in one direction are sufficient and provide a strong vestibular stimulus. The normal response is deviation of the eyes and head opposite the direction of rotation. The Doll's eye phenomenon usually persists for the first 2 weeks of life in full-term neonates and up to six weeks in the full-term baby small for gestational age. Premature babies may have persistent Doll's eye responses until three months of age. Gradually, as vestibular

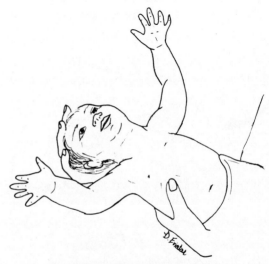

Figure 8D–4   Moro reflex.

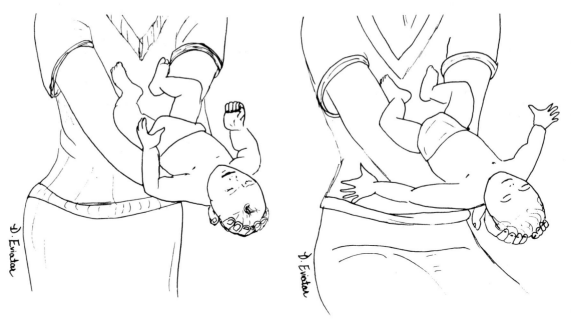

Figure 8D–5 Vertical acceleration.

responses mature, nystagmus is superimposed with a quick component in the direction of rotation. This response can be recorded with electronystagmography. In most cases it is sufficient to observe the response visually during and following rotation.

Group 2: Four to Six Months

Babies in this age group vary in terms of their developmental achievements. Many

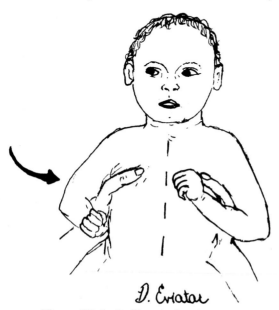

Figure 8D–6 Doll's eye phenomenon.

normal infants will still have residual primitive tonic neck reflexes, while in others righting responses will appear. Both conditions are normal.

Group 3: Six to 18 Months

This is a period of rapid motor and sensory development. Myelination of the pyramidal tract proceeds, as do dendritic arborization of the cerebral cortex and cerebellar cortical differentiation. Integration of visual, labyrinthine, and proprioceptive stimuli occurs, resulting in more elaborate motor responses to changes in head position called righting reflexes. Righting reflexes are elicited by an abrupt tilt of the patient and change in his center of gravity. The acceleration imposed on the labyrinth elicits stimuli that bring on righting of the head and protective reactions of the extremities in the direction of tilt. Since optical and vestibular righting responses are identical, the individual must be tested blindfolded in order to eliminate visual cues.

The most important reflexes are the head-righting responses. They can be obtained by picking up the infant from the prone or supine position and bringing him to the upright position or by tilting the seated infant sideways, frontward, or backward (Fig. 8D–7). Every abrupt change of the head position in space will elicit vestibular head-righting responses whereby the mouth and eyes of the

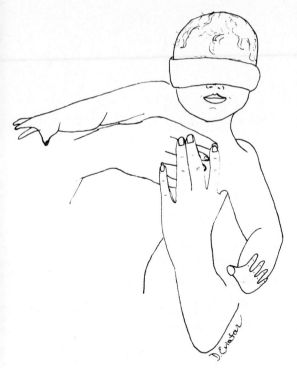

Figure 8D–7 Head righting in vertical suspension.

protective body mechanism that remains present throughout life. During the testing procedure, the baby is held under his armpits with his back toward the examiner, and vertical downward acceleration toward the examining table is applied. The normal response consists of extension and abduction of the arms with extension of fingers as well as righting of the head.

Hopping Reaction (Fig. 8D–9). This reflex appears in the normal full-term infant by eight to 10 months of age. The baby is tested in the standing position with the examiner holding him around the chest and gently tilting him sideways, frontward, or backward. A normal response consists of the initiation of a few steps in the direction of tilt, accompanied by righting of the head. Acquisition of this reflex is preparatory for independent walking.

infant will become parallel to the ground. At the same time, propping reactions of the extremities may be noted, especially in the sitting position. The presence of this reflex will enable the child to maintain his equilibrium in sitting (Fig. 8D–8).

Parachute Reflex. This reflex is also called a sentinel reaction because it is a basic

EQUILIBRIUM RESPONSES: AGES FOUR YEARS TO ADULT

Although equilibrium reactions may be present before age four, it is difficult to test them in the very young child, who may be too frightened to cooperate and relax when major changes in his center of equilibrium are made. The equilibrium responses are essentially more sophisticated and highly integrated righting reactions involving the whole body. They can be tested in the sitting

Figure 8D–8 Head righting in sitting position (buttress response).

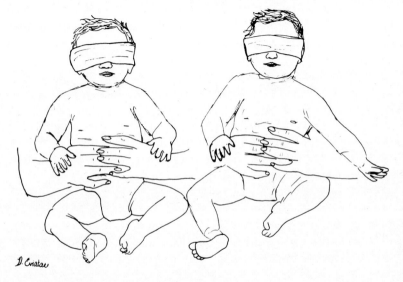

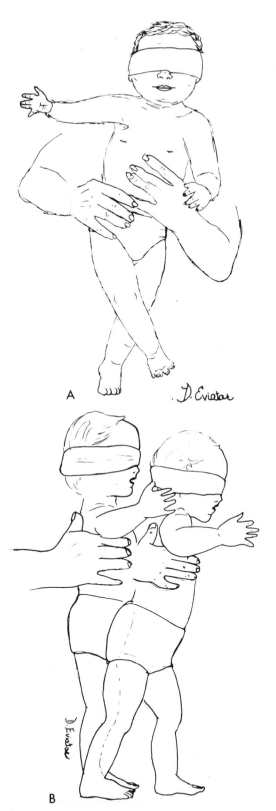

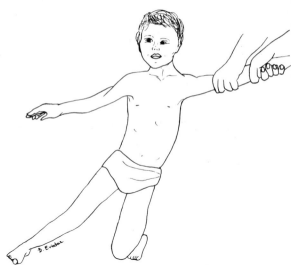

Figure 8D–10   Equilibrium response (kneeling).

position or the kneeling position with the examiner pulling the child by his arm sideways (Fig. 8D–10). The normal response consists of righting of the head and extension with abduction of the extremities on the side opposite the direction of tilt. Postural reactions can also be elicited by tilting the patient either prone (Fig. 8D–11) or supine (Fig. 8D–12) on a tilting board. The angle of tilt of the board is about 45 degrees sideways, and the examiner looks for righting responses of the head and extension with abduction reactions of the extremities.

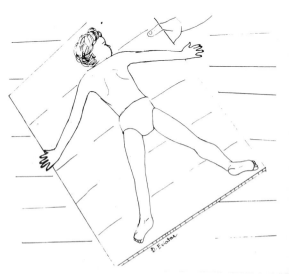

Figure 8D–9 *A*, Hopping reaction (sideways). *B*, Hopping reaction (forward).

Figure 8D–11   Equilibrium response on the tilt board (prone).

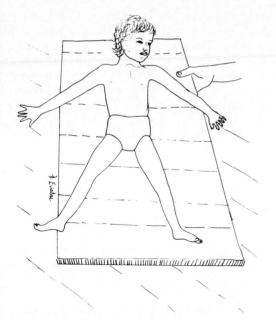

Figure 8D–12 Equilibrium response on the tilt board (supine).

ELECTRONYSTAGMOGRAPHY

Electronystagmography is a method of recording nystagmic eye movements elicited by positional testing or during labyrinthine stimulation by rotation and caloric irrigation (Table 8D–4). The test is performed in a partially darkened room with the patient blindfolded in order to eliminate fixation of gaze or optokinetic nystagmus. It is beyond the scope of this paper to discuss in detail the rationale of this method and the equipment that can be used. Several good monographs on the subject are available (Barber and Stockwell, 1976; Yongkees and Philipson, 1964). For routine clinical testing, a one-channel AC dinograph recorder is sufficient.

Table 8D–4 ELECTRONYSTAGMOGRAPHY

I. Positional test: prone, supine, right lateral, left lateral
   1. Sitting—head right
              head left
              ventroflexed 30°
              dorsiflexed 30°
II. Perotatory (torsion swing)
III. Ice-cold caloric irrigation (10 sec)
IV. Bithermal caloric irrigation (only children older than 4 years)
V. Pendulum tracking from 6 months
VI. Optokinetic stimulation from 6 months

Microelectrodes are applied bitemporally for recording of eye movements, and a neutral electrode is applied on the nasion. A position test is first performed with the infant in supine, right lateral, and left lateral positions. In the older child, a position test is also done in the sitting position.

The perotatory stimulation is provided by a commercially available torsion swing with the application of manual force. In order to obtain a constant angle of 90 degrees, markers are applied to the swing. A constant velocity is maintained by counting the number of excursions between the markers per time unit. The time for a 90 degree excursion in one direction is approximately nine seconds, and the speed is maintained for the same time and degree in the opposite direction as in the torsion swing stimulation procedure previously described (Eviatar, 1970). The excursions are made to the right and to the left of the patient. Two perotatory stimulations are usually recorded with a five minute interval in between the two stimulations.

The stimulus provided by the torsion swing elicits good oculomotor responses and provides the type of stimulation that closely mimics the physiologic conditions encountered in daily situations. Young infants are seated in their mothers' laps on the torsion swing. The mother's right hand maintains the baby's head flexed 30 degrees over the body in order to align the lateral semicircular canals parallel to the ground. Her left hand props the baby's trunk in the vertical position, close to her chest, so the axis of rotation is through the baby's head. The torsion swing is a nonthreatening experience for children, who like to be rocked back and forth and, in most cases, cooperate well throughout the test. Recording of eye movements is done during stimulation with the torsion swing. In the majority of cases, the response ceases with cessation of perotatory stimulation.

In the very young infant, a sinusoidal curve may be the only response obtained, recording the conjugate eye movements in the direction opposite the direction of rotation (Doll's eye), over which slowly will be superimposed a few nystagmoid beats, changing direction with the direction of rotation. As the response fully matures, a good alternating nystagmus is obtained. The response thus recorded is the result of a summation of responses elicited from both labyrinths. About 50 per cent of infants develop nystagmus during perotatory stimulation within the first 10 to 20 days of postnatal life. The majority of infants (95 per cent) have nystagmus in response to perotatory stimulation within the first 20 to 30 days of life. Premature infants, however, have a significant delay (up to 90 days) in the appearance of perotatory evoked nystagmus (Eviatar et al., 1974). These maturational factors, which are correlated with gestational age and weight at birth, are taken into account when evaluating the perotatory response in such infants as those treated with aminoglycosides. Indeed, one of the effects produced by aminoglycoside treatment may be a delay in acquiring perotatory responses (Eviatar and Eviatar, 1980).

In normal infants and children, values for the speed of the slow component, amplitude, and number of beats per torsion swing excursion are identical for the right- and left-beating nystagmus. The total number of beats of nystagmus to right or left is also identical. The nystagmus is not considered to have directional preponderance until the total number of beats in one direction exceeds by 25 per cent the number of beats in the other direction. A directional preponderance may be found in the presence of a strong positional nystagmus and may be secondary to it. When present, it suggests vestibular dysfunction.

There is no significant increase over time in the mean values of amplitude or number of beats per torsion swing excursion of the perotatory nystagmus. The speed of the slow component of perotatory nystagmus increases from the time of its appearance until age four years, from a mean of 35.0 degrees per second to an average of 40.0 degrees per second. Sleep and drowsiness can inhibit responses significantly (Eviatar et al., 1979).

Ice Cold Caloric (ICC) Irrigation

Additional testing with ICC irrigation of each ear canal may be performed in order to evaluate the response from each labyrinth individually.

The test is performed with the blindfolded baby in the supine position, restrained on a papoose board with his head ventroflexed 30 degrees. A 10 sec irrigation with ice water is the stimulus used (temperature of the water at the spout is about 5 degrees C). Recording of the oculomotor response starts at the onset of irrigation. The direction of nystagmus will be opposite the ear stimulated. As soon as a good response appears, the baby is turned to the prone position, and the direction of nystagmus is reversed if the labyrinth is intact. As soon as this new response begins to fade, the baby is turned back to the supine position. The direction of nystagmus reverts to the initial direction, away from the ear stimulated. If the child is sleepy or very irritable during the test, the response may be inhibited or incomplete (a response only in the supine and prone positions, for instance). The test is performed in three positions (supine, prone, and back to supine) with each irrigation in order to eliminate false responses, such as intensification of a latent nystagmus or a response from the other labyrinth (Eviatar and Eviatar, 1974). Ten minutes should elapse before stimulating the other ear canal with ice cold water.

The ICC stimulation is a crude method in that it tests for a response to a vigorous, nonphysiologic stimulus. It is thus performed only in cases where serious doubts exist relative to the function of the vestibular apparatus, such as when there is significant delay in the development of head and postural control, when there are abnormal responses to torsion swing, when there is a history of ingestion of ototoxic drugs, or in the congenitally deaf child in whom abnormal vestibular function is suspected. Twenty-five per cent of the full-term infants tested in our laboratory had a positive response to the caloric test within the first 10 to 20 days of life, and the majority of infants responded within the first month. About 40 per cent of the small-for-date babies responded by a month of age, while the majority responded by six to eight weeks of life. Many premature babies did not respond until three months of age (Eviatar et al., 1974). It is thus important not to confuse the absence of positive response due to delayed maturation with the lack of response due to acquired or congenital vestibular damage. When a positive response is present, the quality of the response becomes an indicator of the maturity and integrity of vestibular responses.

There is a maturational pattern in the development of the caloric evoked nystagmus response: An increase in the number of beats per 10 seconds, in the amplitude, and in the speed of the slow component is apparent in the first three months of life for all gestational groups. The intensity of nystagmus is directly proportional to gestational age and weight at birth (Eviatar et al., 1979). Full-term babies, appropriate or large for gestational age, acquire a mature pattern of nystagmus within three to six months of birth. Premature and small-for-date babies, however, show progressive maturation of caloric responses throughout the first year of life. The frequency and speed of the slow component are the most reliable variables in the qualitative evaluation of induced caloric nystagmus. These variables are directly proportional to gestational age and weight at birth in the first six months of life.

While the intensity of evoked nystagmus increases with age, the latency of the response decreases in direct relation to the length of gestation and weight at birth. Latency provides a good estimate of the maturity of vestibular responses. Because of the method used, the total duration of evoked nystagmus is poorly correlated with the degree of maturation. However, since normative values are available, estimates of dysfunction can be made by evaluating the total duration of the response (Eviatar and Eviatar, 1979b).

Optokinetic Stimulation

Optokinetic nystagmus can be evaluated in most children within three to six months of birth. As the children grow older and pay more attention to the content of images seen, better responses are obtained by projecting a rotating filmstrip on a screen. The nystagmus can be recorded in response to two speeds of rotation: 3 degrees and 16 degrees per second, respectively. The frequency, amplitude, and speed of the slow component can be analyzed in response to the two rotation speeds. Abnormalities of tracing may be related to ocular problems, damage to optic tracts, optic radiation, or frontal or cerebellar lesions. The information obtained is helpful in the evaluation of the overall quality of neurovestibular function.

Bithermal Caloric Irrigation

Bithermal irrigation of the external auditory meatus for 30 sec with 30 degrees C and 44 degrees C water is used in children ages four years and older. A 10 min interval is allowed between two consecutive irrigations. The intensity of nystagmus, represented by the speed of the slow component at the culmination of nystagmus, is used for calculation. Calculation of labyrinthine preponderance (Jongkee's formula) is as follows.

$$\frac{(R30 \text{ degrees} + R44 \text{ degrees}) - (L30 \text{ degrees} + L44 \text{ degrees}) \times 100}{R30 \text{ degrees} + R44 \text{ degrees} + L30 \text{ degrees} + L44 \text{ degrees}}$$

A difference between the two labyrinths of more than 22 per cent suggests labyrinthine preponderance.

Calculation of directional preponderance is done using the following formula.

$$\frac{(R_{30} \text{ degrees} + L_{44} \text{ degrees}) - (R44 \text{ degrees} + L30 \text{ degrees}) \times 100}{R_{30} \text{ degrees} + L_{44} \text{ degrees} + R_{44} \text{ degrees} + R_{30} \text{ degrees}}$$

A difference of more than 18 per cent suggests directional preponderance.

This procedure lasts about 45 minutes and requires the child's cooperation and patience. It cannot, therefore, be used in children less than four years of age. The significance of directional and labyrinthine preponderance in children has been discussed elsewhere (Eviatar and Wassertheil, 1971; Eviatar and Eviatar, 1977).

REFERENCES

Baloh, R. W., and Honrubia, V. 1979. Clinical neurophysiology of the vestibular system. *In* Pulm, F., and McDowell, F. (Eds.) Contemporary Neurology Series, Vol. 18. Philadelphia, F. A. Davis Co., pp.115–118.

Barber, H. O., and Stockwell, C. W. 1976. Manual of Electronystagmography. St. Louis, The C. V. Mosby Co.

Bergstrom, L. 1969. Electrical parameters of the brain during ontogeny. *In* Robinson, R. J., et al. (Eds.) Brain and Early Behavior Development in the Fetus and Infant. CASDS Study Group on Brain Mechanisms of Early Behavior Development. New York, Academic Press, pp. 15–37.

Carpenter, B. 1974. Core Text of Neuroanatomy. Baltimore, Williams & Wilkins.

Cogan, D. G. 1972. Neurology of the Ocular Muscles. Springield, IL, Charles C Thomas.

Cratty, B. T. 1970. Perceptual and Motor Development in Infants and Children. London, Macmillan.

de Morsier, J. 1938. Contribution à l'étude des centres

vestibulaires corticaux et des hallucinations illiputienes. Encephale, *33*:57.

Eviatar, A. 1970. The torsion swing as a vestibular test. Arch. Otolaryngol., *92*:437.

Eviatar, A., and Eviatar, L. 1974. A critical look at the cold calorics. Arch. Otolaryngol., *99*:361–365.

Eviatar, L., and Eviatar, A. 1977. Vertigo in children: Differential diagnosis and treatment. Pediatrics, *59*:833–835.

Eviatar, A., and Eviatar, L. 1980. Vestibular Effect of Aminoglycosides in Humans. Chicago International Symposium on Aminoglycosides. Boston, Little, Brown and Co.

Eviatar, A., and Wassertheil, S. 1971. The clinical significance of directional preponderance concluded by electronystagmography. J. Laryngol. Otol., *85*:355.

Eviatar, L., and Eviatar, A. 1979. The normal nystagmic response of infants to caloric and perrotatory stimulation. Laryngoscope, *89*:1036–1045.

Eviatar, L., Eviatar, A., and Naray, I. 1974. Maturation of neurovestibular responses in infants. Dev. Med. Child. Neurol., *16*:435–446.

Eviatar, L., Miranda, S., Eviatar, A., et al. 1979. Development of nystagmus in response to vestibular stimulation in infants. Ann. Neurol., *5*:508–514.

Fregly, A. R. 1974. Vestibular ataxia and its measurement in man. *In* Kornhuber, H. H. (Ed.) Handbook of Sensory Physiology, Vol. 6, Part 2. New York, Springer-Verlag.

Fukuda, T. 1959. The stepping test: Two phases of the labyrinthine reflex. Acta Otolaryngol., *50*:95.

Gesell, A., and Amatruda, C. S. 1945. The Embryology of Behavior: The Beginning of the Human Mind. New York, Harper.

Hamilton, W. T., and Mossman, H. W. 1972. Human Embryology: Prenatal Development of Form and Function, 4th ed. Cambridge, Hoffer.

Hooker, D. 1952. The Prenatal Origin of Behavior. Lawrence, KS, University of Kansas Press.

Humphrey, T. 1969. Postnatal repetition of human prenatal activity sequences with some suggestions of their neuroanatomical lesions. *In* Robinson, R. J., et al. (Eds.) Brain and Early Behavior Development in the Fetus and Infant. CASDS Study Group on Brain Mechanisms of Early Behavioral Development. New York, Academic Press, pp. 43–84.

Paine, R. S., and Oppe, T. E. 1966. Neurological examination of children. Clin. Dev. Med., 20/21, 98–142.

Penfield, W., and Jasper, H. 1954. Epilepsy and the Functional Anatomy of the Human Brain. Boston, Little, Brown and Co.

Penfield, W., and Kristiansen, D. 1951. Epileptic Seizure Patterns: A Study of the Localizing Value of Initial Phenomena in Focal Cortical Seizures. Springfield, IL, Charles C Thomas.

Schulte, F. T., Linke, I., Michaelis, E., et al. 1969. Excitation, inhibition and impulse conduction in spinal motoneurones of preterm, term and small for date newborn infants. *In* Robinson, R. J., et al. (Eds.) Brain and Early Behavior Development in the Fetus and Infant. CASDS Study Group on Brain Mechanisms of Early Behavioral Development. New York, Academic Press.

Stein, B. M., and Carpenter, M. D. 1967. Central projections of portions of the vestibular ganglia innervating specific parts of the labyrinth in the Rhesus monkey. Am. J. Anat., *120*:281–318.

Yongkees, L. B. W., and Philipson, A. T. 1964. Electronystagmography. Acta Otolaryngol., Suppl. 189.

Chapter **9A**

OTALGIA

Werner D. Chasin, M.D.

INTRODUCTION

This chapter discusses otologic and nonotologic causes of ear pain. Referred pain and the multiple sensory innervation of the ear lead to problems in localizing pain; indeed, disorders of various parts of the head and neck may result in pain being perceived in or about the ear (Table 9A–1). The skin, perichondrium, and periosteum of the external ear, the tympanic membrane, the lining of the middle ear, and the mastoid periosteum all possess rich sensory innervation (Warwick and Williams, 1973h).

The nerves that contribute to this complex innervation originate from several segments of the brain and spinal cord and include the trigeminal, facial, glossopharyngeal, vagus, and spinal accessory nerves and the cervical plexus (C_2–C_3). Tremble (1965) has described the specific portions of the ear that are innervated by the various nerves and has related these to the evaluation of otalgia.

The manner in which children react to otalgia is a function of their ages, level of maturation, and personalities. Infants may not be able to localize the pain and may simply cry and be irritable, although some will manipulate the ear. An infant with ear pain due to a middle ear infection is likely to act as if he or she is ill and has a fever. If the otalgia is referred, as during teething, the manifestations may be similar, but the fever is absent. As the child becomes more verbal he or she is apt to tell the parent that there is pain in the ear, or the child may continue to "act out" the pain by crying and scratching the ear. Children, like adults, have varying pain thresholds and may fail to give any indication of a localized discomfort even when suffering from acute otitis media. They may simply act listless, reject food, may vomit,

and develop some fever. By the time they reach school age, however, most children can describe their ear pain clearly to their parents. A symptom that is most useful in helping to differentiate otalgia due to middle ear inflammation from that which is referred is that of a feeling of fullness, blockage, or pressure in the ear. This symptom, when present, however, can be elicited only from

Table 9A–1 CAUSES OF OTALGIA IN CHILDREN

Intrinsic	
I. External Ear	
A. External otitis	E. Insects
B. Foreign body	F. Myringitis
C. Perichondritis	G. Trauma
D. Preauricular cyst or sinus	H. Tumor
II. Middle Ear, Eustachian Tube, and Mastoid	
A. Barotrauma	F. Aditus block
B. Middle ear effusion	G. Masked mastoiditis
C. Negative intratympanic pressure	H. Intracranial complication
	I. Tumor
D. Acute otitis media	J. Histiocytosis X
E. Mastoiditis	K. Wegener's granuloma

Extrinsic	
I. Trigeminal	*IV. Vagus*
A. Dental	A. Laryngopharynx
B. Jaw	B. Esophagus
C. Temporomandibular joint	C. Thyroid
D. Oral cavity	
II. Facial	*V. Cervical Nerves*
A. Bell's palsy	A. Lymph nodes
B. Tumors	B. Cysts
C. Herpes zoster	C. Cervical spine
	D. Neuralgia
III. Glossopharyngeal	*VI. Miscellaneous*
A. Tonsil	A. Migraine
B. Oropharynx	B. Aural neuralgia
C. Nasopharynx	C. Salivary gland
	D. Paranasal sinuses
	E. Central nervous system

213

older children. The author continues to remain surprised that many children, even those as old as 6 or 7 years, will not admit to a feeling of blockage in an infected ear or in one harboring an obvious effusion, even when they are questioned directly.

EVALUATION OF A CHILD WITH OTALGIA

History

When evaluating a child with ear pain, the physician should first obtain an accurate history. In addition, the physician should have and keep in mind (1) an understanding of the principle of referred pain, (2) a knowledge of the multiple sensory innervation of the ear, and should (3) ask appropriate questions to differentiate intrinsic from referred otalgia. (For example, when the pain is aggravated by chewing of food or gum, this would lead one to evaluate carefully the temporomandibular joints and the teeth.)

Examination of the Ears

The examination of the ears must be thorough. Both the cranial and lateral surfaces of the auricle, as well as the postauricular areas, should be inspected for traumatic or inflammatory lesions. Special attention must be paid to the sites of possible sinus tracts in front of the root of the helix and in the cranial surface of the superior half of the auricle. The external auditory canal should be inspected for anomalies, such as a duplicated external auditory canal.

The tympanic membrane should be inspected next for disorders intrinsic to the drumhead as well as for signs of those middle ear disorders that it may reflect. The author has found the Hallpike-Blackmore monocular ear microscope with a pneumatic attachment and 6x magnification to be the most useful otoscope for routine clinical use in examining the ears of infants and children. This instrument has excellent coaxial illumination and specula that are atraumatic and that afford a perfect pneumatic seal. The otologic examination may need to be supplemented by a tympanometric evaluation to detect possible negative intratympanic pressure, which can be a subtle cause of intrinsic otalgia (Chap. 8A).

Evaluation for Referred Otalgia

When the otologic evaluation fails to disclose the cause of otalgia, a seriatim examination guided by an appreciation of the multiple sensory innervation of the ear must be performed. The temporomandibular joint, a common focus for referred otalgia even in children, should be evaluated. The function of the trigeminal nerve should be assessed by examining the oral cavity, teeth, gums, and, if necessary, the sinuses. (Usually radiographs are necessary to evaluate the sinuses fully.) The seventh cranial nerve is an uncommon mediator of otalgia. The glossopharyngeal and vagus nerves and the cervical plexus may be evaluated systematically by examining the various structures supplied by these nerves. If the clinical examination performed according to this format fails to disclose the cause of the otalgia, and if the symptom persists, then additional radiologic studies are required. These may include films of the mastoids (plain radiographs and possibly polytomographs), paranasal sinuses, nasopharynx, bony and soft tissue structures of the neck, and an evaluation of the esophagus with barium contrast. In the past two years the author has found computerized tomography to be useful in disclosing the presence of deep lesions of the neck and skull bone that may cause otalgia (Chap. 8C).

In the opinion of this author, the cause of otalgia can be discovered in the vast majority of patients with this symptom. Seldom indeed should the diagnosis be made of "otalgia of undetermined etiology."

OTALGIA DUE TO INTRINSIC EAR DISEASE

External Ear

When ear pain is due to a disorder of the external ear, this should be obvious on clinical examination. The pain is localized to the ear with little radiation elsewhere, and an abnormality is seen in either the auricle, the external auditory canal, or both. Some common causes of such pain in children are listed in Table 9A–1 and include external otitis (dermatitis — bacterial, fungal, or allergic), foreign bodies, perichondritis of the auricle, infected preauricular cyst, insects and maggots, herpes zoster, myringitis bullosa, fractures of the tympanic ring, and tumors of the external auditory canal. The management of these disorders is fairly direct and is described in Chapter 15.

The pain-sensitive structures of the external ear include the skin of the auricle and the external auditory canal, the perichondrium of the auricle, and the outer portion of the external auditory canal.

Middle Ear

The pain-sensitive structures of the middle ear and mastoid include the tympanic membrane, periosteum of the mastoid cortex, the visceral middle ear mucosa, and the mucoperiosteum of the middle ear and mastoid. The osseous structures of the middle ear and the other parts of the temporal bone do not appear to be supplied with pain receptors. The factors that stimulate these receptors are (1) stretching, (2) pressure, (3) toxic products of infection, and (4) direct nerve invasion (by tumors) (Chap. 16).

When a disease process involves the middle ear and mastoid system, there exists potentially a large constellation of symptoms in addition to the pain itself. This constellation is broader in the older child who can express them adequately. The infant expresses middle ear otalgia by crying, irritability, and sometimes scratching the ear, sticking the finger into it, or pulling it. He or she may have associated systemic symptoms such as fever, vomiting, and a toxic manifestation. As the child becomes older and more verbal, the physician may be able to elicit the description of such additional symptoms as blockage or fullness in the ear (or ears), "popping," "bells ringing," diminished hearing, and noise intolerance. In general, the more symptoms that exist and that are referable directly to the ear, the more likely it is that the otalgia is due to intrinsic disease of the ear rather than being referred. For example, in an older child with otalgia as the only ear symptom, the pain will, after suitable evaluation, probably turn out to be referred. On the other hand, if the primary complaint of otalgia is accompanied by symptoms of ear blockage, popping, and hearing loss, it becomes much more likely that the otalgia is a symptom of intrinsic ear disease.

The causes and characteristics of otalgia due to intrinsic disease of the middle ear, mastoid, and deeper portions of the temporal bone include acute otitis media, an incom-

petent eustachian tube, chronic middle ear effusions, negative middle ear pressure, mastoiditis, aditus block syndrome, masked mastoiditis, tympanomastoiditis, tumors of the ear, histiocytosis, and Wegener's granulomatosis; each of these will be discussed further.

Acute otitis media is, of course, the most common cause of otalgia due to intrinsic ear disease in the pediatric age group.

Acute environmental pressure changes in the presence of an *incompetent eustachian tube* may cause otalgia. This is seen in children, usually with a history suggestive of eustachian tubal incompetence, when they develop otalgia during flights, auto rides up or down significant land elevations, or when diving into the water. The otologic findings may be negative or may show an acute hemorrhagic otitis with a red or blue tympanic membrane, with or without evidence of a middle ear effusion or hemorrhage as detected by pneumatic otoscopy. If hemorrhagic otitis is present and if the child is old enough to be tested with tuning forks or audiometry, a conductive hearing loss will be found. The pain is most likely due to the sudden intratympanic and intramastoid pressure changes with resultant pressure or tension on the mucosa.

Children with *chronic middle ear effusions* are subject to episodes of otalgia. These may be due either to pressure changes, as in barotrauma, or to bacterial infection of the middle ear effusion. These two different causes of otalgia in middle ear effusions may be difficult to differentiate. Generally, pain due to superinfection is more persistent and may be accompanied by the other symptoms of acute otitis media (fever, toxicity, and vomiting, for instance), and with a well developed superinfection, the tympanic membrane is apt to be full or even bulging, with vesicular surface changes. In cases of middle ear effusion without infection, the drumhead is retracted and no inflammatory changes are noticeable.

In some children, the cause of otalgia is intrinsic in the ear, but the otoscopic examination is quite negative. The pain may be due to simple *negative pressure* without a middle ear effusion and can be diagnosed with the aid of the acoustic impedance bridge.

The pain of *mastoiditis* accompanying an obvious case of otitis media is usually felt behind the ear in the vicinity of the mastoid antrum and tip. The physician should also watch for the possible breakdown of cellular partitions and for the appearance of an abscess between the mastoid cortex and its periosteum — a subperiosteal abscess, which is recognized as a tender and painful postauricular swelling. A clue that mastoiditis is developing is swelling of the skin of the superior and posterosuperior walls of the osseous portion of the external auditory canal, otherwise known as sagging of the canal wall skin. This condition must be differentiated from a circumscribed otitis externa and must be treated surgically.

Some patients continue to complain of ear pain despite an apparent resolution of the otitis media and return of the drumhead to a normal or near normal appearance. These children have developed a sequestered infection of the mastoid known as the *aditus block syndrome*: the narrow communication between the middle ear and mastoid segments has become blocked by mucosal edema. This diagnosis is made by demonstrating radiologic changes consistent with mastoiditis.

Masked mastoiditis is due to an incomplete suppression of the infection of the middle ear and mastoid segment. It may be due to inadequate treatment, to the partial effectiveness of a bacteriostatic antimicrobial, or because the child has an inadequate immune system (due to an immunodeficiency state, diabetes, or suppression of immunity by corticosteroids being administered for an unrelated disorder). A child with masked mastoiditis may have no otologic symptoms until the antibiotic has been discontinued, when the symptoms of otitis media and mastoiditis recrudesce (Chap. 17).

When complications of *tympanomastoiditis* occur, the nature of the pain may change and additional symptoms may appear. Meningitis will become manifest by a generalized headache, signs of meningeal irritation, and the appearance of severe toxicity. A sigmoid sinus thrombophlebitis will be marked by the appearance of mastoid pain and manifestations of septicemia. Brain abscesses and encephalitis, after a quiescent stage, are heralded by severe headache and profound neurologic changes. The pain of Gradenigo syndrome (periapical meningitis) is felt in the ear and behind the ipsilateral eye and is accompanied by diplopia due to a neuritis of the sixth cranial nerve (Chap. 18).

Tumors of the ear, such as rhabdomyosarcoma, lymphoma, and leukemic infiltration, may also cause ear pain and must be differentiated from otitis media (Chap. 22).

The ear may become involved by *histiocytosis* X.

Wegener's granulomatosis, which may sometimes be seen in older pediatric patients, is heralded by what appears to be a common otitis media (Karmody, 1978). The physician should suspect Wegener's granuloma when otitis media does not respond to myringotomy and vigorous antibiotic therapy. The diagnosis is made by submitting mastoid tissue for pathologic examination, or it may be made clinically if the patient develops concomitant involvement of the respiratory tract (granulomatous changes in the nose, nasopharynx, larynx, trachea, or lungs).

OTALGIA REFERRED VIA THE TRIGEMINAL NERVE

The auriculotemporal branch of the mandibular division of the trigeminal nerve supplies sensory innervation to the anterior part of the auricle, the tragus, anterior and superior canal walls, and anterior portion of the tympanic membrane (Fig. 9A–1). According to the principle of referred pain, diseases affecting structures innervated by the mandibular division, as well as those involving structures innervated by the maxillary and ophthalmic divisions, may result in pain referred to areas innervated by the mandibular division. Under most circumstances, pain is referred to other sites only when the irritation persists for more than several minutes.

In order to be guided as to where to search for pain referred via the trigeminal nerve, one must consider the areas of the head and neck, besides the ear, that are innervated by the sensory branches of the trigeminal nerve (Warwick and Williams, 1973g). Because these are many, the search for trigeminal-mediated referred otalgia must be extensive.

Dental Disorders

Dental diseases, such as carious teeth, periapical infections, impacted teeth, unerupted teeth, and disorders of the gingivae, irritate trigeminal fibers of the mandibular or maxillary divisions and hence may cause referred otalgia. A consultation with a dentist may be required to evaluate patients with this problem. Infants and young children with such otalgia may give no clue that would direct the

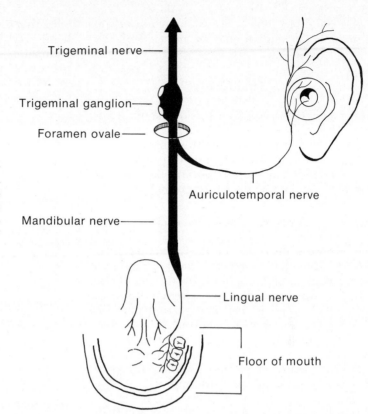

Figure 9A–1   Referred otalgia mediated by the trigeminal nerve may be caused by intraoral disorders such as carious teeth, impacted wisdom teeth, or a calculus in the duct of the submandibular salivary gland.

attention of the parents to the mouth: they fuss instead with their ears. If there has been a past problem with otitis media, the parents naturally assume that the present episode is another attack of otitis media (Chap. 43).

Disorders Involving the Jaw

Inflammatory and neoplastic disorders, as well as disorders of unknown cause such as histiocytosis X, may involve the jaws, giving rise to referred otalgia. The diagnosis may require appropriate radiographs of the mandible and maxilla, including dental films, to demonstrate the alveolar processes to the best advantage.

Temporamandibular Joint

Disorders of the temporomandibular joint and its associated muscles are among the most common forms of referred otalgia in children as well as in adults. True arthritic disorders of this joint are uncommon and are usually seen only in patients with a background of a systemic arthritis such as rheu-

matoid arthritis. Other types of intrinsic joint disease that are also uncommon include post-traumatic alterations and septic arthritis. The more common disorders, which are somewhat inaccurately categorized under the heading of "temporomandibular joint syndrome," involve the muscles and ligaments associated with the temporomandibular joint. These structures, under certain conditions, may cause pain as a result of being abused, stretched, and irritated. The situation is entirely analogous to the muscular pain that occurs in other parts of the body when a muscle is contracted excessively (as in muscle tension headaches).

In children, these periarticular structures may be irritated by bruxism, excessive gum chewing, dental malocclusion, and sometimes merely as a result of clenching of the teeth. The history may suggest that the otalgia is aggravated by movement of the jaw. The diagnosis is made by eliciting tenderness of the temporomandibular joint in front of the tragus and through the anterior cartilaginous external canal wall. Painful spasm of the pterygoid muscles can be diagnosed by palpating these muscles intraorally between the zygomatic arch and the coronoid process of the mandible. The forward excursion of the mandibular condyle may be reduced on the side with otalgia.

Oral Cavity

The diagnosis of disorders of the oral cavity that cause referred otalgia should be straightforward. Such lesions may include herpetic stomatitis, inflammatory and traumatic lesions of the tongue and floor of the mouth, and embedded foreign bodies.

Salivary Gland Disorders

Whereas disorders of the submandibular and sublingual glands are not common in children, diseases of the parotid gland are seen frequently. The most common disorder besides mumps is that of recurrent parotitis due to sialectasia (chronic punctate parotitis). Although the pathologic ectasia of the ductal system is usually bilateral, the clinically apparent, recurrent parotid swelling with pain in and around the ear is often unilateral. The diagnosis is based upon the results of sialography, which usually demonstrates ectasia of the major and minor intraglandular ducts and pooling of contrast material in them. The episodes of parotid inflammation tend to decrease in frequency as the child gets older. Some of these children subsequently develop systemic autoimmune disorders, such as Sjögren's disease, and must therefore be observed over an extended period of time.

Paranasal Sinuses

The paranasal sinuses are innervated by the trigeminal nerve, principally the maxillary division. Inflammatory disease and, less commonly, neoplastic disorders in children can result in otalgia. The otalgia is due to two mechanisms that sometimes act jointly: otalgia may be referred via the trigeminal nerve, or otalgia may be due to an intrinsic aural disease that is secondary to the primary sinus disorder. An example of the latter is tubo-tympanitis caused by infectious secretions from the maxillary sinus as they pass over the torus tubarius in the nasopharynx.

Other

When the cause of otalgia is not apparent, the physician must consider the remote possibility that the trigeminal roots or ganglion are being irritated intracranially by a tumor, an anomalous artery, or by a demyelinating process. A careful neurologic evaluation must therefore be performed in such cases.

REFERRED OTALGIA MEDIATED BY THE FACIAL NERVE

Although the facial nerve is primarily a motor nerve, there exists evidence that it contains several somatic sensory elements that innervate the posterior portion of the tympanic membrane and part of the posterior wall of the external auditory canal (Warwick and Williams, 1973c,d).

Bell's palsy, or idiopathic facial paralysis, is usually accompanied by pain in the ear or, more commonly, behind the ear in the area of the tip of the mastoid process. The otoscopic findings are usually negative. Occasionally, an imminent idiopathic facial paralysis may be preceded for several days by postauricular pain. Keeping in mind this possibility, the physician should reevaluate children with otalgia of undetermined cause after a period of a few days.

Tumors involving the facial nerve in its intracranial course or in its temporal bone course may also cause pain in and around the ear. Such tumors are fortunately uncommon in the pediatric population.

Herpes zoster oticus, or the *Ramsay Hunt syndrome,* is a viral neuritis of the facial nerve that may also involve the fifth and eighth cranial nerves. Patients with this disorder have severe otalgia and vesicular eruption in the ear canal. Once the acute inflammatory changes have subsided and the vesicles have disappeared, otalgia may persist for many weeks. In obscure cases of otalgia, a history should be sought about a vesicular eruption in and about the ear. Chorda tympani nerve function and stapedius muscle function should be checked (Chap. 13).

REFERRED OTALGIA MEDIATED BY THE GLOSSOPHARYNGEAL NERVE

The ninth or glossopharyngeal cranial nerve exits from the base of the skull through the jugular foramen in company with the vagus and spinal accessory nerves. It subsequently is distributed to the tonsils, pharynx, eustachian tube, and posterior third of the tongue (Warwick and Williams, 1973e). A branch ascends into the middle ear as the nerve of Jacobson, ramifies on the promontory, and exits from the anterior part of the middle ear as the lesser superficial petrosal nerve (Warwick and Williams, 1973h). The latter reaches the otic ganglion and supplies preganglionic, special visceral motor fibers to the parotid gland. The nerve provides general somatic sensory fibers to the posterior portion of the external auditory meatus and canal and to the posterior portion of the external surface of the drumhead. The glossopharyngeal nerve also probably supplies most of the sensory innervation of the mucosa of the middle ear, mastoid air cells, and eustachian tube. The glossopharyngeal nerve is one of the most common mediators of deep ear pain referred from the pharynx (Fig. 9A–2).

Tonsillar Diseases

In pediatric patients, inflammatory diseases of the tonsils, mainly acute tonsillitis, peritonsillitis, and peritonsillar abscess, are the main causes of referred otalgia mediated by the ninth cranial nerve. The diagnosis of this type of referred ear pain is made readily upon inspection of the pharynx. Referred otalgia is so universal after tonsillectomy that patients should be advised to expect it so that they do not confuse posttonsillectomy otalgia with a bout of otitis media. Referred otalgia is not as commonly seen after adenoidectomy alone (Chap. 48).

Oropharyngeal Diseases

Because of the widespread sensory distribution of the glossopharyngeal nerve, pharyngeal disorders other than those involving the tonsils also may cause referred otalgia. These include lingual tonsillitis, retropharyngeal abscess, and foreign bodies embedded in either the tongue base or other portions of the pharynx. These diagnoses can be made by careful pharyngeal examination aided by a lateral radiograph of the neck. Tumors of the pharynx, another potential cause of otalgia referred via the glossopharyngeal nerve, fortunately are uncommon in the pediatric age group. An uncommon cause of otalgia is an infection in the pharyngeal end of a branchial cyst or fistula. Glossopharyngeal tic, a cause of severe otalgia in adults, is rare in the pediatric age group (Chap. 47).

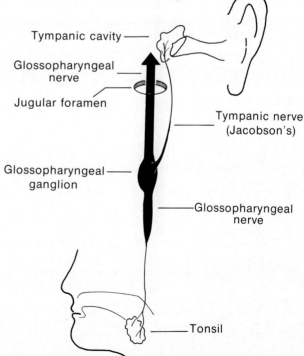

Figure 9A–2   Referred otalgia mediated by the glossopharyngeal nerve may be caused by tonsillitis, peritonsillar abscess, or by neural irritation after tonsillectomy.

Nasopharyngeal Sources of Referred Otalgia

The nasopharynx derives its sensory innervation partly from the glossopharyngeal nerve and partly from the maxillary division of the trigeminal nerve (Warwick and Williams, 1973f). Both of these nerves, as has already been pointed out, can mediate referred otalgia. The nasopharynx must be examined in cases of obscure otalgia, although it is not a common source of otalgia in children.

Nasopharyngeal disorders that might cause otalgia include nasopharyngitis, adenoiditis, a foreign body lodged in the nasopharynx, and, rarely, a neoplasm such as a lymphoma, epithelial malignancy, or mesenchymal tumor. A hypertrophic adenoid may occasionally cause otalgia when it causes intermittent obstruction of the eustachian tube, which results in negative middle ear pressure. When such an adenoid becomes infected as part of a pharyngitis, it may cause a salpingitis or tubotympanitis, which in turn causes otalgia.

REFERRED OTALGIA MEDIATED BY THE VAGUS NERVE

In the ear the sensory fibers of the vagus are distributed by the nerve of Arnold. They supply a portion of the cavum conchae, posterior wall of the external auditory canal, and posterior portion of the external surface of the drumhead (Fig. 9A–3). The vagus nerve also supplies the sensory innervation of the entire larynx, esophagus, trachea, and thyroid gland (Warwick and Williams, 1973i). According to the principles of referred pain, disorders in these structures may be a source of pain that is referred to the ear. In general, vagus-mediated causes of otalgia are not seen as commonly in pediatric patients as they are in adults. When they occur, the local manifestations usually predominate over referred otalgia, which tends to be a secondary symptom.

Laryngeal Disorders

Laryngeal injuries and foreign bodies of the larynx or pyriform sinus may be a source

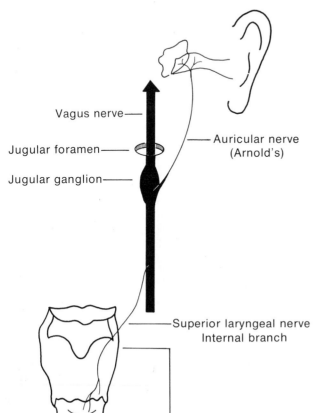

Vagus nerve——

Jugular foramen——

Jugular ganglion——

—— Auricular nerve (Arnold's)

———Superior laryngeal nerve Internal branch

Figure 9A–3   Referred otalgia mediated by the vagus nerve may be caused by such laryngopharyngeal disorders as retropharyngeal abscess, epiglottitis, esophagitis around an impacted foreign body, or a sharp foreign body in the pyriform sinus.

of otalgia. The diagnosis is made by laryngoscopic examination aided by radiographs. Otalgia is usually found in patients with epiglottitis and epiglottic abscess, but the laryngeal symptoms dominate the clinical picture.

Esophageal Disorders

Pediatric esophageal disorders with referred otalgia include impacted foreign bodies and burns of the esophageal mucosa. As in the case of laryngeal disorders, the local esophageal symptoms predominate over the otalgia.

Thyroiditis

The thyroid gland receives its sensory innervation via the vagus nerve. An occasional cause of occult otalgia is the occurrence of thyroiditis (usually de Quervain's), which causes symptoms of throat and neck discomfort and otalgia as a prominent symptom. The diagnosis is often a clinical one based upon the finding of a tender, somewhat swollen thyroid gland, which upon palpation usually evidences otalgia. Childhood thyroiditis must also always be considered as a possible cause of recurrent throat discomfort, often misdiagnosed as pharyngitis or tonsillitis. Such patients should be referred to a pediatric endocrinologist.

REFERRED OTALGIA MEDIATED BY CERVICAL NERVES

The upper cervical nerves, especially the great auricular nerve, supply a significant somatic sensory distribution to the external ear and postauricular area. These nerve endings are distributed in the posterior half of the lateral aspect of the auricle and some of the skin of the cavum conchae (Warwick and Williams, 1973a,b). These cervical nerves also innervate the skin and muscles of the neck and spine. They therefore can mediate pain referred to the ear from a variety of disorders of the neck and cervical spine.

When a patient has otalgia referred from a disease affecting a structure innervated by the sensory fibers of the cervical plexus, the otalgia is usually only one component of a constellation of symptoms. Nevertheless, the parents tend to emphasize the otalgia component of the symptoms and minimize the other symptoms that would indicate the neck as a source of the ear pain.

Lymph Nodes

Cervical lymphadenitis, in addition to causing local neck discomfort, may also cause referred otalgia. This is most commonly seen in the case of inflamed nodes in the upper neck, including the jugulodigastric area, parotid nodes, and postauricular and occipital nodes. The management of such pain, of course, rests in pursuing the cause of the lymphadenitis and treating it (Chap. 76).

Infected Cysts of the Neck

Infected branchial cysts, including those of the second arch and preauricular sinuses, may cause otalgia. The management of such pain depends on appropriate treatment of the cyst (Chap. 74).

Cervical Spine

Injuries, infections, and tumors of the cervical spine are possible but relatively uncommonly seen causes of referred otalgia in children.

A condition that is occasionally seen in children is the Grisel syndrome (Martin, 1942), which consists of painful torticollis due to subluxation of the atlantoaxial joint. The condition follows upper respiratory tract infections and adenoidectomy and is thought to be due to an inflammatory softening of the perivertebral ligaments. These children present with torticollis, a lateral cervical "mass," and pain in the ear. The condition, which may be confused with cervical lymphadenitis, can be diagnosed by obtaining an anterior–posterior radiograph of the upper cervical spine and identifying a lateral shift of the atlas relative to the axis and odontoid process.

Neuralgias

Neuralgias involving the occipital nerves are uncommon causes of otalgia in the pediatric age group.

MISCELLANEOUS

Migraine

Migraine headaches may occur in children. Ear pain is usually a nondominant component of the constellation of symptoms characterizing the various forms of cranial migraine in children. As has been mentioned in several places in this chapter, parents are sometimes so fearful of ear disease that they may overemphasize the otalgia component of the symptoms that turn out on careful evaluation to represent migraine or some other disorder.

Aural Neuralgia

In attempting to diagnose obscure cases of otalgia, the physician should consider an uncommon form of ear pain, intrinsic aural neuralgia (Ballantyne and Groves, 1971). This ailment presents as a ticlike, brief, sharp pain localized deep in the ear without radiation beyond the ear. The cause of this condition, as with most other tic syndromes, is not known. The author has made this diagnosis once in 15 years of practice. As suggested by Golding-Wood (Ballantyne and Groves, 1971) this patient, aged 9 years, was relieved of the pain by a tympanic neurectomy.

SUMMARY

The diagnosis of the cause of otalgia is one of the most challenging in the area of diseases of the head and neck. Nevertheless, the pursuit of the cause of ear pain can be systematized by an understanding of the sensory neuroanatomy of the ear and by evaluating logically on this basis. In this manner, the precise cause of intrinsic or referred otalgia can be discovered in the majority of patients presenting with this symptom.

REFERENCES

Ballantyne, J., and Groves, J. 1971. Tympanic Plexus Neuralgia. *In* Diseases of the Ear, Nose and Throat, 3rd ed., Philadelphia, J. B. Lippincott Co. Vol. 3, pp. 335–338.

Karmody, C. S., 1978. Wegener's granulomatosis: Presentation as an otological problem, Trans. AAOO, July–Aug.

Martin, R. C. 1942. Atlas-axis dislocation following cervical infection. J.A.M.A., *118*:874–875.

Tremble, G. E. 1965. Referred pain in the ear. AMA Arch. Laryngol., *81*:57–63.

Warwick, R., and Williams, P. L. 1973a. Auricle innervation. *In* Gray's Anatomy, 35th British ed. Philadelphia, W. B. Saunders Co., p. 1136.

Warwick, R., and Williams, P. L. 1973b. Cervical plexus. *In* Gray's Anatomy, 35th British ed. Philadelphia, W. B. Saunders Co., pp. 1034–1036.

Warwick, R., and Williams, P. L. 1973c. Facial nerve, sensory portion. *In* Gray's Anatomy, 35th British ed. Philadelphia, W. B. Saunders Co., p. 1012.

Warwick, R., and Williams, P. L. 1973d. Facial nerve, cutaneous fibres. *In* Gray's Anatomy, 35th British ed. Philadelphia, W. B. Saunders Co., p. 1015.

Warwick, R., and Williams, P. L. 1973e. Glossopharyngeal nerve. *In* Gray's Anatomy, 35th British ed. Philadelphia, W. B. Saunders Co., pp. 1017–1019.

Warwick, R., and Williams, P. L. 1973f. Pharyngeal innervation. *In* Gray's Anatomy, 35th British ed. Philadelphia, W. B. Saunders Co., p. 1249.

Warwick, R., and Williams, P. L. 1973g. Trigeminal nerve. *In* Gray's Anatomy, 35th British ed. Philadelphia, W. B. Saunders Co., pp. 1001–1010.

Warwick, R., and Williams, P. L. 1973h. Tympanic and mastoid innervation. *In* Gray's Anatomy, 35th British ed. Philadelphia, W. B. Saunders Co., pp. 1145–1146.

Warwick, R., and Williams, P. L. 1973i. Vagus nerve. *In* Gray's Anatomy, 35th British ed. Philadelphia, W. B. Saunders Co., pp. 1019–1023.

OTORRHEA

Melvin D. Schloss, M.D.

Otorrhea, or discharge from the ear, indicates a disturbance in normal ear function. The clinical approach to this problem is of utmost importance in determining its cause, and the following observations should be made when examining a patient presenting with otorrhea.

FEATURES OF OTORRHEA

Apparent Source

Adequate visualization of the external auditory canal and tympanic membrane are imperative. An aural discharge may be secondary to disease of the external ear, middle ear, or inner ear. Purulent discharge is usually secondary to disease involving the external or middle ear, whereas a clear discharge usually indicates pathologic conditions within the inner ear (Chap. 8A).

Presence of Pulsation

A pulsating discharge is usually due to a disease involving the middle ear or, rarely, the inner ear. Pulsating otorrhea secondary to pathologic conditions of the external auditory canal is unusual.

Odor of the Discharge

A foul-smelling discharge is indicative of infection. Otorrhea, which is nonfoul-smelling, may be inflammatory or noninflammatory in nature.

Associated Signs and Symptoms

Pain. A painful discharge is generally associated with disease of the external ear. The pain of acute suppurative otitis media is relieved when the tympanic membrane perforates spontaneously or following myringotomy, and the discharge that follows is painless. Pain and otorrhea associated with middle ear disease suggest that a complication, either otologic or intracranial, is present.

Local Signs. Swelling of the auricle or external auditory meatus may suggest an otitis externa. Of course, one must always be aware that an underlying neoplastic process frequently causes swelling as well.

Protrusion of the auricle, swelling and tenderness over the mastoid bone, and sagging of the posterosuperior bony meatal wall, in addition to persistent otorrhea, are signs of acute coalescent mastoiditis.

Regional lymphadenitis is usually present with inflammatory processes of the external or middle ear.

Signs and Symptoms of a Complication. There are essentially two major categories of complications that result from middle ear infections — otologic and intracranial. Persistent fever, pain, vertigo, drowsiness, headache, diplopia, and facial nerve paresis are indicative of a complication (Chaps. 17 and 18).

Most complications are amenable to medical or surgical therapy, but results of therapy are usually in direct proportion to the speed

223

with which these are recognized, thus assuring proper medical therapy as soon as possible.

Character of the Discharge

Only by careful examination of the discharge can the cause of otorrhea be diagnosed. The easiest method is to collect the discharge in a clear glass tube, which should be examined first with the naked eye and then, if possible, under the microscope. Essentially five types of discharges may be seen: (1) serous, (2) mucoid, (3) bloody, (4) purulent, and (5) clear (Paparella, 1976). All except the clear discharge (which is usually cerebrospinal fluid) are results of pathologic conditions of the external and middle ear.

By analyzing the type of discharge, the clinician should be able to establish the correct etiology of the otorrhea, and since the character of the otorrhea is so readily established at the time of examination, this step is an efficient way in which to establish the differential diagnosis of otorrhea.

Each of the five types of fluid will be discussed separately.

SEROUS FLUID

Clinically this fluid is a pale yellow transudate resembling serum. It is clear with no mucous strands present.

Mucoid Fluid

Clinically this is a white, cloudy exudate. This fluid may be tenacious, resembling glue; thus the term "glue ear" is used to describe this condition. Numerous mucous strands are present accompanied by some cells, mostly phagocytes.

Serous and mucoid fluids have been proposed to be closely related to other conditions (Paparella and Shumrick, 1973): (a) adenoid hypertrophy, (b) cleft palate, (c) tumors, (d) barotrauma, (e) inflammation and antibiotics, (f) allergy, (g) iatrogenic effects (inadequate antibiotic therapy, radiation therapy, or trauma), (h) immunologic deficiencies, and (i) metabolic disturbance.

Serous and mucoid fluids are usually seen at the time of paracentesis of a middle ear effusion, and rarely are they a spontaneous discharge. The causes of these types of otorrhea are multiple (Table 9B–1).

PURULENT FLUID

A purulent aural discharge is the type of otorrhea most commonly encountered.

This type of fluid is the result of an inflammatory process affecting the external or middle ear (Table 9B–1). Examination of the fluid reveals many neutrophils with mucous strands and a moderate number of cellular remnants. The determination of the bacteriologic components of the fluid is worthwhile in most cases presenting with purulent otorrhea (Healy and Teele, 1977).

Although purulent discharge resulting from infections of the external ear is usually secondary to gram negative bacilli, routine cultures are unnecessary except for infections resistant to the usual therapy.

In middle ear infections, cultures are accurate if proper aspiration is done and if the external ear canal has been properly cleansed. These cultures are particularly important for infections resistant to the standard therapy and for those individuals who are compromised hosts (for example, those with immunologic deficiencies).

Diseases of the External Ear

Purulent otorrhea is caused by purulent inflammatory processes or inflammation secondary to other pathology of the external auditory canal (Table 9B–1). Pain associated with a purulent discharge is almost always secondary to inflammation involving the external auditory canal, and pain produced by pressure to the external auditory canal, pulling on the auricle, or pressing on the tragus indicates disease of the external auditory canal.

Purulent otorrhea may be present as a result of infection of a congenital anomaly. For instance, a fistula of the first branchial cleft may be presented to the physician as a draining ear.

The fissures of Santorini, which are fibrous channels in the cartilaginous portion of the external auditory canal, may transmit infection between the parotid gland and the external canal (Chap. 15).

Table 9B–1   CAUSES OF OTORRHEA

A. Serous, Mucoid, and Purulent
1. congenital anomalies
   a. first branchial cleft fistula
   b. salivary flow through fissures of Santorini
2. inflammatory
   a. external ear
      i. keratosis obturans
      ii. benign necrotizing osteitis of the meatus
      iii. foreign bodies
      iv. otitis externa
         1. furunculosis
         2. diffuse otitis externa
      v. otomycosis
      vi. otitis externa hemorrhagica (bullous myringitis)
      vii. herpes zoster oticus
      viii. herpes simplex
      ix. seborrheic dermatitis
      x. neurodermatitis
   b. middle ear
      i. acute otitis media
         1. acute suppurative otitis media
         2. acute necrotizing otitis media
         3. acute mastoiditis
         4. acute petrositis
      ii. chronic otitis media
         1. chronic suppurative otitis media
            a. tubotympanic disease
               i. permanent perforation syndrome
               ii. persistent mucosal disease
            b. atticoantral disease
         2. tuberculous otitis media
         3. syphilis of the ear
         4. histiocytosis X
3. tumors
   a. external ear
      i. benign
         1. adenoma
            a. sebaceous adenoma
            b. ceruminoma
         2. osteoma
         3. exostoses
      ii. malignant
         1. squamous cell carcinoma
         2. basal cell carcinoma
         3. adenocarcinoma
         4. metastatic

   b. middle ear
      i. benign
         1. adenoma
         2. neurofibroma
         3. glomus jugulare tumors
      ii. malignant
         1. squamous cell carcinoma
         2. metastatic

B. Bloody
1. congenital anomalies
   a. high, dehiscent jugular bulb
   b. anomalous internal carotid artery
2. inflammatory
   a. external ear
      i. otitis externa
         1. furunculosis
         2. diffuse otitis externa
      ii. otitis externa hemorrhagica (bullous myringitis)
   b. middle ear
      i. acute otitis media
      ii. chronic otitis media
3. traumatic
   a. temporal bone fractures
   b. self-inflicted (e.g. cotton swab injuries)
   c. foreign body
   d. iatrogenic
      1. myringotomy
      2. tympanocentesis
      3. curetting to remove wax
4. tumors (e.g., glomus tympanicum)
5. coagulation defects (e.g., leukemia)

C. Clear
1. congenital anomalies
   a. spontaneous perilymph fistula
   b. first branchial cleft fistula
   c. salivary flow through fissures of Santorini
2. traumatic
   a. skull fracture
   b. surgical trauma
3. tumors
   a. intracranial
   b. extracranial

Diseases of the Middle Ear

These are by far the most common causes of purulent otorrhea (Table 9B–1) (Chaps. 16 & 17).

Acute Suppurative Otitis Media

In the stage of suppuration, the tympanic membrane may be perforated spontaneously or by myringotomy. There is characteristically a copious drainage of hemorrhagic or serosanguineous fluid that soon assumes a mucopurulent character. It is usually odorless and is accompanied by loss of pain. The otorrhea will continue until the inflammation of the middle ear has settled; as a rule the acute processes resolve within several weeks. If the disease progresses to acute coalescent mastoiditis, the discharge will persist longer than two or three weeks and will become more profuse and foul-smelling.

Pain and persistent discharge following a simple mastoidectomy usually signify acute petrositis (Shambaugh, 1967).

A foul-smelling discharge devoid of mucus is often a first symptom of acute, necrotizing otitis media (Shambaugh, 1967).

Chronic Suppurative Otitis Media

With chronicity the suppuration produces irreversible damage to the middle ear mucosa and underlying bone. This results clinically in otorrhea that is scanty or profuse, painless, and usually accompanied by some hearing impairment. Pain in middle ear disease is a sign of a complication, in contrast to disease of the external auditory canal of which pain is an early symptom. Because the onset of chronic otitis media is often insidious, the patient may not consult the otologist until the symptoms of a complication occur.

By careful examination and documentation of the otorrhea, the state of the chronic ear disease can be ascertained (Paparella and Shumrick, 1973), an essential step in planning the proper therapy. The active state of chronic disease is characterized by a steady purulent discharge, while the quiescent or inactive state is characterized by intermissions between discharges, and the healed state is the period during which the perforation of the tympanic membrane is healed or repaired.

It is of utmost importance to determine whether the ear being examined has "dangerous" or "benign" middle ear disease (Paparella and Shumrick, 1973). "Dangerous" means that the chronic ear disease could produce early complications. If the ear disease is potentially dangerous, then urgent surgical intervention is indicated.

"Benign" middle ear disease is due to pathologic conditions involving the eustachian tube and middle ear cleft. It is helpful to divide this "benign" disease into two stages.

Permanent perforation is a persistent perforation of the pars tensa of the tympanic membrane (Ballantyne and Groves, 1971). The margins of the perforation are completely covered with healed epithelium, and the ear may remain dry for long periods or may discharge intermittently because of water entering the middle ear cleft via the external auditory canal. Another route for the infection to spread to the middle ear is via the eustachian tube after blowing the nose. The discharge is mucoid or mucopurulent, profuse, and has no odor.

Chronic tubotympanic mucositis is a more active disease state within the middle ear. There may be a prolonged or even persistent mucoid or mucopurulent discharge, which becomes profuse with an upper respiratory infection. On careful examination of the ear there is a large, nearly total defect of the tympanic membrane. The exposed mucosa is thickened and red. Polyps may be present due to marked swelling of the tympanic mucosa.

"Dangerous" chronic ear disease is due to a pathologic condition extending into the attic and antrum (Ballantyne and Groves, 1971). This usually signifies a congenital cholesteatoma, primary acquired cholesteatoma, or occlusion of the attic floor by a chronic non-cholesteatomatous process. The otorrhea is often not profuse, and usually there is a foul odor to the discharge. A bloody discharge may occur from trauma to the granulation tissue or polyps.

Tuberculous Otitis Media

Tuberculous involvement of the middle ear produces a purulent otorrhea, but the discharge is generally less copious than that seen in chronic suppurative otitis media. Tuberculous otitis media is generally painless, although it is associated with surrounding lymphadenopathy. The involved ear occasionally demonstrates a profound hearing loss, with otorrhea being a late sign in this disease. Otoscopy reveals multiple minute tympanic membrane perforations with little surrounding reaction.

Other Specific Diseases of the Middle Ear

Syphilis and histiocytosis X may present with otorrhea. These diseases are rare but must be included in the differential diagnosis of a purulent aural discharge.

BLOODY FLUID

There are many causes of bleeding from the ear.

(a) It may be secondary to lacerations or abrasions of the skin of the external auditory canal. The trauma causing the injury may be self-inflicted, for instance by a cotton swab, secondary to foreign bodies, or iatrogenic (as by a wax curette).

(b) Tumors of the external auditory canal

and middle ear, for instance glomus tympanicum, may present with a bloody aural discharge (Chap. 22).

(c) Bleeding from the ear can be secondary to acute inflammatory processes of the external auditory canal and middle ear. Bloody otorrhea is commonly seen secondary to bullous myringitis.

(d) Profuse bleeding may occur following a myringotomy and tympanocentesis. This is possible in cases involving a congenital vascular anomaly within the middle ear (with a high, dehiscent jugular bulb and anomalous internal carotid artery, for instance), with tumors in the middle ear (as mentioned), or with coagulation defects (as in leukemia).

(e) Bleeding from the ear is one of the most frequent symptoms of middle ear damage from head injury. Hough has described a triad of signs characteristic of a temporal bone fracture (Hough and Stuart, 1968): hearing loss, bleeding from the ear, and unconsciousness. If temporal bone fractures are characterized as transverse or longitudinal, it is the longitudinal type that results in bleeding from the ear. The duration of the bleeding may be short or prolonged for days and may be from the mouth or nose due to flow through the eustachian tube. The bleeding most often ceases spontaneously.

CLEAR FLUID

A clear discharge from the ear is assumed to be cerebrospinal fluid until proven otherwise (Shambaugh, 1967).

Skull trauma resulting from a temporal bone fracture is the most common cause of clear otorrhea. Surgical defects following mastoidectomy or posterior craniotomy are less common. Intracranial or extracranial tumors and congenital anomalies are uncommon causes of clear otorrhea.

Trauma

To locate the site of leakage secondary to skull trauma is a diagnostic challenge. A detailed history and physical examination are the cornerstones in diagnosis and are aided by relatively simple office or bedside procedures. Since cerebrospinal fluid has a high glucose concentration, there is a strongly positive reaction with simple glucose oxidase test paper. Occasionally, cerebrospinal fluid

otorrhea presents as rhinorrhea, the transit from the ear to the nasopharynx being via the eustachian tube, in which case the positive reaction with simple glucose oxidase test paper may be invalid because of the reducing substance in lacrimal gland secretions.

Routine skull radiographs or, if necessary, polytomes of suspected areas may show the fracture site. A leak from the middle or posterior cranial fossa may be demonstrated on posterior fossa myelography. Radioactive tracers or color dyes, e.g., fluorescein, are often successful in demonstrating the leak (Duckert and Mathog, 1977; Shapiro, 1972) (Chap. 21).

Congenital Anomalies

Congenital anomalies are interesting but uncommon causes of clear otorrhea. The otorrhea may be purulent, serous, or clear, depending upon the etiology.

Spontaneous clear otorrhea has been described as a result of perilymphatic fistulas and dural defects secondary to congenital anomalies. It is termed spontaneous otorrhea when there is no apparent cause, and it generally goes undetected until the time of stapedectomy. The classification of this clear discharge as cerebrospinal fluid or perilymph has been rather confusing in the medical literature due to the controversy regarding the origin of perilymph, which is cerebrospinal fluid, at least in part. The fluid reaches the inner ear via the cochlear aqueduct (the bony channel connecting the scala tympani of the basal cochlear turn with the subarachnoid space of the posterior cranial cavity), and perilymph is also thought to be secreted by the blood vessels of the inner ear. A perilymph leak should always be suspected in a patient having congenital footplate fixation (Farrior and Endicott, 1971; Glasscock, 1973); spontaneous perilymphatic fistulas have been reported without any surgical intervention (Chap. 14).

An uncommon cause of clear otorrhea is discharge through the fissures of Santorini connecting the parotid gland and the external auditory canal.

SUMMARY

In summary, otorrhea is an important sign of ear disease. There are basically five types of aural discharge: (1) serous, (2) mucoid, (3) bloody, (4) purulent, and (5) clear. A combination of two or more types is the usual clinical presentation. If otorrhea is approached by the clinician in an organized manner, a correct diagnosis will be established and the proper therapy will be instituted.

SELECTED REFERENCES

Glasscock, M. E. 1973. The stapes gusher. Arch. Otolaryngol., *98*(2):82–91.

This is an excellent review of spontaneous cerebrospinal fluid otorrhea. It is an article related specifically to congenital abnormalities.

Paparella, M. 1976. Middle ear effusions: definitions and terminology. Ann. Otol. Rhinol. Laryngol. Supp. 25,*15*(2):8–11.

Clearly outlines and defines fluid in the middle ear.

Hough, J. V. D., and Stuart, W. D. 1968. Middle ear injuries in skull trauma. Laryngoscope, *78*:899–937.

Classical reference for skull trauma related to middle ear injuries.

REFERENCES

Ballantyne, J., and Groves, J. 1971. Scott-Brown's Diseases of the Ear, Nose and Throat, 3rd ed. London, Butterworks, Chs. 4, 6, and 8.

Duckert, L. G., and Mathog, R. H. 1977. Diagnosis in persistent CSF fistulas. Laryngoscope, *87*:18–25.

Farrior, J. B., and Endicott, J. H. 1971. Congenital mixed deafness: cerebrospinal fluid otorrhea. Ablation of the aqueduct of the cochlea. Laryngoscope, *81*(5):684–699.

Glasscock, M. E. 1973. The stapes gusher. Arch. Otolaryngol., *98*(2):82–91.

Healy, G. B., and Teele, D. W. 1977. The microbiology of chronic middle ear effusions in children. Laryngoscope, *87*:1472–1478.

Hough, J. V. D., and Stuart, W. D. 1968. Middle ear injuries in skull trauma. Laryngoscope, *78*:899–937.

Paparella, M. 1976. Middle ear effusions: definitions and terminology. Ann. Otol. Rhinol. Laryngol. Supp. 25,*15*(2):8–11.

Paparella, M., and Shumrick, D. A. 1973. Otolaryngology. Philadelphia, W. B. Saunders Co., Vol. 2, Sec. 2.

Shambaugh, E., Jr. 1967. Surgery of the Ear, 2nd ed. Philadelphia, W. B. Saunders Co.

Shapiro, S. L. 1972. Cerebrospinal otorrhea. Eye, Ear, Nose, Throat Man., *51*(5):192–196.

Chapter *10*

HEARING LOSS

Kenneth M. Grundfast, M.D.

Much of a child's learning is dependent upon information received from listening to speech and other sounds in the environment. As children grow and develop, they continually acquire and refine their communicative skills, cognitive abilities, and skills in social interaction. Since hearing is so important in the process of developing these skills, significant impairment in a child's hearing ability may affect various related aspects of development.

Realizing the importance of hearing in the context of a child's overall development, it can be seen that a child who is suspected of having a hearing loss needs thorough evaluation. To delay and temporize can be detrimental, whereas an evaluation that leads to a finding of normal hearing either may allay a parent's fears about possible deafness or may lead to the conclusion that there is dysfunction somewhere in the nervous system other than in the auditory portion.

Depending upon the age of the child, an evaluation to determine if manifest symptoms are due to hearing impairment can be difficult. In the sense that hearing is perceptual, involving psychoacoustic phenomena, there is an element of subjectivity inherent in the meaningful perception of auditory stimuli. Although we can make inferences from observing a child's response to auditory stimuli, only the child is actually aware of the type of information that is ultimately received from auditory stimuli. Younger children are less able than older children to verbalize about abnormalities in the perception of sound and to cooperate for behavioral audiometric tests. However, recent advancements in nonbehavioral (objective) audiometric testing now make it feasible at least to estimate the hearing ability of young children and

even of newborn infants (Chap. 8B). *No child is too young to be tested or too young to be evaluated when there is the suspicion that hearing ability may be impaired.*

Since it is not always easy to know where to begin an evaluation for the symptom of hearing loss, an orderly approach is helpful. The complete process of evaluation and management can be subdivided into the initial phase of collecting core information, then proceeding with four tasks that are undertaken in a sequential, stepwise fashion. As a memory aid, the initial phase and succeeding tasks are all described with words beginning with the letter "C," and, thus, the five "Cs" constitute the rudiments of evaluation and management for a child with hearing impairment.

EVALUATION AND TASKS

1. CORE information. Information gleaned from history taking and physical examination combined with results of appropriate laboratory and radiographic studies constitute "core information."
2. CONFIRM that hearing impairment exists.
3. CHARACTERIZE the type of hearing impairment, and quantify the degree of impairment.
4. CAUSE. Attempt to discover the pathophysiologic process that caused the hearing loss.
5. CARE. A plan needs to be formulated for habilitation or rehabilitation, education, and periodic reassessment of the hearing-impaired child.

Collecting the core information, that is, establishing the data base, is fairly routine and is done in much the same way for children in all age groups. However, the method to be chosen for accomplishing the succeeding four tasks depends upon the age of the child. Audiometric test techniques, diagnostic possibilities, and management modalities utilized for the neonate with suspected hearing loss differ markedly from those that are appropriate for a preadolescent child who develops difficulty in hearing. Regarding the symptom of hearing loss, then, it must be realized that the pediatric population is somewhat heterogeneous. Conceptually dividing the childhood years into five age categories makes it possible to develop several different approaches, each of which is more or less specifically suited for use with children in a certain age category. The age categories utilized in this chapter are (1) neonate, birth to four weeks; (2) infant, four weeks to two years; (3) preschool age, two years to five years; (4) school age, five years to 10 years; and (5) preadolescent, 10 years to 14 years.

Keeping in mind these arbitrary age categories and the sequential tasks previously mentioned, one is able to develop an age-specific, task-oriented approach to the evaluation and management of hearing loss in children. To demonstrate how this approach is utilized, the five "C" tasks are described, and then methods for accomplishing the tasks are described for each of the five age categories. Since the method of acquiring "core information" is much the same for children of all ages, separate descriptions are not given in each age category. Rather, the detailed description of a method for acquiring "core information" is intended to be utilized for children in all age categories. Methods for accomplishing the remaining tasks, i.e., *confirm, characterize, cause,* and *care,* are described in subsequent separate sections corresponding to the five arbitrary age categories (Chap. 8A).

Core Information — Data Base

Whereas hearing impairment manifesting during the later adult years usually is the result of degenerative processes, hearing impairment during childhood can be caused by any of a number of factors. Therefore, significant unilateral or bilateral hearing impairment discovered during childhood should be viewed as a specific pathologic process involving one sensory system. Childhood hearing loss may be the result of a common disorder such as otitis media with effusion, or it could represent the initially discovered manifestation that leads to later diagnosis of a syndromal or neurologic disorder. To commence the evaluation of a child with hearing impairment, a detailed history and physical examination are warranted as well as certain appropriate diagnostic studies.

Confirm

Not all children who are suspected of having hearing loss actually have impairment of hearing ability. Recently, the importance of early detection has been widely publicized and, consequently, many types of screening programs have been developed. Even where screening programs are nonexistent, parents, educators, and day care center personnel have become sufficiently cognizant of the importance of early detection to notice young children who may possibly have hearing impairments. As a result, it is becoming common for infants and children to be referred to a physician, medical center, or audiologist for further evaluation of hearing ability. The first task, then, is to confirm the presence of and measure the amount of hearing loss with a test procedure that is appropriate for the chronologic age and developmental level of the child.

Characterize

Next, it is important to characterize the type of hearing impairment as being one of the following.

Conductive. Impairment of hearing by air conduction can be due to any condition that interrupts transmission of sound through the external auditory canal or transmission of vibrations from the tympanic membrane through the ossicular chain to the oval window.

Sensorineural. When hearing by bone conduction is impaired, the malfunction is in the cochlea, the cochlear portion of the eighth cranial nerve, or both. In the purist sense, if the impairment of function is solely in the cochlea, then the hearing loss should be termed "sensory," and if the abnormality is only in the cochlear nerve, then it should be termed "neural" hearing loss. Practically speaking, these distinctions are rarely made, and it is usually considered adequate to identify a hearing loss as being "sensorineural."

Mixed. When hearing by both air and bone conduction is impaired, the loss is termed "mixed." The malfunction in such cases is in the middle ear transformer mechanism and in the cochlea or the cochlear nerve, or at some or all of these sites.

Retrocochlear. A retrocochlear hearing loss involves impaired neuronal transmission somewhere in the cochlear nerve, brain stem auditory pathways, or both, with presumably normal function in the cochlea.

Central. When a hearing loss is central in nature, the middle ear transformer mechanism, the cochlea, and the cochlear nerve function properly, but there is abnormal processing of auditory signals within the brain.

Determining the type of hearing impairment that a child has helps to localize the portion of the auditory system that is not functioning normally. In turn, this helps in the diagnosis and management of the hearing-impaired child.

Cause

An attempt should be made to discover the pathophysiologic process that has caused hearing impairment. Since severe hearing impairment can be such a devastating handicap for a child, attention is often focused on the hearing threshold itself rather than considering the hearing loss as a symptom that requires a complete evaluation in order to discover the pathophysiologic mechanisms involved. The fact that a child has difficulty hearing means that some portion of the auditory pathway is not functioning properly. While hearing loss in adults can usually be attributed to degenerative changes in the cochlea, such is not the case with children. The child with sensorineural hearing impairment should be viewed as a child with a significant pathologic process in one sensory system. Then, further investigation is warranted to determine the etiologic factors involved and to determine whether other sensory systems or even other organ systems also may have been affected by a common etiologic factor. There may be an inherent abnormality in a single portion or several portions of the auditory system, or there may have been an inflammatory, degenerative, neo-

plastic, metabolic, or traumatic process that affected some aspect of the auditory system.

In a broad sense, childhood hearing impairment may be thought of as being congenital, acquired, or of unknown etiology. A detailed history and thorough medical evaluation combined with audiometric tests and laboratory and radiographic studies yield the information that is necessary for formulating a reasonable hypothesis of causality.

Finally, even though inferences regarding causality can be made based on certain information and observations, a greater understanding of the cause of a given hearing impairment can be achieved by histopathologic examination of the involved temporal bone. That is, the damaged or malfunctioning portion of the auditory pathway may involve the ossicles, the basilar membrane, the hair cells, the eighth nerve, the temporal lobe, or any other area in the complex sensory system that enables meaningful perception of auditory stimuli. Since biopsy of middle and inner ear structures is not really feasible, there is a need to locate the temporal bones of people who have had hearing impairment during childhood so that histopathologic examinations can be made and the pathophysiology of childhood hearing impairment can be elucidated. Many major medical centers throughout the world have temporal bone laboratories where detailed examinations can be made on temporal bone specimens that have been donated.

Care

After a child's hearing impairment has been characterized and quantified and an attempt has been made to discover the etiology, then a plan must be established for helping the child function optimally despite the hearing handicap. Depending upon the severity of the hearing impairment, a child may require a hearing aid, preferential seating in school, or some special type of education. It may be necessary to provide the child with assistance in developing communication skills. The child may require assistance in making various psychologic and social adjustments. The family of a hearing-handicapped child may also need assistance in making adjustments. Genetic counseling for the parents may be advisable.

The child with impaired hearing will require frequent assessments of hearing ability to make sure that the hearing is not worsening. Also, there will be a continual need for otologic evaluation.

METHOD FOR ACQUIRING CORE INFORMATION — APPLICABLE TO ALL AGES

An appropriate physical examination and relevant history-taking are essential. The most common cause of hearing loss in children is otitis media with effusion. When there is a history of frequent ear "infections" and it seems likely that persistent middle ear effusion could be causing a conductive hearing loss, then it is important to determine the nature and frequency of prior ear "infections." In doing this, the term "infection" must be defined. Often a parent may report that the child has had four or five "ear infections" in the past several months. When questioned further, it becomes evident that the child has had no fever or otalgia, but a physician who periodically examines the child has noticed fluid in the child's ear and the mother was told that the child had an "infection." Rather than using the term "infection," it is helpful to decide from the history whether the otologic problem is frequent acute otitis media, persistent otitis media with effusion, or chronic suppurative otitis media (Chaps. 16 & 17).

When there is no history suggestive of frequent or persistent otitis media with effusion and it is suspected that the hearing impairment is sensorineural, then history-taking should attempt to discover causative perinatal or genetic factors (Chap. 19).

Gestational History

It is important to identify those factors that may have acted during fetal development to cause impaired hearing after birth. The human embryo is most susceptible to factors that can cause major morphologic abnormalities from about three weeks through 10 weeks of gestation; until 20 weeks of gestation, certain physiologic defects and minor morphologic abnormalities may occur (Moore, 1977). Prenatal infections, such as rubella, toxoplasmosis, influenza, cytomegalovirus infection, or syphilis, can cause

changes in the embryo that will ultimately result in some form of hearing impairment (Bergstrom and Stewart, 1971; Bergstrom, 1974). Subclinical rubella infection in the mother can cause rubella embryopathy; this can occur even if the mother has had a previous attack of rubella, since immunity is not necessarily permanent (Karmody, 1968). Although the evidence is not entirely conclusive, it is probable that certain medications taken during pregnancy can have a deleterious effect upon portions of the developing inner ear. Streptomycin, especially in the dihydro form, quinine, and chloroquine phosphate have all been described as causing sensorineural hearing loss by damaging neural elements in the developing ear of the embryo. Thalidomide embryopathy, on the other hand, is due to a widespread involvement of the auditory apparatus, including the auricles and osseous structures of the middle and inner ear (Partsch and Maurer, 1963; Rosendal, 1963; Kittel and Saller, 1964).

Finally, there have been reports that endocrine diseases of the mother, such as pseudohypoparathyroidism (Hinojosa, 1958) or diabetes mellitus (Kelemen, 1958; Jorgensen, 1961) may predispose her children to congenital hearing loss.

Thus, the prenatal history must be reviewed for any factor, infectious or otherwise, that may have had a deleterious effect upon the developing middle or inner ear in the embryo.

Perinatal History

Certainly, the birth process and the adaptation to extrauterine life can be stressful for the neonate. Intrapartum asphyxia and anoxia may lead to hearing loss through toxic damage to the cochlear nuclei as well as through the production of hemorrhages into the inner ear (Fisch, 1955; Hall, 1964). There is some evidence that the auditory system is selectively vulnerable to brief episodes of asphyxia at birth (Hall, 1964). Early injury to brain stem auditory pathways can interfere with the development of normal auditory processing and can cause impaired language development. Kernicterus may also cause damage to the cochlear nuclei or other central auditory pathways (Crabtree and Genrard, 1950; Haymaker et al., 1961). Although there is no definite evidence, it is logical to assume that events such as intrauterine hemorrhage, placenta previa, prolonged labor, instrument delivery, and possibly cesarean section may cause damage to the middle ear, inner ear, or central auditory pathways of the newborn. In addition to these factors, it has been observed that a relatively high number of premature infants develop hearing impairment.

Family History

Approximately half of all congenital deafness discovered during childhood is caused by genetic factors (Nance and Sweeney, 1975). Of the inherited types of deafness, 75 to 88 per cent are recessively inherited, and about 10 per cent are dominantly inherited (Chung, 1959). Inherited sensorineural hearing loss can be present and manifest at birth, it may be discovered later in childhood, or it may not be discovered until adult life. The hearing loss that is inherited in a dominant manner tends to worsen progressively, whereas the recessively inherited hearing loss usually remains stable. There are more than 50 types of hereditary hearing impairment that are characterized according to the type of hearing loss, age at onset, severity, genetic mode of transmission, and associated clinical findings (Rose et al., 1976). Despite the multiplicity of named syndromes, the great majority of cases of sensorineural hearing loss due to single-gene mendelian inheritance, whether dominant or recessive, are clinically undifferentiated (Fraser, 1976). That is, the hearing impairment does not constitute part of a recognizable syndrome in which it is associated with visible malformations or in which other organs and body systems are involved.

The family history provides information concerning the mode of inheritance. When two or more siblings are affected while the parents and other relatives are not, recessive inheritance is likely, although when the children with hearing loss are exclusively males, it may be difficult to differentiate the X-linked from the autosomal variety. When the parents are consanguineous, it can be presumed that inheritance is autosomal recessive, and this is true whether there is only one or several affected children. When one or more siblings are affected and, in addition, relatives such as parents, uncles, aunts, grandparents, or cousins are deaf, then iden-

tification of a specific mode of inheritance may be extremely difficult. However, the presence of unilateral or mild bilateral sensorineural hearing loss in relatives is suggestive of dominant inheritance.

Even though one is persistent in acquiring information about family members who developed hearing impairment early in life, it may be difficult to construct a meaningful pedigree. Hearing impairment can be defined in social as well as biological terms, and persons who are mildly or unilaterally affected may not consider themselves hearing impaired, or they may even be totally unaware of the hearing impairment. As audiometric test methods improve and as mandatory screening tests become more prevalent, children will be discovered who are labeled as having significant sensorineural hearing impairment, although the same degree of hearing impairment in their parents or in previous generations may have remained undetected throughout life. In fact, it is not uncommon for such mild hearing loss in parents and other relatives to be identified for the first time during the family investigation initiated because of the failure of a child to pass a school screening test (Fraser, 1976).

No examples are known of conductive autosomal recessive deafness that is not part of a syndrome. Therefore, familial conductive hearing loss that is not part of an obvious syndrome is likely to be inherited in an autosomal dominant or, more rarely, X-linked recessive manner. The most common type of dominant, clinically undifferentiated conductive hearing loss is otosclerosis, but this usually does not affect young children.

Physical Examination

Significant abnormalities detected during a physical examination may indicate that an observed hearing loss is part of a syndrome. In Table 10–1, physical abnormalities are listed with their corresponding syndromes or diseases and the type of associated hearing loss. In examining the ears, the external canals should first be cleansed of debris, then inspected. It is best to use a pneumatic otoscope to test eardrum mobility and to gain information about the presence or absence of fluid in the middle ear. Also, the examiner should be aware that there are anatomic

Text continued on page 239

Table 10–1   PHYSICAL ABNORMALITIES AND THEIR ASSOCIATED SYNDROMES
RELATED TO HEARING LOSS

Physical Exam	Physical Abnormality	Disease or Syndrome	Type of Hearing Loss
Skull	Macrocephaly	Osteopetrosis (Albert-Schönberg disease)	PSN or PC*
		Osteogenesis imperfecta	PSN or PC
	Abnormal shape	Apert syndrome	CC
		Crouzon disease	CC and/or CSN
		Craniostenosis	CC
		Craniometaphysial dysplasia (Pyle disease)	CSN and/or CC
		Cranial clefts	CC
		Osteitis deformans (Paget disease)	PSN or PC
	Failure of fontanelle to close	Cleidocranial dysostosis	CSN
Hair	White forelock	Waardenburg syndrome	CSN
	Low posterior hairline	Turner, and Klippel-Feil syndrome	CSN
	Twisted hair	Recessive pili torti	CC
Face	Hemifacial atrophy	First branchial arch syndrome	CSN
		Goldenhar syndrome	CC
	Facial clefts		
	Leonine facies	Generalized cortical hyperostosis (Van Buchem syndrome)	PSN
	Dysplasia of supraorbital ridges	Osteopetrosis	PSN or PC
		Frontometaphysial dysplasia (Gorlin-Hart syndrome)	CSN and CC
	Prominence of frontal bone and coarse facial features	Hurler syndrome	CC
	Frontal bossing	Otopalatodigital syndrome	CC
	Narrow face in region of orbits and flattening of midface	Otofacial cervical syndrome	CC
	Flattened cheeks and coloboma of eyelids	Treacher Collins syndrome	CC and/or CSN
	Facial paralysis	Möbius syndrome	CC
	Strabismus	Möbius syndrome	CC
		Duane syndrome	CC
Eyes	Hypertelorism		CC and CSN
	Eyelid abnormalities		
	Coloboma of eyelids, slant, epicanthal fold, ptosis		
	Lateral displacement of medial canthi	Waardenburg syndrome	CSN
	Adherent	Cryptophthalmus	CC
	Microphthalmus		CSN

Region	Abnormality	Syndrome	Type
Cornea	Dystrophy	Fehrs dystrophy	PSN
	Clouding or keratoconus		CC and CSN
Sclera	Epibulbar dermoids	Oculoauriculovertebral dysplasia (Goldenhar syndrome)	CC
	Blue	Osteogenesis imperfecta	PSN or PC
Iris	Heterochromia	Waardenburg syndrome	CSN
Lens	Cataracts	Congenital rubella	CSN
	Fundus abnormalities	Flynn-Aird syndrome	PSN
		Usher, etc. syndrome	CSN, PSN
	Blindness	Norrie disease	PSN
		Primary testicular insufficiency	PSN
		Congenital lues	CC
Ears	Pinna malformations	Marshall syndrome	CC and CSN
	Atresia		CSN
	Preauricular sinuses (dominant)		CSN
Nose	Saddle	Medial facial cleft	CSN
	Bifid		CC
Mouth	Cleft lip, nose		CC
	Midline cleft lip	Oral-facial-digital syndrome (Mohr II)	CC
	Microstomia	Otopalatodigital syndrome	CSN, CC
Teeth	Pegged incisors	Trisomy 18 syndrome	CSN and PSN
	Abnormal dentine	Congenital lues	PSN and/or PC
	Coniform teeth and dominant onychodystrophy	Osteogenesis imperfecta	CSN
Palate	Cleft palate	Otopalatodigital syndrome	CC
		Pierre Robin syndrome	CC and/or CSN
		Other syndromes	CC
	Bifid uvula		CC
Neck	Goiter (recessive)	Pendred syndrome	CSN
	Goiter (recessive) and stippled epiphyses		CSN
	Short (torticollis)	Klippel-Feil syndrome	CSN and/or CC
		Wildervanck syndrome	CSN and/or CC
Chest	Absent clavicles	Cleidocranial dysostosis	CC
	Narrowing of shoulders	Otofacial-cervical syndrome	CC
	Webbing	Turner syndrome	CSN and/or CC
	Pigeon breast	Marfan syndrome	CSN
		Goiter and stippled epiphyses	CSN and/or CC
		Trisomy 18	CSN and/or CC

Table continued on the following page

Table 10–1   PHYSICAL ABNORMALITIES AND THEIR ASSOCIATED SYNDROMES RELATED TO HEARING LOSS *(Continued)*

Physical Exam	Physical Abnormality	Disease or Syndrome	Type of Hearing Loss
Lungs	(None)		
Heart	Murmur	Ventricular septal defect with congenital rubella	CSN
	Murmur of congenital pulmonary stenosis	Lewis syndrome	CSN
	Murmur of mitral insufficiency	Forney syndrome	CC
Abdomen	Hepatomegaly	Wilson disease	CSN
Extremities			
Hands	Knuckle pads and leukonychia		CSN and/or CC
	Small fissured nails	Dominant onychodystrophy and conform teeth	CSN
	Small fissured nails	Recessive onychodystrophy and strabismus	CSN
Hands and feet	Congenital flexion contractions of fingers and toes	"Hand-hearing" syndrome	CSN
	Clubfoot	Diastrophic dwarfism	CSN
	Split hand-foot	Wildervanck syndrome	CSN
	Flexion contracture of fingers	Hurler syndrome	CC
	Absent joint of fingers	Symphalangism and strabismus syndrome	CC
	Exaggerated space between thumb and index fingers	Otopalatodigital syndrome	CC
	Lobster claw hands and feet	Cockayne syndrome	CC
	Stiff joints	Arthrogryposis	CC
Legs	Short lower legs	Absence of tibia	CSN
	Bowing of legs	Osteogenesis imperfecta	CSN and/or CC
Arms	Limited elbow motion	Frontometaphysial dysplasia	CSN
	Limited radial abduction of arm and hand	Madelung deformity	CC
Spine	Scoliosis		CC
Dwarf	Achondroplasia		CC and/or CSN
Skin	Albinism-dominant		CSN
	Small hyperpigmented lesion, especially head and neck	Dominant lentigines	CSN
	Hypopigmentation spots, especially head and arms	Hereditary piebaldness	CSN

	Leopard-like spots of hypo- and hyperpigmentation	Sex-linked pigmentary abnormalities	CSN
	Ichthyosis of arms but not legs	Recessive atypical atopic dermatitis	CSN
	Inability to sweat	Dominant anhidrosis (ectodermal dysplasia)	CSN
	Xeroderma pigmentosum (with neurologic disease)	DeSanctis-Cacchione syndrome	CSN
	Urticaria, nephritis, and amyloidosis	Muckle-Wells syndrome	PSN
	Ota's nevus		
	Neurofibromatosis	von Recklinghausen disease	PSN and CC
Neurologic Epilepsy	Photosensitive epilepsy	Hyperprolinemia Type I (major part)	PSN
	Progressive familial myoclonic epilepsy and progressive cerebral degeneration (minor part)	Herrmann syndrome	PSN
		Unverricht disease	PSN
Mental status Retardation from birth	And ataxia and hypogonadism	Richard-Rundel syndrome	CSN
	And coarse facies and spine and digit bone changes	Hurler syndrome	CSN
	And muscular wasting and recessive retinal detachment	Small syndrome	CSN
	And hyperprolinemia Type I (minor part)	Shafer syndrome	PSN
	And hereditary nephritis, epilepsy, diabetes	Herrmann syndrome	CSN
	And retinitis pigmentosa and obesity and polydactyly	Lawrence-Moon-Biedl syndrome	CSN
	And retinal malformation	Norrie disease	PSN
	And homocystinuria (one case)		
Mental deterioration	And retinitis pigmentosa and dwarfism	Cockayne syndrome	PSN
	And myopia	Flynn-Aird syndrome	CSN
	And encephalopathy, subcortical	Shilder disease	
Motor abnormalities	Cerebral palsy		CSN
	Spasticity and optic atrophy	Opticocochleodentate degeneration	CSN
	Ataxia	Spinocerebellar degeneration (Friedreich ataxia)	PSN

Table continued on the following page

Table 10-1 PHYSICAL ABNORMALITIES AND THEIR ASSOCIATED SYNDROMES RELATED TO HEARING LOSS *(Continued)*

Physical Exam	Physical Abnormality	Disease or Syndrome	Type of Hearing Loss
		Richard-Rundel syndrome	CSN
		Herrmann syndrome	PSN
		Vestibulocerebellar and retinitis pigmentosa (Hallgren syndrome)	CSN
		Hyperuricemia and renal insufficiency (dominant in Rosenberg's progressive ataxia)	PSN
	Childhood Huntington chorea (rare part)		CSN and PSN
Sensory neuropathy	Dominant sensory radicular neuropathy		PSN
Motor neuropathy	Polyneuropathy, ichthyosis, and retinitis pigmentosa	Refsum syndrome	PSN
	Peripheral neuropathy and skeletal anomalies and dominant myopia	Flynn-Aird syndrome	CSN
	Familial polyneuropathy (resembling Charcot-Marie-Tooth disease) with nerve deafness seen with optic atrophy, or nephritis, or neurofibromatosis, or achalasia		
Myopathy	And mental deficiency and ataxia	Richard-Rundel syndrome	CSN
	And growth failure and chronic lactic acidemia		
	Muscle wasting and retinal detachment and mental retardation	Small syndrome	CSN
	Facioscapulohumeral dystrophy associated with nerve deafness		
Endocrine	Goiter	Pendred syndrome	CSN
	Hypogonadism and blindness		CSN
	Obesity and diabetes, retinal degeneration	Alström syndrome	CSN
	Obesity and polydactyly and retinitis pigmentosa	Laurence-Moon-Biedl syndrome	CSN
Multiple Physical Changes		Trisomy 13–15 (Patau syndrome, trisomy D_1)	CSN and CC
		Trisomy 18 (trisomy E)	CSN and CC
No Physical Findings			

*CC, congenital conductive; PC, progressive conductive; CSN, congenital sensorineural; PSN, progressive sensorineural. Modified and reprinted with permission from Jaffe, B. F. (Ed.) 1977. Hearing Loss In Children: A Comprehensive Text. Baltimore, University Park Press.

differences between the eardrum of a neonate and that of an older child (Chap. 8A).

Laboratory Studies

Although several investigators (Bergstrom, 1974; Jaffe, 1977) have analyzed the problem of defining an appropriate test battery, there is really no specific set of tests that has proved to be of exceptional diagnostic value in the evaluation of all children with hearing losses. Most often, a laboratory test will tend to confirm or negate a tentative diagnosis. It is best to order whatever specific studies seem to be appropriate rather than attempt to discover an underlying etiology with a battery of tests. The following list of laboratory studies may be helpful.

TORCH Studies. TORCH is an acronym used to describe the group of specific IgM antibody assays for *TO*xoplasmosis, *R*ubella, *C*ytomegalovirus, and *H*erpes virus. Usually an immunoassay for syphilis is done along with the TORCH study. Results are reported as titer values, and it is important to know the normal titers for the laboratory where the serum was analyzed. The TORCH studies can help to determine whether or not an intrauterine infection may have caused a hearing impairment in a neonate.

In infants with congenital rubella, hemagglutination inhibition (HAI) and complement fixation (CF) titers remain elevated during the first few years of life, since these include fetally produced antibodies (IgM). In unaffected infants, serial rubella titers show a decline and disappearance at about six months of age, since the majority of the antibody is maternally produced IgG. In congenital rubella, the virus may be cultured from the infant up to three years of age in spite of the presence of rubella antibodies (Michaels, 1969).

In evaluating a congenitally deaf child for intrauterine infection, serial antibody studies are necessary. If a hearing loss is diagnosed or suspected shortly after birth, blood should be obtained for serum gamma globulin determinations and for specific hemagglutination inhibition and complement fixation antibody titers to suspected agents. If the IgM levels are elevated, specific fluorescent antibody tests should be done if available. Although an elevated IgM level is highly suggestive of intrauterine infection, a normal level does not exclude it. Cultures for rubella and cytomegalovirus may also be obtained from the urine, nasopharynx, and throat. At 10 to 12 months of age, these titer determinations should be repeated. Persistent elevation is highly suggestive of an intrauterine infection.

It is possible that the rubella vaccine may aid in the late diagnosis of congenital rubella as a cause of hearing loss. It has been reported that about 19 per cent of children with known congenital rubella have no demonstrable antibody titer by five years of age (Florman et al., 1970). When these children are given the rubella vaccine, only 10 per cent reconvert to seropositive. Although more work needs to be done in this area, the failure of a deaf child to develop antibodies after receiving the rubella vaccine may suggest rubella as the etiology of the hearing loss (Bergstrom and Stewart, 1971).

VDRL-FTA (Venereal Disease Research Laboratory-Fluorescent Treponemal Antibody) Tests. These are the best tests for detecting syphilis, whether congenital or acquired. The VDRL test should be requested routinely for evaluation of a neonate with hearing impairment, and the FTA test can be requested for highly suspicious cases with a negative VDRL test or when results of the VDRL test are equivocal. Also, since hearing impairment caused by congenital syphilis may not be present or apparent at birth, it is worthwhile to request the VDRL-FTA test in any child who is discovered to have sensorineural hearing loss without any evident etiology.

Urinalysis. Protein found in the urine may indicate that hearing impairment is part of a syndrome such as Alport syndrome (hereditary nephritis and progressive sensorineural hearing loss) or Muckle-Wells syndrome (nephritis with recurrent urticaria and deafness). Since hearing loss can occur in children with mucopolysaccharide abnormalities, a urine screen for inborn errors in metabolism can be helpful if a metabolic or mucopolysaccharide abnormality is suspected.

Thyroid Function Tests. An abnormal T4 uptake or perchlorate discharge test may help to confirm the suspicion that hearing loss is part of Pendred syndrome (congenital defective binding of iodine by the thyroid gland associated with sensorineural hearing loss).

Electrocardiogram (EKG). A prolonged Q–T interval, when associated with syncopal episodes and congenital sensorineural hearing loss, is indicative of Jervell and Lange-Nielsen syndrome. EKG abnormalities, such as increased P–Q interval, nodal and auricular extrasystoles, and alteration in the QRS complex, are seen in about a third of children with Refsum syndrome (retinitis pigmentosa, hypertrophic peripheral neuropathy, and sensorineural hearing loss) (Richterich et al., 1965). In some cases of Friedreich ataxia (ataxia, speech impairment, lateral curvature of the spinal column, peculiar swaying and irregular mannerisms, and paralysis of muscles, especially of the lower extremities), both sensorineural hearing loss and cardiomyopathy may be present.

Vestibular Function Tests. In evaluating the child with sensorineural hearing loss, vestibular function tests are not of great diagnostic value. However, such tests may reveal concomitant abnormalities of the nonacoustic labyrinth. Abnormal caloric responses have been found in children with cretinism (Costa et al., 1964), Hallgren syndrome, Klippel-Feil malformation (Proctor and Proctor, 1967), onychodystrophy (Feinmesser and Zelig, 1961), Pendred syndrome (Black et al., 1971), in unilateral congenital deafness (Black et al., 1971), in Waardenburg syndrome (Matalon et al., 1970), in the cervico-oculoacusticus syndrome of Wildervanck (Black et al., 1971), and in 26 of 33 ears with various disorders reported by Valvassori, Naunton, and Lindsay (1969). Electronystagmography (ENG) is a newer, more precise tool for evaluating the vestibular system that can be done in children as young as six years of age. Electronystagmographic abnormalities reportedly have been detected along with congenital deafness in three patients with familial hyperuricemia and ataxia (Rosenberg et al., 1970). Also, electronystagmographic abnormalities have been reported in one patient with rubella and central nervous system involvement (Bergstrom and Stewart, 1971). Absent vestibular function was found in two rubella patients in whom electronystagmograms were obtained (Alford, 1968). This suggests pathologic change more extensive than the classic cochleosaccular degeneration traditionally reported in rubella. Results of vestibular tests can help to distinguish dominant from recessive congenital severe deafness. It is advisable to test vestibular function in children with sensorineural hearing impairment who are having difficulty in walking or maintaining their equilibrium. Also, although it has never been proved, it has been suspected that young children with middle ear effusions may, at times, develop difficulties with equilibrium and postural control. When parents of a child with hearing impairment remark that the child seems excessively clumsy, awkward, or intermittently unable to maintain an upright posture, then some assessment of vestibular function is warranted (Chap. 8D).

Other Tests. Additional tests, such as chromosomal analysis, dermatoglyphics, electroretinography, amino acid screen, blood urea nitrogen determination, platelet count, serum pyrophosphate determination, and uric acid assay, may be of diagnostic value in certain instances, especially in confirming the tentative diagnosis of a syndromal type of hearing impairment.

Radiographic Studies

In most cases of childhood hearing impairment, radiographic studies do not provide information that is essential for decision-making. Further, negative findings on radiographic studies do not exclude the possibility that congenital middle or inner ear malformations exist because minor abnormalities may not be radiographically demonstrable even with modern polytomographic techniques. Several types of radiographic studies can be used for evaluating otologic disorders. The mastoid series can be of value in determining whether or not cholesteatoma is present and in assessing the extent of bone erosion involving the lateral wall of the epitympanum (scutum) or the ossicles. Transorbital views of the internal auditory canals enable a screening type of comparative measurement of size of the right and left internal auditory canals. Since eighth nerve tumors can cause bone erosion, a difference in width between the internal auditory canals can be indicative of a vestibular schwannoma (acoustic neuroma). Temporal bone polytomography demonstrates the minute anatomic structures of the temporal bone. The ossicles, semicircular canals, facial nerve canal, oval and round windows, and internal auditory canals can be visualized.

In cases of sensorineural hearing impairment, polytomography can aid in assessing relative development of the cochlea so that malformations involving the otic capsule can be categorized. In cases of conductive hearing impairment, especially those with external canal atresia, temporal bone polytomography can be extremely helpful in determining the status of the ossicular chain and in assessing the suitability of a given ear for reconstructive surgery. Also, polytomography is helpful in locating the position of the facial nerve in a child who will be operated upon for reconstruction of the middle ear. When the diagnosis of vestibular schwannoma is being considered, temporal bone polytomography provides the best noninvasive method for detecting characteristic widening of an internal auditory canal. When findings on polytomography suggest that there could be an eighth nerve tumor present, then a CT scan or posterior fossa myelogram can be utilized to demonstrate a mass at the cerebellopontine angle or at the porus of the internal auditory canal. If a perilymph fistula is considered the likely cause of a sensorineural hearing loss, then polytomography can demonstrate abnormalities within the otic capsule or a widely patent cochlear aqueduct (Wtodyka, 1978; Dorph et al., 1973), both of which are known sometimes to be associated with perilymph fistulae (Grundfast and Bluestone, 1978) (Chap. 8C).

AGE-SPECIFIC TASKS

Utilizing the age-specific, task-oriented approach for the evaluation of hearing loss, let us first consider the seemingly awesome challenge of evaluating a neonate who is suspected of having impaired hearing.

Neonate

Confirm

For those who believe that early detection and intervention are key factors in enabling a child to cope successfully with a hearing handicap, the ultimate goal is detection of significant hearing impairment at birth. Accordingly, it is logical to attempt to test the hearing ability of neonates soon after birth and before discharge from the hospital in which the neonate was born. In a sense, while neonates are still in the hospital, they are part of a captive population, whereas when they are discharged to their respective homes, it becomes more difficult to identify and test those children suspected of having hearing impairment. Thus, much attention has been

focused on in-hospital hearing screening programs for neonates.

Although there is general agreement that such screening is worthwhile, different investigators advocate different methods for identifying neonates who have impaired hearing. Some experts have felt that all newborn infants should undergo a screening procedure that is designed to identify hearing loss. Indeed, several such procedures were developed, including tests that monitor the neonate's reflexive body movements, blink, or altered respiratory or heart rate in response to a sound stimulus of specific intensity. Although such all-encompassing screening procedures were in vogue for a while, results of large-scale programs appeared to indicate that testing all neonates was not an efficient, cost-effective way of identifying newborn children with hearing impairments. Rather, in an attempt to identify those newborns who are most likely to have impaired hearing, it is now becoming common to define and utilize a so-called "high risk register." This registry is composed of neonates who manifest any or all of a list of characteristics that are likely to be associated with hearing impairment in neonates.

Once the infants in the high-risk category are identified, they are tested by some screening method. Evidence that there is now a trend toward more selective screening procedures lies in the recommendation of the Joint Committee on Newborn Hearing Screening. This committee was established in 1969 by the American Speech and Hearing Association, the American Academy of Ophthalmology and Otolaryngology, and the American Academy of Pediatrics. In 1974, the Committee stated that there was not yet available any satisfactory mechanized technique to screen the hearing of all newborn infants reliably (Northern and Downs, 1978; ASHA report, 1974). Further, the committee recommended that infants at risk for hearing impairment be identified by history and physical examination. If the answer to any one of the following five questions is "yes," there is a chance that the newborn may have impaired hearing and should therefore be evaluated further (Sarno and Clemis, 1980).

1. Is there a family history of hearing loss, especially a genetically determined childhood hearing impairment?
2. Did intrauterine fetal infections occur, such as rubella, cytomegalovirus, herpes virus, or syphilis?

3. Are there any congenital anomalies of the skull or face, such as an abnormally shaped skull or aberrant facial bone development, malformed or absent pinnae, cleft lip or palate, or submucous cleft palate?
4. Was the birth weight low (under 1500 gm)?
5. Is the bilirubin level potentially toxic (greater than 15 mg per 100 ml serum)?
6. Was there significant hypoxemia or asphyxia at birth, with serum pH equal to or lower than 7.3?

A clever mnemonic that can be used to help remember these perinatal risk factors has been described (Downs and Silver, 1972). It is called the "ABCD'S" of congenital deafness: A, *A*ffected family member; B, *B*ilirubin (greater than 15 mg per 100 ml); C, *C*ongenital rubella or other intrauterine infection; D, *D*efects of ear, nose, and throat; S, *S*mall at birth (weight less than 1500 gm).

As experience with use of the high-risk register has been accrued, it has been determined to be a useful, cost-effective method for screening infant hearing. In fact, widespread acceptance and use of the high-risk register led to a National Maternal and Child Health Conference on "Guidelines for Early Screening" (Conference on Hearing Screening Services, 1977), where the following additional suggestions were made.

1. Audiologic follow-up of the high-risk infants should be made "as soon as possible, but certainly by seven months."
2. The mother-child relationship in the first four months should be safeguarded by education and carefully supplied information.
3. Information on what to look for in later infancy should be given.
4. The development and implementation of adequate identification and diagnostic procedures related to hearing impairments should be undertaken by public health agencies.

Once it has been determined that a newborn child is at risk of having impaired hearing or when a parent or referring physician has the impression that a child has a hearing impairment, further evaluation is warranted.

The first step is to *confirm* the impression that there is impairment of hearing and to assess the degree of hearing loss. Not long ago, it was nearly impossible to test a neonate's hearing reliably. Now, however, non-behavioral (objective) tests such as the stapedial reflex test, electrocochleography, and the auditory brain stem electric response (ABR) test are available (Chap. 8B). Although these tests may not actually be tests of hearing per se, they are helpful indicators of significant functional impairment in the neural pathways serving the auditory system. As for quantifying hearing loss, it is virtually impossible to measure precise hearing thresholds in the neonate. Despite this, nonbehavioral tests can be used to estimate a relative magnitude of hearing impairment. That is, test results can be interpreted as being nearly normal, indicative of significant hearing impairment, or indicative of moderate to severe hearing impairment. Although such information may not be precise, it can be helpful in identifying those newborn children who will need close follow-up, further evaluation, and possibly early hearing amplification.

Characterize

Unless there is obvious ear canal atresia or other aural deformity, it is extremely difficult to differentiate conductive from sensorineural hearing impairment in the neonate. Observations made on ABR test patterns can be helpful (Chap. 8B). Delayed appearance of the first wave with normal interwave latencies may be indicative of a conductive type of hearing loss. Elevated thresholds without a delay in the appearance of the first wave and with normal interwave latencies indicate that sensorineural impairment is likely. When interwave latencies are abnormal, some central nervous system abnormality may be responsible for the hearing impairment. Again, these parameters are helpful diagnostic indicators, but they are not as precise or reliable as a battery of sophisticated behavioral tests. However, in dealing with neonates, it is of primary importance to know whether or not a significant hearing impairment is present; characterization of the type of hearing loss is of secondary importance. Once it has been established that a neonate has poor hearing, further testing and evaluation during the first two years of life will usually elicit the information that is needed to proceed with proper diagnosis and management.

Cause

Hearing impairment that is discovered during the neonatal period is most likely the result of some untoward circumstance that occurred during fetal development or at birth. Hereditary factors need to be considered, and a detailed family history should be obtained. A thorough physical examination should reveal abnormalities characteristic of one of the previously described syndromes with which hearing loss is associated (Table 10–1). TORCH studies and the VDRL-FTA tests are helpful in determining whether intrauterine infection may have been a causal factor. A urine sample tested for protein and inborn errors in metabolism may be helpful in diagnosing syndromes that include nephritis or abnormalities of mucopolysaccharide metabolism. If thyroid enlargement is apparent, then Pendred syndrome should be considered, and a T4 uptake and perchlorate discharge test are indicated. If there is a family history of Usher syndrome or if the neonate appears to have eye abnormalities, then electroretinography may be of diagnostic value. An electrocardiogram is probably not often helpful, although the Jervell and Lange-Nielsen syndrome can be diagnosed early in life when profound congenital deafness is found in association with a prolonged Q–T interval. Routine mastoid films and temporal bone polytomography are probably not warranted in the evaluation of neonates with hearing impairment because radiographic findings will be of little value in formulating plans for management of the neonate with impaired hearing.

After information has been gathered and analyzed, it may be possible to discover the cause of a neonate's hearing impairment. Of course, in order to recognize syndromal types of hearing impairment, one must have some familiarity with the syndromes that include hearing loss. Syndromes that can include hearing impairment are listed in Tables 10–2, 10–3, and 10–4.

Even though it is possible to conceive of numerous factors that may cause hearing impairment in the neonate, it may be difficult to detect specific etiology in individual cases unless the neonate has a clear family pedigree of inherited hearing loss or unless there are obvious abnormalities characteristic of a non-mendelian malformation syndrome known to include morphologic or functional aberrations in the auditory system. Further, making a differentiation between truly congenital hearing loss, i.e., that which is present at birth, and acquired hearing loss is extremely

difficult during the neonatal period. George R. Fraser (1976) has succinctly summarized the problem of determining the cause of neonatal hearing loss as follows.

It is clear that the relationship between perinatal problems and subsequent deafness is an exceedingly complicated one and, while in some cases a specific circumstance, such as hemorrhage into the inner ears as a result of birth injury, the administration of ototoxic drugs, or kernicterus due to Rhesus incompatibility, may be identified as the proximate cause of hearing loss, in many others multiple factors must be taken into consideration; these may arise as a result of interaction between both genetic and environmental variables.

Thus, it can be seen that finding the cause for hearing loss detected in a neonate may be a complex and difficult problem. Nonetheless, an attempt should be made to find the factors that are most likely to have caused an observed hearing impairment.

Care

Once it has been established that a neonate has impaired hearing, management must be planned. Otologic surgery is not warranted during the neonatal period, and usually the infant must be more than two months old before he or she can be considered for fitting of a hearing aid. Early steps will have to be taken to assist the child with a congenital hearing loss to learn speech and language. It is most important to help the parents understand and adjust to the problem of having a hearing-impaired child. Also, if the family is indigent or inadequately covered by medical insurance, it will be necessary to involve appropriate agencies so that the family can continue to provide the medical care and special education that the child may require.

Infant

Confirm

Once a child is beyond the neonatal period, concerns about hearing ability usually come from a parent or an observant primary care physician. The parent or another family member initially tends to become concerned when the infant appears not to respond in an appropriate way to sounds in the environment. A parent will remark that the infant is not startled by loud noises or that the infant does not awaken or appear disturbed when a

Text continued on page 248

Table 10-2   SKELETAL AND CRANIAL DEFECTS ASSOCIATED WITH HEARING IMPAIRMENT

Syndrome	Characteristics	Mode of Inheritance	Type of Hearing Loss		
			SN	Conductive	Mixed
Osteogenesis imperfecta	Brittle bones Blue sclerae	Recessive	X	X	X
Hurler syndrome	Mental retardation, cloudy corneas, blindness, thick eyebrows, onset of skeletal deformities after first year of life	Recessive (X-linked form is known as Hunter syndrome)	X	X	
Morquio disease	Dwarfism, normal-sized head, long extremities, short trunk	Recessive			
Otopalatodigital syndrome	Frontal bossing, prominent occiput, ocular hypertelorism, antimongoloid slant of eyes, fish mouth, pseudowinged knobby scapulae, broad distal phalanges of hands and feet, cleft palate	Recessive		X	
Albers-Schönberg syndrome	Brittle bones, intermittent facial palsy, optic atrophy, hydrocephalus, ocular nystagmus, exophthalmos	Recessive	X	X	X
Klippel-Feil syndrome	Fused cervical vertebrae, low posterior hairline; spina bifida and external canal atresia may be present	Recessive	X	X	X
Cervico-oculoacusticus syndrome	Fused neck vertebrae, spina bifida occulta, abducens palsy of eye, possible radiographic evidence of underdevelopment of the cochlea or labyrinth	Recessive	X		
Crouzon disease	Synostosis of cranial sutures, shallow orbits with secondary proptosis (frog eyes), hypoplasia of maxilla with relative prognathism, parrot nose, possible atresia of external auditory canal	Dominant	X (Usually conductive)	X	X
Cleidocranial dysostosis	Fontanelles fail to close, facial bones underdeveloped, high arched palate, absence of clavicles	Dominant	X		

Syndrome	Characteristics	Inheritance			
Treacher-Collins syndrome	Malformations of malar and other facial bones, antimongoloid slant of eyes with notching of lids (colobomata), high palate, external auditory canal and pinna malformations, middle ear ossicular abnormalities	Dominant	X	X	
Pierre-Robin syndrome	Cleft palate, small mandible, glossoptosis; may have atresia of ear canal, microtia of auricles, middle ear anomalies, or digital abnormalities	Dominant	X	X	
Apert syndrome	Acrocephaly (tower skull), fused digits (lobster-claw hands), shallow orbits, underdeveloped maxillae, fixation of stapes footplate	Dominant		X	
Achondroplasia	Dwarfism with normal sized trunk, large head and shortened extremities, saddle nose, and frontal mandibular bone protrusions	Dominant	X	X°	X
Marfan syndrome	Long, spidery fingers, scoliosis, hammer toe, pigeon breast, dolichocephaly, low hairline, tall, thin body structure	Dominant	X	X	X
Branchial anomalies (Karmody-Feingold)	Cervical fistulae, malformed external ears, preauricular pits, preauricular appendages	Dominant	X	X	X
Myositis ossificans	Formation of true osseous tissue in skeletal muscles, microdactyly of great toes, shortened thumbs	Dominant	X	X	X
Symphalangism	Fusion of proximal and middle phalanges of fingers and toes giving characteristic "stiff finger and toe" appearance, prominence on medial and lateral sides of foot at level of navicular and fifth metatarsal bones	Dominant		X	

*Due to middle ear effusions.
(Modified from Black, F. O., Bergstrom, L., Down, M., et al. 1971. Congenital Deafness: A New Approach to Diagnosis Using a High Risk Register. Boulder, CO, Associated University Press.)

Table 10-3   EYE ABNORMALITIES ASSOCIATED WITH HEARING IMPAIRMENT

Syndrome	Characteristics	Mode of Inheritance	Type of Hearing Loss		
			SN	Conductive	Mixed
Usher syndrome	Retinitis pigmentosa, vestibulocerebellar ataxia, mental retardation	Recessive	X		
Cockayne syndrome	Retinal atrophy, motor disturbances, mental retardation, dwarfism	Recessive	X		
Alström syndrome	Obesity, diabetes mellitus, retinal degeneration	Recessive	X		
Hallgren syndrome	Retinitis pigmentosa, vestibulocerebellar ataxia, nystagmus, sometimes mental retardation	Recessive	X		
Laurence-Moon-Biedl-Bardet syndrome	Retinitis pigmentosa, polydactyly, hypogenitalism, obesity, mental retardation	Recessive	X		
Refsum syndrome (heredopathia atactica polyneuritiformis)	Retinitis pigmentosa, cerebellar ataxia, polyneuritis, electrocardiographic abnormalities, ichthyosis-type skin disorder	Recessive	X		
Duane syndrome	Ocular palsy (congenital fibrous replacement of rectus muscle), auricular malformations, meatal atresia, cervical rib, torticollis, cervical spina bifida	Recessive		X	
Möbius syndrome	Facial diplegia, lateral and/or medial rectus palsy bilaterally, auricular malformation, micrognathia, absence of hands, feet, fingers, or toes, tongue paralysis, mental retardation	Recessive	X	X	X

(Modified from Black, F. O., Bergstrom, L., Downs, M., et al. 1971. Congenital Deafness: A New Approach to Diagnosis Using a High Risk Register. Boulder, CO, Associated University Press.)

Table 10-4 PIGMENTARY ABNORMALITIES ASSOCIATED WITH HEARING IMPAIRMENT

Syndrome	Characteristics	Mode of Inheritance	Type of Hearing Loss		
			SN	Conductive	Mixed
Albinism-deafness syndrome	Fair skin and hair; absence of pigment in iris, sclera, and fundus	Recessive or X-linked	X		
	Fair skin, fine hair; eyes not affected (blue irides)	Dominant	X		
Partial albinism or piebaldness	Areas of skin depigmentation, light blue clumps of pigment throughout the retina, good vision	Dominant	X		
Waardenburg syndrome	Heterochromic irides, broad nasal root, thick eyebrows, lateral displacement of medial canthi, white forelock, dappling of skin	Dominant	X		

(Modified from Black, F. O., Bergstrom, L., Downs, M., et al. 1971. Congenital Deafness: A New Approach to Diagnosis Using a High Risk Register. Boulder, CO, Associated University Press.)

sibling in the same room is crying loudly. Or, parents may be concerned that the child of about two years is not speaking words while they remember that an older sibling was saying three-word phrases by the age of 18 months. If an infant has had meningitis or a severe infection that required the administration of potentially ototoxic medications, then an astute pediatrician or family physician may want to have the infant's hearing evaluated.

Even though an infant is brought for evaluation by parents who seem overly impatient about speech development, it is not advisable simply to perform rudimentary tests of hearing in the office, then attempt to reassure the parents that their child's hearing is normal. In the present era of advanced medical technology, observing an infant's response to the loud clapping of hands cannot be considered the definitive test for determining the presence or absence of hearing impairment. When a pediatrician, family physician, or anyone who knows an infant well becomes concerned about an infant's hearing ability, then a full evaluation, including audiometric testing, is warranted.

The infant from two through 24 months of age progressively becomes more easy to condition for play audiometry. Whereas audiometric testing in the neonate necessarily relies on nonbehavioral test methods, it becomes increasingly feasible to utilize behavioral techniques as the child grows and develops during infancy. Around the age of one year, an infant develops the ability to localize sound, and this enables the use of visual reinforcement audiometry. Also, beyond the age of one year, development of the bony tympanic ring makes the ear canal less pliable and more rigid. This means that tympanometry can more readily be utilized to provide accurate information about physical properties of the eardrum and middle ear.

A more detailed discussion of methodology for audiometric testing in infants can be found in Chapter 8B. It should be emphasized here, however, that methods are available for identifying hearing thresholds in infants. Although some audiologists may not have the requisite equipment or specific skills for testing infants, there is usually some nearby medical or diagnostic facility where the testing can be done. Whenever there is a suspicion that an infant has a hearing impairment, it is imperative that the infant undergo

appropriate audiometric testing. There is no reason for delaying such tests until the later childhood years.

Characterize

As the infant becomes older and able to be tested with behavioral techniques, it becomes possible to perform the audiometric tests that will help to characterize the type of hearing impairment.

Conductive, sensorineural, and mixed hearing losses are the types that will most often be discovered during infancy. Although it is conceivable that auditory brain stem electric response audiometry may help in the early diagnosis of central and retrocochlear types of hearing loss, such hearing difficulties are relatively rarely discovered during infancy. At one time, it may have been sufficient merely to detect hearing impairment during infancy. Now, however, with the newer audiometric test techniques that are available, it is imperative to attempt to determine the nature of the hearing impairment.

Auditory brain stem response (ABR) testing, tympanometry, and acoustic reflex testing can be helpful in characterizing the type of hearing loss.

When considering the types of hearing loss that can be seen in infancy, conductive hearing loss due to otitis media with effusion deserves specific mention. When otitis media with effusion is discovered in the infant who has been referred for evaluation of hearing impairment, it should not be assumed that effusion in the middle ear is the sole reason for the hearing loss. Audiometric tests should be obtained to determine whether or not a previously undetected sensorineural hearing loss is also present. Further, if tympanostomy tubes are inserted as treatment for a chronic effusion, then a repeat audiogram several weeks after myringotomy should be obtained when the middle ear is aerated, that is, when no effusion is present. If it had been possible to obtain an air conduction and bone conduction pure tone audiogram prior to insertion of a tympanostomy tube, then a repeat audiogram following the tube insertion should reveal air conduction thresholds that have returned to normal. If a conductive hearing loss persists after the insertion of a tympanostomy tube with aeration of the middle ear, then the infant may have a congenital ossicular abnormality. If it had not been possible to obtain an air conduction and bone conduction audiogram prior to insertion of the tympanostomy tube, then a persistent hearing loss following insertion of the tube may be entirely sensorineural or mixed, or the residual conductive loss may be associated with an ossicular abnormality. Recently, it has been discovered that children with Down syndrome not only are prone to developing otitis media with effusion but also may have congenital middle ear ossicular abnormalities (Balkany et al., 1979).

The ABR test combined with myringotomy and insertion of tympanostomy tubes under general anesthesia may help to differentiate the type of hearing loss an infant has. Comparing characteristics of the ABR pattern before and after the insertion of a tympanostomy tube gives helpful clues about the type of hearing loss that is present. There is no doubt that as more experience is gained with electrocochleography and ABR testing, their usefulness in evaluating infants with hearing loss will be expanded.

Although it may not always be possible to characterize an infant's hearing loss accurately, some attempt should be made to discover the type of hearing loss that is present. Certainly, the diagnostic possibilities and plans for management will vary according to the type of hearing impairment that is discovered.

Cause

Hearing loss discovered during infancy can be thought of as being either congenital or acquired. Cases of congenital hearing loss that were not discovered during the neonatal period will often become manifest during the infant years. Of course, where the high-risk register and selective neonatal hearing screening programs are utilized, there is less likelihood that a neonate will leave the hospital where he or she was born with an undetected congenital hearing impairment.

When evaluating an infant with hearing loss, it is advisable to obtain copies of the medical record from the hospital where the infant was born. The records can then be reviewed to see if excessive jaundice (greater than 15 mg per 100 ml) for a prolonged period, infection, or ototoxic medications could have been factors in the pathogenesis of the hearing impairment.

Next, it is helpful to question the parents carefully about how the suspicion of hearing loss arose. Some helpful questions follow.

1. Do you think that your child was born with normal hearing?
2. When did you first become suspicious that your infant has difficulty hearing?
3. What has it been that gives you the impression that your child has a hearing loss?
4. Did your baby babble and coo? Has the babbling activity ceased? If so, when? What is the level of the infant's speech development?
5. Did meningitis, measles, a high fever, seizures, an exanthematous disease, a viral infection, or any other disorder immediately precede the noticeable hearing problem?
6. Have there been frequent bouts of otitis media? If so, what characterized each episode, and how were they treated?

Answers to these questions may help to determine whether the hearing loss is congenital or whether it is causally related to some other event. Often, the infant born with a severe hearing impairment will experiment with verbalization, making several speech sounds; then at about eight months of age, lacking the reinforcement of hearing his or her voice and lacking the stimulation of hearing others speak, the infant will eventually stop experimenting with speech. Thus, language development sometimes offers a clue about the time of onset of hearing impairment.

In contrast to the difficulty of uncovering the cause of congenital hearing loss, when it can be determined that the hearing loss was acquired after birth, a more direct cause-and-effect relationship may be discernible. For example, bacterial meningitis is a common cause of sensorineural hearing impairment acquired after the perinatal period (Teng et al., 1962; Nadol, 1978). Obviously, if an infant appeared to be developing speech normally and then hearing difficulty was noticed after the occurrence of bacterial meningitis, it can reasonably be assumed that meningitis was a factor in causing the hearing loss, especially if there had been no suspicion of a hearing loss preceding the meningitis infection. Although parents often recall that a high fever, a viral syndrome, or some minor head trauma immediately preceded the noticeable hearing loss, it is difficult to prove that such common entities actually are the cause of hearing loss. Still, it is worthwhile to ask the questions and find out what the parents think was the time of onset and cause of their infant's hearing loss. Understanding the parents' concept of the cause for their infant's hearing loss can be of help in counseling the parents and in mollifying the lingering sense of guilt that they may harbor. Further, it is worthwhile to collect whatever information seems relevant so that a retrospective analysis can be undertaken and relative probability of causality can be ascribed to events that appear to have caused the hearing loss. As the pathogenesis of childhood hearing loss is elucidated, it may be discovered that certain seemingly unrelated factors play a role in the pathogenesis of hearing impairment.

Physical examination adds additional information that can be helpful in determining the cause of hearing loss. Subtle abnormalities that were not noticed at birth may become evident when the infant who presents with a hearing loss undergoes a thorough examination. Special attention must be directed to the pinnae, ear canals, eardrums, the retinae, the facial bones, the neck, and to testing of the cranial nerves. Many of the laboratory studies suggested for the evaluation of the neonate (pp. 242–243) are useful for evaluation of nonsyndromal infants who present with a hearing loss of unknown etiology. Radiographic studies are usually not warranted during infancy.

As already mentioned (p. 232), otitis media with effusion cannot always be assumed to be the sole cause of a confirmed significant hearing impairment.

If it appears that genetic factors are not responsible for the hearing impairment, then a hypothesis should be formulated based on review of all collected information. In many cases, there will be no clear etiology to explain the hearing loss discovered during infancy.

Care

When a significant hearing impairment is discovered during infancy, habilitative measures can be taken. If persistent bilateral otitis media with effusion is discovered, then the hearing may be improved simply by aspirating the fluid and inserting tympanostomy tubes. Almost all infants born with cleft palate have abnormal eustachian tube function and a consequent tendency to develop recurrent or persistent otitis media with effusion. The palate deformity itself makes it difficult for these infants to learn speech. Therefore, every attempt must be made to provide them with keen auditory acuity so that they will be able to hear clearly the subtleties of speech enunciation that they will try so hard to imitate. Early insertion of tympanostomy tubes is advisable and may conveniently be done in conjunction with the first plastic surgery repair of a cleft lip deformity or as a brief surgical procedure for the infant born with an isolated cleft palate deformity.

When an infant without a craniofacial defect is found to have hearing impairment because of frequently recurring or persistent middle ear effusions, the decision to perform a myringotomy with insertion of tympanostomy tubes should be based on the severity and duration of a measurable hearing loss and the inability to eradicate the effusions with medical therapy. In some instances, it will be advisable to insert tympanostomy tubes more as a means of diminishing a sizable conductive hearing loss than as a therapeutic measure aimed at reducing the frequency of middle ear infections.

When all available evidence seems to indicate that there is a significant conductive hearing loss being caused by a factor other than middle ear effusion, then therapeutic measures should be aimed at providing amplification of sound and assistance in learning speech. Surgical procedures to improve hearing deficits due to malformations or fixation of the ossicles usually are not undertaken during infancy. Rather, ossicular reconstruction of the congenitally malformed ear is better undertaken later in childhood.

If the hearing impairment is more sensorineural than conductive, then the infant should undergo complete developmental and neurologic evaluation. The infant discovered to have a moderate or severe sensorineural hearing impairment may also have other previously undetected impairment of central nervous system function. That is, it is important to determine whether the sensorineural hearing loss is an isolated problem or whether it is occurring along with visual impairment, mental retardation, or delayed motor development. If the hearing impairment is an isolated problem, then early sound amplification and speech training should be provided. If the sensorineural hearing impairment is one of a constellation of problems, then the benefit to be derived from early hearing amplification will have to be considered relative to the child's capabilities and other handicaps. However, it is best not to consider an infant too young or unsuitable for a hearing aid until after the infant has been seen and evaluated by a skilled audiologist (Whetnall and Fry, 1964). In fact, when formulating a plan for the management of a severely hearing-handicapped infant, it is best to make sure that a pediatrician, otolaryngologist, audiologist, and a social worker are all involved initially and that each is kept informed of the infant's progress.

It is important to realize that young children can experience serious deficiency in language and communicative skills even if an intensive preschool program is initiated by age three years. For maximal effectiveness, intervention should be achieved before age three, at which time the child with normal hearing is attuned to the sound environment and has become a functionally communicative individual, able to express desires and exchange ideas (Horton, 1975). Therefore, the infant years before age three should be viewed as a critical time for effecting change in the course of development of children with severe sensorineural hearing impairment. During these all-important infant years, training in a structured classroom situation or even an informal nursery-kindergarten setting is not appropriate. It is the parents, the child's natural teachers, who can provide the best educational experience. Parents should be taught methods of capitalizing on the innumerable ways in which auditory training and language acquisition can occur on a daily basis in the child's own home.

The fundamental assumptions that the people most important to a young child are his or her parents and that the place most important to the child is the home have led some speech and hearing centers to institute programs focusing on the role of the parents in the home (Horton, 1975). While some centers send specially trained teachers into the child's home on a regular basis to provide instruction to the parents, others have developed a "model home" for all families to utilize. The model home enables concurrent parent teaching, audiologic assessment, and the use of videotape and sophisticated audiovisual equipment in order to facilitate parent teaching while closely monitoring the child's development.

In summary, the primary concern in management of a severely hearing-impaired infant should be the acquisition of communicative skills and the inculcation of a positive attitude toward learning. As the child develops during the infant years, his or her potential will become manifest. Some hearing-handicapped children will show a remarkable ability to function nearly normally, whereas others will have difficulty communicating. By the time a hearing-impaired child reaches three years of age, the parents and educators should be able to determine the educational mode that will most suit the child. Essentially, the alternatives for education will be a school for the deaf, a special class in a regular public school, or an ordinary public school class. The more information that is accrued during the infant years regarding a child's capabilities, the more appropriate will be the choice of an educational program for future learning. Further, the earlier that special training is begun and the more sophisticated and intensive the training, the greater will be a child's chance for integration into a regular public school system. Early aggressive appropriate intervention yields the best results.

Preschool Child

The main difference between the preschool child and the infant is that a child aged two to five years old is able to complain of difficulty in hearing. Also, preschool age children begin to become involved in group play and social interactions in which auditory acuity is important.

Confirm

It is becoming common for state and local health agencies to encourage or require screening hearing tests for nursery school children and children about to enter elementary school. As a result, increasing numbers of young children are being referred for otologic examination and confirmative audiometric testing. Of the children who fail screening tests, some actually have hearing impairment while others do not. In an attempt to identify those children who have significant hearing impairment, the following questions should be asked:
1. Was the screening test merely a tympanogram or was it a pure tone audiogram?
2. Was the screening test administered to several children simultaneously in a classroom, or was each child tested individually in a soundproof booth?
3. Did the child have an upper respiratory

tract or ear infection at the time that the screening test was administered or within the week prior to the test?

4. Prior to failing the screening test, was there any suspicion of the child's having abnormal hearing?

5. Is there a history of frequently recurring acute otitis media or persistent otitis media with effusion?

With the information gained from the answers to these questions, it is possible to formulate an impression quickly regarding the validity and meaningfulness of the screening procedure in each case. Pneumatic otoscopy can then be performed in order to gain additional information about the status of the eardrum and middle ear. Tuning fork tests may be helpful in older preschool children, but often young children find it difficult to comprehend the instructions they are given for comparing the relative loudness of tuning fork tones. Obviously, the definitive way of confirming an apparent hearing loss is to obtain a complete air and bone conduction pure tone audiogram, to test speech reception thresholds, and possibly to obtain tympanograms.

Surprisingly often, repeat audiometric tests will reveal normal hearing in a child who has been referred for having failed a screening test. There are several reasons for this. First, the screening examinations may have been done where noise conditions were less than optimal and where children could be distracted or tempted to trick the examiner. Second, the child may have had an upper respiratory tract infection accompanied by a transient otitis media with effusion at the time that the screening test was administered; such children may have essentially normal hearing as soon as the infection resolves. Children with mild forms of eustachian tube dysfunction often tend to develop an otitis media with effusion when they have an upper respiratory tract infection. Thus, a child who recently failed a hearing screening test and then appears to have normal hearing when a more complete audiogram is obtained may be a child with borderline abnormal eustachian tube dysfunction. Third, it should be realized that screening programs utilizing only tympanometry are not testing hearing per se. Such programs are supposedly designed to identify children who have previously undiagnosed otitis media with effusion. Since the tympanogram is really measuring acoustic impedance rather than hearing, children with normal hearing and various eardrum or middle ear pressure abnormalities are likely to be identified as "abnormal" and referred for further evaluation. Thus, when an abnormal tympanogram was the main reason for referral, obtaining a reliable air and bone conduction audiogram along with speech reception thresholds should differentiate children with significant hearing problems from those who have innocuous types of tympanogram abnormalities.

Characterize

Once it has been established that a preschool child has a significant hearing impairment, a variety of audiometric tests can be utilized to determine the type of hearing loss that is present. Around the age of two years, it becomes possible to condition children to respond to pure tone signals. Also, since the normal two year old child has developed some receptive and expressive language skills, it is possible to explain and have the child follow simple, explicit instructions. Both speech and pure tone testing can be utilized. Children can be asked to identify familiar pictures as the loudness is varied for the words describing the pictures. Also, audiometers are available that route a speech signal to a bone vibrator so that a bone conduction speech threshold can be obtained.

Although speech testing in younger children may differentiate conductive from sensorineural hearing loss, pure tone testing is required in order to yield information about hearing ability at specific frequencies. Usually, an air and bone conduction audiogram can be obtained when a child is able to be conditioned to respond to a pure tone signal by dropping an object into a box, placing rings on a peg, or performing some other simple task. Further information about the type of hearing impairment can be gained with the ABR test. With a cooperative child, the ABR test can be done awake. In children that are not cooperative, sedation or general anesthesia can be used. Tympanometry, of course, can be useful in assessing the functional status of the eardrum and ossicular chain.

Thus, it should be possible to characterize a hearing impairment in the young child as being conductive, sensorineural, or mixed. From the test results it might be difficult to distinguish a retrocochlear type of hearing loss from a sensorineural one, but analysis of the ABR test pattern, word discrimination scores (if obtainable), and other clinical information should be helpful in making the differentiation. Although retrocochlear lesions such as vestibular schwannomas (acoustic neuromas) are rarely seen in young children, they can occur in this age group.

Cause

Otitis media with effusion is the most common cause of conductive hearing loss in preschool-age children. Mild to moderate conductive hearing losses due to congenital ossicular chain abnormalities may also be discovered in children of this age.

Children with congenital bilateral severe sensorineural hearing losses are usually identified before two years of age, but in some cases the hearing impairment may go unnoticed until the third year of life. When a bilateral moderate to severe sensorineural hearing loss is first discovered in a child between age two and three years, the question often arises as to whether the child was born with poor hearing or whether hearing progressively worsened in the first few years of life. A clue to the time of onset of the hearing loss lies in the child's ability to speak. Those children who were born with little or no hearing ability usually have considerable difficulty learning to speak, whereas those who could hear initially tend to have better speech.

Whether the hearing impairment was present at birth or developed in the first years of life, genetic factors may be the cause. There are at least 16 types of hereditary hearing loss with no associated abnormalities (Konigsmark and Gorlin, 1976). In the early-onset type of inherited hearing loss, the auditory impairment can begin during the preschool years. The family pedigree, shape of the audiogram, severity of the hearing loss, and age at onset of hearing impairment help to separate one type of inherited hearing loss from another when there are no associated abnormalities to aid in identifying a genetic or other etiologic factor.

The three most common inherited syndromes that include hearing loss are Pendred, Usher, and Lange-Jervell-Nielsen syndromes. Since all three syndromes can first present during the preschool years, it is worthwhile to look specifically for goiter, retinitis pigmentosa, or electrocardiographic abnormalities in young children who are being evaluated for sensorineural hearing losses.

If it appears that hereditary factors are not responsible for the hearing loss, then the search for an identifiable (acquired) etiologic factor begins with a careful prenatal and perinatal history. A history of meningitis or any other severe infection during infancy may be significant. If the child had been hospitalized for any reason, it is worthwhile to obtain the hospital records to see if ototoxic medications were administered. Review of the family history may reveal a hereditary hearing problem. After the physical examination has been completed, VDRL-FTA tests and urinalysis should be ordered. Results of thyroid function studies and an electrocardiogram may also be helpful. Routine mastoid films are sufficient for demonstrating the presence or absence of the cochlea, but temporal bone polytomography is necessary for the diagnosis of certain ossicular chain abnormalities and malformations of the otic capsule.

Care

Conductive and sensorineural hearing losses require different types of management. Hearing impairments discovered in children of preschool age are usually conductive and tend to be less severe than sensorineural hearing impairments. Management of the child who has unilateral or bilateral middle ear effusion with associated conductive hearing loss has not been universally agreed upon. Audiologists, educators, and medical practitioners hold variant opinions on the timing and types of intervention that are warranted (Chap. 16). Divergent opinions notwithstanding, it should be realized that impairment of hearing may adversely affect language development and cognitive function in young children (Hanson and Ulvestad, 1979). In order to avoid or minimize the adverse effect, a child with middle ear effusion and concomitant hearing loss should be seen frequently and should undergo sequential audiometric tests. If it is determined that the child has hearing significantly worse than normal (speech receptional threshold greater than 20 dB in both ears) most of the time, then measures should be taken to improve hearing. Although decongestant medication is often prescribed to promote and quicken the resolution of otitis media with effusion, the efficacy of such medication for this purpose has never been scientifically proved. Tympanocentesis with aspiration of fluid from the middle ear space can provide quick disappearance of the conductive hearing loss caused by a middle ear effusion. Insertion of tympanostomy tubes is widely accepted as a method of assuring that an aspirated middle ear effusion will not recur. Although there may be controversy regarding the efficacy of tympanostomy tubes in reducing the frequency of bouts of acute otitis media, it should be realized that myringotomy and insertion of tympanostomy tubes is one effective method of removing middle ear effusion, preventing its recurrence, and abolishing the conductive hearing loss associated with the effusion. If for some reason it is deemed inappropriate to utilize tympanostomy tubes, then use of a hearing aid can be considered.

While the goal in managing children who have hearing losses due to otitis media with effusion is eradication of the hearing deficit, for those children with entirely sensorineural or predominantly sensorineural mixed hearing losses, management is directed more toward finding optimal ways to cope with a given hearing impairment. When a significant sensorineural hearing loss is discovered in a preschool child, attention is focused on methods for enabling the child to develop communicative skills, and plans must be made for selecting an appropriate educational environment.

The preschool years are exceptionally important in a child's overall development. It is a time during which the child develops concept formation and methods for problem solving. The child's natural curiosity and eagerness to explore the environment make the preschool years most fertile for educational experiences. The nurture and reinforcement — or seeming neglect — of the child's earliest attempts to interact with others constitute the experiences that form the child's impression of the world. Pleasant experiences enable the child to trust himself or herself and others in the competitive business of everyday life with siblings, playmates, and adults. The quality of parent-child interaction and the timing and intensity of parental responses to the young child's activities combine to determine whether the child will realize full potential in developing social skills and intellectual prowess or will regress to more immature behavior because of frustra-

tion and feelings of inadequacy (Erikson, 1963; Mowrer, 1960; Northcott, 1975).

Since much of the learning experience for the preschool child is derived from activities at home with the family, parental participation is of utmost importance in fostering optimal development for the hearing-impaired child. Therefore, once it is established that a preschool child has hearing impairment, a comprehensive program should be undertaken to counsel and provide guidance and teaching for the parent(s). Emotional and psychological support is often warranted to help parents cope with the concept of having a handicapped child and to aid in resolving feelings of guilt. Parents need to be taught how to utilize maximally a child's residual hearing for linguistic stimulation during play and other home activities. If the child has no residual hearing, the parent must learn the methods of communicating with the deaf child that will enable behavior management and lead to the child's developing a sense of self-reliance through the acquisition of daily living skills. Also, parents require factual information regarding sources for financial assistance, local and regional education centers for hearing-impaired children, and special preschool nursery school programs suited for hearing-impaired children. Parents should be made aware of the fact that special laws have lowered or eliminated the minimal age for enrollment in publicly funded special education programs (Ebenson, 1963).

In 1975, Public Law 94-142 was passed. This statute emphasizes the right of handicapped children to free public education. Under the provisions of P.L. 94-142, state and local education agencies are required to develop and administer suitable programs for these children. The age specifications of P.L. 94-142 vary for the different provisions of the law. Amendments to P.L. 94-142 and other similar laws have lowered or eliminated the minimal age for enrollment in special programs, and many states grant a school district the authority to contract for services with public, private, or voluntary agencies (Northcott, 1975). This allows the placement of a preschool hearing-impaired child in a regular nursery school with children of his or her own age who have normal hearing.

A major innovation of P.L. 94-142 is the requirement that an individualized education program be prepared for each child identified as handicapped and that this plan be monitored and updated annually (Palfrey et al., 1978). In a sense, the legislation virtually assures that a hearing-handicapped child can attend a regular public school, provided that a suitable individualized educational program can be developed and annual evaluations indicate that the child is learning adequately. Thus, the options for educating a child with significant hearing impairment have been expanded. As a result, the matter of selecting an appropriate educational setting has become somewhat controversial. In the past, it was traditional for severely hearing-impaired and deaf children to attend schools that were specifically equipped and staffed to educate these children (deaf schools) instead of the "regular" public schools. Now, however, some parents and educators are in favor of having children with severe hearing impairments educated in the regular public school system. This newer concept of integrating hearing-impaired children and children with normal hearing is known as "mainstreaming." Proponents of mainstreaming believe that the earlier a hearing-impaired child is surrounded by people with normal hearing, the earlier he or she will learn to cope with real life problems. They believe that proper assistance and preparation will enable the hearing-impaired child to receive a solid education without having to attend a special school. Opponents of the mainstreaming concept believe that the hearing-impaired child's total education and general sense of well-being may suffer when the hearing-impaired child, surrounded by normal-hearing children, is forced to try to learn from teachers who are not specifically trained in methods of educating the hearing-impaired.

There is probably no single best way to educate a severely hearing-impaired child. The child should be placed in the educational setting that best accommodates his or her individual capabilities and needs. In general, children born with severe hearing impairments or total deafness require more specialized types of training. When a severe hearing impairment is discovered late in the preschool years and the child has not yet developed a facility with communication skills, attempts to have the child attend a regular public school may be ill-advised. On the other hand, when the hearing impairment was discovered early and specific habilitative measures were undertaken, the child may have developed receptive and expressive skills suf-

ficient to enable his or her placement in a regular classroom with children who have normal hearing.

Thus, the most important aspect of management when dealing with a preschool child who has significant sensorineural hearing impairment is education. Once an appropriate hearing aid has been provided, attention should be focused on development and preservation of language skills. The decision regarding where and how the child will receive an education is one that should be made with liberal advice from an audiologist, a psychologist, parents, educators, and others.

Additional services that are important in such cases are genetic counseling for parents and maintenance of otologic care for the hearing-impaired child. When the child's hearing impairment is clearly hereditary, the parents should be apprised of the probabilities that another offspring will be hearing-impaired. Children who utilize hearing aids need frequent otologic and audiometric reevaluation to make sure that the hearing aid functions properly and that the ear mold is not causing skin excoriation or ulceration and to detect changes in hearing thresholds or to uncover symptoms of intermittent middle ear disorders that could superimpose a conductive hearing loss on the sensorineural impairment already present.

School-Age Child

Confirm

Hearing tests are almost universally required, either prior to school enrollment or during the first school year. When questions arise as to a child's hearing ability, the parents are informed, and it is usually requested that the child be evaluated by an audiologist, a medical practitioner, or both. Thus, large numbers of children are being referred for further evaluation after having "failed" a school screening audiogram.

With the increasing awareness of hearing problems in children, the likelihood is diminishing that significant hearing impairment in a school-age child will go undetected. In fact, many of the hearing screening test procedures are designed to have high sensitivity and only moderately high specificity. The underlying philosophy is that it is better to accept the fact that some children with entirely normal hearing will be referred for further testing than to accept the risk of not identifying all children with significant hearing impairment.

Almost all school-age children are able to cooperate for some type of behavioral audiometric test that will enable an accurate assessment of hearing ability. However, there are some children who are frightened by earphones, the soundproof booth, or generally are uncooperative in other ways. These children who are slightly difficult to test may have failed a screening procedure done in a test situation where time allotted, space, and personnel did not accommodate the child's specific needs. Children with slightly lower than normal intelligence or those who are emotionally immature may not perform well on a screening hearing test, but then when the child is tested individually in more optimal surroundings, it can be determined that hearing actually is not impaired.

When a child fails a screening hearing test but is found on later testing to have normal hearing, it is advisable to obtain additional information about the child's hearing. A history of frequent otalgia and otitis media probably means that the child has some form of eustachian tube dysfunction with variations in middle ear pressure and possibly intermittent otitis media with effusion. At the time of the screening test, the child may have had otitis media with effusion, which then resolved spontaneously prior to further evaluation and more definitive audiometric tests. When there is suspicion that variations in middle ear pressure or effusion are causing intermittent hearing difficulty, it is best to have the child return for audiometric tests in one or two months and to instruct the parent to return with the child whenever it seems that the child is having difficulty hearing.

Children who appear to have difficulty learning in school should undergo hearing evaluation. Children who are having difficulty with reading may have subtle hearing deficits. Aware of the importance of auditory acuity in the learning process, many educators and specialists in developmental psychology are now referring children for hearing evaluation as part of a total evaluation for learning disability. When assessing these children, it is important to bear in mind that a child's ability to respond to pure tone signals at normal threshold levels does not entirely rule out auditory pathway problems as a contributing factor in the learning disability;

it may be necessary to obtain tests of central auditory processing.

Characterize

Most school-age children are able to cooperate for the behavioral and impedance tests that will enable assessment of the severity and diagnosis of the type of hearing impairment that is present. Many of the tests used for adults are adapted for use with children. A pure tone audiogram and speech reception thresholds can be obtained with conditioning and play audiometry. Simple word lists can be used to assess hearing discrimination ability. As more attention is focused on learning disabilities, newer tests are being developed for assessing central auditory function in children. Thus, once it is confirmed that a school-age child has a hearing impairment, tests are available to characterize and quantify the hearing loss.

Hearing impairment that is newly discovered during the early school years usually will be conductive or of the mild sensorineural type. Children with more severe types of hearing impairment often have difficulty with language development, which usually leads to recognition of the hearing deficit prior to the child's reaching school age. On the other hand, children with unilateral moderate to severe sensorineural hearing losses may learn to speak without difficulty and appear to have normal hearing until the time that they enter school. Then a screening test may uncover the hearing deficit, or difficulty in listening to the teacher may make the child aware of the hearing impairment.

Cause

Conductive. Most of the inherited forms of conductive hearing impairment will be discovered before a child enters school. A large proportion of children who develop hearing impairment during the school years have eustachian tube dysfunction or middle ear disorders, such as effusion, negative pressure, or both. As the child who has been prone to developing otitis media with effusion gets older, the tendency to develop effusions usually diminishes, and hearing tends to improve. However, some children develop sequelae that adversely affect hearing. Children who have had chronic middle ear effusions and numerous bouts of acute otitis media can develop a nonhealing eardrum perforation, tympanosclerosis, erosion of portions of the ossicular chain, or even cholesteatoma. The lenticular process of the incus is the portion of the ossicular chain that is most vulnerable to damage from acute and chronic types of otitis media. Also, trauma must be considered as an etiologic factor. School-age children may poke objects in the ear canal, causing damage to the eardrum, the ossicles, or even the inner ear. Also, blunt head trauma, as in an auto accident, can cause dislocation of the ossicles and can result in a conductive hearing loss. Tumors involving the temporal bone are rare. Benign neoplasms such as osteomata or fibrous dysplasia can affect hearing depending upon the location of the lesion, or malignant lesions such as rhabdomyosarcoma may cause hearing loss when portions of the auditory system are destroyed.

Sensorineural. When it is discovered that a school-age child has a sensorineural hearing impairment, it must be established whether the loss is stable or progressive, and an attempt must be made to discover the etiology. Even though it is not detected in the first five years of life, genetic factors cannot be excluded when attempting to discover the etiology of a sensorineural hearing loss. There is a type of dominant, high-frequency, progressive sensorineural hearing loss that begins to appear after age five years and rapidly worsens up to the third decade (Huizing et al., 1966). A list of other types of inherited progressive sensorineural hearing losses with no associated anomalies follows (Konigsmark and Gorlin, 1976).

1. Dominant, autosomal, low-frequency hearing loss — onset of hearing loss can be in infancy; but progression is not usually seen until adulthood.
2. Dominant, mid-frequency hearing loss — onset of hearing loss in childhood with early progression.
3. Dominant, autosomal, progressive, early-onset sensorineural hearing loss — moderate to severe hearing loss by adolescence, considerable variation in expressivity.
4. Recessive, early-onset neural hearing loss — onset early in childhood with progression to a plateau of marked severity by mid to late childhood.
5. X-linked, early-onset neural hearing loss — progressive deafness after attainment of speech.
6. X-linked, moderate hearing loss — slowly progressive hearing loss in males.

Nongenetic causes of sensorineural hearing loss in school-age children include infections, such as syphilis (congenital), meningitis, or mumps. Administration of ototoxic medications can cause sensorineural hearing loss. All the aminoglycoside antibiotics can affect the inner ear. Dihydrostreptomycin and kanamycin mostly affect the auditory system while streptomycin and gentamycin mostly affect the vestibular system. Neomycin affects both systems about equally. Diuretics such as furosemide and ethacrynic acid can affect hearing, and salicylates can cause a reversible type of hearing impairment. Recently, it has been reported that the intravenous administration of erythromycin lactobionate can be associated with reversible sensorineural hearing loss (Karmody and Weinstein, 1978). Also, it has recently been found that children can develop fistulae at the oval or round window membrane with leakage of perilymphatic fluid and associated sensorineural hearing impairment (Grundfast and Bluestone, 1979). Usually the children who have a perilymphatic fistula have some history of barotrauma, blunt head trauma, or predisposing conditions such as a widely patent cochlear aqueduct or an anomaly involving the temporal bone.

If the family history gives no clues as to the etiology of a hearing loss and if the child has no history of exposure to ototoxic agents that could have caused an observed sensorineural hearing loss, it may be worthwhile to test the urine for protein. If there is a palpably enlarged thyroid, then thyroid function studies are indicated. Transorbital views of the internal auditory canals will be helpful if there is retrocochlear-type hearing impairment and an acoustic neuroma is suspected. Then, if transorbital views of the internal auditory canal show an abnormality, temporal bone polytomography, CT scan, or even posterior fossa myelography may be of diagnostic value. When a perilymph fistula is suspected as the cause of the hearing loss, it is worthwhile to perform the fistula test as well as to obtain electronystagmography, including positional tests.

Finally, it should be emphasized that the diagnosis and management of a sudden or fluctuating sensorineural hearing loss are different from those of a stable or slowly progressive sensorineural loss. In general, otologists view sudden-onset and fluctuating hearing losses as potentially treatable disorders. Although there are numerous approaches to treatment of a patient with sudden hearing loss, no single therapeutic regimen is universally effective. Similarly, no single approach to the management of patients with fluctuating hearing losses has been shown to be optimal. Despite the lack of a proven therapeutic regimen, it is advisable immediately to pursue complete evaluation of any child who suddenly develops a sensorineural hearing loss or who has documented variations in sensorineural hearing.

Care

Management of the school-age child with a hearing loss depends on the type and severity of the hearing impairment. The discussion concerning management of preschool children with middle ear disorders pertains as well to school-age children. However, while younger children are prone to develop otitis media, the incidence of middle ear disease decreases as a child grows older. Hence, the child who has had frequent middle ear disease as a young child with sequelae of impaired conductive hearing may be a candidate for tympanoplasty with ossicular reconstruction as an older child. Reconstructive otologic surgery is best undertaken whenever it appears that problems with otitis media and inadequate ventilation of the middle ear have subsided.

Unilateral sensorineural hearing loss usually does not require hearing amplification. However, it is advisable to notify school authorities that a child with a unilateral loss of hearing should have preferential seating toward the front of the classroom with the better-hearing ear toward the teacher.

When a child develops a bilateral moderate to severe sensorineural hearing loss during the school years, a hearing aid may be necessary, and sometimes measures may have to be taken to assure that loss of auditory feedback does not result in deterioration of the child's ability to articulate and enunciate properly.

Although sensorineural hearing loss is generally considered not to be reversible with otologic surgery, sensorineural hearing loss associated with a perilymphatic fistula may be an exception. Reports have appeared describing restoration of hearing following identification and surgical repair of a perilymphatic fistula (Healy, 1978).

Preadolescent

Confirm

Preadolescence can be a turbulent time emotionally. It is a time during which endocrinologic changes occur, and there tends to be an increased sense of body awareness. In contrast to younger children, the preadolescent child is more likely to complain of difficulty in hearing rather than to have an unnoticed hearing deficit uncovered through screening testing. With younger children, the task of confirming a suspected hearing loss involves selection of an audiometric test procedure that will manifest the hearing deficit. A cooperative preadolescent child should be entirely capable of providing valid responses to air and bone conduction pure tone signals and to speech and discrimination testing. However, it is sometimes necessary to consider the use of tests for nonorganic or functional types of hearing loss in the process of evaluating the preadolescent child.

Another point to remember is that the preadolescent child may be subject to noise-induced temporary threshold shifts. Nowadays, with many children listening to or participating in rock bands, the possibility arises that a hearing loss may be induced by acoustic trauma. In confirming the presence of a hearing loss, it may be important to consider that certain types of hearing impairment can be transient.

Characterize

Audiometric testing for a preadolescent child should be a relatively straightforward matter. Air and bone conduction pure tone audiograms with speech reception threshold tests are sufficient in most cases. Where retrocochlear pathology is suspected, discrimination tests and other sites-of-lesion audiometric tests may be warranted. When nonorganic hearing loss is suspected, acoustic reflex testing and such tests as the Stenger, Doerfler-Stewart, or delayed auditory feedback test may be indicated.

Cause

By the time they reach the preadolescent years, most children have outgrown troublesome middle ear disorders. Ossicular damage or adhesive changes caused by early childhood middle ear disease can cause conductive hearing loss that persists into a child's later years. Otospongiosis, an early form of otosclerosis, can cause conductive hearing loss in children around the age of 11 to 14 years.

Although unusual, it is possible for an inherited sensorineural hearing loss to become manifest in a preadolescent child. Endolymphatic hydrops (Meniere disease) can account for a sensorineural hearing loss when associated with tinnitus and vertigo (Meyerhoff et al., 1978). Multiple sclerosis can cause transient sensorineural hearing loss as well as vertigo during adolescence (Molteni, 1977). Inadequately treated or previously undiagnosed congenital syphilis can cause sensorineural hearing loss in late childhood. Acoustic trauma should also be considered as a possible cause of sensorineural hearing loss.

When sensorineural hearing loss develops in late childhood and no etiology is apparent, acoustic neuroma must be considered, especially if inordinately poor discrimination scores are obtained.

Other than serologic tests for syphilis, urinalysis, and possibly temporal bone radiographs, special studies are not usually helpful in the evaluation of sensorineural hearing loss that presents late in childhood. Unless there have been syncopal episodes, an electrocardiogram will probably be superfluous. Unless there is a palpably enlarged thyroid gland and a family history of goiter, thyroid function tests and the perchlorate discharge test will probably not be helpful. When a child has had middle ear disease early in childhood and then developed a conductive hearing loss, temporal bone polytomography can be helpful in assessing the status of the ossicles or the location of cholesteatoma. At times, the tomograms can provide information that is helpful in choosing an operative approach or planning reconstruction of the middle ear. Finally, when there is a question of retrocochlear pathology or a demyelinating disorder, the ABR test can provide helpful information.

Care

In comparison to the potentially devastating effect of hearing loss in early childhood, the hearing loss of later childhood tends to present fewer problems in management. By the time a child has reached the preadolescent years, language and communication skills are well developed. Although it is usually inadvisable to attempt ossicular reconstruction during a child's younger years when otitis media with effusion is most prevalent, around the time of adolescence there is diminution of the tendency to develop otitis media with effusion, and it is reasonable to attempt otologic surgery that may improve certain conductive hearing deficits. For children who develop a sensorineural loss late in childhood, hearing amplification, speech preservation training, and counseling are appropriate.

REFERENCES

Alford, B. R. 1968. Rubella — la bete noire de la medecine. Laryngoscope, 88:1623–1659.

American Speech and Hearing Association, American Academy of Ophthalmology and Otolaryngology, and American Academy of Pediatrics. 1974. Supplementary statement of joint committee on infant hearing screening. ASHA, 16:160.

Balkany, T. J., Downs, M. P., Jafek, B. W., et al. 1979. Hearing loss in Down's syndrome. A treatable handicap more common than generally recognized. Clin. Pediatr., 18:(2):116–118.

Bergstrom, L. 1974. Hearing loss in children. In Northern, J. L., and Downs, M. P. (Eds.) Hearing in Children. Baltimore, Williams and Wilkins.

Bergstrom, L., and Stewart, J. 1971. New concepts in congenital deafness. Otolaryngol. Clin. North Am., 4(2):431–443.

Black, F. O., et al. 1971. Congenital Deafness: A New Approach to Early Detection of Deafness Using a High Risk Register. Boulder, CO, Associated University Press.

Chung, C. S., Robinson, O. W., and Morton, N. E. 1959. A note on deaf mutism. Ann. Hum. Genet., 23:357–366.

Conference on Hearing Screening Services for Preschool Children. Columbus, Ohio, 1977. Maternal and Child Health Bureau, HEW, Washington, DC

Costa, A., Cottino, F., Mortara, M., et al. 1964. Endemic cretinism in Piedmont. Panminerva Med., 6:250–259.

Crabtree, N., and Genrard, J. 1950. Perceptive deafness associated with severe neonatal jaundice. J. Laryngol., 64:482–506.

Dorph, S., Jensen, J., and Olgaard, A. 1973. Visualization of canaliculus cochleae by multidirectional tomography. Arch. Otolaryngol., 98:121–123.

Downs, M. P., and Silver, H. K. 1972. The ABCD's to H.E.A.R.: Early identification in nursery, office, and clinic of the infant who is deaf. Clin. Pediatr., 11:563–566.

Ebenson, A. (Ed.) 1963. Legal change for the handicapped through litigation. State-Federal Clearinghouse for Exceptional Children. The Council for Exceptional Children, Arlington, VA.

Erikson, E. 1963. Childhood and Society. New York, W. W. Norton.

Feinmesser, M., and Zelig, S. 1961. Congenital deafness associated with onychodystrophy. Arch. Otolaryngol., *74*:507–508.

Fisch, L. 1955. The etiology of congenital deafness and audiometric patterns. J. Laryngol., *69*:479.

Florman, A. L., et al. 1970. Response to rubella vaccine among seronegative children with congenital rubella. Am. Pediatr. Soc. Abstr., May.

Fraser, G. R. 1976. The causes of profound deafness in childhood. Baltimore, Johns Hopkins University Press.

Grundfast, K., and Bluestone, C. D.: 1978. Sudden or fluctuating hearing loss and vertigo in children due to perilymph fistula. Ann. Otol. Rhinol. Laryngol., *87*:761–772.

Hall, J. 1964. Cochlea and cochlear nuclei in asphyxia. Acta Otolaryngol. (Stockh.) Suppl., 194.

Hanson, D. G., and Ulvestad, R. F. (Eds.) 1979. Otitis media and child development — speech, language, and education. Ann. Otol. Rhinol. Laryngol., *88*, Suppl. 60 (5).

Haymaker, et al. 1961. Pathology of Kernietenic and Postleteric Encephalopathy; Kernicterus. Springfield, IL, Charles C Thomas, pp. 22–230.

Healy, G. B., Friedman, J. M., and DiTrola, J. 1978. Ataxia and hearing loss secondary to perilymphatic fistula. Pediatrics, *61*:238–241.

Hinajosa, R. 1958. Pathohistological aural changes in the progeny of a mother with pseudohypoparathyroidism. Ann. Otol. Rhinol. Laryngol., *67*:964.

Horton, K. B. 1975. Early intervention through parent training in sensorineural hearing loss in children. Otolaryngol. Clin. North Am., *8*:143–157.

Huizing, E. H., Van Bolhuis, A. H., and Odenthal, D. W. 1966. Studies on progressive hereditary perceptive deafness in a family of 335 members. Acta Otolaryngol., *61*:35–41.

Jaffe, B. F. (Ed.) 1977. Hearing Loss in Children — A Comprehensive Text. Baltimore, University Park Press.

Jorgensen, M. B. 1961. Influence of maternal diabetes on the inner ear of the foetus. Acta Otolaryngol. (Stockh.), *53*:49.

Karmody, C. S. 1968. Subclinical maternal rubella and congenital deafness. N. Engl. J. Med., *278*:809–814.

Karmody, C. S., and Weinstein, L. 1978. Reversible sensorineural hearing loss with intravenous erythromycin lactobionate. Ann. Otol. Rhinol. Laryngol., *87*:761–771.

Keleman, G. 1958. Maternal diabetes. Changes in the hearing origin of the embryo — additional observation. Arch. Otolaryngol., *71*:921.

Kittel, G., and Saller, K. 1964. Ohrmissbildungen in Beziehung zu Thalidomid. Z. Laryngol. Rhinol., *43*:469.

Konigsmark, B. W., and Gorlin, R. J. 1976. Genetic and Metabolic Deafness. Philadelphia, W. B. Saunders Co.

Matalon, R., Jacobson, C. B., and Dorfman, A. 1970. Prenatal diagnosis of the mucopolysaccharidoses by a chemical method. American Pediatric Society Abstracts, First Plenary Session, May.

Meyerhoff, W. L., Paparella, M. M., and Shea, D. Meniere's disease in children. Laryngoscope, *88*:1504–1511.

Michaels, R. H. 1969. Immunologic aspects of congenital rubella. Pediatrics, *43*:339–350.

Molteni, R. 1977. Vertigo as a presenting symptom of multiple sclerosis in childhood. Am. J. Dis. Child., *131*:553–554.

Moore, K. L. 1977. The Developing Human: Clinically Oriented Embryology. Philadelphia, W. B. Saunders Co.

Mowrer, O. H. 1960. Learning Theory and Behavior. New York, John Wiley and Sons.

Nadol, J. 1978. Hearing loss as a sequela of meningitis. Laryngoscope, *88*:739–755.

Nance, W. E., and Sweeney, A. 1975. Genetic factors in deafness of early life in sensorineural hearing loss in children: Early detection and intervention. Otolaryngol. Clin. North Am., *8*:1.

Northcott, W. H. 1975. Normalization of the preschool child with hearing impairment. Otolaryngol. Clin. North Am., *8*:159–186.

Northern, J. L., and Downs, M. P. (Eds.) 1978. Hearing in Children. Baltimore, Williams and Wilkins.

Palfrey, J. S., Mervis, R. C., and Butler, J. A. 1978. New directions in the evaluation and education of handicapped children. N. Engl. J. Med., *298*:819–824.

Partsch, J., and Maurer, H. 1963. Zur formalen Genese von Ohrmussbildungen bei der Thalidomid — Embriopathis. Arch. Ohr-Nas-Ukelk-Heilk, *182*:594.

Proctor, C. A., and Proctor, B. 1967. Understanding hereditary nerve deafness. Arch. Otolaryngol., *85*:23–40.

Richterich, R., Van Mechelen, P., and Rossi, E. 1965. Refsum's disease (heredopathia atactica polyneuritiformis). Am. J. Med., *39*:230–236.

Rose, S. P., Conneally, P. M., and Nance, N. E. 1976. Genetic analysis of childhood deafness. *In* Bess, F. H. (Ed.) Childhood Deafness. New York, Grune and Stratton.

Rosenberg, A. L., Bergstrom, L., Troost, B. T., et al. 1970. Hyperuricemia and neurologic deficits — a family study. N. Engl. J. Med., *282*:992–997.

Rosendal, T. 1963. Thalidomide and aplasia-hypoplasia of the otic labyrinth. Lancet, *1*:724.

Sarno, C. N., and Clemis, J. D. 1980. A workable approach to the identification of neonatal hearing impairment. Laryngoscope, *90*:1313–1320.

Teng, Y. C., Liu, J. H., and Hsu, Y. H. 1962. Meningitis and deafness. Clin. Med. J., *81*:127–130.

Valvassori, G. E., Naunton, R. F., and Lindsay, J. R. 1969. Inner ear anomalies: Clinical and histopathological considerations. Ann. Otol. Rhinol. Laryngol., *78*:929–938.

Whetnall, E., and Fry, D. B. 1964. The Deaf Child. Springfield, IL, Charles C Thomas, pp. 14–31.

Wtodyka, J. 1978. Studies on cochlear aqueduct patency. Ann. Otol. Rhinol. Laryngol., *87*:22–28.

Chapter 11

VERTIGO

Sidney N. Busis, M.D.

Dizziness is not an infrequent complaint in childhood. Although at first glance the symptom may seem to be frivolous and insignificant, it is of concern to the patient and the family and deserves careful consideration. Evaluation of the patient complaining of dizziness is also important since vague symptoms of this nature or balance disturbances may be due to an organic vestibular disorder or a serious neurologic disease (Harrison, 1962; Busis, 1976; Beddoe, 1977).

True vertigo may be described as a sensation of disorientation in space combined with an illusion of motion, which is usually rotary but may be linear. Lesions within the labyrinth of the inner ear produce this "true" vertigo, whereas lesions elsewhere, along the eighth nerve or in the central nervous system, may produce other symptoms sometimes described as "dizziness." These symptoms include complaints such as lightheadedness, syncope, disturbed consciousness, headache, or pressure in the head and are usually not primarily vestibular in origin. On the other hand, vague descriptions or objective evidence of loss of fine balance, (called dysequilibrium), may indicate primary vestibular disease. Vertigo of labyrinthine end-organ origin is characterized by acute episodes, and between attacks, there may or may not be mild difficulty with balance. Disturbed balance or sensations of dizziness due to primary central nervous system disease may be continuous and persistent.

The evaluation of children complaining of dizziness should include a history and physical examination and tests of hearing and balance. Following the basic examination, further special studies, such as roentgenography, evoked response audiometry, computerized axial tomography, and pediatric or neurological consultations, may be considered (Chap. 87).

A carefully obtained history is essential and invaluable but very difficult to get at times, especially when dealing with very young children. However, it is important to try to extract a subjective report from the child and to acquire an objective description from the family of what the child's problem is. Specific symptoms are frequently difficult to elicit because even older children are sometimes shy and vague. Yet, at times, the child's account may be quite vivid and detailed. In addition, the parents may be able to explain the symptoms as outlined by the patient. An objective description of the child's symptoms may be elusive because the parents may have witnessed few, if any, of the episodes of dizziness. If this is the case, the parents should be advised to record future episodes in detail. They should also be instructed to observe the child for nystagmus during a period of dizziness.

Historical information is helpful in deciding whether or not the child has an organic lesion. The following symptoms or observations suggest that the child has an organic vestibular lesion.

1. Obvious fright, alarm, pallor, perspiration, nausea, or vomiting during an attack.
2. Objective alteration of balance, with ataxia or falling.
3. Alteration in the level of consciousness or loss of consciousness. If there is definite loss of consciousness, the lesion is located in the central nervous system.
4. The presence of seizures or bizarre turning or circling movements suggests temporal lobe disease.
5. Abnormal tilting of the head or twisting

261

of the neck in infants suggests the possibility of paroxysmal torticollis which may be due to vestibular dysfunction.

6. Abnormal eye movements during an attack of dizziness, as witnessed by the family, suggests nystagmus indicative of organic disease.

Other sets of historical data that are less specific but still helpful in determining the etiology of the dizziness include the following.

1. Chronology of symptoms: Are they progressive, increasing, or decreasing in frequency and intensity? Has the child had any similar complaints in the past that cleared spontaneously?

2. Headache or pain may be reflections of tension but may also suggest vascular or central nervous system disease.

3. Recurrent ear symptoms, such as hearing loss, tinnitus, autophony, or ear infections, suggest the possibility of an otologic etiology.

4. Physical trauma, drugs, and exposure to toxic fumes or chemicals each could cause dizziness.

5. The general state of health of the child and his family is important to ascertain. There may be similar symptoms in other members of the family, suggesting that an environmental factor is present or that the symptoms represent some hereditary disorder.

6. Interpersonal relationships and the child's performance in school and at home should be explored, since problems in these areas may generate anxiety in the patient or the family.

7. Another factor to consider is any litigation or possible litigation connected with the child's case. If such exists, the physician should be aware that this may influence the symptoms.

The physical examination includes a complete otorhinolaryngologic examination and a scan of the cranial nerves (Busis, 1973). Hearing should be tested by tuning forks and by complete audiologic evaluation. Evoked response audiometry, especially brainstem and cortical audiometry, may be helpful.

The vestibular examination includes examination for nystagmus in various directions of gaze and in different head and body positions and testing of balance by evaluating gait and by administering the Romberg test. Special tests of vestibular function should be performed. Considering that a cerebral cortical disorder might be present, it has been suggested that all children with vertigo should have an electroencephalogram (Eviatar and Eviatar, 1977).

A very young child, even an infant held in his mother's lap, may be turned in a rotating chair to evaluate the vestibular system; the presence of postrotatory nystagmus indicates vestibular activity. Electrical recording of nystagmus by electronystagmography may be accomplished in school-age children and in many preschool children as well. Most children will cooperate well enough to allow recording of pursuit movements by visually following a pendulum, or optokinetic drum, or both. In addition, recordings can be made to determine if there is any spontaneous nystagmus in various directions of gaze or nystagmus elicited by changing position. Caloric testing with recording of the induced nystagmus can usually be performed even in the young child. Children normally have calorically induced nystagmus that is somewhat dysrhythmic and of wider amplitude and slower velocity than that found in adults. Examples of these patterns are pictured in Figures 11–1 and 11–2. This response may be due to incomplete maturation of central nervous system pathways, perhaps with incomplete myelination. The new technique of posturography (Black et al., 1977), which involves computer analysis of the Romberg test on a posture platform, may also be helpful in evaluating the child experiencing dizziness.

Dizziness may be the primary symptom or an accompanying symptom of the following, each of which will be discussed in greater detail: (1) middle ear disease, (2) benign paroxysmal vertigo of childhood, (3) Meniere disease (hydrops of the labyrinth), (4) labyrinthine fistula, (5) disturbance of the vestibular cortex, (6) labyrinthine trauma, (7) migraine, (8) paroxysmal torticollis in infancy, (9) multiple sclerosis, and others.

MIDDLE EAR DISEASE

Eustachian tube dysfunction, with or without *otitis media with effusion* (secretory or serous otitis media), is perhaps the most common cause of vestibular disturbance in children. Children with otitis media with effusion, which is usually characterized by an auditory disorder, seldom complain of distinct vertigo.

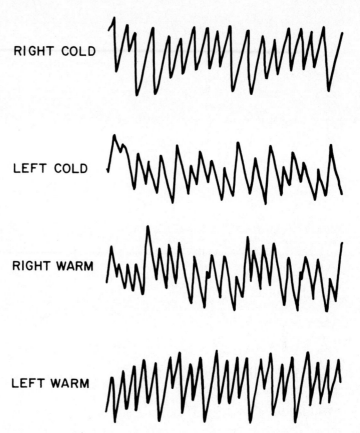

RIGHT COLD

LEFT COLD

RIGHT WARM

LEFT WARM

Figure 11–1 Electronystagmographic recording of an alternate bithermal caloric test in an adult. The order of stimuli, top to bottom, is right cold (left-beating nystagmus); left cold (right-beating nystagmus); right warm (right-beating nystagmus); left warm (left-beating nystagmus). This is a normal tracing with regular, equal, and symmetrical responses from each ear. The slow-phase velocity averages 42 degrees/second.

However, they frequently have abnormal balance as evidenced by awkwardness, clumsiness, and occasional falling (Chap. 16).

These symptoms are due to altered middle ear pressure secondary to eustachian tube dysfunction. Since this abnormality can be documented most consistently by tympanometry (Bluestone et al., 1973; Cantekin et al., 1977), every child who has any apparent vestibular disturbance should undergo tympanography. If the test is normal on the initial examination, it should be repeated in a few weeks if symptoms persist. The symptoms of otitis media with effusion or negative middle ear pressure can be relieved by medical or surgical treatment. Indwelling, ventilating tympanostomy tubes are usually effective.

Acute or chronic purulent otitis media may produce secondary serous labyrinthitis with associated vestibular symptoms. In these patients, if response to medication is not prompt or drainage is not adequate, a wide myringotomy should be performed. If there are signs or symptoms of an associated mastoiditis, the patient should also have a mastoidectomy. Rarely, purulent otitis media may be followed by purulent labyrinthitis, which is accompanied initially by vertigo with subsequent complete loss of auditory and vestibular function (Chaps. 17 & 18).

The occurrence of a *cholesteatoma* is not uncommon in children. Although the cholesteatoma is often very invasive, it seldom produces a fistula into the labyrinth, which would cause balance disturbance. However, in the vertiginous child with a chronically discharging ear, this possibility must be considered, and a careful microscopic examination, including a fistula test, should be performed. If a cholesteatoma is demonstrated to be present, aggressive surgical removal is essential.

BENIGN PAROXYSMAL VERTIGO OF CHILDHOOD

Benign paroxysmal vertigo of childhood appears to be a distinct entity that frequently causes dizziness in children. It usually occurs in early childhood between the ages of one and three years but also may occur in the older child and young teenager. The attacks, which are often mistaken for seizures (Gomez

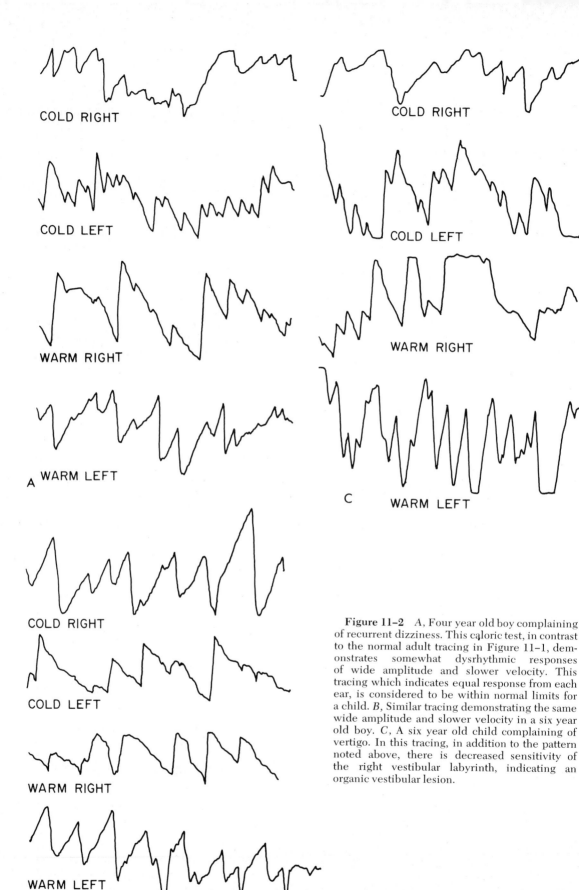

COLD RIGHT

COLD LEFT

WARM RIGHT

A WARM LEFT

COLD RIGHT

COLD LEFT

WARM RIGHT

WARM LEFT

B

COLD RIGHT

COLD LEFT

WARM RIGHT

C WARM LEFT

Figure 11–2 *A,* Four year old boy complaining of recurrent dizziness. This caloric test, in contrast to the normal adult tracing in Figure 11–1, demonstrates somewhat dysrhythmic responses of wide amplitude and slower velocity. This tracing which indicates equal response from each ear, is considered to be within normal limits for a child. *B,* Similar tracing demonstrating the same wide amplitude and slower velocity in a six year old boy. *C,* A six year old child complaining of vertigo. In this tracing, in addition to the pattern noted above, there is decreased sensitivity of the right vestibular labyrinth, indicating an organic vestibular lesion.

and Klass, 1972), are most likely due to vestibular dysfunction analogous to vestibular neuritis in adults. Spontaneous, complete recovery usually takes place over a period of several months to a year or two.

As described by Basser (1964), Koenigsberger et al. (1970), and Chutorian (1972), the clinical features of benign paroxysmal vertigo include sudden, abrupt attacks of dizziness that only last for a few seconds to a few minutes. These episodes, in which the child may cry out and lose balance, cause the child great fright and alarm. Concomitant autonomic symptoms, such as pallor and vomiting, may occur. Some children are vivid in their descriptions of sensations of rotation and turning. Nystagmus may be present and discernible to an observer; the parents should be told about this possibility so that they can look for nystagmus in subsequent episodes and thus help to confirm the diagnosis.

Children with benign paroxysmal vertigo have normal hearing, normal electroencephalograms, and normal roentgenograms. However, vestibular testing may indicate decreased sensitivity of one vestibular system. Koenigsberger et al. (1970) compared a group of affected children with controls and found that there was a consistent bilateral or unilateral decrease of caloric response in children with the disorder.

Every child in whom the diagnosis of benign paroxysmal vertigo is suspected should have a caloric test with electronystagmographic recording. Unilateral, decreased response in the presence of normal hearing and a normal neurologic examination is essentially diagnostic for this disorder.

MENIERE DISEASE

Infrequently, Meniere disease may occur in children (Meyerhoff et al., 1978), and there are several reports of its occurrence in preschool and early elementary school-age children. It is more likely to occur in children over the age of ten years, and in a small percentage of patients the disease may be bilateral (Kitahara et al., 1978).

As in adults, Meniere disease in children is characterized by a triad of symptoms: dizziness, hearing loss, and tinnitus.

The dizziness occurs in clusters of acute attacks, each marked by severe vertigo, frequently accompanied by autonomic symptoms of pallor, perspiration, nausea, or vomiting. Between these acute episodes, the patient may have adjunctive symptoms of vague balance disturbance, referred to as dysequilibrium.

The hearing loss is a sensory loss, frequently accompanied by paracusis (distorted hearing) and diplacusis (hearing a different pitch in each ear at the same time). The hearing loss characteristically fluctuates in degree. It has been reported that an essential difference between Meniere disease in children and in adults may be that children are more likely to recover auditory function than are adults.

Tinnitus is usually low-pitched and roaring, frequently likened to the sound of a seashell held against the ear. The tinnitus may change in pitch or intensity prior to an attack and so serve as an aura preceding vertigo. This is not usually reported by children.

Objective evidence, if attainable, includes a flat, low-tone, sensory hearing loss upon audiologic examination, with the results of special tests indicating a cochlear disorder. Vestibular testing by electronystagmography may reveal spontaneous nystagmus and decreased function of one vestibular labyrinth. These abnormalities may not be present and are not essential for the diagnosis. However, vestibular dysfunction may be manifested by the presence of nystagmus during an attack of vertigo. The child's family and teacher should be alerted to this possibility, since it is unlikely that the physician will have the opportunity to observe the child during an attack.

In addition to reassurance, treatment consists of vestibular suppressant medication. In some instances, vertiginous episodes may continue and become incapacitating. In these patients, Meyerhoff et al. (1978) have reported gratifying success with endolymphatic mastoid shunt operations. Before considering surgery, however, it is imperative that the child be completely reevaluated pediatrically, neurologically, and radiologically, as well as otologically, to be as certain as possible that the diagnosis is correct.

LABYRINTHINE FISTULA

It is well recognized that perilymphatic fistulae can account for hearing loss and dizziness in adults. An increasing number of instances have occurred in which fistulae have been demonstrated as the cause of dizziness and ataxia as well as hearing loss in children (Stroud and Calcaterra, 1970; Grundfast and Bluestone, 1978). It is therefore important to be aware of this possibility when making a diagnosis in the child experiencing dizziness.

Labyrinthine membrane ruptures may occur not only at the inner ear–middle ear interface, producing a fistula (usually of the oval or round window), but may also occur within the labyrinth itself, probably in Reissner's membrane and possibly in the basilar membrane as well. Breaks within the labyrinth most likely account for hearing loss by allowing a mixing of endolymph and perilymph to occur (Simmons, 1978). A leak of perilymph into the middle ear causes balance disturbance, ataxia, and vertigo as well as hearing loss.

A fluctuating sensorineural hearing loss may be explained on the basis of repeated, small, intralabyrinthine breaks that heal spontaneously. On the other hand, persistent balance disturbance (with or without hearing loss) may be explained on the basis of a continuous leakage of perilymph into the middle ear.

Membrane ruptures may occur spontaneously or may follow physical strain or stress (Goodhill, 1971) in which an increase in intralabyrinthine pressure occurs. This may be due to an increase in pressure either within the cranial cavity or within the middle ear space. The former, described as "explosive" by Goodhill et al. (1973), may follow elevated cerebrospinal fluid pressure, which causes an increase in perilymphatic pressure, or elevated cranial venous pressure. The latter, described as "implosive" by Goodhill et al. (1973), may follow an alteration in middle ear pressure, such as that occurring in barotrauma (Knight, 1977).

There may be at least two routes for transmission of cerebrospinal fluid pressure to the perilymph. Some pressure transmission may take place through the internal auditory canal, but the primary route for transmission of pressure is through the cochlear aqueduct. Since it has been demonstrated that the infantile cochlear aqueduct is larger and more patulous than the adult cochlear aqueduct, it is understandable that, in some children, pressure differentials will enhance the probability of a membrane rupture within the labyrinth secondary to increased cerebrospinal fluid pressure. Since a great many children are subjected to frequent great physical

stresses and suffer no ill effects, there must be an individual predisposition (such as a congenital abnormality of the ear) to account for the formation of fistulae in certain children.

Dizziness due to a labyrinthine fistula may occur alone, as episodes of vertigo and balance disturbance, or perhaps more frequently with an associated sensory hearing loss. There are no symptoms pathognomonic of a labyrinthine fistula; however, several features of the history are suggestive.

1. A history of head injury, physical strain or stress, exposure to sudden alterations in environmental pressure (for example, diving or flying), or marked alteration in middle ear pressures (for example, violent sneezing or laughing or blowing a wind instrument).

2. Continuous dizziness, which may be increased by postural change, continuous poor balance or ataxia, especially following any of the preceding.

3. "Sudden" sensory hearing loss, however, the "suddenness" may be difficult to define, since children frequently are unable to express a specific onset or time frame. This sensory loss fluctuates in intensity.

4. A sensation of a "pop" in the ear followed by a hearing loss or dizziness.

5. A prior history of recurrent meningitis, convulsions, or aural discharge suggestive of cerebrospinal fluid otorrhea.

6. The complaint that loud sounds produce dizziness. This may be explained on the basis of the stapedial reflex increasing an oval window leak.

Certain physical findings are suggestive of the diagnosis of a labyrinthine fistula.

1. Continuous vestibular dysfunction as evidenced by the following.

    a. Persistent spontaneous nystagmus noted with eyes open or on electronystagmographic recording with eyes closed; nystagmus produced by position change.

    b. Poor balance, ataxia, or both on physical examination (Healy et al., 1978). The patient may demonstrate an abnormality on the Romberg or sharpened Romberg test or on gait testing. With a labyrinthine disorder, the patient tends to fall to one side and has more difficulty maintaining balance in the dark. In cerebellar ataxia, the tendency to fall in one direction and the influence of darkness are less marked. Ataxia due to proprioceptive dysfunction may be similar to labyrinthine ataxia. However, in the former there is usually some other manifestation of a proprioceptive deficit, such as disturbed sense of position.

2. A unilateral sensory hearing loss that may be moderate in degree and associated with very poor speech discrimination (if testable) or a profound loss of auditory function.

3. A positive fistula test may be elicited by a pneumatic otoscope or a tympanometer. To be positive, a fistula test response must include not only the patient's report of dizziness but also the presence of eye movements. The detection of these can be facilitated by electronystagmography. Occasionally, head movements may also occur following a pressure change in the external canal.

4. Caloric testing responses recorded by electronystagmography may demonstrate a decreased response of one vestibular labyrinth. If this unilateral depression of vestibular function is combined with spontaneous and positional nystagmus, the likelihood of a fistula is greater.

If a labyrinthine fistula is suspected, the immediate treatment is complete bedrest with the head elevated and careful observation. Hearing may gradually return to normal, and vertigo may gradually subside. If this occurs, no further treatment is necessary. However, if this does not occur and some of the risk factors noted above are present, tympanotomy should be performed. Closure of a perilymphatic leak usually controls the dizziness and may improve hearing (Chap. 17).

DISTURBANCE OF THE VESTIBULAR CORTEX

Although there may be additional cortical vestibular representation, the main vestibular projection area is on the anterior end of the supratemporal gyrus of the temporal lobe. Therefore, cortical dysfunction in this area is likely to be associated with vertiginous symptoms. The dysfunction may be due to epilepsy, a tumor, or concussion.

In a detailed study of 666 patients with temporal lobe epilepsy, Currie et al. (1971) reported that 12 per cent of those studied

were under the age of 10 years and 14 per cent were under the age of 15 years; the youngest patient was 1 year old. The incidence of vertigo as an associated symptom in the total series was 19 per cent, but as an isolated symptom it was much less frequent.

The diagnosis of temporal lobe epilepsy (sometimes called psychomotor epilepsy) in a child experiencing dizziness is suggested by the presence of other symptoms or signs. Over 75 per cent of these patients have loss of consciousness during seizure, and others have altered consciousness with disturbance in thinking. There is a high incidence of associated visceral complaints, such as abdominal discomfort. Special sensory symptoms, such as visual or auditory hallucinations (or both) and unpleasant olfactory or gustatory sensations, frequently occur. There may also be motor phenomena, speech disorders, and emotional components. The results of electroencephalography may be helpful in making the diagnosis. However, a child with temporal lobe epilepsy may have a normal electroencephalogram. Nystagmus is not a feature of temporal lobe epilepsy, which is due to a primary abnormal cortical discharge and which does not involve the brainstem directly. On the other hand, vestibulogenic epilepsy, in which epileptiform attacks are precipitated by stimulation of the labyrinth, is accompanied by nystagmus since the brainstem is involved. Idiopathic vestibulogenic temporal lobe seizures are rare. They may follow vestibular testing.

In the study of Currie et al. (1971), 9.5 per cent of all children with temporal lobe epilepsy were found to have tumors. Schneider et al. (1968, 1978), in a study of 46 patients who were operated on for the treatment of intractable temporal lobe seizures, found 12 temporal lobe tumors. Seven of the patients who had tumors had vertigo either as a presenting complaint or as a conspicuous symptom. In several cases, the vertigo had begun in early childhood. These young patients frequently exhibited bizarre turning patterns and associated auditory and visual hallucinations. Some experienced altered consciousness with trance-like states, memory impairment, and aphasia. Since vertigo may be a prominent symptom early in the course of a temporal lobe tumor, it is important to consider this possibility, especially if there is any suggestion of other temporal lobe dysfunction as described previously.

Head injury, particularly a blow to the

occiput, may produce a contrecoup injury to the temporal lobe vestibular cortex as it strikes the sphenoid ridge. This may account for postconcussion syndrome vertigo. In the study of Currie et al. (1971), a series of 666 patients with temporal lobe epilepsy, 7 per cent were found to have a significant head injury which was considered to have some relationship to the etiology of the problem. The possibility of temporal lobe concussion is being recognized more frequently by specialists in sports medicine, and it is suggested that clinical traumatic syndromes that include dizziness may, at times, be neurologic rather than otologic in origin.

LABYRINTHINE TRAUMA

Head injury, in addition to possibly causing a labyrinthine fistula or temporal lobe concussion, may produce a concussion of the labyrinth. This is accompanied by acute vertigo and followed subsequently by postural dizziness. Labyrinthine concussion is most likely to occur if there is a temporal bone fracture, especially a longitudinal fracture, without loss of cochlear function. However, concussion may also be present without a fracture or any other obvious, objective abnormality such as nystagmus. Therefore, if a labyrinthine concussion is suspected, special vestibular tests, such as electronystagmography and posturography, should be performed. For example, on electronystagmography, nystagmus may be discovered with the eyes closed and would confirm the diagnosis of labyrinthine disorder. Special testing is especially important if there is a legal aspect to the case (Chap. 21).

MIGRAINE

Migraine has been reported to occur in children much more frequently than was originally suspected (Gomez and Klass, 1972; Watson and Steele, 1974; Saper, 1978). Since vertigo may be a feature of classic migraine or migraine equivalent, the diagnostic possibility of migraine should be considered in the child experiencing dizziness. Classic migraine is accompanied by headache, whereas migraine equivalent may not be.

Watson and Steele (1974) studied 286 children with migraine, of whom 66 experienced true vertigo. Of these, 43 had accompanying headache and other neurologic signs and symptoms of classic migraine, and 23 had migraine equivalents without headache. Over half of those children with classic migraine had basilar artery migraine accompanied by signs and symptoms of brainstem dysfunction. These included weakness and paresthesias of the extremities, diplopia, and other visual disturbance.

The diagnosis of vertigo due to migraine without headache is tenable if the patient has accompanying transient neurologic disturbances, such as weakness of the extremities, slurred speech, sensory changes, or hallucinations. Episodes of dizziness, which may be abrupt, lasting several minutes, are associated with prostration, pallor, nausea and vomiting, and frequently abdominal pain. A family history of migraine is strongly supportive of this diagnosis in the child.

The symptom complex of migraine equivalent may be similar to that of psychomotor epilepsy. With epilepsy there is more likely to be altered consciousness, whereas with migraine there may be a strong family history. Motor phenomena may occur with either.

Since there is also similarity between these episodes and benign paroxysmal vertigo of childhood, migraine equivalent may be related to or, in fact, be a cause of, benign paroxysmal vertigo.

PAROXYSMAL TORTICOLLIS IN INFANCY

Paroxysmal torticollis is an unusual syndrome occurring in infants and may be due to vestibular dysfunction (Gourley, 1971). There are episodes in which the infant holds the head tilted to one side or the other, frequently rotating it to the opposite side. At the onset there may be vomiting and pallor, and the baby may appear to be quite agitated, especially when an attempt is made to straighten the head. The episodes are brief and self-limited and may recur over a period of several months, or, in some children, a few years.

Snyder (1969) reports a series of 12 cases in which the attacks lasted from 10 minutes to 14 days, recurring for varying lengths of time. In children in whom the attacks lasted until speech was present, four complained that they were dizzy and that the "house was turning."

Aside from torticollis, a physical examination usually reveals no abnormalities in these children. It appears likely that this ailment is a variant of the benign paroxysmal vertigo which occurs in older children. However, it has also been reported that paroxysmal torticollis may be related to gastroesophageal reflux and hiatal hernia (Sandifer syndrome) (Ramenofsky et al., 1978). In infancy, reflux of gastric contents into the esophagus may occur in a significant number of infants. Normally the pH of the esophagus should be neutral, thus acid stomach contents are irritating, and this stimulus in the esophagus and in the pharynx may reflexly produce torticollis. In suspected cases, a pH determination of the upper esophagus should be obtained to ascertain whether or not this possibility exists.

MULTIPLE SCLEROSIS

Vertigo may be a presenting symptom of multiple sclerosis. Molteni (1977) reported that in a series of 14 cases of childhood multiple sclerosis, vertigo was a presenting symptom in four. When combined with the findings of others, this suggests that the incidence of vertigo as the presenting symptom in multiple sclerosis is approximately 20 per cent. In the evaluation of the child with unexplained dizziness, the possibility of multiple sclerosis should be considered.

Vertigo in multiple sclerosis is due to an area of demyelination or plaque formation in the region of the vestibular nucleus. Nystagmus and ataxia are likely to accompany vertigo; however they more frequently occur independently. Because of the exacerbation and remission pattern characteristic of multiple sclerosis, the episodes of vertigo may be relatively brief, sporadic, and isolated, and are likely to be attributed to other causes. This type of vertigo is not accompanied by hearing loss or tinnitus, although associated syncope or convulsions may occur on rare occasions.

Although multiple sclerosis is a rare diagnosis in pediatric practice, childhood onset of this disease has been estimated to occur in 0.4 to 10 per cent of all cases of multiple sclerosis (Molteni, 1977). Physicians should be alert to the possibility that an isolated episode of dizziness without associated symptoms or signs could be the first evidence of this disease.

OTHER DIAGNOSTIC CONSIDERATIONS

In the school-age child especially, dizziness may be a manifestation of anxiety, tension, hyperventilation, or drug ingestion. Recognizing that certain drugs may be toxic to the vestibular system and that others such as barbiturates may also frequently cause nystagmus, one must attempt to obtain a drug history in the child experiencing dizziness, especially if nystagmus is present on examination. Epidemic vertigo on a viral basis has also been reported (Williams, 1963).

In a child with disturbed balance but without clear-cut episodes of vertigo, the possibility of familial ataxia, a pontine tumor, or cerebellar disease should be considered. Also, balance disturbance may be present in hydrocephalus. In these patients, Painter (1978) notes that there may be pressure on the cerebellar afferent pathways as they sweep around the lateral horns (Chap. 22).

Children who wear hearing aids may experience dizziness due to an excessively high sound pressure level. This is likely to occur if amplification is above 120 decibels in an ear with a sensory hearing impairment.

SELECTED REFERENCES

Currie, S., Heathfield, K. W. G., Henson, R. A., et al. 1971. Clinical course and prognosis of temporal lobe epilepsy. Brain, *94*:173–190.
Extensive survey of 660 patients, mostly adults, with temporal lobe epilepsy. Clinical features, including the types of components of seizures, electroencephalographic findings, etiologic factors, managements, and outcome are discussed.

Grundfast, K. M., and Bluestone, C. D. 1978. Sudden or fluctuating hearing loss and vertigo in children due to perilymph fistula. Ann. Otol. Rhinol. Laryngol. *87*(6):761–771.
Illustrative case presentations followed by a detailed discussion of the pertinent literature and current attitudes toward diagnosis and treatment.

Koenigsberger, M. R., Chutorian, A. M., Gold, A. P., et al. 1970. Benign paroxysmal vertigo of childhood. Neurology, *20*:1108–1113.
A study of 17 children with paroxysmal vertigo and a control group. A thoughtful review of the literature and discussion of an entity that is clinically recognizable but perhaps not as frequent as originally thought.

Schneider, R. C., Calhoun, H. D., and Crosby, E. C. 1968. Vertigo and rotational movement in cortical and subcortical lesions. J. Neurol. Sci., *6*:493–516.
A pioneering clinical study that emphasizes the importance of thinking of possible temporal lobe disease in

patients with vertigo and balance disturbance. In 26 patients operated upon for intractable temporal lobe seizures, 12 were found to have temporal lobe tumors. Of these, 7 had vertigo either as a presenting complaint or as a prominent symptom. Temporal lobe trauma as a possible cause of postconcussion vertigo is also discussed. An important paper stressing the relationship between cortical dysfunction and balance disturbances.

Watson, P., and Steele, J. C. 1974. Paroxysmal dysequilibrium in the migraine syndrome of childhood. Arch. Otolaryngol., *99*:177–179.

A study of 286 children with migraine, 66 of whom experienced true vertigo. Of these, 43 had accompanying headache and other neurologic signs and symptoms of classic migraine, and 23 had migraine equivalents without headaches. An excellent review of migraine in childhood.

REFERENCES

Basser, L. S. 1964. Benign paroxysmal vertigo of childhood. Brain, *87*:141–152.

Beddoe, G. M. 1977. Vertigo in childhood. Otolaryngol. Clin. North Am., *10*:139–144.

Black, F. O., O'Leary, D. P., Wall, C. III, et al. 1977. The vestibulospinal stability test: Normal limits. Trans. Am. Acad. Ophthalmol. Otolaryngol., *84*:549–560.

Bluestone, C. D., Beery, Q. C., and Paradise, J. L. 1973. Audiometry and tympanometry in relation to middle ear effusions in children. Laryngoscope, *83*:594–604.

Busis, S. N. 1973. Diagnostic evaluation of the patient presenting with vertigo. Otolaryngol. Clin. North Am., *6*:3–23.

Busis, S. N. 1976. Vertigo in children. Pediatr. Ann., *5*:478–481.

Cantekin, E. I., Bluestone, C. D., Saez, C. A., et al. 1977. Normal and abnormal middle ear ventilation. Ann. Otol., Rhinol. Laryngol., *86*(41):1–15.

Chutorian, A. M. 1972. Benign paroxysmal vertigo of childhood. Dev. Med. Child Neurol. *14*:513–515.

Currie, S., Heathfield, K. W. G., Henson, R. A., et al. 1971. Clinical course and prognosis of temporal lobe epilepsy. Brain, *94*:173–190.

Eviatar, L., and Eviatar, A. 1977. Vertigo in children: Differential diagnosis and treatment. Pediatrics, *59*:833–838.

Gomez, M. R., and Klass, D. W. 1972. Seizures and other paroxysmal disorders in infants and children. Curr. Probl. Pediatr., *2*:3–37.

Goodhill, V. 1971. Sudden deafness and round window rupture. Laryngoscope, *81*:1462–1472.

Goodhill, V., Brockman, S. J., Harris, I., et al. 1973. Sudden deafness and labyrinthine window ruptures. Ann. Otol. Rhinol. Laryngol., *82*:2–12.

Gourley, I. M. 1971. Paroxysmal torticollis in infancy. C. M. A. Journal, *105*:504–505,

Grundfast, K. M., and Bluestone, C. D. 1978. Sudden or fluctuating hearing loss and vertigo in children due to perilymph fistula. Ann. Otol. Rhinol. Laryngol., *87*(6):761–771.

Harrison, M. S. 1962. Vertigo in childhood. J. Laryngol., *76*:601–616.

Healy, G. B., Friedman, J. M., and DiTroia, J. 1978. Ataxia and hearing loss secondary to perilymphatic fistula. Pediatrics, *61*:238–241.

Kitahara, M., Matsubara, T., Takeda, T., et al. 1978. Bilateral Meniere's disease. Abstracts, Barany Society Ordinary Meeting in Uppsala, Sweden, June 1–3, pp. 39–40.

Knight, N. J. 1977. Severe sensorineural deafness in children due to perforation of the round-window membrane. Lancet, *8046*:1003–1005.

Koenigsberger, M. R., Chuntorian, A. M., Gold, A. P., et al. 1970. Benign paroxysmal vertigo of childhood. Neurology, *20*:1108–1113.

Meyerhoff, W. L., Paparella, M. M., and Shea, D. 1978 Meniere's disease in children. Presented at the Southern Section of the American Laryngological, Rhinological and Otological Society, Inc., Houston, Texas, January 13.

Molteni, R. A. 1977. Vertigo as a presenting symptom of multiple sclerosis in childhood. Am. J. Dis. Child., *131*:553–554.

Painter, M. J. 1978. Personal communication regarding balance disturbance associated with hydrocephalus.

Ramenofsky, M. L., Buyse, M., Goldberg, M. J., et al. 1978. Gastroesophageal reflux and torticollis. J. Bone Joint Surg., *60A*:1140–1141.

Saper, J. R. 1978, Migraine. J.A.M.A., *239*:2380–2382.

Schneider, R. C. 1978. Personal communication regarding temporal lobe concussion.

Schneider, R. C., Calhoun, H. D., and Crosby, E. C. 1968. Vertigo and rotational movement in cortical and subcortical lesions. J. Neurol. Sci., *6*:493–516.

Simmons, F. B. 1978. Fluid dynamics in sensorineural hearing loss. Otolaryngol. Clin. North Am., *11*:55–61.

Snyder, C. H. 1969. Paroxysmal torticollis in infancy. Am. J. Dis. Child., *117*:458–460.

Stroud, M. H., and Calcaterra, T. C. 1970. Spontaneous perilymph fistulas. Laryngoscope, *80*:479–487.

Watson, P., and Steele, J. C. 1974. Paroxysmal dysequilibrium in the migraine syndrome of childhood. Arch. Otolaryngol., *99*:177–179.

Williams, S. 1963. Epidemic vertigo in children. Med. J. Aust., *2*:660–661.

Chapter 12

TINNITUS IN CHILDREN

Gerald Leonard, M.D.
F. Owen Black, M.D.
Victor L. Schramm, Jr., M.D.

"Why is it that the buzzing in the ears ceases if one makes a sound? Is it because the greater sound drives out the less?"

Hippocrates (c. 400 B.C.) Book 32, paragraph 961–A.

Tinnitus may be defined as sounds heard in the absence of extracranial sound stimuli that are loud enough to affect conscious thought. It is the most common auditory complaint encountered in clinical practice.

Malfunctions causing tinnitus will be classified generally into disorders arising outside the auditory system (objective) and disorders arising within the auditory system (subjective).

OBJECTIVE TINNITUS

Tinnitus arising outside the auditory system but inside the body or its cavities may be termed "objective." The mechanical activity giving rise to this type of tinnitus is generated within the patient's body and stimulates the auditory system by either normal air or bone conduction mechanisms. The sound that stimulates the inner ear, however, has no external orienting or communicative meaning and, consequently, is regarded as a nuisance by the subject. In a strict sense, this type of tinnitus should be classified as objective (particularly from the patient's point of view) regardless of whether or not the examiner can hear it. The auditory system under these circumstances is functioning normally. Thus, the first determination to be made by the examiner is identification of the sound source — a difficult task indeed. To illustrate the complexity of the problem, consider the sudden onset of a maximum conductive hearing loss, which yields a reduction of 50 dB in auditory sensitivity but leaves the cochlea and its neural connections intact. (A mild form of conductive loss can be produced by sticking your index fingers into your external auditory meati. Try it while you read the remainder of this paragraph.) Many otherwise normal persons will immediately perceive pulsations, roarings, or breathing sounds — a host of possible sounds depending upon the individual. Most are objective forms of tinnitus, perceivable only by the subject. Subjective tinnitus, e.g., high-pitched ringing or complex noise, may also be perceived only in the presence of a conductive hearing loss. In this case, a noise originating and already present in the auditory system was unmasked by the sudden reduction of external sounds that constantly enter the ear under normal circumstances. (Environmental sounds, even in quiet, average 60 to 70 dB in intensity.) The latter type of tinnitus is *really* subjective because it arises within the subject's own auditory system and cannot be transmitted to an examiner, but its perception was prevented, before the conductive loss, by the overriding environmental noise. Objective noises, such as the subject's own voice or joint and muscular noises, may be perceptible or imperceptible for the same reasons. To demonstrate, hum or read a portion of this paragraph aloud for a moment before taking your fingers out of your ears.

SUBJECTIVE TINNITUS

Tinnitus arising within the auditory system, even in the absence of a conductive impairment, may also result from some change in the acoustic signal auditory system noise ratio. This type of tinnitus is called subjective because only the patient will be able to hear the sound. A conductive hearing loss may attenuate external auditory signals, thereby unmasking abnormal (e.g., drug induced) noise in other parts of the auditory system. This type of tinnitus is very common in children with conductive hearing losses (e.g., serous middle ear effusions) who are receiving aspirin.

Fowler (1965) subdivided subjective head noises into (1) vibratory and (2) nonvibratory. He further subdivided the vibratory class into intrinsic and extrinsic and the nonvibratory class into peripheral and nonperipheral. There have been some subsequent misinterpretations of his classification in the literature, and authors have equated Fowler's vibratory tinnitus with what is commonly described as objective tinnitus.

HISTORY AND PHYSICAL EXAMINATION

Complaints of tinnitus from children are rare. When they do occur as isolated auditory symptoms, they are usually difficult to assess. If the child is unable to describe the sound perceived, localization of the underlying pathology may be rendered very difficult in the absence of abnormal physical or auditory test findings. The fact that tinnitus is a rare complaint in children may be due to the fact that tinnitus is usually transient; alternatively, a child may not complain of a persistent tinnitus until adolescence or until his body-image consciousness is developed (Fowler and Fowler, 1955). If possible, the history should be taken from both the parents and the child, depending upon the child's age.

A thorough history will occasionally provide a presumptive diagnosis. The patient should be asked simply if he knows the cause. The query should include questions about severity (intensity), location, whether monaural or binaural, pitch (frequency), whether sounds are pulsating or continuous, and if the sound sensations are altered by factors such as stress, rest, or exercise.

In obtaining a history from the child who has tinnitus, it is important to find out if other symptoms exist. Hearing loss, vertigo, pain, or diplopia will point the physician in respective directions of investigation. It may prove difficult, particularly in a child, to determine temporal characteristics of the tinnitus. One should ask the patient if the tinnitus is continuous (always present) or discontinuous (intermittent). If the tinnitus is continuous, further questioning should elicit whether or not the symptom changes in intensity in the presence or absence of an environmental masking noise, body position, or activity. If the noise is discontinuous, it is usually present only in quiet surroundings (in the absence of masking environmental sounds) and is usually associated with a partial (frequency band limited) hearing loss. Discontinuous tinnitus may also be associated with exercise, which suggests a vascular etiology or an exacerbation of a disease, such as serous middle ear effusion.

The patient should be questioned carefully about the frequency characteristics of the head noise. It is often necessary to explain to the patient the difference between pitch and intensity of sound; often these terms are not familiar to the patient, especially to a child. If possible, an attempt to discern whether the noise is perceived as broad or narrow frequency bands should be made. Broad frequency band noises tend to be associated with medications or other chemical toxins, severe advanced hearing loss, or acute sensorineural hearing loss. Narrow-band (band-limited) noise is usually associated with partial hearing loss, such as noise-induced hearing loss. Both broad-band and narrow-band tinnitus may be continuous or discontinuous. A diagrammatic summary is included in Figure 12–1.

The pathophysiologic basis for most types of auditory tinnitus is unknown. Tinnitus may or may not be associated with a hearing loss. The pattern of hearing loss may be correlated with tinnitus in some cases (Kiang et al., 1970). It is also possible that the essential factor underlying the tinnitus of sensorineural deafness is the existence of distinctly different distributions of activity in adjacent elements of the auditory nerve; the tinnitus that typically occurs at the lower frequency of a noise-induced hearing loss occurs at 3000 Hz.

When a patient presents with tinnitus, the physician must be prepared to search extensively for the etiology, but he should always caution the patient and parents at the outset

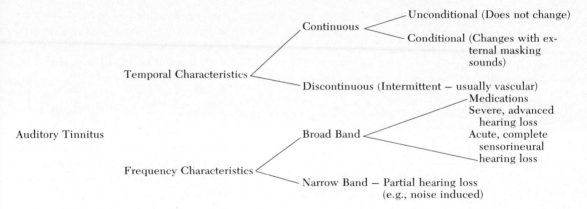

Figure 12–1 Characteristics of auditory (subjective) tinnitus.

of any investigation that a cause may not be found.

There are innumerable causes of tinnitus. The ear contains every basic tissue type present elsewhere in the body, in addition to its encasement in ossified primitive cartilage (otic capsule). Consequently, any general condition affecting a tissue type can also affect the hearing organ.

The history should be followed by a thorough examination of the ears, nasopharynx, palate, mouth, and pharynx. Occasionally, the cause of the tinnitus may be obvious, e.g., impacted external auditory canal cerumen or fluid in the middle ear cleft. If a sound is subjectively pulsatile or intermittent, the physician should determine if it is synchronous with the arterial pulse. More subtle or unusual causes will require systematic investigations for identification (Chap. 8A).

AUDITORY SYSTEM EVALUATION

Following the history and physical examinations, the audiologist should be asked to do the following procedures.

1. Demonstrate the characteristics of any existing hearing loss or auditory disorder.
2. Determine if the tinnitus can be masked (a) ipsilaterally, (b) contralaterally, or (c) not at all. If the tinnitus can be masked ipsilaterally, there is a strong possibility that the causative pathology is peripheral. If the tinnitus sensation can be masked contralaterally, the causative pathology may be either central or peripheral, and if it cannot be masked, the tinnitus is probably located within the auditory neural projections.

3. Match the tinnitus, if possible. The pitch of a tinnitus typically varies with listening conditions and with various causes. In endolymphatic hydrops (Meniere disease), for example, the tinnitus pitch is usually centered at 320 Hz with a range of 90 to 900 Hz. In most conductive (middle ear) hearing losses, the tinnitus averages 490 Hz with a range of 90 to 1450 Hz, and for tinnitus associated with most sensorineural hearing losses, the average frequency is 3900 Hz with a range of 545 to 7500 Hz (Nodar and Graham, 1965) (Chap. 8B).

ETIOLOGIC CLASSIFICATION OF TINNITUS

Objective or Nonauditory Tinnitus. Nonauditory tinnitus can arise from any normal or abnormal bodily function capable of generating motions in the frequency range of auditory function. The most common type in this group is tinnitus arising from transmission of normal or abnormal vascular pulsations to the cochlea. Though the sound stimulus producing the tinnitus is arising outside the auditory system, a defect within the auditory system (e.g., a conductive hearing loss) can exacerbate or cause tinnitus.

Tinnitus of vascular origin has been divided by some researchers into two categories (Hentzer, 1968): (a) tinnitus caused by an anomaly within the arteries of the head and neck and (b) essential tinnitus, which constitutes a category for which no reasonable explanation can be found. However, it is felt by many researchers that the cause of this latter type of tinnitus is to be searched for

Table 12–1 CAUSES OF VASCULAR TINNITUS

Arterial aneurysms
Arterial malformations
Arteriovenous malformation
Stenosis of the carotid or other cerebral arteries
Arteriosclerosis of the basilar artery
Transmitted cardiac murmur
Inflammatory hyperemia of the ear
Hemangioma of the head and neck
Chemodectomas of the head and neck

within the venous return from the head (Ward et al., 1975).

1. *Arterial Causes.* The more common causes of vascular tinnitus are listed in Table 12–1. Some examples of the conditions are described, as well as the management of the conditions and the eventual outcome following treatment (Hentzer, 1968). In· most cases, according to Hentzer, the anomalies within the arterial system can be demonstrated by angiography.

2. *Essential Tinnitus.* This type of tinnitus may be characterized by a lack of distinctive symptoms and by the fact that it has been impossible to demonstrate a cause (Graf, 1952). Certain criteria should be fulfilled before a diagnosis of essential tinnitus can be made: the tinnitus must be of sudden onset and must be unrelated to any demonstrable disease or injury. The character of tinnitus can change in pitch and intensity. However, essential tinnitus should be persistent and unchanging for a year or more. There should be pronounced lateralization, and the sound should be synchronous with the arterial pulse.

Various factors indicate that the cause should be searched for within the venous system of the head and neck and, in keeping with the vascular nature of the condition, the tinnitus should have certain relations to altered head positions. Turning the head away from the side of the tinnitus typically increases the intensity of the sound, possibly owing to some internal jugular vein compression by the ipsilateral sternocleidomastoid muscle.

As previously stated, the condition has not been associated with any other disease or injury and, therefore, does not occur with increased intracranial pressure, pulsating exophthalmos, or abnormalities of extracranial arteries.

Less common causes are described by others (Rossberg, 1967; Wengraf, 1967; Ward et al., 1975). Some of these are:

a. Arteriovenous malformations between the branches of the occipital artery and the transverse sinus. These types of malformations are relatively more common in the posterior cranial fossa but may occur in the middle cranial fossa between the posterior branch of the middle meningeal artery and the greater petrosal sinus.

b. Abnormalities occurring between the internal maxillary artery and vein resulting from trauma or lesions in that region.

c. Cerebral or cervical angiomas and giant cell tumors of the mandible.

Also of serious importance are arteriovenous communications (fistulas) between the internal carotid artery and the cavernous sinus, which occur following head trauma. The pulsatile tinnitus associated with these vascular fistulas may often be detected by both the patient and the physician. Palpation of the eye often reveals a thrill, and upon auscultation a bruit may be heard (see Table 12–2).

3. *Myogenic Causes of Nonauditory Tinnitus.* Tinnitus resulting from rhythmic contractions of the soft palate was first described by Politzer in 1878. Since then, tinnitus of myogenic origin has been described by many others and has been classified according to the three main muscle groups affected (Yamamoto, 1958): soft palate muscles, eustachian tube muscles, and intratympanic muscles.

4. *Palatal Myoclonus.* Palatal myoclonus occurs as involuntary rhythmic contractions of the soft palate and pharyngeal musculature, including the tensor veli palatini, levator veli palatini, salpingo-

Table 12–2 DIAGNOSTIC CRITERIA FOR ESSENTIAL (OBJECTIVE) TINNITUS

Sudden onset, unrelated to other disease or injury
Persistence, unchanged for more than a year
Pronounced lateralization
Synchrony with the pulse
Related to altered head position
No symptoms of increased intracranial pressure
No pulsation exophthalmos
No abnormalities of extracranial arteries
Normal cerebral angiogram

pharyngeus, and superior constrictor muscles. These pathologic contractions commonly affect younger people and are associated with an audible clicking. The patient may volunteer the information that he has rhythmic contractions occurring somewhere in the oropharynx or oral cavity and that they are associated with a disturbing sound.

Examination of the mouth and pharynx in these cases reveals a rhythmically contracting pharyngeal musculature associated with an audible click. The contraction may not be present with the mouth widely open and may have to be viewed endoscopically. The symptoms are usually continuous and do not cease during sleep.

Palatal myoclonus has been thoroughly reported (Heller, 1962; MacKinnon, 1968), including a discussion of probable causes and the pathologic anatomy associated with the condition (Chadwick and MacBeth, 1953). In 1886, Spencer described "pharyngeal nystagmus" in a 12 year old boy who had a tumor of the cerebellar vermis. Others have described the condition in association with cerebral and cerebellar pathology (Grunwald, 1903; Pfeiffer, 1919). Pathological correlation has been possible in other cases, and most of the lesions that were thought to have caused the condition were found in the pons, brain stem, and cerebellar regions (Klein, 1907; Graeffner, 1910; Wilson, 1928; Van Bogaert and Bertrand, 1928). The causative lesions are located in a triangular area within the midbrain bounded by the red nucleus, inferior olivary and accessory nuclei, and the contralateral dentate nucleus (Guillain and Mollaret, 1931; Guillain et. al., 1933). Palatal myoclonus has also been associated with brain stem infarctions, multiple sclerosis, brain stem tumors, trauma, syphilis, malaria, and other degenerative processes. Thus, it appears that any destructive lesion within this anatomical triangle can result in palatopharyngeal myoclonus (see Table 12–3).

The cause of palatal myoclonus has been thoroughly explored. Despite this, however, the most common type is idiopathic, cases in which there is no obvious underlying cause.

5. *Tinnitus Arising from Abnormal Contraction of Intratympanic Muscles.* Intermittent tin-

Table 12–3 CAUSES OF PALATAL MYOCLONUS

Moderate or severe cerebrovascular insufficiency
Myocardial infection and diabetes
Progressive cerebellar degeneration of multiple
  sclerosis
Brain stem tumors
Trauma
Syphilis
Malaria
Following surgical clipping or ligation of the posterior
  inferior cerebellar artery
Familial tremor associated with palatal myoclonus
Cerebellar tumors
Idiopathic

nitus during recovery from facial paralysis due to facial nerve dysfunction has been reported (Watanabe et al., 1974). The tinnitus typically occurred in association with both voluntary or involuntary facial muscle contractions. The tinnitus in these eight cases was relieved by cutting the stapedial tendon.

Rhythmic contractions of the tensor tympani are usually associated with palatal myoclonus. Among the many biologic factors considered to be related to this type of tinnitus are:

a. propagation of muscle contraction noise
b. periodic vibration of the tympanic membrane
c. stimulation of the tympanic plexus
d. temporal variation of inner ear pressure or cochlear microphonic potentials.

Each of these was considered (Watanabe et al., 1974), but a conclusion could not be reached concerning the genesis of the tinnitus.

6. Nasopharyngeal sounds may be transmitted via a patient's eustachian tube to the middle ear space. Occasionally, vascular tumors, such as nasopharyngeal angiofibromas, may transmit sounds to the auditory system via the eustachian tube or via bone conduction.

7. Nonauditory tinnitus may also arise from crepitation in the temporomandibular joint.

Auditory (Subjective) Tinnitus. Auditory tinnitus arises within the auditory receptor system or nervous system pathways. This kind of tinnitus, except for drug-induced types, is rare in children. It is postulated that any irritation or loss of sensory or neural

Table 12–4   OTOTOXIC AGENTS CAUSING TINNITUS

Analeptics
  Caffeine
	Antineoplastics
	  Nitrogen mustard

Analgesics
  Acetylsalicylic acid
    (Aspirin)
  Salicylic acid
  Sodium salicylate
	Antiparasitics
	  A-16612 (rare)
	  Oil of chenopodium (rare)

Anesthetics
  Cocaine
  Lidocaine
  Procaine
  Tetracaine
	Antituberculous Agents
	  Ethambutol
	  Isoniazid
	  Para-aminosalicylic acid (PAS)

Antibiotics
  Chloramphenicol (rare)
  Dihydrostreptomycin
  Framycetin
  Gentamicin
  Kanamycin
  Neomycin
  Polymyxin B
  Streptomycin
  Viomycin
	Cardiovascular Agents
	  Chromonar
	  Digitalis (rare)
	  Hexadimethrine bromide
	  Propranolol (rare)
	  Quinidine (rare)

Anticonvulsants
  Diphenylhydantoin
	Diuretics
	  Acetazolamide
	  Ethacrynic acid
	  Furosemide

Antimalarials
  Chloroquine
  Quinine
  16-126 RP
	Heavy Metals
	  Cobalt
	  Mercury (rare)
	
	Sedatives and Tranquilizers
	  Droperidol

elements from the auditory end organ to the cerebral cortex may result in tinnitus. As noted previously, the difference between nonauditory and auditory tinnitus is that the nonauditory type represents a normal auditory system response to external sound pressure wave energy introduced into the auditory system, rather than a sound sensation arising from a malfunction within the auditory system (Ward et al., 1975). The subjective character of this complaint hinders the study of the auditory types of tinnitus and renders objective evaluation and investigation almost impossible.

Subjective tinnitus may or may not be associated with a sensorineural hearing loss. If a hearing loss is present, the tinnitus is usually centered at the corner frequency of the hearing loss (i.e., the frequency at which there is a significant change in hearing ability or at which hearing sensitivity is decreased). No correlations can be drawn between the severity of the hearing loss and the type of tinnitus. Likewise, the type of tinnitus (or whether it is present at all) cannot be correlated with location of the loss, whether sensory or neural.

The most common cause of this type of tinnitus in children is as a drug side effect, especially of aspirin. A list of the more com-

mon ototoxic drugs is given in Table 12–4. A more complete review of ototoxic agents is available in the Index Handbook of Ototoxic Agents 1966–1971. When this type of tinnitus develops in an otherwise asymptomatic child who is not taking drugs, it is usually caused by a central nervous system lesion, e.g., a tumor, demyelinating disease, or hereditary neuropathic disease, especially if the onset of the tinnitus is mild, progressing to a more severe tinnitus.

Summary.   Because hearing loss is a common complaint in childhood, it is probable that the symptom of tinnitus is much more frequent in children than has previously been supposed, particularly since, as mentioned previously, body-image consciousness is not fully developed in childhood. The most common cause of intermittent, fluctuating tinnitus in children occurs during conductive hearing losses associated with otitis media with middle ear effusions, especially if a child is taking aspirin. Continuous and persistent tinnitus is usually associated with loss of sensory or neural auditory function and may be associated with systemic nervous system diseases. If tinnitus is associated with nonauditory complaints or physical findings, the critical path to diagnosis may be simplified considerably. When vertigo and hearing loss occur with tinnitus, the patient's problem is most likely located within or near the temporal bone. If involvement of other cranial nerves, headaches, or other systemic symptoms are present, a search for central nervous system or general system disease, respectively, should be instituted.

SELECTED REFERENCES

Chadwick, D. L., and MacBeth, R. 1953. Rhythmic palatal myoclonus. J. Laryngol., 67:301–311.
  This paper reports four cases of palatal myoclonus and incorporates an excellent literature review. An attempt to correlate the pathologic and clinical findings is also made.

Hentzer, E. 1968. Objective tinnitus of the vascular type. Acta Otolaryngol., 66:273–281.
  The author describes 24 cases of tinnitus of vascular origin and classifies them into two groups: those caused by arterial anomalies within the head and neck and those that probably arise within the venous system of the head and neck. He gives guidelines for the best form of treatment based on his extensive experience.

REFERENCES

Chadwick, D. L., and MacBeth, R. 1953. Rhythmic palatal myoclonus. J. Laryngol., 67:301–311.
Fowler, E. P., and Fowler, E. P., Jr. 1955. Somatopsychic

and psychosomatic factors in tinnitus, deafness, and vertigo. Ann. Otol. Rhinol. Laryngol. *64*:29–37.

Fowler, E. P. 1965. Subjective head noises (Tinnitus Aurium). Laryngoscope, *75*:1610–1618.

Graeffner, A. 1910. Berl. Klin. Wschr. *47*:1081.

Graf, W. 1952. Kraniala Blas Jud. Nord. Med., *28*:2499.

Grunwald, L. 1903. Hyperkinetic disturbances of the pharynx. *In* Atlas and Epitome of Diseases of the Mouth, Pharynx and Nose, 2nd ed. W. B. Saunders Co., 186.

Guillain, G., and Mollaret, P. 1931. Deux cas de myoclonies synchrones et rhythmees velo-pharyngo-laryngo-oculo-diaphragmatiques. Rev. Neurol., *2*:545.

Guillain, G., Mollaret, P., and Bertrand, I. 1933. Sur la lesion responsable du syndrome myoclonique du troie cerebrae. Rev. Neurol., *2*:666.

Heller, M. F. 1962. Vibratory tinnitus and palatal myoclonus. Acta Otolaryngol., *55*:292–298.

Hentzer, E. 1968. Objective tinnitus of the vascular type. Acta Otolaryngol., *66*:273–281.

Hippocrates. Book 32. Paragraph 961–A.

Index Handbook of Ototoxic Agents 1966–1971. 1971. Baltimore, The Johns Hopkins University Press.

Kiang, N. Y. S., Moxon, E. C., and Levine, R. A. 1970. Auditory nerve activity in cats with normal and abnormal cochleas. *In* Sensorineural Hearing Loss, Churchill and Co., 241–273.

Klein, H. 1907. Neurol. Zentrabl., *26*:245.

MacKinnon, D. M. 1968. Objective tinnitus due to palatal myoclonus, J. Laryngol., *82*:369–374.

Nodar, R. H., and Graham, J. T. 1965. An investigation of frequency characteristics of tinnitus associated with Meniere's disease. Arch. Otolaryngol., *82*:28–31.

Pfeiffer, R. A. 1919. Mschr. Psychiat. Neurol., *45*:96.

Politzer, A. 1878. Lehrbuch der Ohren hal kunde, Stuttgart.

Rossberg, G. 1967. Pulsierende Ohrerausche bei anomalie der arteria carotis und arteria occipitalis externa. J. Laryngol. Rhinol., *46*:79–84.

Spencer, H. R. 1886. Pharyngeal and laryngeal "nystagmus." Lancet, *2*:702.

Van Bogaert, L., and Bertrand, I. 1928. Sur les myoclonies associees synchrones et rhythmiques par lesionsen foyer du trone cerebrale. Rev. Neurol., *1*:203.

Ward, P. H., Babin, R., Calcaterra, T. C., et al. 1975. Operative treatment of surgical lesions with objective tinnitus. Ann. Otol. Rhinol. Laryngol., *84*:473–482.

Watanabe, I., Kumagami, H., and Tsuda, Y. 1974. Tinnitus due to abnormal contraction of stapedial muscle. Otorhinolaryngol., *36*:217–226.

Wengraf, C. 1967. A case of objective tinnitus. J. Laryngol. *81*:143–146.

Wilson, S. A. K. 1928. Case of palato-laryngeal nystagmus. Brain, *51*(1):119.

Yamamoto, T. 1958. Objective tinnitus. Otolaryngol. (Tokyo), *30*:708.

Chapter 13

FACIAL PARALYSIS IN CHILDREN

Mark May, M.D.

INTRODUCTION

Because the most common cause of facial paralysis is a lesion within the temporal bone (Cawthorne, 1953), the otolaryngologist should best be able to handle problems of this nature. However, most clinicians have not had sufficient opportunities of dealing with facial paralysis to accumulate a knowledgeable approach to these cases and must rely on scattered journal reports — frequently representing conflicting or controversial opinions on the subject — to formulate a plan of management of these patients.

This chapter presents the author's approach to facial paralysis, which has been developed during 15 years of evaluating and treating 700 patients with this problem. Of these patients, 153 were between the ages of birth and 18 years (Table 13–1). With few exceptions, all the patients had complete medical otoneurologic evaluations and were followed for six months or longer.

ANATOMY OF THE FACIAL NERVE

A fundamental knowledge of the anatomy of the seventh cranial nerve is essential for localizing the level of the lesion and is helpful in arriving at the diagnosis (Fig. 13–1; Table 13–2). Further, locating the site of the lesion

Table 13–1 CAUSES OF FACIAL PARALYSIS IN 153 PATIENTS BETWEEN BIRTH AND 18 YEARS OF AGE

Causes	Number of Patients	Per Cent	Causes	Number of Patients	Per Cent
Bell Palsy	69	45	*Miscellaneous* Herpes zoster oticus – 4 Leukemia – 3	19	12
Trauma Birth – 7	27	18	Polio – 3 Chicken pox – 3		
Otitis Acute – 19 Chronic – 3	22	14	Sickle cell – 1 crisis (Central VII) Hypothyroid – 1		
Congenital	11	7	Guillain Barré syndrome – 1 Melkersson-Rosenthal syndrome – 1 Sarcoidosis – 1		
Tumors Neurinoma – 2 Glioma – 2 Cholesteatoma – 1 (Congenital)	5	3	Cause unknown – 1 (incomplete evaluation)		

DIAGRAM OF FACIAL NERVE ANATOMY

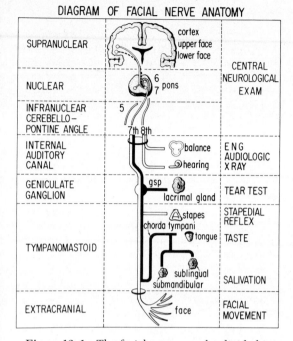

Figure 13–1 The facial nerve may be divided into three segments for anatomic study: The supranuclear, nuclear and infranuclear segments. The infranuclear segments have been further divided (as shown in the left hand column of this figure). Each level can be identified by employing tests listed in the column on the right and signs detailed in Table 13–2.

is critical for the surgical approach in instances of nerve compression by infection, neoplasms, or fractures.

The course of the facial nerve, for the sake of this discussion, may conveniently be divided into three segments: supranuclear, nuclear, and infranuclear. The infranuclear segment is further subdivided into the cerebellopontine angle, internal auditory canal, and labyrinthine, tympanic, mastoid, and extracranial segments (Fig. 13–1). Pathologic conditions at any particular level may be diagnosed by special tests, detailed in Figure 13–1.

Supranuclear Segment. In the cortex, the tracts to the upper face are crossed and uncrossed. The tracts to the lower face are crossed only; therefore the forehead is bilaterally innervated, and a lesion in the facial area on one side of the cortex would spare the forehead. However, one must not rely solely on sparing of the forehead to differentiate supranuclear from infranuclear lesions, since sparing of the forehead or other parts of the face can occur with lesions involving a more distal portion of the nerve. In addition to an intact upper face, supranuclear lesions are characterized by the presence of facial tone, spontaneous facial expression, and loss

Table 13–2 SIGNS AND PROBABLE DIAGNOSES RESULTING FROM LESIONS OF THE FACIAL NERVE AT VARIOUS LEVELS AS DETAILED IN FIGURE 13–1

Level	Signs	Diagnosis
Supranuclear		
Cortex Internal capsule	Tone and upper face intact, loss of volitional movement with intact spontaneous expression, slurred speech (tongue weakness), hemiparesis (arm greater than leg) on side of facial involvement	Lesion of motor cortex or lateral capsule on opposite side of facial involvement. Paresis upper extremity (middle cerebral artery). Paresis lower extremity (another cerebral artery)
Extrapyramidal	Increased salivary flow, spontaneous facial movement impaired, volitional facial movement intact	Tumor or vascular lesion of basal ganglion
Midbrain	Involvement of face and oculomotor roots — loss of pupillary reflexes, external strabismus, and oculomotor paresis on opposite side of facial paresis	Unilateral Weber syndrome (vascular lesion)
	Bilateral facial paresis with other cranial nerve deficits, emotional lability, hyperactive gag reflex, marked hyperflexia associated with hypertension	Pseudobulbar palsy — associated with multiple infarcts
Nuclear		
Nuclear Pons	Involvement of cranial nerves VII and VI on side of lesion, with gaze palsy on side of facial paresis. Contralateral hemiparesis, ataxia, cerebellovestibular signs	Involvement of pons at level of cranial nerves VII and VI nuclei by pontine glioma, multiple sclerosis, encephalitis, infections, or polio

Table continued on the following page

Table 13–2 SIGNS AND PROBABLE DIAGNOSES RESULTING FROM LESIONS OF THE FACIAL NERVE AT VARIOUS LEVELS AS DETAILED IN FIGURE 13–1 (*Continued*)

Level	Signs	Diagnosis
Nuclear (continued)	Cranial nerves VII and VI involved with other anomalies noted at birth	Congenital facial palsy, Moebius syndrome, and thalidomide toxicity
Infranuclear Intracranial	Involvement of cranial nerve VIII (decreased tearing and taste, stapes reflex decay, decreased discrimination), facial motor deficit (late sign)	Acoustic neuroma
Cerebello-pontine angle	Cranial nerves VIII and VII involved in succession, beginning with facial pain or numbness. Computerized axial tomography scan positive for pathology, enhanced with contrast	Meningioma
	Cranial nerves VII and VIII involved successfully, beginning with facial twitching, appearance of an erosion or lysis on plain radiographs of the temporal bone	Cholesteatoma arising in temporal bone
Skull Base	Cranial nerves VII, VIII, IX, X, XI and XII involved in succession; pulsatile tinnitus, purple-red pulsating mass noted bulging through the tympanic membrane	Glomus jugulare tumor
	Same as above with cranial nerve involvement	Glomus jugulare tumor extending to petrous apex and involving middle fossa
	Conductive or sensorineural hearing loss, acute or recurrent Bell palsy, positive family history by skull radiograph	Osteopetrosis
	Multiple cranial nerves involved in rapid succession	Carcinomatous meningitis, leukemia, Landry-Guillain-Barré syndrome, mononucleosis, diphtheria, tuberculosis, sarcoidosis
Infranuclear Transtemporal Bone	Same as listed under Cerebellopontine angle	Same as listed under Cerebellopontine angle
Internal Auditory Canal	Ecchymoses around pinna and mastoid prominence (Battle sign); hemotympanum with sensorineural hearing loss by tuning fork (lateralizes to normal side); vertigo, nystagmus (fast component away from involved side); sudden, complete facial paralysis following head trauma	Transverse fracture of temporal bone
Geniculate Ganglion	Dry eye, decreased taste, and decreased salivation; erosion of geniculate ganglion area or middle fossa as demonstrated by polytomography of temporal bone	Neurinoma, meningioma, cholesteatoma, ossifying hemangioma, malformation arteriovenous
	Pain, vesicles on pinna, dry eye, decreased taste and salivary flow; sensorineural hearing loss, nystagmus, vertigo, red chorda tympani nerve	Herpes zoster oticus (Ramsey-Hunt syndrome)

Table 13–2 SIGNS AND PROBABLE DIAGNOSES RESULTING FROM LESIONS OF THE FACIAL NERVE AT VARIOUS LEVELS AS DETAILED IN FIGURE 13–1 (*Continued*)

Level	Signs	Diagnosis
Geniculate Ganglion (*continued*)	Same as above without vesicles and no cause can be found (keep in mind, if no recovery in six months, dealing with tumor at geniculate ganglion which may require exploration for confirmation)	Bell palsy (viral inflammatory-immune disorder)
	Ecchymoses around pinna and mastoid (Battle sign), hemotympanum; conductive hearing loss by tuning fork (lateralizes to involved ear, bone greater than air), no vestibular involvement	Longitudinal fracture of temporal bone. May be proximal or at geniculate ganglion (dry eye), or distal to geniculate ganglion (tears symmetrical)
Infranuclear Transtemporal Bone / Tympanomastoid Segment	Involvement at this level characterized by decreased taste and salivation and loss of stapes reflex. Tearing is normal. There is sudden onset of facial paralysis which may be complete or incomplete and may progress to complete	
	Pain and vesicles present, red chorda tympani	Herpes zoster oticus
	Pain without vesicles, red chorda tympani	Bell palsy
	Red, bulging tympanic membrane, conductive hearing loss; usually a history of upper respiratory infection; lower face may be involved more than upper	Acute suppurative otitis media
	Foul drainage through perforated tympanic membrane; history of recurrent ear infection, drainage and hearing loss	Chronic suppurative otitis media, most likely associated with cholesteatoma
	Pulsatile tinnitus, purple-red pulsatile mass noted through tympanic membrane	Glomus tympanicum or jugulare
	Recurrent facial paralysis, positive family history, facial edema, fissured tongue; may present with simultaneous bilateral facial paralysis	Melkersson-Rosenthal syndrome
Extracranial	Incomplete involvement of facial nerve (usually one or more major branches spared); hearing, balance, tearing, stapes reflex, taste, and salivary flow spared	Penetrating wound of face; postparotid surgery; malignancy of parotid; tonsil, or oronasopharynx
	Uveitis, salivary gland enlargement, fever	Sarcoidosis (Heerfordt syndrome), lymphoma
Sites Variable	Facial paralysis, especially simultaneous bilateral facial paralysis with symmetrical ascending paralysis, decreased deep tendon reflexes, minimal sensory changes. Abnormal spinal fluid (protein and few cells, albuminocytologic dissociation)	Landry-Guillain-Barré syndrome

°Gratitude is extended to Richard Kasden, M.D., for his assistance in developing this table. Material relating to signs of facial nerve involvement in supranuclear and nuclear regions. (Based on Crosby, E. C., and De Jonge, B. R. 1963. Experimental and clinical studies of the central connections and central relations of the facial nerve. Ann. Otol. Rhinol. Laryngol., 72:735–755.)

of volitional facial movement. Most importantly, there are usually other neurologic signs of central nervous system involvement. The fact that involuntary movement is spared with supranuclear lesions is thought to be due to sparing of the extrapyramidal system, which is considered to be responsible for involuntary or emotional facial movement. With nuclear and infranuclear lesions, there is loss of both involuntary and voluntary movement.

Nuclear Segment. From its nucleus in the pons, the facial nerve begins a circuitous journey around the sixth nerve nucleus before emerging from the brain stem. Because of this relationship between the sixth and seventh cranial waves, a lesion in the region of the pons that caused a facial paralysis of the peripheral type would most likely be accompanied by a sixth cranial nerve palsy and would result in inability to rotate the eye to the side of the facial paralysis.

Cerebellopontine Angle. At the cerebellopontine angle, the eighth cranial nerve joins the facial nerve, and they enter the internal auditory canal together. Lesions in this area would be associated with vestibular and cochlear as well as seventh nerve deficits. Large lesions filling the cerebellopontine angle might compress other cranial nerves and cause deficits of the fifth cranial nerve and later the ninth, tenth, and eleventh cranial nerves.

Internal Auditory Canal. The motor facial nerve and the intermedius nerve are loosely joined together as they enter the internal auditory meatus with the acoustic nerve. The acoustic nerve enters the internal auditory canal inferiorly, while the facial nerve runs superiorly along the roof of the internal auditory canal. The intracranial segment of the facial nerve from the brain stem to the fundus of the internal acoustic meatus is covered only by a thin layer of glia, which makes it quite vulnerable to any type of surgical manipulation but quite resistant to a slow process of stretching or compression. The facial nerve in this region can become quite elongated and spread out over the surface of a sizable but slow-growing vestibular nerve schwannoma without any gross evidence of facial weakness. Although it is unusual to see facial nerve motor involvement in this instance, there is often evidence of such involvement in disruption of tearing, taste, and salivary flow owing to compression of the intermedius nerve. If the intermedius

nerve is considered part of the facial nerve, then the facial nerve is the most common cranial nerve involved with vestibular schwannomas.

Labyrinthine Segment. At the fundus of the internal auditory meatus, the facial nerve is physiologically "pressed" into the fallopian canal. The facial and intermedius nerves carry with them a continuation of the dura mater and periosteum from the internal acoustic meatus, and this dural continuation forms a well-defined and tough fibrous sheath that covers these nerves all the way to the terminal branches of the facial nerve in the face and neck. The portion of the facial nerve from its entrance into the fallopian canal to the geniculate ganglion is designated the labyrinthine segment because it runs between the cochlear and vestibular labyrinths. This segment lies beneath the middle fossa and is the shortest and narrowest part of the fallopian canal, averaging 5 mm in length and 0.68 mm in diameter (Fisch, 1977b). Since this is the narrowest part of the facial canal, it is reasonable to suspect that this is the most vulnerable part of the facial nerve when there are inflammatory changes within the canal. The facial nerve in the labyrinthine segment is further jeopardized by any process that causes further limitation of this very narrow space by the fact that the blood supply to the nerve in this region is unique: This is the only segment of the facial nerve in which there are no anastomosing arterial arcades (Blunt, 1956).

The labyrinthine segment of the facial nerve includes the geniculate ganglion, from which arises the first branch of the facial nerve, the greater superficial petrosal nerve (Fig. 13–2). This nerve carries secretory motor fibers to the lacrimal gland. The second branch from the geniculate ganglion is a tiny thread that forms the lesser superficial petrosal as it is joined by fibers of the tympanic plexus, contributed by the ninth cranial nerve. This nerve carries secretory fibers to the parotid gland.

Tympanic Segment. At the geniculate ganglion the facial nerve makes a sharp angled turn backward, forming a knee or genu, to enter the tympanic or horizontal portion of the fallopian canal. The proximal end of the tympanic portion is marked by the geniculate ganglion, from which point the facial nerve courses peripherally 3 to 5 mm, passing posterior to the cochleariform process and the tensor tympani tendon. The distal end of the

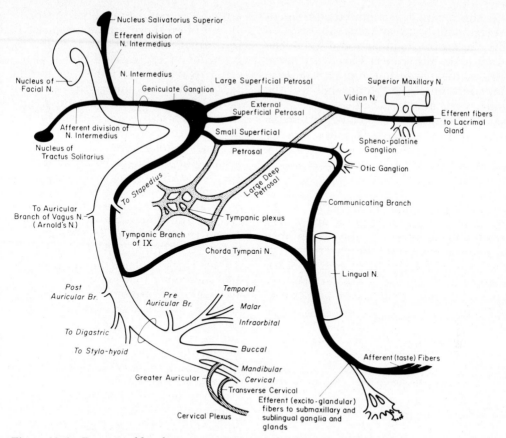

Figure 13–2 Diagram of facial nerve connections with other nerves. The facial nerve connects with the fifth cranial nerve through the large superficial and large deep petrosal nerves, which join the vidian nerve. The small petrosal passes through the otic ganglion. The chorda tympani joins the lingual nerve. The tympanic branch of the cranial nerve in the middle ear (Jacobsen nerve) connects with the facial nerve. The auricular branch of the vagus (Arnold nerve) connects with the facial nerve. The cervical plexus connects with the peripheral branches of the facial nerve in the neck and lower face. (Modified from Warwick, R., and Williams, P. L., 1979. Gray's Anatomy, 36th ed. Philadelphia, W. B. Saunders Co.

tympanic segment of the facial nerve lies just above the pyramidal eminence, which houses the stapedius muscle. This segment is approximately 12 mm long. At the beginning of the tympanic segment, the fallopian canal forms a prominent, rounded eminence between the bony horizontal semicircular canal and the niche of the oval window. The tympanic wall of this part of the fallopian canal is thin and easily fractured. In addition, there are frequent dehiscences present, allowing contact between the nerve and the tympanic mucoperiosteum. In some patients, the uncovered nerve is prolapsed into the oval window niche, partly or completely concealing the footplate of the stapes and, therefore, subject to trauma during stapes surgery. (The surgeon must look for this anomaly when there is a congenital deformity of the incus

and stapes superstructure. It is also worthwhile to palpate the horizontal segment of the facial nerve in performing middle ear or tympanomastoid surgery in order to determine whether the nerve is covered by bone or if there is a dehiscence in the fallopian canal.)

Just distal to the pyramidal eminence, the fallopian aqueduct makes another turn downward, the second genu. The second genu is another area where the facial nerve may be injured during mastoid surgery. The nerve emerges from the middle ear between the posterior canal wall and the horizontal semicircular canal, just beneath the short process of the incus. In the presence of chronic infection, where granulation tissue is present, one must be very careful not to confuse a pathologic dehiscence of the facial nerve in this region with a mound of granulation tissue. The best way to avoid this is to identify the nerve proximal and distal to the area that looks suspicious. The facial nerve gives off its third branch, the motor nerve to the stapedius muscle, at the distal end of the tympanic segment.

Mastoid Segment. The fallopian canal aqueduct proceeds vertically down the anterior wall of the mastoid process to the stylomastoid foramen. The distance from the second genu to the foramen averages 13 mm.

The chorda tympani nerve, which is the fourth branch of the facial nerve and its last sensory branch and thus the terminal branch of the intermedius nerve, usually arises from the distal third of the mastoid segment of the facial nerve, runs upward and anteriorly over the incus and under the malleus, and crosses the tympanic cavity through the petrotympanic fissure to join the lingual nerve. The chorda tympani contains secretory motor fibers to the submaxillary and sublingual glands: it also contains sensory fibers from the anterior two-thirds of the tongue (taste) and from the posterior wall of the external auditory meatus (pain, temperature, and touch).

Extracranial Segment. The facial nerve leaves the fallopian canal at the stylomastoid foramen, lateral to the styloid and vaginal processes. In newborns and in children up to two years of age, the facial nerve as it exits the skull is just deep to the subcutaneous tissue underlying the skin; after two years of age, as the mastoid tip and tympanic ring form, the facial nerve takes a deeper position up to 2 cm from the level of the skin.

Beyond the age of two years, the facial nerve is protected by the tympanic bone, the mastoid tip, the ascending ramus of the mandible, and the fascia between the parotid and cartilaginous external canal. In this region there are branches from the occipital artery and a venous plexus, which account for brisk bleeding when this area is entered in the process of approaching the facial nerve. (Meticulous hemostasis during surgery can be achieved without injuring the facial nerve, which lies deep to these vessels by employing a bipolar cautery.) As the nerve exits the stylomastoid foramen, nerve branches to the digastric and stylohyoid and postauricular muscles are given off. The seventh nerve communicates with branches from the ninth and tenth cranial nerves as well as with the auriculotemporal branch of the fifth nerve. In addition, there are anastomoses between the great auricular and lesser occipital branches of the cervical plexus (Fig. 13–2). After exiting the stylomastoid foramen, the facial nerve runs anteriorly for about 2 cm before bifurcating into an upper and lower division; both divisions run through the substance of the parotid gland, passing over the external jugular vein. After emerging from the parotid gland, the facial nerve passes over the fascia of the masseter muscle, and although its course in this region is variable, there are some relationships that are relatively constant. There are communications between the upper and lower divisions in the majority of patients (Anson and Donaldson, 1973), which explains the faulty regeneration that sometimes follows injuries to the nerve in this region. (Symptoms of faulty regeneration include synkinesis, evidenced by mouth movement with blinking or eye closure with smiling.) This undesirable complication can be discouraged to a great extent by dividing and clipping these anastomotic branches during reanimation surgery.

In the newborn and infant, the marginal mandibular nerve, which innervates the lower lip, courses over the mandible and is very superficial and quite vulnerable to injury. This is in contrast to the course of this branch in the adult, where the nerve is up to 2 cm or more below the angle of the jaw (Sammarco et al., 1966).

The upper division of the facial nerve courses over the fascia covering the *zygomatic arch* and is anterior to the *superficial temporal artery and vein.* The branches to the midface cross over the buccal compartment and deep to the facial muscles. At this point, there is widespread intermingling of nerve fibers with duplication of fibers innervating the same areas. This duplication allows for injuries in the periphery to recover by peripheral sprouting without any noticeable deficit. In addition, it allows surgically for borrowing from the extra branches for cross-face reinnervation.

There are also free communications between the peripheral segments of each of the branches of the facial nerve with each of the divisions of the trigeminal nerve. This free intermingling between the fifth and seventh nerves has been proposed as a mechanism for spontaneous return of facial nerve function following unrepaired peripheral injuries to the nerve. Based on clinical and laboratory

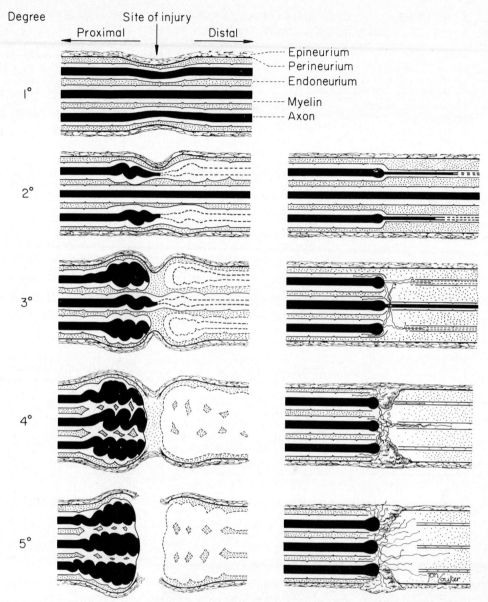

Figure 13–3   Facial nerve injuries may be classified by the extent of the lesion, from first-degree (1°) to fifth-degree (5°). 1°—compression; 2°—interruption of axoplasm; 3°—disruption of myelin; 4°—perineurium, myelin, and axons disrupted; and 5°—nerve transected. 1° to 3° injuries can occur with compressive lesions such as Bell palsy, infection, and temporal bone fractures. Recovery is complete in 1°, complete in 2° but it takes longer; and incomplete in 3° with recovery taking two to six months. 4° to 5° injuries occur with direct trauma, as with surgery or temporal bone fractures. Recovery is unlikely without surgical treatment.

experiments, it is generally agreed that the only possible regenerative role of these anastomoses is in providing available roots for the facial nerve to regrow through aberrant and communicating pathways, eventually to reach the denervated facial muscles. There has been no evidence to support the fifth nerve nucleus and its axonal extensions as an alternate system for facial mimicking and expressive functions.

PATHOPHYSIOLOGY OF INJURY AND CLASSIFICATION OF FACIAL FUNCTION RECOVERY

Nerve injuries due to Bell palsy and other compressive lesions may result in a first-, second-, or third-degree injury to the nerve (Fig. 13–3, Table 13–3). There will be complete recovery with a first-degree injury (Fig. 13–4), fair return with a second-degree injury

Table 13–3 NEUROPATHOLOGY AND SPONTANEOUS RECOVERY CORRELATED WITH DEGREE OF INJURY TO THE FACIAL NERVE

Degree of Injury	Pathology	Neural Recovery	Clinical Recovery Begins	Spontaneous Recovery— Result One Year Post-injury
1	Compression, damming of axoplasm No morphologic changes (neuropraxia)	No morphologic changes noted	1–3 weeks	Group I Complete, without evidence of faulty regeneration
2	Compression persists Increased intraneural pressure Loss of axons but endoneurial tubes remain intact (axonotmesis)	Axons grow into intact, empty myelin tubes at a rate of 1 mm/day, which accounts for longer period for recovery in 2° injuries compared to 1°; less than complete recovery is due to some fibers with a 3° injury	3 weeks and 2 months	Group II Fair (some noticeable difference with volitional or spontaneous movement, minimal evidence of faulty regeneration
3	Intraneural pressure increases—loss of myelin tubes (neurotmesis)	With loss of myelin tubes the new axons have an opportunity to get mixed up and split, causing mouth movement with eye closure, referred to as synkinesis	2–4 months	Group III Moderate to poor (obvious incomplete recovery to crippling deformity—with moderate to marked complications)
4	Above plus disruption of perineurium (partial transection)	In addition to problems caused by 2° and 3° injuries, now the axons are blocked by scars, impairing regeneration	4–18 months	Group IV Recovery less than Group III and complications of faulty regeneration more severe
5	Above plus disruption of epineurium (transection)	Complete disruption with a scar-filled gap presents an insurmountable barrier to regrowth and neuromuscular hook-up	None	Group V None

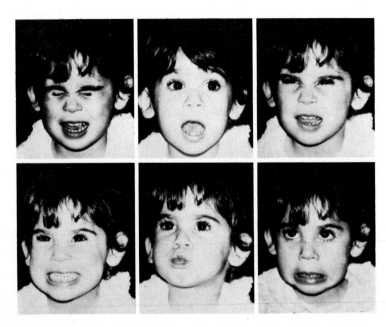

Figure 13–4 Example of fair recovery six months following Bell palsy. Upper photographs suggest complete recovery. Lower photographs taken at same time demonstrate incomplete recovery. This series of photographs stresses the importance of including pictures of facial movement that are exaggerated in order to give accurate evaluation.

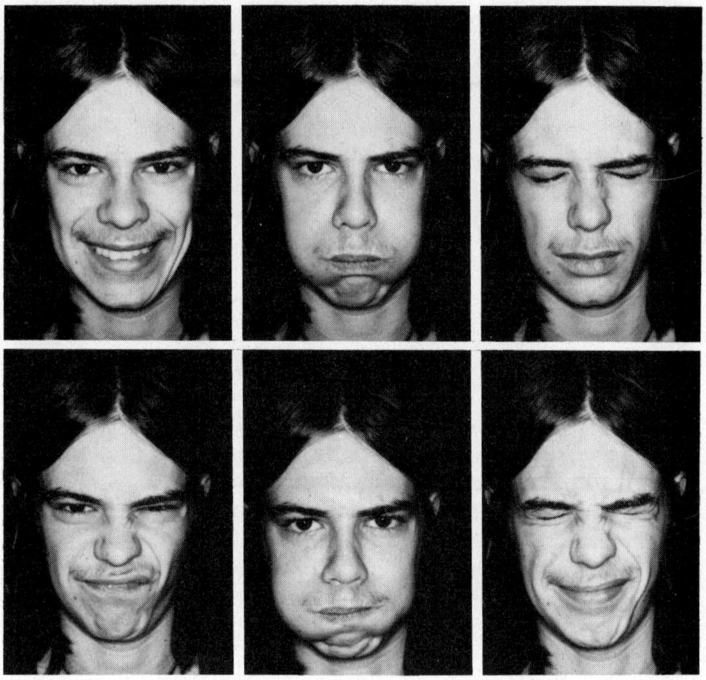

Figure 13–5 This figure shows recovery from a second-degree injury to the facial nerve.

(Fig. 13–5), and a poor return of facial function with a third-degree injury (Fig. 13–6).

Complete recovery is defined as no perceptible difference between the involved and the normal side of the face and no evidence of faulty regeneration as demonstrated by tic, spasm, or synkinesis (Fig. 13–4). Incomplete recovery can be fair or poor. *Fair return* implies incomplete recovery of facial motor

function that is just noticeable and with very mild complications, causing minimal functional and cosmetic impairment (Fig. 13–5). *Poor return* implies markedly incomplete return of facial motor function that is easily noticeable and is accompanied by severe complications of faulty regeneration, such as tic, spasm, and synkinesis (Fig. 13–6).

The final evaluation of the degree of facial

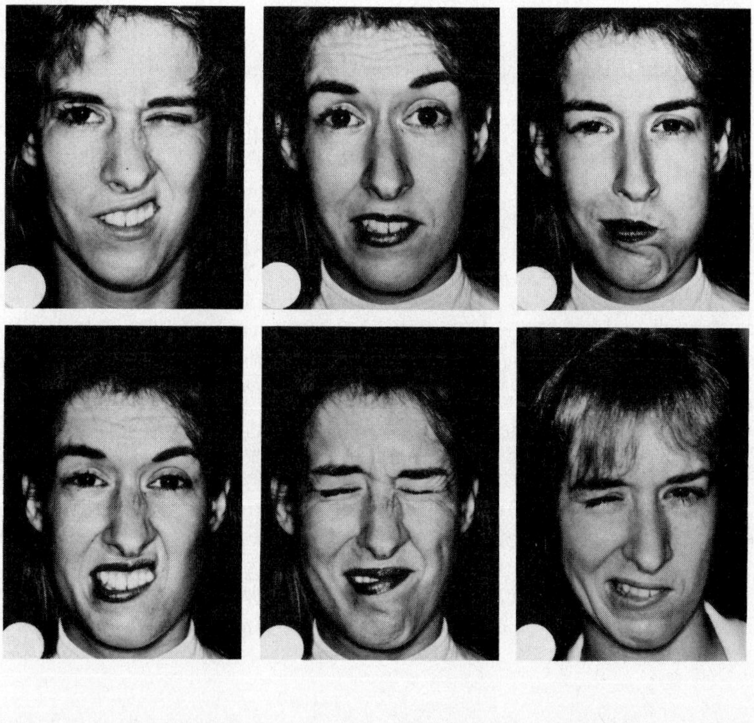

Figure 13–6 Example of poor recovery six months following Bell palsy. The injury in this case was third-degree. (Courtesy of Laryngoscope).

motor recovery in the first three degrees of injury requires a minimum follow-up period of six months after onset of the paralysis to be valid.

Fourth- and fifth-degree neural injuries (Fig. 13–3, Table 13–3) repaired following a tear or transection require a longer follow-up period for evaluation of results. These patients should be followed for a minimum of two years before final evaluation since recovery will continue over this length of time following repair of severed nerves. The classification system used for evaluating return of function of these injuries describes them as: (1) *excellent* when symmetry, eye closure, and mouth movement return; (2) *good* when symmetry and either eye closure or mouth movement return; (3) *fair* when only facial symmetry returns; and (4) *poor* when there is no change in facial symmetry, eye closure, or mouth movement and the patient has a flaccid face.

PROGNOSTIC TESTS

Evaluation of the Intermediate Nerve of Wrisberg

Tear Test

A marked reduction or absolute absence of tear production on the involved side is one of the most accurate topognostic and prognostic determinations in a patient with peripheral facial nerve paralysis. The pathologic decrease or absence of tears on the involved side indicates a lesion at or proximal to the geniculate ganglion. Ninety per cent of our patients with Bell palsy who had loss of tearing on the involved side had severe degeneration and faulty regeneration, which resulted in facial crippling (May and Hardin, 1978).

Tear production must be tested since a history of a dry eye is not reliable. Newborns and young children can be evaluated reliably by observing them during crying: If there is no tear production on the involved side, this is a pathologic sign, and no further testing is required.

Evaluation of tear production may lead to erroneous results if not carefully performed. An excess of tearing might often be more apparent than real, owing to the effects of the pathologic condition. For instance, Horner's muscle, which dilates the lacrimal sac, may be paralyzed, or there may be outward displacement of the opening of the nasolacrimal duct due to orbicularis oculi muscle weakness, which results in ectropion. Possibly lack of muscle tone of the lower lid might allow it to fall slightly away from the globe, producing an increased volume of the inferior conjunctival cul-de-sac; or an excess of tears may be caused by irritation of the exposed eye. Finally, paralysis of the orbicularis oculi muscle causes a defect in the lacrimal pump, inactivating the fine slips of muscle that lie just under the skin along the upper and lower eyelids and that insert on the medial canthus and close the lid; this allows tears to pass across the edges of the lids toward the superior and inferior canaliculi. The opening and closing of the eyelids as a result of contraction and relaxation of the orbicularis oculi muscle dilate and contract the lacrimal sac, which is thought to be responsible for emptying the tears into the nose and then drawing the tears into the sac.

A method to quantify tearing was based on the nasolacrimal reflex. Filter paper strips (Schirmer test strips) can be purchased from the Crookes-Barnes Laboratories, Inc., Wayne, New Jersey, or can be fashioned so that they are 3.5 cm long and 0.5 cm wide. These strips are then folded at one end so that the folded tab can be placed over the lower lid, in the conjunctival sac, leaving 3 cm to absorb the tears produced. Placing the filter paper strip in the normal side first is advised since if the paper is placed in the paralyzed side first, the irritation of the paper will cause a reflex contraction on the normal side, leading to difficulty placing the paper slip in the normal eye; these strong reflex contractions do not occur on the paralyzed side. It is important to empty the sacs with a piece of cotton prior to inserting the strips to avoid erroneous results from pooled or excess tears that may be present in the involved side prior to the start of a test. Once the strips are in place, the patient is asked to take a sniff of fresh spirits of ammonia, which sets up a nasolacrimal reflex. The filter paper strips are left in place for a period of three minutes or until one strip is completely moistened, at which time the strips are removed and the amount of liquid on each is noted. The test results are considered abnormal if the strip from the affected side has 25 per cent or less liquid than the strip from the normal side.

The tear test is most accurate if absolutely no tears are produced on the involved side over a period of three minutes. This is considered to represent a dry eye, and portends a poor prognosis. Over 90 per cent of the patients we have seen with Bell palsy or herpes zoster oticus and a dry eye had faulty recovery of facial nerve function and suffered a crippling facial defect. Surgical decompression of the geniculate and labyrinthine segments of the facial nerve before loss of response to electrical stimulation was the only form of therapy that favorably altered the outcome.

Salivation Test

The submandibular salivary flow test is the most useful prognostic indicator in cases of acute peripheral facial paralysis since salivary flow, like tear flow, may become reduced within two days of onset of the paralysis in patients who are likely to develop denervation. Since results of electrical tests do not become altered until later, it is important to perform the salivary flow test in order to intervene before the results of denervation become irreversible.

The salivation test can be done in the office with inexpensive material: lemon juice, lacrimal punctum dilators (Wilder, long taper, medium taper, and short taper, and Ruedeman dilator); No. 50 polyethylene tubing; and the wire stylet that comes with a No. 5 suction tip. The flow of saliva is measured by cannulating Wharton's duct on each side with the No. 50 polyethylene tube. First, the area in the region of the salivary puncta is infiltrated submucosally with 1 per cent xylocaine and 1:100,000 epinephrine. The ducts may be found in either side of the frenulum at the anterior extreme of the plica sublingualis by drying the mucosa with compressed air to identify them by the first drop of saliva as it forms. By probing gently with the long, tapered slider dilator, the ducts may be enlarged for cannulation. Care must be taken not to form a false channel. If this technique is not successful, an operating binocular microscope may help to identify the ducts; when even this fails, the coruncle with the punctum and the meatus may be nipped off to allow easy identification of the submandibular salivary gland duct. The duct should be cannulated by passing the polyethylene tube over the stylet that is used to clean the No. 5 suction tube, allowing the stylet to protrude several millimeters beyond the polyethylene tube. When the stylet has been placed in the duct, the polyethylene tube may be twisted

off the stylet into the duct and the stylet removed. When both salivary ducts have been cannulated, a piece of cotton saturated with lemon juice is placed in the mouth. The tubes are held in place by the patient's closed lips and crossed so that the tube in the right side comes out of the left side of the mouth, and the one in the left duct comes out of the right side of the mouth. This prevents kinking of the tubes against the mucosa of the ducts. One must see a flow of saliva from both tubes in order to be sure that a false channel has not been created and that the tubes are properly placed in the ducts. The test is recorded as a percentage of normal obtained by dividing the number of drops of saliva on the involved side by the number of drops on the normal side and multiplying by 100. Once the drops begin to flow following stimulation with the lemon juice, they are counted from each side for 60 seconds or until the combined total of drops from both sides equals 20. This is repeated three times, and the results are averaged. When salivary flow was reduced to 25 per cent or less, 88 per cent of the patients had incomplete return of facial nerve function. When salivary flow was 26 to 49 per cent of normal, 66 per cent of the patients had incomplete return, and when salivary flow was 50 per cent or greater on the involved side, only 22 per cent of the patients had incomplete return of facial function (May et al., 1976a). Salivary flow is a very useful prognostic indicator when the patients are seen within the first few days after the onset of facial palsy and before electrical tests become altered. Once electrical tests become altered, the salivary flow test has no significance (May et al., 1976a).

Evaluation of Facial Motor Fibers by Electrical Tests

The problem for the clinician who sees a patient with facial paralysis of recent onset is to determine whether the involved nerve is mildly compressed and is in a state of first-degree injury from which it will recover spontaneously, or whether there is beginning, second-degree injury which will go on to third-degree injury involving the entire nerve trunk if pressure is not relieved. There are three electrical tests that are useful clinically: the maximal percutaneous excitability test (MST), electroneurography, and electromyography. The first two tests are capable of detecting early or ensuing degeneration, while the last test becomes useful once degeneration has occurred. The first two tests are useful in the first week following onset of facial nerve paralysis, while the last test becomes useful by the tenth to the fourteenth day following the onset of paralysis.

Maximal Stimulation Test

This test is based upon the fact that a motor nerve will conduct in response to an electrical stimulus applied distal to a lesion, even though the lesion blocks volitional movement, provided the nerve is morphologically intact distal to the lesion (i.e., the injury is first-degree). When the injury is second-degree, causing damage to the axon, an increase in the intensity of the stimulus is required to cause a muscle twitch. If the myelin and axon distal to the lesion degenerated, as with a third-degree injury, then no conduction will occur no matter how intense the stimulus. It has been shown that a completely sectioned nerve may continue to conduct distal to the section for as long as 48 to 72 hours after the injury. For this reason, the MST has limited value until 48 to 72 hours after the onset of the paralysis. In addition, MST is only of value as long as the nerve remains intact. Once the nerve degenerates and response to electrical excitability is lost, the test is no longer useful. Duchenne (1872), who first suggested the excitability test, stated that when excitability is lost after degeneration, it returns in only a minority of cases, even if there is recovery and return of volitional movement. Another limitation of this test is the need to compare the results of the involved side to the normal side, which acts as a control. Thus, in cases of recurrent palsy or alternating bilateral involvement the test has limited value.

The excitability test can be performed with any electrical stimulus in which the strength and duration can be varied. The Hilger nerve stimulator is especially designed to test the facial nerve. (Model 2r with a rechargeable battery is favored by the author: the instrument is conveniently portable, allowing for bedside consultation, and testing can be performed in several minutes without discomfort to the patient.) The test is performed by setting the intensity at 5 ma, or the highest setting tolerated by the patient without undue discomfort. An area of the patient's skin between the sideburns and the eyebrow and extending down over the cheek, jaw, and neck is wiped with electrode conduction paste. Then the stimulating probe is passed slowly over this area. The responses over the forehead, eye, nose, mouth, lower lip, and neck are noted and recorded as equal, decreased, or absent on the involved side, as compared to the normal side. The test is repeated by stimulating at the area of the stylomastoid foramen, between the mastoid tip and the ascending ramus. Since degeneration proceeds from proximal to distal, evidence of degeneration might be detected a couple of days earlier by testing at the site where the facial nerve exits the temporal bone. The nerve is tested more peripherally in order to evaluate each major branch, which cannot be done by testing only in the area of the stylomastoid foramen.

The maximal stimulation test, as described, was more reliable and became altered earlier than did the percutaneous electrical stimulation test, which depends upon looking for a 3.5 ma difference in excitability between the two sides (May et al., 1971). The maximal stimulation test, although quite useful, was not completely accurate in predicting the patient's ultimate degree of recovery. When the response to maximal stimulation was equal, 12 per cent of the patients had incomplete return and when the response to MST was decreased, 73 per cent of the patients had incomplete return of facial function. The test was most accurate when MST was lost: In this case all patients had incomplete return with marked evidence of faulty regeneration (May et al., 1976a).

The rationale for testing each major facial motor area supplied by the nerve is based on the orientation of the facial nerve fibers as they course through the temporal bone (May, 1973). Certain fibers can be affected more than others depending upon the nature, location, and severity of the lesion. (We have observed a first-degree injury in one part of the face and a third-degree injury in another part.) This has been noted in acute cases as well as during the phase of recovery (May, 1973). Electrical evidence of denervation involving any part of the nerve is an indication for surgical exploration, and one should not wait for the entire nerve to become involved. In acute involvement of the facial nerve, as with paralysis following trauma or infection, ideally the electrical test should be repeated daily until the response to MST becomes abnormal or return of volitional facial movement is noted.

Electroneurography (ENoG)

ENoG is the recording of evoked summation potentials and was popularized by Fisch and Esslen (1972). In principle, it is similar to the maximal stimulation test (MST) except that, instead of depending upon visual observation of the degree of muscle twitch elicited, evoked summating potentials (SP) are recorded on a graph produced by a sophisticated electrodiagnostic apparatus, the direct recording electromyograph. The amount of degeneration is related to the difference in amplitude of the measured SP's on the normal and involved sides.

The great advantage of ENoG over the simple observation of facial movements as described under maximal stimulation is the precise quantitative assessment of the response available with ENoG.

Fisch (1977b) recommended surgical exposure of the intratemporal portion of the facial nerve (1) in traumatic lesions when the amplitude of the SP became reduced to 10 per cent or less of the normal side within six days after the onset of the palsy; (2) in idiopathic (Bell) palsy as soon as the SP became reduced to 10 per cent or less of the normal side within two weeks of onset of the palsy or in the presence of a lesser reduction when inner ear symptoms are present; and (3) in acute otitis media when there is a reduction to 10 per cent or less in spite of paracentesis and antibiotic treatment.

ENoG is a welcome contribution to help document accurately the·electrical changes in an injured nerve, but unfortunately it has the same disadvantages as have been noted with MST. Furthermore, waiting until the SPs become reduced to 10 per cent of normal may preclude intervention at an appropriate time to reverse nerve damage. We suggest considering surgery for those patients who show a reduction to 25 per cent or less of normal in an effort to effect complete recovery of facial nerve function. This cannot be achieved if one waits until there is reduction to 10 per cent as suggested by Fisch and Esslen (1972).

Electromyography (EMG)

EMG is indispensable once degeneration occurs, as a measure of damage to the nerve.

A denervated muscle, being hyperirritable, produces spontaneous electrical potentials, referred to as fibrillation potentials, which can be measured. Usually, these fibrillation potentials do not appear until 10 to 21 days after degeneration occurs. Although the time delay is a major limitation in the application of EMG, it is the most reliable test to determine nerve degeneration since it samples motor unit activity. When the motor unit is intact, a motor unit potential can be detected with volitional movement. When this is demonstrated following trauma, nerve transection can be ruled out. Reappearance of motor unit potentials after degeneration of a nerve is one of the first signs of regeneration. Often, this can be detected before volitional movement is noted.

Other Prognostic Indicators

Prognostic evaluation of a particular case of facial paralysis must be based, in addition to tear, salivary flow, and electrical tests, on the history of onset, the duration of palsy, and the completeness of the paralysis. The progression of paresis to complete paralysis over a period of 3 to 10 days is a poor prognostic sign. Seventy-five per cent of the patients with this type of history developed degeneration with incomplete return (May et al., 1976a). The maintenance of some facial movement, or the early return of facial movement within the first two weeks of onset, indicates a very favorable prognosis for spontaneous recovery in spite of the presence of abnormal prognostic indicators such as abnormal tear and submandibular salivary flow or electrical tests.

DIAGNOSIS AND PROGNOSIS BY TOPOGNOSTIC TESTS

Localizing the site of involvement is a great aid in determining the diagnosis. Specific neurologic signs (listed in Table 13–2) and the results of topognostic tests outlined in Figure 13–1 will help in this process. Once the lesion has been localized and its severity determined from the results of the tearing, salivary flow, maximal stimulation, and electroneurography tests, it will be possible to establish a prognosis.

Tschiassny (1953) proposed a scheme designed to localize eight levels of involvement on the basis of distinctive syndromes associated with facial paralysis. Tschiassny's scheme, designed over 20 years ago, still has validity today but must be revised to incorporate new concepts and observations. For instance, Tschiassny suggested that supranuclear syndromes are distinguished mainly by sparing of the forehead musculature, but there are many signs other than sparing of the forehead that are more reliable in pinpointing a cortical lesion; in addition, sparing of the forehead alone is not an exclusive sign of a cortical lesion (May, 1973).

The major limitations of Tschiassny's (1953) scheme for involvement of the facial nerve at the level of the nucleus and more peripherally are based upon the following: (1) the facial nerve anatomy is not constant, but rather variable; (2) lesions involving the facial nerve may not be sharply localized; (3) lesions may not affect all components of the facial nerve at a particular level to an equal extent; and (4) it is difficult to evaluate the adequacy of the stapedial reflex, lacrimation, and even salivation because of technical problems. Tschiassny (1953), commenting on the limitations of his scheme, noted that it could be applied with reliability only to early lesions. Further, it should be kept in mind that, as a lesion evolves, some functions may be lost while others initially lost may be recovering and that each function may become altered at different times in the course of an individual disease.

Topognostic tests are most valid for localizing lesions that occur with severe injuries, such as tumors or trauma, and are least reliable with diffuse lesions that may ascend or descend and vary in intensity and progression over 5 to 10 days, as with Bell palsy and herpes zoster oticus.

Attempts to localize the site of a lesion by looking for neurologic signs and testing hearing, balance, tearing, the stapes reflex, taste, and salivary flow, as well as electrical testing by maximal stimulation or electroneurography, are more than academic exercises. Such evaluations are done routinely on patients suffering from facial nerve paralysis because they represent the absolute minimum that can be done to evaluate and formulate a plan for managing such patients.

MANAGEMENT OF FACIAL PARALYSIS: GENERAL PRINCIPLES

The patient with facial paralysis or his or her family usually asks three questions: (1) What caused the facial paralysis? (2) When can recovery be expected? (3) What can be done to bring about recovery at the earliest possible time? These three questions can be translated into the medical tasks of: (1) making a diagnosis, (2) determining the prognosis, and (3) recommending treatment.

Diagnosis

The diagnosis can be made in a majority of cases by a careful history and physical examination, as well as by neuro-otologic evaluation. It should be emphasized that *Bell palsy is a diagnosis of exclusion* and should be used only when all other causes of facial paralysis have been eliminated.

Facial paralysis due to acute and chronic suppurative infection usually can be diagnosed by the presence of ear pain and by a bulging, red tympanic membrane in acute suppurative otitis media and a fetid mucoid discharge or evidence of a *cholesteatoma* in chronic otitis media.

Facial paralysis associated with a closed head injury is diagnostic of a *temporal bone fracture*. Tuning forks can distinguish between a conductive and a sensorineural hearing loss: a conductive hearing loss usually indicates a longitudinal fracture with sparing of the one capsule, whereas a sensorineural hearing loss is diagnostic of a transverse fracture with violation of the otic capsule.

A tumor as a cause of facial paralysis should be suspected if (1) the paralysis is slowly progressive beyond three weeks; (2) the paralysis is recurrent on the same side; or (3) there is no recovery from an acute facial paralysis after six months. Examination of the nasopharynx, tonsil, parotid, and neck, as well as of the area between the ascending ramus and mastoid tip, might discover a neoplasm that could involve the facial nerve.

The presence of vesicles on the pinna, face, or oral mucosa suggests herpes zoster oticus, which may also be associated with dysequilibrium and a sensorineural hearing loss. The onset of a simultaneous bilateral facial paralysis excludes Bell palsy and suggests Guillain-Barré syndrome, bulbar palsy, sarcoidosis, or some other systemic disorder. A detailed, general neurologic examination usually reveals other neurologic signs in such patients.

Pregnancy, especially in the third trimester, is significant in the evaluation of facial paralysis. It has been reported by Adout et al. (1978) that facial paralysis of the Bell palsy type has a three to four times higher incidence among pregnant women, particularly those in the third trimester, than in nonpregnant women of the same age group. Further, the prognosis for spontaneous recovery of facial function is not as good in pregnant as in nonpregnant women.

Recurrent facial paralysis occurs in 10 per cent of patients with Bell palsy, but when it recurs on the same side the presence of a tumor must be considered. Melkersson-Rosenthal syndrome is characterized by the presence of a fissured tongue, alternating bilateral facial palsy associated with facial edema, and a positive family history.

Bell palsy is the likely diagnosis when other causes have been excluded and in those patients with one or more of the following: (1) a positive family history of facial paralysis; (2) a viral prodrome; or (3) the presence of a red chorda tympani nerve. Of the patients we treated, 13 per cent who were diagnosed as having Bell palsy had a positive family history for that illness; 60 per cent had had a viral prodrome; and a red chorda tympani nerve was noted in 40 per cent of those patients whose chorda tympani nerve was visible (May, 1974).

Although Bell palsy has been thought of as a mononeuropathy, there is clinical evidence that many nerves are involved (May and Hardin, 1978). This impression is supported by decreased or lost corneal sensation; presence of pain or numbness over the side of the head, ear, face, neck, and shoulder; and numbness of the tongue in patients with Bell palsy (Fig. 13–7). The loss of corneal sensation may be due to direct involvement of the fifth nerve endings innervating the conjunctiva or due to exposure hypesthesia. The changes in sensation may be explained by involvement of nerves that connect with the facial nerve. These include branches of the cervical plexus, ninth nerve, tenth nerve, and fifth nerve (Fig. 13–2).

The presence of intact, symmetrical upper facial movements has been noted with acute suppurative otitis media, temporal bone fractures, and lower motor neuron lesions such as Bell palsy and therefore is not an exclusive diagnostic sign of a central lesion (May, 1973).

Prognosis

Once the diagnosis has been established, the prognosis can be made with 90 per cent accuracy, even in patients seen within the first

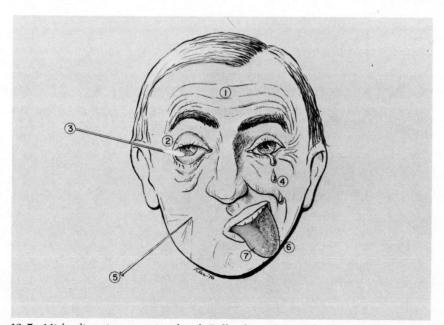

Figure 13–7 Misleading signs associated with Bell palsy: (1) intact forehead, (2) Horner syndrome (constricted pupil and ptosis of upper eyelid), (3) loss of corneal sensation, (4) tearing only on uninvolved side, (5) loss of skin sensation, (6) apparent tongue deviation, (7) loss of taste papillae. (Courtesy of Laryngoscope.)

Table 13–4   PERIPHERAL FACIAL PARALYSIS: CORRELATION OF NEUROPATHOLOGY, PROGNOSTIC TESTS RESULTS, RECOMMENDED TREATMENT, AND NATURAL HISTORY IN THOSE LESIONS INVOLVING THE FACIAL NERVE

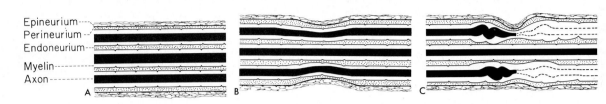

		Group I	Group II
Neuropathology		(ONSET TO THIRD DAY)	(THIRD TO FIFTH DAY)
EPINEURIUM			
PERINEURIUM			
ENDONEURIUM	NORMAL		
MYELIN		1°	2°
AXON	Figure A	Figure B	Figure C
Seddon classification		Neurapraxia	Neurapraxia-axonotmesis
Sunderland classification		First degree	First to second degree
Histologic findings		Damming of proximal and distal flow of axoplasm	Disruption of axons
Prognostic Tests			
Lacrimation		≥ 70%	≤ 25%
Salivation		≥ 70%	≤ 25%
Maximal stimulation		Equal =	↓
Electroneurography		Equal =	≥ 50%
Recommended Treatment		Eye care, sedation, no steroids Analgesics, reassurance Incomplete paralysis: reevaluate in one week; if becomes complete return immediately for reevaluation Complete paralysis: reevaluate and retest every other day until recovery noted or tests indicate Group II	Supportive care as Group I Surgical decompression to labyrinthine segment
Natural History		Complete recovery beginning 7–10 days	Fair recovery: incomplete recovery with minimal cosmetic and functional impairment, beginning 3 weeks to 2 months.
Surgical Results			
Technique Open to endoneurium proximal and distal to lesion before loss of electrical response			Complete recovery beginning 7–10 days after surgery

Epineurium
Perineurium
Endoneurium
Myelin
Axon
A   B   C

Table 13-4 PERIPHERAL FACIAL PARALYSIS: CORRELATION OF NEUROPATHOLOGY, PROGNOSTIC TESTS RESULTS, RECOMMENDED TREATMENT, AND NATURAL HISTORY IN THOSE LESIONS INVOLVING THE FACIAL NERVE (*Continued*)

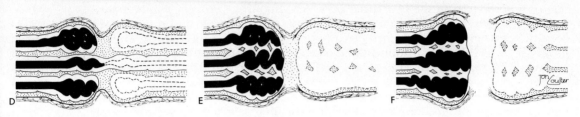

	Group III	Group IV	Group V
	(FIFTH TO FOURTEENTH DAY)		
	3° Figure D	4° Figure E	5° Figure F
	Axonotmesis-neurotmesis	Neurotmesis	Neurotmesis
	Second to third degree	Third to fourth degree	Fifth degree
	Disruption of axons and myelin tubes	Disruption of perineurium, myelin tubes and axons	Disruption of epineurium, perineurium, myelin, and axons
	Dry eye	Absent if lesion at or proximal to geniculate ganglion	
	≤ 25%	≤ 25%	
	↓ ↓ /0	Response lost 2–3 days	
	≤ 25%	Response lost 3–5 days	
	Same as Group II: surgical decompression to labyrinthine segment	Ideally, explore and repair immediately or within 30 days	
	Poor recovery: obvious incomplete recovery with marked complications of faulty regeneration—tic, spasms, synkinesis—beginning 2–4 months	If nerve is completely severed, some spontaneous recovery may occur in rare instances. If incompletely severed, recovery may occur but results in marked facial weakness with no recovery of parts of face and mass movement	
	Fair recovery beginning 3 weeks to 2 months	Surgical repair within 30 days (90%): excellent (symmetry, eye and mouth movement); or good (symmetry, eye or mouth movement), beginning 4–10 months	

few days after onset of facial paralysis. The determination of tear production and sub-mandibular salivary flow are the most accurate prognostic tests in the first three days. A reduction in tear production or salivary flow below 25 per cent of normal portends a poor prognosis, which has been found to be accurate in over 90 per cent of cases (May, 1978a, 1978b).

The presence or absence of taste or pain has not been of prognostic value. The presence of a stapes reflex is a favorable sign provided the lesion is not distal to the pyramidal segment of the facial nerve as noted with trauma or tumor involving the facial nerve in the vertical segment or in the extra-temporal bone region. Loss of stapes reflex did not have prognostic significance since it was commonly lost in patients with complete loss of facial movement and half of these patients had complete recovery without treatment.

After the first few days, electrical tests become valuable. Although they usually become altered by the third day in a transected nerve, they may not become altered until the fifth to the tenth day in a dynamic, slowly progressive lesion, such as is noted with Bell palsy, or a slowly compressive lesion due to infection or following trauma. When the response to maximum stimulation, electro-neurography, or both becomes reduced to 25 per cent or less of the normal side, in our experience the prognosis is poor for spontaneous, complete recovery.

The natural history of Bell palsy, the most common type of facial paralysis, has been established. Peiterson (1977), at the Facial Nerve Symposium held in Pittsburgh, reported the natural history of Bell palsy in 778 subjects. He divided the patients into three groups. Seventy per cent had complete recovery, 15 per cent had fair recovery, and 15 per cent had poor recovery from Bell palsy. These results have been confirmed by others as well as by our own studies (Olsen, 1975; May et al., 1976b). From these findings we have learned that 70 to 85 per cent of patients afflicted with Bell palsy will have complete to satisfactory recovery of facial nerve function.

The time that recovery is first noted is one of the most useful late prognostic indicators: (1) if recovery begins between the tenth day and the third week, with few exceptions, recovery will be complete; (2) if recovery does not begin until after three weeks but before two months, the majority of these patients will have fair recovery of function; and (3) if recovery does not begin until two to four months, recovery will be poor.

Progression and completeness of palsy during the first three weeks after onset have been found to have prognostic significance (May et al., 1976a). There are four distinct patterns of facial motor involvement that are almost evenly divided among all the patients with Bell palsy: (1) those with complete paralysis at onset have a 50 per cent chance of having incomplete recovery; (2) those with incomplete paralysis at onset and whose palsy does not progress will recover completely; (3) those with incomplete paralysis that progressed (but not to complete paralysis) will have complete recovery; and, finally, (4) those that present with incomplete paralysis that progresses to complete paralysis will have an incomplete recovery in 75 per cent of the cases.

These guidelines, which were derived from treating patients with Bell palsy, have been found to be just as valid for other disorders that cause compressive lesions of the facial nerve.

Treatment

Contrary to the opinion of most primary physicians, who see only an occasional case of facial paralysis that resolves without treatment, facial paralysis is a potential medical-surgical emergency. On occasion a patient who presents with a facial paralysis has an underlying, life-threatening disorder, and others spend their lives as facial cripples because treatment was not offered until death of the facial nerve was established by electrical tests. In Bell palsy, nerve death may occur between the fifth and tenth day after onset of paralysis, and in most severe cases denervation may occur as early as the first or second day. Treatment can be effective only if the nerve is treated at the earliest possible moment following onset of the paralysis. Therefore, facial paralysis is truly an emergency.

The rationale for treatment and expected results for the various lesions causing facial paralysis is based upon the existing neuropathology in each case (Table 13–4).

Eye. Considerations for management of the eye in patients with facial paralysis were discussed in detail by Levine (1974, 1979).

There are two major problems that result when eye closure is impaired: The eye becomes irritated owing to exposure, and this irritation is significantly compounded when tear production is impaired. Treatment is thus directed toward protecting the eye from exposure and drying. This can be accomplished by having the patient instill artificial tears every hour during waking hours and a bland ointment at night. The eye may also be protected by a moisture chamber* that either may be secured with a band or that may fit on the eyeglasses. A half-moon cutout of skintone micropore surgical tape acts as an effective splint for the upper eyelid, it should be placed with the dome toward the fold in the upper eyelid and the base along the eyelash margin. This often allows the patient to overcome the pull by the superior levator muscle and affords natural protection for the eye.

Eye care should be continued until return of spontaneous eye closure. Patients with acute facial paralysis who have a favorable prognosis can be managed adequately by the conservative treatment suggested. On rare occasions, surgical measures are necessary for patients who are developing eye complications in spite of conservative treatment, and especially when the prospects for recovery are very poor. The surgical techniques used involve reestablishing eye closure as well as tightening up the sagging lower eyelid.

*Optical Associates, Inc., 203 N. Meramac St., Clayton MO 63105. Phone 800–325–4160. Large with band (adult). small with band (child), clip-on-left or right for use with eyeglasses.

Pain. Patients with pain, particularly that associated with herpes zoster oticus or Bell palsy, often require analgesic medication for the first week and sometimes longer.

Depression. The emotional impact of facial palsy can be quite significant, particularly in the first few weeks, and must not be neglected. Reassurance may be offered to those patients who are expected to have a complete or satisfactory recovery, but if the prognosis is unfavorable, the patient should be advised of this possibility so that he or she does not develop an attitude of denial that leads him or her to deal unrealistically with residual deformity.

It is reassuring to patients with facial palsy of the acute compressive type, such as Bell, herpes zoster oticus, or acute otitis media, to learn that the face will not remain completely paralyzed, since some recovery is expected even in the most severe cases. The depression that accompanies the onset of the facial paralysis is often relieved by the prediction of a favorable outcome, as well as by a prediction as to when the recovery may be noted. Occasionally, temporary treatment with sedatives is helpful. Reassurance and support can be offered by arranging for the patient to share experiences with another person who had facial paralysis. If the depression persists in spite of this counseling, then psychiatric consultation should be considered.

Medications. Medications, such as vitamins or antihistamines, have no efficacious influence on the natural history of Bell palsy but may serve as psychological support. Patients often feel better when they know that

Table 13–5 STEROIDS INEFFECTIVE FOR BELL PALSY

Author(s)	Patients	Steroid Dose (mg/14 days)	Recovery Complete* Steroids	Controls	Comments
Peitersen (1977)	Consecutive 778	—		70%	Results represent natural history
May et al. (1976a)	Double blind Randomized 51	400	60%	65%	Difference not statistically significant
Wolf et al. (1978)	Randomized 239	760	88%	80%	Difference not statistically significant
Devriese (1977)	Consecutive 76	570	66%		Results not significantly better than achieved without treatment

*Studies quoted were controlled; patients were evaluated within 7 days, the majority within 3 days; and complete recovery was defined similarly as full volitional activity and absence of distortion at rest or upon volitional movement.

Table 13–6 POOR PROGNOSTIC INDICATORS FOR RECOVERY FROM FACIAL PARALYSIS

Test	Results
Tears*	≤25%
Submandibular flow	≤25%
Maximal stimulation test**	↓↓/0
Electroneurography	≤25% (75% degeneration)

*≤25% = reduced to 25% or less compared to the normal side.
**↓↓ = markedly decreased response
0 = no response.

SPECIAL CONSIDERATIONS IN MANAGING FACIAL PARALYSIS IN YOUNG CHILDREN

The principles involved in managing facial paralysis are the same for patients of all ages, perhaps excepting very young children (newborn to age five years). Facial paralysis noted at birth can be due to trauma or to a developmental anomaly. The distinction is important since the prognosis and treatment of each differs. Traumatic paralysis may require immediate surgical decompression or nerve repair, whereas the congenital type presents no urgency. Isolated involvement of the marginal mandibular branch of the facial nerve, noted at birth, might be associated with other congenital anomalies as reported by Pape and Pickering (1972). These authors stress that asymmetric crying facies, as evidenced by the lack of pulling down of the lower lip on the involved side, may signal the presence of congenital anomalies in the skeletal, genitourinary, respiratory, or cardiovascular systems.

Isolated unilateral paralysis, as noted with involvement of the marginal mandibular branch in a young child, may be associated with acute, suppurative otitis media (Fig. 13–8) and should be treated by myringotomy and administration of an appropriate antibiotic.

Prepubescent children, particularly those under 5 years of age, rarely are reliable in relating historical factors, such as alterations in sensation, hearing, balance, taste, tear production, or the presence of vesicles, all of which may be helpful in making a diagnosis.

they are taking a medication rather than relying on the physician's predictions alone. My personal preference is to prescribe vitamins to patients with a favorable prognosis. Steroids have no place in the management of facial paralysis, may cause serious complications, and often delay appropriate management. Table 13–5 summarizes the studies that demonstrate that the administration of steroids to patients with Bell palsy did not have any influence on recovery of facial function.

Surgery. Surgical exploration in acute cases is recommended for those patients who have an unfavorable prognosis determined by the presence of one or more unfavorable prognostic indicators (Table 13–6). The general principles that influence the decision for surgery as well as the procedure employed are outlined in Table 13–7.

Table 13–4 gives a summary of the general principles involved in evaluating and managing facial paralysis.

Table 13–7 RECOMMENDED MANAGEMENT OF BELL PALSY (PATIENTS EVALUATED WITHIN TEN DAYS OF ONSET OF FACIAL PARALYSIS)

	Medical Treatment	Surgical Treatment	Too Late
Tears	≥20%*	≤25%†	Response to ENOG and MST lost. Wait four to six months; if no recovery, explore to rule out tumor.
Submandibular flow	≥20%	≤25%	
Maximal stimulation test (MST)	=/↓**	↓↓‡	
Electroneurography (ENOG)	20%	≤25%	
	Eye care	Total surgical decompression	
	Analgesic	Transmastoid extralabyrinthine subtemporal	
	Sedative (no steroids)	or	
		Combined transmastoid middle fossa approach	

*≥ Equal to or greater than normal side
**=/↓ Equal or slightly decreased response
†≤ Equal to or less than normal side
‡↓↓ Marked decreased response

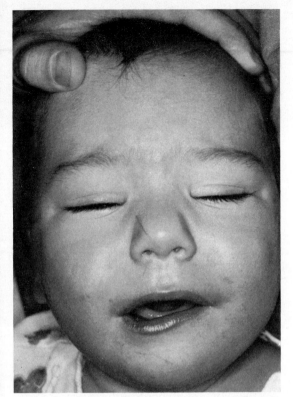

Figure 13–8 Palsy of left lower lip associated with acute suppurative otitis media involving the left ear.

This information might be obtained by questioning the parents, but it is interesting that even the most concerned parents are not always reliable historians. This observation is supported by evaluating young children with mild facial weakness that was not noted by the parents but was picked up by friends or teachers. However, some parents can provide useful information and must be questioned carefully regarding the time of onset of the crooked cry or whether tears formed on the involved side during crying. This is quite helpful in dating the onset of the paralysis as well as in assessing the involvement of tear production. Old photographs are another useful aid in documenting the presence of facial asymmetry that might have gone unnoticed.

Tests requiring subjective responses, such as audiometry and taste perception, may not be reliable in the young child. Measurement of evoked auditory brain stem potentials, however, may help to overcome these problems since the measurements depend on objective responses.

Evaluation of facial motor function is possible with children as young as 2 years of age who are very expressive and who will mimic facial expressions (Fig. 13–4). Although most require observation while spontaneous emotions are displayed, play therapy, tickling, and at times provoking crying, such as might occur with electrical testing, are quite useful in the evaluation of facial motor function and of tear production.

Taste testing may not be a reliable method of evaluating the integrity of the chorda tympani nerve in the young child. However, since the taste papillae in children are very prominent, one may easily note by inspection if the papillae have atrophied on the involved side, which implies that the chorda tympani nerve has been interrupted. A lesion involving the chorda tympani nerve that causes atrophy of the taste papillae may be the result of a disorder located anywhere between the middle ear and the brain stem.

Electrical tests may be used if the stimulus is kept below the pain threshold. Usually a stimulus in the range of 2 to 3 ma is tolerated by young children.

Maximal stimulation, electroneurography, and electromyographic testing have not been used successfully in young children without sedation or general anesthesia. This is usually true for the salivation test as well, although it has been successfully performed in a child as young as 6 years of age.

Eye care is usually not required in children. The exact reason for this is not known, but children born with facial paralysis who are unable to close the eye, and even those who suffer loss of tear production, rarely develop eye complications even without additional moisture or protection for the eye. It is interesting to note that young children (those between birth and age 5 years) blink very infrequently and that the ratio of the area of the iris to that of the sclera is greater in the younger than in the older child; thus, perhaps something is unique in the tear content or production of young children that allows them to avoid most eye problems associated with facial paralysis in adults.

SURGICAL TREATMENT: GENERAL PRINCIPLES

Compressive Lesions

The treatment of benign, compressive lesions, such as occur with acute and chronic infection, viral inflammatory disorders such as Bell palsy, and trauma or tumors, may require surgical decompression of the facial nerve.

Indications. In cases evaluated within 21 days of onset of the facial palsy, one or more of the following criteria indicate impending degeneration and the need for surgical decompression: (1) loss of tearing on the affected side (May and Hardin, 1978; May, 1978a); (2) salivary flow 25 per cent or less (May, 1978a, 1978b; May et al., 1976a); and (3) evidence of an abnormal response to electrical testing (May and Hawkins, 1972; May, 1978a, 1978b; Fisch and Esslen, 1972).

Surgical Technique. (1) Surgical decompression, to be effective, may require reaching the internal auditory canal, depending upon the response to direct electrical stimulation of the exposed facial nerve or location of the lesion by topognostic test results (May, 1978a).

(2) To achieve ideal results, decompression must be applied prior to loss of the electrical response (May and Hawkins, 1972; Groves and Gibson, 1974) and proximal to the area of compression as determined by intraoperative, direct electrical stimulation at the time of exploration (May 1978a; Fisch and Esslen, 1972).

Transected Nerve

In cases where the nerve has been interrupted by tumor or trauma, a variety of approaches are available. The decision to use any approach is based upon the cause and location of the lesion, the status of hearing, and the length of time since paralysis was first noted (Fisch, 1977b).

The ideal technique for facial reanimation achieves facial symmetry at rest and spontaneous facial expression with mouth movement and eye closure. The techniques include, in order of preference, (1) end-to-end anastomosis; (2) cable interposition grafts; (3) cross-over graft from normal facial nerve to the paralyzed nerve (Samii, 1977; Fisch, 1977a; Anderl, 1977); (4) grafting the hypoglossal or spinal accessory nerve to the paralyzed nerve (Fisch, 1977b; Conley, 1977a, 1977b); (5) muscle-nerve pedicle grafting from the ansa hypoglossal nerve (Tucker, 1977); (6) free-muscle grafting with neural or neurovascular anastomosis (Thompson, 1971; Thompson and Gustavsson, 1976; Anderl, 1977; Hakelius, 1977); (7) temporalis or masseter muscle swings (Conley and Gullane,

1978; Rubin, 1976); (8) facial suspension or (9) combinations of the preceding.

Tucker (1978) discussed the management of extracranial facial nerve injuries and proposed pertinent considerations in the choice of an approach to the repair of such injuries.

INFECTION

Acute otitis media is not a rare cause of facial paralysis in children; it was the second most common cause in our series. Paralysis due to acute otitis media is not benign since 7 of 19 children in our study had incomplete recovery of facial function, and one of the seven had an extremely poor return of function.

Acute Otitis Media

Pathophysiology. The pathophysiology of facial paralysis associated with acute otitis media was described by Tschiassny (1944) and included thinness of the outer wall of the fallopian canal as it bends around the oval window, persistence of dehiscences of the fallopian canal, which are normally present only during the first year of life, anatomic connections of the nerve with the tympanic cavity, and pathways into the fallopian canal from the stapedius nerve, the chorda tympani, and the posterior tympanic artery. Further, the fact that the facial nerve is enclosed in a bony fibrous conduit makes it vulnerable to increases in its volume as a result of exudate, edema, congestion, or hemorrhage. Toxins, as well as osteitis of the mastoid associated with acute infection, may be additional factors in facial paralysis.

Botman and Jongkees (1955) reported that facial paralysis complicating acute otitis media increases in severity when there is osteitis surrounding the nerve.

Management. Since 1944, electrical diagnostic studies such as maximal stimulation, electroneurography, and electromyography have been developed to correlate changes occurring in the nerve with the pathologic state of the nerve. By employing these electrical tests and determining lacrimal and submandibular salivary flow, an accurate prognosis can be made prior to complete degeneration of the nerve. Therefore, it is no longer justified to rely on antibiotics and myringotomy alone for treatment of acute otitis media. Nor has it been found that all patients with acute otitis media recover completely without surgery. With these accurate prognostic tests available, it is no longer acceptable to reserve surgery for those who show no recovery over a period of six weeks or to withhold surgery until there is loss of response to electrical tests.

Hof (1977) supported the concept that facial paralysis associated with acute otitis media is not rare and that it is not a benign process. He stated that, according to statistics, acute otitis media was the most frequent cause of facial palsy in children and that paracentesis and placement of a ventilating tube was not sufficient treatment to arrest the increasing degeneration of facial nerve fibers in some cases. A mastoidectomy with surgical decompression of the fallopian canal was recommended as an emergency procedure when the response to electroneurography was reduced to 10 per cent or more of the normal side within six days from the onset of the palsy. In this manner, intraoperative-evoked electromyography could be employed in determining the precise site of the lesion. This was a significant contribution to surgery for acute otitis media, as it insured that the surgical exploration would approach the lesion proximally. With this approach, recovery of function was obtained in all instances.

Patient Analysis. An analysis of our data from 19 patients with facial paralysis associated with acute otitis media supported the recommendations of Hof (1977). Although the material obtained from our experience is based on a retrospective, uncontrolled, and nonrandomized group of patients, there seem to be significant clinical trends that are worth reporting.

Medical Treatment. Antibiotics and myringotomy are the recommended treatments of choice for acute otitis media and are thought to be effective in the great majority of cases. It was of interest to note that four patients treated for acute suppurative otitis media with an appropriate antibiotic developed complete peripheral facial paralysis two to five days following the start of the antibiotics. Facial nerve function in four patients degenerated following antibiotics and myringotomy therapy. Each of these had incomplete recovery, and in one of these the final return of facial nerve function was poor.

These observations suggest that in some cases the infectious process progresses to damage the facial nerve in spite of medical therapy. For this reason, prognostic tests

must be employed to determine if the facial nerve is being threatened. In this way surgery can be carried out at the earliest appropriate moment, hopefully before there is degeneration.

Surgical Treatment. Suppurative mastoiditis was confirmed in 10 of 19 patients operated upon. The surgical findings consisted of granulation tissue lying against an exposed nerve in the horizontal segment in five ears, and in three patients there was soft, osteitic bone around the vertical segment in addition to the granulation tissue found in the horizontal segment. In two ears the findings were limited to osteitic bone around the vertical segment. In each of these cases, the nerve was exposed and the sheath opened. Twelve patients had complete recovery, six fair, and one had poor recovery of facial nerve function.

Two patients were initially treated with penicillin and myringotomy and operated upon after electrical response was lost. One had complete recovery, and the other had fair recovery of facial nerve function.

Seven patients were operated upon before response to electrical stimulation was lost. Surgery was performed on the basis of one or more of the following being present: salivary flow reduced to 25 per cent or less of normal; a marked decrease in response to maximum stimulation; or evidence of progressive decrease in response to maximum stimulation. Three patients who were operated upon when their response to electrical stimulation was equal on both sides recovered completely; four patients who were operated upon after there was marked decrease in electrical response had fair recovery.

Opening Nerve Sheath. Two patients in our series were operated upon for peripheral facial paralysis associated with acute otitis media and mastoiditis. The recovery was complete in each case. Both patients presented approximately a year later with acute otitis media and suppurative mastoiditis. Keeping in mind that the facial nerve had been decompressed and the sheath opened, it was surprising to note that the facial paralysis did not recur. These observations suggest that surgical decompression prevents recurrent peripheral facial paralysis due to acute suppurative otitis media and that removing the bone and opening the sheath around the nerve does not place the nerve in jeopardy from the present infection or future infections. Surgery may not only allow the nerve to recover but also may protect it from possible future compressive processes.

Recommended Treatment. The goal in managing facial paralysis associated with acute otitis media is not only to treat the infection but also to insure complete recovery of facial function. Adequate doses of an appropriate antibiotic and a wide myringotomy is effective treatment in most cases. As long as there is paresis with some residual facial movement, complete recovery can be expected. If there is complete loss of facial movement and one or more of the poor prognostic indicators listed in Table 13–6 is present, then transmastoid surgical exploration and facial nerve decompression should be performed without delay. In our opinion, the surgery is not complete unless the sheath is opened (Chap. 16).

Chronic Otitis Media

There is little controversy regarding treatment for facial paralysis associated with chronic otitis media and mastoiditis, particularly when it is associated with cholesteatoma. Whereas conservative treatment is the order of the day for acute suppurative otitis media, surgical intervention at the earliest possible moment is recommended for facial paralysis associated with chronic infection. The mechanism in chronic infection is extraneural compression from cholesteatoma, usually in the region of the cochleariform process. This is the only point in the middle ear where cholesteatoma can impinge on the facial nerve and this process. The pathophysiologic events in chronic infection are less acute, and the results, provided the surgery is done prior to the loss of electrical response and within the first 24 to 48 hours after onset, have been uniformly excellent (Chap. 17).

TRAUMA

Traumatic facial paralysis occurred in 27 (18 per cent) of the patients in this series, as shown in Table 13–1. The variety of causes of traumatic paralysis are listed in Table 13–8. Each will be discussed in terms of diagnosis and management (Chap. 21).

Birth

Facial paralysis noted at birth can be traumatic or congenital in origin. There are factors that aid in differentiating one from the

Table 13–8   TRAUMATIC FACIAL PARALYSIS

Number of Cases	Causes		
1	*Central* Fell out of tree		
7	*Peripheral* Birth	Forceps	No Forceps
	Total paralysis	2	2
	Marginal branch	1	2
8	*Iatrogenic* Otologic 4 Parotid 4		
9	*Temporal Bone Fracture* Longitudinal 7 Transverse 2		
2	*Extracranial* Shotgun wound 1 Laceration 1		
27	*Total*		

other (Table 13–9). The presence of other congenital anomalies, facial diplegia, or upper face palsy suggests a congenital cause, whereas the absence of these signs and the presence of a history of a prolonged labor in a primipara mother, high-forceps delivery, evidence of forceps marks over the area of the ear, or a hemotympanum suggest birth trauma. Congenital facial paralysis does not improve, whereas paralysis due to birth trauma may. With recovery following trauma, there is usually some evidence of faulty regeneration such as a tic, synkinesis, or spasm. This does not occur with paralysis of the congenital type.

Patients must be evaluated within a few days of birth for traumatic causes of facial paralysis to be documented, as the clues suggesting trauma disappear quickly.

The differential diagnosis of facial paralysis at birth is quite important, since effective treatment for the traumatic type requires early intervention, ideally before the peripheral nerve degenerates. Since the nerve is usually compressed in the temporal bone and not transected, decompression will usually give excellent results if performed before the nerve degenerates. This can be determined by employing the same prognostic indicators (Tables 13–6 and 13–7) discussed under management of facial paralysis. In the rare case in which the nerve has been transected, neural repair or grafting performed within

Table 13–9 FACIAL PALSY AT BIRTH – DIFFERENTIAL DIAGNOSIS

Characteristics of Congenital Causes	Method of Differentiation	Characteristics of Traumatic Causes
Illness in first trimester No recovery of facial function after birth Family history of facial and other anomalies	History	Total paralysis at birth with some recovery noted subsequently
Other anomalies, facial diplegia (bilateral palsy)	Physical Examination	Hemotympanum, ecchymoses, tics, syskinesis
Anomalous (external, middle, or inner ear)	Radiograph of temporal bone	Fracture
Response ↓/0 without change	MST° ENOG°°	Normal at birth, then decreasing response may be lost
Reduced or absent response, no evidence of degeneration	EMG†	Normal at birth, then loss of spontaneous motor units and fibrillations 10 to 21 days later

°MST = Maximal Stimulation Test
°°ENOG = electroneurography
†EMG = electromyography

the first three weeks after injury will yield excellent results; results of these procedures will become progressively less satisfactory as the time between injury and repair lengthens.

Temporal Bone Fractures

Incidence. Mitchell and Stone (1973) reported the incidence of facial paralysis among 1015 children who presented with head injuries over a two-year period to the Hospital for Sick Children in Toronto. Of the total, 71 patients had temporal bone fractures, and 21 per cent of these had facial paralysis.

Pathophysiology. A longitudinal fracture, the most common type of temporal bone fracture, usually courses along the long axis of the pyramid, down the squamous bone, across the mastoid cortex, and through the posterior canal wall and involves the facial nerve at the second genu; or if the fracture crosses the mastoid tegmen, the facial nerve is usually compressed or torn in the area of the geniculate ganglion. This type of fracture is usually associated with a hemotympanum and may cause disruption of the ossicular chain. An excellent review of middle ear injuries with skull trauma was reported by Hough and Stuart (1968). There may or may not be a tear of the tympanic membrane. Vertigo will be present along with spontaneous nystagmus if the stapes is subluxed into the vestibule. Longitudinal fractures usually involve the middle ear, and facial paralysis

occurs in approximately 25 per cent of these patients. Cerebrospinal fluid leaks are associated with longitudinal fractures but are more common with transverse fractures.

Transverse fractures are caused by a more severe injury than are longitudinal fractures, and loss of consciousness is common. The fracture is usually across the occiput and up the posterior wall of the pyramid, through the internal auditory canal and the otic capsule. Facial paralysis occurs in 50 per cent of such cases and rarely spares the inner ear.

Diagnosis. Peripheral facial paralysis following a head injury usually indicates a fractured temporal bone. The fracture may be longitudinal, transverse, or a combination of these two. The types can be differentiated by the use of a tuning fork. A conductive hearing loss usually indicates a longitudinal fracture, and a profound sensorineural hearing loss indicates a transverse fracture.

Location of the fracture can be determined by tear testing. Loss of tearing indicates that the fracture is at or proximal to the geniculate ganglion, while the injury is usually distal to the geniculate ganglion if tearing is normal. Testing for tearing and response to tuning forks have been found to be more accurate for defining the type of fracture and its location than have sophisticated radiographic techniques such as polytomography of the temporal bone. Further, tuning forks can differentiate a hemotympanum from an ossicular dissociation. If the Weber test lateralizes to the injured ear but air conduction is greater than bone conduction with a 512 cycle tuning fork then an ossicular chain disruption is unlikely.

Management. Once the status of the patient's central nervous system and general condition have been stabilized, attention is directed toward injuries within the temporal bone. These include, in the order of priority, vertigo, facial paralysis, cerebrospinal fluid leak, a tear of the tympanic membrane, and ossicular discontinuity. Schneider and Boles (1968) discuss the neurosurgical and neuro-otologic problems in head trauma. Our discussion will be limited to facial paralysis since the other aspects will be covered in another section.

Otologic consultation is encouraged as soon as possible following a head injury when there is associated facial paralysis. Patients with immediate onset of facial paralysis should undergo exploratory facial nerve surgery as soon as they are able to tolerate general anesthesia. Those patients with a delayed onset of facial palsy that becomes complete should be followed by daily tear, salivary flow, and electrical testing. Surgical exploration should be recommended if there is evidence of one or more poor prognostic indicators (Table 13–6). In cases of trauma, the patient should undergo surgery if salivary flow becomes reduced to 40 per cent or less of normal (May et al., 1973).

Surgical Approach. The surgical approach selected is dependent upon the status of the hearing and the presence or absence of tearing. A transmastoid approach is indicated for a patient with intact hearing and tearing. A middle fossa approach is indicated for a patient with intact hearing and loss of tearing, although a transmastoid, extralabyrinthine, subtemporal approach is an alternative in these cases (Fig. 13–9). A translabyrinthine approach is indicated for a patient with loss of hearing and tearing.

Finally, surgical exploration of the facial nerve in temporal bone fractures must include the labyrinthine segment in longitudinal fractures and the portion in the internal auditory canal in transverse fractures. This recommendation is based upon the frequency of involvement at the level of the geniculate ganglion or proximal to the ganglion in temporal bone fractures (Fisch, 1974).

Facial nerve surgery for managing facial paralysis due to a fractured temporal bone is most challenging. The surgeon must be capable of exploring the facial nerve through its entire transtemporal course and must be pre-

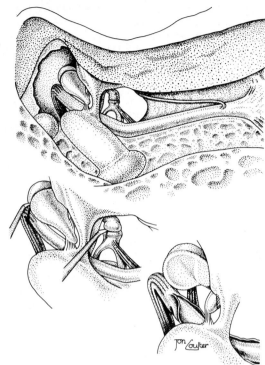

Figure 13–9 Transmastoid, extralabyrinthine, subtemporal approach to the right facial nerve can reach the labyrinthine segment while avoiding a middle fossa craniotomy. Top drawing illustrates posterior tympanotomy looking at the mastoid and tympanic segment of the facial nerve. The bottom two drawings show that by disarticulating the incus and rotating it forward with its attachment to the fossa incudis, the surgeon can reach the geniculate ganglion and labyrinthine segment of the facial nerve. The incus is replaced in its anatomic position at completion of the procedure.

pared to employ a translabyrinthine or middle fossa approach, disassemble or reconstruct the ossicular chain, repair a torn tympanic membrane, seal a cerebrospinal fluid leak, or take a donor nerve from the neck or leg to place a nerve graft between the freshened ends of a transected facial nerve.

IATROGENIC CAUSES OF FACIAL PARALYSIS (OTOLOGIC SURGERY)

Introduction

Facial nerve injuries in otologic surgery continue to occur, even with the most experienced surgeons. The facial nerve runs through the temporal bone between the middle ear and the mastoid, and congenital anomalies as well as distortions due to chronic infection, tumors, and trauma make the facial nerve vulnerable to injury during surgery.

The possibility of an injury to the facial nerve must always be included as part of informed consent whenever surgery is performed on any part of the temporal bone or parotid gland. Positive identification of the facial nerve during all stages of surgery is the best method of avoiding injury. Anatomic landmarks that help to identify the facial nerve in the temporal bone have been described by Rulon and Hallberg (1962) and by Glasscock (1971).

Management

Nonsurgical. The authors suggest that facial paralysis following a temporal bone procedure does not require reexploration if the nerve (1) was positively identified; (2) was purposely decompressed proximal and distal to where it was exposed; and (3) responded to direct electrical stimulation prior to completion of the procedure. Nothing can be gained by exploring the nerve that is intact. The only reason for reexploring the facial nerve in such a case would be to rule out traumatic interruption of the nerve. Immediate paralysis following an otologic procedure can be due to the influence of the local anesthesia, but this should not last beyond two hours. The postoperative dressing might put pressure against an exposed nerve and should be removed in the event that postoperative facial paralysis is noted.

Surgical. In the event that unexpected facial paralysis follows a surgical temporal bone procedure and the nerve was not identified, exploration of the nerve is mandatory.

This can best be performed the following day when the surgeon is free from fatigue and stress and the patient and family have been fully advised of the situation. This time period also allows for careful reevaluation to confirm that there is total facial paralysis. Further, this allows an opportunity for consultation.

If the nerve is intact, then only decompression above and below the area of involvement is necessary. If the sheath is frayed but the endoneural contents are grossly intact, then reapproximation is better than a graft. If the nerve is transected, the ends should be freshened, and an interposition graft should be placed. The anticipated results can be predicted by the degree of injury (Fig. 13–3, Table 13–3). With an intact nerve, the injury can be of first- to third-degree severity; if the nerve is frayed or transected, then the

injury is usually of the fourth- to fifth-degree level.

Parotid Surgery

Prevention. Surgery in or around the parotid gland in the young child is hazardous. The nerve fibers are extremely small and often require magnification for identification. Benign lesions, such as hemangiomas or cystic hygromas, frequently send out finger-like projections that envelop the facial nerve, making dissection difficult and placing the facial nerve fibers in great jeopardy. These benign lesions should thus be managed conservatively.

In the event that surgery in this region becomes necessary, great experience and skill are required not to injure the facial nerve. Not only is the use of the microscope helpful, but identification of the major branches of the facial nerve as they emerge from the parotid gland over the masseter fascia also may be useful to follow the nerve branches back into the tumor region. In some instances it is helpful to identify the facial nerve in the temporal bone and follow it out to the parotid substance. Surgery of the parotid gland requires positive identification of the facial nerve in order to avoid injuring it; the adage, "if you don't see it, you won't injure it," is not only untrue but also dangerous. Familiarity with the anatomic variations of the facial nerve in the young child is essential in order to avoid injuring the facial nerve. The lack of development of the mastoid tip, the narrow tympanic ring, and lack of subcutaneous tissue in young children place the main trunk of the facial nerve just beneath the skin as it emerges from the temporal bone in the young child. As compared to its much deeper position in the adult, the lower division of the facial nerve in the young child runs over the mandible and is quite superficial. It is in these two locations, the exit site from the temporal bone and over the mandible, that the facial nerve is most often injured by an incorrectly placed incision.

Management. Ideally, injury to the facial nerve should be avoided, but in the event that it is injured the nerve should be treated as outlined in the section discussing injury of the facial nerve in the temporal bone. The facial nerve should be identified during the procedure and stimulated when the procedure is completed prior to closing the wound at its most proximally exposed segment. This is usually near its exit from the temporal bone. If all parts of the face move, the surgeon can be certain that the nerve is intact. Even if the patient awakens with facial paralysis, no further treatment is required, and recovery can be expected. On the other hand, if the face does not respond to stimulation following this procedure, the fibers should be followed out to their termination in an effort to locate the area of injury. If the nerve is still intact, then nothing further need be done. The injury is due to stretching, and recovery, although it may be delayed two to four months, is usually satisfactory. In the event that branches have been severed, they should be repaired. If part of the nerve has been removed and the ends cannot be approximated, an interposition graft should be placed. The grafting technique consists of fascicular anastomosis with the aid of the otomicroscope. Ten-0 nylon sutures are used. The epineurium is trimmed back, and the sutures are placed through the perineurium and endoneurium, approximating the ends of the fascicles of the donor and recipient nerves. Immediate grafting will yield excellent results (Chap. 51).

FACIAL WOUNDS

Management of injuries to the extracranial segment of the facial nerve should be explored as soon after the injury as possible so that one can use the nerve stimulator to find the distal branches. These branches will continue to respond to stimulation up to three days following transection. If the wound is clean, primary repair or interposition grafting should be carried out. In case the wound is contaminated, such as occurs with a shotgun injury, the distal ends of the nerve should be tagged with nonabsorbable sutures. The proximal end can always be found as it emerges from or within the temporal bone. The wound should be drained and allowed to granulate and heal. Secondary repair of the nerve can be accomplished within three weeks with practically the same results as one might achieve with immediate repair.

CONGENITAL CAUSES OF FACIAL PARALYSIS

Many authors discuss congenital causes of facial paralysis (Paine, 1957; Harrison and Parker, 1960; Parker, 1963; Masaki, 1971; Garcin et al., 1976).

In our series of patients with facial palsy, 18 patients (12 per cent) were born with facial paralysis. The paralysis was congenital in 11 and traumatic in 7. The diagnosis was established in each case by employing the factors listed in Table 13–9 (Chap. 14).

Associated Anomalies

The most common finding associated with congenital facial paralysis was the presence of one or more other anomalies. This was noted in 9 of the 11 patients. There were five patients with an anomaly of the maxilla, making this the most common site of defect. A cleft palate was noted in two, a hypertrophied maxilla in one, a hypoplastic maxilla in another, and an accessory palate containing teeth and a tongue-like structure was present in the maxilla in one patient.

Three patients had skeletal deformities: two involved the cervical spine and one had spina bifida. One patient had a gastrointestinal anomaly, and another had a cardiac defect.

Multiple Anomalies

Eight patients had multiple congenital anomalies. Multiple congenital anomalies were noted in two of three patients with paralysis of the lower lip on one side. One of these two patients eventually died as a result of the multiple anomalies.

There were three patients with a hearing loss: two with a sensorineural type and one with a congenital conductive defect.

Two patients had an anomaly of the external pinna on the paralyzed side, but both patients had normal hearing.

Family History

There were two patients with a positive family history of congenital facial paralysis. One involved nine members of the same family covering three generations. Each member of this family who had facial paralysis had identical facial involvement as well as the same congenital defects. The defects consisted of hypertrophy of the maxilla, hypertelorism, and a congenital conductive hearing loss. The other patient with a positive family history of congenital facial paralysis had an older brother with an identical anomaly involving the same side of the face and associated malformation of the nares on the involved side.

Möbius Syndrome

Four of the patients in this series had Möbius syndrome. One had involvement of the sixth and seventh nerves bilaterally and lacked tear production. Another had involvement of only the seventh nerve with preservation of taste papillae and tear production. A third had bilateral involvement of the seventh and sixth nerves, as well as unilateral twelfth nerve involvement, a cleft palate, and absence of tearing. The fourth had bilateral involvement of the sixth and seventh nerves, cervical fusion, an anomaly of the external pinna, a naso-orbital sinus, and an accessory palate. A report by Rubin (1976) is recommended for an excellent discussion of Möbius syndrome.

Significance of Lower Lip Involvement

There were two patients with multiple congenital anomalies with involvement of only the lower lip on one side. It is important to look for other anomalies in the presence of congenital facial paralysis, even if the paralysis involves only the lower lip (Pape and Pickering, 1972). The significance of lower lip involvement in assessing the patient for other, more serious anomalies is borne out by the fact that the one patient who died as a result of serious multiple anomalies was one with facial nerve involvement of the lower lip only.

Management of Congenital Facial Paralysis

The presence of nerve and muscle must be determined prior to planning facial rehabilitation surgery. This can be determined by the presence of spontaneous movement or by electromyography determinations. In the absence of spontaneous movement or electrical evidence of the presence of muscle, the muscle should be explored and samples should be obtained for histologic evaluation.

Improvement of facial function may be accomplished in patients with a congenital facial paralysis by careful analysis of the defect and by the use of appropriate, combined surgical approaches discussed under the section on general principles of surgical treatment.

TUMORS

Although tumors are an unusual cause of facial paralysis in children, they did account for facial paralysis in four patients (3 per cent) in this series. A tumor involving the facial nerve should be considered in patients regardless of age if there is one or more of the following findings: (1) facial paralysis does not resolve after six months; (2) paralysis progresses slowly beyond three weeks; (3) paralysis recurs on the same side; (4) there is facial weakness associated with twitching; or (5) there is facial paralysis associated with other neurologic signs.

The four patients in our series exemplified each of these presentations that are classic for tumors involving the facial nerve, and yet there was a significant delay between onset of symptoms and appropriate diagnosis and treatment. A plea is made to evaluate carefully all patients with facial nerve disorders so that the natural history of the causative disease can be arrested and the patient can be treated with a minimum of morbidity.

REFERENCES

Anderl, R. 1977. Cross-face nerve grafting up to twelve months of seventh nerve disruption. In Rubin. I.. R. (Ed.) Reanimation of the Paralyzed Face. St. Louis. The C. V. Mosby Co., pp. 241–277.

Anson, B. J., and Donaldson, J. A. 1973. Surgical Anatomy of the Temporal Bone and Ear, 2nd ed. Philadelphia, W. B. Saunders Co., pp. 363–364.

Blunt, M. J. 1956. The possible role of vascular changes in etiology of Bell's Palsy. J. Laryngol. Otol., 70:701–713.

Botman, J. W. N., and Jongkees, L. B. W. 1955. Results of Intratemporal Treatment of Facial Palsy. Pract. ORL., 17:80–100.

Cawthorne, T. 1953. Surgery of the temporal bone. Hunterian lecture. J. Laryngol. Otol., 67:437–448.

Conley, J. 1977a. Hypoglossal crossover – 122 cases. Trans. Am. Acad. Ophthalmol. Otolaryngol., 84: 763–768.

Conley, J. 1977b. Panel on rehabilitation of the face. In Fisch, U. (Ed.): Facial Nerve Surgery. Birmingham, Ala., Aesculapius Publishing Co., pp. 241–243.

Conley, J., and Gullane, P. J. 1978. Facial rehabilitation with temporal muscle – new concepts. Arch. Otolaryngol., 104:423–426.

Crosby, E. C., and De Jonge, B. R. 1963. Experimental and clinical studies of the central connections and central relations of the facial nerve. Ann. Otol., Rhinol. Laryngol., 72:735–755.

Devriese, P. P. 1977. Prednisone in idiopathic facial paralysis (Bell's palsy). ORL, 39:257–271.

Duchenne, G. B., 1872. De I electrisation localisée, 3rd ed. Paris, France, Baillere, pp. 864–870.

Fisch, U. 1974. Facial paralysis in fractures of the temporal bone. Laryngoscope, 84:2141–2154.

Fisch, U., and Esslen, E. 1972. Total intratemporal

exposure of the facial nerve; pathologic findings in Bell's palsy. Arch. Otolaryngol., 95:335–341.

Fisch, U. (Ed.) 1977a. Special techniques of facial nerve repair, 204–226. Rehabilitation of the face by seventh nerve substitute, 227–250. New concepts in rehabilitation of the long standing facial paralysis, 251–284, In Facial Nerve Surgery. Birmingham, Ala., Aesculapius Publishing Co.

Fisch, U. 1977b. Total facial nerve decompression and electroneurography. In Silverstein, H., and Norrell, H. (Eds.) Neurological Surgery of the Ear, Birmingham, Ala., Aesculapius Publishing Co.

Garcin, M., Magnan, F. X. L., and Bremond, G. 1976. Facial paralysis in children, review of 82 cases. J. Franc. Oto-rhino-laryngol., 25:435–443.

Glasscock, M. E. 1971. Unusual facial nerve problems. Some thoughts on identifying the nerve in the temporal bone. Laryngoscope, 81:8669–8683.

Groves, J., and Gibson, W. P. R. 1974. Bell's palsy: The nerve excitability test in selection of case for early treatment. J. Laryngol. Otol., 88:581–584.

Hakelius, L. 1977. Free muscle and nerve grafting in the face. In Rubin, L. R. (Ed.) Reanimation of the paralyzed face. St. Louis, C. V. Mosby Co., pp. 278–293.

Harrison, M., and Parker, N. 1960. Congenital facial diplegia. Med. J. Australia, 1:650–653.

Hof, E. 1977. Facial palsy of infectious origin in children. In Fisch, U. (Ed.) Facial Nerve Surgery. Birmingham, Ala., Aesculapius Publishing Co., pp. 414–418.

Hough, J. V. D., and Stuart, W. D. 1968. Middle ear injuries in skull trauma. Laryngoscope, 78:899–937.

Levine, R. E. 1974. Management of the eye in facial paralysis. Otolaryngol. Clin. North Am., 7:531–544.

Levine, R. E. 1979. Management of the eye after acoustic tumor surgery. In House, W. F., and Laetje, C. M. (Eds.) Acoustic Tumors, Vol. II, Management. Baltimore, University Park Press, pp. 105–149.

Masaki, S. 1971. Congenital bilateral facial paralysis. Arch. Otolaryngol., 74:259–263.

May, M., Harvey, J. E., Marovitz, W. F., et al. 1976. The prognostic accuracy of the maximal stimulation test compared with that of the nerve excitability test in Bell's palsy. Laryngoscope, 81:931–938.

May, M., and Hawkins, C. S. 1972. Bell's palsy: Results of surgery: Salivation test versus nerve excitability test as a basis of treatment. Laryngoscope, 82:1337–1348.

May, M. 1973. Anatomy of the facial nerve (spatial orientation of fibers in the temporal bone). Laryngoscope, 83:1311–1329.

May, M., Lucente, F. E., Harvey, J. E., et al. 1973. Salivation testing in traumatic facial paralysis. Ann. Otol. Rhinol. Laryngol. 82:17–22.

May, M. 1974. Red chorda tympani nerve and Bell's palsy. Laryngoscope, 84:1507–1513.

May, M. 1976. Red chorda tympani nerve and herpes zoster oticus. Laryngoscope, 86:1572.

May, M., Hardin, W. B., Sullivan, J., et al. 1976a. Natural history of Bell's palsy; The salivary flow test and other prognostic indicators. Laryngoscope, 86:704–712.

May, M., Hardin, W. B., Sullivan J., et al. 1976b. The use of steroids in Bell's palsy: A prospective controlled study. Laryngoscope, 86:1111–1122.

May, M. 1978a. Bell's palsy: Progressive ascending paralysis, therapeutic implications. Laryngoscope, 88:61–72.

May, M. 1978b. Submandibular salivary flow test in facial paralysis. Ann. Otol. Rhinol. Laryngol., 87:279–281.

May, M., and Hardin, W. B. 1978. Facial palsy: Interpretation of neurologic findings. Laryngoscope, 88:1352–1362.

Mitchell, D. P., and Stone, P. 1973. Temporal bone fracture in children. Can. J. Otolaryngol., 2:(2):156–162.

Olsen, P. Z. 1975. Prediction of recovery in Bell's palsy. Acta Neurol., Suppl. 61, 52:1–121.

Paine, R. S. 1957. Facial paralysis in children. Review of the differential diagnosis and report of ten cases treated with cortisone. J. Pediatr. 19:303–316.

Pape, R. E., and Pickering, B. 1972. Asymmetric crying facies: An index of other congenital anomalies. J. Pediatr., 81:21–30.

Parker, N. 1963. Dystrophia myotonica presenting as congenital facial diplegia. Med. J. Australia, 2:939–944.

Peitersen, E. 1977. Incidence, natural history, progression and functional impairment of facial paralysis. Presented at the First Facial Nerve Symposium in the United States. Pittsburgh, Pa. June 19–23, 1977.

Rubin, L. R. 1976. The Möbius syndrome: Bilateral facial diplegia. Clin. in Plast. Surg. 3:625–636.

Rulon, J. T., and Hallberg, O. E. 1962. Operative injuries to the facial nerve. Explanation for its occurrence during operations on the temporal bone and suggestions for its prevention. Arch. Otolaryngol., 76:131–139.

Samii, M. 1977. Panel on rehabilitation of the face. In Fisch, U. (Ed.) Facial Nerve Surgery. Birmingham, Ala., Aesculapius Publishing Co., pp. 243–245.

Sammarco, J. G., Ryan, R. F., and Longenecker, C. G. 1966. Anatomy of the facial nerve in fetuses and stillborn infants. Plast. Reconstr. Surg., 37:566–574.

Schneider, R. C., and Boles, R. 1968. Combined neuro-otologic and neurosurgical problems in head trauma. Laryngoscope, 78:955–972.

Thompson, N. 1971. Autogenous free grafts of skeletal muscle. Plast. Reconstr. Surg., 48:11.

Thompson, N., and Gustavsson, E. H. 1976. The use of neuromuscular free autografts with microneural anastomosis to restore elevation of the paralyzed angle of the mouth in cases of unilateral facial paralysis. Chir. Plastics (Berlin), 3:165.

Tschiassny, K. 1944. Facial palsy, when complicating a case of acute otitis media, indicative for immediate mastoid operation? Cincinnati J. Med., No. 25, 262–266.

Tschiassny, K. 1953. Eight syndromes of facial paralysis and their significance in locating the lesion. Ann. Otol. Rhinol. Laryngol., 62:677–691.

Tucker, H. M. 1977. Selective reinnervation of paralyzed facial muscles by the nerve muscle pedicle technique. In Fisch, U. (Ed.) Facial Nerve Surgery, Birmingham, Ala., Aesculapius Publishing Co., pp. 276–284.

Tucker, H. M. 1978. The management of facial paralysis due to extra-cranial injuries. Laryngoscope, 88:348–354.

Wolf, S. M., Wagner, J. H., Davidson, S., et al. 1978. Treatment of Bell's palsy with prednisone; a prospective randomized study. Neurology, 28:158–161.

Chapter 14

CONGENITAL ANOMALIES OF THE EXTERNAL AND MIDDLE EAR

Isamu Sando, M.D.

Susumu Suehiro, M.D.

Raymond P. Wood, II, M.D.

INTRODUCTION

We owe a great debt for our knowledge of congenital anomalies of the ear to the early students of otohistopathology and their successors. Guild, Nager, Reudi, and Lindsay stand out in any list of distinguished investigators in temporal bone pathology. At the time when much of their work was done, the surgical techniques for correction of middle ear anomalies did not exist. The period of rapid development of otosurgical techniques that began in the early 1950s has continued to the present. Although much of this work has been focused on the treatment of chronic infectious disease, an important result of such study has been the development of procedures applicable to the correction of middle ear anomalies.

From studying the temporal bones of patients who suffered from many varied diseases, we know that congenital anomalies of the ear may be caused by genetic (familial) factors, chromosomal alterations *in utero,* and maternal infectious diseases. Agents that are related to the production of congenital anomalies may have an effect either on genetic material or directly upon the developing otocyst anlagen. In many cases, congenital an-

omalies are of unknown origin, but by comparing the nature and extent of the anomaly and the normal embryonic development of the ear, we can in some cases determine the point in gestation at which the insult occurred.

The clinician must be cognizant of the association of certain anomalies with others. Where one congenital anomaly is found, others must be sought. The use of a high-risk register for deafness is helpful in this regard.

For the otologic surgeon, knowledge of the associated occurrence of structural anomalies is imperative. Failure to realize that, in an ear with an anomaly the presence of a normal fallopian canal on tomographic radiographs does not mean that the facial nerve lies within the canal, has resulted in many surgical disasters.

The purpose of this chapter is to make the physician aware of the possibility of encountering external and middle ear anomalies during examinations and surgery. To do this, the anomalies are reviewed and discussed by grouping them according to their etiology (Classification I) and according to the anatomic structures involved (Classification II). A brief section is devoted to the current surgical techniques for correction of external and middle ear anomalies and hearing improvement. In certain cases, most notably Down syndrome, our failure to achieve satisfactory hearing improvement surgically probably reflects our imperfect understanding of the factors involved in the hearing loss rather than the absence of appropriate surgical techniques.

CLASSIFICATION OF DISEASES WITH EXTERNAL AND MIDDLE EAR ANOMALIES BY THEIR ETIOLOGIC FACTORS (CLASSIFICATION I)

The diseases associated with external and middle ear anomalies can be classified by their origins into five divisions.

DISEASES OF UNKNOWN ETIOLOGY
DISEASES WITH HEREDITARY CHARACTERISTICS
DISEASES ASSOCIATED WITH PRENATAL INFECTIONS
DISEASES OF IATROGENIC OTOTOXICITY
DISEASES ASSOCIATED WITH ENVIRONMENTAL FACTORS

Each of these classifications will be dealt with in turn.

Table 14–1 is a list of the diseases by eponym and pathologic name to assist the reader.

DISEASES OF UNKNOWN ORIGIN

1. Without Associated Anomalies

External Ear Anomaly

(1)* CRYPTOTIA (E)+ (SILCOX, 1967)**

Cryptotia is of unknown etiology and is present at birth. It may be observed alone. This anomaly is rare. The auricle demonstrates fusion of the superior portion with the scalp.

---

*The numbers in parentheses are the numbers of the diseases as we have designated them throughout the chapter.
+The following notations are used throughout the chapter:
   (D) Dominant hereditary disease;
   (R) Recessive hereditary disease;
   (E) Anomalies observed in the external ear;
   (M) Anomalies observed in the middle ear;
   (I) Anomalies observed in the inner ear;
   (O) Anomalies observed in other parts of the body.
(Some diseases have more than one etiologic factor or more than one mode of hereditary transmission. Only one representative description is selected for each disease.)
**Some of the information listed for the diseases in Classifications I and II may not be annotated by the reference listed. Only one reference was permitted for each category of disease and anatomic structural anomaly. An attempt was made to select papers with the latest literature review as the representative reference for each disease in Classification I.

Table 14–1 DISEASES WITH EXTERNAL AND MIDDLE EAR ANOMALIES LISTED BY THEIR PATHOLOGIC DEFECTS AND BY THEIR TRADITIONAL NAMES

Eponym	Pathologic Name
(11)* Turner syndrome	Gonadal aplasia
(12) Patau syndrome	Trisomy 13–15 syndrome
(13) Edward syndrome	Trisomy 18 syndrome
(14) Down syndrome	Trisomy 21 syndrome
(17) Apert syndrome	Acrocephalosyndactylia
(20) Klippel-Feil syndrome	Brevicollis
(22) Pierre Robin syndrome	Cleft palate, micrognathia, and glossoptosis
(24) Möbius syndrome	Congenital facial diplegia
(26) Crouzon disease	Craniofacial dysostosis
(27) Pyle disease	Craniometaphyseal dysplasia
(29) Duane syndrome	Duane's retraction syndrome
(31) Hurler syndrome	Gargoylism
(35) Treacher-Collins syndrome	Mandibulofacial dysostosis
(37) Fanconi syndrome	Multiple congenital anomalies
(38) Mohr syndrome	Orofaciodigital syndrome II
(39) Paget disease of bone	Osteitis deformans
(40) Van der Hoeve syndrome	Osteogenesis imperfecta tarda
(41) Albers-Schonberg disease	Osteopetrosis
(47) DiGeorge syndrome	Third and fourth pharyngeal pouch syndrome

*The number in parentheses indicates the disease as it is listed in the classification system in the first section of this chapter.

(2) MACROTIA (E) (SILCOX, 1967)

Macrotia is of unknown etiology and may be observed alone. This anomaly is uncommon. Associated anomalies are rare.

Middle Ear Anomaly

(3) *ANOMALIES OF OSSICLES§ (M) (KOIDE ET AL., 1967)

This is a disorder of unknown etiology, although some cases are reported to be autosomally dominant. This is considered a rare condition and is present at birth.

Ossicular anomalies can be observed alone. Malleolar anomalies include absence of the malleus, deformed malleolar head, triple bony union of the malleolar handle with the long process of the incus and head of the stapes, and bony fusion of the incudomalleolar joint. Incudal anomalies include absence of the incus, bony fusion of the short process of the incus with the horizontal semicircular canal wall, shortening of the long process of the incus, malformed long process of the incus, absence of the incudostapedial joint, bony fusion of the incudostapedial joint, and fibrous union of the incudostapedial joint. Stapes anomalies include absence of the stapes, absence of the head and crura of the stapes, small or fetal form of the stapes, a columella-type stapes, bony fusion of the stapes head to the promontory, and stapes footplate fixation.

The major anomalies of the middle ear associated with ossicular anomalies include facial nerve anomalies and absence of the stapedial muscle, stapedial tendon, and pyramidal eminence. It may be worthwhile to note that in cases of a congenitally fixed stapes footplate, an abnormally

§The asterisk (*) before a disease indicates that there are reports that describe the temporal bone histopathology in this disease.

patent cochlear aqueduct may be present, which results in a geyser of cerebrospinal fluid if the footplate is removed at surgery.

Audiometric testing of individuals with ossicular anomalies reveals a unilateral or bilateral, nonprogressive, moderate to severe, flat type of conductive hearing loss.

(4) *ABERRANT FACIAL NERVE (M)
(BASEK, 1962)

The etiology of an aberrant facial nerve is unknown. This condition is felt to be rare and present at birth. It may be observed alone.

Many facial nerve anomalies have been reported. The nerve may be displaced anteroinferiorly, with or without the fallopian canal, and pass through the middle ear on either side of the stapes. It may run in a canal on the promontory inferiorly from the geniculate ganglion. Also, the nerve may be seen to split into two or three branches that continue separately in the descending (mastoid) portion of the nerve; this condition is frequently associated with hypoplasia of the nerve. Stapes anomalies, atresia of the external auditory canal, malformations of the auricle, and other anomalies may be seen with anomalies of the facial nerve.

There are no specific audiometric findings in cases of facial nerve aberrations.

(5) ANOMALOUS INTERNAL CAROTID
ARTERY IN MIDDLE EAR (M)
(RUGGLES AND REED, 1972)

This is a disorder of unknown origin. It is rare; six cases have been described — five in females and one in a male — and it is present at birth. The condition is usually unilateral.

The middle ear shows a vascular mass in the inferior portion of the tympanum behind the tympanic membrane. There are no associated anomalies.

Clinical findings include pulsatile tinnitus with a bruit heard in the external auditory canal. The carotid arteriogram shows a small internal carotid artery coming up through the posterior hypotympanum, turning abruptly forward beneath the stapes and the fallopian canal to head toward the area of the eustachian tube. Tomograms do not show a normal carotid canal, and indentations are seen on the promontory. A conductive or mixed type of hearing loss may be present.

This condition may be confused with an aneurysm of the carotid artery.

(6) INTERNAL CAROTID ARTERY
ANEURYSM (M) (STALLINGS AND
McCABE, 1969)

This is a disorder of unknown etiology and unknown prevalence; however, it is rare. It presents as a pulsatile smooth mass in the anterior inferior portion of the tympanic cavity. There are no known associated anomalies. It is sometimes symptomatic, with the patient complaining of pulsatile tinnitus. The diagnosis is aided by carotid arteriograms with subtraction studies. No specific treatment is required.

(7) HERNIATION OF JUGULAR BULB
(M) (STEFFEN, 1968)

This is a disorder of unknown origin and unknown prevalence. This middle ear anomaly is present at birth as a jugular bulb in the middle ear, occurring just below the oval window through the dehiscent floor of the middle ear. There are no associated anomalies and no audiometric findings. There is no specific treatment.

(8) CONGENITAL ABSENCE OF ROUND WINDOW (M) (HARRISON ET AL., 1966)

This anomaly is of unknown origin and is rare. It is present at birth and can be observed alone. The audiometric configuration of round window closure by itself is indistinguishable from that observed with oval window closure; there is a nonprogressive, moderate, flat, conductive hearing loss.

2. With Associated Anomalies

(9) CONGENITAL CHOLESTEATOMA OF THE MIDDLE EAR (EPIDERMOID OF MIDDLE EAR) (E,M,O) (HOENK ET AL., 1969)

This is a lesion of unknown origin that is usually acquired but is occasionally congenital.

The middle ear findings include an epidermoid mass in the middle ear. The ossicles and bony walls of the tympanum may be eroded by this growth. Cholesteatoma has been described in connection with atresia, appearing behind an atretic bony plate, and also in association with cup-ears.

Mastoid radiographs and petrous pyramid tomograms show areas of bony erosion by cholesteatoma. A conductive hearing loss may result from involvement of the tympanic membrane or ossicles.

(10) *CONGENITAL HEART DISEASE (M,I,O) (EGAMI ET AL., 1979)

Congenital heart disease is of unknown origin but is frequently found associated with trisomies 13–15, 18, and 21, although no regular relationship between the chromosomal and cardiac anomalies has yet been established. Any major congenital heart defect may be associated with ear anomalies. Findings are present at birth. External and middle ear anomalies include a bulky incus, wide angle of the facial genu, persistence of the stapedial artery, a high jugular bulb, dehiscence of the facial canal, and remnants of mesenchymal tissue present in the middle ear.

Inner ear anomalies observed include a shortened cochlea, thickened trabecular bone at the cribriform base of the cochlea, absence of the helicotrema, patent utriculoendolymphatic valve, complete absence of all semicircular canals, and simple outpouching of the lateral semicircular canal.

Other associated anomalies include scleral dermoid, cleft of the soft palate, Meckel diverticulum, duodenal atresia, absence of the spleen, supernumerary pulmonary lobulation, and absence of the kidney.

(11) GONADAL APLASIA (TURNER SYNDROME) (E,M,O) (SZPUNAR AND RYBAK, 1968)

Turner syndrome is a chromosomal aberration in which the patients are sex chromatin-negative in 80 per cent of the cases with a chromosomal configuration of XO. The prevalence is 1 in 5000 live births.

External and middle ear anomalies include low-set ears with large lobes, poor development of the mastoid air cell system, and developmental malformation of the stapes.

Other anomalies and clinical findings include short stature, disturbance of the organs of sight, webbing of the neck, various bony dysplasias, malformations of the heart, and deformed kidney.

Hearing loss of a sensorineural or mixed type may be present.

(12) *TRISOMY 13–15 SYNDROME
(PATAU SYNDROME) (E,M,I,O) (SANDO
ET AL., 1975)

Trisomy 13–15 is a chromosomal aberration in which the somatic cells have an extra chromosome in the 13–15 group. The lesions are present at birth. The prevalence of this syndrome is 0.45 per 1000 births.

External and middle ear findings include low-set, malformed ears, stenotic external auditory canal, small tympanic membrane, thick manubrium of the malleus, distorted incudostapedial joint, deformed stapes, small facial nerve, wide angle of the facial genu, absence of the stapedial muscle and tendon, persistence of the stapedial artery, dehiscence of the facial canal, absence of the pyramidal eminence, absence of the antrum, a small antrum, and a small mastoid.

Inner ear anomalies include a distorted and shortened cochlea, absence of the hook portion of the cochlea, malformed apical turn of the cochlea, absence of the modiolus, underdevelopment of the modiolus, malformed Rosenthal canal, scala communis between apical and middle cochlea turns, scala communis between middle and basal cochlea turns, underdevelopment of the osseous spiral lamina, malformed scala vestibuli with moderately small space in the basal turn, displacement and encapsulation of the tectorial membrane, large and patent cochlear aqueduct, unusual shape of the macule of the utricle, shortened utriculoendolymphatic valve, direct communication between the utricle and saccule, partial absence of the lateral limb of the superior semicircular canal, partial absence of the membranous superior semicircular canal, wide bony lateral semicircular canal, large ampulla of the membranous lateral semicircular canal, nearly flat crista of the membranous lateral semicircular canal, narrow lumen of the bony posterior semicircular canal, short and straight endolymphatic duct, shallow and wide internal auditory canal, spiral ganglion cells serving the basal turn located in the fundus of the internal auditory canal, and the singular nerve entering the otic capsule from the posterior fossa via a separate canal.

Individuals with trisomy 13–15 syndrome may have other associated anomalies: microcephaly, arhinoencephaly, multiple eye anomalies, hypertelorism, cleft lip and palate, intraventricular septal defect, abnormal palm print, simian creases, and hyperconvexity of the nails.

The diagnosis is proved by the karyotype, which shows 47 chromosomes with an extra chromosome in the 13–15 group. It arises as a result of nondisjunction of the chromosomes.

(13) *TRISOMY 18 SYNDROME
(EDWARD SYNDROME) (E,M,I,O)
(SANDO ET AL., 1970)

The symptoms of trisomy 18 syndrome are due to the presence of an extra chromosome in the 16–18 group. The findings are present at birth. The prevalence is 0.23 to 2 per 1000 births. It appears to be more common in infants born of older mothers.

External and middle ear anomalies include low-set, deformed ears, atretic external auditory canals, deformed malleus and incus, malformed stapes of the columella type or of a fetal form, a split tensor tympani muscle in separate bony canals, exposed stapedial muscle in the middle ear cavity, absence of the stapedial tendon, underdevelopment of the facial nerve, abnormal course of the facial and chorda tympani nerves, and absence of the pyramidal eminence.

Inner ear anomalies include incompletely developed modiolus, scala communis between apical and middle turns, underdeveloped cystic stria vascularis, absence of the utriculoendolymphatic valve, absence of the lateral limb of the superior semicircular canal and crista, absence of the lateral limb of the lateral semicircular canal, a flat, macula-like crista of the lateral semicircular canal, an enlarged endolymphatic duct, and a double singular nerve.

Other associated anomalies include ptosis of the eyelids, a high arched palate, micrognathia, flexion deformities, such as the index finger overlapping the third finger, and hypertrophy of the pancreatic tissue. These patients generally show failure to thrive, mental retardation, and hypertonicity and have a very poor prognosis.

Audiometric testing shows a failure to respond to sound.

(14) *TRISOMY 21 SYNDROME (DOWN SYNDROME) (E,M,I,O) (IGARASHI ET AL., 1977)

The trisomy 21 syndrome is due to a chromosomal aberration in which the somatic cells have an extra chromosome in the 21–22 group. The findings are present at birth. The prevalence is 0.1 to 1.0 per 1000 births.

The external and middle ear findings include low-set ears, deformed stapes, slightly distorted crura of the stapes, and poor development of the mastoid air cells.

Associated anomalies in the inner ear include a shortened cochlea, absence of the utriculoendolymphatic valve, hypogenesis of the posterior semicircular canal, and an enlarged bony posterior canal ampulla.

Other associated anomalies include hypertelorism, epicanthic fold, slanting eyes, strabismus, narrowing of the nasal space, impaired development of the paranasal sinuses, protruding tongue, a high palate, and cardiovascular malformations, such as a ventricular atrial septal defect, patent ductus arteriosus, and situs inversus.

Audiometric tests show the presence of a sensorineural, mixed, or conductive hearing loss.

DISEASES WITH HEREDITARY CHARACTERISTICS

1. Without Associated Anomalies

(15) *OTOSCLEROSIS (D,M) (LARSSON, 1962) (SCHUKNECHT, 1974)

Otosclerosis is a disorder inherited as an autosomal dominant trait. The penetrance appears to be 40 to 50 per cent with a clinically apparent prevalence of 1 in 500 persons in the United States. According to pathologic studies of the temporal bone, the prevalence is 1 in 8 among Caucasian adult females and 1 in 15 among Caucasian adult males; it is much less common in Orientals and Negroes. The clinical onset is usually postpubertal (average age 20 to 25 years), and the disease is exacerbated by pregnancy. The main surgical finding is fibrous or bony fixation of the stapedial footplate to the otic capsule owing to invasion by the otosclerotic focus. Both ears are affected in the majority of patients.

Histopathologically, abnormal changes are first seen in the enchondral bone of the otic capsule, in which the normal bone is replaced by a network of newly formed web-like bone. This bone has a mosaic pattern. The sites of predilection are the oval window and round window areas. A primary focus may be present in the stapes footplate. The physical examination is usually normal, although there may be a pinkish color to the promontory as seen through the intact tympanic membrane (Schwartze sign). Otosclerosis has been related to van der Hoeve disease and Paget disease, but the characteristics of these diseases are in fact quite different.

The audiometric findings in individuals with otosclerosis include a low-frequency conductive loss sometimes associated with a sensorineural loss. Uncommonly, a sensorineural hearing loss alone is seen (cochlear otosclerosis). Caloric tests are usually normal. The treatment is usually surgical (stapedectomy), but these patients frequently obtain good results from hearing aids.

2. With Associated Anomalies

(16) *ACHONDROPLASIA (CHONDRODYSTROPHIA FETALIS) (D,M,I,O) (SCHUKNECHT, 1967)

Achondroplasia is a hereditary dominant disorder with many sporadic cases and is probably the result of mutation. It is also seen as a recessive trait in rare instances. The onset of the anomalies occurs in fetal life. The disorder occurs in 1 of 10,000 newborn infants and 1 of 50,000 in the general population.

The middle ear anomalies associated with achondroplasia include fusion of the ossicles to the surrounding bony structures and the appearance of dense, thick trabeculae without islands of cartilage in the endochondral bone and periosteal bone.

Associated anomalies of the inner ear include a deformed cochlea and thickened intercochlear partitions. Other associated anomalies include dwarfism due to imperfect ossification within the cartilage of the long bones, which results in shortening of the extremities, with the proximal bones being more affected than the distal bones. Many of these patients die at birth or shortly thereafter. The hearing loss associated with this disorder has been described as being either conductive or mixed.

(17) *ACROCEPHALOSYNDACTYLIA (APERT SYNDROME, ACROBRACHYCEPHALY, ACROKRANIODYSPHALANGIE, SPHENAKROKRANIOSYNDAKTYLIE, ACRODYSPLASIA) (D,M,I,O) (LINDSAY ET AL., 1975)

This disorder is apparently transmitted as an autosomal dominant trait. It appears to be associated with a high mutation rate and has been related to increasing parental age. The malformation occurs in 1 in 100,000 to 1 in 160,000 live births, and the manifestations are present at birth. There are no reports of external ear anomalies. The middle ear anomaly associated with this disorder is fixation of the stapedial footplate. Inner ear anomalies include a patent cochlear aqueduct, an enlarged internal auditory canal, and an unusually large subarcuate fossa that connects to the middle fossa dura.

Other associated anomalies reported include craniofacial dysostosis, brachiocephaly, hypertelorism, bilateral proptosis, saddle nose, high arched palate, spina bifida, ankylosis of the joints, and syndactyly.

The audiometric findings are usually those of a flat conductive hearing loss, although a sensorineural component is suspected in some cases.

(18) *ANENCEPHALY (R,E,M,I,O) (ALTMANN, 1957)

This anomaly is a hereditary recessive disorder and consists of complete or incomplete absence of the forebrain and midbrain. Anencephaly accompanies acrania, which is described as holocrania or meroacrania on the basis of the degree of the osseous changes. The prevalence of this disease is 1 in 1000 births.

External and middle ear anomalies include a small stapes footplate, exposed facial nerve, hypoplasia of the intratympanic muscles, a persistent stapedial artery, dehiscence of the facial canal, and a small oval window.

Inner ear anomalies include a shortened cochlea, an underdeveloped modiolus, scala communis between middle and basal cochlea turns, communication between the bony lateral canal and the posterior canal, and an unusually narrow or wide internal auditory canal.

Other associated anomalies reported are spina bifida and amelia.

(19) *ATRESIA AURIS CONGENITA (D,E,M,I,O) (HIRAIDE ET AL., 1974)

Atresia is inherited as an autosomal dominant and is present at birth. It can be either unilateral or bilateral, partial or complete, and with or without deformities or absence of the auricle.

Middle ear anomalies associated with atresia include a misshapen tympanic membrane, replacement of the tympanic membrane by a bony plate, absence of the malleus and incus, fused malleus and incus, misshapen malleus and incus, lack of an incudostapedial connection, absence of the stapes head and crura, a deformed stapes and crura, stapes footplate fixation, anomalous course of the chorda tympani nerve, absence of the lesser superficial petrosal nerve, hypoplastic and displaced tensor tympani muscle, persistent stapedial artery, a hypoplastic tympanic cavity, and absence of the tympanic cavity.

Inner ear anomalies include all degrees of deformity of the cochlea, vestibule, semicircular canals, and internal auditory meatus.

Associated conditions include epilepsy, mental retardation, internal hydrocephalus, posterior choanal atresia, mandibulofacial dysostosis, and cleft palate.

Audiometric testing shows the presence of a nonprogressive maximum conductive loss with variable degrees of sensorineural loss, including total absence of hearing.

(20) *BREVICOLLIS (KLIPPEL-FEIL SYNDROME) (R,E,M,I,O) (McLAY AND MARAN, 1969)

Brevicollis is a hereditary disorder that appears to be due to a recessive gene. Females are predominantly affected, and the disease is rare. External and middle ear anomalies include microtia, presence of a preauricular appendage, atresia of the external auditory canal, narrowing of the external auditory canal, a slit-like malleoincudal joint, short process of the incus fused to the floor of the attic, long process of the incus attached to the stapes by fibrous tissues without any sign of a lenticular process, and an elongated stapes with its anterior crus fused to the cochleariform process.

Inner ear anomalies include a rudimentary cochlea (a short, curved, single tube extending from the vestibule), a rudimentary modiolus, a poorly developed and shallow internal auditory canal, internal auditory canal more superiorly positioned than normal, absence of statoacoustic nerve in the internal auditory canal, and a vestigial inner ear.

Associated anomalies include congenital deformity of the cervical spine due to a fusion or reduction in the number of cervical vertebrae, spina bifida, and Sprengel scapular deformity. There is a very short, almost immobile neck with prominent soft tissue and the hairline going down to the back.

Deafness is the second most common finding in this disorder and is of the sensorineural or mixed type. There is frequently an absence of vestibular function.

(21) CHEMODECTOMA OF THE MIDDLE EAR (NONCHROMAFFIN TYMPANOJUGULAR PARAGANGLIOMA, GLOMUS TYMPANICUM AND JUGULARE TUMOR, CAROTID BODY TUMOR) (D,M,O) (ROSEN, 1952)

Middle ear chemodectoma is a hereditary autosomal dominant tumor with low penetrance and variable expressivity. It is uncommon, and 70 per cent of these middle ear tumors occur in women. The tumor becomes clinically evident in adulthood, frequently quite late.

Middle ear anomalies include a fleshy red tumor of the middle ear arising from the jugular bulb or from the tympanic plexus (Jacobsen nerve) on the promontory. The tumor is sometimes seen to fill the middle ear space and to surround the ossicles. The lesion may be associated with ipsilateral or contralateral carotid body tumors of the neck. These middle ear tumors do not produce epinephrine. The lesion bleeds easily and blanches on compression with a pneumatic otoscope (Brown sign). The patient may report pulsatile tinnitus.

Diagnostic studies include retrograde jugular venography and carotid arteriography with subtraction studies.

The audiometric findings are those of a conductive hearing loss when the tumor impairs tympanic membrane mobility or the function of the ossicular chain. The cold water caloric response may be decreased. Treatment is usually excision of the tumor after controlling the blood supply.

(22) *CLEFT PALATE, MICROGNATHIA, AND GLOSSOPTOSIS (PIERRE ROBIN SYNDROME) (D,E,M,I,O) (IGARASHI ET AL., 1976)

This is a hereditary disorder that may also result from an intrauterine insult in the first trimester. If it is hereditary, the syndrome is probably inherited as an autosomal dominant with variable penetrance. The prevalence is 1 in 30,000 live births. The findings are present at birth.

External ear anomalies include cup-ears and low-set ears. Middle ear anomalies include thickened stapes crura and footplate, a small facial nerve, dehiscence of the facial canal, and absence of the middle ear.

Inner ear anomalies observed are a scala communis between the apical and middle cochlear turns, an underdeveloped modiolus, an abnormally narrow communication between the crus commune and the utricle, superior dislocation of the crus commune and the posterior semicircular canal, and a small internal auditory canal.

Other associated findings include mental retardation, hydrocephalus, microcephaly, microphthalmia, myopia, congenital cataracts, esotropia, retinal detachment, sixth nerve palsy, Möbius syndrome, cleft palate, hypoplasia of the mandible, the tongue being displaced backward and downward, congenital heart anomalies, spina bifida, hip dislocation, syndactylia, and clubfoot.

A conductive hearing loss has been found to be associated with this disorder.

(23) CLEIDOCRANIAL DYSOSTOSIS (D,E,M,O) (FØNS, 1969)

This is a hereditary autosomal dominant disorder. The findings are present at birth.

External and middle ear anomalies include a small auricle, atresia of the external auditory canal, a narrow external auditory canal, small ossicles, absence of the manubrium of the malleus, absence of the long process of the incus, fixation of the stapes footplate, and a small tympanic cavity.

Associated anomalies include aplasia of the clavicle, overdevelopment of the transverse diameter of the cranium, and retardation of ossification of the fontanels.

Audiometric tests may reveal a sensorineural hearing loss.

(24) CONGENITAL FACIAL DIPLEGIA (MÖBIUS SYNDROME) (D,E,M,I,O) (LIVINGSTONE AND DELAHUNTY, 1968)

This is a disorder that may be either genetic or nongenetic in etiology; on a genetic basis it appears to be of the autosomal dominant type. Parental consanguinity and the possibility of recessive inheritance have also been suggested. Most patients have no family history of the disease. It is rare.

External ear anomalies include microtia and slight atresia of the external auditory canal. Some form of auricular malformation is seen in 15 per cent of patients. Middle ear anomalies include an ossicular mass without a clearly identifiable stapes, oval window, or round window at surgical exploration.

Inner ear anomalies that have been observed radiologically include a dilated vestibule and canal system.

Other associated anomalies are absence of the abductors of the eye, aplasia of the brachial and thoracic muscles, anomalies of the extremities, and involvement of the cranial nerves, especially of the oculomotor, trigeminal, facial, and hypoglossal nerves.

Audiometrically, deafness has been reported in 15 per cent of individuals with this syndrome.

(25) CONGENITAL HEART DISEASE, DEAFNESS, AND SKELETAL MALFORMATION (D,E,M,O) (FORNEY ET AL., 1966)

This disorder is inherited as an autosomal dominant. Its prevalence is unknown. External and middle ear anomalies include a narrowed and oblique external auditory canal and fixation of the stapes footplate to the oval window. Associated anomalies and clinical findings include fusion of the carpal and tarsal bones and mild to moderate mitral insufficiency. Audiometric tests show a moderate congenital conductive hearing loss.

(26) *CRANIOFACIAL DYSOSTOSIS (CROUZON DISEASE) (D,E,M,O) (KONIGSMARK AND GORLIN, 1976)

Craniofacial dysostosis is a hereditary autosomal dominant disorder. It is a rare condition. The main features of this disease consist of skull deformity, hypoplasia of the maxilla, ocular malformations, and aural malformations.

External ear anomalies reported to be associated with this disease are atresia and stenosis of the external auditory canal. Middle ear anomalies include absence of the tympanic membrane, ankylosis of the malleus to the outer wall of the epitympanum, a deformed stapes with bony fusion to the promontory, distortion and narrowing of the middle ear space, a narrow round window niche, underdevelopment of the periosteal portion of the labyrinth, and a greatly reduced periosteal layer of the petrous bone.

This disease includes anomalies of the skull with exophthalmos; cranio-synostosis involving the coronal, sagittal, and lambdoidal sutures; small maxillae; a hypoplastic mandible; and facial abnormalities with ocular hypertelorism, a parrot-beaked nose, a short upper lip, and mandibular prognathism.

Audiometric findings reveal that approximately one third of the patients with this syndrome have a hearing loss that is usually nonprogressive and conductive in nature.

(27) CRANIOMETAPHYSEAL DYSPLASIA (PYLE DISEASE) (D,M,I,O) (KONIGSMARK AND GORLIN, 1976)

This hereditary autosomal disorder is quite rare; some cases have appeared to be inherited as an autosomal recessive. The disorder becomes evident clinically in early childhood and is progressive.

Middle ear anomalies include encasement of the malleus in bone from the promontory, a deformed incus fixed by bone to the promontory, a stapes head in an oval window filled with bone, and enlargement of the chorda tympani nerve.

The inner ear anomaly most frequently observed is constriction of the internal auditory meatus.

Associated anomalies and clinical findings include hypertelorism, deformity of the nasal dorsum, saddle nose, prognathism, posterior choanal atresia, defective dentition, metaphyseal widening of the long bones, nystagmus, optic atrophy, seventh nerve palsy, narrowing of the nasal passage, obliteration of the paranasal sinus, and obstruction of the nasolacrimal duct.

Audiometric tests have shown a sensorineural, high-frequency sloping loss with an associated large conductive loss. No results of vestibular tests on such individuals have been reported.

(28) DOMINANT PROXIMAL SYMPHALANGISM AND HEARING LOSS (D,E,M,O) (VASE ET AL., 1975)

This disease is inherited as an autosomal dominant with variable penetrance. External and middle ear anomalies include stenotic external auditory meatus, an elongated long process of the incus, and fusion of the stapes to the petrous bone.

Associated anomalies include symphalangism involving the proximal interphalangeal joints, most marked at the ulnar digits. Audiometric tests reveal a conductive hearing loss.

(29) DUANE RETRACTION SYNDROME (DUANE SYNDROME) (D,E,M,O) (PFAFFENBACH ET AL., 1972)

This syndrome involves autosomal dominant inheritance, but some cases seem to be inherited recessively and to be X-linked. Thalidomide has also been implicated in the etiology of this disorder. External and middle ear anomalies include microtia, atresia of the external auditory canal, fusion of the ossicles, lack of contact of the fused ossicles with the oval window, closure of the oval window by a thin membrane, and an ossicular mass that does not connect to the stapes.

Also seen in this disorder are limitation or absence of abduction, restriction of adduction, retraction of the globe upon adduction, and narrowing of the palpebral fissure on adduction. The condition is usually unilateral.

It is more frequent in females and most often occurs on the left side. The hearing loss is said to be conductive.

(30) *EAR MALFORMATION, CERVICAL FISTULAS OR NODULES, AND MIXED HEARING LOSS (D,E,M,I,O) (FITCH ET AL., 1976)

This is a hereditary autosomal dominant disease. External and middle ear anomalies include a preauricular sinus, a preauricular appendage, malformations of the auricle, an enlarged incus, a bony mass in place of the ossicles, and an inferiorly located tympanic cavity. Inner ear anomalies include a broad base of the modiolus, deformed stria vascularis, a deformed vestibule, a large vestibular aqueduct, a misshapen utricular macula, a large endolymphatic duct, a wide nonampullated end of the superior semicircular canal, and an underdeveloped lateral semicircular canal.

Other associated anomalies include cervical fistulas or nodules and renal dysplasia. Audiometric tests reveal a mixed hearing loss.

(31) *GARGOYLISM (HURLER SYNDROME) (R,E,M,O) (KELEMEN, 1966a)

Gargoylism is inherited as an autosomal recessive, sometimes X-linked, disorder and was the first of the genetic mucopolysaccharidoses to be recognized. The clinical findings become manifest by one year of age.

The external ear anomaly usually included in this syndrome is low-set ears. Middle ear anomalies include absence of the incudomalleolar joint, fibrous tissue invasion into the otic capsule with the presence of "gargoyle cells," multiple bony outgrowths into the middle ear, a small middle ear space filled with mesenchymal tissue, obliteration of the oval window and round window areas by mesenchymal tissue, a small mastoid antrum, poor development of the mastoid air cell system, and hypertrophy of the mucosa.

Other associated anomalies and clinical findings include dwarfism, hepatosplenomegaly, corneal clouding, and mental deficiency. These patients frequently have large, deformed heads with hypertelorism, prominent eyebrows, a saddle nose, wide nostrils, a long mouth, a high palate, thick lips and tongue, widely spaced teeth, and a prominent chin. Also seen are optic nerve atrophy, hypertrichosis, a short neck, a deformed thorax, lumbar kyphosis, a prominent abdomen, hernia limitation of joint movements, and broad hands with stubby fingers.

The diagnosis is made on the basis of the presence of mucopolysaccharides (chondroitin sulfate B and heparitin sulfate) in the urine. These same substances may be seen in the tissues. In the autosomal recessive type, deafness is seen in 5.2 per cent of individuals. In the X-linked recessive type, which is rare, deafness is seen in 43 per cent of individuals.

(32) HALLUX SYNDACTYLY — ULNAR POLYDACTYLY — ABNORMAL EAR LOBE SYNDROME (D,E,O) (GOLDBERG AND PASHAYAN, 1976)

This disorder is inherited as an autosomal dominant. External ear anomalies associated with this syndrome include a deep horizontal groove or a nodule on the ear lobe.

Other associated anomalies include webbed toes, partial toe syndactyly, and absence of the middle phalanx. Neither audiometric nor vestibular test results have been reported in such cases.

(33) LETTERER-SIWE DISEASE
(R,E,M,I,O) (COHN ET AL., 1970)

This is a hereditary autosomal recessive disorder of unknown prevalence, although it is uncommon. The onset is early in childhood. External and middle ear findings include bony destruction of the external auditory canal; partial destruction of the ossicles, fallopian canal, and tympanic membrane; the occurrence of remnant ossicles; and the middle ear being filled by tissue containing many histiocytes.

Associated anomalies in the inner ear include destruction of the bony cochlea and internal auditory canal. Hydrops of the scala media, rolling of the tectorial membrane into the inner sulcus, spiral ganglion cell loss, and replacement of the inner ear spaces by either growth or fibrous tissue are other inner ear findings reported.

Associated findings include ulcerative tonsillitis, stomatitis, hepatosplenomegaly, diffuse lymph node enlargement, anemia, thrombocytopenia, and leukopenia.

The hearing loss is of either the conductive or the mixed type, and vestibular function is depressed or absent.

(34) KNUCKLE PADS, LEUKONYCHIA, AND DEAFNESS (D,M,O) (BART AND PUMPHREY, 1967)

This disease is inherited as an autosomal dominant. The knuckle pad manifestation appears in childhood. Middle ear anomalies include absence of the ossicles and facial nerve, a high jugular bulb, and absence of the facial canal. Audiometric and vestibular examinations reveal sensorineural and mixed hearing losses and hypoactive vestibular responses.

(35) *MANDIBULOFACIAL DYSOSTOSIS (TREACHER-COLLINS SYNDROME) (D,E,M,I,O) (KONIGSMARK AND GORLIN, 1976)

Mandibulofacial dysostosis is a hereditary disorder. It is of dominant inheritance by a gene or group of genes and is present at birth.

Anomalies in the external ear include various auricular deformities and atresia or stenosis of the external auditory canal. Middle ear anomalies include replacement of the tympanic membrane by a bony plate, and deformities of the malleus, incus, and stapes. Other anomalies are absence of the tensor tympani muscle, stapedius muscle, tendon of the stapedius muscle, pyramidal eminence, cochleariform process, and mastoid antrum. The facial nerve has been seen to course directly lateral in this disorder with no tympanic or mastoid portions. The chorda tympani, and superficial petrosal nerves also have been reported to be absent. The epitympanum and sometimes the mesotympanum are said to be small, irregular, and filled with fibrous tissue.

Inner ear anomalies include a huge cochlear aqueduct and a blind-pouch horizontal canal.

Other associated anomalies include antimongoloid slant of the eyes with colobomas of the lower lids, absence of eyelashes medially, micrognathia, a short palate, and hypoplasia of the malar bones and infraorbital rims. Cleft lip and cleft palate are sometimes present. Clinodactylia and sternal deformities have also been reported.

Audiometric tests show sensorineural and nonprogressive conductive hearing losses that involve the high frequencies especially.

(36) MIXED HEARING LOSS, LOW-SET MALFORMED EARS, AND MENTAL RETARDATION (R,E,M,O) (MENGEL ET AL., 1969)

This very rare disorder is inherited as an autosomal recessive.

External and middle ear anomalies are present at birth and include a low-set, malformed auricle; a single ossicle shaped like a malleus and placed posteriorly; absence of the incus, stapes superstructure, and footplate; and absence of the round window niche.

Associated anomalies and clinical findings include mental retardation, a high arched palate, a systolic murmur, and small stature.

The hearing loss is mainly of the conductive type, with some sensorineural loss. Vestibular tests may be normal.

(37) MULTIPLE CONGENITAL ANOMALIES WITH HYPOPLASTIC ANEMIA (FANCONI SYNDROME) (R,E,M,O) (McDONOUGH, 1970)

Fanconi syndrome consists of congenital abnormalities and aplastic anemia. This is a hereditary autosomal recessive disorder.

External ear anomalies include atresia of the external ear. Middle ear anomalies include fixation of the stapedial footplate. Other associated anomalies include skin pigmentation, skeletal deformities, renal anomalies, and mental retardation.

(38) OROFACIODIGITAL SYNDROME II (MOHR SYNDROME) (R,M,O) (RIMOIN AND EDGERTON, 1967)

This is a hereditary autosomal recessive disorder. Its prevalence is unknown.

Middle ear anomalies include blunting of the long process of the incus and absence of the incudostapedial joint.

Associated anomalies include facial deformities with widely spaced medial canthi, a flat nasal ridge, a high arched palate, a hypoplastic body of the mandible, a lobulated tongue, and digital abnormalities, including polydactylia, syndactylia, and brachydactylia. Audiometric tests reveal a conductive hearing loss.

(39) *OSTEITIS DEFORMANS (PAGET DISEASE OF BONE) (D,E,M,I,O) (LINDSAY AND SUGA, 1976)

Osteitis deformans is inherited as an autosomal dominant with variable penetrance. The onset of symptoms occurs in middle age, and the disease is seen in 3 per cent of those older than 40 years of age.

The external ear anomaly usually reported is narrowing of the external bony auditory canal. Middle ear anomalies observed are pagetic bone growth in the epitympanum, pagetic changes in the stapes superstructure, thickening of the stapes footplate, footplate fixation, ossification of the stapedial tendon, and vascular spaces in the periosteal layer. These mosaic (pagetic) bony changes may involve any part of the temporal bone, the endochondral bone being most resistant.

Associated anomalies in the inner ear include loss of spiral ganglion cells, atrophy of the organ of Corti, atrophy of the stria vascularis, sarcomatous degeneration, and fractures of the temporal bone.

Other features include an enlarged skull, progressive kyphosis with shortening of stature, and pagetic involvement of the spine, femur, and fibula. Headaches are one of the most common and constant features of this disease, and vertigo is likewise a common complaint.

Radiographs originally show osteolytic lesions that are succeeded in several years by osteoblastic lesions. The semicircular canals and labyrinth are more visible on radiographic examination than usual. Audiometric findings show an early conductive loss, which progresses to a mixed loss, which may become profound. Responses to vestibular testing range from normal to those representative of canal paresis.

(40) *OSTEOGENESIS IMPERFECTA (D,M,I,O) (BERGSTROM, 1977)

Osteogenesis imperfecta is a hereditary autosomal dominant disease. It is present at birth, but symptoms of the tarda form (van der Hoeve syndrome) appear later in childhood. It is characterized by defective synthesis of connective tissue, including bone matrix. Middle ear anomalies include an abnormally shaped stapes head and crura; they may be very delicate and are sometimes replaced by fibrous tissue. The remainder of the temporal bone may show areas of skein-like bone throughout its structure.

Other associated anomalies and clinical findings include blue sclerae (in 95 per cent of patients), skein-like bone replacing lamellar bone throughout the body, multiple bone fractures, weak joints, prominence of the occiput, and abnormal tooth dentin with caries and dental fractures. Deformities such as kyphoscoliosis and pectus excavatum are common, and internal hydrocephalus, nerve root compression, cardiovascular and platelet lesions, and thin and atrophic skin also occur with this syndrome.

The audiogram usually shows a conductive hearing loss, although a sensorineural loss may occur in the high frequencies.

(41) OSTEOPETROSIS (ALBERS-SCHÖNBERG DISEASE) (R,M,O) (KONIGSMARK AND GORLIN, 1976)

Osteopetrosis is a hereditary disorder that is usually recessive but occasionally dominant. The onset is in early infancy or fetal life. Middle ear anomalies include a stapes of fetal form with an abnormal malleus and incus, persistence of the stapedial artery, a small middle ear space, lack of pneumatization of the antrum, and abnormally basophilic enchondral bone.

Associated deformities and clinical findings include macrocephaly, blindness due to optic nerve atrophy, absence of the paranasal sinuses, choanal atresia, facial paralysis, hepatosplenomegaly, bone fractures due to brittleness of the bones, and severe anemia.

The hearing loss is mainly of a sensorineural type.

(42) OTOPALATODIGITAL SYNDROME (R,M,O) (KONIGSMARK AND GORLIN, 1976)

This is a hereditary autosomal recessive disorder. The middle ear anomalies associated with this syndrome include crudely shaped ossicles that resemble their fetal forms.

Associated deformities include a characteristic facies consisting of frontal and occipital bossing, hypertelorism, a broad nasal root, a small mandible, and cleft palate. Mild dwarfism and skeletal abnormalities, including retardation of ossification in the carpal and tarsal centers, also occur. There are abnormalities of the hands with widely spaced first and second digits and a shortened first digit. Mental retardation may also be associated with this disease.

The hearing loss is of the conductive type.

(43) RECESSIVE MICROTIA, MEATAL ATRESIA, AND HEARING LOSS (R,E,M,O) (KONIGSMARK ET AL., 1972)

This is an autosomal recessive disorder. External and middle ear anomalies include microtia, atresia of the external auditory canal, and malformed ossicles.

Associated anomalies include pectus excavatum and duplication of the thumb.

The hearing loss associated with this syndrome is said to be conductive.

(44) RECESSIVE RENAL, GENITAL, AND MIDDLE EAR ANOMALIES (R,E,M,O) (WINTER ET AL., 1968)

This is a hereditary autosomal recessive condition. External and middle ear anomalies include small, low-set ears with a stenotic external ear canal, fixation of the malleus and incus in the attic, and a deformed or absent incus. Also a part of this syndrome is renal agenesis or atresia and variable involvement of the genital system, occasionally with atrophic ovaries, tubes, or vagina. The hearing loss is reported to be conductive in nature.

(45) *SICKLE CELL DISEASE (D,M,O) (MORGENSTEIN AND MANACE, 1969)

Sickle cell disease is a hereditary dominant disorder. It is said that it affects 7 to 8 per cent of African blacks.

Middle ear anomalies include resorption of the body and long process of the incus and the head of the stapes.

Other associated anomalies include hemolytic anemia, extramedullary hemopoiesis, and hyperplastic bone marrow.

Audiometric tests may reveal a sensorineural hearing loss.

(46) THICKENED EAR LOBULE AND INCUDOSTAPEDIAL MALUNION (D,E,M) (ESCHER AND HIRT, 1968)

This is a hereditary dominant, non-X-linked autosomal anomaly of rare occurrence. It is present at birth. External and middle ear anomalies include a hypertrophic, thickened ear lobule, malformation of the long process of the incus, absence of the lenticular process of the incus, presence of a fibrous connection from the stapes to the incus, and absence of the stapes head.

A conductive hearing loss should be present. No vestibular studies have been reported.

(47) *THIRD AND FOURTH PHARYNGEAL POUCH SYNDROME (DIGEORGE SYNDROME, PARTIAL DIGEORGE SYNDROME) (R,E,M,I,O) (ADKINS AND GUSSEN, 1974a,b)

This is a hereditary autosomal recessive defect. The anomalies are present at birth. The prevalence of this syndrome is quite low. External and middle ear anomalies include a malformed, low-set auricle; atresia of the external auditory canal; absence of the malleus, incus, and stapes; a small facial nerve; absence of the stapedial muscle; partial atresia of the tympanic cavity; and absence of the oval window. Inner ear anomalies include absence of the apical portion of the modiolus, absence of the horizontal semicircular canal, and hypoplastic seventh and eighth cranial nerves.

Other anomalies include absence or hypoplasia of the thymus, abnormalities of the aortic arch, patent ductus arteriosus, agenesis of the thyroid, acrania, microcephaly, and micrognathia.

DISEASES ASSOCIATED WITH PRENATAL INFECTIONS

(48) *CONGENITAL RUBELLA SYNDROME (M,I,O) (HEMENWAY ET AL., 1969)

Maternal rubella is an infectious viral disorder. Its manifestations are present at birth. Middle ear anomalies include an anomalous stapes with a rudimentary thickened head, neck, crura, and footplate; cartilaginous fixation of the stapes footplate; and persistence of fetal mesenchymal tissue in the middle ear.

Associated features in the inner ear include depression of the Reissner membrane, cystic dilatation of the stria vascularis, rolling of the tectorial membrane into the inner sulcus, hair cell degeneration, spiral ganglion cell loss, and collapse of the saccular membrane with adherence to the saccular macula.

Other associated anomalies and clinical findings are mental retardation, microcephaly, microphthalmia, retinitis, congenital cataracts, thrombocytopenia, cardiovascular deformities, and deformities of the lower extremities. Confirmatory tests include the presence of fluorescent antibodies in the serum, serum hemagglutination, and positive viral cultures of the stool and throat.

Audiometric testing reveals sensorineural and conductive hearing losses.

(49) *CONGENITAL SYPHILIS (M,I,O) (KARMODY AND SCHUKNECHT, 1966)

Congenital syphilis is an infection of the fetus by *Treponema pallidum* that passes the placenta. Symptoms may begin in childhood, but 50 per cent of individuals first develop symptoms between the ages of 25 and 35 years. The middle ear findings reported are thickening of the malleus as a result of bony hyperplasia, fusion of the malleolar head to the body of the incus, spongy appearance of the long process of the incus, and abnormalities of the stapes. Histopathology of the temporal bones reveals primary osteitis with mononuclear leukocytic infiltration and obliterative endoarteritis of the otic capsule with secondary labyrinthitis characterized by endolymphatic hydrops and degeneration of the membranous labyrinth end-organs. Other associated findings are a perforated nasal septum, interstitial keratitis, and Hutchinson teeth.

The diagnosis is made by the history and verifying tests, including serum and cerebrospinal fluid tests for syphilis. However, these tests are not always positive. Audiometric findings include a typical sensorineural type of hearing loss with a flat audiometric curve in 38 per cent of the patients with congenital syphilis. Sometimes the curve shows a conductive component if the middle ear is involved. The onset of hearing loss in childhood is usually sudden, bilaterally symmetrical, severe to profound, and unaccompanied by marked vestibular symptoms. In adults, deafness begins abruptly, and a partial, asymmetric, flat, sensorineural hearing loss is accompanied by episodes of vertigo. Tinnitus may be present. Treatment involves the administration of large doses of penicillin and steroids.

DISEASES OF IATROGENIC OTOTOXICITY

(50) *THALIDOMIDE OTOTOXICITY (E,M,I,O) (JØRGENSEN ET AL., 1964)

Thalidomide ototoxicity is an iatrogenic, drug-induced congenital disorder that occurs following the administration of thalidomide to a pregnant woman. The probability of malformation following exposure is unknown. Twenty per cent of the children suffering from thalidomide-induced anomalies show ear anomalies. External and middle ear anomalies include a deformed or absent auricle, complete or partial atresia of the external auditory canal, a deformed tympanic membrane, a fixed malleus, a displaced long process of the incus, absence of the stapes, absence of the facial nerve and chorda tympani nerve, persistence of the stapedial artery, a slit-shaped tympanic cavity, and absence of the oval window. Inner ear anomalies include aplasia of the inner ear and absence of the facial nerve and statoacoustic nerve in the internal auditory canal.

Associated anomalies include shortening, deformity, or absence of the long bones; capillary hemangiomas of the forehead, nose, and lips; colobomas; microphthalmia; congenital heart disease; intestinal atresia; and renal hypoplasia or agenesis.

Approximately 75 per cent of the infants affected can be expected to have a moderate to profound sensorineural hearing loss, and 25 per cent have a maximal conductive hearing loss. Absence of vestibular function has also been reported.

DISEASES ASSOCIATED WITH ENVIRONMENTAL FACTORS

(51) ENDEMIC CRETINISM (M,I,O) (WARKANY, 1971)

This disease is caused by environmental factors. The external and middle ear anomalies associated with endemic cretinism include plump ossicles, thickened periosteal parts of the stapes, a small mastoid process, and thickened periosteal layers of the otic capsule.

Other anomalies include a brachiocephalic cranium, brachydactyly with shortness of the thumb, and abnormal hip joint. These individuals often have a hearing loss.

CLASSIFICATION OF THE EXTERNAL AND MIDDLE EAR ANOMALIES BY THEIR INVOLVED ANATOMIC STRUCTURES (CLASSIFICATION II)

In order to enhance the reader's understanding of external and middle ear anomalies, the various kinds of anomalies that occur in the external and middle ear are classified according to the anatomic structures that are involved in the anomaly.

CONGENITAL EXTERNAL EAR ANOMALIES

(A) **Auricular Anomalies (1)****, **(2), (9), (11)–(14), (18)–(20), (22)–(24), (29)–(32), (35), (36), (43), (44), (46), (47), (50)**

1. AURICULAR ANOMALIES (IN GENERAL) (1), (2), (9), (11)–(14), (18)–(20), (22)–(24), (29)–(31), (35), (36), (43), (44), (47), (50)

   a. Absence of auricle — anotia (Altmann, 1951a)
   b. Superior portion of the auricle buried in the scalp — cryptotia (Altmann, 1951a)
   c. Double ear (Altmann, 1951a)
   d. Auricle smaller than normal — microtia (Altmann, 1949)
   e. Auricle larger than normal — macrotia (Altmann, 1951a)
   f. Auricle located on the upper anterior cervical region near the midline of the neck — synotia (Black et al., 1973)
   g. Ear located on the cheek — melotia (Altmann, 1951a)
   h. Lack of aural ascent due to underdevelopment of the mandibular area — low-set ear (Altmann, 1957)
   i. Other (Altmann, 1951a)

2. LOBULAR ANOMALIES (32), (46)

   a. Absence of lobule (Altmann, 1951a)
   b. Adherent lobule (Altmann, 1951a)
   c. Split lobule (Altmann, 1951a)
   d. Deep horizontal groove on the lobule (Goldberg and Pashayan, 1976)
   e. Hypertrophic and thickened lobule (Escher and Hirt, 1968)
   f. Nodule on the lobule (Goldberg and Pashayan, 1976)

3. HELIX ANOMALIES

   a. Auricle folded forward and downward in varying degrees from above and behind — cat's ear (Altmann, 1951a)
   b. Helix with sharp angle on its tip portion — cercopithecus ear (Altmann, 1951a)
   c. Small projection from the descending part of the helix — Darwin tubercle (Altmann, 1951a)

4. ANTHELIX ANOMALIES (9)

   a. Absence of anthelix (Hoenk et al., 1969)
   b. Poor development of the anthelix — lop ear (Converse et al., 1955)
   c. Small projection from the descending part of the helix – Darwing tubercle (Altmann, 1951a)
   d. Enlarged portion of the anthelix connecting with the helix — Mozart ear (Altmann, 1951a)
   e. Crus extending from the helix to the cymbae — Stahl ear (Altmann, 1951a)

5. TRAGUS ANOMALY (19) — RUDIMENTARY TRAGUS (ALTMANN, 1949)

**Numbers in parentheses refer to the diseases listed in Classification I.

6. CONCHAL ANOMALY — VERTICAL CARTILAGINOUS RIDGE IN THE CONCHA — CRUS CYMBAE (ALTMANN, 1951a)

7. APPENDAGE (20), (30)

    a. Numerous appendages — Polytia (Altmann, 1951a)
    b. Preauricular appendage (Altmann, 1951a)

8. FISTULA (30)

    a. Colloaural fistula (Altmann, 1951a)
    b. Preauricular fistula (Altmann, 1951a)
    c. Postauricular fistula (Altmann, 1951a)
    d. Prehelical pit (Melnick et al., 1975)

(B) External Auditory Meatus Anomalies (9), (11)–(13), (18)–(20), (22)–(26), (28), (29), (35), (37), (39), (43), (44), (47), (50)

    a. *Atresia auris (Altmann, 1949) (Fig. 14–1)
        i. *membranous atresia*
        ii. *bony atresia*
    b. *Stenotic external auditory meatus (Kelemen, 1966a)
    c. *Short bony external auditory meatus (Altmann, 1957)
    d. Long bony external auditory meatus (Stratton, 1965)

CONGENITAL MIDDLE EAR ANOMALIES

(A) Tympanic Membrane Anomalies (9), (12), (19), (26), (30), (35), (50)

    a. *Tympanic membrane replaced by bony plate (Sando et al., 1968)
    b. Tympanic membrane replaced by fibrous tissue (Schuknecht, 1974)
    c. *Small tympanic membrane (Bordley and Hardy, 1969)
    d. *Distorted tympanic membrane (Sando et al., 1970)

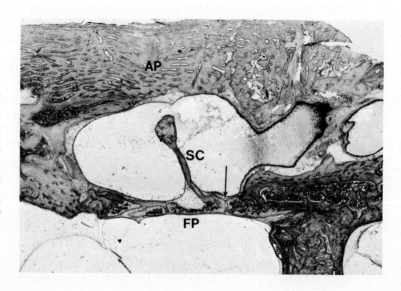

Figure 14–1 Horizontal section of the left temporal bone from a patient with Treacher-Collins syndrome with the following middle ear anomalies: columella-type stapes (*SC*) with a single crus attached to an underdeveloped footplate (*FP*), which was partially ankylosed anteriorly (arrow); absence of the malleus and incus, which were probably included in the bony atresia plate (*AP*), which replaced the area of the tympanic membrane. H&E stain. × 22.

(B) Ossicular Anomalies (3), (9)–(20), (22)–(31), (33)–(51)

1. OSSICULAR ANOMALIES (IN GENERAL) (16), (24), (29), (30), (33), (42)

    a. *Remnant ossicle (Cohn et al., 1970)
    b. *Fusion of three ossicles (Hough, 1963)
    c. Thickening of ossicles (Buran and Duvall, 1967)

2. MALLEUS ANOMALIES (3), (9), (12), (13), (19), (20), (23), (26), (27), (34)–(36), (41)–(44), (47), (49)–(51)

    a. Absence of:
        i. *malleus (Ruedi, 1954) (Fig. 14–1)
        ii. manubrium (Herberts, 1962)
        iii. lateral process (Hoenk et al., 1969)
        iv. head (Herberts, 1962)
    b. Bony fusion of:
        i. *malleolar head to epitympanic wall (Ritter, 1971)
        ii. anterior malleolar ligament to tympanic ring (McGrew and Gregg, 1971)
    c. Other anomalies:
        i. *displacement of malleus (Ruben et al., 1969)
        ii. long manubrium (Hough, 1963)
        iii. shortening of manubrium (Buran and Duvall, 1967)
        iv. cartilaginous fusion between malleus and Meckel cartilage (Zonis, 1969)

3. INCUS ANOMALIES (3), (10), (12), (13), (19), (20), (23), (27), (28), (30), (31), (34)–(36), (38), (41)–(47), (49)–(51)

    a. Absence of:
        i. *incus (Sando et al., 1968) (Fig. 14–1)
        ii. long process (Føns, 1969)
        iii. *lenticular process (McLay and Maran, 1969)
    b. Bony fusion of:
        i. *incus to malleus (Altmann, 1949)
        ii. incudomalleolar joint (Maran, 1965)
        iii. *short process to floor of aditus ad antrum (McLay and Maran, 1969)
        iv. short process to horizontal canal wall (Koide et al., 1967)
    c. Other anomalies
        i. *displacement of incus (Ruben et al., 1969)
        ii. shortening of short process (Jaffee, 1968)
        iii. shortening of long process (Maran, 1965)
        iv. *dislocation of long process (Sando et al., 1970)
        v. resolution of body and long process (Morgenstein and Manace, 1969)

4. STAPES ANOMALIES (3), (9), (11)–(15), (17)–(20), (22)–(28), (34)–(43), (45)–(51)

    a. Absence of:
        i. stapes (Fernández and Ronis, 1964)
        ii. *incudostapedial joint (Altmann, 1955)
        iii. *head (Altmann, 1955)
        iv. *crus (Altmann, 1957)
        v. *footplate (Jørgensen et al., 1964)

    b. Rudimentary form of stapes
        i. *columellar-type stapes (Kelemen, 1966b) (Fig. 14–1)
        ii. *doughnut-type stapes (Hough, 1963)
        iii. *thickening of stapes (Sando et al., 1970)
        iv. *two-layer footplate (Lindsay et al., 1960)
    c. Bony fusion of:
        i. incudostapedial joint (Hough, 1958)
        ii. head to promontory (Hough, 1963)
        iii. *head to facial canal (Altmann, 1949)
        iv. *crus to cochleariform process (McLay and Maran, 1969)
        v. *crus to oval window bony wall (Altmann, 1955)
        vi. *crus to promontory (Jørgensen et al., 1964)
        vii. crus to pyramidal eminence (Buran and Duvall, 1967)
        viii. *footplate to otic capsule (Altmann, 1957)
    d. Other anomalies
        i. adherence of stapes to facial nerve (Durcan et al., 1967)
        ii. *fibrous connection of incudostapedial joint (McLay and Maran, 1969)
        iii. displacement of incudostapedial joint (Black et al., 1971)
        iv. *resolution of head (Morgenstein and Manace, 1969)
        v. degeneration of crus into fibrous threads (Opheim, 1968)
        vi. *small bone on footplate (Bergstrom et al., 1972)

(C) Nerve Anomalies (4), (10), (12), (13), (18), (19), (21), (22), (27), (30), (34), (35), (47), (50)

    1. FACIAL NERVE ANOMALIES (4), (10), (12), (13), (18), (22), (30), (34), (35), (47), (50)

    a. *Absence (Jørgensen et al., 1964)
    b. Poor development (Henderson, 1939)
    c. Abnormal course
        i. *wide angle of facial genu (Egami et al., 1979)
        ii. *runs laterally from geniculate ganglion and leaves temporal bone immediately (Sando et al., 1968)
        iii. runs inferiorly from geniculate ganglion (Caparosa and Klassen, 1966)
        iv. *runs more inferiorly than normal (Adkins and Gussen, 1974a)
        v. *absence of second genu (Sando et al., 1970)
        vi. facial nerve located medial to stapedial muscle (Sando et al., 1970)
    d. Other — *exposed facial nerve (Altmann, 1957)

    2. CHORDA TYMPANI NERVE ANOMALIES (13), (19), (27), (35), (50)

    a. *Absence (Sando et al., 1968)
    b. Abnormal course
        i. *runs out of temporal bone (Altmann, 1949)
        ii. runs from the area of the geniculate ganglion (Fowler, 1961)
        iii. *runs more vertically than normal (Sando et al., 1970)
        iv. bifurcation (Durcan et al., 1967)
    c. Other anomalies
        i. enlargement (Hough, 1958)
        ii. chorda tympani with bony sleeve at posterior edge of external auditory meatus (Kraus and Ziv, 1971)

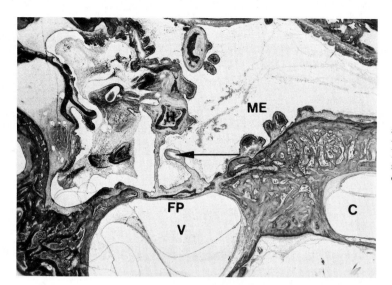

Figure 14–2 Persistent stapedial artery (arrow) observed in a patient with trisomy 13 syndrome. *C*, cochlea; *V*, vestibule; *FP*, footplate of stapes; *H*, head of stapes; *ME*, middle ear. H&E stain. × 15.

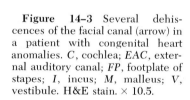

Figure 14–3 Several dehiscences of the facial canal (arrow) in a patient with congenital heart anomalies. *C*, cochlea; *EAC*, external auditory canal; *FP*, footplate of stapes; *I*, incus; *M*, malleus; *V*, vestibule. H&E stain. × 10.5.

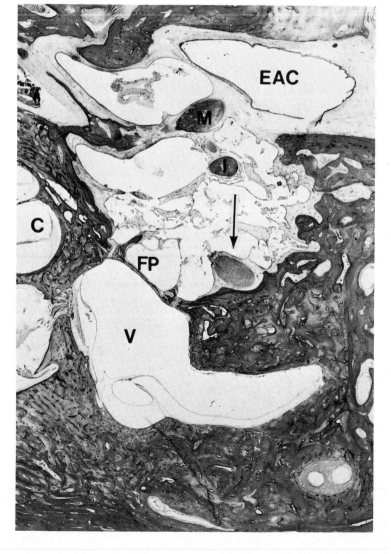

3. SUPERFICIAL PETROSAL NERVE
ANOMALIES (19), (35)

    a. *Absence of greater superficial petrosal nerve (Sando et al., 1968)
    b. *Absence of lesser superficial petrosal nerve (Altmann, 1949)

4. JACOBSON NERVE ANOMALY
(21) — PARAGANGLIOMA (VON DER
BORDEN, 1967)

**(D) Intratympanic Muscular Anomalies (11)–(13), (18),
(19), (35), (39), (47)**

1. TENSOR TYMPANI MUSCLE AND
TENDON ANOMALIES (31), (18), (19), (35)

    a. Absence of muscle and tendon (Sando et al., 1968)
    b. Abnormal course
        i.   abnormal course without connection to cochleariform process and malleus (Ruben et al., 1969)
        ii. abnormal course without connection to cochleariform process (Hiraide et al., 1974)
        iii. *split in muscle (Kos et al., 1966)

2. STAPEDIUS MUSCLE AND TENDON
ANOMALIES (11)–(13), (18), (35), (39), (47)

    a. *Absence of muscle and tendon (Sando et al., 1968)
    b. *Huge muscle exposed in the middle ear (Sando et al., 1970)
    c. Two muscles (Wright and Etholm, 1973)
    d. Absence of tendon (Jaffee, 1968)
    e. Atrophy of tendon (Tabor, 1961)
    f. Ossification of tendon (Hough, 1958)
    g. Tendon attached to lenticular process (Pou, 1963)
    h. Tendon attached to head or posterior crus (Hough, 1958)

3. OTHER ANOMALIES
(12) — *SUPERNUMERARY OR ECTOPIC
MUSCLES (DRUSS, 1952)

**(E) Vascular Anomalies (5)–(7), (10), (12), (18), (19),
(34), (41), (50)**

1. INTERNAL CAROTID ARTERY
ANOMALIES (5), (6)

    a. Existence in middle ear (Goldmann et al., 1971)
    b. Existence of aneurysm in the middle ear (Steffen, 1968)

2. STAPEDIAL ARTERY ANOMALY (10),
(12), (18), (19), (41), (50)– *Persistence
(Altmann, 1947) (Fig. 14–2)

3. JUGULAR BULB ANOMALIES (7), (10),
(34)

    a. Herniation of jugular bulb into the middle ear (Steffen, 1968)
    b. *High jugular bulb (Egami et al., 1979) (Fig. 14–3)

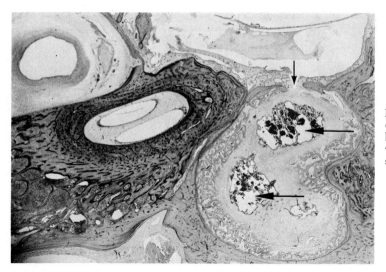

Figure 14–4 High jugular bulb (large arrows), accompanied by dehiscence (arrow) of the medial bony wall of the tympanic cavity. H&E stain. × 11.

(F) **Tympanic Cavity Anomalies (9), (10), (12), (13), (18)–(20), (22), (23), (26), (30), (31), (33)–(35), (41), (47), (50)**

    a. Absence of:
        i. tympanic cavity (Gnanapragasam, 1975)
        ii. *cochleariform process (Sando et al., 1968)
        iii. *facial canal (Altmann, 1957)
        iv. *pyramidal eminence (Sando et al., 1970)
    b. Dehiscence of:
        i. *facial canal (Altmann, 1957) (Fig. 14–4)
        ii. floor (Steffen, 1968)
        iii. *tegmen tympani (Sando et al., 1968)
    c. Rudimentary form:
        i. *small tympanic cavity (Jørgensen et al., 1964)
        ii. *small tympanic cavity with fetal connective tissue (Jørgensen et al., 1964)
    d. *Bony mass in promontory (Sando et al., 1968)
    e. Others:
        i. *congenital cholesteatoma (Hoenk et al., 1969)
        ii. *H-shaped tympanic cavity (Ruben et al., 1969)
        iii. large facial canal (Fernández and Ronis, 1964)

(G) **Window Anomalies (8), (18), (24), (26), (36), (47), (50)**

    1. OVAL WINDOW ANOMALIES (18), (24), (47), (50)

        a. *Absence (Jørgensen et al., 1964)
        b. *Calcification of annular ligament (Davis, 1968)
        c. *Filled with fetal connective tissue (Kelemen, 1966a)
        d. Thin membranous window (Livingstone and Delahunty, 1968)

    2. ROUND WINDOW ANOMALIES (8), (24), (26), (36)

        a. Absence (Hough, 1963)
        b. Round window partitioned by bony bar (Livingstone and Delahunty, 1968)

    c. Displacement of round window (Hough, 1958)
    d. Absence of niche (Hough, 1958)
    e. Connective tissue obstruction of niche (Ruedi, 1954)
    f. Narrow niche (Baldwin, 1968)

(H) Otic Capsule Anomalies (15), (16), (26), (31), (39)–(41), (49), (51)

    a. *Achondroplasia (Schuknecht, 1967)
    b. *Fibrous resorption focus in two external layers due to gargoylism (Kelemen, 1966a)
    c. *Osteitis due to syphilis (Goodhill, 1939)
    d. *Osteitis deformans (Davis, 1968)
    e. *Osteogenesis imperfecta (Altmann, 1962)
    f. *Osteopetrosis (Myers and Stool, 1969)
    g. *Otosclerosis (Schuknecht, 1974)
    h. Thickened periosteal layer due to endemic cretinism (Warkany, 1971)
    i. *Underdevelopment of periosteal layer due to craniofacial dysostosis (Baldwin, 1968)

(I) Mastoid Anomalies (11), (12), (14), (31), (35), (51)

    a. *Absence of mastoid antrum (Sando et al., 1968)
    b. *Poor development of mastoid antrum (Ruedi, 1954)
    c. *Poor development of mastoid air cells (Ruedi, 1954)
    d. *Small mastoid process (Ruedi, 1954)

(J) Eustachian Tube Anomalies (19)

    a. Absence (Altmann, 1951b)
    b. Abnormally narrow (Altmann, 1949)
    c. Diverticula of eustachian tube (Von Kostanecki, 1887, quoted by Altmann, 1951b)
    d. Congenital tumor (polyp) (Henke, 1924, quoted by Altmann, 1951b)

DISCUSSION

External and middle ear anomalies are of major importance to both the patient and the otologist. When they are bilateral and associated with significant hearing loss from birth, they result in poor speech and language development or failure of such development. Children thus afflicted are sometimes mistakenly classified as being mentally retarded and are needlessly condemned to a lifetime of institutionalization and intellectual deprivation. Also, cosmetic anomalies of the external ear may produce severe psychologic trauma in children. Early correction of deformities is essential in assuring normal development of speech and is also helpful to the psychologic development of the patient who is affected by the anomaly. Correction of congenital anomalies represents a challenge to the surgical ingenuity of the otologist, but the fact that a hearing loss is frequently correctible by modern otomicrosurgical techniques should be encouraging to the patient, his or her family, and the otologist. As has been mentioned, surgical misadventures may result from encountering unexpected anatomic variations. A study of the nature of the anomaly often provides the otologist with some clue as to the period of embryonic development when the insult occurred and, thus, to what other anomalies might be encountered during corrective surgery.

From a review of the literature on this subject and from study of temporal bones, certain trends are evident.

1. External and middle ear anomalies that occur in the absence of associated an-

omalies usually are of unknown origin and occur in the absence of any family history of anomalies.

2. External and middle ear anomalies that occur with other anomalies usually are of known etiology or are associated with a positive family history.

3. Of the middle ear anomalies that occur without other anomalies, those most frequently encountered include ossicular anomalies and anomalies of the facial nerve. There is a tendency for middle ear anomalies to occur together, such as facial nerve and ossicular anomalies, especially those involving the stapes. This, of course, reflects their interdependent embryonic development.

4. In the case of external and middle ear anomalies associated with other anomalies, the association of branchial arch anomalies with external and middle ear anomalies is clear. Because of the small number of histopathologic reports available regarding the temporal bone, it is not yet possible to compile a comprehensive list of associated anomalies.

5. Routine audiometric testing does not provide any clue as to the nature of the anomaly.

Some findings do provide us with diagnostic clues.

1. A positive family history of congenital malformations is important.

2. A maternal history of infectious disease during pregnancy and drug ingestion or exposure to ionizing irradiation before or during pregnancy should be sought.

3. A history of a nonprogressive, usually unilateral, conductive hearing loss present since birth suggests an anomaly of the external auditory meatus or ossicles, or both.

4. A history of retarded or absent speech development suggests a congenital hearing loss.

5. The presence of any other congenital anomalies makes imperative a complete physical and audiometric examination.

In studying suspected congenital external and middle ear anomalies, we would make the following suggestions.

1. A careful family history must be taken, with emphasis on congenital anomalies, ear infections, hearing aid use, and hearing loss.

2. The maternal history of drug ingestion, exposure to ionizing radiation, or utiliza-

tion of chelating agents or antimetabolites before or during pregnancy as well as a history of infectious diseases, especially viral, during pregnancy are important.

3. For differential diagnosis, a history of postnatal infections, perinatal trauma, or postnatal injury or surgery may provide information as to the origin of the anomaly.

4. Polytomographic studies may reveal anomalies of the external auditory meatus, middle ear, and inner ear.

5. The result of testing a child with an anomaly with the acoustic impedance bridge may make possible a differential diagnosis between ossicular fixation and ossicular discontinuity.

6. Chromosomal analysis may be helpful in making a differential diagnosis.

7. Surgical exploration, aided by radiographic findings, provides the only definitive diagnosis and also the treatment for these conditions.

8. During the surgery to correct conductive hearing losses of unknown origin, extreme care must be exercised in order to avoid injuring anatomic structures, such as the facial nerve, that may be located in other than their usual locations in anomalous ears. A knowledge of embryology provides the surgeon with some information as to where these structures are likely to be found when they are not in their normal locations.

An intensive campaign should be carried out to obtain the temporal bones from all patients with known anomalies of the ear, other associated anomalies, or conductive and sensorineural hearing loss of unknown origin so that histopathologic studies of the temporal bone can be carried out.

TREATMENT AND REHABILITATION OF PATIENTS WITH CONGENITAL ANOMALIES OF THE EXTERNAL AND MIDDLE EAR

The variety and seriousness of anomalies of the external and middle ear range from minor variations from the normal and no functional disability to total absence of identifiable structures and of hearing. Even within any one disease category, the degree of abnormality and the nature of the anomaly (i.e., the structures affected) may vary widely.

Consequently, such patients cannot be managed by a "cookbook" approach. Because many of the anomalies found at surgery are unsuspected preoperatively (many of them occurring without any other associated anomalies) or the surgeon encounters hitherto undescribed anatomic variations in the middle ear, it is necessary to understand the *principles* of correction and to have a broad knowledge of the myriad of possibilities for creating a satisfactory mechanism for conducting sound to the cochlea. In some instances, surgical correction of an anomaly simply will not be possible.

Many of the conditions discussed are associated with mild to severe or even total sensorineural hearing losses. At the present time, no satisfactory medical or surgical treatment exists for a sensorineural hearing loss, except perhaps in the case of otosclerosis (Shambaugh and Causse, 1974). There are some as yet unpublished reports on the stabilization of progressive sensorineural hearing losses in patients with Mondini-type (shortened cochlea) cochlear deformities using the endolymphatic shunt operation. Direct electrical stimulation of the cochlear nerve by cochlear electrode implantation, which is currently under investigation, may be beneficial to patients in whom there is essentially total sensory hearing loss but the fibers of the cochlear nerve are intact.

The role of any physician who undertakes the care of patients with congenital anomalies is to remedy their problems in whatever manner is feasible. When dealing with anomalies of the ear, this includes restoration of hearing or at least improvement of hearing to as near normal levels as possible and the prevention or correction of any speech and language disorders that may accompany the hearing loss. The physician's responsibility goes beyond that, however, and now includes the determination and remediation of any learning disabilities which may be associated with the hearing loss and its resultant speech and language disorders.

The process of treatment must begin with a determination of the extent of the disability. In many medical centers, in addition to the routine neonatal examination which will, hopefully, discover many visible congenital anomalies, a high-risk register (Northern and Downs, 1978) for hearing loss is used to determine which babies should receive neonatal hearing screening; determinations are based upon family history, prenatal history, conditions surrounding the birth, and early neonatal history. Some centers do routine hearing screening on all newborn infants.

Once an infant has been placed in the high-risk category by virtue of the register criteria, repeated physical examinations and hearing screening are performed in the first few months of life until it is determined that the hearing is normal.

For those children in whom a hearing loss is strongly suspected or proved, remediation is begun at once. It is the policy at the University of Colorado Medical Center to fit any infant suspected of having a hearing loss greater than 20 dB bilaterally with a hearing aid. The earliest fittings have been at about one month of age. Air conduction aids are used whenever possible; in cases of external atresia, bone conduction aids are used. Very close follow-up with frequent hearing retesting is carried out until accurate estimations of the hearing can be obtained. Speech and language development are closely observed, and special education is provided when necessary. In cases of multiple anomalies in which mental and motor retardation may be present, it is difficult to determine the child's developmental potential early in the course.

In cases in which the association between certain anomalies and hearing loss is very high (e.g., cleft palate and middle ear effusion), a myringotomy will be performed and middle ear ventilation tubes placed as soon as possible (Paradise, 1975).

In other cases, as soon as the nature and severity of the hearing loss (i.e., conductive, sensorineural, or mixed loss) have been determined, a course of action is decided upon. Those children with sensorineural losses will continue to use hearing amplification. When a conductive loss is accompanied by a middle ear effusion, a myringotomy is performed, and ventilating tubes are placed. The hearing must be carefully monitored after tube placement, since the first clue to an otherwise unsuspected middle ear anomaly frequently is the failure of the hearing to improve after tube placement. (Normally, if a hearing loss is caused by a middle ear effusion, the hearing will improve quickly following myringotomy.)

Patients who are known to have anomalies, such as aural atresia, and those with severe conductive and mixed hearing losses are further studied using polytomographic studies of the temporal bone to evaluate the condition of the external ear canal, the presence of an atretic bony plate, the size and condition of the middle ear space and ossicular chain, and the cochlea, vestibule, semicircular canals, and internal auditory meatus. The locations of the carotid artery, sigmoid sinus, and fallopian canal are also determined by these studies.

Following these studies, a decision is made as to the feasibility of surgery to improve hearing and to correct cosmetic deformities.

THE SURGICAL CORRECTION OF CONGENITAL ANOMALIES OF THE EXTERNAL EAR AND MIDDLE EAR

Auricle

Surgery to correct anomalies of the auricle has been carried out for many years; however, there has been a difference of opinion as to the efficacy of different types of surgical management of some of the anomalies. It is generally agreed that minor deformities of the auricle can be repaired surgically with quite acceptable cosmetic results, but severe deformities with few normal structures frequently still appear distinctly abnormal, even to casual view, after multiple operative procedures. In such cases, the question arises as to whether or not a better alternative might not be excision of the minor skin tags and fitting with a good cosmetic prosthesis rather than the trauma of multiple operations resulting in an equivocal cosmetic result (Jensen and Terkildson, 1967; Lowenstein, 1966).

The simplest auricular anomaly to correct is an outstanding (protruding) auricle. With the exception of failure of formation of the anthelical rim and sometimes an exceptionally deep concha, the auricle is well-formed. Although the standard surgical procedures (Becker, 1952; Converse et al., 1955) for correcting such deformities yield excellent results in the best of hands, the cartilaginous incisions can result in unpleasant, sharp demarcations that are visible from the anterior and lateral aspects. In recent years, we have instead used the simpler technique of Mustarde (1963).

Next in complexity is the repair of cryptotia. In this disorder, the superior portion of auricular cartilage is buried beneath the scalp. Usually a relatively simple operative procedure to release the buried cartilage framework and overlying skin from the side of the head and to place a split-thickness graft to the posterior aspect of the auricle and postauricular area will yield a satisfactory result. Some minor revisions may be necessary (Pollock, 1969).

Far more serious problems are encountered in the correction of anotia and microtia. These conditions represent a continuum of deformity ranging from total absence of any identifiable auricular structures (anotia), to the presence of primordial hillocks (microtia Type III) barely recognizable as auricular structures, to the existence of a curving elevation representing a deformed helix (microtia Type II), and finally to the presence of a small auricle that is deformed but possesses the essential structures (microtia Type I) (Fig. 14–5). In all these anomalies, the structures may be displaced downward and anterior to their usual locations. Although many surgical procedures have been described for the correction of these conditions, it is the authors' opinion that anotia and Type III microtia are better handled by excision of any vestigial tags and fitting of a good cosmetic prosthesis.

Microtia Types I and II may be repaired by the procedures described by Converse (1964), sometimes with very acceptable results.

External Auditory Meatus and Middle Ear

For those interested in the well-being and development of the child with bilateral congenital atresia of the external auditory meatus, there is a moral and medical dilemma. Although there are mild forms of this condition, manifested only by abnormally narrow external auditory meatuses without any associated conductive hearing loss and requiring no correction or only minor treatment (such as frequent cleaning or canaloplasty), the more serious forms involve total or partial absence of the external canal. These are normally accompanied by a maximum conductive hearing loss in the range of 60 to 70 dB. This is compounded by the inability to fit an air conduction hearing aid and, frequently, lack of an auricle or the presence of a deformed or misplaced auricle. Also associated are anomalies of the middle ear ranging from minor anomalies of the

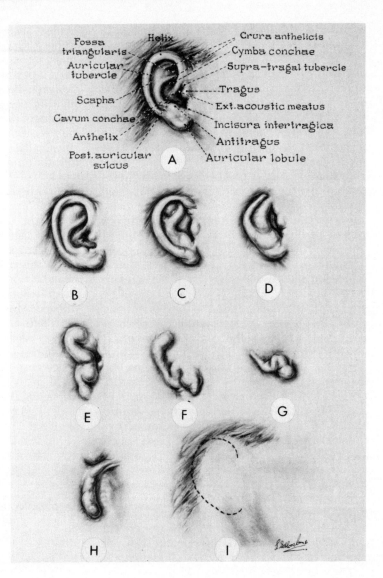

Figure 14–5 Examples of auricular malformations. *A*, normal adult pinna. *B*, example of a minor malformation. The pinna reveals regular overall dimensions and position, but incomplete differentiation. *C* and *D*, examples of microtia type I: the auricle is smaller, rudimentary, and often located in an abnormal position. The different parts of the pinna are still discernible. *E* and *F*, examples of microtia type II: the auricle, besides being smaller and often in an abnormal position, is represented by a vertical curving ridge, resembling a primitive helix. *G* and *H*, examples of microtia type III: the rudiment of the auricle has no resemblance to any portion of the pinna. *I*, example of anotia. (From Nager, G. T. 1973. *In* Paparella, M. M., and Shumrick, D. A. (Eds.) Otolaryngology, Vol. 2, Philadelphia, W. B. Saunders Co., p. 10).

ossicles to absence of the mastoid and middle ear cleft. There may also be anomalies of the inner ear ranging from minor malformations of the labyrinth to absence of the inner ear. The surgical correction of the more serious anomalies presents a risk to hearing and facial nerve function.

The presence of anomalies of the auricle and the external auditory meatus makes imperative a careful examination of the patient to determine the extent of the deformities. This involves first a physical examination to determine if other anomalies are present. Next, audiometric testing must be performed in a center that is equipped to do neonatal testing. Even in the immediate postnatal period, reasonably accurate behavioral test results may be obtained. Localization, howev-

er, may be difficult to determine. Next, radiographic studies must be performed. In planning the surgical correction of atresia, anteroposterior and lateral polytomographic roentgenograms of the external auditory meatus, mastoid, middle ear, inner ear, and internal auditory meatus are mandatory. In order to obtain adequate data from these tests in infants, general anesthesia is frequently necessary.

Once these studies are completed, a plan may be formulated for the surgical management of the patient's deformities. It is the authors' opinion that if the atresia is unilateral and the hearing is normal in the opposite ear, *no* surgical correction is indicated other than cosmetic until the patient reaches the age of consent so that he or she may decide whether to undertake the risk inherent in surgical correction of severe malformations. In the case of bilateral atresia, there is a question as to which ear should be operated upon. Before any operation, it should be determined that the patient has hearing in the opposite ear so that the patient would have functional hearing should there be a sensorineural hearing loss secondary to the surgery.

Evaluation of the polytomograms includes establishing the presence of a normal internal auditory canal and cochlea. Next, the presence of a middle ear cleft and mastoid air cell system must be determined. The condition of the ossicular chain must be evaluated, and the presence of a fallopian canal may be determined on lateral views. (It must be remembered, however, that the presence of the bony canal *does not* mean that the nerve is lying within it.) If possible, the canal is traced to its point of exit from the temporal bone. (It must be remembered that in normal infants the nerve exits laterally behind and below the external auditory meatus because the mastoid tip is not yet developed.) The location and condition of the oval window niche, round window, and the horizontal semicircular canal are determined. The examiner must also look for replacement of the tympanic membrane by a bony atresia plate. Lastly, the external auditory meatus is examined to determine if the atresia is made up of soft tissue or bone and to establish the relative position of the mandibular condyle, which may be displaced posteriorly, occupying the normal position of the external auditory meatus.

The more normal ear should be operated upon first. Then, if an auricular deformity has occurred in addition to the canal deformity, the staging of surgery must be decided with whomever will operate to correct the external deformity. Usually, the middle ear and canal correction will be done first to locate the new ear canal, although there are differences of opinion on this aspect. The auricle can then be relocated to place it over the canal.

The surgical procedure to correct ear deformities has several goals. The first is to create a patent external auditory meatus and is accomplished by removing the stenotic soft tissue of the existing canal. If the medial portion of the canal is bony, this must be drilled away to create a large meatus, which is then lined with a split-thickness graft. Next, if a bony atresia plate is present, this must be drilled away carefully so as not to transmit unnecessary trauma to the stapes. Most authors recommend disarticulating the incus and stapes prior to drilling in this region. It is desirable to create a shelf of bone approximating the annulus onto which one can lay the drum prosthesis. In some cases, the posterior position of the mandibular condyle will drastically alter the position of the external auditory meatus (Figs. 14–6, 14–7, and 14–8).

The condition of the ossicular chain is then ascertained; fixation of the malleus and incus to the bony atretic plate is not uncommon. If this is the case, it must be determined if the ossicles can be salvaged or if they must be sacrificed. It is best to save them if possible, but if the risk of refixation seems great, they must be removed. The condition of the stapes superstructure and footplate is then determined. Most importantly, mobility of the footplate must be established.

The recreation of the sound-conducting mechanism is the next step. If the middle ear ossicles are relatively normal and mobile, a fascia graft is placed beneath the manubrium of the malleus in the usual fashion. If not,

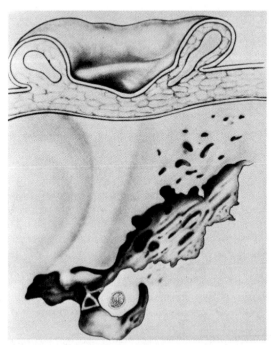

Figure 14–6 Sagittal section of the temporal bone illustrating absent bony external auditory meatus with malleus-incus complex fused to bony atresia plate. (From Jahrsdoerfer, R. A. 1978. Congenital atresia of the ear. Laryngoscope, 88, Suppl. 13.)

grafting may be accomplished with fascia or with a homograft tympanic membrane–ossicular prosthesis. We believe the homograft will become more commonly used in time. The attachment to the stapes may be carried out at the first operation or in a later reconstruction, depending upon the situation encountered. In the absence of an incus, either a homograft ossicle or an alloplastic strut may be used. Our personal experience with alloplastic struts in middle ear reconstruction has not been entirely favorable, and hence we prefer to use autograft or homograft ossicles.

Lastly, the external auditory meatus is lined with a split-thickness skin graft. Preferably, no external canal stent is used, as we believe this may cause further stenosis.

The results of surgery for congenital atresia have not been uniformly good (or else there would have been considerably more enthusiasm for it); however, recent reports have been encouraging. The chief problems have been damage to the facial nerve, stenosis

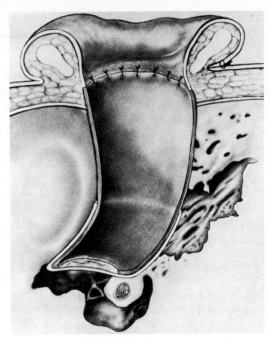

Figure 14–8 In this drawing, a split-thickness skin graft with a hole over the neotympanum graft has been placed to line the bony external auditory meatus. (From Jahrsdoerfer, R. A. 1978. Congenital atresia of the ear. Laryngoscope, 88, Suppl. 13.)

of the external auditory meatus, poor hearing results (for unknown reasons), and sensorineural hearing loss. For a complete review of the problem, its analysis, and treatment, we refer readers to the excellent articles by Jahrsdoerfer (1978) and Crabtree (1968).

Middle Ear

The exact nature of middle ear anomalies is seldom known prior to surgical exploration. In children in the early years of life, when middle ear effusions and recurrent suppurative otitis media are common, and in those with a predisposition to eustachian tube malfunction (e.g., those with cleft palates), one would anticipate poorer surgical results than in patients whose eustachian tube function is normal. Consequently, the surgeon must weigh the possibility of complications resulting from impaired eustachian tube function against the benefits of early improvement in hearing. Entering into this is the frequent refusal of some children to wear hearing aids.

Owing to the diverse nature of middle ear

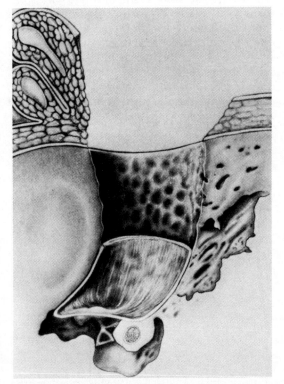

Figure 14–7 Drawing illustrating newly created bony external auditory meatus with a fascia graft placed over the ossicular chain and the facial ridge, lining a portion of the external canal walls. (From Jahrsdoerfer, R. A. 1978. Congenital atresia of the ear. Laryngoscope, 88, Suppl. 13.)

anomalies, there is no single operative procedure for the restoration of hearing. In some circumstances, no feasible way to improve hearing may be found.

It is beyond the purview of this text to discuss all the possible methods for recreation of the sound-conducting mechanism of the middle ear; however, some examples will be given. The principle involved is to create a mobile ossicular chain with good contact between a mobile tympanic membrane and a mobile stapes footplate (Figs. 14–9, 14–10, and 14–11) (Tabor, 1971). In turn, for this system to be effective there must be a normal round window membrane. In rare instances (where an oval window niche is not present or is covered by an aberrant facial nerve), sound must be conducted to other than the stapes footplate; usually the horizontal semicircular canal is fenestrated in such cases (Shambaugh, 1967).

The most straightforward operative procedure for the treatment of a congenital conductive hearing loss is the performance of a stapedectomy to correct the effects of otosclerosis. In this instance, the fixed footplate and stapes are removed, the oval window is covered by a tissue graft such as perichondrium, and a wire is placed from the incus to the oval window to transmit sound (Fig. 14–12).

Summary

Minor abnormalities of the auricle can usually be corrected by simple operative pro-

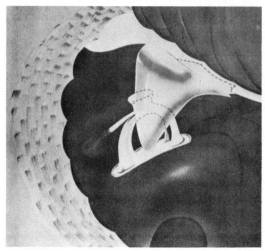

Figure 14–10 Drawing illustrating transposition of the incus with the short process on the stapes footplate between the superstructure and the promontory. The articular surface of the incus is placed medial to the malleus manubrium. (From Tabor, J. R. 1971. Methods of Ossiculoplasty. Springfield, Ill., Charles C Thomas Co.)

cedures that give quite acceptable cosmetic results. Where only vestigial auricular structures are present, surgical reconstruction through many operative procedures frequently yields unacceptable cosmetic results. In these cases, a well-made auricular prosthesis is preferable.

When a child presents with atresia in which there is considerable distortion of the normal anatomy of the external auditory meatus,

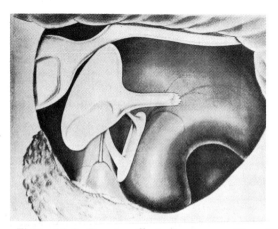

Figure 14–9 Drawing illustrating transposition of the incus between the malleus long process and the stapedial head with the incudal head flat on the stapedial head. (From Tabor, J. R. 1971. Methods of Ossiculoplasty. Springfield, Ill., Charles C Thomas Co.)

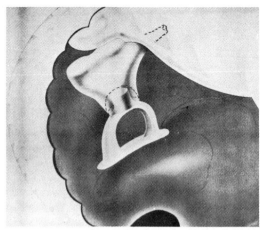

Figure 14–11 Drawing illustrating incus transposition in which a cup that has been drilled in the short process of the incus is placed over the head of the stapes. The long process of the incus is placed beneath the medial aspect of the malleus manubrium. (From Tabor, J. R. 1971. Methods of Ossiculoplasty. Springfield, Ill., Charles C Thomas Co.)

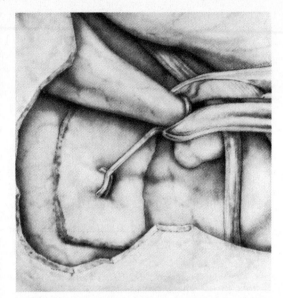

Figure 14–12 A House wire stapes prosthesis being crimped over the long process of the incus. The loop is resting upon tissue (compressed fat, vein, fascia, perichondrium) which seals the oval window. (From Goin, D. W. 1976. *In* English, G. M. (Ed.) Otolaryngology, a Textbook, Hagerstown, Md., Harper and Row, p. 154.)

middle ear, and sometimes inner ear, sophisticated roentgenographic studies must be made to determine the feasibility of reconstructing the existing ear. Care must be exerted to avoid damage to the facial nerve and cochlea, which would result in a sensorineural hearing loss. Ultimately one of the most difficult problems encountered in this type of reconstruction is in the prevention of postoperative external meatus stenosis.

Anomalies of the middle ear sound-conducting mechanism may very frequently be corrected by modern otomicrosurgical techniques. The exact nature of the anomaly is almost never known until surgical exploration is carried out. At that time, hitherto unsuspected anomalies, such as those of the facial nerve and carotid artery or a persistent stapedial artery, may be encountered. Nowhere is the experience and flexibility of the otologic surgeon of greater import than in the correction of these anomalies: using accepted surgical principles, he or she must often remedy previously undescribed conditions.

The responsibility of the otologist does not end with the surgical correction of otic anomalies. This practitioner must be aware of the social, psychological, and educational consequences of these anomalies and the speech and language delays that may result from the associated hearing loss. It is incumbent upon the physician to be responsible for seeing that the appropriate rehabilitative measures are instituted. Likewise, in those cases of sensorineural hearing loss or conductive hearing loss that are not amenable to surgical correction, it is the responsibility of the otologist to oversee an appropriate amplification treatment program.

SELECTED REFERENCES

Crabtree, J. A. 1968. Tympanoplastic techniques in congenital atresia. Arch. Otolaryngol., *88*:89–96.
This article is particularly valuable for its explanation of the surgical approach to congenital atresia.

Hough, J. V. D. 1958. Malformations and anatomical variations seen in the middle ear during the operation for stabilization of the stapes. Laryngoscope, *68*:1337–1379.
This report on anomalies and variations in middle ear structures encountered during stapes surgery is valuable, especially for its description of a number of interesting cases and for the colored photomicrographs and illustrations that accompany these descriptions.

Jahrsdoerfer, R. A. 1978. Congenital atresia of the ear. Laryngoscope, *88*, Suppl. 13.
This article gives an excellent, complete review of the problem, analysis, and treatment of congenital atresia of the ear.

Konigsmark, W., and Gorlin, R. J. 1976. Genetic and Metabolic Deafness. Philadelphia, W. B. Saunders Co.
This textbook is a valuable reference source for information on many types of hereditary hearing losses.

Schuknecht, H. F. 1974. Pathology of the Ear. Cambridge, MA, Harvard University Press.
This textbook should be extremely helpful to both researchers and clinicians who concern themselves with the function of hearing in association with external and middle ear anomalies.

Tabor, J. R. 1971. Methods of Ossiculoplasty. Springfield, IL, Charles C Thomas Co.
This textbook discusses clearly and concisely the principles of ossicular chain reconstruction in various situations that may be encountered in the middle ear.

The authors are grateful to Professor Bruce Jafek, M.D., Department of Otolaryngology, University of Colorado Medical Center, for the use of the Center's cases for some of the figures in this chapter.

The authors wish to express their deep gratitude to Professor E. N. Myers, M.D., Department of Otolaryngology, University of Pittsburgh School of Medicine, for encouraging them to study this subject and for giving helpful criticism during the preparation of this chapter.

The authors are also grateful to Mrs. Ruth Anderson for her assistance.

REFERENCES

Adkins, W. Y., Jr., and Gussen, R. 1974a. Oval window absence, bony closure of round window, and inner ear anomaly. Laryngoscope, *84*:1210–1224.

Adkins, W. Y., Jr., and Gussen, R. 1974b. Temporal bone findings in the third and fourth pharyngeal pouch (DiGeorge) syndrome. Arch. Otolaryngol., *100*:206–208.

Altmann, F. 1947. Anomalies of the internal carotid artery and its branches. Laryngoscope, *58*:313–339.

Altmann, F. 1949. Problem of so-called congenital atresia of the ear. Arch. Otolaryngol., *50*:759–788.

Altmann, F. 1951a. Malformations of the auricle and the external auditory meatus (A Critical Review). Arch. Otolaryngol., *54*:115–139.

Altmann, F. 1951b. Malformations of the Eustachian tube, the middle ear, and its appendages (A Critical Review). Arch. Otolaryngol., *54*:241–266.

Altmann, F. 1955. Congenital atresia of the ear in man and animals. Ann. Otol. Rhinol. Laryngol., *64*:824–858.

Altmann, F. 1957. The ear in severe malformations of the head. Arch. Otolaryngol., *66*:7–25.

Altmann, F. 1962. The temporal bone in osteogenesis imperfecta congenita. Arch. Otolaryngol., *75*:486–497.

Baldwin, J. L. 1968. Dysostosis craniofacialis of Crouzon. Laryngoscope, *78*:1660–1677.

Bart, R. S., and Pumphrey, R. E. 1967. Knuckle pads, leukonychia and deafness. A dominantly inherited syndrome. N. Engl. J. Med., *276*:202–207.

Basek, M. 1962. Anomalies of the facial nerve in normal temporal bones. Ann. Otol. Rhinol. Laryngol., *71*:382–390.

Becker, O. J. 1952. Correction of protruding deformed ear. Brit. J. Plast. Surg., *5*:187.

Bergstrom, L., Hemenway, W. G., and Sando, I. 1972. Pathological changes in congenital deafness. Laryngoscope, *82*:1777–1792.

Bergstrom, L. 1977. Osteogenesis imperfecta. Otologic and maxillofacial aspects. Laryngoscope, *87*, Suppl. 6.

Black, F. O., Sando, I., Wagner, J. A., et al. 1971. Middle and inner ear abnormalities, 13–15 (D$_1$) trisomy. Arch. Otolaryngol., *93*:615–619.

Black, F. O., Myers, E. N., and Rorke, L. B. 1973. Aplasia of the first and second branchial arches. Arch. Otolaryngol., *98*:124–128.

Bordley, J. E., and Hardy, J. M. B. 1969. Laboratory and clinical observations on prenatal rubella. Ann. Otol. Rhinol. Laryngol., *78*:917–928.

Buran, D. J., and Duvall, A. J. 1967. The oto-palato-digital (OPD) syndrome. Arch. Otolaryngol., *85*:394–399.

Caparosa, R. J., and Klassen, D. 1966. Congenital anomalies of the stapes and facial nerve. Arch. Otolaryngol., *83*:420–421.

Cohn, M., Statloff, J., and Lindsay, J. R. 1970. Histiocytosis X (Letterer-Siwe disease) with involvement of the inner ear. Arch. Otolaryngol., *91*:24–29.

Converse, J. M., Nigro, A., Wilson, F. A., et al. 1955. A technique for surgical correction of lop ears. Plast. and Reconstr. Surg., *15*:411–418.

Converse, J. M. (Ed.) 1964. Reconstructive Plastic Surgery: Principles and Procedures in Correction, Reconstruction and Transplantation, Vol. 3. Philadelphia, W. B. Saunders Co.

Crabtree, J. A. 1968. Tympanoplastic techniques in congenital atresia. Arch. Otolaryngol., *88*:89–96.

Davis, D. G. 1968. Paget's disease of the temporal bone. Acta Otolaryngol. (Stockh.) Suppl., *242*.

Druss, J. G. 1952. Supernumerary muscle of middle ear. Arch. Otolaryngol., *55*:206–209.

Durcan, D. J., Shea, J. J., and Sleeckx, J. P. 1967. Bifurcation of the facial nerve. Arch. Otolaryngol., *86*:619–631.

Egami, T., Sando, I., and Myers, E. N. 1979. Temporal bone anomalies associated with congenital heart disease. Ann. Otol. Rhinol. Laryngol. *88*:72–78.

Escher, F., and Hirt, H. 1968. Dominant hereditary conductive deafness through lack of incus–stapes junction. Acta Otolaryngol. (Stockh.), *65*:25–32.

Fernandez, A. O., and Ronis, M. L. 1964. Congenital absence of the oval window. Laryngoscope, *74*:186–197.

Fitch, N., Lindsay, J. R., and Srolovitz, H. 1976. The temporal bone in the preauricular pit, cervical fistula, hearing loss syndrome. Ann. Otol. Rhinol. Laryngol., *85*:268–275.

Føns, M. 1969. Ear malformations in cleidocranial dysostosis. Acta Otolaryngol. (Stockh.), *67*:483–489.

Forney, W. R., Robinson, S. J., and Pascoe, D. J. 1966. Congenital heart disease, deafness, and skeletal malformations: A new syndrome? Pediatr., *68*:14–26.

Fowler, E. P., Jr. 1961. Variations in the temporal bone course of the facial nerve. Laryngoscope, *71*:937–946.

Gnanapragasam, A. 1975. Bilateral symmetrical maldevelopment of the external ear and middle ear cleft with pharyngeal and soft palate defects. J. Laryngol., Otol., *89*:845–851.

Goldberg, M. J., and Pashayan, H. M. 1976. Hallux syndactyly–ulnar polydactyly–abnormal ear lobes: A new syndrome. Birth Defects, *12*(5):255–266.

Goldman, N. N., Singleton, G. T., and Holly, E. H. 1971. Aberrant internal carotid artery. Arch. Otolaryngol., *94*:269–273.

Goodhill, V. 1939. Syphilis of the ear: A histopathologic study. Ann. Otol. Rhinol. Laryngol., *48*:676–706.

Harrison, W. H., Shambaugh, G. E., Jr., and Derlacki, E. L. 1966. Congenital absence of the round window: Case report with surgical reconstruction by cochlear fenestration. Laryngoscope, *76*:967–978.

Hemenway, W. G., Sando, I., and McChesney, D. 1969. Temporal bone pathology following maternal rubella. Arch. Klin. Exp. Ohr. Nas. Kehlk. Heilk., *193*:287–300.

Henderson, J. L. 1939. The congenital facial diplegia syndrome: Clinical features, pathology and aetiology. A review of sixty-one cases. Brain, *62*:381–403.

Herberts, G. 1962. Otological observations on the "Treacher-Collins syndrome." Acta Otolaryngol, (Stockh.), *54*:457–465.

Hiraide, F., Nomura, Y., and Nakamura, K. 1974. Histopathology of atresia auris congenita. J. Laryngol. Otol., *88*:1249–1256.

Hoenk, B. E., McCabe, B. F., and Anson, B. J. 1969. Cholesteatoma auris behind a bony atresia plate. Arch. Otolaryngol., *89*:470–477.

Hough, J. V. D. 1958. Malformations and anatomical variations seen in the middle ear during the operation for mobilization of the stapes. Laryngoscope, *68*:1337–1379.

Hough, J. V. D. 1963. Congenital malformations of the middle ear. Arch. Otolaryngol., *78*:335–343.

Igarashi, M., Filippone, M. V., and Alford, B. R. 1976. Temporal bone findings in Pierre Robin syndrome. Laryngoscope, *86*:1679–1687.

Igarashi, M., Takahasi, M., Alford, B. R., et al. 1977. Inner ear morphology in Down syndrome. Acta Otolaryngol. (Stockh.), *83*:175–181.

Jaffee, I. S. 1968. Congenital shoulder-neck-auditory anomalies. Laryngoscope, *78*:2119–2139.

Jahrsdoerfer, R. A. 1978. Congenital atresia of the ear. Laryngoscope, *88*, Suppl. 13.

Jensen, P. V., and Terkildson, K. 1967. Prosthetic reconstruction of external ear defects. Acta Otol., *64*:492–499.

Jørgensen, M. B., Kristensen, H. K., and Buch, N. H. 1964. Thalidomide-induced aplasia of the inner ear. J. Laryngol. Otol., *78*:1095–1101.

Karmody, C. S., and Schuknecht, H. F. 1966. Deafness in congenital syphilis. Arch. Otolaryngol., *83*:18–27.

Kelemen, G. 1966a. Hurler's syndrome and the hearing organ. J. Laryngol. Otol., *80*:791–803.

Kelemen, G. 1966b. Rubella and deafness. Arch. Otolaryngol., *83*:520–532.

Koide, Y., Kato, I., Yamasaki, H., et al. 1967. Congenital anomalies of the ossicles without deformities of the external ear. Jap. J. Otol., *70*:1358–1366.

Konigsmark, W., Nager, G. T., and Haskins, H. L. 1972. Recessive microtia, meatal atresia and hearing loss. Arch. Otolaryngol., *96*:105–109.

Konigsmark, W., and Gorlin, R. J. 1976. Genetic and Metabolic Deafness. Philadelphia, W. B. Saunders Co.

Kos, A. O., Schuknecht, H. F., and Singer, J. D. 1966. Temporal bone studies in 13–15 and 18 trisomy syndromes. Arch. Otolaryngol., *83*:439–445.

Kraus, P., and Ziv, M. 1971. Incus fixation due to congenital anomaly of chorda tympani. Acta Otolaryngol. (Stockh.), *72*:358–360.

Larrson, A. 1962. Genetic problems in otosclerosis. *In* Schuknecht, H. (Ed.) Henry Ford Symposium on Otosclerosis. Boston, Little, Brown, and Co., pp. 109–118.

Lindsay, J. R., Sanders, S. H., and Nager, G. T. 1960. Histopathologic observations in so-called congenital fixation of the stapedial footplate. Laryngoscope, *70*:1587–1602.

Lindsay, J. R., Black, F. O., and Donnelly, W. H. 1975. Acrocephalo-syndactyly (Apert's syndrome). Temporal bone findings. Ann. Otol. Rhinol. Laryngol., *84*:174–178.

Lindsay, J. R., and Suga, F. 1976. Paget's disease and sensorineural deafness. Temporal bone histopathology of Paget's disease. Laryngoscope, *86*:1029–1042.

Livingstone, G., and Delahunty, J. E. 1968. Malformation of the ear associated with congenital ophthalmic and other conditions. J. Laryngol. Otol., *82*:495–504.

Lowenstein, H. 1966. Long-term observations on ear and nose prostheses. Br. J. Plast Surg., *19*:385–390.

Maran, A. G. D. 1965. Persistent stapedial artery. J. Laryngol. Otol., *79*:971–975.

McDonough, S. R. 1970. Fanconi anemia syndrome. Arch. Otolaryngol., *92*:284–285.

McGrew, R. N., and Gregg, J. B. 1971. Anomalous fusion os the malleus to the tympanic ring. Ann. Otol. Rhinol. Laryngol., *80*:138–140.

McLay, K., and Maran, A. G. D. 1969. Deafness and the Klippel-Feil syndrome. J. Laryngol. Otol., *83*:175–184.

Melnick, M., Bixler, D., Sil, K., et al. 1975. Autosomal dominant branchio-oto-renal dysplasia. Birth Defects, *11*(5):121–128.

Mengel, M. C., Konigsmark, B. W., Berlin, C. I., et al. 1969. Conductive hearing loss and malformed low-set ears, as a possible recessive syndrome. J. Med. Genet., *6*:14–21.

Morgenstein, K. M., and Manace, E. D. 1969. Temporal bone histopathology in sickle cell disease. Laryngoscope, *79*:2172–2180.

Mustarde, J. C. 1963. The correction of prominent ears using simple mattress sutures. Br. J. Plast. Surg., *16*:170.

Myers, E. N., and Stool, S. E. 1969. The temporal bone in osteopetrosis. Arch. Otolaryngol., *89*:460–469.

Northern, J. L., and Downs, M. P. 1978. Hearing in Children. Baltimore, Williams and Wilkins Co., pp. 204–211.

Opheim, O. 1968. Loss of hearing following the syndrome of van der Hoeve-De Kleyn, Acta Otolaryngol. (Stockh.), *65*:337–344.

Paradise, J. L. 1975. Middle ear problems associated with cleft palate. Cleft Palate J., *12*:17–22.

Pfaffenbach, D. D., Cross, H. E., and Kearns, P. K. 1972. Congenital anomalies in Duane's retraction syndrome. Arch. Ophthalmol., *88*:635–639.

Pollock, W. J. 1969. Technique for correction of cryptotia. Plast. Reconstr. Surg., *44*:501–503.

Pou, J. W. 1963. Congenital absence of the oval window. Laryngoscope, *73*:384–391.

Rimoin, D. L., and Edgerton, M. T. 1967. Genetic and clinical heterogeneity in the oral-facial-digital syndrome. J. Pediatr., *71*:94–102.

Ritter, F. N. 1971. The histopathology of the congenital fixed malleus syndrome. Laryngoscope, *81*:1304–1313.

Rosen, S. 1952. Glomus jugulare tumor of middle ear with normal drum: Improved biopsy technique. Ann. Otol. Rhinol. Laryngol., *61*:448–451.

Ruben, R. J., Toriyama, M., Dische, M. R., et al. 1969. External and middle ear malformations associated with mandibulo-facial dysostosis and renal abnormalities: A case report. Ann. Otol. Rhinol. Laryngol., *78*:605–624.

Ruedi, L. 1954. The surgical treatment of atresia auris congenita: A clinical and histological report. Laryngoscope, *64*:666–684.

Ruggles, R. L., and Reed, R. C. 1972. Symposium on ear surgery. V. Treatment of aberrant carotid arteries in the middle ear: A report of two cases. Laryngoscope, *82*:1199–1205.

Sando, I., Hemenway, W. G., and Morgan, W. R. 1968. Histopathology of the temporal bones in mandibulo-facial dysostosis (Treacher-Collins syndrome). Trans. Am. Acad. Ophthalmol. Otol., *72*:913–924.

Sando, I., Bergstrom, L., Wood, R. P., II, et al. 1970. Temporal bone findings in trisomy 18 syndrome. Arch. Otolaryngol., *91*:552–559.

Sando, I., Leiberman, A., Bergstrom, L., et al. 1975. Temporal bone histopathological findings in trisomy 13 syndrome. Ann. Otol. Rhinol. Laryngol., *84*, Suppl. 21.

Schuknecht, H. F. 1967. Pathology of sensorineural deafness of genetic origin. *In* McConnell, F., and Ward, P. H. (Eds.) Deafness in Childhood. Nashville, Vanderbilt University Press, pp. 69–90.

Schuknecht, H. F. 1974. Pathology of the Ear. Cambridge, MA, Harvard University Press.

Shambaugh, G. E., Jr. 1967. Surgery of the Ear. Philadelphia, W. B. Saunders Co., p. 525.

Shambaugh, G. E., and Causse, J. 1974. Ten years experience with fluoride in otosclerotic (otospongiotic) patients. Ann. Otol. Rhinol. Laryngol., *83*:635–643.

Silcox, L. *In* Rubin, A. (Ed.) Handbook of Congenital Malformation. Philadelphia, W. B. Saunders Co., pp. 227–247.

Stallings, J. O., and McCabe, B. F. 1969. Congenital middle ear aneurysm of internal carotid. Arch. Otolaryngol., *90*:39–43.

Steffen, T. N. 1968. Vascular anomalies of the middle ear. Laryngoscope, *78*:171–197.

Stratton, H. J. M. 1965. Gonadal dysgenesis and the ears. J. Laryngol. Otol., *79*:343–346.

Szpunar, J., and Rybak, M. 1968. Middle ear disease in Turner's syndrome. Arch. Otolaryngol., *87*:34–40.

Tabor, J. R. 1961. Absence of the oval window. Arch. Otolaryngol., *74*:515–521.

Tabor, J. R. 1971. Methods of Ossiculoplasty. Springfield, Charles C Thomas Co.

Van der Borden, J. 1967. Bilateral non-chromaffin tympano-jugular paraganglioma. J. Laryngol. Otol., *81*:445–448.

Vase, P., Prytz, S., and Pedersen, P. S. 1975. Congenital stapes fixation, symphalangism and syndactylia. Acta Otolaryngol. (Stockh.), *80*:394–398.

Warkany, J. 1971. Congenital Malformations: Notes and Comments. Chicago, Year Book Medical Pub., pp. 401–416.

Winter, J. S. D., Kohn, G., Mellman, W. J., et al. 1968. A familial syndrome of renal, genital and middle ear anomalies. J. Pediatr., *72*:88–93.

Wright, J. L. W., and Etholm, B. 1973. Anomalies of the middle ear muscles. J. Laryngol. Otol., *87*:281–288.

Zonis, R. D. 1969. Meckel's cartilage remnant. Laryngoscope, *79*:2012–2015.

Chapter 15

DISEASES OF THE EXTERNAL EAR

LaVonne Bergstrom, M.D.

ANATOMY AND PHYSIOLOGY

Certain features of form and function are important to an understanding of diseases of the external ear.

The external ear is composed of a flexible, potentially mobile auricle and attached external auditory canal formed of fibrous tissue and elastic cartilage. These elements are in continuity with the osseous external canal, which medially ends in a tympanic ring incomplete superiorly. It contains the annular or tympanic sulcus into which the tympanic membrane inserts. The mobile, lateral one third of the canal inserts by fibrous bands on the external surface of the osseous canal. The cartilaginous canal contains slitlike fissures of Santorini, which communicate with the parotid gland. An inconstant hiatus may occur in the floor of the osseous canal (Anson and Donaldson, 1967; Hollinshead, 1968). Over this skeletal framework the skin is applied tightly, especially over the lateral surface of the pinna where the skin is immobile. It is thin over the pinna where blood vessels are superficial, and it is unprotected by a layer of fat except for small amounts on the mastoid surface where the skin is slightly mobile. The skin becomes thicker over the meatus and cartilaginous canal, where there are coarse hairs in the auditory meatus and, just within the meatus, modified sweat or cerumen glands. Medially the skin becomes very thin and inseparable from the periosteum over the osseous canal, and it contains no skin adnexae. Finally its squamous layer continues on over the lateral tympanic membrane surface (Hollinshead, 1968).

In adult life and later childhood the os-seous canal comprises about two thirds of the depth of the canal. In infancy, however, the bony canal consists only of the tympanic ring and hence is very shallow. Furthermore, the ring, into which the tympanic membrane inserts, is nearly horizontal when the infant is held erect so that the membrane is nearly horizontal (Hollinshead, 1968). Its superior portion is quite close to the external meatus so that an ear speculum that is too small may touch or nearly touch this important area of the drumhead, exposing it to possible damage.

The vascular supply to the external ear is ample, coming from the posterior auricular, superficial temporal, and deep auricular branches of the external carotid circulation (Hollinshead, 1968). The terminal arterioles of these vessels supply skin, subcutaneous tissue, and perichondrium, but cartilage itself is avascular, extracellular fluid being replaced by solid cartilaginous matrix (Ham, 1957).

The venous drainage is via the superficial temporal, the posterior auricular, and the mastoid emissary veins to the external and internal jugular veins and sigmoid sinus. Lymphatic channels go to the preauricular parotid nodes, superficial cervical nodes along the external jugular vein, and postauricular nodes (Hollinshead, 1968).

The normal external canal is longer anteriorly to inferiorly in both infant and adult to accommodate to the obliquely inward slant of the drum membrane. The anterior osseous canal bulges, sometimes prominently, and thus serves somewhat to obscure the view of the anterior drum margin and adjacent external canal sulcus.

Cerumen varies both qualitatively and

347

quantitatively. Most Caucasians have wet, sticky, brown cerumen, which is considered to be a dominant genetic trait, whereas most Mongoloid races, including the American Indian, have dry, brittle, light grey, "rice-bran" cerumen. Wet cerumen contains one third as much protein as the dry type but three times as much lipid. Dry cerumen occurs frequently in individuals who have Down syndrome, or "mongolism." Preliminary work suggests that dry cerumen is higher in lysozyme than wet cerumen and that there may be differences in immunoglobulin content, but this has been contested (Matsunaga, 1962; Hyslop, 1971; Petrakis et al., 1971). Studies using the scanning electron microscope suggest that the mode of cerumen secretion is both apocrine and eccrine (Main and Lim, 1976).

The squamous epithelium of the tympanic membrane and external canal skin desquamates keratin, but in the normal ear the epithelium migrates centrifugally so that keratin debris is mobilized out of the ear canal together with cerumen (Litton, 1963).

The normal flora of the external canal consists of *Staphylococcus epidermidis*, *Corynebacteria* ("diphtheroids") *Micrococci* species, and occasionally *Staphylococcus aureus* and *Streptococcus viridans*. The contributory factors that may initiate the process that renders the skin of the canal vulnerable to infection are excessive wetness (swimming, bathing, or increased environmental humidity), excessive dryness (previous infection, dermatoses, or insufficient cerumen), and trauma (digital or foreign body). Once the preinflammatory stage has been set, endogenous bacteria assume pathogenic characteristics, or virulent exogenous bacteria may propagate in the canal (Chap. 16).

CERUMEN IMPACTION

In some individuals spontaneous cerumen removal does not occur. Ultimately physical discomfort and conductive hearing loss bring the person to the doctor. Chandler studied obstruction of the human ear canal experimentally and established that the perception of high frequency sound is affected first, and even after lower frequencies are involved the loss is greater in higher frequencies (Chandler, 1964). Predisposing factors in cerumen impaction may include small or collapsing ear canals, unusual properties of the

cerumen itself, increased production of cerumen, or a combination of these factors (Peterkin, 1974). However, in most patients cerumen impaction results from ill-advised attempts at removal by the patient or from nervous digital ear canal manipulation, which shoves the bolus of cerumen deeper into the osseous canal. Children may introduce foreign bodies into the ear canal, thus pushing cerumen deeper.

Cerumen removal may be accomplished in a variety of ways. In preschool children in whom a small, firm plug partly obscures the view of the tympanic membrane it may be removed quickly, deftly, and unobtrusively during the ear examination with head mirror and hand-held speculum, thus, obviating some of the fears and objections that often occur if the ear loop or curet is displayed and an explanation is offered. However, if the ear canal is completely obstructed a simple, step-by-step explanation is given and the child is positioned under the microscope for removal. In skilled hands the otoscope or head mirror and hand-held speculum may be substituted for the microscope. For a somewhat apprehensive but inquisitive child, allowing him or her a preliminary opportunity to look through the microscope or otoscope at the examiner's hand or the parent's ear may then permit uneventful cerumen removal, which is accomplished using suction for soft cerumen and the curet, loop, or small cup forceps. The noise of the suction must be explained and demonstrated before introducing it into the ear canal because it is fairly loud and frightening there. Skilled help to steady the child's head is essential, as is the reassuring presence of the parent nearby where the child can see him or her.

Mechanical cerumen removal is preferred when the ear is symptomatic, as in cases of a documented hearing loss or when the ear is painful. Such removal should be accomplished, if at all possible, when the patient first presents. However, under circumstances in which the ear examination is for routine purposes and immediate removal proves difficult or in which the child is incapable of cooperation, it is better to take a more leisurely course, which may involve using mineral oil or oily otic drops at home until the cerumen comes out spontaneously or can be removed easily. It may be possible to use body temperature irrigation to remove the cerumen, but it is this author's preference not to use this at the first examination of a patient, as instances have been known in which pain occurred owing to an unforeseen tympanic membrane perforation. In one instance, concurrent transient facial palsy occurred. A suitable irrigation solution is one containing lactated Ringer's solution mixed in equal parts of isopropyl alcohol, but a variety of other solutions are satisfactory, provided the ear is carefully dried afterward. Commercial detergents for removing cerumen may be quite irritating or may provoke an allergic response in the skin of the ear canal and probably should be used, if at all, only in adults. After cerumen removal the canal should be inspected carefully for minor skin abrasions. If there has been any canal wall trauma, medicinal otic drops should be used for a few days.

SPECIFIC INFLAMMATORY DISORDERS OF THE EXTERNAL EAR

External otitis may be divided into five types: (1) acute diffuse, (2) acute circumscribed, (3) chronic, (4) eczematous, and (5) malignant. In the pediatric age group acute external otitis and eczematous otitis externa are the most commonly seen.

Acute Otitis Externa. Acute otitis externa may be divided into bacterial and fungal types. Bacterial otitis externa usually occurs as a result of getting and retaining water in the external ear canal, frequently when swimming and more frequently in hot, humid weather. At first the ear itches, and the patient scratches, traumatizing the ear canal and introducing organisms into macerated skin. The superficial epithelium absorbs moisture and desquamates to expose a raw wet surface that is easily infected. The pH of the ear canal changes from a normal pH of 5 to 7 to alkaline. The ear canal fills with wet debris, itself a good culture medium. Pus exudes; edema of the ear canal and mild perichondritis of the ear canal may ensue so that the ear is quite painful when touched, manipulated, or during chewing. Foul-smelling or sour-smelling exudate is noted by the patient or the parents. On physical examination frank pus may be seen, and the canal may be very edematous or even closed so that cleaning and culture may be difficult or impossible initially (Senturia, 1957, 1973). *Pseudomonas* species are found in one half to two

thirds of instances. Other organisms seen include *Proteus* species, *Escherichia coli*, *S. epidermidis*, *S. aureus*, streptococci, diphtheroids, *Enterobacter aerogenes*, *Klebsiella pneumoniae*, and *Citrobacter*. In patients under age 21 the proportion of those with severe involvement is greater than in any other age group. There is a correlation between severity of external otitis and the organisms found: gram negative organisms tend to be found in severe infections and gram positive organisms are found in milder infections. Gram negative organisms are found in 74 per cent of affected patients under age 21 as compared with 64 per cent in the older age group, and *Pseudomonas* species account for most of the positive bacterial cultures (Cassisi et al., 1977).

Probably the most important aspect of management of acute diffuse external otitis is thorough cleaning of the ear canal to remove all debris. This can be done with suction, gentle wiping with small, soft cotton pledgets, or irrigation with a solution at body temperature. Appropriate irrigants include 3 per cent saline, alcohol in a spray bottle attached to compressed air so that the canal can be dried, boro-alcohol solution, or a solution made up of alcohol and acetic acid, 3 to 5 per cent. If the ear canal is too swollen to permit cleaning, then a wick soaked in steroid-containing medication should be inserted gently into the canal. All of these procedures are painful, and the usual local anesthetic block of the ear may not be successful because the pH change of infection does not allow the chemical reaction of local anesthetic agents in the tissues to occur. A field block around the pinna might be helpful, but often it is as efficacious to explain that the procedure will be uncomfortable briefly but will help make the ear feel better shortly. The ear should be cleaned and medicated daily. Drops containing neomycin or polymyxin and steroid in an acid vehicle can be administered as soon as the ear canal opens. Tampons or cotton pledgets medicated with cream containing similar compounds can be inserted into the ears of older children or adolescents, but this generally causes too much discomfort or apprehension in younger children. In children who wear hearing aids or who need pressure-equalizing tubes placed in the tympanic membrane, the need for prompt control and prevention is especially urgent. Prevention of otitis externa may involve abstaining from swimming or placing Domeboro or VōSol drops containing an acetic acid solution in the ear immediately after swimming (McLaurin, 1973; Senturia, 1973; Templer, 1976; Cassisi, et al., 1977).

Other forms of acute diffuse otitis externa include erysipelas, which usually involves only the pinna; bullous myringitis, in which hemorrhagic bullae involve the canal and tympanic membrane skin; herpes simplex, which involves primarily the pinna and responds to 10 per cent carbamide peroxide in anhydrous solution; and herpes zoster oticus (Shambaugh, 1967; McLaurin, 1973; Templer, 1976).

Acute fungal otitis externa or otomycosis occurs in fewer than 10 per cent of patients in the United States (McLaurin, 1973), and may occur as part of generalized or regional fungal disorders. Otomycosis is said to occur most frequently in tropical climates and is usually due to *Aspergillus, Phycomycetes, Rhizopus, Actinomyces, Penicillium,* or yeasts. Hyphae may be seen in the ear canal as a dark or greenish-yellow mass (Beneke, 1970). *Aspergillus* causes about 90 per cent of the fungal infections. Fungi may find a more favorable environment where tissues are rich in glucose, as in uncontrolled diabetics. It is even possible that ordinarily saprophytic *Mucor* species of the *Phycomycetes* group, residing in the external ear, may infect the middle ear and mastoid of diabetics (Bergstrom et al., 1970). Patients receiving immunosuppressive medications such as steroids or azathioprine, those who have been receiving long-term antibiotic therapy, or those who are immunodeficient may also be subject to fungal otitis externa. An interesting disorder is mucocutaneous candidiasis, found in immunodeficient children. The infecting organism is *Candida albicans.* The pinna, external canal, and even the middle ear may be infected (Fig. 15–1). Nails, skin, mouth, pharynx, larynx, trachea, bronchi, and esophagus may also be infected. Other fungal infections of adjacent skin and scalp may also involve the pinna and external canal, but this is extremely rare.

The causative organism can often be identified from scrapings or aspirated material on a 20 per cent potassium hydroxide preparation. At times culture on Sabouraud's media or even biopsy may be needed to establish the diagnosis (Beneke, 1970).

Treatment may consist of topical medications such as nystatin, amphotericin B, 1 per cent gentian violet, 1 per cent iodine, or 10 per cent resorcin; gentian violet and iodine may be unacceptable because of their staining

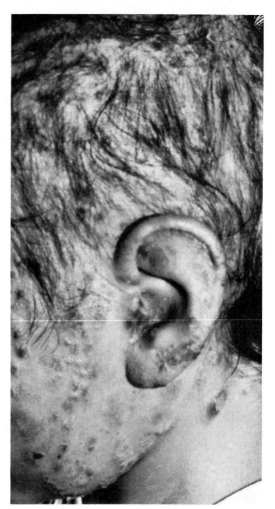

Figure 15–1   The affected scalp and pinna of a child who has chronic mucocutaneous candidiasis. The patient is immunodeficient, has similar lesions in the external auditory canal, and has otitis media as well. The last condition may be due to monilial nasopharyngitis that also involves the contiguous oropharynx, mouth, hypopharynx, and larynx.

properties (Beneke, 1970). Systemic agents such as griseofulvin or even amphotericin B may rarely be indicated. The usual measures of ear cleaning and aural hygiene are essential, and general improvement of health, control of diabetes, and discontinuing or lowering the doses of systemic antibiotics and immunosuppressants (when possible) should also be tried. If amphotericin B is used the patient must be pretested for sensitivity and renal function must be monitored closely. If the fungus is deeply seated or if the patient requires, but cannot tolerate, amphotericin B, surgery may be indicated to remove diseased tissue (Bergstrom et al., 1970).

Actinomycosis and blastomycosis cause granulomatous lesions of the pinna that may need to be biopsied or drained but that respond to chemotherapy (McLaurin, 1973).

Acute Circumscribed External Otitis. Acute circumscribed external otitis is synonymous with furuncle. These lesions, which are usually small, are pustules associated with a hair follicle, and the infecting organism is usually staphylococcus. The pain is severe. Local heat and systemic antibiotics will usually lead to resolution of the problem, although incision and drainage may be necessary. Often an ointment-impregnated wick will provide some symptomatic relief and possibly protect the rest of the ear canal from infection. Frank cellulitis of the ear canal, usually due to streptococci or staphylococci, can be treated with penicillin or similar appropriate systemic antibiotics.

Chronic External Otitis. Chronic external otitis seldom occurs in children, but when it does occur it may be quite stubborn. The author treated one young school-age patient who had cleft palate and a considerable conductive hearing loss resulting from persistent serous otitis media and nearly constant debris in the ear. Itching was a severe problem. After six months of frequent ear cleanings, a variety of topical and systemic medications, rigid adherence to aural hygiene and, fortunately, having a most cooperative patient and mother, the condition cleared and cultures, which had grown out *Pseudomonas,* cleared. The hearing loss was still significant, and middle ear ventilating tubes were successfully placed. Frequent visits were essential to keep the ears clear of debris that seemed to cause considerable itching. The tubes remained patent, the middle ear was free of infection, and the tubes were still in place after more than a year had elapsed, without complications. Presumably in stubborn cases surgery, such as the Proud procedure, might be required (Proud, 1967). It would also be important to rule out underlying systemic disease.

Other forms of chronic external otitis are granulomatous, such as tubercular (Sinha, 1969), luetic, and that due to yaws, leprosy, or sarcoidosis (McLaurin, 1973).

Eczematous Otitis Externa. Eczematous otitis externa may accompany typical atopic eczema, but it also occurs in association with seborrheic dermatitis, psoriasis, lupus erythematosus, neurodermatitis, sensitivities to topical medications, contact dermatitis, purulent otitis media, and infantile eczema. The pinna is often involved, and fissuring, weeping, and inflammation are seen in the various crevices and creases, particularly in the postauricular sulcus. Pruritus is extreme and secondary infection is common. In the canal scaling, crusting, oozing, vesicles, and even hives may be seen. Nervous or emotionally disturbed children and adolescents greatly worsen the situation or even provoke it by unnecessary rubbing and scratching of the area. The specific cause is usually found by taking a history and by using the visual recognition so essential to dermatologic diagnosis. At times biopsy or patch testing may be valuable. Oral antipruritics, antihistamines, analgesics, or tranquilizers are useful as general measures. Various topical agents, including solutions of aluminum acetate 8 per cent, lead subacetate 5 per cent and 5 per cent glycerin in water, acetic acid 2 per cent in aluminum acetate buffered to an acid pH, or Burrow's solution for acute oozing or weeping, are followed by steroid creams, lotions, or ointments as the acute phase abates. Occasionally, boric acid powder can be helpful. However, only topical preparations specifically suited for the ear canal should be used there. Eliminating from use around the ear common contact irritants such as spray colognes, hair sprays, certain shampoos, or soaps is essential but needs to be tailored to the particular patient. It may be necessary to keep gloves on the patient at night to lessen scratching and contamination with organisms found under the fingernails (McLaurin, 1973; Templer, 1976).

Necrotizing "Malignant" External Otitis. "Malignant" external otitis is generally considered a disease of elderly, diabetic, or debilitated adults (Chandler, 1968, 1977). However, cases have been reported in children (Giguere and Rouillard, 1976). "Malignant" external otitis in children must be differentiated from a virulent otitis media, at times caused by *Pseudomonas* that has secondarily infected the external canal. Such a distinction can readily be made if the ear canal is carefully cleaned first (Chandler, 1977).

Malignant external otitis does not respond to measures generally successful for the usual varieties of external otitis. The usual infecting organism is *Pseudomonas*, which in this instance gains access to the deeper tissues of the ear canal and causes a localized vasculitis, thrombosis, and necrosis of the tissues. The bone and cartilage of the external ear canal, parotid gland, mastoid, facial nerve, regional lymph nodes, and skin are often involved by direct extension. Malignant external otitis can spread to the middle ear, sigmoid sinus, jugular bulb, cranial nerves in the jugular foramen, bone of the petrous pyramid, and adjacent base of the skull or to the meninges, brain, and brain stem substance. The external canal will often show granulation tissue at the junction of the osseous and cartilaginous canals, and the mastoid process may be red, tender, and swollen. Multiple cranial nerves may be involved, and the onset of symptoms may be delayed (Dinapoli and Thomas, 1971). Widespread central nervous system involvement and death may ensue. Permanent facial paralysis is frequent (Chandler, 1977). Bilateral malignant external otitis necessitating multiple hospital admissions and surgical explorations occurred in a 10 year old girl; the course of the disease covered nearly one year and resulted in permanent diabetes insipidus and permanent unilateral facial palsy. She had apparently been healthy prior to the onset of the illness (Giguere and Rouillard, 1976).

Successful treatment requires hospitalization, supportive measures, workup for underlying systemic disease, ear cleaning and debriding of devitalized tissue, topical and systemic treatment with gentamicin and carbenicillin intravenously for 4 to 6 weeks or longer, careful monitoring of renal function, and, in some instances, mastoidectomy, facial nerve decompression, removal of the infected clot from the affected dural sinuses, ligation of the internal jugular vein, removal of the jugular bulb, and removal of sequestra of osteomyelitic bone. The blood levels of antibiotics need to be followed closely; a sensitive organism will likely respond to a concentration of gentamicin of 1 μg per ml or less and of less than 32 μg per ml of carbenicillin, although sensitivity may need to be reassessed by tube dilution methods if the patient is not responding satisfactorily (Chandler, 1977). Vestibular and auditory baseline and follow-up testing should be done. Caloric tests using water are contraindicated in the presence of external otitis, but iced ear drops or air calorics might be substituted. Audiometric thresholds may need to be tested by bone conduction only or free-field testing, as pain, swelling, and drainage may preclude the use of earphones unless they are hand-held. The ear canal should have been cleaned just before audiometry to minimize the amount of conductive hearing loss. Vestibular function can to some degree be followed by having the patient stand with feet in a heel-to-toe position or by using posturography, where that is available; at present it is still a research tool with limited availability.

The most difficult aspect of treatment is keeping the patient in the hospital for weeks of antibiotic treatment after ear pain and drainage have ceased. However, the recurrence rate after inadequate treatment is 100 per cent, and the mortality rate is significant.

OTHER INFLAMMATORY CONDITIONS OF THE EXTERNAL EAR

A potentially serious complication of external otitis, surgical procedures on the ear, hematoma, trauma to the ear, frostbite, or burns is perichondritis of the pinna, sometimes extending into the cartilaginous external auditory canal. Perichondritis at its most severe results in suppurative destruction of ear cartilage which in turn finally causes a deformed ear, sometimes leaving but a nubbin of pinna. The pinna first becomes exquisitely tender and swollen and, if untreated, fluctuation and spontaneous but inadequate drainage occurs. Causative organisms are usually gram negative, commonly *Pseudomonas,* but *Staphylococcus* may also be a cause (Martin et al., 1976).

After culture, treatment should be begun without waiting for fluctuation, using through-and-through irrigation of the area. Small catheters or open Penrose drains should be threaded just superficial to the cartilage through stepladder incisions on both the anterior and posterior surfaces; the incisions should be concealed in creases and under ridges of the pinna as well as possible (Fig. 15–2). The irrigation solution may be acetic acid in propylene glycol diacetate, benzethonium chloride, or sodium acetate. Systemic antibiotics may be required as well. This treatment must continue for several weeks to be efficacious. Sometimes removal of necrotic cartilage is required (Wanamaker, 1972; McLaurin, 1973; Templer, 1976; Martin et al., 1976).

Recently, acupuncture in or near the pinna has been used as a treatment for deafness, tinnitus, and obesity. Perichondritis has occurred as a complication (Baltimore and Moloy, 1976).

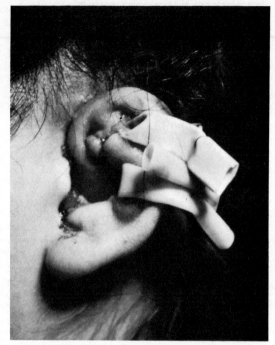

Figure 15–2 This teenager underwent a tympanomastoidectomy via a postauricular incision. Perichondritis caused by *Pseudomonas aeruginosa* developed in the postoperative period. It gradually resolved after intensive treatment, which included irrigations with topical gentamicin along the Penrose drains.

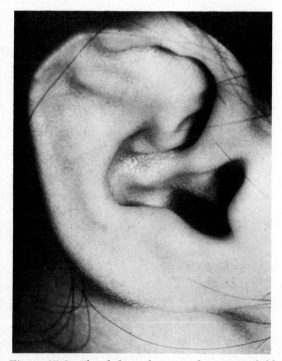

Figure 15–3 The deformed pinna of a young child who has diastrophic dwarfism. This represents fairly minimal involvement.

A peculiar type of problem, the pathogenesis of which is uncertain, occurs in patients who have the autosomally recessive syndrome of diastrophic dwarfism (diastrophic nanism syndrome). In early infancy the pinnae develop cystic swellings, thought to represent a hemorrhagic phase because from these swellings serosanguineous fluid can be aspirated. The condition is apparently painless, but the ears become deformed with calcification and eventual ossification (Fig. 15–3) (McKusick, 1972; Gorlin et al., 1976; Smith, 1976). Mesomelic dwarfism, deformed extremities, and scoliosis are other prominent features. Conductive hearing loss, probably not directly related to the pinna degeneration, has been observed.

Relapsing polychondritis is another disorder included in the differential diagnosis of perichondritis. It is of uncertain etiology but probably is an autoimmune disorder, since tests for antinuclear antibody and rheumatoid factor are positive in some patients, and it has been observed in association with connective tissue disorders (McKenna et al., 1976; McCaffrey et al., 1978). Inflammatory degeneration of various cartilages occurs, including those of the pinna, ribs, and joints and the nasal, laryngeal, tracheal, and eustachian tube cartilages. Systemic symptoms also may occur (Schuknecht, 1974). Persons in their late teens have been afflicted with this disorder (McCaffrey et al., 1978). The ear may be the first visible area involved (Odkvist, 1970), and hence the exact nature of the problem may not at first be apparent. The pinna becomes painful, erythematous, and edematous, but the pain is not as excruciating as in bacterial perichondritis, and in some instances pain is not present but the ear may be tender. Hemolytic complement factor may be decreased in fluid aspirated from the pinna (McKenna et al., 1976). Eventually the ear may acquire a cauliflower configuration. Conductive hearing loss due to damage to the eustachian tube may occur; sensorineural hearing loss and vertigo are also reported. The pathogenesis of this disease is unknown (Schuknecht, 1974).

Ear piercing is occasionally complicated by mild inflammation, cellulitis, or abscess, and since ear piercing is done in infancy in some cultures infection is possible and made even more likely should otitis media with otorrhea occur. Sometimes infection recurs every time the earrings are reinserted. It is alleviated by topical or systemic antibiotics or changing to an earring of a different metal. Eventually, if desired, the earring holes could be closed surgically, although the cosmetic problem is not significant.

Hepatitis may complicate either acupuncture or ear piercing (Johnson et al., 1974; Baltimore and Moloy, 1976).

Irradiation of the head and neck area, pituitary, or brain stem may include the external, middle, and inner ears in the field. Fairly commonly the skin and its appendages within the ear canal may show inflammatory changes, some apparently permanent (Schuknecht, 1974). However, necrosis and breakdown of ear canal skin occur less frequently with cobalt 60 and other newer types of radiation than was true with orthovoltage radiation (Borsanyi et al., 1961). The production of cerumen ceases; the canal wall becomes edematous, the skin is dry and flaky, and material collects in the external canal with resulting pruritus and at times secondary bacterial infection due to scratching. Telangiectatic skin changes may be seen in the pinna.

DERMATOSES AFFECTING THE PINNA

Some of the allergic and scaly dermatoses have already been mentioned as they contribute to chronic external otitis. However, other disorders may produce other manifestations in or on the external ear.

Epidermolysis bullosa simplex produces cutaneous and mucosal blisters as early as birth. The condition is due to autosomal recessive inheritance. Stenosis of the ear canal may occur but apparently responds surprisingly well to surgical excision, canal drill-out, and skin grafting (Thawley et al., 1977). Another bullous lesion, pemphigoid or benign pemphigus, may also cause discrete rather than diffuse lesions in the ear canal and may occur in young persons (Rook et al., 1968).

Lipoid proteinosis of the skin and mucosa is a recessively inherited disease affecting the larynx, pharynx, mouth, lips, tongue, nose, and skin. On the pinna waxy, hyperkeratotic deposits occur, and the pinna may lose its normal contours. The lesions are apparently neither painful nor pruritic, but those on the mucosa of the upper airway and mouth can cause considerable disruption of function (MacKinnon, 1968).

STENOTIC LESIONS OF THE EAR CANAL

Acquired canal stenosis is more common than the congenital variety and generally results from surgery, trauma, or infection. It may occur as a complication of chronic external otitis (Proud, 1967), perichondritis, bullous lesions (Thawley et al., 1977), chronic otitis media, tuberculosis of the pinna and external auditory canal (Sinha, 1969), irradiation, and relapsing polychrondritis. Surgical excision alone or with the addition of a long-term stent postoperatively is the treatment of choice unless the patient's general condition does not permit it. However, surgery should be deferred until the causative lesion is inactive or as quiescent as possible. Surgery on young children for this problem would preferably be deferred, but upon suspicion of cholesteatoma behind the obstruction it might need to be done sooner.

THE EXTERNAL EAR AND CANAL IN SYSTEMIC DISEASE

Gardner syndrome, an autosomal dominant disorder, is characterized by gastrointestinal polyps and multiple skin lesions, including epidermal inclusion cysts, fibromas, desmoids, and osteomas that occur primarily in craniofacial bones. They may occur in the external auditory canal, and keratin debris may become trapped behind them when they are large, leading to canal infection (McKusick, 1975; Smith, 1976).

In Weber-Osler-Rendu disease (hereditary telangiectasia), mild forms may occur with only mild cutaneous telangiectasia. The pinna is a common site.

In alkaptonuria or ochronosis of recessive inheritance, cartilages and other tissues of collagen origin turn black. In the pinna, the cartilage is just under the skin and the black color shines through. A characteristic laboratory finding is that urine turns dark when alkaline and left standing (McKusick, 1975).

SELECTED REFERENCE

Senturia, B. H. 1957. Diseases of the External Ear. Springfield, Ill., Charles C Thomas.
This small book, although 25 years old, is still the classic work to which all others refer. Senturia's completeness and synthesis of material relating to these common but often poorly managed problems has not been surpassed.

REFERENCES

Anson, B. J., and Donaldson, J. A. 1967. The Surgical Anatomy of the Temporal Bone and Ear, 1st ed. Philadelphia, W. B. Saunders Co.

Baltimore, R. S., and Moloy, P. J. 1976. Perichondritis of the ear as a complication of acupuncture. Arch. Otolaryngol., 102:572–573.

Beneke, E. S. 1970. Human Mycoses. Kalamazoo, Mi, Upjohn Co., pp. 17–20, 38–41.

Bergstrom, L., Hemenway, W. G., and Barnhart, R. A. 1970. Rhinocerebral and otologic mucormycosis. Ann. Otol. Rhinol. Laryngol., 79:70–79.

Borsanyi, S., Blanchard, C. L., and Thorne, B. 1961. The effects of ionizing radiation on the ear. Ann. Otol. Rhinol. Laryngol., 70:255–262.

Cassisi, N., Cohn, A., Davidson, T., et al. 1977. Diffuse otitis externa, clinical and microbiologic findings in the course of a multicenter study on a new otic solution. Ann. Otol. Rhinol. Laryngol., 86:Suppl. 39.

Chandler, J. R. 1964. Partial occlusion of the external auditory meatus: its effect upon air and bone conduction hearing acuity. Laryngoscope, 74:22–54.

Chandler, J. R., 1968. Malignant external otitis. Laryngoscope, 78:1257–1294.

Chandler, J. R. 1977. Malignant external otitis: further considerations. Ann. Otol. Rhinol. Laryngol., 86:417–428.

Dinapoli, R. P., and Thomas, J. E. 1971. Neurologic aspects of malignant external otitis: report of three cases. Mayo Clin. Proc., 46:339–344.

Giguere, P., and Rouillard, G. 1976. Otite externe maligne bilatérale chez une fillette de 10 ans. J. Laryngol., 5:159–166.

Gorlin, R. J., Pindborg, J. J., and Cohen, M. M. 1976. Diastrophic dwarfism. In Syndromes of the Head and Neck, 2nd ed. New York, McGraw-Hill Book Co., pp. 250–252.

Ham, A. W. 1957. Histology, 3rd ed. Philadelphia, J. B. Lippincott Co., pp. 250–253, 860–866.

Hollinshead, W. H. 1968. Anatomy for Surgeons, Vol. 1, 2nd ed. New York, Hoeber Medical Division, Harper and Row, pp. 183–192.

Hyslop, N. E., Jr. 1971. Ear wax and host defense. N. Engl. J. Med., 284:1099–1100.

Johnson, C. J., Anderson, H., Spearman, J., and Madson, J. 1974. Ear piercing and hepatitis: nonsterile instruments for ear piercing and subsequent onset of viral hepatitis. J.A.M.A., 227:1165.

Litton, W. B. 1963. Epithelial migration over tympanic membrane and external canal. Arch. Otolaryngol., 77:254–257.

MacKinnon, D. M. 1968. Hyalinosis cutis et mucosae (lipod proteinosis). Acta Otolaryngol. (Stockh.), 65:403–412.

Main, T., and Lim, D. 1976. The human external auditory canal secretory system — an ultrastructural study. Laryngoscope, 86:1164–1176.

Martin, R., Yonkers, A. J., and Yarington, C. T. 1976. Perichondritis of the ear. Laryngoscope, 86:664–673.

Matsunaga, E. 1962. The dimorphism in human normal cerumen. Ann. Hum. Genet., 25:273–286.

McCaffrey, T. V., McDonald, T. J., and McCaffrey, L. A. 1978. Head and neck manifestations of relapsing polychondritis. "A review of 29 cases." Trans. Am. Acad. Ophth. Otolaryngol. 86:473–478.

McKenna, C. H., Luthra, H. S., and Jordon, R. E. 1976. Hypocomplementemic ear effusion in relapsing polychondritis. Mayo Clin. Proc., 51:495–497.

McKusick, V. A. 1972. Heritable Disorders of Connective Tissue, 4th ed. St. Louis, The C. V. Mosby Co., pp. 772–775.

McKusick, V. A. 1975. Mendelian Inheritance in Man, 4th ed. Baltimore, The Johns Hopkins Press, pp. 272–273, 343–344.

McLaurin, J. W. 1973. Trauma and infections of the external ear. In Paparella, M. M., and Shumrick, D. A. (Eds.): Otolaryngology, Vol. II. Philadelphia, W. B. Saunders Co., pp. 24–32.

Odkvist, L. 1970. Relapsing Polychondritis. Acta Otolaryngol. (Stockh.), 70:448–454.

Peterkin, G. A. G. 1974. External otitis. J. Laryngol. Otol., 88:15–21.

Petrakis, N. L., Doherty, M., Lee, R. E., et al. 1971. Demonstration and implications of lysozyme and immunoglobulins in human ear wax. Nature (London). 229:119–120.

Proud, G. O. 1967. Surgical treatment of chronic otitis externa. Pac. Med. Surg., 75:186–187.

Rook, A., Wilkinson, D. S., and Ebling, F. J. G. 1968. Textbook of Dermatology, Vol. II. Oxford, Blackwell Scientific Publications, pp. 1183–1188.

Schuknecht, H. G. 1974. Pathology of the Ear. Cambridge, MA, Harvard University Press, pp. 266–267, 311–312, 487–488.

Senturia, B. H. 1957. Diseases of the External Ear. Springfield, Il., Charles C Thomas Co.

Senturia, B. H. 1973. External otitis, acute diffuse. Evaluation of therapy. Ann. Otol. Rhinol. Laryngol., 82:Suppl. 8.

Shambaugh, G. E., Jr. 1967. Surgery of the Ear, 2nd ed. Philadelphia, W. B. Saunders Co., pp. 229–232.

Sinha, S. N. 1969. Lupus vulgaris of the pinna and soft palate. Eye, Ear, Nose, Throat Monthly, 48:471–473.

Smith, D. W. 1976. Recognizable Patterns of Human Malformation, 2nd ed. Philadelphia, W. B. Saunders Co., pp. 202–203.

Templer, J. W. 1976. Infections and inflammatory diseases of the external ear and external auditory canal. In English, G. M. (Ed.) Otolaryngology. New York, Harper and Row, pp. 122–125.

Thawley, S. E., Black, M. J., Dudek, S. E., et al. 1977. External auditory canal stricture secondary to epidermolysis bullosa. Arch. Otolaryngol., 103:55–57.

Wanamaker, H. H. 1972. Suppurative perichondritis of the auricle. Trans. Am. Acad. Ophth. Otol., 76:1289–1291.

Chapter 16

OTITIS MEDIA WITH EFFUSION, ATELECTASIS, AND EUSTACHIAN TUBE DYSFUNCTION

Charles D. Bluestone, M.D.
Jerome O. Klein, M.D.

Otitis media is the most frequent diagnosis recorded for children who visit physicians because of illness. Children suffer not only from the signs and symptoms of the acute episode but also from the sequelae of infection of the middle ear, most important of which is persistent effusion. During the past decade, there has been a wealth of new information from otolaryngologists, pediatricians, epidemiologists, biochemists, microbiologists, immunologists, and physiologists that has markedly increased our understanding of the disease and its most appropriate management. In this chapter, we summarize the results of recent investigations, integrate this information with that available previously, assess the current state of the art, and consider optimal choices for management of the various stages of otitis media.

DEFINITIONS AND CLASSIFICATION

During the past century, a multitude of terms has been used to describe various inflammatory conditions of the middle ear. This has resulted in confusion and misunderstanding among clinicians and investigators in their attempt to evaluate published reports, since interpretation of the results of these investigations depends upon definition of the specific disease entity being studied. In

defense of our well-meaning predecessors, the natural history, etiology, and pathogenesis of otitis media are better understood today than in the past. In an effort to eliminate ambiguity, the authors will employ terminology that they believe meets current understanding of the disease process and organizes the information in a manner that will aid the clinician's understanding of otitis media. In order to do this, the terminology used will be defined, and a classification of otitis media and its complications and sequelae will be presented.

Terminology and Definitions

Otitis media is an inflammation of the middle ear without reference to etiology or pathogenesis.

Otitis media with effusion is an inflammation of the middle ear in which a collection of liquid is present in the middle ear space. (No perforation of the tympanic membrane is present.)

Middle ear effusion is liquid in the middle ear. The effusion may be either *serous*, a thin, watery liquid; *mucoid*, a thick, viscid, mucus-like liquid; or *purulent*, a pus-like liquid.

Atelectasis of the tympanic membrane, which may or may not be associated with otitis media, is collapse or retraction of the tympanic membrane. Collapse implies passivity, whereas retraction implies active pulling inward of the tympanic membrane, usually from negative middle ear pressure.

A *retraction pocket* is a localized area of atelectasis of the tympanic membrane.

Otorrhea is a discharge from the ear.

In describing and classifying otitis media, the temporal relation of the disease is important, and, therefore, the terms *acute, subacute,* and *chronic* will be used. The separation of these intervals of time is arbitrary but is based on the natural history of the disease. *Acute* otitis media implies rapid and short onset of signs and symptoms of inflammation of the middle ear, which may last approximately three weeks. From three weeks to three months, the acute process may be in the state of resolution or in a *subacute stage*. An otitis media that persists longer than three months is considered to be *chronic*.

Classification

The classification presented here is derived from our present knowledge of the disease, but it is often difficult to determine by history and visual inspection of the tympanic membrane the specific type and stage of otitis media confronting the clinician. The physician usually arrives at a presumptive diagnosis of the variety of otitis media present in the individual patient from limited data, but a more definitive diagnosis can be determined by the following:

1. Knowledge of the condition of the middle ear prior to onset of the present illness differentiates acute, subacute, and chronic forms. A child may have signs and symptoms of acute otitis media, but whether or not the middle ear was effusion-free prior to the onset of this episode may not be known.
2. Tympanocentesis determines the characteristics of the middle ear effusion, i.e., serous, mucoid, or purulent, and appropriate cultures of the effusion establish the microbiologic origin.
3. Biopsy of the middle ear mucosa, although rarely necessary for care of the patient in the clinical setting, defines the middle ear pathology.

Table 16–1 shows the classification of otitis media, which is a modification of that proposed by Senturia et al. (1980a). Inflammation of the middle ear that is not associated

Table 16–1   CLASSIFICATION OF OTITIS MEDIA

Otitis Media without Effusion (or perforation)
  Acute
  Subacute
  Chronic
Otitis Media with Effusion (without perforation)
  Acute
    Serous
    Purulent
  Subacute
    Serous
    Mucoid
    Purulent
  Chronic
    Serous
    Mucoid
    Purulent
Otitis Media with Perforation
  Without Discharge
    Acute
    Subacute
    Chronic
  With Discharge
    Acute
      Serous
      Purulent
    Subacute
      Serous
      Mucoid
      Purulent
    Chronic
      Serous
      Mucoid
      Purulent

with effusion may occur initially in acute otitis media but also may be rarely found in subacute and chronic forms. Tympanocentesis performed in the earliest stages of acute otitis media may fail to reveal purulent material. Likewise, after myringotomy for chronic otitis media (without perforation) in infants with unrepaired cleft palate, investigators have occasionally found a chronically inflamed tympanic membrane and middle ear mucosa without effusion (Bluestone, 1971). However, the most common varieties of ear disease found in infants and children are the various types of otitis media with effusion. Many synonyms have been used for acute otitis media with effusion in the past, such as *acute suppurative* or *bacterial otitis media with effusion* (Table 16–2). Chronic otitis media with effusion has had many more synonyms than the acute form, such terms as *serous, secretory,* and "glue ear" being the most common. Many of these names were introduced as descriptive terms, whereas others implied the etiology or pathogenesis of otitis media, such as "salpingitis" and *eustachian tube ob-*

Table 16–2 SYNONYMS COMMONLY USED IN THE PAST FOR ACUTE AND CHRONIC OTITIS MEDIA WITH EFFUSION

Acute Otitis Media with Effusion	Chronic Otitis Media with Effusion
Purulent	Serous
Suppurative	Secretory
Nonsuppurative	Allergic
Serous	Catarrhal
Bacterial	Nonsuppurative
	Mucoid
	Secondary
	Tubotympanic catarrh
	Hydrotubotympanum
	Exudative catarrh
	Tubotympanitis
	Tympanic hydrops
	Glue ear
	Fluid ear
	Middle ear effusion

struction, however, they have only contributed to the confusion in understanding otitis media with effusion.

Knowledge of the stages of disease or type of effusion or both is helpful in determining appropriate management. On occasion, a straw-colored effusion that is known to be of sudden onset can be visualized behind a translucent tympanic membrane. The presumptive diagnosis would be acute serous otitis media with effusion. Likewise, a child with acute onset of fever, otalgia, and hearing loss is found to have a bulging, opaque, and immobile tympanic membrane by pneumatic otoscopy. The presumptive diagnosis would be acute purulent otitis media with effusion. However, without direct inspection of the middle ear effusion (by tympanocentesis), only a presumptive diagnosis can be made.

Since the tympanic membrane can spontaneously perforate at any time during an episode of otitis media, the classification must include otitis media with perforation. The middle ear may be inflamed in the presence of perforation, but no discharge (otorrhea) is visible. More commonly, a discharge is present, which may be either serous, mucoid, or purulent and either in the acute, subacute, or chronic stage. However, a persistent or preexistent perforation of the tympanic membrane in which inflammation of the middle ear is *absent* should be considered a complication of otitis media, and the often-used label of "chronic suppurative otitis media" in such a circumstance is inappropriate.

Atelectasis of the tympanic membrane (retraction or collapse) is not included in this classification, since it is not strictly a type of otitis media but is a related condition. It may be present prior to, concurrent with, or after an episode of otitis media with effusion. It also may be present in some patients without evidence of otitis media and, if persistent and progressive, can lead to one or more of the complications or sequelae commonly attributed to otitis media, such as hearing loss, ossicular chain discontinuity, or cholesteatoma.

Eustachian tube dysfunction may cause otologic symptoms without an apparent middle ear effusion or even atelectasis of the tympanic membrane. The complications and sequelae of otitis media and these related conditions are divided into those that occur within the middle ear and temporal bone and those that occur within the intracranial cavity. It should be noted that these conditions are considered complications and sequelae of otitis media, but they also may develop from causes other than otitis media. For example, ossicular chain discontinuity may occur, among other possible etiologies, as the result of trauma to the middle ear. On the other hand, several of these conditions listed may be complications or sequelae not of otitis media but of a related condition. An example of this situation would be the presence of atelectasis of the tympanic membrane without otitis media in which a discontinuity of the ossicular chain occurs or an acquired cholesteatoma develops (Bluestone et al., 1977b, 1978). The term "chronic suppurative otitis media" is not included in this classification, since it can be confused with cholesteatoma. An acquired cholesteatoma may have a purulent discharge secondary to inflammation within the confines of the sac-like structure, but the middle ear is not inflamed; therefore, the term "chronic suppurative otitis media" would be inaccurate. On the other hand, a cholesteatoma that is present in association with chronic inflammation of the middle ear would be defined as chronic "suppurative" otitis media with cholesteatoma and purulent discharge. However, the term chronic suppurative otitis media is in common usage and is included as a sequela of otitis media (p. 526).

EPIDEMIOLOGY

Epidemiology is the study of health and disease in defined populations. Whereas the physician is concerned with information about each patient, the epidemiologist is concerned with information about a group or community. The epidemiologist considers various factors that may be relevant to illness: host factors — age, sex, race, social and cultural characteristics, hygiene, nutrition, special habits (such as smoking or breast-feeding), family history, vocations or avocations, and immune or anatomic defects; environmental factors — climate, season, geology, places of work, study, play, worship, or other communal (gathering) areas, sources of food and water, and animal and plant contacts; and suspected etiologic agents — microorganisms, allergens, or toxins.

Few studies have been designed specifically to provide epidemiologic information about middle ear disease in children. Many reports of clinical experience, therapeutic trials, and microbiologic studies also provide some information that can be used to calculate incidence and prevalence rates and other epidemiologic data about otitis media. Incidence is the frequency of occurrence of new or separate episodes of illness in a defined population over a specific period of time. New cases of otitis media in children observed in a physician's practice in one year would be representative of an incidence study. In contrast, prevalence is the frequency of illness in a defined population at a given time. An example of a prevalence study would be a survey of children for middle ear disease in a school or village performed by a team in one or a few days. Unfortunately, most reports do not provide appropriate epidemiologic information; the studies are incomplete because the authors do not provide satisfactory criteria for the disease or do not adequately describe the characteristics of the population surveyed.

Longitudinal studies that provide information about children over a long period of time are an excellent source of information about the epidemiology of otitis media. Reports of three longitudinal studies of middle ear disease in children are available: The Arctic Health Research Center conducted a long-term cohort study of middle ear disease in Eskimo children living in Alaska (Reed et al, 1967; Kaplan et al., 1973); two pediatricians, Drs. Virgil Howie and John Ploussard of Huntsville, Alabama, have studied the natural history of otitis media in children seen in their office practice (Howie, 1975; Howie et al., 1975); a prospective study of otitis media in 2565 children observed from birth by

pediatricians in the greater Boston area is now in progress (Teele et al., 1980b). These longitudinal studies and selected data from other reports are the basis for this review of the epidemiology of otitis media in children.

Historical Perspective

It is likely that humans have always suffered from acute infection of the middle ear and its suppurative complications. Studies of 2600-year-old Egyptian mummies reveal perforations of the tympanic membrane and destruction of the mastoid (Lynn and Benitez, 1974). Evidence of middle ear disease was also evident in skeletal material from a prehistoric Iranian population (1900 to 800 B.C.) (Rathbun and Mallin, 1977). Prior to the introduction of antimicrobial agents, otitis media either resolved spontaneously (via central perforation of the tympanic membrane or evacuation of the middle ear contents through the eustachian tube) or came to the attention of a physician who drained the middle ear by means of myringotomy. Purulent otitis media was a frequent reason for admission to a hospital. In 1932, purulent otitis media accounted for 27 per cent of all pediatric admissions to Bellevue Hospital (Bakwin and Jacobinzer, 1939). Mastoiditis and intracranial complications were common.

Incidence of Otitis Media

Otitis media is one of the most common infectious diseases of childhood. A survey of the office practices of physicians who provide medical care to children showed that otitis media was the most frequent diagnosis for illness and the most frequent reason, after well baby and child care, for office visits (Koch and Dennison, 1974). A survey of the frequency of infectious diseases during the first year of life in 246 children in Rochester, New York, indicated that otitis media was second only to the common cold as a cause of illness (Hoekelman, 1977). In addition, recurrent episodes of otitis media add substantially to the number of visits to physicians for the child. During the first two years of life, Boston children with little or no ear disease had an average of 10 office visits as compared with children with recurrent episodes of otitis media, who had 20 visits to the physician (Teele and Klein, unpublished data). Otitis

Table 16–3 OTITIS MEDIA IN CHILDREN SEEN IN A "WALK-IN" PEDIATRIC CLINIC BOSTON CITY HOSPITAL, OCTOBER–NOVEMBER, 1973[*]

Age	Number Examined	Number with Otitis	Percentage with Otitis
0–3 mos.	325	27	8.3
4–6 mos.	221	56	25.3
7–12 mos.	576	124	21.5
13–24 mos.	902	141	15.6
25–36 mos.	215	23	10.7
3–5 yrs.	958	99	10.3
> 5 yrs.	3340	141	4.1

[*]From Klein, J. O., and Bratton, L. 1973. Unpublished data.

Table 16–4 INCIDENCE OF ACUTE OTITIS MEDIA IN BOSTON CHILDREN[*]

Age (mos.)	Percentage of Children Observed with Indicated Number of Episodes of Otitis Media		
	0	1 or 2	> 3
6	75	25	0
12	53	38	9
24	35	40	24
36	29	38	33

[*]2565 children enrolled at birth.

From Teele, D. W., Klein, J. O., and Rosner, B. A. 1980. Epidemiology of otitis media in children. Ann. Otol. Rhinol. Laryngol., 89(68):5–6.

media was the most frequent diagnosis (22 per cent) for visits of children to the Medical Emergency Clinic at Children's Hospital in Boston in a six week survey from March through April, 1960 (Bergman and Haggerty, 1962). A review of the causes of visits to the Ambulatory Clinic of the Boston City Hospital revealed that 19 per cent of children between 4 and 24 months of age had a diagnosis of otitis media (Klein and Bratton, unpublished data) (Table 16–3).

Howie et al. (1975) found that two thirds of children seen in their office practice had at least one episode of otitis media by their second birthday and one in seven children had more than six episodes. The Boston study showed similar trends; 71 per cent of children had one or more episodes, and 33 per cent had three or more episodes of otitis media by three years of age (Table 16–4).

Both the incidence and the severity of middle ear disease in Eskimo children are great. Studies done at the Arctic Health Research Center indicate that 76 per cent of these children had one or more episodes of otorrhea and that approximately half had

three or more episodes by 10 years of age (Kaplan et al., 1973). Children with recurrent episodes of otorrhea had the onset of the first episode early in life, before the age of two years (Table 16–5).

These longitudinal studies suggest that children may be categorized into three groups relative to acute infections of the middle ear. One group is free of ear infections; a second group may have occasional episodes of otitis, and a third group is "otitis-prone," subject to repeated episodes of acute middle ear infections.

Few studies dealing with the incidence or prevalence of chronic middle ear infection or persistent middle ear effusion have been done. Pelton et al. (1977) found that approximately one third of children with acute otitis media had middle ear effusions that persisted for four or more weeks. Persistence of middle ear effusion was very frequent in Boston children (Teele et al., 1980b). After the first episode of otitis media, 70 per cent of the children still had effusion at two weeks, 40 per cent had effusion at one month, 20 per cent had effusion at two months, and 10 per cent had effusion at three months. Breast-feeding had a significant effect on time spent with effusion (pp 364–365); but other varia-

Table 16–5 EPISODES OF OTORRHEA IN ALASKAN ESKIMO CHILDREN[*]

Age at Onset of First Episode	No. of Children	Average No. of Episodes/Child	Percentage of Children with ≥ 3 Episodes
0–2 yrs	291	4.8	61%
2 yrs	83	2.2	29%

[*]479 children were surveyed—birth to 10 years of age. Of these, 76 per cent had one or more episodes of otorrhea.

From Kaplan, G. J., Fleshman, J. D., Bender, T. R., Baum, C., and Clark, P. S. 1973. Long-term effects of otitis media: A ten-year cohort study of Alaskan Eskimo children. Pediatrics, 52:577–585.

bles, including sex, race, birth weight, family history of allergy, or season at the time of diagnosis, did not affect time spent with effusion

Age

In the newborn infant, otitis media may be an isolated infection, or it may be associated with sepsis, pneumonia, or meningitis. The incidence of otitis media in newborn infants is uncertain. Warren and Stool (1971) examined 127 consecutive infants whose birth weights were under 2300 gm and found three with infections of the middle ear (at 2, 7, and 26 days). Jaffe et al. (1970) examined 101 Navajo infants within 48 hours of birth and identified 18 with impaired mobility of the tympanic membrane. Balkany and coworkers identified effusion in the middle ear of 30 per cent of 125 consecutively examined infants who were admitted to a neonatal intensive care unit. The clinical diagnosis was corroborated by aspiration of middle ear fluid. Nasotracheal intubation for more than seven days was correlated with presence of effusion (Balkany et al., 1978)

Otitis media is very common in infants following the neonatal period (after 28 days of age). In the study of children in Boston, 13 per cent had at least one episode of otitis media by three months of age, 25 per cent had one or more episodes by six months of age, and 65 per cent experienced otitis media by 24 months of age (Table 16–4). These data and those of Howie et al. (1975) suggest that the highest incidence of episodes of acute otitis media occurs between 6 and 24 months of age. Subsequently, the incidence of otitis media declines with age except for a limited reversal of the downward trend between five and six years of age, the time of entrance into school. Otitis media is less common in children seven years of age and older. Virolainen and coworkers (1980) examined 1207 Turku school children aged seven to eight years and identified 51 (4.2 per cent) with serous or secretory otitis media, seven with signs of acute otitis media, and nine with adhesive otitis media.

Pelton et al. (1977) found that persistent effusions of the middle ear were more likely in young children. Approximately 50 per cent of children two years of age or younger had effusions that lasted for four weeks or more after an episode of acute otitis media, whereas only 20 per cent of children more than two years of age had persistent effusions.

Although the incidence of acute otitis media is limited in adults, a survey by the National Disease and Therapeutic Index published in 1970 found that there are almost four million visits by adults each year to private physicians for this infection (NDTI Review, 1970).

Sex

In most studies, the incidence of acute episodes of otitis media was not significantly different in boys from that in girls, but in the Boston study, males had significantly more single and recurrent (three or more) episodes (Teele et al., 1980b). Males have more myringotomies and tympanoplasties than do females, a fact suggesting that chronic or severe infections of the middle ear may be more common among males (Solomon and Harris, 1976).

Race

Studies of American Indians and Alaskan and Canadian Eskimos indicate that there is an extraordinary incidence of infection of the middle ear and that the disease is severe in these groups. Otorrhea is frequent, but chronic otitis and persistent effusion are uncommon. The following examples illustrate the extent and severity of ear disease in these populations. Zonis performed a prevalence study of an Apache community of 500 people of all ages; evidence of present or past ear infection was found in 23 per cent (draining ear, 5.6 per cent; perforation, 2.8 per cent; healed perforation or tympanosclerosis or both, 13.1 per cent; serous otitis, 1 per cent; and acute otitis media, 0.4 per cent; Zonis, 1968). Shaw and colleagues designed a cohort study of children from various tribes on four Arizona reservations (Shaw et al., 1979). The incidence of acute otitis media was similar to that noted for Boston children: By two years of age, 71 per cent had at least one episode, and 29 per cent had three or more episodes. Arctic Health Research Center investigators found a high rate of otorrhea in Alaskan Eskimo children. By one year of age, 38 per cent had at least one episode, and 20 per cent of all children had two or more episodes; by four years of age, 62 per cent of children had one or more episodes of otorrhea, and 40 per cent of the children had two or more episodes (Reed et al., 1967). Ling and colleagues (1969) found that 31 per cent of Canadian Eskimo children 10 years of age or younger living on Baffin Island had draining ears at the time of examination. None of the children were febrile or had evidence of acute otitis media (Ling et al., 1969).

The severity of middle ear infection has also been noted in African children living in primitive conditions and in Australian aboriginal children. A form of disease termed *necrotizing otitis media*, which is rarely seen in children living in developed areas, is seen in these children. An episode of acute middle ear infection progresses to perforation of the tympanic membrane with profuse discharge. Necrosis of the tympanic membrane follows, leaving a large central perforation that may persist for many years. This ear is termed a "safe ear" because the perforation allows for drainage of the middle ear infection, and intracranial complications rarely occur even without use of antimicrobial agents. However, there may be destruction of the ossicular chain, and deafness may result (Clements, 1968; Dugdale et al., 1978). Parents in these areas accept otorrhea as a way of life.

Timmermans and Gerson (1980) described a more indolent form of otitis media in Inuit Eskimo children, which they termed "chronic granulomatous otitis media." After one or more episodes of acute otitis media (usually treated with antimicrobial agents), there is a sudden onset of otorrhea without pain or fever. The discharge may persist for years, interspersed with periods of variable length in which the ear is dry. A large central perforation of the tympanic membrane is present, and granulomatous tissue fills the middle ear cavity. Resolution occurs with a scarred tympanic membrane and a mild to moderate hearing deficit.

Thus, the studies of children in different geographic and climatic areas suggest that the incidence of disease may be, in general, similar in children from developed and underdeveloped areas, but the severity of disease represented by chronic otorrhea, destruction of the tympanic membrane and ossicles, and other forms of a necrotizing process in the middle ear is much more frequent in (at present, almost unique to) the underdeveloped areas

Kessner and coworkers (1974) found a higher incidence of ear pathology and hearing impairment in white children as compared with black children aged 6 months through 11 years who lived in Washington, D.C. On examination, ear pathology was noted in 35 per cent of 112 white children and 18 per cent of 2031 black children. Hearing was tested in children 4 to 11 years of age; 20 per cent of 82 white children and 6 per cent of 1545 black children had significant impairment of hearing. The predominance of ear disease in white children was unexpected and not readily explained. The results may be related to the relatively small size of the sample of white children or to socioeconomic factors unique to the white children living in a predominantly black community. In a second study in the Washington, D.C., area, investigators observed a tenfold difference in the incidence of acute otitis media in white and black children. The disease rate in children less than 15 years of age with at least one encounter with acute otitis media was 155 per 1000 children attending a clinic in an affluent, predominantly white suburb and was 15 per 1000 children attending a clinic in a blue-collar area of northeast Washington, D.C., in which nearly all of the patients were black. Although the difference in disease incidence may be real, the authors note that other explanations must be considered, including differences in the perception of ear infection by parents, basis for visits to the physician, basis of payment for medical services, and diagnostic acumen or style of the clinic physicians (Bush and Rabin, 1980).

In the Boston study (Teele et al., 1980b), white children had a higher incidence of otitis than did black children, but "other," including Hispanic, children had the highest incidence. These data suggest that race is one determinant of the likelihood that a child will develop otitis media

In the study of persistence of middle ear effusions after acute episodes of otitis media, Pelton et al. (1977) also noted a higher incidence of persistent effusions in white or Hispanic children as compared with black children (21 per cent of 42 black children and 51 per cent of 51 white children)

The higher incidence of ear disease in white children is not readily explained. Of interest are the studies of Doyle of the position of the bony eustachian tube in skulls of American Negroes, Americans of Caucasian ancestry, and American Indians (Doyle, 1977). Significant differences were present in the length, width, and angle of the tube in the groups, implicating an anatomic basis for racial predisposition to, or protection from, otitis media.

Further information about possible mechanisms was provided by Beery and associates, who studied eustachian tube function in Apache Indians living in Arizona (Beery et al., 1980). The results of inflation-deflation tests indicated that the Indians had lower forced opening pressures than had been measured previously in a group of Caucasians (with perforations secondary to chronic otitis media). The eustachian tube function of the American Indian was functionally different from that of the Caucasians previously studied and was characterized by comparatively abnormal, low passive tubal resistance, which may be considered to facilitate ventilatory function but to impair the protective function of the tube. The authors speculated that the difference may account for the high prevalence of otitis media with perforation (and the low incidence of cholesteatoma) in this population.

Few interracial studies have been done, and we cannot therefore fully evaluate the significance of the extent and severity of ear disease in different racial groups. Poverty is a common factor among many of the nonwhite populations that have been studied. Other variables include extremes of climate (temperature, humidity, altitude), crowding in the homes, inadequate hygiene, poor sanitation, and lack of medical care.

Social and Economic Conditions

Cambon and coworkers (1965) noted a strong relationship between middle ear disease and poor socioeconomic conditions among Indians of British Columbia. The specific reasons for the high incidence and severity of disease were not identified. Factors suggested include crowded living conditions, poor sanitation, and inadequate medical care. "The running ear is the heritage of the poor" (Cambon et al., 1965) may be as true today as in the past, but we still do not understand the reasons for the high incidence and marked severity of disease among the underprivileged. In the Boston study, children living in households with many members were more likely to have otitis media than were children living in households with fewer members (Teele et al., 1980b).

Season

The seasonal incidence of infections of the middle ear parallels the seasonal variations of upper respiratory tract infections. Acute episodes peak during the winter and spring and occur less frequently in the summer and early fall. The incidence of episodes of otitis media also increases during outbreaks of viral infections of the respiratory tract in children; these are most likely to occur in the winter and spring seasons (Henderson et al., 1977).

The prevalence of middle ear effusion in asymptomatic children of various ages has been determined by use of tympanometry combined, in some cases, with physical examination. Four to five year old New Orleans children had a different prevalence of middle ear effusion in winter and fall; 29 per cent of children tested in February and 6 per cent of those tested in September had effusion (Sly et al., 1980). A one year study of 389 seven year old Danish school children used tympanometry on 8 to 10 occasions during the year to test for the presence of middle ear effusions. Twenty-six per cent of the children had evidence of middle ear effusion on one or more tests during the year. The prevalence varied from 5.7 per cent in August, 1978, to 9 per cent in November through April and dropped to 2.4 per cent in August, 1979. Of the episodes of middle ear effusion, 78 per cent resolved during the year; 65 per cent of cases of effusion were present for two consecutive months, 12 per cent for a period of three to five months, and 12 per cent for six months or longer (including one case with effusion for 12 months). Middle ear effusion occurring in the winter months persisted longer than effusion occurring in the summer months. Since medical intervention was minimal, spontaneous improvement occurred in all but a few of the seven year old asymptomatic children (Lous and Fiellau-Nikolajsen, 1981).

Genetic Factors

Genetic predisposition to middle ear infection was suggested by data from the Boston study (Teele et al., 1980b) and by a study of Apache children living on a reservation as well as those who were adopted and living outside the Indian community (Spivey and Hirschhorn, 1977). Children enrolled in the Boston study who had single or recurrent episodes of otitis media were more likely to have siblings with histories of significant middle ear infections than were children who had had no episodes of otitis media. Adopted Apache children had more episodes of acute otitis media than their non-Apache siblings and had an illness rate similar to that of Apache children who remained on the reservation.

Breast-feeding

Breast-feeding has been suggested as an important factor in prevention of respiratory and gastrointestinal infections in infancy. Does breast-feeding prevent otitis media? Various investigators have attempted to answer the question in different geographic and cultural populations. Schaefer (1971) surveyed Canadian Eskimo children in five areas, including an urban center (Frobisher Bay), village settlements, and hunting camps (Table 16–6). There was an increase in the incidence of middle ear disease in children who lived in urban centers compared to those living in villages or camps, but in each area there was an inverse relationship of incidence of middle ear disease and duration of breast-feeding. Children who were breast-fed for 12 or more months had significantly less ear pathology related to otitis media than did infants who were bottle-fed at birth or within the first month.

Timmermans and Gerson (1980) conducted a prevalence study of ear disease in a small Inuit Eskimo community in Labrador. The number of children with evidence of otitis media (defined as acute otitis media or wet or dry perforation) was inversely related to the age at onset of bottle-feeding. History of infant feeding was obtained by interview of the mother at the time of the prevalence study. Children who were bottle-fed at or soon after birth had significantly more disease (67 of 160 children, 42 per cent) than did children who had been bottle-fed only after six months of breast-feeding (0 of 21 children).

Chandra (1979) reported a significant decrease in episodes of otorrhea (observed or recorded by a nurse-midwife) among 35 infants who lived in a rural community in India and were breast-fed for at least two months when compared with 35 bottle-fed infants matched for socioeconomic status and family size.

Cunningham (1977) reviewed the medical records of infants who were born at the Mary Imogene Bassett Hospital in Cooperstown, New York, and who were seen regularly in the pediatric clinic in the first year of life. A significant difference in acute lower respiratory tract infections occurred in infants who were breast-fed for at least four and one half months when compared with infants who were bottle-fed. The incidence of otitis media was lower in the breast-fed infants, but the difference was not statistically significant.

These studies suggest that breast-feeding does have a protective effect against infections of the middle ear in some populations, but the question remains uncertain because one or more significant defects in design is present in each of the studies, including retrospective analysis of records, otoscopic examination at one point in time to determine prior disease history, lack of uniform criteria for diagnosis, lack of standardization, absence of multivariable analysis or failure to control adequately for other variables, and insufficient sample size to provide appropriate analysis of confounding variables.

The study of Boston children (Teele et al., 1980c) was designed to avoid these defects in

Table 16–6 MIDDLE EAR DISEASES IN CANADIAN ESKIMOS: OTOSCOPIC FINDINGS RELATED TO HISTORY OF INFANT NUTRITION*

Type of Settlement	Breast-Fed		Bottle-Fed	
	No. Examined	Middle Ear Pathology (%)	No. Examined	Middle Ear Pathology (%)
Camps	197	1.5	17	17.6
Villages	117	6.8	20	35.0
Urban areas	89	11.2	29	62.1
TOTAL	403	5.2 (average)	66	42.4 (average)

*From Schaefer, O. 1971. Otitis media and bottle-feeding. An epidemiological study of infant feeding habits and incidence of recurrent and chronic middle ear disease in Canadian Eskimos. Can. J. Public Health, 62:478–489.

Table 16–7 ASSOCIATION OF BREAST FEEDING AND DURATION OF MIDDLE EAR EFFUSION FOLLOWING FIRST ATTACK OF ACUTE OTITIS MEDIA*

Feeding Method	No. Patients	Percentage with Middle Ear Effusion by Days After Diagnosis of First Acute Otitis Media			
		30 Days	*60 Days*	*90 Days*	*120 Days*
Bottle (always)	770	40	22	15	11
Breast (ever)	241	30	13	8	5
Breast (180+ days)	93	25	8	4	2

*From Teele, D. W., Klein, J. O., and the Greater Boston Collaborative Otitis Media Program. 1980. Beneficial effects of breastfeeding on the duration of middle ear effusion after the first episode of acute otitis media. Pediatr. Res., *14*:494.

design. The children were followed prospectively from birth with frequent examinations and frequent assessments of the mode of feeding. A large number of children was studied (1565), and multivariable analysis was performed. Breast-feeding did not protect from acute infection of the middle ear. The number of episodes of otitis media was similar in breast-fed and bottle-fed infants. Breast-feeding did shorten significantly the duration of middle ear effusion. Longer periods of breast-feeding (six or more months) were more beneficial than shorter periods (Table 16–7).

These studies do not provide reasons for the effect of infant feeding on disease resulting from middle ear infection. Is breast-feeding beneficial or is bottle-feeding harmful? A number of hypotheses has been suggested:

1. Immunologic factors of value are provided in breast milk that prevent various bacterial and viral infections. These immunologic factors may prevent infection in some populations and may play a role in promoting resolution of middle ear fluid after the occurrence of infection.
2. The facial musculature of breast-fed infants develops differently from that of bottle-fed infants. The muscles may affect eustachian tube function and assist in promoting the drainage of middle ear fluids.
3. Aspiration of fluids into the middle ear occurs during bottle-feeding because the bottle-fed infant is required to produce high negative intraoral pressure, whereas breast-feeding involves nipple massage and reflex "letdown" of milk.
4. The breast-fed infant is maintained in a vertical or semivertical reclining position, whereas the bottle-fed infant is placed in a reclining or horizontal position. The horizontal position may result in reflux of milk through the wide and horizontal eustachian tube. The practice of propping a bottle in bed has been criticized because fluids are forced under pressure into the oral cavity with possible reflux into the middle ear.
5. Allergy to one or more components in cow or formula milk may result in alteration of the mucosa of the eustachian tube and middle ear.

Effect of Altered Host Defenses or Underlying Disease

Although the vast majority of children have no obvious defect responsible for chronic otitis media with effusion, a small number may have altered host defenses, including anatomic changes (cleft palate, cleft uvula, submucous cleft), congenital or acquired immunologic deficiencies (immunoglobulin deficiencies, chronic granulomatous disease), presence of malignancies or use of drugs that suppress immune processes, or alteration of normal physiologic defenses (patulous eustachian tube or barotrauma). Some patients may have disease states that lead to otitis media, such as nasopharyngeal tumors or connective tissue disorders. These conditions probably do not significantly affect epidemiologic studies of large numbers of patients but should be considered in the management of individual patients.

Summary

Otitis media is a very common infectious disease of early childhood. The incidence of acute episodes is highest among infants 6 to 24 months of age. Although some children never have middle ear infections, a large group (as high as one third in some studies) have multiple episodes of acute infections. Many children have persistent effusions in the middle ear after episodes of acute infection.

Some racial groups, such as American Indians and Canadian and Alaskan Eskimo children, have high rates of infection and severe middle ear disease. Poverty, with its accompanying factors of crowding, poor sanitation, and inadequate medical facilities, is common to these children. Whether other factors specifically related to race or culture are involved remains unknown. Preliminary data from studies of urban children suggest that the incidence of ear pathology is lower among black children than among white children of similar socioeconomic status. Black children have fewer episodes of acute otitis media and a shorter time spent with middle ear effusion after an episode of acute otitis media.

Other features important in the epidemiology of the disease include males affected more frequently than females, increased incidence during periods of viral infections in winter and spring when compared with summer and fall, and clusters of cases of otitis in families.

Data about the role of breast-feeding in middle ear infections are inconsistent. Some studies show no effect, whereas others suggest that the breast-fed infant, when compared with the bottle-fed infant, has fewer episodes of acute disease or a shorter period spent with middle ear effusion after an episode of acute otitis media.

ANATOMY OF THE NASOPHARYNX–EUSTACHIAN TUBE–MIDDLE EAR SYSTEM

The eustachian tube connects the middle ear and mastoid air cells to the nasopharynx. The nasal cavities and palate also constitute part of this system and may influence the function of the eustachian tube. In the adult, the anterior two thirds of the eustachian tube are cartilaginous and the posterior third is bony; in the infant, the bony portion is relatively longer. In adults, the tube lies at an angle of 45 degrees in relation to the horizontal plane, whereas in infants this inclination is only 10 degrees (Proctor, 1967) (Fig. 16–1).

The lumen of the eustachian tube is shaped like two cones, with the apex of each directed toward the middle. The aural orifice of the

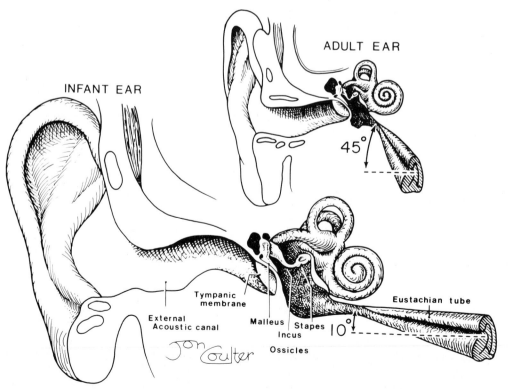

Figure 16–1   The difference in the angle of the eustachian tube between infants and adults.

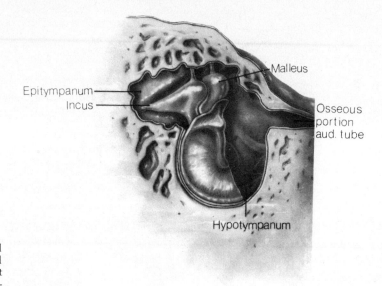

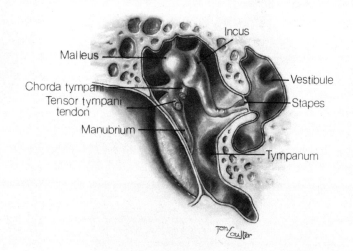

Figure 16–2 The anatomy of the aural portion of the eustachian tube as viewed from the external canal (upper). Note that the orifice of the eustachian tube is relatively high in the middle ear. Coronal section through middle ear (lower).

tube is oval, measuring 5 mm high and 2 mm wide in the adult (Fig. 16–2). The nasopharyngeal orifice in the adult is a vertical slit at right angles to the base of the skull, but in the infant this opening is oblique owing to the more horizontal position of the cartilage. The diameter of the orifice is 8 to 9 mm in the adult and 4 to 5 mm in the infant. In the newborn, the nasopharyngeal orifice lies in the plane of the hard palate, but in the adult it is situated 10 mm above this plane (Fig. 16–3).

The middle portion, or isthmus, of the eustachian tube is not sharply constricted but is relatively long, with gradual widening at each end to form the aural and nasopharyngeal orifices. The diameter of the isthmus in the adult is 1 to 2 mm, but in the infant it is somewhat larger.

The mucosal lining of the eustachian tube and middle ear is similar to mucosa elsewhere in the respiratory tract, including mucus-producing gland cells, ciliated cells, and plasma cells. The cartilaginous portion is similar to that of the nasopharynx and contains mucous glands. The mucosa in the bony portion of the eustachian tube is similar to that of the middle ear and contains both mucus-producing elements and ciliated cells.

Usually the eustachian tube is closed, but it opens during swallowing, yawning, and sneezing, permitting the air pressure in the middle ear to equalize with atmospheric pressure. This opening mechanism is muscular and involves the cartilaginous portion. As elucidated by Rich (1920), the levator palatini, palatopharyngeus, internal pterygoid,

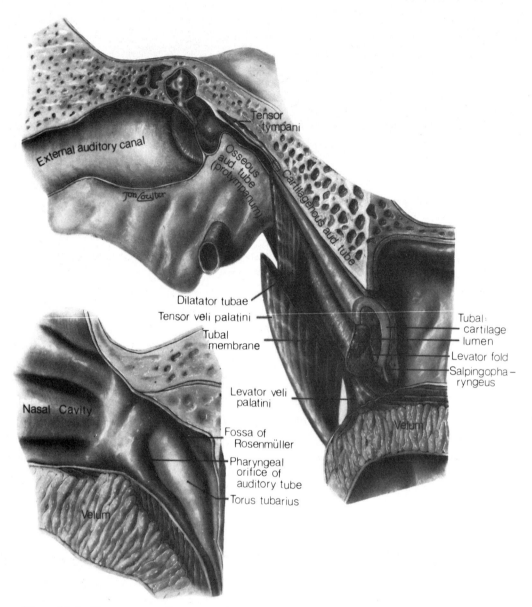

Figure 16–3 The anatomy of osseous and cartilaginous portions of the eustachian tube (upper) and pharyngeal end of the eustachian tube (lower).

and superior constrictor muscles have no influence on the patency of the orifice or the lumen of the tube. The tensor veli palatini is the *only* muscle related to active tubal opening (Cantekin et al., 1979a; Honjo et al., 1979). No constrictor muscle of the tube has ever been demonstrated, and closure has been attributed to the relaxation of the tensor muscle with passive return of the tubal walls to a condition of approximation. However, the internal pterygoid muscle may have some constrictor function (Cantekin et al., 1979a).

The tensor veli palatini muscle is composed

of two bundles of muscle fibers divided by a layer of fibroelastic tissue. The bundles lie lateral to the eustachian tube, in a superficial-deep relationship to one another (Fig. 16–4). The fibers of the superficial bundle run in an inferosuperior direction from their attachment in the inferior margin of the sphenoid bone, around the hamulus, to an attachment along the posterior border of the hard palate. The fibers of the deep bundle run from an inferolateral attachment in the fibroelastic layer to a superomedial attachment on the lateral membranous tubal wall, forming an

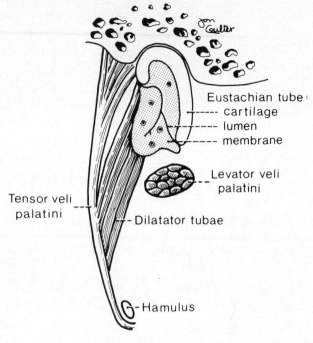

Figure 16–4 Diagrammatic representation of the relationship between the superficial muscle bundle (tensor veli palatini) and the deep bundle (dilatator tubae) to the lateral wall of the eustachian tube.

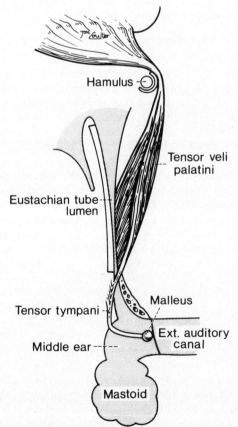

Figure 16–5 Diagrammatic representation of the tensor veli palatini muscle attachment along the lateral wall of the eustachian tube, its course around the hamulus of the pterygoid bone, and its attachment into the posterior margin of the hard palate.

acute angle with the wall. The tendinous portion of the deep bundle passes around the hamulus and inserts along the posterior mar-1978) (Fig 16–5) The anatomy of the middle ear is described in Chapter 6.

PHYSIOLOGY, PATHOPHYSIOLOGY, AND PATHOGENESIS

Abnormal function of the eustachian tube appears to be the most important factor in the pathogenesis of middle ear disease. This hypothesis was first suggested more than 100 years ago by Politzer (1862). However, later studies by Zollner (1942), Suehs (1952), Senturia et al. (1958), and Sadé (1966) suggested that otitis media was a disease primarily of the middle ear mucous membrane, that is, due to infection or allergic reactions in this tissue, rather than related to dysfunction of the eustachian tube. Related to this hypothesis is the concept that nasopharyngeal infection spreads up the mucosa of the eustachian tube to the middle ear. Figure 16–6 is an attempt to incorporate these hypotheses and thus to resolve the controversy.

The vast majority of patients with otitis media and related conditions have (or have had in the past) abnormal function of the eustachian tube that may have caused secondary mucosal disease of the middle ear, that is, inflammation. A much smaller number of

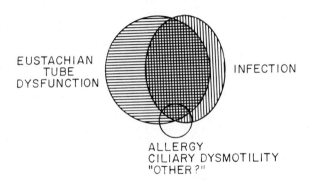

Figure 16–6   Etiology and pathogenesis of otitis media. (From Bluestone, C. D., and Cantekin, E. I.: Current clinical methods, indications and interpretation of eustachian tube function tests. Ann. Otol. Rhinol. Laryngol., *90*:552, 1981.)

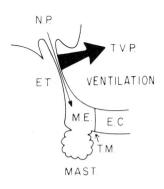

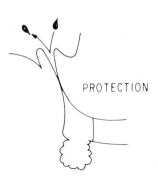

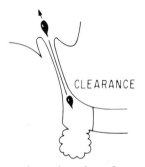

Figure 16–7   Three physiologic functions of the eustachian tube in relation to the middle ear. NP, nasopharynx; ET, eustachian tube; TVP, tensor veli palatini muscle; ME, middle ear; MAST, mastoid; TM, tympanic membrane; EC, external canal.

patients may have primary mucosal disease as a result of infection, allergy, or more rarely, an abnormality of the mucociliary transport system, such as Kartagener syndrome (Fischer et al., 1978). Hematogenous spread of bacteria to the middle ear may also result in otitis media. However, an abnormality of the mucous membrane can affect eustachian tube function, and abnormalities of eustachian tube function can cause otitis media and certain related conditions.

Physiology and Pathophysiology

The eustachian tube has at least three physiologic functions with respect to the middle ear (Fig. 16–7): (1) protection from nasopharyngeal sound pressure and secretions, (2) clearance into the nasopharynx of secretions produced within the middle ear, and (3) ventilation of the middle ear to equilibrate air pressure in the middle ear with atmospheric pressure and to replenish oxygen that has been absorbed. Assessment of these functions has been helpful in understanding the physiology and pathophysiology of the eustachian tube, as well as in the diagnosis and management of patients with middle ear disease.

Protective and Clearance Functions

The clearance or drainage function of the eustachian tube has been assessed by a variety of methods in the past. By means of radiographic techniques, the flow of contrast media from the middle ear (tympanic membrane not intact) into the nasopharynx has been assessed by Welin (1947), Aschan (1952, 1955), Compere (1960, 1970), Parisier and Khilmani (1970), Bluestone (1971), Bluestone et al. (1972a, 1972c), and Ferber and Holmquist (1973). Rogers et al. (1962) instilled a solution of fluorescein into the middle ear and assessed the clearance function by subsequently examining the pharynx with an ultraviolet light. Lafaye et al. (1974) utilized a radioisotope technique to monitor the flow of saline solution down the eustachian tube. Bauer (1975) assessed clearance by observing methylene blue in the pharynx after it had been instilled into the middle ear. Elbrond and Larsen (1976) assessed middle ear–eustachian tube mucociliary flow by determining the time that elapsed after saccharin had been placed on the mucous membrane of the middle ear until the subject reported tasting it. Unfortunately, all of these methods are qualitative and actually test eustachian tube patency rather than measure the clearance function of the tube quantitatively.

Even though abnormalities of the protective function are directly related to the pathogenesis of otitis media, this function has been assessed only by radiographic techniques and only by Bluestone and coworkers (Bluestone, 1971; Bluestone et al., 1972a, 1972c) by a test that was a modification of a tubal patency test described by Wittenborg and Neuhauser (1963).

Combined Radiographic Studies

The protective and clearance functions of the eustachian tube have been assessed by a combined radiographic technique (Bluestone et al., 1972a, 1972c). Radiopaque material was instilled through the nose of patients so that the retrograde flow of the medium from the nasopharynx into the eustachian tube could be observed (Fig. 16–8). Patients were considered to have normal protective function when radiopaque material entered only the nasopharyngeal or isthmic portion of the tube and did not enter the bony portion of the tube or middle ear cavity during swallowing. The normal eustachian tube protected the middle ear from the contrast material even when the liquid was under increased nasopharyngeal pressure during closed-nose swallowing (Fig. 16–9). If, during the retrograde study, contrast medium traversed the entire eustachian tube and refluxed into the middle ear during swallowing, the tube was considered to have increased distensibility and poor protective function (Fig. 16–10).

The effectiveness of the eustachian tube in clearing the radiopaque medium instilled into the middle ear was taken as an indication of the effectiveness of the eustachian tube in the clearance of secretions. Rapid and complete clearance of the medium into the nasopharynx was considered to indicate normal drainage function, while failure of the contrast material to drain from the middle ear into the nasopharynx indicated mechanical obstruction of the eustachian tube (Fig. 16–11), especially when contrast material also failed to enter the nasopharyngeal portion of the tube during the retrograde study (Fig.

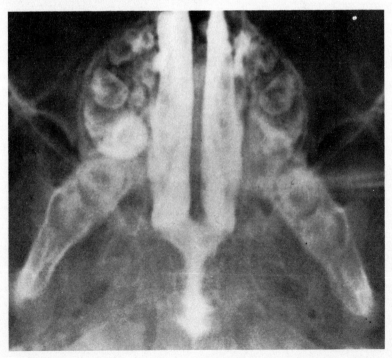

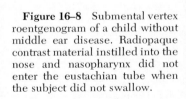

Figure 16–8 Submental vertex roentgenogram of a child without middle ear disease. Radiopaque contrast material instilled into the nose and nasopharynx did not enter the eustachian tube when the subject did not swallow.

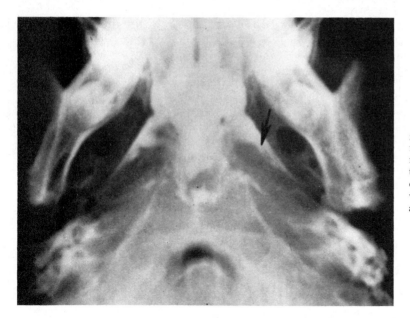

Figure 16–9 Normal retrograde function. During both open-nose and closed-nose swallowing, radiopaque contrast material filled the nasopharyngeal portion of the eustachian tube (arrow) of a child with normal tympanic membranes and a negative otologic history.

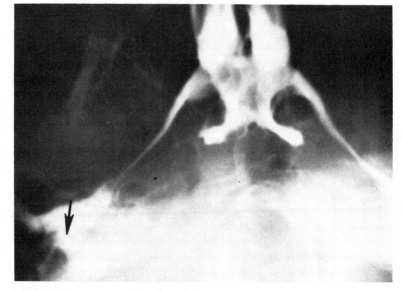

Figure 16–10 Retrograde reflux. Radiograph of a six year old boy with recurrent otitis media with effusion. On open-nose swallowing, contrast material traversed the entire eustachian tube and refluxed into the middle ear and mastoid (arrow).

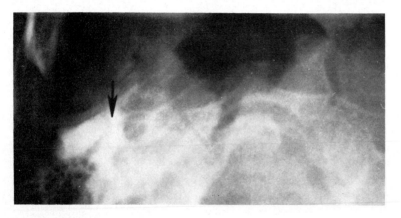

Figure 16–11 Roentgenogram showing prograde obstruction at the middle ear end of the isthmus of the eustachian tube (arrow). Radiopaque contrast material failed to flow from the middle ear into the nasopharynx.

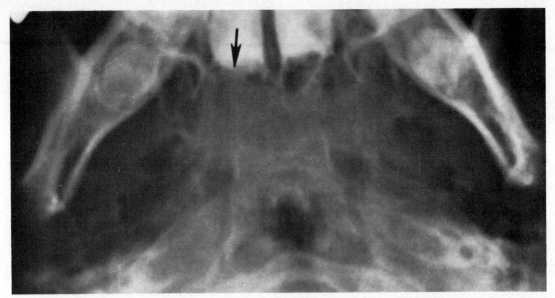

Figure 16–12 Retrograde obstruction. Radiograph of a five year old boy with otitis media. Radiopaque medium failed to enter the nasopharyngeal portion of the eustachian tube during both open-nose and closed-nose swallowing. Note enlarged adenoids (arrow).

16–12). These abnormal functions of the tube were found in patients with otitis media and were not found in a small group of normal subjects.

Model of Protective and Clearance Functions

The understanding of these radiographic studies can be enhanced if a model of the system is constructed (Bluestone and Beery, 1976). The eustachian tube, middle ear, and mastoid–air cell system can be likened to a flask with a long, narrow neck (Fig. 16–13). The mouth of the flask represents the nasopharyngeal end; the narrow neck, the isthmus of the eustachian tube; and the bulbous portion, the middle ear and mastoid air chamber. When a small amount of liquid is instilled into the mouth of the flask, liquid flow stops somewhere in the narrow neck owing to capillarity within the neck and the relative positive air pressure that develops in the chamber of the flask. This basic geometric design is considered to be critical for the protective function of the eustachian tube–middle ear system. Reflux of liquid into the body of the flask occurs if the neck is excessively wide. This is analogous to the abnormally patent eustachian tube in the human, in which there is not only free flow of air from the nasopharynx into the middle ear but also free flow of nasopharyngeal secretions, which can result in "reflux otitis media." Fluid flow is also dependent upon the length of the narrow neck and the viscosity of the liquid.

The position of the flask in relation to the liquid is another important factor. In the human, the supine position enhances liquid flow into the middle ear; thus, infants are at particular risk for developing reflux otitis media because they are frequently supine.

Reflux of a liquid into the vessel also occurs if a hole is made in the bulbous portion of the flask, since this prevents the creation of slight positive pressure in the bottom of the flask, which deters reflux. This hole is analogous to a perforation of the tympanic membrane or the presence of a tympanostomy tube that could allow reflux of nasopharyngeal secretions as a result of the loss of the middle ear–mastoid air cushion. Similarly, following a radical mastoidectomy, a patent eustachian tube could cause troublesome otorrhea (Bluestone et al., 1978).

If negative pressure is applied to the bottom of the flask, the liquid is aspirated into the vessel. In the clinical situation represented by the model, high negative middle ear air pressure could lead to the aspiration of nasopharyngeal secretions into the middle ear. If positive pressure is applied to the mouth of the flask, the liquid is insufflated into the vessel Nose blowing, crying, closed-nose swallowing, diving, or descent in an airplane could create a high positive nasopharyngeal pressure and could result in a similar condition in the human system.

One of the major differences between a flask with a rigid neck and a biologic tube

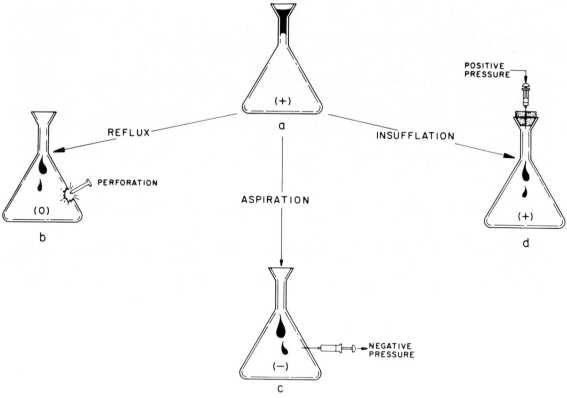

Figure 16–13   Fluid flow into a flask. *A*, Model of normal function. *B*, Effect of perforation. *C*, Effect of negative pressure on the bottom of the flask. *D*, Effect of positive pressure on the mouth of the flask.

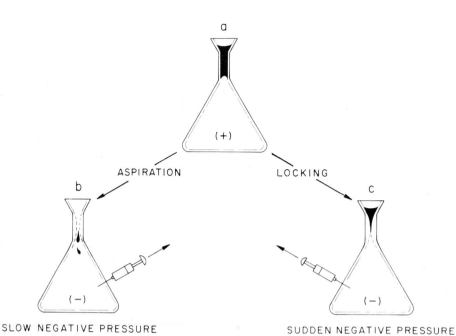

Figure 16–14   Fluid flow through a flask with a compliant neck. *A*, Fluid stopped in the neck of the flask. *B*, Effect of negative pressure applied slowly to the bottom of the flask. *C*, Effect of negative pressure applied suddenly to the bottom of the flask.

such as the eustachian tube is that the isthmus (neck) of the human tube is compliant. Application of positive pressure at the mouth of a flask with a compliant neck distends the neck, enhancing fluid flow into the vessel. Thus, less positive pressure is required to insufflate liquid into the vessel. In humans, insufflation of nasopharyngeal secretions into the middle ear occurs more readily if the eustachian tube is abnormally distensible (has increased compliance). The effect of applied negative pressure in the flask with a compliant neck is shown in Figure 16–14; liquid flow through the neck does not occur until a negative pressure is slowly applied to the bottom of the flask. In this case, fluid flow occurs even if the neck is collapsed; if the negative pressure is applied suddenly, however, temporary locking of the compliant neck prevents flow of the liquid. Therefore, the speed with which the negative pressure is applied as well as the compliance in such a system appears to be a critical factor in the results obtained. Clinically, aspiration of gas into the middle ear is possible, since negative middle ear pressure develops slowly as gas is absorbed by the middle ear mucous membrane. On the other hand, sudden application of negative middle ear pressure such as occurs with rapid alterations in atmospheric pressure (as in the descent in an airplane, in an ascent after diving, or during an attempt to test the ventilatory function of the eustachian tube) could lock the tube, thus preventing the flow of air.

Certain aspects of fluid flow from the middle ear into the nasopharynx can be demonstrated by inverting the flask of the model (Fig. 16–15). In this case, a liquid trapped in the bulbous portion of the flask does not flow out of the vessel because of the relative negative pressure that develops inside the chamber. However, if a hole is made in the vessel, the liquid drains out of the flask, since the suction is broken. Clinically, these conditions occur in cases of middle ear effusion; pressure is relieved by spontaneous rupture of the tympanic membrane or by myringotomy. Inflation of air into the flask could also relieve the pressure, which may explain the frequent success of the Politzer or Valsalva method in clearing a middle ear effusion.

The foregoing description of fluid flow through a flask only presents some of the mechanical aspects of the physiology of the human middle ear system. Other factors that probably affect the flow of liquid and air

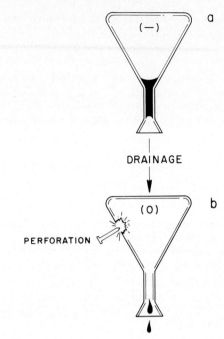

Figure 16–15 Fluid flow from an inverted flask. *A,* Fluid trapped by relative negative pressure in the chamber. *B,* Effect of perforation of the chamber.

through the middle ear include (1) the mucociliary transport system of the eustachian tube and middle ear, (2) contraction of the tensor tympani muscle and tympanic membrane movement, (3) active tubal opening mechanisms, and (4) surface tension factors.

Ventilatory Function of the Eustachian Tube

Classic Methods of Assessment

Until about 1960, most tests of the ventilatory function of the eustachian tube were in reality only assessments of the tubal patency. The classic methods of Valsalva, Toynbee, and Politzer for assessing the eustachian tube are still in use today, as is catheterization of the eustachian tube.

Valsalva Test

The effect of high positive nasopharyngeal pressures on the eustachian tube can be evaluated qualitatively by the Valsalva test. The test results are considered to be positive when the eustachian tube and middle ear can be inflated by a forced expiration, that is, with the mouth closed and the nose held by the thumb and forefinger. The amount of overpressure thus created is quite variable and may be as much as 2000 mm H_2O.

When the eardrum is intact, the overpressure in the middle ear can be observed as a bulging tympanic membrane by visual inspection of the tympanic membrane with a pneumatic otoscope or, more precisely, with the aid of the otomicroscope and a nonmagnifying Bruenings or Siegle otoscope. The tympanic membrane moves inward when positive canal pressure is applied, but outward mobility in response to applied negative canal pressure is decreased or absent if positive pressure is present within the middle ear (Bluestone and Shurin, 1974).

The most accurate method of assessing changes in middle ear pressure is by tympanometry, but since the positive pressure created in the middle ear for such a test may only be momentary — inflation followed by immediate equilibration prior to tubal closing — the alteration in middle ear pressure may not be visualized or recorded by tympanometry. When the tympanic membrane is not intact, the sound of the air entering the middle ear can be heard with a stethoscope or with the Toynbee tube. However, these methods are outmoded, and measurements now are made with a manometric system, preferably one equipped with a strip chart recorder.

Unfortunately, regardless of the testing technique or method of assessment, the Valsalva test by itself is not a reliable test of eustachian tube function. When positive, it indicates only an anatomically patent and probably distensible eustachian tube. Indeed, without inflation of the middle ear during this test, no useful information concerning tubal function is obtained. Elner et al. (1971d) found that 85 per cent of 101 adults with normal ears had positive results on the Valsalva test.

TOYNBEE TEST

In performing the Toynbee test, the subject is asked to swallow when the nose is manually compressed (Fig. 16–16). This maneuver usually creates a positive pressure within the nasopharynx, followed by a negative pressure phase (Perlman, 1951). If the eustachian tube opens during the test, the middle ear pressure changes; the way in which it changes is determined by the timing of the tubal opening and the nasopharyngeal pressure gradient.

Change in middle ear pressure is assessed on the Toynbee test in the same way that it is assessed on the Valsalva test. If negative pressure is present within the middle ear, the tympanic membrane will be retracted and will not move inward to applied positive pressure with the pneumatic otoscope. It will move outward to applied negative pressure if the pressure applied exceeds the negative pressure within the middle ear.

The test results are usually considered positive when there is an alteration in the middle ear pressure. Negative middle ear pressure after the Toynbee test or only momentary negative middle ear pressure followed by ambient pressure usually indicates good tubal function, since it shows that the eustachian tube can open actively (the tensor veli palatini

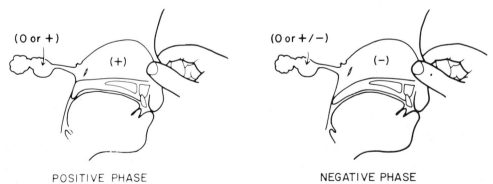

POSITIVE PHASE   NEGATIVE PHASE

Figure 16–16 The Toynbee test of eustachian tube function. Closed-nose swallowing results in first positive pressure in the nose and nasopharynx, followed by a negative pressure phase. When positive pressure is in the nasopharynx, air may enter the middle ear, creating positive pressure. During or after the negative pressure phase, negative pressure may develop in the middle ear, or positive pressure may still be in the middle ear (no change in middle ear pressure during negative phase), or positive pressure may be followed by negative middle ear pressure, or ambient pressure will be present if equilibration takes place before the tube closes. If the tube does not open during either the positive or negative phase, no change in middle ear pressure will occur (see text).

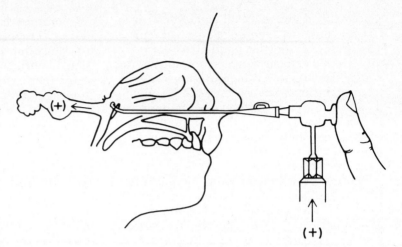

Figure 16–17 Catheterization of the eustachian tube to test patency of the tube.

muscle contracts) and that the tubal structure is sufficiently stiff to withstand nasopharyngeal negative pressure (as noted by absence of temporary tubal locking). However, some abnormal eustachian tubes that are either patulous or have very low tubal resistance may transfer gas from the middle ear into the nasopharynx during the Toynbee test (as they may with sniffing). The finding of only positive middle ear pressure signifies tubal patency but does not have the same significance as does even transitory negative pressure.

Unfortunately, the absence of any alteration in middle ear pressure during the Toynbee test does not indicate poor eustachian tube function. Zollner (1942) and Thomsen (1958b) reported that 30 per cent of the adults with normal ears that they examined had negative results on the Toynbee test. Elner et al. (1971d) reported that in 21 per cent of 94 normal adults, middle ear pressure did not change during the Toynbee test. Cantekin et al. (1976) found that only two of 49 children with tympanostomy tubes inserted for otitis media with effusion could open their eustachian tubes during the Toynbee maneuver.

POLITZER TEST

The Politzer test is performed by compressing one naris into which the end of a rubber tube attached to an air bag has been inserted while the opposite naris is compressed with finger pressure. The subject is asked to repeat the letter K or is asked to swallow to close the velopharyngeal port. When the test is positive, the overpressure that develops in the nasopharynx is transmitted to the middle ear, thus creating positive middle ear pressure. Assessment of the mid-

dle ear pressure and the significance of the test results are the same as with the Valsalva test in that a positive result indicates only tubal patency. However, both the Valsalva and Politzer methods can be of benefit as a treatment when effusion or high negative pressure is present within the middle ear if the child can successfully inflate the middle ear.

EUSTACHIAN TUBE CATHETERIZATION

Transnasal catheterization of the eustachian tube with the classic metal cannula has been used to assess tubal function for over a century (Fig. 16–17). Cannulation can be performed by blindly rooting for the orifice of the tube, by indirect visualization with a nasopharyngoscope or transoral right-angle telescope. Successful transferring of applied positive pressure from the proximal end of the cannula into the middle ear signifies only tubal patency. However, the use of this method as a test or treatment is limited in children, since it can be frightening and difficult to perform.

Tests of Ventilatory Function

The ventilatory function of the eustachian tube can be assessed by manometry, sonometry, and tympanometry. Not yet perfected, sonometry is available for investigation only in the laboratory, but the other two tests can be used in the clinical setting. Some of the manometric tests of eustachian tube function are technologically complicated and are available only in the laboratory; others are quite simple and are available to the clinician.

MANOMETRY

Manometric measurements of tubal function have been conducted for the past 100 years. The simplest techniques involve the placement of an ear canal catheter, with an airtight connection, between a pressure monitoring device and the middle ear cavity. If the tympanic membrane is not intact, the middle ear pressure is measured directly (intratympanic manometry) but if the tympanic membrane is intact, then the middle ear pressure must be inferred from the pressure change in the ear canal (extratympanic manometry). In both cases, it is a closed pneumatic system.

Recordings obtained by this method when the tympanic membrane is intact are of little value for assessing tubal function because atmospheric pressure changes, the system volume, and the effects of temperature on the system are much more significant than are the small volumes displaced by the tympanic membrane with changes in middle ear pressure. On the other hand, this technique is a valuable tool for intratympanic applications when the tympanic membrane is not intact. In such cases, a middle ear pressure application device, such as a syringe or an air pump, is connected to the ear canal through a valve. Using this arrangement, different levels of middle ear pressure can be generated, and the equilibration capacity of the eustachian tube can be recorded directly as pressure drops after the subject swallows.

The first quantitative tubal function study performed by intratympanic manometry was the systematically conducted inflation-deflation test (Ingelstedt and Ortegren, 1963). Later, numerous investigators employed the same technique to determine tubal function (Miller, 1965; Holmquist, 1969a). The next improvement in this technique was the addition of a flow meter to the manometric system in order to involve pressure-flow

relationships during eustachian tube function testing (Flisberg, 1966). The evaluation of tubal function was limited to the assessment of active function (owing to the contractions of the tensor veli palatini muscle) until Bluestone et al. (1972a, 1975a, 1975b) introduced a modified inflation-deflation test by which passive function could also be described by parameters like forced opening pressure and closing pressure of the tube. Later, a device similar to the ear canal catheter was developed for use with the modified inflation-deflation test so that nasopharyngeal pressure could be measured (Cantekin et al., 1976). Recently, a new testing procedure, the forced-response test, was developed to test eustachian tube function in the clinical setting when the tympanic membrane is not intact (Cantekin et al., 1979b). This technique seems to discriminate between normal and abnormal eustachian tube function without the overlap encountered in the inflation-deflation test. With the forced-response test, it has also been possible to make a distinction between tubal dysfunction that stems from inefficient active opening of the tube and that which is the result of structural properties of the eustachian tube.

Nonintact Tympanic Membrane

Inflation-Deflation Test. When a perforation of the tympanic membrane or a tympanostomy tube is present, inflation-deflation tests to measure the ventilatory function of the eustachian tube can be performed in the clinical setting with the pump-manometer portion of an impedance bridge (Bluestone et al., 1972a) (Fig. 16–18) or a controlled syringe pump and manometer (Bluestone et al., 1977a) (Fig. 16–19).

Figure 16–20 is a simplified explanation of

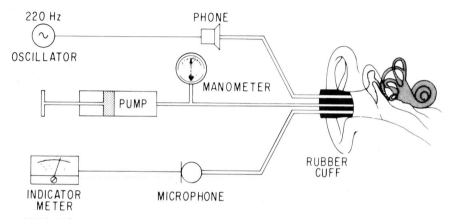

Figure 16–18 Electroacoustic impedance instrument in which a pump-manometer system is employed for eustachian tube function tests when the tympanic membrane is not intact (see text).

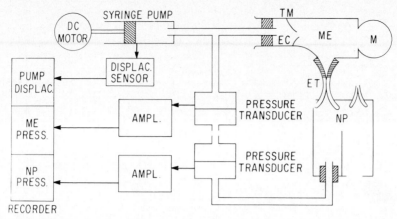

Figure 16–19 Instrumentation employed to test inflation-deflation eustachian tube function when the tympanic membrane is not intact. TM, tympanic membrane; EC, external canal; ME, middle ear; M, mastoid; ET, eustachian tube; NP, nasopharynx. A closed air pressure system is sealed into the external auditory meatus (ear canal) and into one naris by means of a double-lumen balloon catheter (modified Foley). A constant-speed syringe pump is used for inflation and deflation of the middle ear. The pump delivers constant airflow to the external canal. The volume of airflow is monitored by the piston displacement sensor. The rate of applied pressure is 20 to 30 mm H$_2$O per sec, depending upon the subject's middle ear–mastoid volume and the starting position of the pump piston. Middle ear pressure is measured by a pressure transducer; nasopharyngeal pressure is measured simultaneously by another pressure transducer. Pressure signals are amplified and recorded onto heat-sensitive paper (Bluestone, Cantekin, and Beery, 1977; Bluestone et al., 1977).

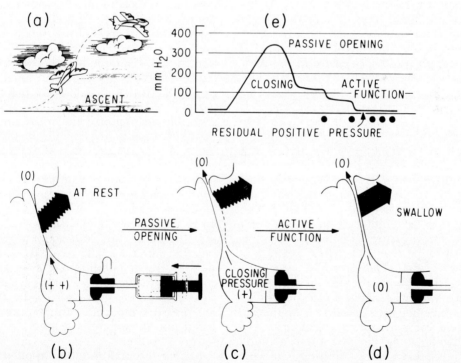

Figure 16–20 Test of passive and active function of the eustachian tube following application of positive middle ear pressure. *A,* Analogous ascent in an airplane. *B,* Assessment of passive function. *C,* Closing pressure. *D,* Assessment of active function (swallowing). *E,* Strip chart recording showing an example of normal pressure tracing. Black circles represent swallows.

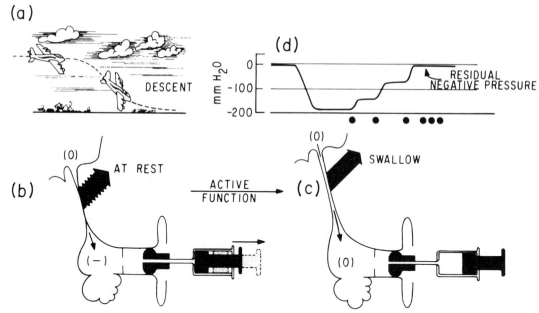

Figure 16–21 Deflation phase of eustachian tube testing. *A*, Analogous descent in an airplane. *B*, Application of low negative pressure to the middle ear. *C*, Equilibration by active tubal opening. *D*, Strip chart recording showing an example of a normal tracing. Black circles represent swallows.

the combined passive and active function test when positive pressure is applied to the middle ear (inflation). This test is similar to ascending in an airplane until the eustachian tube opens passively. It involves the application of enough positive pressure to the middle ear to force the eustachian tube open The pressure remaining in the middle ear after passive opening and closing is termed *the closing pressure* Further equilibration of pressure is by swallowing (an active function), which is the result of contraction of the tensor veli palatini muscle (Rich, 1920; Honjo et al , 1979; Cantekin et al , 1979a) When the muscle contracts, the lumen of the eustachian tube is opened and air flows down the tube The pressures can be monitored on a strip chart recorder The pressure remaining in the middle ear after passive and active function is termed *the residual positive pressure*

Figure 16–21 shows the deflation phase of the study, which is similar to descent in an airplane. Low negative pressure is applied to the middle ear and is then equilibrated by active tubal opening. The pressure remaining in the middle ear after swallowing is termed *the residual negative pressure.*

In certain instances, the ability of the tube to open actively in response to applied low positive pressure is also assessed (Fig. 16–22). This is similar to ascent in an airplane to an altitude lower than a pressure that would

force the eustachian tube open. The patient is asked to swallow in an attempt to equilibrate the pressure by active function.

Figure 16–23 shows the symbols employed and examples of results obtained in ventilation studies. Example A shows the results of a typical study in a patient with normal eustachian tube function. Following passive opening and closing of the eustachian tube during the inflation phase of the study, the patient was able to completely equilibrate the remaining positive pressure. Active swallowing also completely equilibrated applied negative pressure (deflation). Example B shows the results of a typical study in a child who had had otitis media with effusion. The eustachian tube passively opened and closed following inflation, but subsequent swallowing failed to equilibrate the residual positive pressure. In the deflation phase of the study, the child was unable to equilibrate negative pressure. Inflation to a pressure below the opening pressure but above the closing pressure could not be equilibrated by the active swallowing function.

Failure to equilibrate the applied negative pressure indicates locking of the eustachian tube during the test. This type of tube is considered to have increased compliance or to be "floppy" in comparison to the tube with perfect function. A stiff tube will neither distend in response to high positive pressures

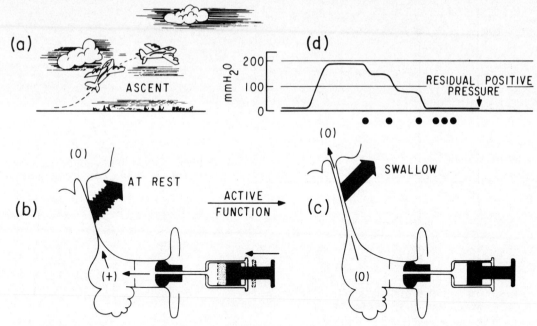

Figure 16–22   Active opening of the eustachian tube to applied positive pressure tested by inflation to a pressure below the opening pressure but above the closing pressure. *A*, Analogous ascent in an airplane. *B* and *C*, Attempt to equilibrate pressure by swallowing. *D*, Strip chart recording showing an example of a normal tracing. Black circles represent swallows.

nor collapse in response to negative pressures; however, a tube that lacks stiffness is collapsed, and this in turn results in functional tubal obstruction. The tube collapses even further and may lock entirely in response to negative pressures; it may not open in response to low positive pressure, but as pressure progressively increases, it opens and may ultimately distend.

The speed of the application of the positive and negative pressure is an important variable in testing eustachian tube function with the inflation-deflation test. The faster the positive pressure is applied, the higher the

Figure 16–23   Examples of results of inflation-deflation ventilation studies that employed a strip chart recorder. *A*, Normal adult with a traumatic perforation. *B*, Four year old boy with a functioning tympanostomy tube who had had a persistent otitis media with effusion.

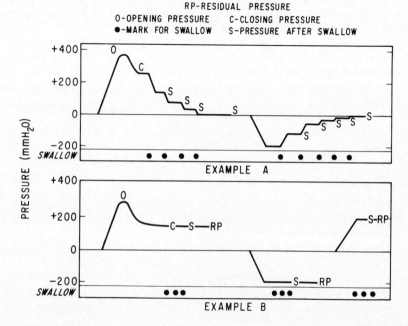

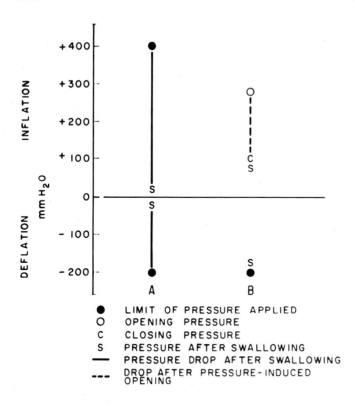

Figure 16-24 Procedure and symbols used in describing ventilatory (inflation-deflation) studies when a strip chart recorder is not employed. Two illustrative examples are shown (*A* and *B*).

opening pressure. During the deflation phase of the study, the faster the negative pressure is applied, the more likely it is that the locking phenomenon will occur.

Figure 16–24 illustrates elements of the procedure and the symbols used in recording the results of ventilatory studies with an electroacoustic impedance bridge when a strip chart recorder is not available, that is, when the pressures are noted on the manometer. Example A in Figure 16–24 is similar to example A in Figure 16–23; in Figure 16–24, however, the tube did not open passively. Depending upon the type of electroacoustic impedance bridge, the pump-manometer may not produce pressures greater than 400 mm H_2O. The mean opening pressure for apparently normal subjects with a traumatic perforation and negative otologic history reported by Cantekin and coworkers (1977) was 330 mm H_2O ($\pm$70 mm H_2O). Many eustachian tubes open at pressures above 400 mm H_2O, which is above the limit of the manometers used in the most commonly available bridges. Again, the opening pressure is dependent on the speed of the pump.

Example B in Figure 16–24 is another example of functional obstruction of the eustachian tube. The diagnosis of total mechanical obstruction of the eustachian tube (air cannot flow out of or into the middle ear) cannot be made if the pressures cannot be elevated above 400 mm H_2O.

During each equilibration, the time interval between each swallow should be approximately 20 sec to avoid strain on the pharyngeal muscles. The subject should swallow "dry," but patients with reduced function of the eustachian tube may need water to swallow.

Figure 16–25 shows the procedures employed in assessing the ventilatory function of the eustachian tube with the instrumentation illustrated in Figure 16–19. The results are based on a four-part test in the following sequence: (a) active opening of the tube, (b) passive opening of the tube during open-nose swallowing, (c) active opening of the tube during closed-nose swallowing (Toynbee maneuver), and (d) the Valsalva test. These tests of ventilatory function are more complete and provide more information than the more simplified testing procedure.

Even though the inflation-deflation test of eustachian tube function is not strictly physiologic, the results are helpful in differentiating normal from abnormal function. If the test results reveal passive opening and closing within the normal range, if residual positive pressure can be completely equilibrated by swallowing, and if applied negative pressure

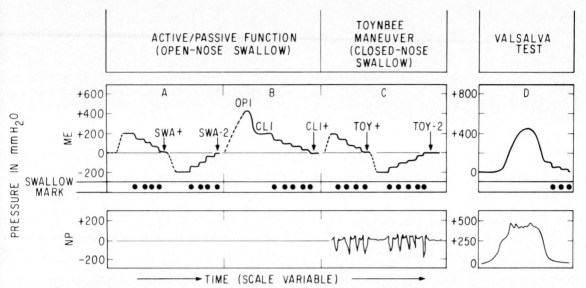

Figure 16–25   Sequence of procedures employed in assessing many aspects of the ventilatory function of the eustachian tube using the instrumentation shown in Figure 16–19. *A*, Active tubal function. After obtaining a hermetic seal in the ear canal, 200 mm H_2O pressure is applied in the middle ear (inflation). The subject is then instructed to swallow to equilibrate. The pressure remaining in the middle ear following five consecutive swallows without a pressure change is termed the residual positive pressure (SWA+). Then −200 mm H_2O is applied in the middle ear (deflation), and the patient is instructed to swallow. The pressure remaining in the middle ear following this test is termed the residual negative pressure (SWA-2). *B*, Passive and active tubal function. The middle ear is inflated with a constant flow of air until the tube spontaneously opens, at which time the syringe pump is manually stopped. The first passive opening of the eustachian tube by middle ear over-pressure is termed the opening pressure (OP1). Following discharge of air through the eustachian tube, the tube closes passively without a further decay in middle ear pressure. This pressure is called the closing pressure (CL1). Then the patient is instructed to swallow for further equilibration. The residual pressure following passive closing and swallowing is termed CL1+. The minimal residual positive pressure (MIN+) is the lowest recorded pressure remaining in the middle ear after active and passive equilibration of middle ear over-pressure (lowest value of CL1+ and SWA+). *C*, The Toynbee test. Active function of the tube during closed-nose swallowing is assessed by applying a positive pressure of 200 mm H_2O in the middle ear and manually compressing the unattached naris. The opposite naris is connected to the pressure transducer in order to record the nasal pressure developed during closed-nose swallowing. The residual positive pressure remaining in the middle ear after closed-nose swallowing (TOY+) is determined. Next, the middle ear pressure is reduced to −200 mm H_2O. The residual negative pressure remaining in the middle ear following closed-nose swallowing (TOY-2) is noted. *D*, Valsalva test. Passive opening of the eustachian tube by nasopharyngeal over-pressure is observed by instructing the subject to blow against obstructed nares — the Valsalva maneuver — while the middle ear pressure is ambient. The nasopharyngeal pressure corresponding to the first detectable change in middle ear pressure is taken as the nasopharyngeal opening pressure of the eustachian tube. If a residual positive pressure remains in the middle ear after the termination of nasopharyngeal over-pressure, equilibration is attempted by open-nose swallowing. Irrespective of eustachian tube opening, the maximal pressure achieved in the nasopharynx is also noted.

can also be equilibrated, the function of the eustachian tube can be considered to have normal function. However, if the tube does not open to 1000 mm H_2O, one can assume that total mechanical obstruction is present. This pressure is not hazardous to the middle ear or inner ear windows if the pressure is applied slowly. An extremely high opening pressure (for example, greater than 500 to 600 mm H_2O) may indicate partial obstruction, whereas a very low opening pressure

(for example, less than 100 mm H_2O) would indicate a semipatulous eustachian tube. Inability to maintain even a modest positive pressure within the middle ear would be consistent with a patulous tube, that is, open at rest. Complete equilibration by swallowing of applied negative pressure is usually associated with normal function, but partial equilibration or even failure to reduce any applied negative pressure may or may not be considered abnormal, since even a normal eustachian tube will lock when negative pressure is rapidly applied. Therefore, inability to equilibrate applied negative pressure may not indicate poor eustachian tube function, especially when it is the only abnormal parameter.

Forced-Response Test.   A new technique has been developed to test eustachian tube function in subjects with nonintact tympanic membranes. Originally, the forced-response test was utilized to evaluate tubal function in the Rhesus monkey animal model for normal and abnormal middle ear ventilation (Cantekin et al., 1977); then the same procedure was used in the assessment of tubal function in human subjects (Cantekin et al., 1979b).

Briefly, this method enables the investigator to study both passive and active responses of the eustachian tube. The active response is due to the contractions of the tensor veli palatini muscle, which displaces the lateral walls from the cartilage-supported medial wall of the tube. Thus, the clinician can determine if tubal dysfunction is due to the material properties of the tube or to a defective active opening mechanism. During this test, the middle ear is inflated at a constant flow rate, forcing the eustachian tube open. Following the forced opening of the tube, the pump continues to deliver a constant airflow, maintaining a steady stream of air through the tube. Then, the subject is instructed to swallow in order to assess the active dilation of the tube.

The method is unique in that it eliminates the "mucous forces" in the eustachian tube lumen that may interfere with the results of the inflation-deflation test when an attempt is made to assess the active opening mechanisms and the compliance of the tube. In this test, the passive resistance is assessed, and the active resistance is determined during swallowing. Patients with nonintact tympanic membranes secondary to chronic perforation or tympanostomy tubes can be distinguished from apparently normal subjects with traumatic perforations of the tympanic membrane and negative otologic histories. The ratio of the passive and active resistance correctly separates a normally functioning eustachian tube from an abnormally functioning one.

Figure 16–26 schematizes the forced-response test in a normal subject and compares the results with two response patterns that are commonly seen in association with defects in active dilation. Studies in a large number of patients with tympanostomy tubes

in place or perforations secondary to otitis media revealed that all the abnormal ears either had poor active function (as demonstrated by weak or absent dilation of the eustachian tube during swallowing activity) or constricted during swallowing. Constriction of the eustachian tube with swallowing was found to occur in most children with cleft palates (Doyle et al., 1980a) and has been attributed to opposing muscle force (Cantekin et al., 1979b). This test was also done with American Indians as subjects; they showed low resistance of the eustachian tube (Beery et al., 1980). The forced-response test appears to be more indicative of the active function of the eustachian tube than is the inflation-deflation test.

Intact Tympanic Membrane

Eustachian tube function in individuals with intact tympanic membranes may also be determined by manometry. Middle ear pressure is measured indirectly by the response to pressure changes in a pressure chamber. Decompression of the chamber creates relative positive pressure in the middle ear, whereas chamber compression results in relative negative pressure in the middle ear.

Investigation of eustachian tube function by means of pressure chambers dates back over a century to 1864, when Magnus first reported his findings on tubal function in a diving bell. By using rising external pressures, Magnus was able to make several observations: (1) he confirmed Toynbee's assumption that the eustachian tube is closed under normal conditions; (2) he realized the importance of deglutition for the opening of the tube; and (3) he noted that if the pressure difference between the middle ear and the bell became too pronounced (relative negative pressure in the middle ear), it could not be equilibrated by swallowing. These findings were confirmed eight years later by Mach and Kessel (1872), when they conducted experiments in a primitive pressure chamber. Their chamber consisted of a wooden box in which the pressure could be varied between −200 and 140 mm H_2O with the aid of an organ pump. Since that time, pressure chambers have been used to test the function of the eustachian tube.

Early volume displacement measurements of the tympanic membrane were done by means of closed manometry in the external ear, with simultaneous direct measurements of middle ear pressure. This was abandoned as a clinical procedure because of the difficulties encountered in direct measurements,

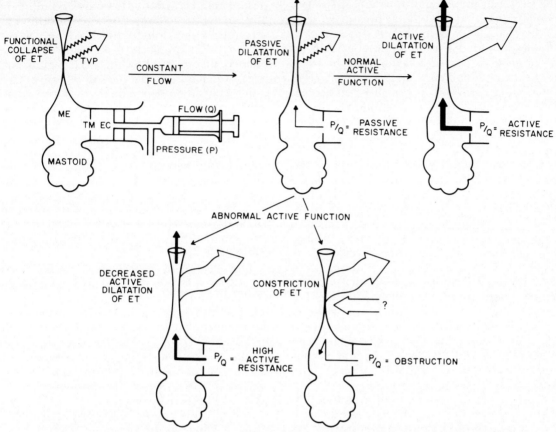

Figure 16–26   Forced-response test for the ventilatory function of the eustachian tube. TVP, tensor veli palatini; ME, middle ear; TM, tympanic membrane; EC, external canal; ET, eustachian tube.

which were usually made by inserting a mandarin needle into the middle ear cavity. More recently, however, tympanic membrane displacements have been recorded using microflow techniques. When the drum is moving, airflow is produced in the external ear canal. This flow is recorded by a flowmeter and then is integrated to give quantitative measurements of volume displacement. Displacements as small as 1 μl have been recorded with up to 95 per cent accuracy.

Microflow Technique.   The microflow method (Ingelstedt et al., 1967a, 1967b; Elner et al., 1971a, 1971b, 1971c) is the only method used to assess normal eustachian tube function quantitatively in adults. This technique permits continuous recording of the volume deviation of the tympanic membrane resulting from changes of ambient pressure and changes of pressure within the middle ear. During the test, the tympanic membrane is in permanent and free contact with ambient air.

Under an otomicroscope, the subject is fitted with a catheter through a rubber disc inserted in the bony part of the ear canal. The rubber disc maintains an airtight seal with the canal walls. The air cushion between the tympanic membrane and the disc is connected to a very sensitive flowmeter via the catheter; the other end of the flowmeter is open to ambient air. An identical flowmeter is connected to a reference volume simulating the air cushion volume between the tympanic membrane and the rubber disc seal. The signal from the reference flowmeter is subtracted from that of the ear canal flowmeter, compensating for the flow changes due to compression or expansion of air in the pressure chamber. This corrected airflow rate is integrated to obtain the volume displacement of the tympanic membrane. Then, by changing the ambient pressure in the chamber, the tympanic membrane displacement as a function of middle ear pressure is obtained.

This procedure in a way calibrates the tympanic membrane as a pressure transducer so that after this measurement has been made the subjects can be tested for their abilities to equilibrate various middle ear pressures created by changes in chamber pressure. Within the elastic limits of the tympanic membrane ($\pm$ 150 mm H_2O pressure differential between the middle ear and ear canal), a very accurate inflation-deflation test can be conducted. However, since this technique requires a pressure chamber and very sophisticated equipment, it is only practical for use in research centers.

Sonometry. Sound conduction through the eustachian tube was first reported by Politzer (1869). He observed that the sound of a tuning fork placed near the nose appeared to increase in amplitude during swallowing. He concluded that this sound must be traveling through the eustachian tube, which opens during swallowing. Politzer's findings were soon forgotten, and it was not until 1932 that sound conduction through the eustachian tube was reported again, this time by Gyergyay. He used various musical instruments to generate a sound that was introduced into the nose. He verified Politzer's experiments but concluded that the eustachian tube opens only intermittently during swallowing.

In 1939, Perlman studied sound conduction through the eustachian tube by introducing a 500 Hz tone through a tube to the nostril of his subjects. By placing a microphone in the ear canal of his subjects and recording the test sound, he was able to detect tubal opening. His results provided some information on tubal opening time but were too varied to be useful. Little work was done until 1951, when Perlman repeated his earlier studies. This time he reduced the tone frequency to 100 Hz, and by recording the output of the microphone he was better able to assess the duration of tubal opening. He observed increases in sound-pressure levels of up to 20 dB during swallowing. These measurements by Perlman were instrumental in the development of sonometry.

Elpern et al. (1964) used a 200 Hz tone as the sound source in experiments in eustachian tube conduction of sound. They catheterized the eustachian tube with a thin polyethylene tube in order to verify that the sound was presented to the tube only and were able to show that the sound indeed traveled through the eustachian tube during swallowing.

In 1966, Guillerm et al. repeated Perlman's procedure using a 100 Hz tone but made one important modification. They varied the pressure in the nasopharynx with the aid of an air pump and recorded the sound conduction and pressure change in the middle ear through a Foley catheter that was sealed at the external ear canal. If the eustachian tube opened during swallowing, both sound and pressure changes were recorded; conversely, if the tube did not open, neither was recorded. This procedure, known as sonomanometry, was used later by Venker (1973) and Pieraggi (1974).

Naunton and Galluser (1967) developed a eustachian tube analyzer that utilized a 200 Hz tone to analyze the theoretic vector of the response. Satoh et al. conducted experiments using 1930 Hz as the test frequency. Then, in 1975, Eguchi constructed a model of the eustachian tube and conducted similar tests using 2000 Hz.

The selection of the test frequency had been somewhat arbitrary up to this point; each experimenter had chosen a frequency that he felt would best overcome the technical difficulties of the measurement, but little thought had been given to selecting the frequency (or frequencies) at which the maximal amount of sound would be transmitted through the open eustachian tube. All of the frequencies used were 2000 Hz or below.

In 1977, Virtanen conducted experiments using a wide set of frequencies. He chose single tones at 1 kHz intervals between 1 and 20 kHz and found that sound conduction through the eustachian tube appeared to be best at 6, 7, and 8 kHz. He also recorded the physiologic noise due to swallowing and found it to be significant up to 5 kHz. This led him to conclude that recordings of sound conduction using test frequencies below 5 kHz were invalid because they are distorted by the physiologic noise of swallowing.

Pilot studies were conducted using white noise as the stimulus (Murti et al., 1980). When white noise is used, no a priori assumptions are made about which test frequencies are most suitable. The results of these pilot studies were in agreement with those of Virtanen (1978). Based on these results, it appears that sound conduction may be a reliable test to indicate tubal function. As more work is done in this area, it should be possible to obtain further information on middle ear status and eustachian tube dynamics by such studies. However, the instrumentation and technique are still experimental and are not available for use in the clinical setting.

Tympanometry. Techniques for determining middle ear pressure and acoustic impedance with electroacoustic impedance equipment were introduced more than 30 years ago (Metz, 1946). These same techniques have been used to perform tympanometry, which is the measurement of the acoustic driving-point admittance as a function of the static pressure in the canal. If low-frequency tones are used for the measurement, the static pressure that produces the maximal acoustic admittance is approximately equal to the pressure in the middle ear.

In 1958, Thomsen (1958a) adapted the acoustic impedance method for use in a pressure chamber. He varied the chamber pressure and measured the percentage of absorption of a tone presented into the ear canal. He found that there was a fall in absorption as the pressure difference between the middle ear and the chamber was increased. The absorption reached a peak when the two pressures were identical.

Unfortunately, Thomsen's technique failed to account for the change in middle ear pressure caused by the measurement procedure. As the pressure in the chamber is varied (in search of maximal loudness or absorption), the tympanic membrane moves from its original position to a new position, thus changing the volume of the middle ear cavity. However, according to Boyle's law, as the volume of the cavity changes, the pressure must also change. Thus, by knowing the volume displacement and "measuring" the final pressure, the original pressure can be deduced.

Tympanometry has been widely used in clinical and basic research investigations. Today, a variety of commercially available instruments allow this method to be used routinely in most clinical settings without a pressure chamber. However, an attempt was recently made to use tympanometry with a pressure chamber to evaluate eustachian tube function in normal children (Ingelstedt and Bylander, 1978). In this method, the resting middle ear pressure is obtained from the initial tympanogram. Then, the chamber pressure is lowered to -100 mm H_2O relative to ambient pressure, and a second tympanogram is obtained, verifying the relative overpressure in the middle ear. Following this, after each deglutition of the subject, a tympanogram is recorded to determine middle ear pressure. The same procedure is repeated with 100 mm H_2O relative over-pressure in the chamber to assess the subject's ability to actively equilibrate relative under-pressure in the middle ear. Using this method, the

inflation-deflation test was conducted on 50 children, and the results were compared with the results of tests that measured tubal function in adults. In this way, the first data base for tubal function in otologically normal children was established.

There are five methods for the clinical evaluation of eustachian tube function by tympanometry. Each of these methods is based on an indirect determination of middle ear pressure under various conditions. The pressure is, of course, obtained by finding the peak in the tympanogram. It must be remembered, however, that only relative qualitative information can be obtained using these methods. If the subject fails to induce pressure changes in the middle ear, tubal function cannot be evaluated. Therefore, there is no truly satisfactory clinical test that is indicative of tubal function in subjects with intact tympanic membranes.

1. Resting Middle Ear Pressure. When the tympanic membrane is intact, tympanometry is a reliable method to determine the middle ear pressure in the absence of a severely distorted tympanic membrane. Figure 16–27 is a tympanogram of a patient with normal middle ear resting pressure. Figure 16–28 is a tympanogram of a patient with high negative middle ear resting pressure, which is indicative of obstruction of the eustachian tube. (Such obstruction may be functional, mechanical, or both.) However, these determinations represent the middle ear pressure only at one moment. A single measurement of normal resting middle ear pressure does not necessarily indicate normal eustachian tube function, but a measurement of negative middle ear pressure is presumptive evidence of eustachian tube dysfunction. Serial determinations are more indicative of the dynamics of tubal function in a single patient. Therefore, the chief drawback of this procedure is that it gives no indication of the ventilating capacity of the eustachian tube under various conditions of middle ear pressure. It is for this reason that the remaining four tests were developed.

2. Toynbee and Valsalva Tests. The second method for measuring eustachian tube function, which involves the Toynbee and Valsalva tests, developed naturally as an extension of the first. This procedure gives a semiquantitative indication of the

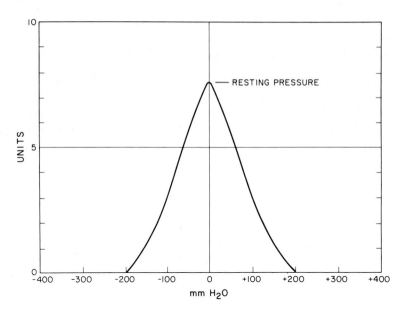

Figure 16–27 Tympanogram in which the resting middle ear pressure is normal.

ability of the eustachian tube to equilibrate established over-pressures and under-pressures in the middle ear (Bluestone, 1975) (Fig. 16–29).

First, a tympanogram is obtained to determine the resting middle ear pressure. Then the subject is asked to perform a Toynbee maneuver, which normally leads to negative pressure in the middle ear. The establishment of this negative middle ear pressure is verified by a second tympanogram. If the second tympanogram fails to record a change in middle ear pressure, the subject is classified as Toynbee negative, indicating possible tubal dysfunction. If the maneuver is successful in inducing negative middle ear pressure, then the subject is asked to swallow in an attempt to equilibrate the negative pressure. A third tympanogram is recorded to determine whether the equilibration was successful and, if so, to what degree. If the equilibration was not complete, the subject is asked to swallow repeatedly. A tympanogram is recorded between each swallow to monitor the progressive equilibration. The pressure remaining in the middle ear after several swallows is termed residual negative pressure. A similar approach is used with the Valsalva (or Politzer air bag) maneuver to test for the tube's ability to equilibrate over-pressure

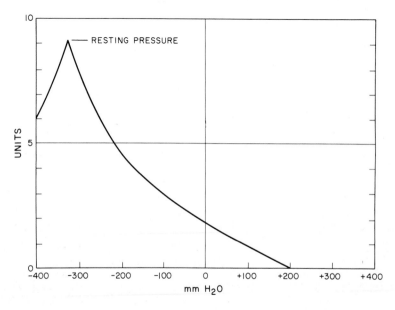

Figure 16–28 Tympanogram of a patient with high negative resting middle ear pressure.

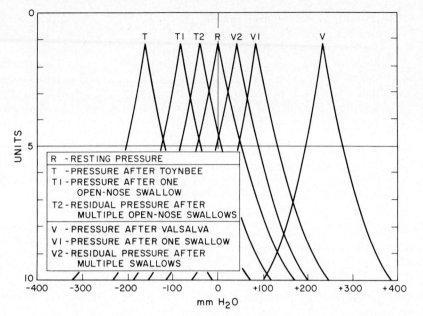

Figure 16–29 Tympanogram of the Toynbee and Valsalva tests of eustachian tube function when the tympanic membrane is intact.

in the middle ear. Figure 16–30 illustrates the results of the Toynbee and Valsalva tests as they appear on a strip chart recorder.

These combined tests are most significant if the subject is able to develop negative pressure within the middle ear during the Toynbee test and then is able to equilibrate the negative pressure to the initial resting pressure. This indicates excellent function of the eustachian tube. However, inability to develop negative middle ear pressure following the Toynbee test or positive intratympanic pressure after the Valsalva test does not differentiate between normal and abnormal tubal function. One obvious problem with these tests is that it is impossible to control the relative amounts of over-pressure and under-

pressure generated in each individual. (In fact, some individuals fail to generate negative pressure during the Toynbee maneuver.) To overcome this difficulty, three other tests were developed.

3. Holmquist Method. The third test, developed principally by Holmquist (1969b, 1972), measures the ability of the eustachian tube to equilibrate induced negative middle ear pressures. The test procedure involves five steps: (1) a tympanogram is recorded to determine the initial middle ear pressure; (2) a negative pressure is created in the nasopharynx by a pressure device connected to the nose, and the subject is asked to swallow in order to establish a negative pressure of about -200 mm H_2O in the middle ear; (3) a second tympanogram is recorded to eval-

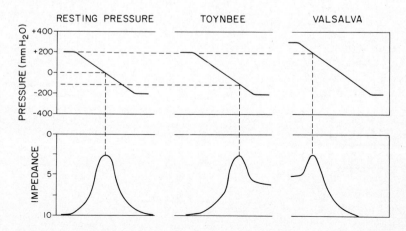

Figure 16–30 Strip chart tympanometric recording of the Toynbee and Valsalva tests of eustachian tube function when the tympanic membrane is intact.

uate the exact negative middle ear pressure achieved; (4) the patient is told to swallow repeatedly (if the tube opens, the pressure is equalized); and (5) a third tympanogram is recorded to register the final middle ear pressure.

Holmquist did not describe a similar procedure for testing equilibrating capacity with induced positive pressures. Siedentop et al. (1978) described the difficulties encountered in using this method to measure tubal function and concluded that many subjects could not be tested by this method even though they had normal tympanic membranes and negative otologic histories.

4. Inflation-Deflation Test. Another method of measuring eustachian tube function, developed by Bluestone (1975), is also called an inflation-deflation test, although

the applied middle ear pressures are very limited in magnitude. Figure 16–31 shows such a study.

If the subject can successfully perform all parts of the test, eustachian tube function is assumed to be excellent; however, failure to alter the middle ear pressure during this testing procedure does not necessarily indicate poor function. Extensive studies of subjects with and without eustachian tube–middle ear disease have not been reported.

5. Patulous Eustachian Tube Test. If a patulous eustachian tube is suspected, the diagnosis can be confirmed by tympanometry when the tympanic membrane is intact. One tympanogram is obtained while the patient is breathing normally, and a second is obtained while the patient holds his or her breath. The fluctuation in

EVALUATION OF EUSTACHIAN TUBE
FUNCTION USING TYMPANOMETRY
(9 STEP PROCEDURE)

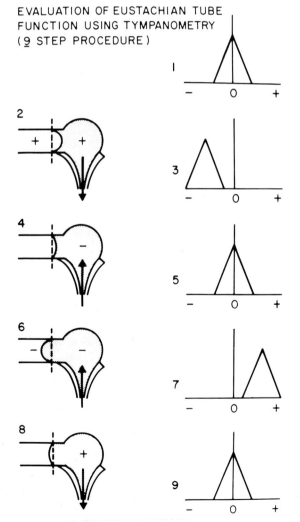

Figure 16–31 The nine step tympanometry procedure may be summarized as follows: (1) Tympanogram records resting middle ear pressure. (2) Ear canal pressure is increased to +200 mm H_2O, causing medial deflection of the tympanic membrane and a corresponding increase in middle ear pressure. The subject swallows to equilibrate positive middle ear pressure; airflow is from the middle ear to the nasopharynx. (3) While the subject refrains from swallowing, ear canal pressure is returned to normal, thus establishing a slight negative middle ear pressure (as the tympanic membrane moves outward). The tympanogram documents established middle ear under-pressure. (4) The subject swallows in an attempt to equilibrate negative middle ear pressure. If equilibration is successful, airflow is from the nasopharynx to the middle ear (see arrow). (5) The tympanogram records the extent of equilibration. (6) Ear canal pressure decreased to −200 mm H_2O, causing a lateral deflection of the tympanic membrane and a corresponding decrease in middle ear pressure. The subject swallows to equilibrate negative middle ear pressure; airflow is from the nasopharynx to the middle ear. (7) The subject refrains from swallowing while external ear canal pressure is returned to normal, thus establishing a slight positive pressure in the middle ear as the tympanic membrane moves medially. The tympanogram records established over-pressure. (8) The subject swallows to reduce over-pressure. If equilibration is successful, airflow is from the middle ear to the nasopharynx. (9) The final tympanogram documents the extent of equilibration.

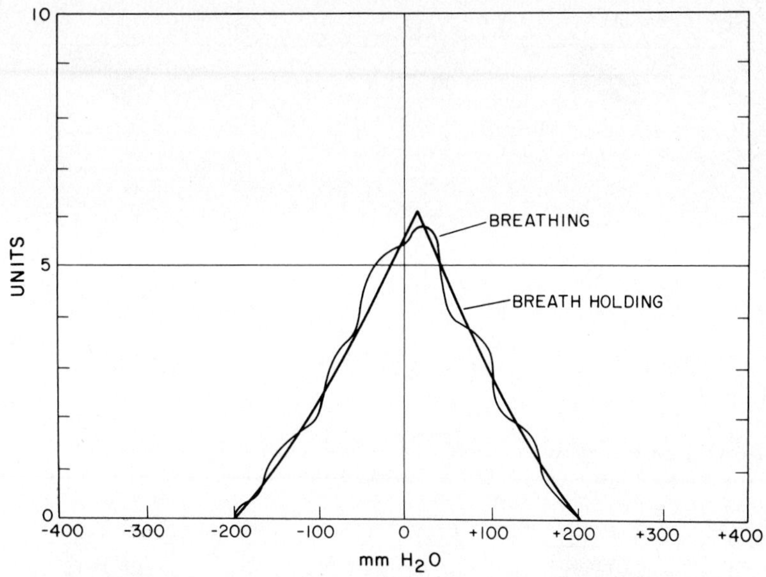

Figure 16–32 Tympanogram of a patient with a patulous eustachian tube. The wavy line was obtained while the subject was breathing; the steady line was recorded when the patient held his breath.

the tympanometric line should coincide with breathing (Fig. 16–32). The fluctuation can be exaggerated by asking the patient to occlude one nostril with the mouth closed during forced inspiration and expiration or by the Toynbee test (Fig. 16–33).

Physiology of the Ventilatory Function

From studies in children, the function of the eustachian tube has been postulated (Bluestone and Beery, 1976). The normal eustachian tube is functionally obstructed or collapsed at rest; there is probably a slight negative pressure in the middle ear (Fig. 16–34). When

the eustachian tube functions ideally, intermittent active opening of the tube maintains near-ambient pressures in the middle ear. It is suspected that when active function is inefficient in opening the eustachian tube, functional collapse of the tube persists. The interval between openings then depends on the establishment of a pressure gradient between the middle ear cavity and the nasopharynx, which passively assists tubal function. Physiologically, this gradient is achieved by the absorption of middle ear gas, which results in the creation of progressive negative middle ear pressure. This type of ventilation appears to be quite common in children, as moderate

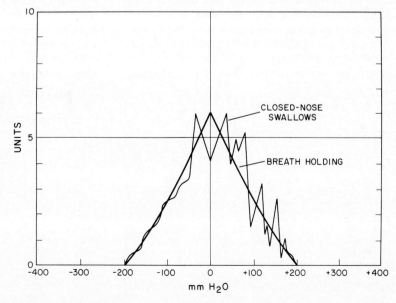

Figure 16–33 Tympanogram of the same patient in Figure 16–32. Wide fluctuations were obtained when the patient swallowed several times with his mouth and nose closed (Toynbee test). The steady line was recorded when the patient held his breath.

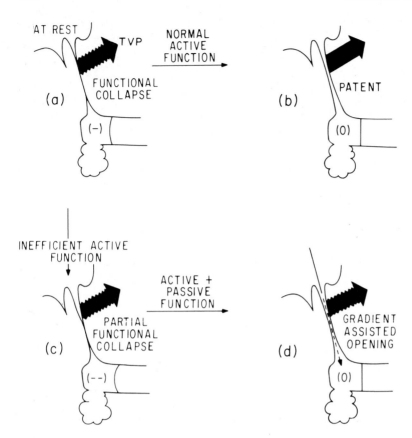

Figure 16–34 Physiologic ventilation of the middle ear during active opening of the eustachian tube by the tensor veli palatini muscle. TVP, tensor veli palatini. *A*, Normal function of the eustachian tube. *B*, Ideal function to maintain near-ambient middle ear pressure. *C*, Partial functional collapse of the tube. *D*, Gradient-assisted opening of tube.

to high negative middle ear pressures have been identified by tympanometry in many children who have no apparent ear disease (Beery et al., 1975).

In an effort to describe normal eustachian tube function by using the microflow technique inside a pressure chamber, Elner et al. (1971d) studied 102 adults with intact tympanic membranes and apparently negative otologic histories. The patients were divided into four groups according to their abilities to equilibrate static relative positive and negative pressures of 100 mm H_2O in the middle ear

(Table 16–8). The patients in group 1 were able to equilibrate pressure differences across the tympanic membrane completely. Those in group 2 equilibrated positive pressure, but a small residual negative pressure remained in the middle ear. The subjects in group 3 were capable of equilibrating only relative positive pressure with a small residual remaining, but not negative pressure, and those in group 4 were incapable of equilibrating any pressure. The Toynbee test was negative and the Valsalva test positive in all patients in groups 3 and 4. These data probably indicate decreased stiff-

Table 16–8 EUSTACHIAN TUBE FUNCTION TEST RESULTS OF 102 OTOLOGICALLY NORMAL ADULTS WITH INTACT TYMPANIC MEMBRANES*

Tubal Function Group	No. of Subjects (%)	Equilibration When Middle Pressure is: (mm H_2O) +100	−100	Toynbee Positive/ No. Tested (%)	Valsalva Positive/ No. Tested (%)
I	74 (72)	Yes	Yes	67/69 (97)	63/73 (86)
II	21 (21)	Yes	Residual	7/18 (39)	16/21 (76)
III	2 (2)	Residual	No	0/2 (0)	2/2 (100)
IV	5 (5)	No	No	0/5 (0)	5/5 (100)
TOTAL				74/94 (79)	86/101 (85)

*Adapted from Elner, A., Ingelstedt, S., and Ivarsson, A. 1971. The normal function of the Eustachian tube: A study of 102 cases. Acta Otolaryngol., 72:320–328.

ness of the eustachian tube in the subjects in groups 2 to 4 when compared with those in group 1. This study also showed that 95 per cent of normal adults could equilibrate an applied positive pressure and that 93 per cent could equilibrate applied negative pressure by active swallowing to some extent. However, 28 per cent of the subjects could not completely equilibrate either applied positive or negative pressure or both.

Bylander (1980) compared the eustachian tube function of 53 children with 55 adults, all of whom had intact tympanic membranes and who were apparently otologically healthy. Employing a pressure chamber, she reported that 53 per cent of the children could not equilibrate applied negative intratympanic pressure (-100 mm H_2O) by swallowing, whereas only 9 per cent of the adults were unable to perform this function. Children between three and six years of age had worse function than the 7- to 12-year-old age group. In addition, she found that children who had tympanometric evidence of negative pressure within the middle ear had poor eustachian tube function.

From these two studies, it can be concluded that even in apparently otologically normal children, eustachian tube function is not as good as in adults, which would contribute to the higher incidence of middle ear disease in children as compared to adults.

In studying the parameters of middle ear pressure, Brooks (1969) determined the resting middle ear pressure by tympanometry in a large group of apparently normal children as being between 0 and -175 mm H_2O. However, pressures outside this range have been reported as normal for large populations of apparently asymptomatic children who were measured for this parameter by screening (Jerger, 1970). High negative middle ear pressure does not necessarily indicate disease; it may indicate only physiologic tubal obstruction. Ventilation occurs, but only after the nasopharynx–middle ear pressure gradient reaches an opening pressure. It has been suggested that these children probably should be considered at risk for middle ear problems until more is learned about the normal and abnormal physiology of the eustachian tube (Bluestone et al., 1973). In normal adults, Alberti and Kristensen (1970) obtained resting middle ear pressures of between 50 and -50 mm H_2O. Again, a pressure outside this range does not necessarily mean that the patient has ear disease.

The rate of gas absorption from the middle ear has been reported to be approximately 1 ml in a 24 hour period by several investigators (Riu et al., 1966; Ingelstedt et al., 1967b; Elner, 1972, 1977). However, since values taken over a short period were extrapolated to arrive at this figure, the true rate of gas absorption over 24 hours has yet to be determined.

The role of the mastoid air cell system in physiology in relation to the middle ear is not fully understood, but the current concept is that it acts as a surge tank of gas (air) available to the relatively smaller middle ear cavity. During intervals of eustachian tube dysfunction, the compliance of the tympanic membrane and ossicular chain (which would affect hearing) would not be decreased owing to reduced middle ear gas pressure, since there is a reservoir of gas in the mastoid air cells. If this concept is correct, then a small mastoid air cell system could be detrimental to the middle ear if abnormal eustachian tube function is present.

Posture appears to have an effect on the function of the eustachian tube. The mean volume of air passing through the eustachian tube was found to be reduced by one third when the body was elevated 20 degrees to the horizontal and by two thirds when in the horizontal position (Ingelstedt et al., 1967a). This reduction in function with change in body position was found to be the result of venous engorgement of the eustachian tube (Jonson and Rundcrantz, 1969).

A seasonal variation in eustachian tube function was reported by Beery et al. (1979). In children who had had tympanostomy tubes inserted for recurrent or chronic otitis media with effusion, serial inflation-deflation studies revealed better eustachian tube function in the summer and fall than in the winter and spring.

Unfortunately, the true physiology of the eustachian tube–middle ear system still remains to be defined.

Eustachian Tube Dysfunction Related to Pathogenesis of Otitis Media and Certain Related Conditions

The major types of abnormal function of the eustachian tube that can cause otitis media appear to be obstruction, abnormal patency, or both (Fig. 16–35). Eustachian tube obstruction can be functional or me-

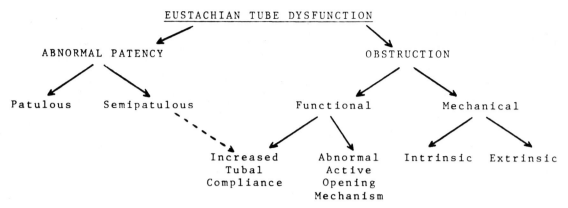

Figure 16–35   Various types of eustachian tube dysfunction.

chanical or both. Functional obstruction results from persistent collapse of the eustachian tube due to increased tubal compliance, an abnormal active opening mechanism, or both. Functional eustachian tube obstruction is common in infants and younger children, since the amount and stiffness of the cartilage support of the eustachian tube are less than in older children and adults. In addition, there appear to be marked age differences in the craniofacial base that render the tensor veli palatini muscle less efficient prior to puberty. Mechanical obstruction of the eustachian tube may be intrinsic or extrinsic. Intrinsic obstruction could be the result of abnormal geometry or intraluminal or mural factors that could compromise the lumen of the eustachian tube; the most common of these is inflammation due to infection or possibly to allergy. Extrinsic obstruction could be the result of increased extramural pressure, such as occurs when the subject is supine or when there is peritubal compression secondary to a tumor or possibly an adenoid mass.

In extreme cases of abnormal patency of the eustachian tube, the tube is open even at rest, i.e., patulous. Lesser degrees of abnormal patency result in a semipatulous eustachian tube that is closed at rest but has low resistance in comparison to the normal tube. Increased patency of the tube may be due to abnormal tube geometry or to a decrease in the extramural pressure, such as occurs as a result of weight loss or possibly as a result of mural or intraluminal factors.

Functional Eustachian Tube Obstruction

Figure 16–36 depicts the chain of events in the pathogenesis of otitis media with effusion

when the eustachian tube is functionally obstructed. This type of obstruction may result in persistent high negative middle ear pressure, and when associated with marked collapse or retraction of the tympanic membrane, it has been termed *atelectasis.* This condition has been demonstrated in an experimental animal model (Cantekin et al., 1977). Following transection of the tensor veli palatini muscle posterior to the hamulus of the pterygoid bone in the rhesus monkey, temporary high negative middle ear pressure and severe retraction of the tympanic membrane were noted to occur and persisted until the muscle healed. If ventilation occurs when there is high negative middle ear pressure, nasopharyngeal secretions can be aspirated into the middle ear and can result in an acute bacterial otitis media with effusion. To test this hypothesis, Cantekin and coworkers (1977) unilaterally transected the tensor muscle in the rhesus monkey. The result was persistent high negative middle ear pressure without effusion, while in the unoperated side, middle ear pressure remained normal. Forty-eight hours after instillation of *Pneumococcus* into the nasopharynx of the monkey, acute otitis media with effusion developed in the ear with the high negative middle ear pressure but not in the unoperated side.

If ventilation does not occur, persistent functional eustachian tube obstruction could result in sterile otitis media with effusion. Cantekin and coworkers (1977) also reproduced this condition in the rhesus monkey by excision of the tensor muscle, which resulted in severe functional eustachian tube obstruction and the development of sterile otitis media with effusion shortly after the procedure. Development of otitis media with effusion at this stage might be dependent upon the degree and duration of the negative pressure as well as middle ear hypoxia or hypercapnia. Since tubal opening is possible in a middle ear with an effusion, aspiration of nasopharyngeal secretions might occur, thus creating the clinical condition in which persistent otitis media with effusion and recurrent acute bacterial otitis media with effusion occur together. All infants with unrepaired palatal clefts and many children with repaired cleft palates have otitis media with effusion as a result of functional obstruction of the eustachian tube (Bluestone, 1971).

Mechanical Eustachian Tube Obstruction

Intrinsic Mechanical Obstruction

Intrinsic mechanical obstruction of the eustachian tube is most commonly the result of inflammation. Obstruction within the bony or protympanic portion of the tube is usually due to acute or chronic inflammation of the mucosal lining, which may also be associated with polyps or a cholesteatoma. Total obstruction may be present at the middle ear end of the tube. However, these conditions are the result of eustachian tube dysfunction and not the initial cause. Stenosis of the

eustachian tube has also been described but is a rare finding.

Figure 16–37 illustrates the sequence of events in which intrinsic inflammation of the cartilaginous portion of the eustachian tube may result in an abnormal middle ear condition. Most ears at risk for developing atelectasis or otitis media with effusion when inflammation is present probably have a significant degree of functional obstruction. An upper respiratory tract infection in children with this condition has been shown to significantly decrease eustachian tube function (Bluestone et al., 1977a). Periods of upper respiratory tract infection may then result in either atelectasis of the tympanic membrane–middle ear, bacterial otitis media with effusion, or a sterile otitis media with effusion due to swelling of the eustachian tube lumen. The mechanisms are similar to those described for functional eustachian tube obstruction. Allergy as a cause of intrinsic mechanical eustachian tube obstruction has not been demonstrated (Bluestone, 1978).

Extrinsic Mechanical Obstruction

Extrinsic mechanical obstruction of the eustachian tube may be the result of extrinsic compression by nasopharyngeal tumors or

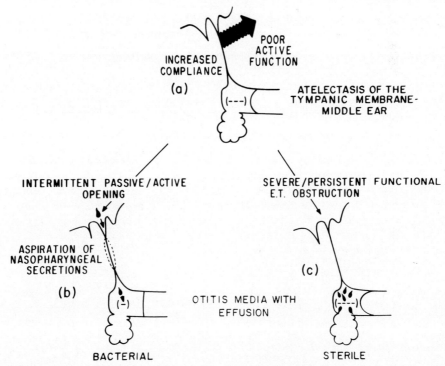

Figure 16–36 Mechanism by which functional obstruction of the eustachian tube can result in atelectasis of the tympanic membrane–middle ear (a) or a bacterial (b) or sterile (c) otitis media with effusion. ET, eustachian tube.

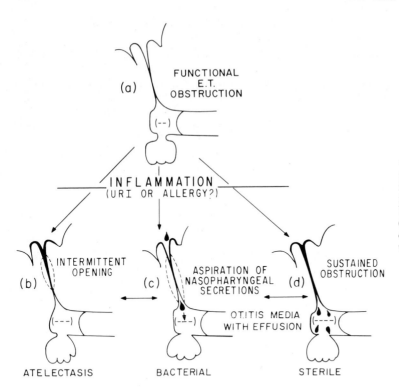

Figure 16–37 Mechanism by which intrinsic mechanical obstruction of the eustachian tube that has functional obstruction (a) can result in atelectasis of the tympanic membrane–middle ear (b) or a bacterial (c) or sterile (d) otitis media with effusion. ET, Eustachian tube; URI, upper respiratory tract infection.

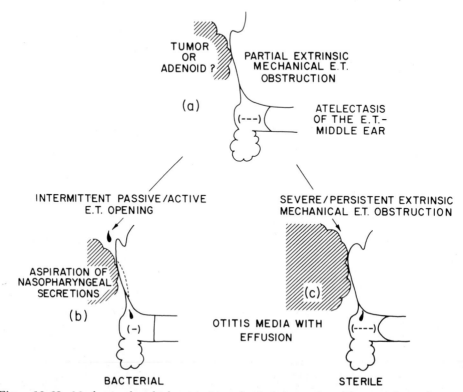

Figure 16–38   Mechanism by which extrinsic mechanical obstruction of the eustachian tube can result in atelectasis of the tympanic membrane–middle ear (a) or bacterial (b) or sterile (c) otitis media with effusion. ET, eustachian tube.

adenoids. In an attempt to improve criteria for the preoperative selection of children for adenoidectomy to prevent otitis media with effusion, Bluestone et al. (1972c) made radiographic studies of the nasopharynx and eustachian tube prior to and following adenoidectomy. The ventilatory function of the eustachian tube has also been studied by the inflation-deflation manometric technique both before and after adenoidectomy in a group of children with recurrent or chronic otitis media with effusion in whom tympanostomy tubes had been inserted (Bluestone et al., 1975a). The results of these studies indicated that following adenoidectomy, eustachian tube function improved in some, remained the same in others, and in a few children worsened. Improvement was related to a reduction of extrinsic mechanical obstruction of the eustachian tube.

Figure 16–38 shows the possible mechanisms by which extrinsic obstruction may result in ear disease. Partial eustachian tube obstruction may result only in atelectasis of the tympanic membrane–middle ear or a bacterial otitis media with effusion, but more severe obstruction could result in a sterile otitis media with effusion. Otitis media with effu-

sion has been produced in animal models when the eustachian tube was mechanically obstructed (Paparella et al., 1970).

Abnormal Patency of the Eustachian Tube

Figure 16–39 depicts the possible sequence of events that can cause an otitis media with effusion when the eustachian tube is abnormally patent. A patulous eustachian tube usually permits air to flow readily from the nasopharynx into the middle ear, which thus remains well ventilated; however, unwanted nasopharyngeal secretions can also traverse the tube and result in reflux otitis media. A semipatulous eustachian tube may be obstructed functionally as the result of increased tubal compliance, and the middle ear may even have negative pressure or an effusion or both. Since the tubal walls are abnormally distensible, nasopharyngeal secretions may readily be insufflated into the middle ear even with modest positive nasopharyngeal pressures, for example, as a result of noseblowing, sneezing, crying, or closed-nose swallowing. If active tubal opening (tensor veli palatini contraction) occurs, resulting in an abnormally patent tube, reflux or insuffla-

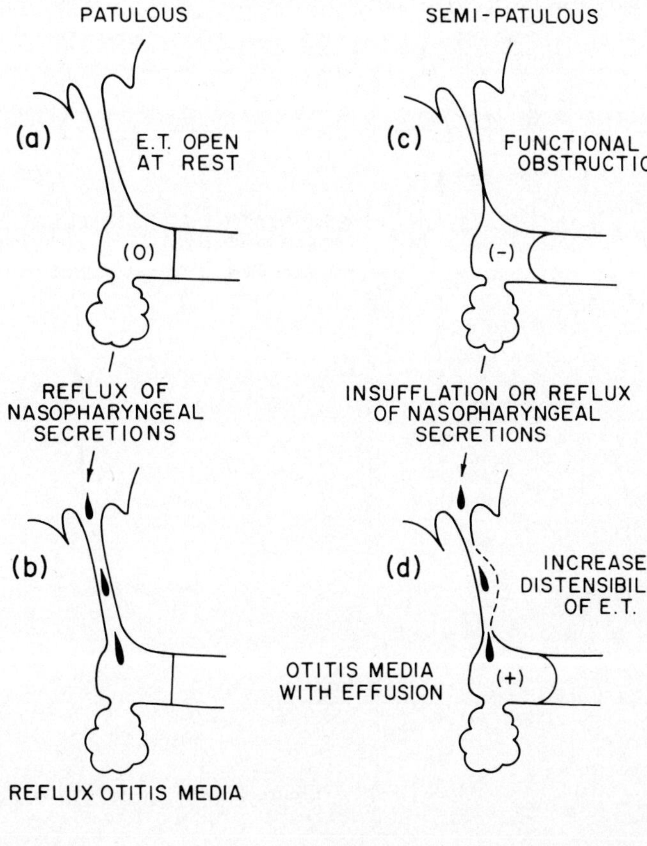

Figure 16–39 Abnormal patency of the eustachian tube. In the patulous condition (a), reflux of nasopharyngeal secretions can result in otitis media (b). If the eustachian tube is semipatulous (c), otitis media may occur following reflux, insufflation, or aspiration of nasopharyngeal secretions (d). ET, eustachian tube.

tion of nasopharyngeal secretions is also likely.

If the eustachian tube has lower resistance than normal but remains functionally obstructed even during attempts at active tubal opening, it is conceivable that nasopharyngeal secretions would enter the middle ear more readily than would air. American Indians have been shown to have tubal resistances that are lower than those of the average Caucasian (Beery et al., 1980). They seem to have an increased incidence of reflux of nasopharyngeal secretion into the middle ear and frequently suffer from recurrent acute otitis media that is often associated with perforation and discharge. However, American Indians have a low incidence of cholesteatoma. This type of eustachian tube function and middle ear disease is different from the types of disease seen in individuals who have a cleft palate.

Nasal Obstruction Related to Eustachian Tube Function

Nasal obstruction may also be involved in the pathogenesis of otitis media with effusion. Swallowing when the nose is obstructed (owing to inflammation or obstructed adenoids) results in an initial positive nasopha-

ryngeal air pressure followed by a negative pressure phase. When the tube is pliant, positive nasopharyngeal pressure might insufflate infected secretions into the middle ear, especially when the middle ear has a high negative pressure (Fig. 16–40); with negative nasopharyngeal pressure, such a tube could be prevented from opening and could be further obstructed functionally (Toynbee phenomenon) (Bluestone et al., 1975a).

Allergy and Eustachian Tube Function

Allergy is thought to be one of the etiologic factors in otitis media with effusion, because otitis media with effusion occurs frequently in allergic individuals (Draper, 1967). The mechanism by which allergy might cause otitis media with effusion remains hypothetical and controversial. Some have assumed that mucosal swelling associated with nasal allergy extends to the eustachian tube and causes intrinsic mechanical obstruction (Paparella and Dickson, 1969). However, even though this seems logical, there are no data available to support this contention. The role of allergy in the etiology and pathogenesis of acute and chronic otitis media with effusion may be one or more of the following mechanisms (Fig. 16–41): (1) the middle ear func-

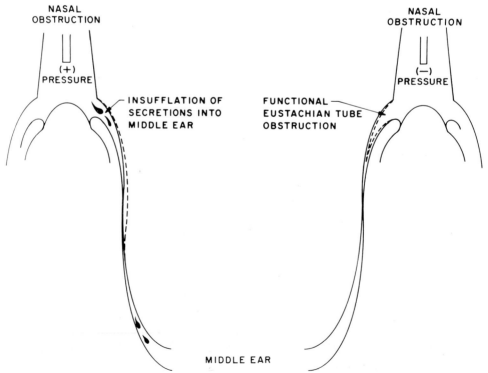

Figure 16–40 Toynbee phenomenon.

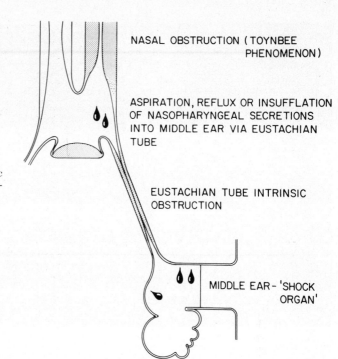

NASAL OBSTRUCTION (TOYNBEE PHENOMENON)

ASPIRATION, REFLUX OR INSUFFLATION OF NASOPHARYNGEAL SECRETIONS INTO MIDDLE EAR VIA EUSTACHIAN TUBE

EUSTACHIAN TUBE INTRINSIC OBSTRUCTION

MIDDLE EAR-'SHOCK ORGAN'

Figure 16–41 Four possible pathogenic mechanisms that could be involved in the relationship between allergy and otitis media.

tioning as a "shock organ," (2) inflammatory swelling of the eustachian tube, (3) inflammatory obstruction of the nose, or (4) aspiration of bacteria-laden allergic nasopharyngeal secretions into the middle ear cavity. The latter three mechanisms would be associated with abnormal function of the eustachian tube. It is obvious that further research is required to establish the relationship of allergy to otitis media with effusion.

Eustachian Tube Function Related to Cleft Palate

Otitis media with effusion is universally present in infants with an unrepaired cleft of the palate (Stool and Randall, 1967; Paradise et al., 1969). Palate repair appears to improve middle ear status, but middle ear disease nonetheless often continues or recurs even after palate repair (Paradise and Bluestone, 1974). Radiographic assessment has shown that infants and children with both unrepaired and repaired cleft palates have abnormal eustachian tube function, which suggests an abnormal opening mechanism in the infants with an unrepaired cleft palate (Fig. 16–42) (Bluestone, 1971; Bluestone et al., 1972a) and either a persistent failure of the eustachian tube to open actively or increased distensibility of the eustachian tube, or both, after repair of the soft palate (Bluestone et al., 1972b).

Inflation-deflation manometric eustachian tube function tests have shown that infants with unrepaired cleft palates have variable degrees of difficulty equilibrating increased middle ear pressure and are unable to equilibrate negative pressure by active function (swallowing) (Bluestone et al., 1975b). Children with repaired cleft palates had either the same type of test results as those with unrepaired palates or had lower opening pressures. Doyle and colleagues (1980a), employing the forced-response test, found that the eustachian tubes of infants and children with cleft palates constricted instead of dilating during swallowing. Animal models in which the palate was surgically split have developed otitis media with effusion (Odoi et al., 1971; Doyle et al., 1980b).

All of these studies indicated that the eustachian tube is functionally obstructed in children with cleft palates, which results in middle ear disease characterized by either persistent or recurrent high negative middle ear pressure, effusion, or both. Cholesteatoma is a frequent sequela in such children; this is not the case in American Indians, in whom the eustachian tube has been shown to be abnormally patent, that is, to have low tubal resistance.

Patients with a submucous cleft of the palate appear to have the same risk of developing middle ear disease as those with an overt cleft. In addition, the presence of a bifid

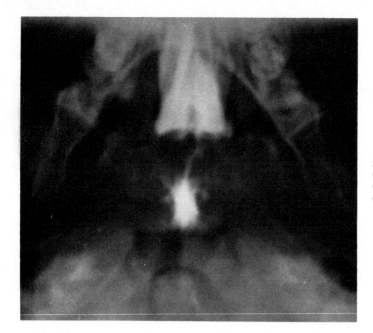

Figure 16–42 Submental vertex roentgenogram of infant with an unrepaired cleft palate showing retrograde flow of contrast material from the nasopharyngeal end of the eustachian tube.

uvula has also been associated with a high incidence of otitis media (Taylor, 1972). Both of these conditions are probably associated with the same pathogenic mechanism for otitis media as is found in patients with overt cleft palates, that is, functional obstruction of the eustachian tube.

Other Causes of Eustachian Tube Dysfunction

There are many other etiologic factors responsible for abnormal function of the eustachian tube. Inflammation of the nose–nasopharynx–eustachian tube–middle ear system has been presented as a major factor in the pathogenesis of otitis media, but there are congenital, traumatic, neoplastic, degenerative, metabolic, and idiopathic conditions that also can result in tubal abnormalities.

Since a cleft of the palate results in functional obstruction of the eustachian tube, any child with a craniofacial malformation that has an associated cleft of the palate will have otitis media or a related condition, one of the more common examples being Pierre-Robin syndrome. However, children with craniofacial anomalies that do not include an overt cleft of the palate also have an increased incidence of middle ear disease. These anomalies include, among others, syndromes such as Down, Crouzon, Apert, and Turner. Even though there have been no reports of formal eustachian tube function studies in

individuals with these and other anomalies, dysfunction of the eustachian tube is the most likely cause of such ear disease. Presumably, a defect related to the abnormal craniofacial complex influences the relation between the eustachian tube and the tensor veli palatini muscle.

Even in the absence of an obvious craniofacial malformation that is associated with otitis media, there is some evidence that children and adults with middle ear disease have a congenital defect that results in a dysfunction of the tube. Such a dysfunction could be abnormal patency or functional obstruction of the tube that is the result of an abnormal relation between the eustachian tube and the tensor veli palatini muscle. Such an assumption is supported by apparent racial differences in the prevalence and incidence of otitis media: Eskimos and American Indians have a higher incidence of otitis media than do whites, while blacks have an incidence of otitis media that is half that in whites. There is also some evidence that otitis media is more prevalent in certain families. In the Boston Collaborative Study (Doyle, 1979), a familial tendency to otitis media has been found.

It has also been observed that patients with dentofacial abnormalities may have otitis media or may develop middle ear disease as a result of these abnormalities. Correction of the defect to relieve the eustachian tube dysfunction would appear to be indicated.

In certain patients with a deviated nasal

septum, impaired eustachian tube function has been reported. This dysfunction is especially apparent during attempts to equilibrate middle ear pressure by the Valsalva maneuver during periods of wide fluctuations in barometric pressure, such as flying in an airplane or diving. In such cases, successful inflation of the middle ear by the Valsalva maneuver has been reported following repair of the deviated nasal septum (McNicoll and Scanlan, 1979).

Trauma to the palate, the pterygoid bone, the tensor veli palatini muscle, or the eustachian tube itself can also result in abnormal eustachian tube function. Injury to the trigeminal nerve, or more specifically, to the mandibular branch of this nerve, can result in either functional obstruction of the eustachian tube or a patulous tube, since the innervation of the tensor veli palatini is from this nerve (Perlman, 1951; Cantekin et al., 1979a). The trauma may be associated with surgical procedures, such as palate or maxillary resection for tumor.

Neoplastic disease, either benign or malignant, that invades the palate and pterygoid bone can interfere with tensor veli palatini muscle function and can result in functional obstruction of the tube. Functional obstruction or abnormal patency of the tube can also occur from involvement of the innervation of the tensor veli palatini muscle. Mechanical obstruction of the eustachian tube can result from direct invasion by neoplasm. Degenerative and metabolic diseases such as myasthenia gravis can alter the eustachian tube by affecting the tubal musculature or by changing the extramural or mural pressures in such a way as would occur with major shifts of extracellular fluids.

Finally, whenever eustachian tube dysfunction is diagnosed and the etiology is obscure, the dysfunction is usually considered to be idiopathic. Most patients with otitis media have been found to have functional obstruction of the eustachian tube with an idiopathic etiology. It should not be forgotten, however, that the cause may be a congenital defect in the anatomy of the base of the skull.

Indications for Testing Eustachian Tube Function

The most direct method available to the clinician today for testing eustachian tube function is the inflation-deflation method. However, a perforation of the tympanic membrane or a tympanostomy tube must be present in order to perform this test. The test uses the simple apparatus described earlier (see Fig. 16–18) with or without the electroacoustic impedance bridge pump manometer system. Since most patients will have either functional obstruction of the eustachian tube or an abnormally patent tube, no other test procedures may be needed. However, if there is a mechanical obstruction, especially if the tube appears to be totally blocked anatomically, then further testing is indicated. In such instances, retrograde-prograde radiographic contrast studies of the eustachian tube should be performed to determine the site and cause of the blockage. Most of the cases in which mechanical obstruction is found have inflammation at the middle ear end of the eustachian tube (protympanic or bony portion), which usually resolves with medical or surgical management. Repeated inflation-deflation studies should show resolution of the mechanical obstruction. However, if no middle ear cause is obvious, roentgenographic studies should be performed to rule out the possibility of a neoplasm in the nasopharynx.

Since resting middle ear pressure may be an indication of how well the eustachian tube is functioning, serial testing of certain patients by tympanometry may be helpful. One of the most important indications for assessing eustachian tube function is the differential diagnosis in a patient who does not have otitis media but has symptoms that might be related to eustachian tube dysfunction (such as fullness, snapping or popping in the ear, fluctuating hearing loss, tinnitus, or vertigo). When the tympanic membrane is intact, a tympanogram that reveals high negative pressure is presumptive evidence of abnormal tubal obstruction, whereas normal resting middle ear pressure is not a diagnostic aid. However, when the resting intratympanic pressure is within normal limits and the patient can develop negative middle ear pressure following the Toynbee test (see Fig. 16–29) or during the deflation test (see Fig. 16–31), the eustachian tube is probably functioning normally. Unfortunately, failure to develop negative middle ear pressure during either or both of these tests does not indicate poor eustachian tube function.

Screening for the presence of high negative pressure in certain high-risk populations (children with known sensorineural hearing losses, developmentally delayed and mentally impaired children, children with cleft palates or other craniofacial anomalies, American Indian and Eskimo children, and children with Down syndrome) appears to be helpful in identifying those individuals who may need to be monitored closely for the occurrence of otitis media (Harford et al., 1978).

Tympanometry appears to be a reliable method for detecting the presence of high negative pressure as well as otitis media with effusion in children (Brooks, 1968, 1971; Beery et al., 1975). The identification of high negative pressure without effusion in children is indicative of some degree of eustachian tube obstruction. These children, as well as those with middle ear effusions, should have follow-up serial tympanograms.

Patients with recurrent acute or chronic otitis media with effusion should have eustachian tube function studies as part of their otolaryngologic and audiologic work-up. The management of such patients may depend on the results of these studies, as mechanical obstruction of the eustachian tube may indicate treatment different from that for functional obstruction. For instance, adenoidectomy may not be indicated in a child with a small adenoid mass and tubal function test results that indicate functional obstruction; however, the operation may benefit the child with marked mechanical obstruction of the eustachian tube (Bluestone et al., 1975a).

Patients in whom tympanostomy tubes have been inserted may benefit from serial eustachian tube function studies. Improvement in function as indicated by inflation-deflation tests might aid the clinician in determining the proper time to remove the tubes. Cleft palate repair (Bluestone et al., 1972b), adenoidectomy (Bluestone et al., 1975a), elimination of nasal and nasopharyngeal inflammation (Bluestone et al., 1977a), or growth and development of a child (Holborow, 1970) may be associated with improvement in eustachian tube function.

Studies of the eustachian tube function of the patient with a chronic perforation of the tympanic membrane may be helpful in determining preoperatively the potential results of tympanoplasty surgery. Holmquist (1970) studied eustachian tube function in adults before and after tympanoplasty and reported that the operation had a high rate of success in patients with good eustachian tube function (those who could equilibrate applied negative pressure) but that in patients without good tubal function, surgery frequently failed to close the perforation.

Bluestone et al. (1979a) assessed children prior to tympanoplasty and found that in addition to inflation-deflation studies in the ear with a perforation, tympanometric assessment of a contralateral ear with an intact tympanic membrane may be helpful in predicting the success of surgery. If the ear with the perforated tympanic membrane gave perfect results on eustachian tube inflation-deflation studies and if the contralateral ear with an intact tympanic membrane gave normal middle ear pressure results on several occasions, tympanoplasty was frequently successful (see Chap. 17).

Even though the testing of eustachian tube function is not an exact science, the methods presently available provide useful information related to the diagnosis and management of otitis media in children.

MICROBIOLOGY OF OTITIS MEDIA

The microbiology of otitis media has been documented by appropriate cultures of middle ear effusions obtained by needle aspiration. Many studies of the bacteriology of acute otitis media have been performed, and the results are remarkably consistent in demonstrating the importance of *Streptococcus pneumoniae* and *Haemophilus influenzae*. Recent studies of asymptomatic children with middle ear effusion indicate that bacterial pathogens are also present in these fluids, suggesting that bacteria may be a factor in the development and persistence of the effusion. Epidemiologic evidence associates viral infection with otitis media, but these organisms are isolated infrequently from middle ear effusions, and their role in the pathogenesis of otitis media is uncertain. Preliminary results of studies using recently developed techniques suggest that anaerobic bacteria and chlamydia may be responsible for some episodes of otitis media. New methods are now available for classifying, differentiating, and identifying microbial agents. These methods have resulted in the creation of new species and nomenclature changes in existing species. Recent changes in terminology of microorganisms of importance in infections of the middle ear are listed in Table 16–9. The purpose of this section is to review the results

Table 16–9 RECENT CHANGES IN TERMINOLOGY OF MICROORGANISMS OF IMPORTANCE IN INFECTIONS OF THE MIDDLE EAR

Old Designation	New Designation
Diplococcus pneumoniae	Streptococcus pneumoniae
Staphylococcus albus	Micrococcus sp.
	Staphylococcus epidermidis
Neisseria catarrhalis	Branhamella catarrhalis
Anaerobic streptococcus	Peptococcus
	Peptostreptococcus
Propionibacterium acnes	Corynebacterium acnes
Eaton agent, PPLO	Mycoplasma pneumoniae
Bedsoniae, TRIC agent	Chlamydiae

of these microbiologic studies and to consider various aspects of the infectious process in the middle ear.

Bacteriology

The results of studies of the bacteriology of otitis media in children from Sweden, Finland, and the United States during the period from 1952 to 1981 are very similar among countries and over time (Table 16–10) *S pneumoniae* and *H influenzae* are the most frequent agents in all age groups Group A

Table 16–10 BACTERIAL PATHOGENS ISOLATED FROM MIDDLE EAR FLUID IN 4675 CHILDREN WITH ACUTE OTITIS MEDIA*

	Percentage of Children with Pathogen	
Microorganism	Mean	Range
Streptococcus pneumoniae	33	26–53
Haemophilus influenzae	21	14–31
Streptococcus, group A	8	0.3–24
Staphylococcus aureus	2	0–3
Branhamella catarrhalis	3	0–8
Gram-negative enteric bacilli	1	0–4
Miscellaneous bacteria	1	0–2
None or nonpathogens	31	2–47

*Twelve reports from centers in United States, Finland, and Sweden, 1952–1981.
Bjuggren and Tunevall, 1952
Lahikainen, 1953
Mortimer and Watterson, 1956
Gronroos et al., 1964
Coffey, 1966
Feingold et al., 1966
Halstead et al., 1968
Nilson et al., 1969
Howie, Ploussard, and Lester, 1970
Kamme, Ageberg, and Lundgren, 1970
Howard et al., 1976
Schwartz, 1981

beta-hemolytic *Streptococci, Staphylococcus aureus,* and gram-negative enteric bacilli are infrequent causes of otitis. No growth, or isolation only of an organism considered to be a contaminant such as *Staphylococcus epidermidis* or diphtheroids, occurs in approximately one third of effusions that are cultured for bacteria.

Streptococcus Pneumoniae

Because *S. pneumoniae* is the most important cause of otitis media, investigators have carefully studied the types responsible for infections of the middle ear. The results of studies of 1837 episodes of acute otitis media indicate that relatively few types are responsible for most disease. The most common types in order of decreasing frequency are 19, 23, 6, 14, 3, and 18 (Kamme et al., 1970; Austrian et al., 1977; Gray et al., 1979) (Table 16–11). All are included in the currently available 14-valent pneumococcal vaccines (Pneumovax, Merck, Sharpe and Dohme; Pnu-Imune, Lederle Laboratories). Reports of multiresistant strains of *S. pneumoniae* from South Africa and the United States suggest the possibility of a major change in the pattern of antimicrobial susceptibility of this organism (see Antimicrobial Agents, p 442)

Table 16–11 DISTRIBUTION OF SEROTYPES OF 1837 STRAINS OF *STREPTOCOCCUS PNEUMONIAE* ISOLATED FROM MIDDLE EAR EFFUSIONS OF CHILDREN WITH ACUTE OTITIS MEDIA*

Serotype	Percentage of Strains
1	2.1
3	8.5
4	3.4
6	12.0
7	2.3
8	1.5
9	2.9
14	10.3
18	5.8
19	23.0
23	12.5
Others	15.7

*Compiled from Kamme, Ageberg, and Lundgren, 1970; Austrian, Howie, and Ploussard, 1977; Gray, Converse, and Dillon, 1979.

Table 16–12 OTITIS MEDIA DUE TO
HAEMOPHILUS INFLUENZAE TYPES
ISOLATED FROM 605
MIDDLE EAR FLUIDS

Type	Percentage
a	0.3
b	9.8
c	0.0
d	0.0
e	1.3
f	0.4
Nontypable	88.1

Haemophilus Influenzae

Otitis media due to *H. influenzae* is associated with nontypable strains in the vast majority of patients (Table 16–12). In approximately 10 per cent, the otitis is due to type b; some of these children appear to be very toxic, and about one quarter of these children have concomitant bacteremia or meningitis (Harding et al., 1973). Until recently, *H. influenzae* appeared to be limited in importance to preschool children; however, new information indicates that this organism is a significant cause of otitis media in older children, adolescents, and adults. Schwartz and colleagues (1977) reported that *H. influenzae* was isolated from middle ear fluids of 36 per cent of children aged five to nine years with acute otitis media. In a subsequent survey, these investigators (Schwartz and Rodriguez, 1981) identified *H. influenzae* as the cause of otitis media in 33 per cent of 18 children aged 8 through 17 years. Herberts et al. (1971) isolated *H. influenzae* from 15 of 45 patients over 16 years of age. Thus, initial antimicrobial therapy of acute otitis media must be effective against *S. pneumoniae* and *H. influenzae* in all age groups. Approximately 15 to 30 per cent of nontypable strains of *H. influenzae* isolated from middle ear effusions of children with acute otitis media produce beta-lactamase that hydrolyzes ampicillin, amoxicillin, and penicillins G and V (see Antimicrobial Agents, p 443)

Groups A and B Streptococci

Group A *Streptococcus* has been a significant pathogen in some studies from Scandinavia, but this has not been the case in most studies from the United States. During the preantibiotic era, middle ear suppuration, often of a very destructive form, was frequently associated with scarlet fever (Clarke, 1962). But the form of streptococcal infection now seems to be less frequent and much less virulent. *Streptococcus hemolyticus* (presumably group A *Streptococcus*) was the most prevalent organism in cultures taken at myringotomy for acute otitis media and was the most frequent cause of mastoid infection coming to mastoidectomy at the Manhattan Eye, Ear, and Throat Hospital during 1934 (Page, 1935).

Group B *Streptococcus* is now, with *Escherichia coli*, the leading cause of sepsis and meningitis in the newborn infant as reported by surveys in the United States and Western Europe (Klein, 1976). Group B *Streptococcus* has been isolated from various body fluids, including middle ear fluid in neonates with otitis media. Bacteremia is frequently associated with otitis media in these infants.

Gram-Negative Enteric Bacilli

Gram-negative enteric bacilli are responsible for about 20 per cent of otitis media in young infants, but these organisms are rarely present in the middle ear effusions of older children with acute otitis media.

A report from Israel describes 33 patients with acute otitis media caused by gram-negative bacilli during the period from 1971 to 1978 (Ostfeld and Rubinstein, 1980). *Pseudomonas aeruginosa* was isolated from middle ear fluids of 23 patients, and indole-positive Proteus sp, were isolated from the fluids in six patients. Seven of the patients were 3 months of age or younger, 16 were 4 to 24 months of age, and 10 were 2 to 80 years of age. Four adult patients had diabetes mellitus, but there were no other patients in the study with significant underlying diseases. The patients had a high rate of complications, including five with acute mastoiditis, three with accompanying bacteremia due to the pathogen isolated from the middle ear, and four adult patients with extensive osteomyelitis of the base of the skull Some patients had prolonged courses that might be better described as chronic otitis media Culture material was obtained from purulent drainage from the middle ear in cases with perforated tympanic membrane, and the bacteriologic results may represent contaminants from the external ear Nevertheless, this series indicates the potential danger of middle ear infection due to gram-negative enteric bacilli

Anaerobic Bacteria

Recent improvements in techniques for isolation and identification of anaerobic bacteria have provided a better understanding of the anaerobic flora of humans and the roles of these organisms in disease. The studies of Brook et al. (1978) suggest that anaerobic bacteria may cause otitis media. Anaerobic bacteria were isolated from the middle ear effusions of 28 per cent of 62 children with acute otitis media. *Peptococcus*, an organism that colonizes the upper respiratory tract and may cause lower respiratory tract disease, and *Propionibacterium acnes*, a part of normal skin flora, were the anaerobic organisms most frequently isolated. These investigators did not cleanse the external canal prior to aspiration, and it is possible that the organisms isolated represent contaminants from the external canal rather than pathogens in the middle ear fluid. A recent study by Brook and Schwartz (1981) indicates a more limited role for anaerobic bacteria in acute otitis media. Twenty-eight infants with acute infection were studied; aerobic bacteria were isolated from the middle ear fluids of 20 children, and cultures from two children yielded mixtures of aerobic and anaerobic bacteria. This study suggests that these organisms are relatively uncommon in infected middle ear effusions.

Branhamella Catarrhalis, Staphylococcus Epidermidis, and Diphtheroids

The roles of *Branhamella* (formerly *Neisseria*) *catarrhalis* (Coffey et al., 1967), coagulase-negative staphylococci (*S. epidermidis*) (Feigin et al., 1973b), and diphtheroids in acute otitis media are uncertain. These organisms are considered commensals and are part of the skin flora of the external ear canal, but some investigators have reported isolation of pure cultures of *B. catarrhalis* or coagulase-negative staphylococci from cases of purulent middle ear effusions after adequate cleansing of the external canal. Organisms were seen in gram-strained materials both free and engulfed by polymorphonuclear leukocytes. The findings suggest that, in some cases, these bacteria may be responsible for suppurative otitis media.

Lewis and colleagues (1979) demonstrated specific antibody to diphtheroids in middle ear effusions and serum of children undergoing myringotomy for chronic otitis media with effusion. Specific IgG antibodies were present in both fluids, whereas IgA antibodies were present in the middle ear effusion but not in the serum of two children. Bernstein et al. (1980) found antibody-coated *S. epidermidis* and diphtheroids in the middle ear of children with chronic otitis media with effusion. The fluids contained specific antibody, and in several cases of *S. epidermidis*, antibody was present in the middle ear fluid but absent from serum. These data indicate that diphtheroids elicit an immune response in the middle ear and cannot be considered as contaminants in all cases. The role of these organisms in middle ear disease, however, remains uncertain. It is possible that they are opportunistic pathogens that invade the middle ear only under certain circumstances such as persistent effusion.

Serologic evidence has recently been provided for a pathogenic role of *B. catarrhalis* in children with acute otitis media. The presence of IgG and IgA antibodies to *B. catarrhalis* in serum and/or middle ear fluid was correlated with isolation of the organism from the middle ear. An increase in titer of antibodies to the organisms between acute and convalescent serum was found in 10 of 19 children with acute otitis media whose middle ear fluid yielded *B. catarrhalis* alone and from none of 14 children with acute otitis media, whose middle ear fluids yielded other pathogens.

Mixed Cultures

Mixed bacterial cultures of middle ear fluid obtained by needle aspiration from children with unilateral or bilateral otitis media have been reported by several investigators. Disparate results occur when the cultures of the two ears in bilateral disease yield different information: Effusion from one ear is sterile, but a bacterial pathogen is isolated from the other ear, or a different bacterial pathogen is isolated from each of the two ears. In some cases, mixed cultures are present: Two types or two species of bacteria are found in the same middle ear fluid. Gronroos et al. (1964) reported 31.6 per cent disparate results of cultures from children with bilateral otitis media. All children had either *S. pneumoniae*, *H. influenzae*, or group A *Streptococcus* recovered from one middle ear fluid sample and sterile fluid in the other. Van Dishoeck et al.

(1959) found that 19 per cent of cultures from children with bilateral otitis media yielded different results. The majority of children had a pathogen recovered from one ear and sterile fluid in the other. Also included were six cases in which cultures of one middle ear fluid sample yielded a single pathogen and the opposite middle ear fluid sample yielded two pathogens. Austrian et al. (1977) recovered different serotypes of *S. pneumoniae* in 18 children, 1.5 per cent of the cases of bilateral pneumococcal otitis media. Pelton et al. (1980) cultured middle ear fluid from both ears of 122 children with bilateral acute otitis media. Disparate results were found in 31 (25 per cent) of the children: In 25 children, a pathogen was present in one ear and the fluid from the other ear was sterile or yielded a nonpathogen; in six children, different pathogens (*H. influenzae* and *S. pneumoniae* in each case) were isolated from the two fluids. Howard and colleagues (1976) noted *S. pneumoniae* and *H. influenzae* together in 20 effusions (5 per cent of those studied). These data indicate that investigative studies of the microbiology of bilateral otitis media must include aspiration of both ears to determine the efficacy of methods of treatment (such as trials of antimicrobial agents) or prevention (such as evaluation of vaccines or drugs).

Sterile Cultures

In all studies of acute otitis media, a significant proportion (approximately one third) of middle ear fluids are sterile after appropriate cultures for bacteria. The etiology of these cases may be one or more of the following: (1) presence of a nonbacterial organism such as a virus, chlamydia, or mycoplasma; (2) presence of fastidious bacterial organisms, such as anaerobic bacteria, that are not isolated by usual laboratory techniques; (3) prior administration of an antimicrobial agent that would suppress growth of a bacterial pathogen; (4) presence of antimicrobial enzymes, such as lysozyme, alone or in combination with immunoglobulins in middle ear fluid that would suppress growth of a bacterial pathogen; and (5) an acute illness in a child who has persistent middle ear effusion from an episode of otitis media sometime in the past. Since children may have middle ear fluids for weeks to months after the onset of acute otitis media (Teele et al., 1980b), an illness due to a separate infectious episode during the time spent with middle ear effusion persisting

from a prior episode of otitis might be assumed by the physician to be a recurrence of otitis media.

Use of the Gram stain is of value in identification of fastidious bacterial organisms and may provide evidence of bacterial infection, although antibiotics or antimicrobial substances inhibit growth of the organism. Techniques for identification of bacterial and viral antigens are also likely to decrease the number of episodes of otitis that are now categorized as "no growth."

Techniques for Identification of Bacterial Antigens

Results of studies using techniques for identification of bacterial antigens provide new insights into the infectious process. Countercurrent immunoelectrophoresis (CIE), latex agglutination, and enzyme linked immunosorbent assay (ELISA) have been used to detect bacterial antigens such as capsular polysaccharides of *S. pneumoniae*, *H. influenzae* type b, *Neisseria meningitidis*, and group B *Streptococci* in blood, urine, cerebrospinal fluid, and other body fluids. These methods are advantageous because of ease of performance, rapidity, specificity, sensitivity (as little as 0.2 ng of polysaccharide capsular antigens can be detected), and ability to identify bacteria whose growth in culture media would be inhibited because of prior administration of antimicrobial agents. Studies of middle ear fluids (Ostfeld and Altmann, 1980; Luotonen et al., 1981) indicate that *S. pneumoniae* is identified by countercurrent immunoelectrophoresis in the vast majority of fluids in which the organism is cultured and in many specimens that have no bacterial growth. Luotonen and colleagues identified pneumococcal capsular polysaccharide in 83 per cent of middle ear fluids from which *S. pneumoniae* was cultured and in about one third of middle ear fluids from which no bacteria were grown. These methods to detect bacterial antigens (and similar methods for viral antigens) add information about the large number of patients who have negative cultures by previously available microbiologic techniques. Thus, the "no growth" category should become smaller than is evident in current studies (Table 16–10).

Viruses

Epidemiologic data suggest that viral infection is frequently associated with acute otitis

Table 16–13   ISOLATION OF VIRUSES IN 663 PATIENTS WITH OTITIS MEDIA*

Virus	No. of Patients
Respiratory syncytial virus	22
Influenzae viruses	4
Coxsackievirus B4	1
Adenovirus 3	1
Parainfluenzae 2	1
Totals	29 (4.4%)
No Growth	634

*622 patients had acute and 41 had chronic otitis media.

From Klein, J. O., and Teele, D. W. 1976. Isolation of viruses and mycoplasmas from middle ear effusions: A review. Ann. Otol. Rhinol. Laryngol., 85(Suppl. 25): 140–144.

media. In a longitudinal study of respiratory illnesses and complications in children 6 weeks to 11 years of age attending a day care and school program, Henderson and colleagues (1977) demonstrated a correlation between isolation of viruses from the upper respiratory tract and clinical diagnosis of otitis media. Virus outbreaks coincided with epidemics of otitis media Adenoviruses, respiratory syncytial viruses, and enteroviruses accounted for the majority of isolates from the upper respiratory tract.

In contrast to this epidemiologic association are the results of studies of fluids obtained for viral cultures from the middle ear effusions of children with acute and chronic otitis media (Klein and Teele, 1976). Viruses were infrequently isolated from the middle ear effusions of children with acute infection of the middle ear; a virus was isolated from only 4.4 per cent of 663 patients (Table 16–13). Respiratory syncytial virus and influenza virus were isolated most frequently. The isolation of these two agents was usually made during periods of epidemic infection in the community.

Otitis media may accompany the exanthematous viral infections, such as measles Invasion of the middle ear by smallpox virus has been demonstrated Guarnieri bodies were present in the tympanic membrane of a three month old Indian child who died of smallpox (Bordley and Kapur, 1972)

The small number of viruses isolated from middle ear fluids does not support the belief that these agents play a significant role in acute otitis media. However, it is possible that viruses were present early in the course of the disease and were no longer present when the patients sought medical attention; or that viruses were present in low concentrations and were not readily isolated from the ear fluids; or that inhibitory materials such as antibody, interferon, or lysozymes prevented successful isolation; or that viruses produced inflammatory changes in the upper respiratory tract but were not present in the effusion fluid.

A recent study by Klein and colleagues (in press) suggests that recently developed techniques for identification of viral antigens may yield more specific information about the role of viruses in middle ear infections. Enzyme immunoassay techniques (ELISA) were used to identify viral antigens. Evidence of viral infection was found in middle ear fluids obtained from approximately one quarter of children with acute otitis media. Respiratory syncytial virus (RSV) was the most frequently identified virus; influenza virus and rotavirus were also identified but were uncommon. The enzyme immunoassay techniques measure viral antigens rather than replicating virions and may detect viral materials that grow poorly or not at all in tissue culture or animal systems. Thus, previous failure to identify viruses in middle ear fluids may have been a result of lack of sensitivity of available techniques.

Mycoplasma

The isolation and identification of mycoplasma from secretions obtained from the upper respiratory tract is now readily accomplished in solid and liquid media. An initial report of a volunteer study suggested a role for these organisms in otitis media. Myringitis, associated with hemorrhage and bleb formation in the more severe cases, was observed in nonimmune volunteers inoculated with *Mycoplasma pneumoniae* (Rifkind et al., 1962). However, the middle ear fluid of a large number of patients (771) has been studied, and *M. pneumoniae* was isolated in only one case (Sobeslavsky et al., 1965). Thus, mycoplasmas do not appear to play a significant role in acute otitis media. Some patients with lower respiratory tract disease due to *M. pneumoniae* may have concomitant otitis media.

Chlamydia

Chlamydia trachomatis is the etiologic agent of a mild but prolonged pneumonitis in infants. Dawson et al. (1967) reported isolation of this organism from the middle ear fluid of a patient with inclusion cell conjunctivitis. This group also reported finding otitis media in 11 of 77 adults infected during an experiment by the ocular route (1967).

Many infants with pneumonia due to *C. trachomatis* have otitis media (Schachter et al., 1979; Tipple et al., 1979). Tipple et al. (1979) isolated the organism from ear aspirates of 3 of 11 infants with chlamydial pneumonia who had myringotomy. However, *C. trachomatis* was not isolated from middle ear fluids obtained at the time of placement of tympanostomy tubes in 68 children nine months to eight years of age. Thus, *C. trachomatis* is associated with acute respiratory infections in young infants (under age six months) and is a cause of acute infection of the middle ear in this age group.

Uncommon Microorganisms

Diphtheritic Otitis

Diphtheritic otitis may accompany diphtheritic croup and nasopharyngitis. Although many cases cannot be differentiated from other forms of purulent otitis, diphtheritic membranes may form and be recognized in the middle ear. Complications are frequent, including destruction of the tympanic membrane and the ossicles and invasive infection of contiguous structures leading to necrosis of the mastoid process, the temporal bone, and the labyrinth (Drury, 1925; Downes, 1959). Thirteen cases of otitis media due to *Corynebacterium diphtheriae* were among 3916 cases reported to the Center for Disease Control of the U.S. Public Health Service for the years 1959 to 1970. Five cases of diphtheritic otitis occurred among 1433 cases of diphtheria seen at the Los Angeles County Hospital during the 10 year period beginning June, 1941 (Naiditch and Bower, 1954).

Tuberculous Otitis

At the turn of the century, tuberculous otitis was occasionally a cause of severe middle ear disease, particularly in the very young. Turner and Fraser (1915) reported a series of cases at the Royal Infirmary in Edinburgh for the period from 1907 to 1914; 51, or 2.8 per cent of cases of otitis, were due to tuberculosis, and 84 per cent of these cases occurred

in the first year of life. Today, the disease is seen in underdeveloped areas of the world, but occasionally cases occur in the United States. Bovine tuberculosis was responsible for 29 cases of chronic otorrhea in children seen in Kampala between 1969 and 1972 (Raikundalia, 1975). Eleven cases of tuberculous otitis were reported in Capetown children between 1967 and 1971 (Sellers and Seid, 1973). Three cases of tuberculous otitis were seen at the Children's Memorial Hospital in Oklahoma City in the same period as the Capetown cases (MacAdam and Rubio, 1977).

When otitis occurs as the only apparent focus of tuberculous infection, the disease is usually due to ingestion of infected cow's milk. The infection may also occur in patients with active pulmonary disease; the middle ear is infected from the upper respiratory tract.

Tuberculous otitis is characterized by a painless, watery otorrhea, enlarged periauricular lymph nodes, and a high incidence of facial paralysis and early hearing loss. Prior to perforation, the tympanic membrane appears thickened and granular. Chemotherapy shortens the course and severity of the disease, but persistent hearing loss is frequent.

Otogenous Tetanus

Otogenous tetanus usually occurs as a sequela of chronic otitis media with perforation. *Clostridium tetani* multiplies in the purulent drainage in the external ear canal and may gain access to the middle ear (Deinard et al., 1980). The organism may be present also in the oropharynx, and it is possible that the infection in the middle ear occurs via the eustachian tube. Fischer et al. (1977) reported the cases of eight children admitted to Children's Hospital in Bangkok with trismus and other signs of tetanus, otitis media, and otorrhea. *C. tetani* was isolated from swabs of the middle ear fluid.

Otitis Due to Ascaris Lumbricoides

The only parasitic infection associated with otitis media is *Ascaris lumbricoides*. Roundworms may be vomited through the mouth or nostrils, enter the eustachian tube, and produce an inflammatory reaction in the middle ear. The worm perforates the tympanic membrane and emerges through the external canal. A recent report describes infection in a 1½ year old child who was brought to a

Bombay clinic with a worm emerging from the ear. Under direct visualization, a 7.5 cm long roundworm, *A. lumbricoides*, was removed from the canal and middle ear (Shah and Desai, 1969).

Bacteriology of Chronic Otitis Media with Effusion

The results of recent studies of the bacteriology of chronic otitis media with effusion suggest new and perplexing questions about the infectious process in the middle ear.

These studies were performed by investigators in Columbus, Ohio (Liu et al., 1975), Boston (Healy and Teele, 1977), Pittsburgh (Riding et al., 1978a; Stanievich et al., 1981), and Minneapolis (Giebink et al., 1979). The protocols were similar: Children with chronic otitis media were investigated; most children were observed to have persistent effusion for at least two months. At the time of myringotomy or placement of tympanostomy tubes, fluid was obtained from the middle ear for culture of bacteria. In each study, 30 to 50 per cent of the children had bacteria in the middle ear fluid. *S. pneumoniae*, *H. influenzae*, or group A *Streptococcus* were isolated from 10 to 22 per cent of the fluids of these asymptomatic children. Anaerobic bacteria were isolated from the middle ear fluids of most patients with chronic otitis media by Brook (1979), but the findings are of uncertain validity because of the failure to adequately cleanse the external canal prior to tympanocentesis. When the canal was adequately cleansed by other investigators (Giebink et al., 1979; Teele et al., 1980a), anaerobic organisms were rarely isolated; *Propionibacterium* was identified in one specimen of 68 fluid samples cultured appropriately for anaerobic bacteria. There were only minimal differences in the rates of isolation of bacteria from serous, mucoid, or purulent fluids. Bacteria were isolated also from washings of the middle ear that had no fluid at myringotomy (Riding et al., 1978a). A higher incidence of respiratory pathogens was noted in children three years of age or younger in the Boston study. Herpesvirus hominis was isolated from one fluid sample (Giebink et al., 1979).

Thus, middle ear fluid of asymptomatic children may harbor respiratory pathogens. The significance of this finding is at present uncertain. The bacteria may be present without provoking an inflammatory response, or they may produce a low-grade or subclinical infection, or the effusion may represent an immune response to the prolonged presence of the bacteria. Specific antibody to the bacteria isolated is present in the middle ear fluid of children undergoing myringotomy for persistent effusion (Lewis et., 1979; Bernstein et al., 1980). These data suggest that the organisms are not passive but elicit an immunologic response and may be involved in the disease process.

Table 16–14 BACTERIAL PATHOGENS ISOLATED FROM 169 INFANTS WITH OTITIS MEDIA DURING THE FIRST SIX WEEKS OF LIFE*

Microorganism	Percentage of Infants with Pathogen
Respiratory bacteria	
Streptococcus pneumoniae	18.3
Haemophilus influenzae	12.4
S. pneumoniae + *H. influenzae*	3.0
Staphylococcus aureus	7.7
Streptococcus, groups A and B	3.0
Branhamella catarrhalis	5.3
Enteric bacteria	
Escherichia coli	5.9
Klebsiella-Enterobacter species	5.3
Pseudomonas aeruginosa	1.8
Miscellaneous	5.3
None or nonpathogens	32.0

*Compiled from Bland, 1972; Tetzlaff, Ashworth, and Nelson, 1977; Berman, Balkany, and Simmons, 1978; Shurin et al., 1978. The report of Berman, Balkany, and Simmons includes some infants 7 to 12 weeks of age.

Otitis Media in the Newborn Infant
(Table 16–14)

The unexplained bacteriology of otitis media in newborn infants is more clear now that data are available from aspiration of middle ear fluids of 169 neonates with otitis media (Bland, 1972; Tetzlaff et al., 1977; Shurin et al., 1978; Berman et al., 1978). *S. pneumoniae* and *H. influenzae* are the bacteria isolated most frequently in the very young, as is the case in older infants and children. However, organisms associated with local and septic infection in the newborn infant, group B *streptococci*, *Staphylococcus aureus*, and gram-negative enteric bacilli, are important pathogens in the newborn infant within a week after birth or from older infants who have remained in the nursery because of risk features (low birth weight or prematurity) or disease (respiratory distress syndrome).

Bacteriology of the External Canal

The microbial flora of the external canal is similar to the flora of skin elsewhere on the body. In various microbiologic studies (Riding et al., 1978a; Pelton et al., 1980; Brook and Schwartz, 1981), there is a predominance of *S. epidermidis, S. aureus*, and diphtheroids, and to a lesser extent, anaerobic bacteria such as *P. acnes*. Pathogens responsible for infection of the middle ear, *S. pneumoniae, H. influenzae,* or *B. catarrhalis,* are uncommonly found in cultures of the external auditory canal when the tympanic membrane is intact. Thus, isolation of *S. epidermidis, S. aureus*, diphtheroids, or certain anaerobic bacteria from cultures of middle ear fluids may represent contamination of the fluid by organisms present in the external canal. Adequate cleansing of the external canal is necessary before tympanocentesis is performed for the purpose of microbiologic diagnosis.

Diseases of the external canal are not considered in this text. The interested reader is referred to a recently published monograph by Senturia et al. (1980b).

Summary and Conclusions

S. pneumoniae and *H. influenzae* are the bacteria most frequently isolated from the middle ear effusions of children with acute signs and symptoms of otitis media. Gram-negative enteric bacilli are isolated from the middle ear effusions of approximately 20 per cent of infants up to six weeks of age. We presume that the isolation of bacteria from the middle ear in children who have acute signs and symptoms of illness indicates that these organisms are responsible for the suppurative disease. However, bacterial pathogens are also isolated from the middle ear fluid of asymptomatic children with persistent effusions. The role of the bacteria in the prolonged effusion, at present, is unexplained.

Preliminary studies of anaerobic bacteria and chlamydia are not adequate to provide indications of the importance of these organisms in otitis media. Viruses and mycoplasmas are associated with otitis media in epidemiologic studies, but the association is not confirmed by studies of cultures of middle ear fluids; viruses were isolated in only 4.4 per cent of 663 middle ear aspirates and *M. pneumoniae* from only one of 771 effusions Thus, the role of viruses and mycoplasmas in the development of acute or chronic otitis media remains uncertain.

IMMUNOLOGY

The middle ear is the site of a secretory immune system similar to those of other areas of the respiratory tract. Local and systemic immune responses occur in patients with acute or chronic otitis media with effusion. In the middle ear, immunologically active antigen interacts with immunocompetent cells in the lamina propria to produce a local immune response. The middle ear effusion that results from acute or chronic infection contains all the major classes of immunoglobulins, complement, cells, immune complexes of antigen and antibody, and various chemical mediators of inflammation. The role of these substances in the course of otitis media with effusion is uncertain. The immune response to various antigens may assist in clearance of the middle ear effusion, may prevent subsequent infection, or may contribute to the accumulation and persistence of fluid in the middle ear cavity.

The immunology of otitis media with effusion is a relatively new area of investigation. Almost all important reports have been published since 1967. At present, our understanding of the immunology of otitis media is incomplete, but this field of investigation is in a dynamic phase, and results of current studies should yield important new information. This chapter is a review of information presently available.

Problems in Methodology

Studies of the immunology of otitis media in the human are based on assays of serum and middle ear effusion (obtained by needle aspiration through the tympanic membrane) and histology and immunochemistry of the mucosa of the middle ear (obtained by biopsy). Problems in methodology and limitations of data must be considered in evaluating the results of these studies.

1. Effusion or mucosa is most readily obtained at operation. Therefore, most initial reports include patients with chronic

disease who required an operative procedure and could also provide materials for study. Only a few reports of patients with acute otitis media with effusion are available.

2. Without information gathered prospectively, the investigator cannot identify the stage of disease when material is obtained. In most reports, the stage of otitis media is identified grossly as acute or chronic or by the characteristic of the middle ear effusion (serous, mucoid, purulent, or hemorrhagic). Few studies have results from more than one specimen or one observation. Thus, there is a paucity of information on the sequence of immune events.

3. Techniques for assay of the same function vary in sensitivity and specificity. New techniques may provide results at variance with previously used methods.

4. The quality and quantity of middle ear fluid obtained by tympanocentesis are limited. The volume of most aspirates is 1 ml or less. Therefore, only a few studies can be performed with each sample. In addition, the liquid may be fibrinous, mucoid, or filled with cellular debris, making homogenization difficult. Trauma may occur during the course of aspiration and may contaminate the effusion with products of blood and tissue.

5. Materials are not usually available from "normal" patients, and controls are difficult to define.

6. The investigator may not be able to identify the origin of the substance in the effusion. The liquid represents the sum of substances derived from serum, inflamed middle ear mucosa, degenerating white blood cells, or other cellular elements.

Experiments in animal models have provided important new information and stimulated new concepts, but significant differences exist between species, and data derived from studies in animals must be viewed with caution. For the purposes of this section, only data derived from studies of humans will be presented.

Immunology of the Pharynx

Immunocompetent lymphoid tissue is present in the mucosa of the upper respiratory tract, the site of initial exposure for ingested and inhaled antigens. The lymphoid tissue of the pharynx includes the palatine tonsils and adenoids, lymphoid tissue at the base of the tongue (lingual tonsil), lymphoid tissue on the posterior wall of the pharynx (pharyngeal tonsil), and a circular ring of lymphoid tissue (Waldeyer's ring). Plasma cells capable of producing all the major classes of immunoglobulins have been identified in the tonsils. The immunology of the tonsils was reviewed recently by Wong and Ogra (1980).

The precise role of the tonsils and adenoids with regard to the middle ear is unknown. Since microbial organisms responsible for infection of the middle ear proliferate first in the throat or nasopharynx, the immunology of these lymph tissues may play a significant role in the host's defense against otitis media. The immunocompetent cells present in the tonsils and adenoids are an important defense in excluding microbial and environmental antigens from the systemic lymphoid system, thus performing a "gatekeeper" function, but the mechanism for defense in these tissues against infection of the middle ear is unknown.

Role of Specific Immunoglobulins

Immunoglobulin A (IgA) and Secretory Immunoglobulin A (SIgA)

Immunoglobulin A (IgA) is secreted by plasma cells in lymphoid tissues lining the gastrointestinal, genitourinary, and respiratory tracts. Secretory component (SIgA) is a nonimmune glycoprotein formed by local epithelial cells that exists in either a bound state with IgA or in a free state in effusion fluids. Two IgA molecules combine with secretory component in the epithelium, and the complex (SIgA) is transported through the cell and into the lumen. The production of SIgA begins when antigen is presented to immunocompetent cells in the mucosa.

IgA is the predominant immunoglobulin in the middle ear effusion. The ratio of IgA to IgG is higher in middle ear effusion than in serum in most patients, and some patients have IgA in middle ear fluid but not in serum. Fluorescent antibody staining of middle ear mucosa demonstrates SIgA in the epithelium. SIgA isolated from middle ear effusions has the same antigenicity and subunit structures as SIgA found in other secretions, including saliva, nasal mucus, and colostrum (Mogi et al., 1976). Small amounts of free secretory component are present, but most secretory component in middle ear effusions is bound to IgA (Mogi et al., 1973).

A specific IgA response takes place in the middle ear following administration of a parenteral antigen. The presence of specific IgA antibody for measles, mumps, rubella, and poliovirus in middle ear fluid and its absence in some specimens of simultaneously obtained serum indicates that local antibody production takes place following systemic infection or immunization (Sloyer et al., 1977). These data require corroboration but suggest that an immunologic response can be expected in the middle ear following a parenteral immunization, such as intramuscularly administered pneumococcal vaccine, and that such a vaccine could be successful in prevention of recurrences of homotypic infection in the middle ear.

Immunoglobulin G (IgG)

Immunoglobulin G is present in the effusions of patients with both acute and chronic otitis media in concentrations suggesting that local development of antibody occurs in some patients.

Immunoglobulin M (IgM)

Although immunoglobulin M is present in the middle ear effusions of patients with both acute and chronic otitis media with effusion, concentrations are lower than in serum, and studies of middle ear mucosa obtained by biopsy in patients with chronic otitis media with effusion suggest that local synthesis of IgM does not occur.

Immunoglobulin D (IgD)

Few investigators have studied IgD in patients with otitis media. Veltri and Sprinkle (1973) found concentrations of IgD in the middle ear effusions of patients with chronic otitis media with effusion in excess of concentrations found in serum. The function of IgD in the middle ear or elsewhere in the body is unknown.

Immunoglobulin E (IgE)

The activity of reaginic antibody resides in IgE. Similar to IgA, IgE is part of the external secretory system of antibody produced in large part by plasma cells in the lymphoid tissue of the respiratory and gastrointestinal tracts. Increased concentration of IgE has been found in serum and secretions of patients with various atopic diseases. IgE antibody when combined with appropriate antigen causes release of histamine, slow-reacting substance, and chemotactic substance from mast cells and basophilic granulocytes.

IgE-producing plasma cells have been identified in biopsy of mucosa of the middle ear, and IgE has been found in the middle ear effusions of patients with both acute and chronic otitis media. The source of IgE in most patients, however, remains uncertain; some investigators present evidence in patients with chronic otitis media with effusion suggesting that IgE is produced locally by middle ear mucosa (Phillips et al., 1974), whereas the data presented by other investigators (Bernstein and Reisman, 1974; Mogi et al., 1974; Lewis et al., 1978) indicate that IgE in the middle ear is a transudate of serum.

Complement

The term *complement* was originally used in reference to a serum factor that acted upon an antibody-coated cell (red blood cell or bacterium) and caused lysis of the cell. We recognize now that complement represents a system including 11 discrete but interacting proteins and possesses a wide variety of activities, including viral neutralization, phagocytosis, immune adherence, chemotaxis, anaphylatoxin activities on smooth muscle and blood vessels, and a cytotoxic effect that may serve a protective function leading to destruction of foreign cells (Ward and McLean, 1978). Activation of complement occurs by the classical or alternate pathways. The classical pathway is usually activated by antigen-antibody complexes and proceeds in sequence from C1 to C9. The alternate pathways do not require immune complex for activation but utilize materials such as endotoxin or bacterial polysaccharide. The early factors of the classical pathway (C1, C2, and C4) are not required, but properdin and C3 are involved in activation.

Evidence for activation of complement in the middle ear effusions of patients with acute and chronic otitis media has been reviewed by Bernstein and colleagues (1978) and Prellner and coworkers (1980). Studies of middle ear effusion indicate that C2, C3,

C4, and C5 are all significantly depressed when compared to the corresponding serum and suggest utilization of complement in the middle ear during the course of otitis. Prellner and colleagues (1980) also demonstrated the presence of complexes of early complement factors indicating complement activation. The complement profile tended to become normal within a few weeks after treatment in patients who remained free of middle ear effusion, suggesting that changes in the complement system reflect the dynamics of the inflammatory process in the middle ear.

Other Host Defense Mechanisms in the Middle Ear (Table 16–15)

Nonspecific Factors Present in Tissue and Blood

A variety of nonspecific factors are present in the middle ear that may play roles in defense against infection. The epithelium of the eustachian tube and middle ear is ciliated with mucus-producing cells that are equipped to trap and expel inhaled particles. The network of fibrin that is present in middle ear effusions, particularly in mucoid and purulent effusions, restricts movement of organisms and facilitates phagocytosis. Destruction of white blood cells and cells lining the mucosa produces lactic acid with a decrease in pH sufficient to kill or inhibit growth of many bacteria.

Lysozymes and Other Enzymes

Lysozyme is a hydrolytic enzyme with bacteriolytic activity that is present in blood, urine, tears, middle ear effusions, and other body fluids. Lysozyme is found in the lysosomes of neutrophils, monocytes, and phago-

cytic cells of the reticuloendothelial system. The molecular basis of the bacteriolytic activity of lysozyme is the ability to solubilize the rigid cell wall common to all bacteria. Lysozyme acts synergistically with complement and specific antibody to achieve its antibacterial effect.

High levels of lysozyme have been found in the middle ear effusions of patients with chronic otitis media with effusion (Veltri and Sprinkle, 1973; Liu et al., 1975; Juhn and Huff, 1976). Lysozyme concentrations in middle ear effusions are higher than in serum and higher in mucoid than in serous effusions (Lang et al., 1976). The high concentration of this antimicrobial substance may explain the bactericidal and virucidal effects of middle ear effusion identified by Siirala and colleagues (1952, 1961).

Enzymes contained in lysozymes, including acid phosphatase, beta glucuronidase and isocitric dehydrogenase, have been identified in the effusion of patients with chronic otitis media. Juhn and Huff (1976) found significant concentrations in the middle ear effusions of lactic dehydrogenase, malate hydrogenase, leucine aminopeptidase, and alkaline phosphatase. Lactic dehydrogenase is an intracellular enzyme liberated during the destruction of tissue. Malate dehydrogenase and the other dehydrogenases of the Krebs cycle are believed to be bound to the inner mitochondrial membrane. In otitis media, proliferation of ciliated cells in the middle ear mucosa occurs. The increase in the number of cells and the increase in mitochondria may result in higher activity of the enzyme in the middle ear fluid than in serum (Juhn and Huff, 1976). Leucine aminopeptidase is a proteolytic enzyme that is present in various tissues and concentrated in leukocytes. Histochemical studies of the location of the enzyme in the middle ear mucosa show increase of activity throughout the mucoperiosteum. The concentrations of all enzymes were higher in middle ear effusions compared to simultaneously obtained serum and were higher in mucoid than in serous middle ear effusions, reflecting the local inflammatory process.

Miscellaneous Substances

In addition to the preceding factors, a variety of substances that take part in immune or inflammatory reactions have been identified in the middle ear effusions of pa-

Table 16–15 SUBSTANCES IDENTIFIED IN MIDDLE EAR EFFUSIONS OF PATIENTS WITH ACUTE OR CHRONIC OTITIS MEDIA WITH EFFUSION

Immunoglobulins	Enzymes
G, A, M, E, D, and	Lysozyme
Secretory IgA	Oxidative enzymes
Complement	Lactic dehydrogenase
Prostaglandins E and F	Malate dehydrogenase
Chemotactic substances	Hydrolytic enzymes
Macrophage inhibitory factor	Leucine aminopeptidase
Transferrin and lactoferrin	Alkaline phosphatase
Alpha$_1$-antitrypsin	Acid phosphatase
Surface active agents	

tients with chronic otitis media with effusion. These include the following:

1. A chemotactic factor for neutrophils (Bernstein, 1976). Chemotactic substances alter the nature of migration of neutrophils so that cells that otherwise would migrate randomly are directed to the vicinity of the chemotactic substance.
2. Macrophage inhibition factor (Bernstein, 1976). Macrophage inhibition factor inhibits the migration of macrophages *in vitro*; *in vivo* it serves to contain macrophages at the site of injury or inflammation. Macrophage inhibition factor augments the capacity of the macrophage to kill certain bacteria.
3. Lactoferrin inhibits growth of iron-dependent bacteria by competing for elemental iron (present in mucoid but not serous effusions) (Bernstein et al., 1972).
4. The functions of prostaglandins E and F include increasing capillary permeability and release of lysozymal enzymes. Bernstein and colleagues (1976) found prostaglandins E and F in middle ear fluids; in some patients, the concentration in middle ear fluid was higher than it was in serum.

Cytology of the Middle Ear and Middle Ear Effusions

Palva et al. (1976) analyzed the cells present in the middle ear effusions of patients with chronic otitis media with effusion. Lymphocytes and neutrophils were the predominant cell types. Monocytes and phagocytes were present but in small numbers in most specimens. Occasionally, giant phagocytes with ingested cells, cell debris, and bacteria were seen. Eosinophils and mast cells were rare. Mucous strands were numerous. Epithelial cells included numerous flat endothelial cells and few ciliated and goblet cells. Similar cell types are found in middle ear mucosa obtained by biopsy of patients with chronic otitis media with effusion. Inflammatory cells in the submucosa were predominantly of the mononuclear type. Plasma cells and small lymphocytes predominated. The presence of IgA and IgG was demonstrated by use of an immunofluorescent stain of mononuclear cells from middle ear effusions; IgM and IgE were uncommonly detected.

The cytologic studies indicate exfoliation of surface cells into the effusion with subsequent disintegration. The large number of neutrophils and lymphocytes indicates infiltration and proliferation of these cells in the submucosa of the middle ear during chronic inflammation.

Immunology of Acute Otitis Media with Effusion

Role of Antibody in Serum

Specific antibody to the infecting strain of *S. pneumoniae* or nontypable *H. influenzae* is present in the acute-stage serum of some children at the time of diagnosis of acute otitis media (Table 16–16). An immune response, reflected in a rise in serum antibody, occurs in a varying number of children after acute infection of the middle ear (Table 16–17) (Howie et al., 1973). Sloyer and colleagues (1974, 1975) identified specific antibody in the acute-stage serum of more than

Table 16–16 ANTIBODY RESPONSE IN SERUM AND MIDDLE EAR EFFUSION TO INFECTING STRAIN OF *STREPTOCOCCUS PNEUMONIAE* OR *HAEMOPHILUS INFLUENZAE* IN CHILDREN WITH ACUTE OTITIS MEDIA

Microorganism	No. of Children Studied	Specimen	No. of Children with Strain-Specific Antibody (%)
*Streptococcus pneumoniae**[*]	49	Acute serum	18 (37)
		Convalescent serum	12 (25)
		Middle ear fluid[‡]	13 (27)
Haemophilus influenzae[†]	29	Acute serum	14 (52)
		Convalescent serum	22 (76)
		Middle ear fluid[‡]	22 (76)

[*]Sloyer et al., 1974.
[†]Sloyer et al., 1975.
[‡]Obtained at same time as acute serum.

Table 16–17 RELATIONSHIP OF SPECIFIC ANTIBODY IN MIDDLE EAR FLUID AND CLEARANCE OF FLUID IN CHILDREN WITH ACUTE OTITIS MEDIA*

| | No. (%) of Middle Ear Effusions with: | | |
Status of Middle Ear Cavity	Antibody Present	Antibody Absent	Totals
Streptococcus pneumoniae isolated			
Middle ear fluid cleared	6 (40)	2 (5)	8
Middle ear fluid not cleared	9 (60)	42 (95)	51
TOTALS	15	44	
Haemophilus influenzae isolated			
Middle ear fluid cleared	17 (68)	7 (25)	24
Middle ear fluid not cleared	8 (32)	21 (75)	29
TOTALS	25	28	

*At second visit two to seven days following diagnosis (Sloyer et al., 1976).

one third of children with otitis media due to *S. pneumoniae* and one half of children with otitis due to *H. influenzae*. Approximately one quarter of the children had a significant antibody response to the infecting organism in the convalescent serum. The immune response to *S. pneumoniae* increased with age; only 12 per cent of children under one year of age had a significant rise in antibody level in the convalescent serum, whereas 48 per cent of the children two years of age or older responded (Sloyer et al., 1974). A majority of children two years of age or younger had a response as a result of acute otitis media due to nontypable strains of *H. influenzae*; of 29 pairs of serum samples from children two years of age or younger that were assayed, 15 acute and 22 convalescent serum samples contained specific antibody (Sloyer et al., 1975). Thus, infants are more likely to respond with serum antibody following acute infection due to *H. influenzae* than when infection is due to *S. pneumoniae*.

Shurin and coworkers (1980b) studied the immune responses of children 2 months to 12 years of age with acute otitis media due to nontypable strains of *H. influenzae*. Eleven per cent of the children had homotypic antibody in the acute-stage serum, but 78 per cent had specific antibody in the convalescent specimen. In contrast to the age-related immune response to *S. pneumoniae*, an immune response to nontypable *H. influenzae* occurred in all age groups.

There is a paucity of data about the role of specific serum antibody in protecting against subsequent homotypic episodes of acute otitis media. Shurin and coworkers (1980b) studied the prevalence of bactericidal antibody to a prototype strain of nontypable *H. influenzae* in children with acute otitis media of varying etiology. None of 28 children with acute otitis media due to nontypable *H. influenzae* (defined by culture of middle ear fluid) had homotypic antibody in acute-stage serum, whereas 18 of 66 children who had acute otitis media due to other agents had antibody to nontypable *H. influenzae* in acute-stage serum. Thus, the presence of bactericidal antibody correlated with protection from infection with nontypable strains of *H. influenzae*, and lack of antibody correlated with susceptibility to infection. Some of the children studied by Sloyer and colleagues had antibody to the infecting strain of *H. influenzae* and *S. pneumoniae* at the time of initial examination. Since the precise time of infection of the middle ear is difficult to determine, it is possible that infection occurred some time prior to initial examination and that sufficient time elapsed between the onset of infection and the time when specimens were obtained to allow for the evidence of an early immune response.

Significant concentrations of IgA, IgM, and IgG are present in the middle ear effusions of children with acute otitis media (Howie et al., 1973). SIgA is also present.

Role of Antibody in Clearance of the Middle Ear Effusion

Clearance of fluid from the middle ear in patients with acute otitis media due to *S. pneumoniae* and *H. influenzae* was significantly associated with the presence and concentration of specific antibody to the infecting strain in the middle ear fluid at the time of diagnosis (Sloyer et al., 1976). Clearing of the middle ear was identified by pneumatic otoscopy and defined as return to an aerated state, free of effusion by the second visit (two to seven days following diagnosis). Clearing of the effusion by the second visit was associated with specific antibody in the middle ear effusion obtained at first visit and was directly associated with the concentration of specific antibody. More children with infection due to *H. influenzae* cleared rapidly (45.3 per cent) than children with infection due to *S. pneumoniae* (13.6 per cent) whether or not antibody was present. Thus, the presence and concentration of antibody in the middle ear effusion at the time of presentation was significantly related to rapid clearing of the effusion and return of the middle ear cleft to a normal air-filled state. The source for the antibody in the effusion at the time of presentation of acute otitis media is uncertain; antibody may have developed after a prior infection or may have developed rapidly after a current infection and was present when the specimen was obtained. If present from a prior infection, type-specific antibody did not protect the patient from a recurrent episode of acute otitis media but reduced the duration of the effusion. Thus, immune response in the middle ear, whether from prior or current infection, reduced the morbidity of the illness as reflected in a shorter period of time spent with middle ear fluid.

Immunology of Chronic Otitis Media with Effusion

Role of Antibody in Middle Ear Fluid

Studies of patients with chronic otitis media with effusion are based on materials obtained at the time of myringotomy and/or placement of ventilating tubes and thus represent varying stages of chronic disease.

All the major classes of immunoglobulins, IgA, IgG, IgM, IgD, and IgE, have been identified in the middle ear effusions of patients with chronic otitis media with effusion. Secretory component, IgA, and IgG are synthesized by the mucosa of the middle ear; synthesis of other immunoglobulins in the middle ear is less certain (Bernstein and Reisman, 1974). Both IgA and IgG are present in

middle ear effusions in concentrations higher than in simultaneously obtained serum, whereas IgM and IgE are present in equivalent or lower concentrations in effusion when compared with serum. The highest concentrations of each of the major classes of immunoglobulins are present in mucoid effusions, the lowest are in serous effusions, and intermediate values are in leukocytic middle ear effusions.

Polymorphonuclear Leukocyte Response

Hill and coworkers (1977) identified defective chemotactic response in selected patients with recurrent episodes of otitis media and diarrhea. Giebink and colleagues (1980) studied the polymorphonuclear leukocyte response in children at the time of myringotomy and/or placement of ventilating tubes and, in a few cases, two to eight weeks later. In some children with chronic otitis media with effusion, there were transient abnormalities of polymorphonuclear leukocyte motility (depressed chemotactic responsiveness), phagocytosis (depressed polymorphonuclear leukocyte bactericidal activity), or intracellular oxidation (depressed polymorphonuclear leukocyte chemiluminescence). Repeat studies performed after surgery in some of the children found these indices to be normal in the majority of children, suggesting that leukocyte dysfunction was transient and probably associated with the inflammatory reaction that elicited the middle ear fluid. The results demonstrating a return to normal after drainage suggest that the polymorphonuclear leukocyte is a consequence rather than cause of the chronic disease.

These data indicate that there is a system of local immune function in patients with chronic otitis media with effusion and suggest that chronic otitis media with effusion is an immune complex disease. Substances available for such an immune complex reaction include the presence of specific antibody, antigen (microbial agents or allergens present in the pharynx), and lysosomal enzymes. Antigen may combine with antibody (locally produced or derived from serum) to form an immune complex. Activation of the complement sequence through the classical or alternate pathways results in the attraction of polymorphonuclear leukocytes and monocytes. With the death of these cells, intracellular enzymes are released, producing local tissue damage and stimulating effusion.

Evidence for this hypothesis is incomplete. The presence of immune complexes in middle ear fluid may represent a normal immunologic reaction as a method of elimination of antigen (Bernstein, 1980). Bernstein noted that immune complex disease is usually manifested by deposition of IgG and C3 in the basement membrane of the epithelium or the blood vessels in the involved tissue, and at present, there is no immunopathologic evidence for such deposits in the middle ear mucosa obtained from patients with otitis media with effusion.

At present, there are too few data to develop a comprehensive theory of the role of the immune response in the acute and chronic phases of otitis media with effusion. More information is needed to define the role of the immune response in the development of fluid in the middle ear after challenge by antigen, the role of the immune mechanism in the resolution of or the persistence of that fluid, and, finally, the protective mechanisms against subsequent invasion by microorganisms of the same or different types.

Children with Defects of the Immune System

Defects of the Immune System

Most children with recurrent episodes of otitis media with effusion have no apparent systemic or local immune defect. These children have normal concentrations of immunoglobulin in serum, normal systemic cell-mediated responses, and normal phagocytic and bactericidal capacity of neutrophils in peripheral blood (Giebink and Quie, 1978). Available data about the immune system of the middle ear in children with recurrent otitis media with effusion indicate that most have the essential elements for immunologic resistance, including B cell responses that are fully operative, T cell systems that are present, macrophages that are available for engulfing and ingesting antigenic material, and appropriate antibody response by the middle ear mucosa (Palva et al., 1980).

However, patients with immune deficiencies that are likely to result in recurrent episodes of bacterial infections may have recurrent episodes of suppurative infections of the middle ear. The major categories for conditions that may affect these children are acquired or congenital deficiencies of immu-

noglobulins and of polymorphonuclear leukocytes. The defect may be quantitative (neutropenia) or qualitative (an abnormality of phagocyte function, such as chronic granulomatous disease, the Chédiak-Higashi syndrome, or myeloperoxidase deficiency). These children are susceptible to local and systemic pyogenic infections, and otitis media is only one of many bacterial diseases that may occur (Berdal et al., 1976).

Reduction in concentration of serum immunoglobulins (IgE, IgM, and IgA) was noted in some children by Karma et al. (1976); all cases that were clinically normal on reexamination also had normal immunoglobulins. Absence or deficiency of IgA has been associated with recurrent pneumonia, chronic bronchitis, and sinusitis, but susceptibility to infections of the middle ear has not been noted in these patients. Many children with deficiencies of IgA are entirely asymptomatic.

Patients with defects in splenic function are susceptible to overwhelming infection due to encapsulated organisms such as *S. pneumoniae* or *H influenzae* type b Such patients, including those with congenital or acquired asplenia and those with sickle cell disease, have not been identified as groups with unusual susceptibility to infections at local sites, such as the skin and soft tissues or middle ear.

The Role of Allergy in Otitis Media with Effusion

The role of allergy as an etiologic factor in otitis media with effusion is uncertain. Few critical studies of appropriate design are available to clarify the relationship of allergy and otitis media with effusion. Available studies are often biased (subjects include children referred for allergy evaluation) and do not include appropriate control patients. However, the association of reaginic antibody with IgE provides a specific measure for precise definition of allergy and has already provided some significant information about the primary or secondary role of allergy in otitis media with effusion.

The evidence for a role for allergy in recurrent otitis media with effusion in some children was discussed by Siegel (1979) and Bernstein (1980) and includes the following: (1) observations that many patients with recurrent otitis media with effusion have concomitant allergic respiratory disease; (2) a history of one or more major allergic illnesses in parents; (3) presence of an increased number of nasal or peripheral eosinophils; (4) a high incidence of positive skin tests to allergens or positive radioallergosorbent (RAST) tests; (5) elevated IgE levels in middle ear effusions and in the serum of some children; and (6) mast cells (some that are degranulating) found frequently throughout the middle ear mucosa.

Evidence against a major role for allergy in otitis media with effusion was summarized by Bernstein (1980): (1) In unselected series of cases of otitis media with effusion, fewer than one third of patients are atopic (2) The seasonal incidence of otitis media with effusion (winter-spring) is contrary to the seasonality when grasses, trees, and pollens cause acute nasal allergy (late spring and early fall). (3) Most studies indicate an absence of, or only small numbers of, IgE-producing cells in middle ear fluids and middle ear mucosa. (4) Failure of patients to improve with aggressive allergic treatment, including hyposensitization and use of antihistamines in spite of improvement in nasal symptoms.

Thus, many patients may be allergic, but there is no substantive evidence correlating nasal allergy with otitis media with effusion. However, it is possible that the allergic response plays a role in some children with otitis media with effusion or in some episodes of otitis media with effusion. The presence of specific IgE on mast cells in middle ear mucosa could result in the release of mediators of inflammation. The allergic reaction might be a predisposing factor, producing congestion of the mucosa of the nose and eustachian tube and leading to obstruction of the tube with retention of fluid in the middle ear. The question of the role of allergy in otitis media with effusion remains unanswered, but the availability of specific markers of the allergic reaction provides a means to better answers in the future.

Use of Bacterial Vaccines for Prevention of Otitis Media

If type-specific serum antibody is correlated with protection from homotypic infection, as suggested by Shurin and colleagues (1980b), bacterial vaccines may be an effective mode of prevention of type-specific otitis

media Among bacterial vaccines currently under investigation, the meningococcal vaccines and the *H. influenzae* type b vaccine are of limited interest because of the infrequency of acute otitis media due to these organisms. A vaccine for nontypable *H. influenzae* is not available. A multitype pneumococcal vaccine is available and is of major interest because of the importance of this organism as a cause of otitis media in all age groups. The clinical and microbiologic results of recent trials of pneumococcal vaccine to prevent recurrences of acute otitis media are presented in the section on immunization (p 470) in this chapter.

Summary and Conclusions

1. Immunology of acute otitis media: Specific antibody to the infecting strain of bacteria is present in the acute-stage serum and in the middle ear effusions of some children at the time of diagnosis of acute otitis media. Many children have a significant type-specific antibody response in serum to the bacteria responsible for acute otitis media. Recent studies suggest that the presence of antibody is correlated with protection from infection and that lack of antibody is correlated with susceptibility to infection; specific antibody in the middle ear effusion at the time of diagnosis of acute otitis media is associated with clearance of fluid and early return to normal of the middle ear.

2. Immunology of chronic otitis media with effusion: All the major classes of immunoglobulins, IgA, IgG, IgM, IgD, and IgE, have been identified in the middle ear effusions of patients with chronic otitis media with effusion. The highest concentration of immunoglobulins is present in mucoid effusions, followed by leukocytic and serous effusions. The data suggest that the immune response may be responsible for the presence and persistence of effusion in the middle ear and that some cases of chronic otitis media with effusion are examples of immune complex disease.

3. Substances in middle ear fluid that may play roles in immune and inflammatory reactions: A variety of mediators of the immune and inflammatory responses have been identified in the middle ear effusions of patients with chronic otitis media with effusion, including complement (usually

in a lower concentration than is present in simultaneously obtained serum), lysozyme and other hydrolytic and oxidative enzymes, lactoferrin and transferrin, chemotactic factors, and prostaglandins. At present, only speculation on the role of these substances in the middle ear based on their activities in other organs or body fluids is possible.

The immunology of otitis media is a new area of investigation. The immune reaction plays a role in the pathogenesis and course of the disease in terms of development of the inflammatory response in the middle ear, recovery of the functional state of the eustachian tube and the middle ear, control of infection, and development and removal of the middle ear effusion. At present, the data are incomplete and, in some cases, inconsistent. Nevertheless, the field of study is dynamic, and answers are forthcoming to the outstanding questions about the role of the immune response in otitis media with effusion.

PATHOLOGY

In the initial stages of classic acute otitis media the mucoperiosteum of the middle ear and mastoid air cells is hyperemic and edematous. This is followed by an exudation of polymorphonuclear leukocytes and serofibrinous fluid into the middle ear. The quantity of fluid increases until the middle ear is filled and pressure is exerted against the tympanic membrane (Fig. 16–43). If the disease progresses, the bulging tympanic membrane may rupture spontaneously. The resultant discharge is at first serosanguineous but then becomes mucopurulent. Throughout the middle ear and mastoid, the mucosa becomes markedly thickened by a mixture of inflammatory cells, new capillaries, and young fibrous tissue. This process may become associated with blockage of the aditus ad antrum, resulting in inadequate drainage of the mastoid air cells and a consequent mastoiditis. Extension beyond the mucoperiosteum may lead to intratemporal complications, such as facial paralysis, laby-

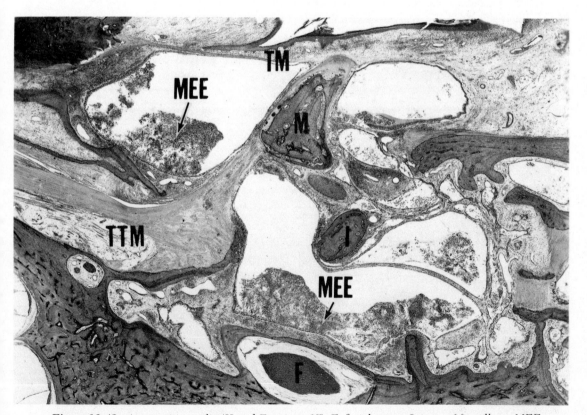

Figure 16–43 Acute otitis media (H and E stain × 15). F, facial nerve; I, incus; M, malleus; MEE, middle ear effusion; TM, tympanic membrane; TTM, tensor tympani muscle. (Courtesy of H. F. Schuknecht, M.D.)

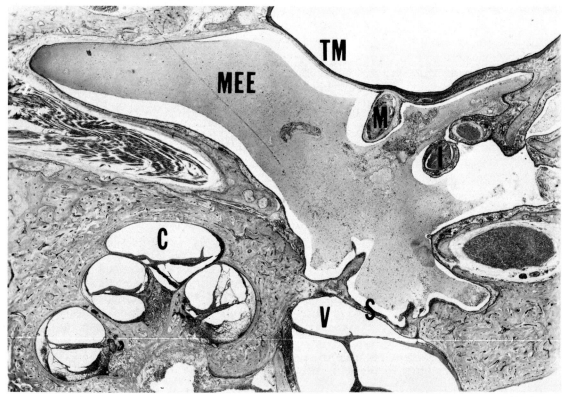

Figure 16–44 Otitis media with serous effusion (H and E stain × 11). C, cochlea; I, incus; M, malleus; MEE, middle ear effusion; TM, tympanic membrane; S, stapes; V, vestibule. (Courtesy of H. F. Schuknecht, M.D.)

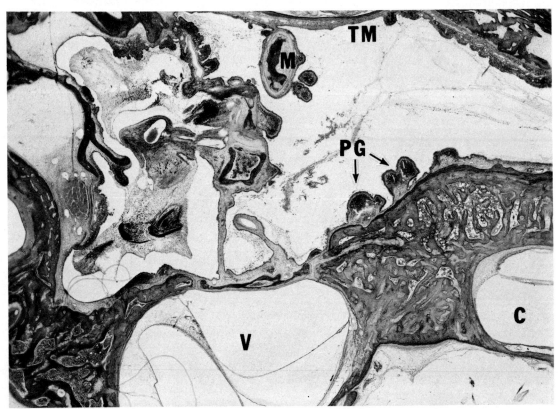

Figure 16–45 Chronic otitis media (H and E stain × 15). C, cochlea; M, malleus; PG, polypoid granulation tissue; TM, tympanic membrane; V, vestibule. (Courtesy of I. Sando, M.D.)

rinthitis, and petrositis, or intracranial complications, which may include lateral sinus thrombophlebitis, meningitis, otitic hydrocephalus, subdural abscess, epidural abscess, and brain abscess.

The pathologic findings associated with the serous (Fig. 16–44) or mucoid type of chronic middle ear effusion are similar. There is an increase in the number of secretory cells, including glands and ciliated cells. The lamina propria or connective tissue layer becomes thickened by edema and infiltration of numerous inflammatory cells consisting of lymphocytes, plasma cells, macrophages, and polymorphonuclear leukocytes. These changes are more striking in the presence of a mucoid effusion than for a pure serous effusion in which tissue edema is the predominant finding, in addition to the presence of chronic inflammatory cells (Fig. 16–45). It is generally believed that mucoid effusions are mainly the result of secretion, whereas serous effusions are mostly transudates. Persistent atelectasis of the middle ear, chronic middle ear effusions, or both are associated with a number of intratemporal complications and sequelae, including hearing loss, tympanosclerosis, adhesive otitis media, perforation with discharge, chronic mastoiditis, and cholesteatoma.

DIAGNOSIS OF OTITIS MEDIA

The methods of examination of a child with ear disease have been extensively described (including pneumatic otoscopy) in Chapter 8; however, the specific diagnostic features that characterize the various forms of otitis media and certain related conditions are presented in this section.

Clinical Description

For the clinician, the diagnosis of otitis media usually depends upon a high index of suspicion and the presence of symptoms, but primarily on the pneumatic otoscopic findings.

Acute Otitis Media

The usual picture of acute otitis media is seen in a child who has an upper respiratory tract infection for several days and suddenly develops otalgia, fever, and hearing loss. Examination with the pneumatic otoscope re-veals a hyperemic, opaque, bulging tympanic membrane that has poor mobility. Purulent otorrhea is usually also a reliable sign. In addition to fever, other systemic signs and symptoms may include irritability, lethargy, anorexia, vomiting, and diarrhea. However, all of these may be absent, and even earache and fever are unreliable guides and may frequently be absent. Likewise, otoscopic findings may consist only of a bulging or full, opaque, poorly mobile eardrum without evidence of erythema. Hearing loss will not be a complaint of the very young or even noted by the parents.

Tympanometry usually reveals an effusion pattern (flat) but may show a pattern that is not classically associated with an effusion.

When performed, tympanocentesis usually is productive of a purulent middle ear aspirate, but in approximately 20 per cent a serous or mucoid effusion is present (Bluestone et al., 1979b). Because of the variability of symptoms, infants and young children presenting with diminished or absent mobility and opacification of the tympanic membrane should be suspected of having acute otitis media.

Chronic Otitis Media with Effusion

Most children with chronic middle ear effusions are asymptomatic. Some may complain of hearing loss and, less commonly, tinnitus and vertigo. In children the attention of an alert parent or teacher may be drawn to a suspected hearing loss. Sometimes the child presents with a behavioral disorder due to the hearing deficit and consequent inability to communicate adequately. More often, the reason for referral is the detection of a hearing loss during a school hearing screening test or when acute otitis media fails to resolve completely. Occasionally, the first evidence of the disease is discovered during a routine examination or in high-risk cases, such as in children with a cleft palate.

Older children will describe a frank hearing loss or, more commonly, a "plugged" feeling or "popping" in their ears. The symptoms are usually bilateral. Unilateral signs and symptoms of chronic middle ear effusion may be secondary to a nasopharyngeal neoplasm such as an angiofibroma or even a malignancy.

Pneumatic otoscopy will frequently reveal either a retracted or full tympanic membrane that is usually opaque, but when it is translucent, an air-fluid level or air bubbles may be visualized, and a blue or amber color is present. The mobility of the eardrum is almost always altered.

It is evident from the preceding clinical description of acute otitis media and chronic otitis media with effusion that there is considerable overlap; hence it is often very difficult for the clinician to distinguish between acute and chronic forms unless the child has been observed over a period of time before the onset of disease or there are associated specific (otalgia) or systemic (fever) symptoms. It may not be possible to distinguish between the two even when the middle ear effusion is aspirated (tympanocentesis), since in both acute and chronic otitis the effusion may be either serous, mucoid, or purulent. In approximately half of chronic effusions, bacteria have been cultured that are frequently found in ears of children with classic signs and symptoms of acute otitis media (Riding et al., 1978a).

Atelectasis of the Tympanic Membrane—Middle Ear and High Negative Pressure

Atelectasis of the tympanic membrane may be acute or chronic, generalized or localized, and mild or severe. The tympanic membrane may be retracted or collapsed. High negative pressure may be present or absent. When middle ear effusion is also present the clinical description is the same as described above when an acute or chronic otitis media is present. In such cases, it is not unusual to visualize through the otoscope a severely retracted malleus in association with a tympanic membrane that is full or even bulging in the posterior portion. The malleus is retracted by concurrent high negative middle ear pressure or chronic inflammation of the tensor tympani muscle or the malleolar ligaments, or both, whereas the hydrostatic pressure of the effusion (not completely filling the middle ear–mastoid air cell system) results in bulging of the most compliant (floppy) portion of the pars tensa, the posterosuperior and posteroinferior quadrants. Frequently an effusion is evident by the presence of an air-fluid level or bubbles behind a severely retracted tympanic membrane.

Just as when there is a middle ear effusion present, there may be a lack of specific otologic symptoms when no effusion is present. The child may have a severely retracted translucent tympanic membrane with evidence of high negative pressure by pneumatic otoscopy (immobile to applied positive pressure and either decreased or absent mobility to applied negative pressure) or a high negative middle ear pressure tracing on the tympanogram. The otoscopist can look through the tympanic membrane and see that there is no effusion present. Some children with such an otoscopic (and tympanometric) examination may not have any complaint, while others may have a feeling of fullness in the ear, otalgia, tinnitus, hearing loss, and even vertigo. The condition may be self-limited and in some it may be physiologic, owing to temporary eustachian tube obstruction. But in others, especially those with symptoms, the condition is pathologic and should be managed in a manner similar to management when an effusion is present.

When there is localized atelectasis or a retraction pocket, especially in the pars flaccida, or posterosuperior portion of the pars tensa of the tympanic membrane, then the condition may be more serious than when only generalized atelectasis is present. The child may be totally asymptomatic, but the retraction pocket may be associated with a significant conductive hearing loss, especially if there is erosion of one or more of the ossicles. Erosion of the long process of the incus may be present when a deep posterosuperior retraction pocket is visualized (Fig. 16–46). It is extremely important to visualize these areas of the tympanic membrane to determine if a retraction pocket is present, and if so, whether there is destruction of one

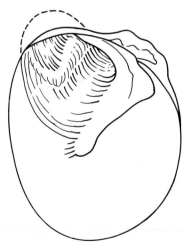

Figure 16–46 Illustration of an atelectatic membrane that has a severe retraction pocket in the posterosuperior quadrant of the pars tensa.

of the ossicles. It is important to distinguish between a retraction pocket and a cholesteatoma. If the otoscopic examination is not adequate to make this differential diagnosis, then the otomicroscope should be used; the clinician should not hesitate to perform otomicroscopic examination under general anesthesia when indicated. Cholesteatoma, like its precursor, the deep retraction pocket, may be without signs and symptoms (other than the otoscopic appearance) unless conductive hearing loss or otorrhea is present.

Eustachian Tube Dysfunction

Some children, especially older ones, will complain of a periodic popping or snapping sound in the ear, which may be preceded or accompanied by a feeling of fullness in the ear, hearing loss, tinnitus, or vertigo. Otoscopic examination may reveal a normal tympanic membrane or possibly slight retraction of the eardrum, but the middle ear pressure is within normal limits. These children have obstruction of the eustachian tube that is not severe enough to cause atelectasis, or a middle ear effusion, but nevertheless may be quite disconcerting. When troublesome, the child should be managed the same as children who have middle ear effusion.

On occasion, older children may complain of autophony (hearing one's own voice in the ear) and hearing their own breathing. The eustachian tube is most likely patulous (abnormally patent), in which case the tympanic membrane will appear normal when visualized through the otoscope. Middle ear pressure will be normal; however, if the child is asked to breathe forcefully through one nasal cavity, the opposite being occluded with a finger, the posterosuperior portion of the tympanic membrane will be observed to move in and out with respiration, which will confirm the diagnosis. Tympanometry may also aid in diagnosis (see section on Tympanometry—Patulous Tube Test, p. 390).

Microbiologic Diagnosis

The correlation between results of bacterial cultures of the nasopharynx or the oropharynx and those of cultures of middle ear fluids is poor. The poor correlation occurs because of the frequency of colonization of the upper respiratory tract with organisms of known pathogenicity for the middle ear and

less commonly because of absence in cultures of the oropharynx or nasopharynx of the pathogen responsible for infection of the middle ear. Thus, cultures of the upper respiratory tract are of limited value in specific bacteriologic diagnosis of otitis media. Specific microbiologic diagnosis is achieved by culture of middle ear fluid, obtained by needle aspiration through the intact tympanic membrane. If the patient is toxic or has a localized infection elsewhere, culture of the blood or the focus of infection should be performed. Bacteremia is rarely associated with otitis media due to nontypable strains of *H. influenzae*, uncommonly associated with otitis media due to *S. pneumoniae*, but frequently associated with otitis media due to type b strains of *H. influenzae* (Harding et al., 1973).

The consistent results of microbiologic studies of middle ear fluid of children with acute otitis media provide an accurate guide to the most likely pathogens. Thus, initial therapy in the uncomplicated case does not require obtaining specimens for bacterial diagnosis. If the patient is critically ill when first seen, or has altered host defenses (as is the case with the newborn infant, the patient with malignancy, or the patient with immunologic disease), or if the patient fails to respond appropriately to initial therapy for acute otitis media, culture of the middle ear fluid and in addition, for the first two examples, culture of the blood, is warranted.

Diagnostic Aspiration of the Middle Ear

When the diagnosis of acute otitis media is in doubt or when determination of the etiologic agent is desirable, aspiration of the middle ear should be performed. Indications for tympanocentesis or myringotomy (Fig. 16–47) include the following:

1. Otitis media in patients who are seriously ill or appear toxic
2. Unsatisfactory response to antimicrobial therapy
3. Onset of otitis media in a patient who is receiving antimicrobial agents
4. Presence of suppurative complications
5. Otitis media in the newborn, the very young infant, or in the immunologically deficient patient, in each of whom an unusual organism may be suspected

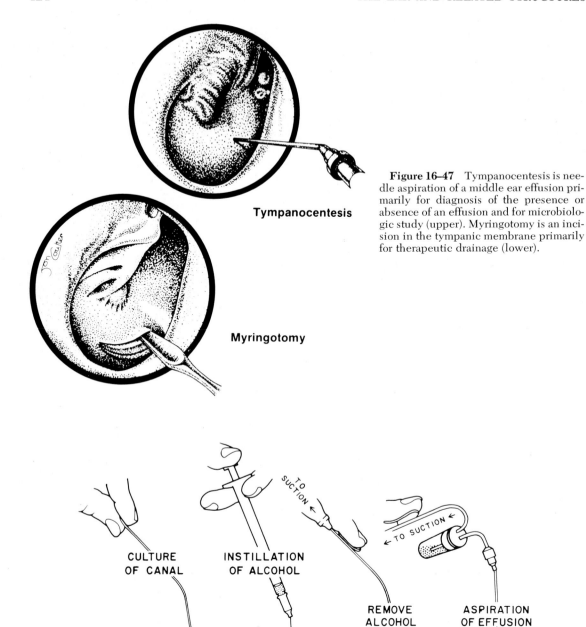

Tympanocentesis

Myringotomy

Figure 16–47   Tympanocentesis is needle aspiration of a middle ear effusion primarily for diagnosis of the presence or absence of an effusion and for microbiologic study (upper). Myringotomy is an incision in the tympanic membrane primarily for therapeutic drainage (lower).

CULTURE OF CANAL

INSTILLATION OF ALCOHOL

TO SUCTION

REMOVE ALCOHOL

TO SUCTION

ASPIRATION OF EFFUSION

CANAL →

TYMPANIC MEMBRANE →

MIDDLE EAR EFFUSION

Figure 16–48   Method recommended for tympanocentesis and aspiration of a middle ear effusion for microbiologic assessment. A culture of the external auditory canal is obtained with a Calgiswab (Falton, Oxnard, CA) that has been moistened with trypticase soy broth. The canal is then filled with 70 per cent ethyl alcohol for one minute, after which as much as possible of the alcohol is removed from the ear canal by aspiration. Tympanocentesis is performed in the inferior portion of the tympanic membrane with an Alden-Senturia trap (Storz Instrument Co., St. Louis, MO) with a needle attached. Care is taken not to close the suction hole in the trap before entering the middle ear.

Both of these procedures can usually be performed without general anesthesia. In certain instances, premedication with a combination of a short-acting barbiturate and either morphine or meperidine, or even a general anesthetic, is advisable. The procedures can be carried out with an otoscope with a surgical head or with the otomicroscope. Adequate immobilization of the patient is essential when a general anesthetic is not used.

Diagnostic aspiration may be performed through the inferior portion of the tympanic membrane employing an 18-gauge spinal needle attached to a syringe or collection trap (Fig. 16–48). Culture of the ear canal and cleansing of the canal with alcohol should precede the procedure. The canal culture is helpful in determining whether organisms cultured are contaminants from the exterior canal or pathogens from the middle ear. When therapeutic drainage is required, a myringotomy knife should be employed and the incision should be large enough to allow for adequate drainage and aeration of the middle ear (see section on Myringotomy, p. 476).

Following tympanocentesis, the effusion caught in the syringe or collection trap is sent to the laboratory for culture. A Gram-stained smear may provide immediate information about the bacterial pathogens.

The external ear swab and the fluid aspirated from the middle ear are inoculated onto appropriate solid media and into broth to isolate the likely organisms. Sensitivities of organisms isolated should be tested by the standard method described by Bauer et al. (1966).

Nasopharyngeal Culture

In an attempt to identify the causative organism in a child with acute otitis media, the results of a nasopharyngeal culture would be less traumatic than a tympanocentesis or myringotomy. The concept is an attractive one, since the bacteria found in middle ear aspirates are the same type found in the nasopharynx of children with acute otitis media. However, the correlation between the organisms found in the middle ear and nasopharynx as reported in the past has not proven to be high enough to warrant the procedure. More recently, Schwartz et al. (1979) reported a technique that improved the correlation of organisms isolated by the nasopharyngeal culture with bacteria identified by culture of middle ear fluid. The method used involved immediate plating of the nasopharyngeal swab on solid media and a semiquantitative estimation of colonies growing on culture plates.

White Blood Cell Count

Although the white blood cell counts are too variable to be helpful in distinguishing the child with otitis media due to a bacterial pathogen from the child with otitis media and a sterile effusion, there are data which suggest that the mean white blood cell count of children with bacterial otitis media is higher than the white blood cell count of children with sterile middle ear effusion. Lahikainen (1953) noted that the mean white blood cell counts (per cu mm) of children with otitis due to S. pyogenes was 13,400; due to S. pneumoniae, 10,500; due to H. influenzae, 11,500; and of children with sterile middle ear effusion, 8700. Mortimer and Watterson (1956) found similar results in children who had a bacterial pathogen in the middle ear effusion, the mean white blood cell count (per cu mm) being 10,300; the mean white blood cell count was 6700 in children with sterile effusions. Feingold and colleagues (1966) found as association of higher white blood cell counts with isolation of bacterial pathogen from the middle ear effusion; of 35 children with white blood cell counts of 15,000 or more, 27 (77 per cent) had a bacterial pathogen grown from the middle ear effusion, whereas of children with a white blood cell count of 9000 or less, 8 of 20 (40 per cent) had a bacterial pathogen grown from the middle ear effusion.

Sedimentation Rate

Lahikainen (1953) found increases in sedimentation rate in children with otitis media and differences among the bacterial pathogens isolated from the middle ear effusion. The mean sedimentation rate for 104 children with otitis media due to S. pyogenes was 43.7; for 171 children with otitis media due to S. pneumoniae, 30.2; for 43 with otitis media due to H. influenzae, 17.3; and for 85 children with sterile effusion, 21.3.

TYMPANOGRAM   TYMPANIC MEMBRANE
PATTERNS   MIDDLE EAR FINDINGS

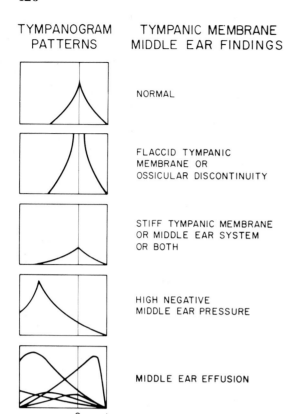

NORMAL

FLACCID TYMPANIC
MEMBRANE OR
OSSICULAR DISCONTINUITY

STIFF TYMPANIC MEMBRANE
OR MIDDLE EAR SYSTEM
OR BOTH

HIGH NEGATIVE
MIDDLE EAR PRESSURE

MIDDLE EAR EFFUSION

−   0   +
mmH₂O

Figure 16–49 Examples of tympanograms related to tympanic membrane compliance and middle ear pressure (mm H₂O).

Tympanometry

The electroacoustic impedance bridge, with which a tympanogram can be obtained, has become an important aid in the diagnosis of otitis media. To perform typanometry, a small probe is inserted into the external auditory canal. A tone of fixed characteristics is presented through the probe, and the compliance of the tympanic membrane is measured electronically while the external canal pressure is artificially varied (see Chapter 8B). The tympanograms produced reflect the dynamics of the entire tympanic membrane–middle ear–eustachian tube system. The patterns shown in Figure 16–49 demonstrate the acoustic compliance of the tympanic membrane on the vertical axis over a range of external canal pressures on the horizontal axis. As is true for eardrum mobility observed visually, acoustic compliance is greatest when pressures that show peaks at zero pressure when middle ear pressure is normal usually

have no effusion. A peak is present in the negative range when middle ear pressure is reduced. In this pattern, an effusion may be present especially if the peak is not sharp. Middle ear effusions are present in most cases in which no impedance peak can be determined.

Audiometry

Audiometry is not a reliable diagnostic aid in the identification of children with middle ear effusions (see Chapter 8B). Bluestone et al. (1973) reported that only half of a group of children with middle ear effusions would have been identified by routine audiologic screening criteria (Fig. 16–50). In addition, audiometry employing standard methods cannot be obtained on infants, in whom the prevalence of the disease is the highest. However, in children and adults, the audiogram may show a mild to moderate flat conductive hearing loss in the range of 10 to 40 dB.

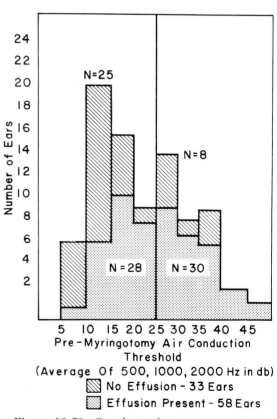

Figure 16–50 Correlation between premyringotomy average air conduction thresholds and myringotomy findings in 55 children (91 ears) (Bluestone, Beery, and Paradise, 1973).

Occasionally a mixed hearing loss may be present. The sensorineural component is thought to be due to increased tension and stiffness of the round window membrane. Generally, both the conductive and sensorineural components disappear when the middle ear fluid or negative pressure is relieved. However, permanent sensorineural hearing loss may result from chronic otitis media (Paparella et al., 1972).

Screening for Otitis Media

Screening for otitis media is a process that is intended to identify children who may have the disease but who would otherwise go undetected. Otitis media is a disease that appears to be important to screen, since it is highly prevalent, is associated with varying degrees of conductive hearing loss, and may lead to other, more serious, complications and sequelae. Otoscopy performed by an expert is an excellent method to identify otitis media and should be employed by professionals who care for children as a routine part of the examination. This is especially important in infants and young children. However, for most screening situations, otoscopy is not feasible. Audiometry, employing the routine audiologic screening criteria, has been shown to identify only half of a group of children with middle ear effusion (Bluestone et al., 1973). In addition, audiometry, employing standard methods, cannot be performed on infants in whom the prevalence of the disease is the highest. However, impedance screening employing tympanometry and possibly the acoustic reflex, is a highly sensitive method of screening for otitis media with effusion. Impedance testing is acceptable to both the child and the health care provider because it is safe, noninvasive, and simply executed. Studies have shown impedance measurements to be reliable, but these studies have not involved subjects of all age groups or all instruments that are available, many of which have been designed specifically for screening purposes.

The validity of referral criteria based on impedance measurements (i.e., their association, singly or in combination, with the presence or absence of middle ear effusion) has not been established completely, and further studies are required. In addition, neither the epidemiology nor the natural history of the disease has been adequately studied in the various age groups affected, which makes most of the methods of management currently employed difficult to evaluate. The disease in many instances spontaneously disappears. Because of these problems, the referral criteria for children who are identified with a middle ear effusion remain controversial. A Task Force convened in 1977 addressed this problem and advised against universal (mass) screening on a routine basis for the detection of middle ear disorders in children of any age group (Harford et al., 1978). Although not recommending mass screening, the Task Force did advise screening employing impedance measurements in small, carefully controlled programs in order to determine the best method for larger screening programs.

The following is a summary of that Task Force's recommendations. Middle ear effusion has its highest prevalence and incidence in the age group between 6 and 36 months. Following episodes of acute infection, asymptomatic otitis media with effusion continues for extended periods in a large number of infants, and there is concern about the possible effects of undetected effusions on their function and development. Below the age of seven months, the relations between tympanometric findings currently employed and middle ear disease are not well understood, although the limited data now available indicate that the sensitivity of tympanometry as usually performed is relatively low. There are also feasibility problems associated with impedance screening of infants. Logistically, it may be difficult to gather infants for testing after they leave their place of birth. Moreover, impedance testing in infants may sometimes be difficult and time consuming. However, if these difficulties can be overcome, impedance testing of infants should be attempted, if feasible.

Even though mass screening of preschool and school-age children by impedance measurements is not recommended at present, screening may be used in small and well-designed programs. The following procedures and criteria have been judged to be minimal:

1. A combination of tympanometry and acoustic reflex measurement should be used.
2. For eliciting the acoustic reflex, a signal of 105 dB HTL should be used in the contralateral mode, or a signal of 105 dB SPL in the ipsilateral mode, or both.

Table 16-18 PROPOSED CLASSIFICATION FOR SCREENING FOR OTITIS MEDIA
EMPLOYING TYMPANOMETRY AND ACOUSTIC REFLEX TESTING

Classification	Initial Screen	Retest	Subject Outcome
I	Acoustic reflex present and tympanogram normal	Not required	Cleared
II	Acoustic reflex absent and/or tympanogram normal	Acoustic reflex absent and/or tympanogram normal	Referred
III	Acoustic reflex absent and/or tympanogram abnormal	Acoustic reflex present and tympanogram normal	At risk—recheck at later date

From Harford, E. R., Bess, F. H., Bluestone, C. D., and Klein, J. O. (Eds.). 1978. Impedance Screening for Middle
Ear Disease in Children. New York, Grune and Stratton.

3. Whether broad-band noise or pure tone is preferable as an eliciting stimulus for the acoustic reflex remains to be established. A pure tone between 1000 Hz and 3000 Hz would be acceptable for this purpose. The stimulus should be specified or described, or both.

4. Acoustic reflex measurements can be obtained either with the ear canal air pressure that results in minimum acoustic impedance, or with ear canal air pressure equal to ambient pressure. The condition used should be specified.

5. For tympanometry, a 220 Hz probe tone is preferred.

6. For tympanometry, an air pressure range of −400 to +100 mm H_2O is preferred. However, a range of −300 to −100 mm H_2O is acceptable. Automatic recording should be used whenever possible, and the rate of air pressure change should be specified.

7. Failure on the initial screening test is denoted by either an absent acoustic reflex or an abnormal tympanogram. An abnormal tympanogram is defined as one that either (a) is flat or rounded (i.e., without a definite peak), or (b) has a peak at, or more negative than, −200 mm H_2O. Flat or rounded tympanograms appear to be more highly correlated with middle ear effusions than do tympanograms with peaks at negative pressure readings.

8. Any child failing the initial screening should be retested in four to six weeks. Parents or guardians should be advised accordingly. Any child who has an acoustic reflex and a normal tympanogram on the initial screening passes and is "cleared."

9. The schema in Table 16-18 is recommended for various screening findings. Classifications I and II should constitute the majority of children in a given population. Referral, when indicated after confirmatory retest, should be made to an appropriate health care provider in the community. Classification III constitutes a group of children who require special monitoring by the agency responsible for the screening program. These "at risk" children should be retested periodically to determine the best possible need for future medical referral.

10. An optimal time and frequency for screening or referring particular populations could not be advised because of lack of adequate information. Future research is needed.

11. The agency responsible for a testing program must have facilities available for referral that include expert management. Prior to the initiation of a screening program, referral and management procedures must be defined.

12. Impedance testing should be supervised by professionals who are qualified by training and experience to perform and interpret impedance measurements.

13. Programs should be designed to gather information of value in defining the role of impedance measurement in screening children for middle ear disease.

Special Populations

Because of high risk, serious consequences, or known high prevalence, certain populations of children warrant special consideration for early detection of, and surveillance for, middle ear disease, beginning soon after birth. These populations include children with known sensorineural hearing loss, developmentally delayed and mentally impaired children, children with cleft palate or other craniofacial anomalies, and native American children (Indian and Eskimo).

It was the conclusion of the Task Force that screening in infants and children should be carried out using the above criteria. However, they did emphasize the need for further research to clarify the epidemiology, natural history, and optimal clinical management of middle ear disease.

High Risk Populations

Cleft Palate

In patients with cleft palate, ear disease and hearing loss have long been recognized as common problems. This association was first reported by Alt in 1878, who noted hearing improvement following treatment of otorrhea associated with cleft palate. Thorington, in 1892, reported increased hearing in a patient following artificial correction of a destroyed palate. In 1893, Gutzmann noted hearing loss in one half of his patients with cleft palate. Lannois, in 1901, reported the association of middle ear disease and hearing loss in patients with cleft palate. In 1906, the need for otologic examination of patients with cleft palate was stressed by Brunck (1906). Since these early descriptions, many reports have appeared in the literature related to the incidence, nature, and degree of hearing loss in patients with cleft palate.

Hearing Loss

The prevalence of hearing loss in the cleft palate population, as reported in the literature, varies considerably. The findings of 35 recent reports are summarized in Table 16–19. These findings range from 0 per cent, reported by Goetzinger et al. (1960), to 90 per cent in the study of Sataloff and Fraser (1952), but of all the studies, the average prevalence is approximately 50 per cent. Even though the criteria of hearing loss were not generally agreed upon, it has been identified as conductive and usually bilateral. Halfond and Ballenger (1956) found that, of the 69 patients tested, 37 (54 per cent) had a hearing loss of 20 dB or greater. Miller (1956) reported that 19 (54 per cent) of 35 children with cleft palate had a hearing loss greater than 30 dB. That the prevalence may be even greater is suggested by Walton

Table 16–19 HEARING LOSS IN PATIENTS WITH CLEFT PALATE: REVIEW OF MORE THAN 20 YEARS' LITERATURE

Investigator(s)	Year	Patients	Per Cent Loss
Sataloff and Fraser	1952	30	90
Means and Irwin	1954	225	59
Holmes and Reed	1955	26	62
Lindsay et al.	1962	390	42
Berry and Eisenson	1956	383	60
Miller	1956	35	54
Halfond and Ballenger	1956	69	75
Whaley	1957	295	25
Pfisterer	1958	54	89
Skolnik	1958	401	39
Linthicum, Body, and Keaster	1959	58	40
Goetzinger et al.	1960	42	0
Drettner	1960	49	63
Masters, Bingham, and Robinson	1960	172	49
Spriesterbach et al.	1962	163	62
Graham and Lierle	1962	43	51
Graham	1963	190	22
Loeb	1964	108	42
Aschan	1966	82	40
Bennett, Ward, and Tait	1968	30	13
Pannbacker	1969	87	61
Yules	1970	69	58
Bennett	1972	100	58
Kaufman	1970	57	62
Heller et al.	1970	63	40
Harrison and Phillips	1971	9	100
Noone et al.	1973	147	47
Walton	1973	93	69
Korsan-Bengtsen	1974	60	32
Bess et al.	1975	40	48
Crysdale	1976	71	57
Bergstrom	1978	51	90
Potsic et al.	1979	138	46
Chaudhuri and Bowen-Jones	1978	100	63
Webster	1980	35	48

(1973), who studied 93 school-age children with cleft palate: one half of those who would have passed conventional audiometric screening at the 20 dB level were found to have air-bone gaps indicative of conductive hearing loss. This contention is supported by the study of Bluestone et al. (1973), who found high-viscosity middle ear effusions in children, including those with cleft palate, who would have passed a 25 dB screening audiogram. Even though a conductive hearing impairment would be expected, Bennett et al. (1968) reported 30 per cent of 100 adults with cleft palate had either sensorineural or mixed hearing loss. This finding might be explained by the work of Paparella et al. (1972), who found sensorineural hearing loss in some patients with otitis media, and ascribed this to directly associated pathologic changes in the inner ear, presumably mediated via the round window. Unfortunately, no information is available in the literature concerning hearing in the infant with cleft palate.

Aural Pathology

INFANTS

Variot, in 1904, was the first to report ear disease in an infant with cleft palate. In 1936, Beatty described "acute tubotympanic congestion frequently found between the ages of three months and two years." Sataloff and Fraser, in 1952, reported that, in their experience, "examination of the ears of very young children with cleft palate reveals a high incidence of pathologic changes, despite the absence of subjective symptoms of otitis media." In 1958, Skolnick reported that only 6 per cent of cleft palate patients below the age of one, and only 27 per cent of those between the ages of one and four years, had aural pathology. Linthicum and coworkers, however, in 1959, discovered ear pathology in 77 per cent of a group of 100 infants and children with cleft palate. In 1967, Stool and Randall reported that middle ear effusion was present at myringotomy in 94 per cent of 25 cleft palate infants. In 1969, Paradise and coworkers, employing standard office otoscopy, diagnosed middle ear disease in 49 of 50 infants with cleft palate. Most had full or bulging, opaque, immobile tympanic membranes, although spontaneous perforations and otorrhea were observed. Subsequent studies by the same team indicate that throughout the first two years of life in infants with unrepaired cleft palate, otitis media is a virtually constant complication (Bluestone, 1971; Paradise and Bluestone, 1971; Paradise and Bluestone, 1974). The otitis is usually characterized by an inflammatory effusion of variable viscosity; suppuration also occurs occasionally (Bluestone, 1971; Paradise, 1980).

OLDER CHILDREN AND ADULTS

Although the criteria of aural pathology in older children and adults with cleft palate vary considerably, its prevalence appears to be quite high. Meissner (1939) examined 213 such patients between the ages of 10 and 35 years and found that 83 per cent had abnormal tympanic membranes. Skolnick (1958) found that the prevalence of aural pathology was 67 per cent in patients above the age of five. Graham and Lierle (1962) found ear pathology in 44 per cent of 29 patients with cleft palate and in 55 per cent of 146 with a cleft of both palate and lip. In a group of 82 patients, Aschan (1966) found that 78 per cent had aural pathology. In a retrospective, longitudinal study of 191 patients with cleft palate between 5 and 27 years of age, Severeid (1972) reported that 83 per cent had a

middle ear effusion confirmed by myringotomy. In Bennett's study (1972) of 100 adults with cleft palate, 30 per cent had aural pathology consisting of signs of eustachian tube obstruction (13 per cent), chronic suppurative otitis media with or without mastoiditis (8 per cent), dry tympanic membrane perforation (6 per cent), and chronic adhesive otitis media (3 per cent).

Schools and Programs for the Deaf

Severely deaf to profoundly deaf children (primarily those whose hearing loss is sensorineural), whether enrolled in a special class in a regular school ("mainstreamed") or in a residential school for the deaf, are of particular concern. Should a conductive hearing loss secondary to chronic or recurrent otitis media with effusion or high negative pressure or both be superimposed on the pre-existing hearing loss, auditory input may be severely affected. This may critically interfere with the education of such children (Ruben and Math, 1978).

The incidence of middle ear problems in deaf children has not been studied systematically, but the few studies that have been reported indicate the incidence to be equal to or possibly higher than that in nondeaf children. Porter (1974) found that 25 per cent of 79 deaf children aged six to ten years had abnormal tympanograms. Brooks (1974) reported that five year old children in a residential school for the deaf in England had a higher incidence of abnormal tympanograms than did nondeaf children. Mehta and Erlich (1978) found a high incidence of otitis media with effusion in children in a school for the deaf. Rubin (1978) reported the incidence of middle ear effusion in children three to six years of age to be 30 per cent. Over a period of one year, Stool and coworkers (1980) conducted otoscopic, tympanometric, and audiometric evaluations on 446 students at the Western Pennsylvania School for the Deaf and reported that the incidence of middle ear effusions was 8 per cent, while that of high negative middle ear pressure was 21 per cent. However, the incidence of otitis media with effusion in this study was 26 per cent in the two to five year age group. In addition, they found that 79 per cent of the students who initially were identified as having high negative middle ear pressure consistently had abnormal negative pressures during the one year observation period.

From these few studies, it is apparent that

continuous surveillance for middle ear disease and early treatment should be part of every program or school for deaf children. This is especially critical for those children with some residual hearing who benefit from amplification, since even the slightest conductive hearing loss may decrease or eliminate the efficacy of amplification. It is recommended that every school for deaf children be afforded appropriate health care professionals who are competent in otoscopy, tympanometry, audiometry, and treatment of otologic disorders to carry out this program. Most schools for the deaf do not have sufficient provisions for such care of the child.

Because the external canals of deaf children are frequently obstructed with cerumen, frequent examination and removal of the cerumen may be extremely beneficial, especially for those who wear a hearing aid (Riding et al., 1978b). This finding alone is reason enough for frequent periodic otologic examination; however, a schedule for screening for otitis media with effusion and high negative pressure should be established. Until a formal long-term study has been completed which will offer recommendations for a screening program in schools for the deaf, we propose the following schedule of examinations of such children, based on the findings of Findlay et al. (1977), Riding et al. (1978b), Craig et al. (1979), and Stool et al. (1980): all children should have an otoscopic, tympanometric, and audiometric examination upon entering the school and periodically during the first school year (Table 16–20). Since infants and young children are at highest risk, they should be examined once a

month by otoscopy (and tympanometry when indicated) during this first year. Older children and adolescents probably can be evaluated upon entry and every three months during the first year, since the incidence of middle ear disease in this age group is less than in the younger age group. All students should be examined during periods of upper respiratory tract infection and whenever there are signs or symptoms related to the ear, such as otalgia or otorrhea. In addition, a child should be examined if the teacher or parent suspects a middle ear problem owing to a noticeable lack of attention, sudden or gradual failure to benefit from amplification, or overt and progressive loss of hearing. After the first year of follow-up the children will usually separate into one of four groups, based on the occurrence of otitis media with effusion or high negative pressure or both: (1) no disease; (2) infrequent disease and when present, of short duration; (3) frequently recurrent disease; and (4) chronic disease. Infants and young children who fit into either of the first two categories based on the examination of the first year, may be examined at less frequent intervals, such as every two to three months during the second year. Older children who have no evidence of disease during the first year probably can be examined once a year, either upon entering in the fall or, more ideally, during the winter months. Older children with infrequent problems during the first year should probably be examined every three months during the second year. All infants and children who have frequently recurrent or chronic middle ear disease during the first year must be

Table 16–20 SUGGESTED SCREENING FOR MIDDLE EAR DISEASE IN PROGRAMS AND SCHOOLS FOR DEAF CHILDREN

	Population Groups				
	Infants and Young Children (also multiply handicapped children of all ages)		Older Children and Adolescents		
First Year Upon Entry					
Frequency of examination	Monthly[*]		Every Three Months[*]		
Experience at the end of the first year	No disease or infrequent and of short duration	Frequently recurrent and/or chronic	No disease	Infrequent and of short duration	Frequently recurrent and/or chronic
Second Year					
And each succeeding year until experience changes	Every 2–3 months[*]	Monthly[*]	Yearly	Every 3 months[*]	Monthly[*]

[*]And with every upper respiratory tract infection and/or otologic signs and symptoms, e.g., otalgia, otorrhea.

examined every month and with each upper respiratory tract infection until they, too, have a year without significant problems. Screening during the succeeding years should be related to the middle ear disease experience in the preceding year. Children who have multiple handicaps, in addition to deafness, are considered to be at high risk for middle ear disease, which can significantly compound their handicap owing to the attendant conductive hearing loss. Therefore, screening for all such students during the first year should be the program recommended for infants and young children.

Ideally, every examination should be conducted by a physician who is expert in the diseases of the middle ear, but this is not always feasible. Therefore, a nurse should be trained to perform routine otoscopy, examination of the nose and throat, and removal of cerumen from the external canal when present. Tympanometry can be performed by the nurse, a technician, or, if available, an audiologist. Even though an otologist cannot examine every child with the frequency recommended, every school for the deaf must have a physician, preferably an otologist, assigned to the school for diagnosis and treatment of those children found to have middle ear disease.

It is important that all children with severe or profound deafness be considered to be at risk for developing middle ear disease. Therefore, they should have regular periodic examinations of the ear by competent health care professionals and appropriate early management instituted so that their educational handicap is not further compromised by a condition that is amenable to medical or surgical management.

Other Possible High-Risk Populations

Infants and children who have parents and/or siblings with otitis media with effusion appear to have a greater risk of developing otitis media with effusion than do those whose parents and/or siblings have no evidence of disease. Teele et al. (1980b) studied 2565 infants from birth to their third birthdays. They found that children who had single or recurrent episodes of otitis media were more likely to have parents and/or siblings with histories of significant middle ear infections than were children who had no episodes of otitis media. Therefore, children whose siblings have had otitis media are at higher risk and should have more frequent

otologic examinations than children whose siblings have not had the disease.

Upper respiratory allergy is thought to be involved in the etiology of otitis media and therefore requires close surveillance. Even though there is no proof that children who have an upper respiratory allergy have a higher incidence of otitis media than do children without such an allergy, they should be examined frequently for possible occurrence of otitis media.

Other possible risk factors, such as prematurity or some other reason for placing the infant in a neonatal ICU (Berman et al., 1978), first episode of otitis media during early infancy (Howie et al., 1975), malnutrition, and child abuse (Downs, 1980), are not proven but warrant consideration for close surveillance until these factors are disproven by further studies.

Radiography

Radiographs of the mastoids are not routinely obtained in patients with acute or chronic middle ear effusions but are indicated when intratemporal or intracranial complications are suspected or present. Longstanding eustachian tube dysfunction is usually associated with a poorly pneumatized mastoid air cell system as visualized on routine mastoid radiographs. Effusion in a well-pneumatized mastoid may appear as clouding of the air cell system but is not indicative of mastoid ("coalescent" mastoiditis) unless there is cell breakdown. Sinus radiographs, including a lateral view of the nasopharynx, are useful in assessing sinusitis and adenoid enlargement, respectively (see Chapter 8C).

Allergy Testing

Allergy testing is indicated in those patients who have recurrent acute or chronic middle ear effusions in association with signs and symptoms of allergy of the upper respiratory tract. Methods are discussed in Chapter 37.

MANAGEMENT

Since the different stages of otitis media with effusion and atelectasis are most frequently a continuum and since it is often

Table 16–21 OPTIONS FOR MANAGING VARIOUS STAGES OF OTITIS MEDIA WITH EFFUSION AND ATELECTASIS OF THE TYMPANIC MEMBRANE

Antimicrobials
Decongestants
Antihistamines
Corticosteroids
Immunization
Hyposensitization (allergy control)
Inflation of eustachian tube–middle ear
Myringotomy with or without tympanostomy tube
Adenoidectomy with or without tonsillectomy
Tympanoplasty
Tympanomastoidectomy
Watchful waiting with or without hearing aid

difficult for the clinician to diagnose the precise stage of a patient's illness accurately, the most common methods of managing these problems will be discussed as they relate to the specific condition. However, before presenting these methods of management in detail, summary of each stage and an overview of the treatment options available will be helpful (Table 16–21).

Acute Otitis Media

At present, antimicrobials are the mainstay of therapy for infants and children with signs and symptoms of acute otitis media. Since most clinicians rarely perform a tympanocentesis or myringotomy initially, the organism causing the otitis is usually not known with certainty before treatment begins. However, the physician can be guided in his selection of the appropriate antibiotic by a knowledge of the pathogenic organisms that have most frequently been aspirated from the ears of children with acute otitis media in the community. The recommended therapeutic dose of the antimicrobial should be administered for 10 days (American Academy of Pediatrics, 1977), although there are no studies available that have shown the most effective duration of antimicrobial therapy. During this period, the parents should be instructed to notify the clinician if the child fails to show a satisfactory clinical improvement. If there is persistence or recurrence of otalgia or fever, or both, then the child should be reexamined before the completion of the antibiotic course. For certain children in whom severe signs and symptoms of acute infection are present, or for social considerations (e.g., poor home environment), it may be more

advantageous to reexamine the child 48 to 72 hours after initiating therapy. However, at this time the appearance of the tympanic membrane alone should not determine a change in the treatment. Almost all children will have a persistent middle ear effusion, and even erythema and bulging of the tympanic membrane may still be present. Persistent pain or fever, or both, would signal the need either for surgical intervention or for selection of another antimicrobial agent, or for both. Tympanocentesis with or without a myringotomy should be offered as a logical management option in such cases, since culture of the middle ear effusion may reveal the presence of an unusual organism. Further antimicrobial treatment should be based on the results of the culture. If surgery is not feasible (the parents or child might refuse surgery, in which case an otolaryngologist should be consulted), then a new antibiotic should be administered. This antibiotic should be chosen to be effective against whatever unusual bacteria have been found to be in the community and have been associated with the treatment failures during the first 10 days. An example of this situation would be the presence of *H. influenzae* that is resistant to ampicillin. In patients with unusually severe earache or toxicity, tympanocentesis and myringotomy may be performed initially in order to provide immediate relief. Tympanocentesis (and possibly myringotomy) should also be performed if the child develops acute otitis media while he has been taking an antimicrobial agent for another condition when the drug he has been taking should have been effective against the common pathogens that cause otitis. When therapeutic drainage is required for the indications that will be outlined, a myringotomy knife should be used and the incision should be large enough to allow for adequate drainage of the middle ear.

During the acute phase of otitis media, a spontaneous perforation with otorrhea may develop, or in some cases the child may present initially with a discharge from the ear. When otorrhea is present, either at the first evaluation or at any time during this phase, meticulous cleaning of the external auditory canal, culture of the discharge from the middle ear, and treatment with instillation of topical antibiotic-cortisone ear drops may be helpful (see Chapter 17, p. 518).

Children may be reexamined at the end of the course of antibiotic therapy, i.e., after 10 to 14 days. At this time, some chil-

Table 16–22   PERCENTAGE OF PERSISTENT MIDDLE EAR EFFUSION AFTER INITIATING ANTIBIOTIC TREATMENT° FOR ACUTE OTITIS MEDIA

Investigator(s)	No. of Subjects	Per Cent with Middle Ear Effusion After:			
		10–14 Days	4 Weeks	8 Weeks	12 Weeks
Roddey, Earle, and Haggerty, 1966	121	35	7	2	—
Herberts et al., 1971	81	10	—	—	—
Pelton, Shurin, and Klein, 1977	93	—	38	—	—
Lorentzen and Haugsten, 1977	190	16 (est)	6	—	—
Shurin, Pelton, and Klein, 1976	33	72	—	—	—
Bluestone et al., 1979b	55	69	—	—	—
Puhakka et al., 1979	90	58	29	—	—
Teele, Klein, and Rosner, 1980	1821	70	40	20	10
Thomsen et al., 1980	75	50	33	—	25
Quarnberg and Palva, 1980	151	50	—	—	—
Schwartz, Rodriguez, and Schwartz, 1981	222	50	23	12	8

°No initial myringotomy performed.

dren will have a persistent middle ear effusion. Table 16–22 shows this proportion to be 16 to 72 per cent of those treated with antibiotics. (This wide range is probably related to one or more of the following sources of inconsistency among various studies reported: age of the child, definition of acute otitis media, mode of treatment, and criteria for persistence of effusion.) Regardless of the exact incidence of such cases, persistent middle ear effusion after a two-week trial of an antimicrobial agent is common (occurring in approximately 50 per cent of children), and this finding alone is not sufficient grounds for performing surgery such as a myringotomy and tympanostomy tube insertion.

Additional supportive therapy, including analgesics, antipyretics, and local heat, will usually be helpful. In some instances, meperidine hydrochloride may also be required for sedation. An oral decongestant, such as pseudoephedrine hydrochloride, may relieve nasal congestion, and antihistamines may help patients with known or suspected nasal allergy. However, the efficacy of antihistamines and decongestants in the treatment of acute otitis media has not been proven. Olsen et al. (1978) failed to show efficacy of an oral decongestant when administered in conjunction with an antibiotic for children with acute otitis media. Complete clearing of the effusion may take six weeks or longer. Within two to three months the tympanic membrane should be entirely normal. If complete resolution has occurred and the episode represents the only known attack, the patient may be discharged. However, periodic follow-up is indicated for patients who have had recurrent episodes.

If the middle ear fluid is persistent after the initial 10 days of antimicrobial therapy, one or more of the following treatment options have been advocated to hasten the resolution of the effusion during the next, *subacute*, phase:

1. A course of an antimicrobial agent different from the initial one, based on the hope that if a resistant organism is present the new antimicrobial agent may be effective
2. A topical or systemic nasal decongestant or antihistamine, or a combination of these drugs
3. Eustachian tube–middle ear inflation employing the method of Valsalva or Politzer
4. A tympanocentesis or myringotomy, or both, for culture of the aspirate and drainage of the middle ear.

Unfortunately, these commonly employed methods appear to be helpful but have not been shown to be effective in randomized, controlled trials of children with subacute otitis media with effusion. At present, the best treatment for children who have asymptomatic otitis media with effusion still present after two weeks is watchful waiting with reexamination of the ears six weeks later, i.e., two months after the initial visit. At this time, most patients should have a middle ear that is effusion-free (Table 16–22). However, treatment with another antimicrobial agent that is effective against possible resistant bacteria is a reasonable alternative, especially if such organisms have been isolated from subacute effusions in the community. If the child still has otitis media with effusion after two or three months, the effusion is chronic and should be treated as described under the heading "Chronic Otitis Media with Effusion," p. 437.

The method of management of acute otitis media may vary with the age of the patient. Acute otitis media during the neonatal period may warrant more aggressive management than such a condition in an older child. Bland (1972) reported that otitis media in neonates was frequently caused by an unusual organism as compared with those which usually cause such problems in older infants and in children, i.e., gram-negative bacilli, or *S. aureus*. Following this report, many authorities advocated treating these babies in the hospital according to protocols for neonatal sepsis, since the infection could be life-threatening. However, since then other investigators (Shurin et al., 1976; Tetzlaff et al., 1977; Schwartz et al., 1978b; Shurin et al., 1978) have shown that the incidence of these unusual organisms is relatively low, especially in neonates who were apparently well when discharged from the hospital following birth and then developed an acute otitis media while at home. For these neonates, the acute otitis media should be treated as described above for older infants and children. However, if the neonate appears to be severely ill and toxic, hospitalization and a tympanocentesis and possibly a myringotomy are indicated. If the baby remains hospitalized because of other medical problems and develops an otitis media, tympanocentesis (and myringotomy) are indicated. Culture of the middle ear aspirate may reveal an unusual organism that would require treatment with an antimicrobial agent different from the antibiotics recommended for treatment of acute otitis media in older children.

The management of acute otitis media may be different in certain infants and children whose underlying condition is known to be associated with otitis caused by an unusual organism. Such children would be primarily those who are immunologically compromised. Tympanocentesis possibly followed by a myringotomy would be indicated in an effort to identify the causative organisms and to promote drainage.

Recurrent Acute Otitis Media

It is not uncommon for an infant to have recurrent bouts of acute otitis media. Some children develop an acute episode with almost every respiratory tract infection, have more or less dramatic symptoms, respond well to therapy, and improve with advancing age. Others may have persistent middle ear effusion and suffer recurrent episodes of acute otitis media superimposed on the chronic disorder. The child with recurrent acute otitis media who completely clears between episodes may be managed as previously outlined. However, if the bouts are frequent and close together, prevention of further attacks is desirable. The patient requires further evaluation. Several avenues of investigation are open: a search for respiratory allergy may prove fruitful; roentgenograms of the paranasal sinuses may reveal sinusitis; immunologic studies may be of value if other organs are involved (the lung, for example). In addition, more thorough physical examination may reveal abnormalities, such as submucous cleft palate or a tumor of the nasopharynx, that require definitive management. If none of the above conditions is present, then one or more of the popular methods of prevention may be attempted; however, the efficacy of these various modalities has yet to be proven in acceptable clinical trials. For infants and children who have frequent episodes (such as three or more episodes within the preceding six months) of acute otitis media without middle ear effusion in between the bouts, the most common nonsurgical and surgical methods currently employed for prevention are (1) chemoprophylaxis with one or more of the following — antibiotics, topical or systemic nasal decongestants, and antihistamines; (2) myringotomy with or without tympanostomy tubes; (3) adenoidectomy with or without tonsillectomy. More recently, the administration of polyvalent pneumococcal vaccine has been advocated, but the vaccine is of limited efficacy in infants, an age group in which recurrent otitis has its highest incidence.

Antimicrobial prophylaxis has been studied in the past and appears to reduce some of the signs and symptoms of acute otitis, i.e., otorrhea, otalgia. In these investigations, sulfonamide (Ensign, et al., 1960; Perrin et al., 1974; Biedel, 1978) and ampicillin (Maynard et al., 1972) have been the antimicrobial agents employed. None of these studies addressed the possibility that an asymptomatic effusion might have been present within the middle ear. However, until further, more convincing, studies are reported, prophylaxis employing an antimicrobial agent seems to be a reasonable option at present. A daily dose of an antimicrobial agent that is effective against the pathogens that are commonly found in the middle ears of children with acute otitis media would be appropriate. Parental and patient compliance in administering and taking the medication daily is a consideration, as are the potential risks of drug toxicity and possible emergence of resistant organisms while on the medication. Since the studies reported in the past have shown that some children still have recurrent episodes of acute otitis media in spite of the preventive dose of the antibiotic, and since there is a possibility that an asymptomatic effusion may be present, infants and children who are receiving antimicrobial prophylaxis should be reexamined at relatively frequent intervals. In addition, signs and symptoms of eustachian tube dysfunction may persist, such as pain, fluctuating hearing loss, and vertigo, or severe atelectasis may develop.

At present, there is no evidence that a topical or systemic nasal decongestant or antihistamine, either alone or in combination, administered daily or at the onset of an upper respiratory tract infection, prevents recurrent acute otitis media. Therefore, the use of such medications for prophylaxis is not recommended until their efficacy is proved.

It has been suggested that a myringotomy performed at the initial onset of an attack of acute otitis media would reduce the recurrence rate of this problem (Diamant and Diamant, 1974); however, this was not shown in a study by Lorentzen and Haugsten (1977). At present, myringotomy as the initial treatment for acute otitis media remains optional and should be considered only in selected patients. Nevertheless, myringotomy with insertion of tympanostomy tubes is commonly performed to prevent recurrent episodes of acute otitis media. The procedure is usually performed after the signs and symptoms of the acute otitis media have resolved, but it may be performed during an acute episode if persistent otalgia or fever, or both, are present in a child who has had frequently recurrent episodes. In some children, insertion of tympanostomy tubes will prevent the severe symptoms of acute otitis media, but recurrent episodes will occur. Systemic antimicrobial agents or ototopical antibiotic-cortisone medication, or both, will usually be effective in resolving the otitis media in the child with tympanostomy tubes in place.

Adenoidectomy with or without tonsillectomy is frequently advocated for the prevention of recurrent acute otitis media, but the randomized, controlled studies reported in the past have not proven the efficacy of these procedures for this condition (Bluestone, 1979). At present, adenoidectomy with or without tonsillectomy, when recurrent otitis media is the only indication, should be considered only of possible benefit until further clinical studies are reported.

In summary, the parents of a child who has frequently recurrent episodes of acute otitis media in whom the effusion appears to clear between bouts should be offered the following management options: (1) antimicrobial treatment of each episode; (2) antimicrobial prophylaxis; (3) myringotomy and tympanostomy tube insertion; or (4) possible polyvalent pneumococcal vaccination if the patient is two years of age or older. The treatment option selected should involve the parents and possibly the child (if old enough) in the decision-making process. A few parents choose to watch and wait if the episodes have been mild or relatively infrequent.* At present, the decision should be between administering an antibiotic in a prophylactic dose or a myringotomy and insertion of a tympanostomy tube. Since neither of these two procedures has been shown to be superior to the other, or even to watchful waiting, the decision should be based upon the parents' and (child's) willingness to have the child take daily medications as a preventive measure or to have surgery performed on the child's ear, which usually involves the administration of general anesthetic. The possibility of an adverse reaction occurring with either method should be discussed fully with the family. Usually a decision in favor of one of the treatment options is arrived at by this method, since some parents are unwilling to give a daily antibiotic or are concerned about the possible side effects of long-term antibiotic treatment, while on the other hand other parents are concerned about the possible complications and sequelae of tympanostomy tube insertion or complications of a general anesthetic, or both. If the parents are undecided, then a trial of antimicrobial prophylaxis can be offered with the option to perform a myringotomy and tympanostomy tube insertion if the chemoprophylaxis fails to prevent recurrent otitis media or the signs or symptoms of eustachian tube dysfunction persist.

---

*Use of pneumococcal vaccine in children 2 years old or older may be considered as an adjunct to these options.

For the rarely encountered child in whom tympanostomy tubes fail to prevent frequently recurrent acute otitis media, i.e., otorrhea through the tube, the combination of both antimicrobial prophlaxis and tympanostomy tubes is usually effective in preventing the recurrent episodes.

The above management options should be offered only to those children in whom chronic middle ear effusion is not present between episodes. If recurrent bouts of acute otitis media are superimposed on the chronic condition, the child should be treated as described below for management of chronic otitis media with effusion.

Chronic Otitis Media with Effusion

A middle ear effusion that has persisted for three months or longer is chronic and treatment should be considered, since there are possible complications and sequelae associated with this stage. However, since little information is currently available regarding the incidence of these complications and sequelae, and since the natural history of these chronic effusions has not been studied completely, some thoughtful clinicians would take a watch-and-wait position and not actively treat such a child. However, hearing loss of some degree always accompanies a middle ear effusion. Although the significance of this hearing loss is still uncertain, such a loss may impair cognitive and language function and result in disturbances in psychosocial adjustment. With these uncertainties in mind, the clinician should decide whether or not to treat or to watch, and, if treatment is decided upon, which treatment option or options appear to be most appropriate in eliminating the chronic effusion in the individual child. Many factors should be considered in this decision-making process. A child with a unilateral, asymptomatic chronic otitis media with effusion, in whom there is only a mild hearing loss and in whom there are no serious secondary changes in the tympanic membrane, *may* be a candidate for watchful waiting. Conversely, a child with bilateral chronic middle ear effusions who has an associated marked hearing loss would be a more likely candidate for active treatment. Important factors that should be considered in addition to hearing loss when deciding to treat or not to treat (and which treatment) would be one or more of the following: (1)

otalgia, especially when associated with recurrent acute otitis media; (2) vertigo; (3) tinnitus; (4) alterations of the tympanic membrane, such as severe atelectasis, especially a deep retraction pocket in the posterosuperior quadrant or the pars flaccida, or both; (5) middle ear changes such as adhesive otitis, tympanosclerosis, or ossicular involvement; or (6) any of the other intratemporal complications or sequelae associated with otitis media with effusion (see Chapter 17).

Before embarking on a nonsurgical or surgical method of management of chronic effusion, a thorough search for an underlying etiology (i.e., paranasal sinusitis, upper respiratory allergy, submucous cleft palate) should be attempted as described previously for children who suffer from recurrent acute otitis media.

Of the many methods of management that are available for chronic otitis media with effusion, none has been shown to be effective in acceptable clinical trials. However, the clinician is forced to make decisions to treat actively or not treat (watchful waiting); and, if treatment is decided upon, which of the surgical or nonsurgical treatment options would be reasonable and most appropriate for the individual child. The most rational approach initially should be a trial of one or more of the nonsurgical methods, and if the effusion is still persistent, then either periodic observation or surgical intervention should be considered. The decision between these latter options should be based upon the signs and symptoms present and should consider the potential complications and sequelae of both.

Of all the medical treatments that have been advocated, a trial of an antimicrobial agent would appear to be most appropriate in those children who have not received an antibiotic recently. Since bacteria similar to those found in acute otitis media have been isolated from a significant proportion of middle ear aspirates in children with chronic otitis media with effusion (Senturia et al., 1958; Liu et al., 1976; Healy and Teele, 1977; Riding et al., 1978a; Stanievich et al., 1981), the antibiotic chosen and duration of treatment should be the same as recommended for children who have acute otitis media. The use of the other popular medical forms of therapy such as topical nasal or oral decongestants, antihistamines, adrenocorticosteroids, immunotherapy, either alone or in some combination, must remain optional at present, since convincing studies are lacking. Middle ear inflation employing the method of Valsalva or Politzer can also be used, but again, proof of efficacy has yet to be shown.

If nonsurgical methods of management fail, then surgical intervention should be considered. Myringotomy with aspiration of the middle ear effusion would appear to be appropriate in those children in whom the procedure can be performed without the aid of a general anesthetic, since a second myringotomy with or without the insertion of a tympanostomy tube would be indicated if the effusion is present soon after the myringotomy incision heals, i.e., if the disease is persistent. It is desirable to avoid the risk of administering a second general anesthetic: if a myringotomy is elected and general anesthesia is required, a tympanostomy tube should be inserted at the time of the initial myringotomy to preclude, if possible, the necessity of performing a second procedure under general anesthesia should a tube later be required. This method of management appears at present to be the most reasonable. The efficacy of adenoidectomy with or without tonsillectomy either alone or in combination with a myringotomy and with or without a tympanostomy tube insertion has yet to be shown. Following spontaneous expulsion of the tympanostomy tube, reinsertion for recurrence of effusion would be indicated only after appropriate nonsurgical treatment options have failed and the effusion has persisted for two to three months.

In some children the procedure must be repeated for several years until the child grows older. For children who have had chronic otitis media with effusion that appears to be resistant to the methods or management described above, mastoidectomy has been advocated (Proud and Duff, 1976), but this procedure is rarely indicated and should be reserved for those children in whom mastoid osteitis or a cholesteatoma is suspected, since almost all chronic effusions are at least temporarily eliminated following tympanostomy tube insertion.

Atelectasis of the Tympanic Membrane–Middle Ear and High Negative Middle Ear Pressure

Atelectasis of the tympanic membrane can be either acute or chronic, localized or generalized, and mild or severe, and it may or may not be associated with abnormal negative middle ear pressure. Retraction of the tympanic membrane may be secondary to the presence of high negative pressure. However, a flaccid, atelectatic tympanic membrane may not be associated with high negative intratympanic pressure: the abnormal negative pressure may have been the original cause of such a condition of the membrane but may no longer be present. Localized atelectasis or a retraction pocket may be seen in the area of a healed perforation or at the site where a tympanostomy tube had been inserted ("atrophic scar" or dimeric membrane). A retraction pocket in the posterosuperior portion of the pars tensa or a pars flaccida retraction pocket is more frequently associated with the development of more serious sequelae (ossicular discontinuity or cholesteatoma) than is a retraction pocket in other areas of the tympanic membrane. These variations should be kept in mind when deciding how to manage atelectasis.

If a chronic middle ear effusion is present concurrently with atelectasis, then the child should be treated as previously outlined for patients with chronic otitis media with effusion. However, whether or not a middle ear effusion is present, if a chronic severe retraction pocket of the posterosuperior area of the pars tensa or of the pars flaccida or both is present, a myringotomy and insertion of a tympanostomy tube should be performed to prevent possible irreversible changes in the middle ear. Following insertion of a tympanostomy tube, the tympanic membrane in the area of the retraction pocket should return to a more neutral position within several weeks or months, but if the retraction area remains adherent to the ossicles or middle ear or both (Fig. 16–51), then adhesive otitis media is present, and a tympanoplasty should be considered to prevent further progression of the disease process (such as ossicular discontinuity or cholesteatoma formation, or both). Even though this method of management has not been tested in appropriately controlled clinical trials and the natural history of retraction pockets in these areas has not been studied adequately, this method of management would appear to be reasonable at present (Bluestone et al., 1977a).

For less severe cases in which the atelectasis of the tympanic membrane is apparently not associated with a middle ear effusion and a retraction pocket is not present in the posterosuperior portion or pars flaccida, the

RETRACTION POCKET-ATELECTASIS

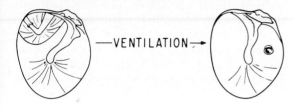

RETRACTION POCKET-ADHESIVE OTITIS

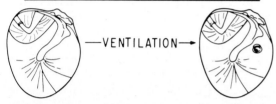

Figure 16–51 When a retraction pocket is in the posterosuperior portion of the pars tensa of the tympanic membrane and adhesive otitis media is not present between the eardrum and ossicles, the insertion of a tympanostomy tube may return the tympanic membrane to the neutral position. However, if adhesive otitis media is present, the retraction pocket will persist in spite of the presence of a tympanostomy tube and middle ear ventilation.

management options become less obvious and more controversial. Generalized atelectasis, or even a localized area that is retracted for only a short time (acute retraction), is usually secondary to transient high negative middle ear pressure associated with an acute upper respiratory tract infection (and occasionally due to barotrauma). This condition is quite common in children and usually is self-limited. No specific treatment should be directed toward the middle ear unless the child complains of severe otalgia, hearing loss, tinnitus, or vertigo. The atelectasis (and high negative intratympanic pressure) and associated symptoms, if present, will usually subside when the acute upper respiratory tract infection disappears. Treatment at this time should be directed toward relief of the nasal symptoms. Topical or systemic nasal decongestants may provide relief of these symptoms and may also decongest the eustachian tube, although their effectiveness in this latter area has not yet been shown. If the symptoms become severe enough, a myringotomy may be necessary to provide relief by returning middle ear pressure to ambient. Inflation of the eustachian tube–middle ear employing the methods of Valsalva or Po-

litzer, or eustachian tube catheterization, has been advocated and has merit from a physiologic standpoint, but controlled trials have not been reported to demonstrate the efficacy of these methods.

When the atelectasis is chronic and there is no evidence of a deep retraction pocket in the posterosuperior quadrant or pars flaccida, a thorough search should be made for an underlying etiology as described previously for recurrent acute or chronic otitis media with effusion. If none is found, then the management options include only watchful waiting and active treatment. The decision for or against treatment should rest on the presence or absence of other, associated symptoms, and whether or not there is abnormal negative pressure within the middle ear. The presence of persistent or transient otalgia, hearing loss, vertigo, or tinnitus that is troublesome to the patient warrants active treatment. For chronic atelectasis in this case, a trial with a topical or systemic nasal decongestant with or without an antihistamine may be helpful; however, this type of treatment is often disappointing. Inflation of the eustachian tube–middle ear may provide temporary relief but usually must be repeated for permanent control of the symptoms and to maintain the tympanic membrane in a more normal position. For most children, a myringotomy with insertion of a tympanostomy tube will usually be necessary to provide long-term relief. The procedure will prevent the sustained or transient high negative pressure secondary to eustachian tube obstruction which is responsible for the active retraction of the tympanic membrane. If the severely atelectatic tympanic membrane does not return to a more normal position after the insertion of the tympanostomy tube or if the tube cannot be inserted owing to lack of a suitable aerated space within the middle ear, a tympanoplasty should be considered.

When a flaccid tympanic membrane is passively collapsed upon the ossicles and middle ear and high negative middle ear pressure is not present, the nonsurgical and surgical management options described above may not be effective in restoring the tympanic membrane to a more normal position. Fortunately, symptoms of high negative middle ear pressure and eustachian tube obstruction are frequently absent so that no treatment may be necessary. Even myringotomy and tympanostomy tube insertion may not be beneficial, since the tympanic membrane is no longer actively being retracted by high negative middle ear pressure. In addition, at this stage, adhesive otitis media may also be present so that portions of the tympanic membrane may be adherent to the middle ear. In such cases there are two management options: tympanoplasty or periodic (once or twice a year) observation (see section on Cholesteatoma (Keratoma) and Retraction Pocket in Chapter 17).

Eustachian Tube Dysfunction

Otitis media with effusion and atelectasis with or without effusion are usually the result of dysfunction of the eustachian tube. However, abnormal function of the eustachian tube may cause otologic symptoms without an apparent effusion or severe atelectasis. The tympanic membrane may have a normal appearance and mobility may be unimpaired when tested by pneumatic otoscopy or by tympanometry. Two types of eustachian tube dysfunction can be present: obstruction or abnormal patency. When the eustachian tube is obstructed but no effusion is present, the tube periodically opens to ventilate the middle ear cavity but at less frequent intervals than normal; in this case high negative intratympanic pressure may be present for relatively long periods. This type of intermittent middle ear ventilation may cause periods of otalgia, a feeling of fullness or pressure, hearing loss, popping and snapping noises, tinnitus, and even vertigo. Management of this situation should be similar to that described for generalized atelectasis of the tympanic membrane. If the condition is present only during an acute upper respiratory tract infection, medical treatment should be directed toward relief of the nasal congestion. If the symptoms are of a chronic nature, a search for an underlying cause should be attempted, and if found, appropriate management instituted. If no underlying cause is uncovered, then a trial with a decongestant or antihistamines or both may be helpful, or eustachian tube–middle ear inflation may be tried. However, if the nonsurgical methods are not successful, then myringotomy and insertion of a tympanostomy tube may be necessary.

At the other end of the spectrum of eustachian tube dysfunction is abnormal patency. In its extreme form, the hyperpatent eustachian tube is open even at rest, i.e., patulous.

Lesser degrees of abnormal patency result in a semipatulous eustachian tube that is closed at rest but has low tubal resistance to airflow in comparison to the normal tube. A patulous eustachian tube may be due to abnormal tube geometry or to a decrease in extramural pressure, such as occurs as a result of weight loss or possibly as a result of mural or intraluminal changes. These latter may be seen when the extracellular fluid is altered by medical treatment of another, unrelated condition. Interruption of the innervation of the tensor veli palatini muscle has also been shown to be a cause of a hyperpatent eustachian tube (Perlman, 1939).

Clinically, a patulous eustachian tube may be present in adolescents and adults but is rarely seen in young children. The patient frequently complains of hearing his/her own breathing in the ear or of autophony. Otoscopic examination reveals a tympanic membrane that moves medially on inspiration and laterally on expiration; the movement can be exaggerated with forced respiration. The condition is relieved when the patient is recumbent, since eustachian tube extramural pressure is increased by paratubal venous engorgement in this position. The patient should therefore be examined in the sitting position. The diagnosis can also be made by measuring the impedance of the middle ear (Bluestone, 1980). A tympanogram should be obtained while the patient is breathing normally and a second one obtained while the patient holds his breath. Fluctuation in the tympanometric line should coincide with breathing. The fluctuation can be exaggerated by asking the patient to occlude one nostril and close the mouth during forced inspiration and expiration, or by performing the Toynbee or Valsalva maneuver.

Management of a patulous eustachian tube depends on first determining the etiology of the problem. If the symptoms are of relatively short duration, the condition may subside without any active treatment. In children and teenagers this condition is usually self-limited and probably related to changes in the structure and function of the eustachian tube and adjacent areas secondary to rapid growth and development. When a medication can be identified as the agent responsible, cessation of the medication usually alleviates the problem. However, in most instances the condition is idiopathic. When the symptoms are disturbing and the condition is chronic, active treatment is indicated. A myringotomy with insertion of a tympanostomy tube may be performed but usually does not alter the symptoms in most cases and occasionally will result in increasing the patient's discomfort. Insufflation of powders into the eustachian tube (the Bezold treatment — insufflation of boric and salicylic acid powder) and instillation of 2 per cent iodine or 5 per cent trichloroacetic acid solution have also been advocated (Mawson, 1974). Infusion of an absorbable gelatin sponge solution has also been suggested (Ogawa et al., 1976), as has injection of polytetrafluoroethylene (Teflon) into the paratubal area (Pulec, 1967), but all of these methods have major disadvantages. Changes produced by these methods are, for the most part, irreversible and may not improve the condition or may provide only temporary relief. Total obstruction of the eustachian tube can also be a complication. Stroud et al. (1974) have suggested the transposition of the tensor veli palatini through a palatal incision, but the procedure has not been shown to be safe and effective in a large number of patients by other investigators.

At present, the most logical choice for relief when the discomfort becomes severe is a procedure that would alleviate the symptoms simply, reversibly, and without untoward reactions. The technique described below has been found to fulfill these criteria and has been successful in relieving the symptoms of patulous eustachian tube. An anterior tympanotomy approach is used to insert an indwelling intravenous catheter with a flared tip (Medicut*) into the protympanic, or bony, portion of the eustachian tube (Fig.

*Argyle Medicut, Sherwood Medical Industries, St. Louis, MO 63013.

16–52). The flared end of the catheter rests in the middle ear end of the eustachian tube. Prior to insertion, the lumen of the catheter is filled with methyl methacrylate to prevent the passage of air through the catheter; thus, the catheter occludes the eustachian tube. Following insertion of the catheter, a tympanostomy tube is inserted into the tympanic membrane to aerate the middle ear through the membrane. Even though spontaneous extrusion of the tympanostomy tube may occur, the middle ear may remain aerated with relief of symptoms and without development of high negative pressure or effusion, or both. The catheter most likely does not totally obstruct the eustachian tube, and adequate ventilation of the middle ear is provided around the catheter. Only a small number of patients have had the procedure, but the results have been gratifying. The indwelling eustachian tube catheter can be removed at any time, especially if and when the etiology of this most perplexing otologic problem is uncovered and a nonsurgical or surgical method of management is shown to be more efficacious. In the meantime, this method to partially obstruct the eustachian tube appears to be effective in providing relief of symptoms of a patulous eustachian tube.

Specific Management Options

Antimicrobial Agents

Decisions about optimal chemotherapy for otitis media are based on information about (1) the bacterial pathogens isolated from middle ear fluids, (2) the *in vitro* activity of antimicrobial agents against these pathogens, (3)

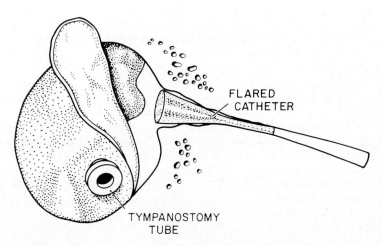

Figure 16–52 Illustration of the technique of placement of an indwelling catheter used to obstruct a patulous eustachian tube.

FLARED CATHETER

TYMPANOSTOMY TUBE

the clinical pharmacology of antimicrobial agents of value, (4) concentrations of drug achieved in middle ear fluid, and (5) the results of clinical and microbiologic studies. These factors in choice of antimicrobial agents and a strategy for management of children with otitis media with effusion will be discussed in this section.

Bacteriology of Otitis Media: Therapeutic Implications

The preferred antimicrobial agent for the patient with otitis media must be active against *S. pneumoniae* and *H. influenzae*, the two most important bacterial pathogens in all age groups. Group A *Streptococcus* and *S. aureus* are infrequent causes of acute otitis media and need not be considered in initial therapeutic decisions. Gram-negative enteric bacilli must be considered when otitis media occurs in the newborn infant, in the immuno-compromised host, and in suppurative complications or postoperative wound infections of the head and neck area. Anaerobic bacteria appear to have a limited role in chronic and probably a minimal role in acute otitis media. *S. epidermidis* and *B. catarrhalis* have been considered commensals, but results of recent studies suggest that they may play a pathogenic role in otitis media. The bacterial pathogens are discussed in the section on Microbiology, p. 402.

STREPTOCOCCUS PNEUMONIAE

S. pneumoniae is markedly susceptible to penicillins, cephalosporins, erythromycin, clindamycin, and the trimethoprim-sulfamethoxazole combination. Chloramphenicol and sulfonamides have moderate activity. Aminoglycosides are relatively ineffective.

Since the introduction of the penicillins more than 35 years ago, almost all strains of *S. pneumoniae* have been uniformly and markedly sensitive to penicillin G and other penicillins. In recent years, however, moderate and high resistance to penicillin G and other antimicrobial agents has appeared and in some cases has been responsible for clinical and microbiologic failure. There are three facets to the problem: strains that are moderately resistant to penicillin G but susceptible to other antimicrobial agents, strains that are highly resistant to penicillin G and resistant to other antimicrobial agents, and strains that are sensitive to penicillin G but resistant to some other antimicrobial agents. The clinical and epidemiologic aspects of antibiotic-resistant pneumococci were reviewed by Ward (1981).

During the past 15 years, an increasing number of strains of *S. pneumoniae* have had decreased susceptibility to penicillins. The susceptibility of most strains of *S. pneumoniae* is less than 0.05 μg per ml, whereas moderately resistant strains are 2 to 20 times less sensitive to penicillin G, requiring 0.1 to 1.0 μg per ml of penicillin G for inhibition (Table 16–23). Since usual dosage schedules of penicillin G or V achieve concentrations of 0.2 to 4 μg per ml in middle ear fluid, infection due to some moderately resistant strains may result in microbiologic and clinical failure (Kamme, 1970; Howard et al., 1976). Clinical and microbiologic failure in cases of pneumococcal meningitis due to moderately resistant strains treated with penicillin G has been reported (Paredes et al., 1976; Mace et al., 1977). Although the number of moderately resistant strains is now low (approximately 3 per cent of pneumococcal isolates tested in our laboratory [Klein, unpublished data] and reported from laboratories in the United States and western Europe), if the incidence of moderately resistant strains increases, physicians will have to reevaluate initial therapy and dosage schedules for treatment of otitis media.

Multiply resistant strains of pneumococci were noted in early 1977 by Applebaum and colleagues (1977). These strains were highly resistant to penicillin G, requiring more than 4 μg per ml for inhibition, and were resistant to other drugs that serve as alternatives to penicillin G in pneumococcal disease, including other penicillins and cephalosporins, tetracyclines, chloramphenicol, erythromycin, clindamycin, sulfonamides, and rifampin. Some children with sepsis and meningitis due to a highly resistant pneumococcus died when treated with penicillin G alone. Since 1977, these strains have continued to appear in South Africa, mainly in Durban and Johannesburg, but have been reported rarely outside that country. Cases appearing elsewhere have usually been in immunosuppressed patients (Cates et al., 1978). The reason for the relative restriction of these strains to South Africa is unknown.

Strains of *S. pneumoniae* sensitive to penicillins but resistant to other antimicrobial agents are not uncommon. Resistance has been noted in some strains to tetracycline, chloramphenicol, sulfonamides, erythromycin, and lincomycin. Susceptibility testing should be considered for strains of *S. pneumoniae* causing disease that does not respond

Table 16–23 SENSITIVITY OF *STREPTOCOCCUS PNEUMONIAE* AND *HAEMOPHILUS INFLUENZAE* ISOLATED FROM MIDDLE EAR EFFUSIONS IN CHILDREN WITH ACUTE OTITIS MEDIA, 1976–1979*

| Antimicrobial Agent | Minimal inhibitory concentration (MIC) (μg/ml), median[+] | | | |
| | S. pneumoniae | | H. influenzae | |
	Sensitive [†]	Resistant [††]	Sensitive [‡]	Resistant [§]
Penicillin G	0.01	0.4	1.6	>100
Penicillin V	0.01	0.4	12.5	>100
Ampicillin	0.03	0.1	0.8	>100
Methicillin	0.1	6.4	3.2	50
Nafcillin	0.01	0.8	25	50
Carbenicillin	0.2	6.4	0.4	>100
Cephalothin	0.1	1.6	25	12.5
Cephalexin	3.2	3.2	100	50
Cefoxitin	1.6	6.4	6.4	6.4
Cefamandole	0.1	1.6	0.4	3.2
Cefaclor	0.4	1.6	12.5	25
Erythromycin	0.05	0.03	3.2	3.2
Clindamycin	0.05	0.05	3.2	6.4
Chloramphenicol	3.2	3.2	0.4	0.8
Tetracycline	0.2	25	0.4	0.4
Amikacin	>100	100	3.2	6.4
Trimethoprim	1.6	3.2	0.8	1.6
Sulfamethoxazole	100	>100	>100	>100
Trimethoprim-sulfamethoxazole[‖]	0.3/6	0.3/6	0.2/3	0.2/3

*From Teele, D. W., Norton, C. C., Klein, J. O.: Unpublished data.
[††]Inocula replicator method; 10^0 dilution for *S. pneumoniae*
    10^{-2} dilution for *H. influenzae*
[†]22 strains with MIC for penicillin G < 0.1 μg/ml
[††]1 strain with MIC for penicillin G ≥ 0.1 μg/ml
[‡]Beta-lactamase–negative strains including 3 type b and 20 nontypable
[§]Beta-lactmase–positive strains including 3 type b and 4 nontypable
[‖]Trimethoprim-sulfamethoxazole = 1 part trimethoprim/19 parts sulfamethoxazole

to an appropriate course of a usually effective antimicrobial agent.

HAEMOPHILUS INFLUENZAE (Table 16–23)

Strains of *H. influenzae* responsible for otitis media may be subdivided on the basis of susceptibility to ampicillin. Ampicillin-sensitive strains are only slightly less susceptible to penicillin G than they are to ampicillin, but they are much less susceptible to penicillin V and the penicillinase-resistant penicillins. Cefoxitin, cefamandole, and cefaclor are the only cephalosporins with significant activity against *H. influenzae* and are effective against both ampicillin-sensitive and ampicillin-resistant strains. Chloramphenicol and tetracycline are also effective against both ampicillin-sensitive and ampicillin-resistant strains, as are less active agents such as aminoglycosides, erythromycins, and clindamycin.

In recent years, ampicillin-resistant strains of both nontypable and type b *H. influenzae* have been reported throughout the United States. The resistance appears to be a new phenomenon; few resistant strains were detected before 1972. Resistance to ampicillin is based on production of penicillinase, a beta-lactamase that hydrolyzes the penicillin nucleus. Thus, all penicillins that are susceptible to beta-lactamase, including penicillin G, penicillin V, ampicillin, amoxicillin, and carbenicillin, are likely to be ineffective against infections caused by these strains (Table 16–23). At present in the United States approximately 10 to 30 per cent of strains of nontypable, and 5 to 20 per cent of type b *H. influenzae* (Ward et al., 1978) isolated from children with disease are beta-lactamase–producing strains. Children with suppurative life-threatening complications of otitis media in which *H. influenzae* may be the etiologic agent, including sepsis, or meningitis, must receive a drug of uniform efficacy, such as chloramphenicol. Chloramphenicol-resistant strains of *H. influenzae* (most of which are susceptible to ampicillin) are uncommon, but meningitis due to such a strain has been reported (Kinmonth et al., 1978). Ampicillin or amoxicillin alone is still appropriate therapy for children with mild to moderately severe disease of the respiratory tract, including otitis media. But if the patient fails to respond favorably, the presence of a resistant strain must be considered and therapy changed to include a drug effective against beta-lactamase–producing *H. influenzae* (a sulfonamide, trimethoprim-sulfamethoxazole, or cefaclor).

GROUP A STREPTOCOCCI

There are no known strains of group A *Streptococci* that are resistant to the penicillins. These streptococci are markedly sensitive to the penicillins, cephalosporins, erythromycin, chloramphenicol, and clindamycin. They are relatively resistant to the aminoglycosides and to sulfonamides. Trimethoprim and sulfamethoxazole in combination are more active than either component alone, but clinical efficacy is uncertain against group A *Streptococci*.

STAPHYLOCOCCUS AUREUS and EPIDERMIDIS

Most strains of *S. aureus* that cause otitis media in hospitalized patients produce penicillinase and are resistant to penicillin G and ampicillin; the number of strains of resistant staphylococci in patients who have community-acquired disease is lower but significant. Thus, the penicillinase-resistant penicillins are the drugs of choice for initial management of the patient with suspected or documented staphylococcal otitis media (Table 16–24). Most cephalosporins are also effective against penicillinase-producing strains. The efficacy of erythromycins, clindamycin, chloramphenicol, and the aminoglycosides is variable, and tests of susceptibility should be used to guide the choice of treatment for the patient who is suspected or known to have a staphylococcal infection and is allergic to penicillin.

Table 16–24 PERCENTAGES OF SELECTED ISOLATES OF *STAPHYLOCOCCUS AUREUS* AND *STAPHYLOCOCCUS EPIDERMIDIS* RESISTANT TO THE INDICATED ANTIBIOTICS*

Antibiotic	S. aureus	S. epidermidis
Penicillin G	90	70
Nafcillin or Oxacillin	2	19
Cephalothin	1	5
Erythromycin	23	32
Clindamycin	17	26
Chloramphenicol	13	9
Vancomycin	1	1
Kanamycin	25	33
Gentamicin	18	18
Tetracycline	9	33

*171 strains of *S. aureus*; 274 strains of *S. epidermidis*. Boston City Hospital: 1977–1978.

Although disease due to methicillin-resistant staphylococci was reported shortly after the introduction of the drug, there have been relatively few cases in the United States. The strains are usually resistant to all penicillinase-resistant penicillins and to most cephalosporins. Bacterial resistance must be considered as a possible cause of therapeutic failure whenever a patient with staphylococcal disease who is on an adequate dosage schedule of a penicillinase-resistant penicillin does not respond favorably. Gentamicin or vancomycin is usually effective for these strains.

S. epidermidis is part of the normal microbial flora of the skin but may be pathogenic in otitis media. Most strains of *S. epidermidis* produce beta-lactamase that inactivates penicillin G, penicillin V, and ampicillin. *S. epidermidis* is also more resistant than *S. aureus* to the penicillinase-resistant penicillins, cephalosporins, erythromycin, and clindamycin (Table 16–24). Thus, initial therapy for disease due to *S. epidermidis* must be considered carefully and reevaluated when results of susceptibility tests are available.

BRANHAMELLA CATARRHALIS

Although most strains of *B. catarrhalis* are susceptible to penicillin G and ampicillin, beta-lactamase–producing strains have been identified. These strains are resistant to ampicillin and other beta-lactamase–susceptible penicillins but are susceptible to various cephalosporins (including cefaclor), erythromycin, chloramphenicol, and trimethoprim-sulfamethoxazole. Methicillin and other penicillinase-resistant penicillins and clindamycin are ineffective. As in the case with *H. influenzae*, the isolation of beta-lactamase–producing strains of *B. catarrhalis* appears to be a recent phenomenon. In 1970, Kamme reported that all 108 strains of *B. catarrhalis* isolated in the Department of Clinical Bacteriology in Lund, Sweden, were highly susceptible to penicillin G and ampicillin. In 1980, Kamme reported that 15 per cent of strains of *B. catarrhalis* isolated in the same laboratory produced beta-lactamase. His *in vitro* studies showed trimethoprim-sulfamethoxazole and erythromycin to be the preferred drugs for beta-lactamase–producing strains.

GRAM-NEGATIVE ENTERIC BACILLI

The choice of antibiotics for infections due to gram-negative bacteria depends on the particular pattern of susceptibility in the hospital or community. These patterns vary in different hospitals or communities and from time to time within the same institution. In most areas, the most effective agents for *E. coli*, Proteus (indole-positive and -negative) species, Klebsiella-enterobacter species, and *P. aeruginosa* are the aminoglycosides tobramycin, gentamicin, and amikacin. Some of the new cephalosporins (cefamandole and cefoxitin, moxalactam, and cefotaxime) have significant activity. Many gram-negative enteric bacilli are resistant to streptomycin, tetracycline, ampicillin, and the early cephalosporins such as cephalothin. Since the susceptibility of gram-negative enteric bacilli is variable and unpredictable, isolates should be tested to determine optimal choice of antimicrobial agents.

ANAEROBIC BACTERIA

Most anaerobic bacteria responsible for infection and disease in the upper respiratory tract, including anaerobic cocci, gram-positive nonsporulating anaerobic bacilli, and anaerobic gram-negative bacilli, are susceptible to penicillin G. Some strains of the gram-negative bacilli, such as *Bacteroides melaninogenicus*, are resistant to penicillin G; *Bacteroides fragilis* is an uncommon pathogen in the respiratory tract but most strains are resistant to penicillin G and susceptible only to clindamycin, chloramphenicol, or carbenicillin of cefoxitin. Finegold (1981) has reviewed therapeutic implications for anaerobic infections in otolaryngology.

Clinical Pharmacology of Antimicrobial Agents of Value in Therapy of Otitis Media and Its Suppurative Complications

The clinical pharmacology of antimicrobial agents of value in otitis media is discussed below. Although suppurative complications of otitis media are considered in subsequent chapters, it is appropriate to discuss also drugs of value for these infections in this section.

THE PENICILLINS

Penicillin G and Penicillin V

It is remarkable that in the more than 30 years that this drug has been in use, some organisms have remained exquisitely sensitive to penicillin G and no resistant strains have emerged. Thus, there are no penicillin G–resistant strains of groups A or B streptococci. In contrast, the vast majority of strains of *S. aureus* and *S. epidermidis* are now resistant to penicillin G, and initial therapy for any disease believed to be due to these organisms must include a penicillinase-resistant penicillin rather than penicillin G.

Several oral and parenteral forms of penicillin G are available. Choice of preparation for the patient is based on the pattern of antimicrobial activity, including the peak and duration of activity in serum and tissues, factors which reflect the absorption, distribution, and excretion of the drug. These characteristics of the penicillins are listed below.

1. Aqueous (water soluble) penicillin G produces high peak levels of antibacterial activity in serum within 30 minutes after intramuscular administration but is rapidly excreted; thus, the concentration in serum is low within two to four hours after administration. If aqueous penicillin G is given by the intravenous route, the peak is higher and earlier and the duration of antibacterial activity in serum is shorter (approximately two hours). Aqueous penicillin G, given intramuscularly or intravenously, is used for severe disease including suspected sepsis and meningitis. In such cases the drug should be given at frequent intervals, usually every four hours, until the infection has been brought under control.

2. Procaine penicillin G given intramuscularly produces lower levels of serum antibacterial activity (approximately 10 to 30 per cent of the peak level achieved by the same dose of the aqueous form) but activity persists in serum for as long as 12 hours. Intramuscular administration of procaine penicillin G should be reserved for the patient with mild to moderate disease who cannot tolerate oral penicillins (patients who are vomiting or have diarrhea, or the comatose patient) or the patient who requires the reliability of parenteral administration although the disease is not severe enough to warrant frequent intramuscular or intravenous doses of aqueous penicillin G.

3. Benzathine penicillin G given intramuscularly is a repository preparation providing low levels of serum activity (approximately 1 to 2 per cent of the peak level achieved by the same dose of the aqueous form). After administration of this drug, low concentrations of penicillin activity are measurable in serum for 14 days or more and in urine for several months. However, a drawback is that most patients complain of significant pain at the site of injection. This form is appropriate only for highly sensitive organisms present in tissues that

are well vascularized so that the drug can diffuse readily to the site of infection. Thus, benzathine penicillin G is suitable for treatment of children with pharyngitis and otitis media due to *S. pneumoniae* but not *H. influenzae*.

4. Oral preparations of buffered penicillin G and phenoxymethyl penicillin (penicillin V) are absorbed well from the gastrointestinal tract; the peak level of serum activity of penicillin V is approximately 40 per cent, and that of buffered penicillin G approximately 20 per cent, of the level achieved by the same dose of aqueous penicillin G administered intramuscularly. Therefore, oral penicillins may be satisfactory for treatment of mild to moderately severe infections due to sensitive organisms. Penicillin V and penicillin G are of approximately equivalent efficacy *in vitro* against gram-positive cocci, but penicillin V is much less effective than penicillin G against *H. influenzae* (see Table 16–23).

All penicillins are excreted by both glomerular filtration and tubular secretion. The tubular excretion of penicillins (and of cephalosporins) can be exploited by use of a drug such as probenecid that blocks tubular excretion of organic acids. Probenecid, when administered concomitantly with a penicillin or cephalosporin, results in higher peak and more sustained levels of antimicrobial activity than does the penicillin alone.

Penicillinase-Resistant Penicillins

Methicillin was the first penicillinase-resistant penicillin to be introduced and is available in parenteral form only. Oxacillin and nafcillin are available in both parenteral and oral preparations and have greater *in vitro* activity against gram-positive cocci. Cloxacillin and dicloxacillin are available in oral forms only and are absorbed more efficiently from the gastrointestinal tract than are the other oral drugs. Differences among these five penicillins include degree of binding to proteins and of degradation by beta-lactamases, and *in vitro* level of susceptibility; however, all are effective for treatment of staphylococcal disease, and clinical studies have shown them to be comparable when used according to appropriate dosage schedules. In addition, all but methicillin have proved to be effective against infections due to *S. pneumoniae* and beta-hemolytic streptococci. Although penicillin G should be considered the drug of choice for disease due to these organisms, the penicillinase-resistant penicillins can be used for initial therapy until the results of culture are available or when the otitis is suspected to be due to *S. aureus*.

Broad-Spectrum Penicillins

Ampicillin and Amoxicillin. Ampicillin and amoxicillin are effective *in vitro* against a wide spectrum of bacteria, including gram-positive cocci (*S. pneumoniae*, beta-hemolytic streptococci, nonpenicillinase-producing strains of *S. aureus*, and oropharyngeal strains of anaerobic bacteria), gram-negative cocci, gram-negative coccobacilli (nonpenicillinase-producing strains of *H. influenzae*), and some gram-negative enteric bacilli (*E. coli* and *Proteus mirabilis*). The broad-spectrum activity of ampicillin and amoxicillin provides the basis for their use as a single agent for treatment of otitis media.

Both drugs are available for oral administration; ampicillin alone is available in a parenteral form. Amoxicillin provides levels of activity in serum that are higher and more prolonged than those achieved with equivalent doses of ampicillin; thus, amoxicillin can be given in lower doses and three times a day rather than four times, as required for ampicillin. An additional advantage of amoxicillin is that absorption is not altered when the antibiotic is administered with food, whereas absorption of ampicillin is decreased significantly when it is given with food.

Cyclacillin and bacampicillin are two new preparations that are similar to ampicillin in chemistry and pharmacology. Cyclacillin is an oral penicillin with a spectrum of activity similar to that of ampicillin. *In vitro* activity of cyclacillin against gram-positive and gram-negative microorganisms, however, is 25 to 50 per cent below that of ampicillin. Cyclacillin is inactivated by the beta-lactamase of *H. influenzae* and *S. aureus*. Peak serum concentrations of cyclacillin are three to four times greater than equivalent doses of ampicillin. Patients who received cyclacillin had fewer side effects, including diarrhea and rash, than did patients who received ampicillin in a double-blind clinical trial involving 2581 patients (Gold et al., 1979).

Bacampicillin is a new semisynthetic ester of ampicillin. After absorption, bacampicillin is completely hydrolyzed to yield ampicillin. The antibacterial activity of bacampicillin is similar to that of ampicillin, and thus it is hydrolyzed by the beta-lactamase of *H. in-*

fluenzae. The drug is rapidly and completely absorbed after oral administration and achieves peak serum levels that are more than twice as high as those of ampicillin and approximately 30 per cent greater than those of amoxicillin. Ingestion with food does not decrease or delay absorption. The peak serum level is achieved earlier than is the case with ampicillin and the duration of activity is more prolonged. As a result of the more prolonged activity, dosage schedules require only two doses per day. Early clinical experience with bacampicillin was summarized in a series of articles published in the January-February, 1981, issue of *Review of Infectious Diseases*. The clinical usage and adverse effects are similar to those of ampicillin.

Carbenicillin and Ticarcillin. These drugs have a unique spectrum of activity among penicillins; they are effective against gram-positive cocci; *H. influenzae*; anaerobic bacteria, including Bacteroides species; and gram-negative enteric bacilli, including Enterobacter species, indole-positive Proteus species, and *P. aeruginosa*. High concentrations of drug are required to inhibit the gram-negative organisms, but this advantage is overcome in part by the low toxicity of the drugs, even when they are given in large intravenous doses. Combination of these penicillins with an aminoglycoside such as gentamicin or tobramycin produces synergistic activity against many gram-negative enteric bacilli. These combinations have been used effectively in initial therapy of sepsis of unknown origin or sepsis suspected to be due to gram-negative enteric bacilli in patients with malignancy or immunosuppressive disease (Kirby, 1970).

Ticarcillin is similar to carbenicillin but is more active against some strains of *P. aeruginosa* and less active against gram-positive cocci. Because of the increased activity, smaller dosages of ticarcillin than of carbenicillin may be used for treatment of disease due to gram-negative organisms (Fuchs et al., 1977).

Although ticarcillin and carbenicillin have no dose-related toxicity, both drugs are disodium salts; the large amounts in which they are given include significant quantities of sodium: 1 gm of carbenicillin contains 4.7 mEq of 108 mg of sodium per gram of drug; 1 gm of ticarcillin contains 5.2 mEq or 120 mg of sodium per gram of drug. The amount of sodium administered may be of concern in the treatment of certain patients with renal or cardiac disease.

For otitis media, the primary role of carbenicillin is in cases of chronic otitis media with perforation and discharge due to *P. aeruginosa* or Proteus species that is unresponsive to other forms of medical treatment, such as ototopical drops.

Toxicity and Sensitization

The penicillins are unique among antimicrobial agents in having low dose-related toxicity. Seizures may occur under circumstances that result in high concentrations of penicillin in nervous tissues: rapid intravenous infusion of single large doses, large dosage schedules for prolonged periods in patients with impaired renal function, high concentrations given by an intrathecal route, or direct application of penicillin to brain tissue, as might occur inadvertently during a neurosurgical procedure. Nephritis has followed administration of some penicillins, most frequently after use of methicillin. The mechanism of the nephrotoxicity is uncertain, but recent data suggest that the renal injury is probably an immunologic reaction and not a direct toxic effect (Barza, 1978). Thrombocytopenia with purpura due to drug-induced platelet aggregation has been noted after use of carbenicillin and penicillin G. These reports indicate a very low incidence of toxicity, so low as to preclude any change in the choice of therapy for the patient with an infection due to susceptible bacteria. However, when patients with impaired renal function are receiving prolonged courses of penicillin therapy (more than one week), the concentration of drug in serum should be determined to make certain that serum levels of the drug are not excessive.

If toxicity is not a significant concern with the penicillins, sensitization is a most important factor. Four types of reactions may occur after administration of a penicillin (or any drug or antigen):

1. *Immediate or anaphylactic reactions* occur within 30 minutes after administration and are life-threatening events. Clinical signs include hypotension or shock, urticaria, laryngeal edema, and bronchospasm. Acute anaphylaxis is rare after administration of penicillin (approximately one case per 20,000 courses of treatment in adults), but a significant number

of fatalities occurs each year because of the extensive usage of these drugs. Children are believed to have fewer systemic reactions than adults, presumably because of less previous exposure to penicillin antigens. Oral preparations are less likely to result in an immediate reaction than are parenteral forms, perhaps because antigens are altered in the gastrointestinal tract, or because of slower absorption.

2. *Accelerated reactions* occur in 1 to 72 hours after administration. The signs are similar to those of the immediate reaction but occur in a less severe form.

3. *Late allergic reactions* usually occur after three days. The major sign is skin rash. This is the most perplexing reaction to penicillin because it is nonspecific, and the rash may also be due to other drugs given at the same time or may be a sign of the infectious disease. Skin rash is associated with approximately 4 per cent of courses of penicillins (up to 7 per cent in the case of ampicillin).

4. *Immune complex reactions* include serum sickness, hemolytic anemia, and drug fever. Penicillin-induced hemolytic anemia is associated with high and sustained levels of penicillin in blood. Circulating red blood cells are coated with a penicillin hapten, the patient makes antibody to the penicillin antigen, the antibody binds to the altered red cell surface, and the cell undergoes lysis or sequestration (Petz and Fudenberg, 1966).

Identification of the patient who will have a significant reaction if penicillin is administered is still difficult. Serologic assays for detection of antibodies to penicillin have been considered; however, such assays lack specificity. Since the immediate reaction is largely mediated by IgE reagin or skin-sensitizing antibody, the patient who may subsequently respond with a life-threatening reaction could be identified by use of intradermal tests with appropriate antigens. Selection of the antigens to be used for skin testing, however, is an uncertain procedure because many different antigens play roles in the allergic reaction: at least 10 metabolic breakdown products of the penicillin nucleus have been identified; macromolecular impurities are present in solutions of the drug and high molecular weight penicillin polymers can be found in poorly buffered penicillin solutions standing for prolonged periods; side chains of the various penicillins may be responsible for reactions; and, finally, bacterial enzymes (amidases) used to prepare semisynthetic penicillins may be a cause of an allergic reaction (Parker, 1972). Thus, investigators have had difficulty in choosing sensitive and specific antigens to use for skin testing purposes.

The most promising studies of skin test antigens have come from the laboratories of Levine (1966) at New York University and of Parker (1972) in St. Louis. Levine identified two materials for use in skin testing, penicilloyl polylysine (Pre-pen, Kremers-Urban Co., Milwaukee, WI) and "a minor determinant mixture," a preparation of a dilute solution of aqueous crystalline penicillin G that includes metabolic breakdown products. In contrast, Parker used four skin test antigens associated with penicillin and its products. A positive test is indicated by a wheal-and-flare reaction in 10 to 15 minutes and suggests a significant chance of reaction on subsequent administration of a penicillin; a negative test suggests that a significant allergic reaction will not take place. Although much effort has gone into clinical tests of these antigens, their prognostic value in children is still uncertain (Green et al., 1977; Levine et al., 1966).

At present, the physician must rely on the patient's history of an adverse reaction after administration of a penicillin to identify the patient who is likely to be allergic. If the reaction appears to be related to the administration of a penicillin, the drug should be avoided for minor infections. If a life-threatening infection should occur and penicillin is clearly the drug of choice, as in the case of overwhelming disease due to *S. pneumoniae*, the physician may choose to administer the drug under carefully controlled conditions. A small dose may be injected initially in an extremity and may be followed by increasingly larger doses given every 30 minutes. Epinephrine, a tourniquet, and a tracheotomy set should be available in the event of a severe reaction during the testing period. All penicillins are cross-reactive in regard to sensitization, and allergy to any one implies sensitization to all.

ANTIMICROBIAL AGENTS USED AS ALTERNATIVES TO PENICILLIN

The Cephalosporins

The cephalosporins have a broad range of activity that includes effectiveness against gram-positive cocci and selected gram-negative enteric bacilli. The cephalosporins are relatively resistant to hydrolysis by beta-lactamases produced by *S. aureus*; resistance to beta-lactamase is not absolute, however, and some cephalosporins, especially cefazolin and cephradine, are hydrolyzed *in vitro* to a variable extent by penicillinase-producing strains. At present, 11 cephalosporins are available in the United States, and several more are undergoing clinical trials. The available products differ from each other in absorption, distribution, and toxicity. The antibacterial spectra of the first six cephalosporins to be introduced (cephalothin, cephradine, cefazolin, cephapirin, cephalexin, and cephaloglycine) were essentially similar (Moellering and Swartz, 1976), but new products such as cefamandole, cefoxitin, cefaclor, moxalactam, and cefotaxime have increased activity for gram-negative enteric bacilli. As of February, 1982, all are approved for usage in infants and children. In addition, the new drugs are the most effective cephalosporins against *H influenzae* (including beta-lactamase–producing strains [Moellering, 1978]), and cefoxitin has significant activity for anaerobic organisms (Kass and Evans, 1979). Cefaclor, the only oral agent among the new cephalosporins, appears to be effective against acute otitis media caused by ampicillin-resistant strains of *H. influenzae,* even though the *in vitro* sensitivity to both sensitive and resistant strains is high (Table 16–23).

Of the oral preparations, cephalexin, cephradine, and cefaclor are absorbed well from the gastrointestinal tract, and the presence of food does not alter absorption significantly.

Cephalothin, cefazolin, cephapirin, cephradine, cefoxitin, cefamandole, moxalactam, and cefotaxime are available for parenteral administration. These drugs may be administered by either intramuscular or intravenous routes. Pain is significant, however, after intramuscular injection of cephalothin and cephapirin; thus, the intravenous route is preferable for these preparations.

As is true for the penicillins, glomerular filtration and tubular secretion are the major modes of excretion of the cephalosporins.

The cephalosporins appear to be safe to use in children. Reports of toxicity in adults include nephrotoxicity in those who received cephalothin in combination with gentamicin (Barza, 1978). Apart from nephrotoxicity, few instances of toxicity have been reported.

The cephalosporins may produce allergic reactions similar to those caused by the penicillins. There is cross-sensitization among the cephalosporins, and allergy to one indicates allergy to all (as is the case with the penicillins). Various degrees of immunologic cross-reaction of penicillins and cephalosporins have been demonstrated *in vitro* and in animal models (Petz, 1978). Patients with a history of penicillin allergy have shown increased reactivity to cephalosporins. However, some patients who are allergic to penicillin have increased incidence of hypersensitivity to unrelated drugs, and it is still uncertain whether or not the penicillin-allergic patient reacts to a cephalosporin because of cross-allergenicity. Most patients who are believed to be allergic to penicillin may be given cephalosporins without an adverse reaction occurring. Although a cephalosporin may be used with caution as an alternative to penicillin in children who have an ambiguous history of skin rash, these cephalosporins should be avoided for the patient with a known immediate or accelerated reaction to a penicillin.

An unusual serum sickness–like reaction has been reported in children who received cefaclor (Murray et al., 1980). The children developed a generalized pruritic rash, similar to erythema multiforme, in some cases accompanied by purpura and arthritis with pain and swelling in knees and ankles. The signs appeared 5 to 19 days after the start of therapy with cefaclor and generally disappeared within four to five days after discontinuing the drug. The children had no prior history of allergy to a penicillin or a cephalosporin. At present, the incidence of this reaction is not known.

The cephalosporins are effective bactericidal drugs for a wide variety of diseases caused by gram-positive cocci and gram-negative enteric bacilli, but their role in the treatment of infectious diseases in children is uncertain. With the exception of the parenteral preparations of cefamandole, moxalactam and cefotaxine, and the oral preparation cefaclor, all currently available cephalosporins have relatively high mean inhibitory concentrations (MICs) *in vitro* for *H. influenzae*. Preliminary data suggest that moxalactam and cefotaxine produce sufficient concentrations of drug in cerebrospinal fluid to treat meningitis due to *H. influenzae* type b, but prior cephalosporins failed to cure children with meningitis due to *H. influenzae*, and some children developed meningitis due to this organism while receiving one of these drugs (Steinberg et al., 1978). The reason for failure of the early cephalosporins in these cases of meningitis is believed to be inadequate concentrations of drug in cerebrospinal fluid. All the cephalosporins are of value as alternatives to penicillin for disease due to *S. aureus, Streptococcus pyogenes, S. pneumoniae* (but excluding cases of meningitis), and selected gram-negative enteric bacilli that are resistant to other drugs and are uniquely susceptible to one of the cephalosporins. The new generation of cephalosporins, including cefoxitin, cefamandole, and cefaclor may extend the list of uses for these drugs in children to include disease other than meningitis due to *H. influenzae*. Treatment of meningitis due to *H. influenzae* with moxalactam and cefotaxine should now be considered investigational.

Erythromycin

For otitis media, erythromycin is effective *in vitro* against the gram-positive cocci, *S. pneumoniae, S. pyogenes*, and penicillinase- and nonpenicillinase-producing strains of *S. aureus* but possesses only moderate activity against *H. influenzae*. Erythromycin is effective for infection due to chlamydia, a cause of otitis in young infants, and for infection due to *S. pneumoniae*, a possible cause of otitis in school age children, adolescents, and young adults who have other respiratory manifestations of disease due to this organism.

Several preparations are available for oral administration. Because the erythromycin base is unstable in the acidic environment of the stomach, better-absorbed products were prepared by adding a protective enteric coating or by altering the chemical structure through formation of salts and esters. The derivatives of erythromycin are absorbed more efficiently from the gastrointestinal tract than is the base form; these derivations include the ethylsuccinate or propionate (esters), the stearate (a salt), and the estolate (salt of an ester). The estolate provides the highest concentration of antimicrobial activity in serum, but there is still controversy about which of the preparations provides the most biologically active drug at the site of infection. Since the base is the active component, all the erythromycin preparations must be hydrolyzed to the base after absorption.

Two erythromycin preparations are available for intravenous administration, the glucoheptonate and the lactobionate forms. Intramuscular administration of these forms is painful and should be avoided. Phlebitis is frequent during intravenous administration and may limit the duration of use of these drugs.

The erythromycins administered by mouth are well tolerated, and all but the estolate are nontoxic. The estolate may give rise to a cholestatic jaundice that is believed to be due to a hypersensitivity reaction. Since this syndrome has been observed less frequently with other forms of erythromycin, the ester is thought to be responsible for the hepatotoxicity. The jaundice has been reported to occur almost exclusively in adults who receive the estolate for more than 14 days and to resolve usually when administration of the drug is stopped. Few cases of jaundice in children have been reported. At present, potential hepatotoxicity is not considered a contraindication to the use of the estolate in children. Nevertheless, physicians prescribing this preparation should limit duration of therapy to 10 days and should be alert for signs of liver toxicity (Braun, 1969).

Erythromycin may be considered for treatment of otitis media due to *S. pneumoniae, S. pyogenes*, and *S. aureus* (mild to moderate disease) in patients who are known or suspected to be allergic to penicillins. Serious disease due to *S. aureus* should be treated with a combination of erythromycin and another effective agent such as chloramphenicol because of the rapid development of resistance to erythromycin when prolonged usage is required. Erythromycin has limited activity against *H. influenzae* and thus should not be relied on as the single antibiotic in treatment of otitis media (Table 16–23). *C. trachomatis* may be an important cause of otitis media in young infants (two weeks to six months of age); this disease appears to respond to therapy with either sulfonamides or erythromycin.

A fixed combination of erythromycin ethylsuccinate and sulfisoxazole is now available. Each 5 ml contains 200 mg of erythromycin activity and the equivalent of 600 mg of the sulfonamide. The combination provides activity against the pneumococcus and ampicillin-sensitive and -resistant strains of *H. influenzae*. The combination drug is of value for children who are allergic to penicillin or who fail initially when treated with ampicillin or amoxicillin and may have infection due to an ampicillin-resistant strain of *H. influenzae*.

Lincomycin and Clindamycin

Both lincomycin and clindamycin are effective *in vitro* against gram-positive cocci, including *S. pneumoniae*, are also active against a wide range of anaerobic bacteria, but have limited activity against *H. influenzae*. Clindamycin provides higher levels of activity in serum than does lincomycin, and, in contrast to lincomycin, its oral absorption is not decreased when the drug is taken with food.

Diarrhea and pseudomembranous enterocolitis may occur after use of clindamycin. Antibiotic-associated colitis has been reported in as many as 10 per cent of patients after treatment with clindamycin. The epithelium of the colon undergoes necrosis, the mucous glands dilate, and an inflammatory plaque forms and adheres loosely to the underlying epithelium. This disease has been associated with other antibiotics that alter intestinal flora including ampicillin (Auritt et al., 1978), tetracycline, chloramphenicol, and lincomycin. Recent studies indicate that overgrowth of toxin-producing strains of *Clostridium difficile* is probably responsible for most cases of antibiotic-associated colitis. The antibiotic suppresses the normal flora in the colon, and the *C. difficile* organisms proliferate and produce an enterotoxin that is responsible for the disease. Most such reactions have occurred in elderly patients, those with severe illness, or those receiving multiple antimicrobial agents (Gorbach and Bartlett, 1977). Clindamycin has been well tolerated by children. Diarrhea is a common side effect, but enterocolitis occurs rarely in this age group.

Clindamycin and lincomycin may be considered as alternatives to penicillin for the patient who is believed to be allergic and has disease due to group A *Streptococci*, *S. pneumoniae*, or *S. aureus*. Clindamycin should also be considered when infection is due to anaerobic bacteria, particularly Bacteroides species. Because of its limited activity against *H. influenzae*, these drugs can be used as initial therapy for otitis only when combined with an agent such as a sulfonamide that is active against this organism.

THE SULFONAMIDES

The first sulfonamide (and the first drug of the modern antimicrobial era), prontosil, was reported in 1935 by Domagk to be effective against infections due to beta-hemolytic streptococci. Sulfapyridine was introduced in 1938 and was the first antimicrobial agent effective against pneumococcal pneumonia. Soon after the introduction of these drugs, however, both streptococci and pneumococci developed some resistance to the sulfonamides. Today, sulfonamides are used in the treatment of a wide variety of infections in children, including otitis media due to nontypable strains of *H. influenzae*, usually in combination with a penicillin or erythromycin to provide coverage for *S. pneumoniae*.

Trimethoprim-sulfamethoxazole is an antimicrobial combination with significant activity against a broad spectrum of gram-positive cocci and gram-negative enteric pathogens. Trimethoprim is more active than the sulfonamide, but the mixture is significantly more effective than either drug alone (see Table 16–24). The drugs act in synergy by blocking the sequence of steps by which folic acid is metabolized: the sulfonamide competes with and displaces para-aminobenzoic acid in the synthesis of dihydrofolate; trimethoprim binds dihydrofolate reductase, inhibiting conversion of dihydrofolate to tetrahydrofolate. The effect of sulfonamide in bacteria is circumvented in the mammal, which obtains folates from food sources. The reaction inhibited by trimethoprim is similar in bacteria and mammals but differs quantitatively in the extent of binding of the drug to the enzyme. Mammalian dihydrofolate reductase is 60,000 times less sensitive to trimethoprim than the enzyme from *E. coli*.

Sulfamethoxazole was chosen as the sulfonamide to use in combination with trimethoprim because the drugs have similar patterns of absorption and excretion. Both are well absorbed from the gastrointestinal tract, and food does not affect absorption. A parenteral preparation is available. Rapid absorption and peak serum activity occur between one and four hours after oral administration; serum activity persists for more than 12 hours, but there is no significant accumulation after repeated doses given at 12 hour intervals.

Adverse reactions to the combination include rashes similar to those previously associated with sulfonamides (maculopapular or urticarial rashes, purpura, photosensitivity reactions, and erythema multiforme bullosum) and gastrointestinal symptoms, primarily nausea and vomiting. Hematologic indices have been carefully evaluated because of the antifolate activity of trimethoprim. Leukopenia, thrombocytopenia, agranulocytosis, and aplastic anemia have been associated with administration of trimethoprim sulfamethoxazole, but the incidence of these adverse reactions appears to be low. Hemolysis may occur in patients with erythrocyte deficiency of glucose-6-phosphate dehydrogenase deficiency.

The combination of trimethoprim and sulfamethoxazole in children has been effective in the treatment of acute otitis media due to *S. pneumoniae* or *H. influenzae* (including beta-lactamase–producing strains (see Table 16–23). However, its lack of efficacy when *S. pyogenes* or *S. aureus* is the causative organism precludes its use as the drug of choice for acute otitis media. It also is not recommended for pharyngitis due to *S. pyogenes*. The combination has been used with success for children who are allergic to penicillins or who fail after an initial course of ampicillin due to beta-lactamase–producing strains of *H. influenzae* (Schwartz and Schwartz, 1980; Teele et al., 1981).

Vancomycin

Vancomycin is a parenterally administered antimicrobial agent with a spectrum of activity limited to gram-positive organisms. It is usually administered by the intravenous route because intramuscular injection causes pain and tissue necrosis. Ototoxicity and nephrotoxicity resulted from high concentrations in serum of early preparations, but improvements in the manufacturing process have resulted in a product that is believed to have lower toxicity. The principal uses in children are treatment of serious staphylococcal disease caused by strains resistant to the penicillinase-resistant penicillins, and sepsis (particularly endocarditis) caused by enterococci in the patient who has a significant history of allergy to penicillin. Vancomycin is one of the few drugs (rifampin, fusidic acid, and bacitracin are others) effective *in vitro* against the highly resistant strains of *S. pneumoniae* isolated recently in South Africa and may be an important therapy if this strain becomes more widespread (Jacobs et al., 1978).

The Tetracyclines

The tetracyclines are effective against a broad range of microorganisms, including gram-positive cocci and some gram-negative enteric bacilli. Tetracycline should not be considered to be a substitute for penicillin for patients with otitis media due to or suspected to be due to gram-positive cocci because a significant proportion of group A streptococci and some strains of *S. pneumoniae* are resistant to this drug.

Seven tetracycline compounds are available for oral administration in the United States: tetracycline, chlortetracycline, oxytetracycline, demethylchlortetracycline, methacycline, doxycycline, and minocycline. Tetracycline, chlortetracycline, doxycycline, and minocycline are also available for intravenous administration. With few exceptions, there are only minor differences in the *in vitro* activity of the different preparations. However, minocycline may be effective against some strains of *S. aureus* and doxycycline may inhibit strains of *B. fragilis* resistant to the other tetracyclines (Neu, 1978).

Tetracyclines are deposited in teeth during the early stages of calcification and cause dental staining. A relationship between the total dose and the degree of visible staining has been established. Tetracyclines cross the placenta and discoloration of teeth has been seen in babies of mothers who received tetracycline or its analogues after the sixth month of pregnancy. The permanent teeth are stained if the drug is administered after six months and before six years of age. Other adverse effects include phototoxicity (particularly with demethylchlortetracycline), nephrotoxicity (with tetracycline hydrochloride, oxytetracycline, and demethylchlortetracycline) and vestibular toxicity (with minocycline).

There are few indications for administering a tetracycline to a young child; other effective drugs are available for almost all infections for which tetracycline might be considered. Therefore, tetracyclines should be avoided unless there is no alternative. The Food and Drug Administration recently withdrew certification of concentrated liquid forms of tetracycline designed for pediatric use (Yaffe, 1975). There is little reason to consider a tetracycline in the treatment of otitis media in children.

Drugs Effective Against Infections Due to Gram-Negative Enteric Bacilli

The Aminoglycosides

The aminoglycosides are drugs of value because they provide broad coverage against gram-negative enteric bacilli and some gram-positive organisms (such as *S. aureus*), are rapidly bactericidal, and are readily absorbed after administration. The major concerns in their use are nephrotoxicity, ototoxicity, and poor diffusion across biologic membranes, including passage into cerebrospinal fluid. The aminoglycosides of current importance include streptomycin, kanamycin, gentamicin, tobramycin, and amikacin.

The *in vitro* activity of these antibiotics

against gram-negative enteric bacilli varies and must be defined for each institution on the basis of current sensitivity tests. Streptomycin is not included in routine disk sensitivity tests nowadays because results for many years indicated that it is ineffective against a significant proportion of gram-negative enteric bacilli. The other aminoglycosides are active against most isolates of *E. coli*, Enterobacter, Klebsiella, and Proteus. At present, gentamicin, tobramycin, and amikacin are the most active of the aminoglycosides against these organisms and also the only aminoglycosides active against *P. aeruginosa*. The spectra of activity of gentamicin and tobramycin are similar, and strains resistant to one are usually resistant to the other. The major advantage of tobramycin is its activity against some strains of *P. aeruginosa* that are resistant to gentamicin. The spectrum of activity of amikacin is similar to that of gentamicin and tobramycin, but there is little cross-resistance, and some gram-negative organisms resistant to gentamicin and tobramycin are sensitive to amikacin.

The aminoglycosides have significant *in vitro* activity against *S. aureus* but are less effective for groups A and B beta-hemolytic *Streptococci* and for *S. pneumoniae*. A combination of a penicillin and an aminoglycoside results in more rapid killing and lower concentration of drug required to inhibit selected strains of gram-negative enteric bacilli and enterococci.

After parenteral administration, the aminoglycosides distribute rapidly in extracellular body water, with slow accumulation in tissues. Peak levels occur in serum between one and two hours after administration, and significant activity persists for six to eight hours. The drugs are excreted unchanged in urine and are filtered almost exclusively by the glomerulus, with limited tubular reabsorption. Penetration across biologic membranes is variable, and diffusion into cerebrospinal fluid is limited (the concentration in cerebrospinal fluid is approximately 10 per cent of the peak serum concentration). Thus, effective therapy of patients with meningitis may require direct instillation into the lumbar space or ventricles.

All aminoglycosides may produce renal injury and ototoxicity. In general, gentamicin and tobramycin are more likely to affect vestibular function, and amikacin and kanamycin are more likely to damage the cochlear apparatus, but both functions may be affected by each drug. The cochlear effect may present as a high-frequency hearing loss or tinnitus; vestibular disturbances include vertigo, nystagmus, and ataxia. Some of the effects may be reversible, but permanent damage is frequent. Nephrotoxicity may present as albuminuria, the presence of white and red blood cells and casts in the urine sediment, or elevation of blood urea nitrogen or serum creatinine. Toxicity appears to be dose-related, although eighth nerve damage has followed the use of relatively small doses in patients with renal failure. Neuromuscular blockage may occur after rapid infusion or when high concentrations of the drug are instilled into the peritoneum or pleura. A curare-like effect may lead to sudden respiratory paralysis. Toxicity has not been a significant problem in children with normal kidney function who were treated with aminoglycosides according to currently recommended dosage schedules. Toxicity has usually been associated with administration of high doses for a long time, previous therapy with other aminoglycosides, administration of drugs to elderly patients or those with impaired kidney function, or concurrent administration of other agents that are potentially nephrotoxic, e.g., the diuretics furosemide and ethacrynic acid.

Patients who receive a prolonged course of aminoglycosides or who have impaired renal function require careful monitoring to determine the safety as well as the efficacy of the aminoglycoside. Studies of absorption and excretion indicate that the concentrations of aminoglycosides in serum are variable and unpredictable. Blood should be obtained to determine drug concentration at the expected peak (one to two hours after parenteral administration) or trough (prior to the next dose, i.e., 8 or 12 hours after last administration). Specimens of blood should be obtained early in the course of therapy (within the first three days) to be certain that effective levels in serum are achieved and at subsequent intervals (every three to four days) to determine that the concentration of aminoglycoside in the serum is below the level of toxicity (Evans et al., 1978). The desired peaks for the aminoglycosides are gentamicin and tobramycin, 5 to 10 μg/ml; kanamycin and amikacin, 15 to 25 μg/ml. The trough should not exceed 2 μg/ml for gentamicin and tobramycin and 10 μg/ml for kanamycin and amikacin. The toxic ranges are considered to be 14 μg/ml for gentamicin and tobramycin and 40 μg/ml for kanamycin and amikacin. Dosage schedules should be modified if concentrations in serum are either too low, and therefore inadequate for optimal therapy, or too high and potentially toxic.

The major use of aminoglycosides for otitis media in children is for serious disease that is due to, or suspected to be due to, gram-negative enteric bacilli; these infections include neonatal sepsis and the suppurative complications of otitis media such as sepsis in the child with malignancy or an immunologic defect. Aminoglycosides are of value when chronic otitis media is due to *P. aeruginosa*.

Although the aminoglycosides are not effective for therapy of infections due to some gram-positive cocci, e.g., *S. pneumoniae* and *S. pyogenes*, they are effective *in vitro* against most strains of *S. aureus* and are used for severe disease due to strains of *S. aureus* that are methicillin-resistant and cross-resistant with other penicillinase-resistant penicillins and cephalosporins. Enterococci are resistant to clinically achievable levels of aminoglycosides, but a combination of a penicillin plus an aminoglycoside may be synergistic, and combined therapy is of value for serious enterococcal disease.

The aminoglycosides may be administered by the intramuscular or intravenous (by slow drip over one to two hours) route. The oral preparations are not absorbed.

Recent symposia should be consulted for more specific information about the pharmacology and clinical uses of gentamicin (Finland and Hewitt, 1971), tobramycin (Finland and Neu, 1976), and amikacin (Finland et al., 1976).

Chloramphenicol

Chloramphenicol is active against many gram-positive and gram-negative bacteria and chlamydiae. Oral preparations are well absorbed. The intravenous route is preferred for parenteral administration, since lower levels of serum activity follow intramuscular use. The drug diffuses well across biologic membranes even in the absence of inflammatory reaction. Approximately 70 per cent of the concentration of chloramphenicol in serum is present in cerebrospinal fluid of patients with meningitis.

The major limiting factor in the use of chloramphenicol is its toxic effect on bone marrow. A dose-related anemia occurs in most patients receiving high-dosage schedules for more than a few days. The anemia is concurrent with therapy, ceases when the drug is discontinued, and is characterized by decreased reticulocyte count, increased concentration of serum iron, and cytoplasmic vacuolization of early erythroid and myeloid precursors in bone marrow (Scott et al., 1965).

Aplastic anemia is a rare (approximately one case per 20,000 to 40,000 courses of treatment) idiosyncratic reaction that is usually fatal. Most cases of aplastic anemia follow use of the oral preparation of chloramphenicol; only four reports have been published of aplastic anemia that followed parenteral administration alone (Domart et al., 1961; Grilliat et al., 1966; Restrepo and Zambrano, 1968; Wallerstein et al., 1969). In some of these cases other drugs or the patient's disease could have been responsible for the aplastic anemia. Since very few patients receive chloramphenicol by the parenteral route only, as compared with the extensive world-wide oral usage of chloramphenicol (particularly in the many countries of Central and South America and Africa where the oral drug is available without a prescription), and since the incidence of aplastic anemia is so low, we cannot be certain that aplastic anemia occurring almost exclusively after oral usage, rather than after parenteral administration, is a true event or one of statistical chance. In any event, very few cases of aplastic anemia follow parenteral administration, and clinicians should not avoid use of intravenous chloramphenicol when it is indicated for serious cases of otitis media, especially when a suppurative complication is present.

Because of the significant proportion of ampicillin-resistant strains of *H. influenzae*, chloramphenicol should be used in the initial treatment of severe and life-threatening complications of otitis media that are due to, or suspected to be due to, *H. influenzae* type b, such as meningitis. The initial regimen should be reevaluated when results of cultures and susceptibility tests are available. Chloramphenicol may also be the only effective drug in the treatment of some cases of otitis media due to gram-negative enteric bacilli.

The Polymyxins

Polymyxin and colistin are highly effective *in vitro* against a broad spectrum of gram-negative enteric bacilli, including *P. aeruginosa*. These drugs do not diffuse well across biologic membranes, however, and are usually effective only when they are applied topically.

Diffusion of Antimicrobial Agents into Middle Ear Fluids (Tables 16–25 to 16–27)

Although studies of concentrations of various drugs in serum and middle ear fluid cited in Tables 16–25 to 16–27 differ in dosage schedules, time of collection, and methods of assay, the results indicate that most antimicrobial agents of value for treatment of acute

Table 16–25 CONCENTRATIONS OF ANTIMICROBIAL AGENTS IN SERUM (S) AND MIDDLE EAR FLUIDS (MEF) OF CHILDREN WITH ACUTE OTITIS MEDIA

Agent	Dosage (mg/kg)	Concentration (μg/ml)*			Reference
		S	MEF	MEF/S	
Penicillin V	13 PO	8.1	1.8	0.22	Kamme, Lundgren, and Rundcrantz, 1969
Ampicillin	10 PO	4.3	1.2	0.28	Lahikainen, Vuori, and Virtanen, 1977
Amoxicillin	10 PO	4.8	2.2	0.46	Howard et al., 1976
Bacampicillin	800 IM†	7.7	2.4	0.31	Virtanen and Lahikainen, 1979
Cefaclor	10 PO	7.0	1.3	0.19	Ginsburg, McCracken, and Nelson, 1981
Cefotaxime	25 IM/IV	5.8	2.1	0.36	Danon, 1980
Erythromycin					Ginsburg, McCracken, and Nelson, 1981
estolate	15 PO	3.6	1.7	0.49	
ethylsuccinate	15 PO	1.2	0.5	0.42	
Sulfonamide (trisulfapyrimadine)	30 PO	13.4	8.3	0.62	Howard et al., 1976

*0.5–2.5 hours after administration.
†Single dose administered to adults.

Table 16–26 CONCENTRATIONS OF ORALLY ADMINISTERED ANTIMICROBIAL AGENTS IN SERUM (S) AND MIDDLE EAR FLUIDS (MEF) OF CHILDREN WITH CHRONIC OTITIS MEDIA

Agent	Dosage	Concentration (μg/ml)*			Reference
		S	MEF	MEF/S	
Penicillin V	10 mg/kg	–	0.2		Nelson et al., 1981
Ampicillin	1 gm	22.4	1.5	0.07	Klimek et al., 1977
Amoxicillin	1 gm	15.3	6.2	0.41	Klimek et al., 1977
Trimethoprim-sulfamethoxazole†					Klimek et al., 1980
Trimethoprim	4 mg/kg	1.9	1.4	0.76	
Sulfamethoxazole	20 mg/kg	40.4	8.2	0.20	
Cefaclor	15 mg/kg	8.0	0.5	0.06	Lildholdt et al., 1981
Erythromycin	10 mg/kg				Nelson et al., 1981
Estolate		–	2.0	–	
Ethylsuccinate		–	0.3	–	

*0.5–2 hours after administration.
†Administered as the combination but assayed separately.

Table 16–27 CONCENTRATIONS (μg/ML) OF CEFACLOR IN SERUM AND MIDDLE EAR FLUIDS OF CHILDREN WITH ACUTE AND CHRONIC OTITIS MEDIA

Disorder	Time After Administration (hours)				
	½	1	2	3	5
Acute Otitis Media*					
Serum (S)	10.5	8.2	1.9	1.3	0.4
Middle Ear Fluid (MEF)	0.4	1.3	0.7	0.2	0.1
MEF/S	0.04	0.16	0.36	0.15	0.25
Chronic Otitis Media†					
Serum (S)	7.2	4.8	1.9	1.5	0.5
Middle Ear Fluid (MEF)	0.2	0.6	1.2	0.8	0.2
MEF/S	0.03	0.13	0.63	0.53	0.40

*Ginsburg, McCracken, and Nelson, 1981.
†Nelson et al., 1981.

otitis media achieve significant concentrations in middle ear fluid. The interested reader will find data about diffusion of the listed antimicrobial agent into middle ear fluid of patients with acute or chronic middle ear infection in these references:

penicillin G	Lahikainen, 1970; Silverstein et al., 1966
penicillin V	Kamme et al., 1969; Howard et al., 1976; Lundgren et al., 1979; Nelson et al., 1981
ampicillin	Coffey, 1968; Klimek et al., 1977; Lahikainen et al., 1977
amoxicillin	Klimek et al., 1977; Nelson et al., 1981
erythromycin estolate	Bass et al., 1971; Ginsburg et al., 1981
ethylsuccinate	Nelson et al., 1981
trimethoprim-sulfamethoxazole	Klimek et al., 1980; Nelson et al., 1981
cefaclor	Ginsburg et al., 1981; Lildholdt et al., 1981; Nelson et al., 1981
bacampicillin	Virtanen and Lahikainen, 1979
cefotaxime	Danon, 1980
oxytetracycline	Silverstein et al., 1966

Significant concentrations of each of the drugs tested appear red promptly in middle ear fluid. The concentrations of drug in the middle ear fluid were, in general, parallel though lower than concentrations of drug in serum. The peak activity in middle ear fluid was delayed when compared with peak activity achieved in serum, but duration of activity was similar in both serum and middle ear fluid (Table 16–26). Concentrations of penicillin V and ampicillin in middle ear fluid of patients with chronic otitis media were lower than concentrations of fluid of patients with acute disease, but concentrations of amoxicillin, erythromycins, and cefaclor were similar in acute and chronic effusions (Table 16–26).

Penicillin V, ampicillin, bacampicillin, and cefaclor achieved concentrations in middle ear fluid that were approximately one fifth to one third of the levels present in serum. Approximately 50 per cent of serum concentrations was achieved in middle ear fluid after administration of amoxicillin, erythromycins, and sulfonamides. Thus, usual dosage schedules of ampicillin, amoxicillin, bacampicillin, cefaclor, and trimethoprim-sulfamethoxazole produced concentrations of antimicrobial activity in middle ear fluid that were sufficient to inhibit *S. pneumoniae* and most strains of *H. influenzae* (excluding beta-lactamase–producing strains in the case of ampicillin, amoxicillin, and bacampicillin). The concentrations achieved in middle ear fluid after administration of penicillin V and erythromycins are sufficient to inhibit *S. pneumoniae* but were not adequate to inhibit most strains of *H. influenzae*.

THE *In Vivo* SENSITIVITY TEST (Table 16–28)

Drs. Virgil Howie and John Ploussard, pediatricians in practice in Huntsville, Alabama, have contributed significant new information about the epidemiology, diagnosis, and management of otitis media. The *in vivo* sensitivity test is one of their most valuable studies (Howie and Ploussard, 1969). The middle ear fluid of children with acute otitis media was aspirated and cultured prior to the start of therapy with various antimicrobial agents. All drugs were prescribed in usual dosage schedules and patients were advised to return in two to five days. If fluid was still present at the second visit, a culture of the fluid was obtained by needle aspiration. The results of these cultures are listed in Table 16–28. Their studies are consistent with expected results based on *in vitro* data (see Table 16–23) and achievable concentrations of drug in middle ear fluid (see Tables 16–25 and 16–27). Penicillins G and V, intramuscular benzathine penicillin G, and erythromycin were successful in eradicating *S. pneumoniae* from middle ear fluid. Sulfonamides and tetracyclines did not eradicate *S. pneumoniae*. *H. influenzae* was eradicated by ampicillin but not by penicillin V, intramuscular benzathine penicillin G, and erythromycin. The high minimum inhibitor concentration of penicillin V for *H. influenzae* and the relatively low concentrations of benzathine penicillin G achieved in serum (and by extrapolation in middle ear fluid) are the probable reasons for failure of these two penicillins to sterilize *H. influenzae* from the middle ear fluid. An oral form of penicillin G was not studied.

Table 16–28 RESULTS OF ANTIMICROBIAL THERAPY IN OTITIS MEDIA:
The "In Vivo Sensitivity Test"

Drug	Number of Patients from whom Organism was Recovered during Therapy*/ Number of Patients with Bacterial Otitis Media	
	Streptococcus pneumoniae	*Haemophilus influenzae*
Phenoxymethyl penicillin	0/2	7/7
Phenoxymethyl penicillin with sulfonamides	0/17	2/6
Ampicillin	1/20	0/17
Benzathine, procaine, aqueous penicillin	1/9	7/7
Erythromycin ethylsuccinate	1/15	17/20
Erythromycin ethylsuccinate plus triple sulfonamide suspension	3/8	2/7
Triple sulfonamide suspension	8/18	3/8

*Two to 10 days after beginning therapy.
From Howie, V. M., and Ploussard, J. H. 1969. The *"in vivo* sensitivity test"': Bacteriology of middle ear exudate during antimicrobial therapy in otitis media. Pediatrics, *44*:940–944.

Results of Clinical Trials

HISTORY

The design of clinical trials for evaluation of efficacy of antimicrobial agents in children with acute otitis media has undergone significant changes in the past 30 years. Prior to 1960, most American studies were performed without tympanocentesis and, thus, without a specific microbiologic diagnosis. Often large numbers of children were enrolled to evaluate two or more drugs, the definition of otitis media was broadly stated and included such signs as inflammation of the tympanic membrane (which most experts now do not accept as a suitable sole criterion for otitis media with effusion), the drugs were assigned by some random method, and results of therapy were presented in general terms such as "good response" or "therapeutic failure." The results were usually ambiguous and demonstrated only minimal differences between the drugs studied (Stickler and McBean, 1964). A review of such articles today would yield little information of value in assessment of use of various antimicrobial agents available for management of acute otitis media.

Tympanocentesis to define the etiologic agent in middle ear fluid of children with otitis media with effusion had been common to early clinical trials by Scandinavian investigators, but became customary in American studies only in the 1960s. About this time, more investigators, both in the private practice of pediatrics and in academic centers, became interested in various aspects of injection of the middle ear, including evaluation of antimicrobial agents. The study designs were more precise — most studies were double-blind; sterilization was defined in some studies by re-aspiration of persisting middle ear fluid; compliance was evaluated by assessment of use of the drug (weighing of returned bottles of medication or assay of urine for antimicrobial activity); the clinical course was followed with precise endpoints; and side effects and toxicity of the antimicrobial agents were carefully assessed by clinical evaluation and laboratory tests. Outcome measures for efficacy of antimicrobial agents and comparison of new and previously used drugs included time to resolution of clinical signs (fever and ear pain), sterilization of middle ear fluid, and incidence of relapse, recurrence, and complications. In recent years, an additional outcome measure has been added — time to clearance of middle ear fluid.

ARE ANTIMICROBIAL AGENTS INDICATED FOR ACUTE OTITIS MEDIA?

Prior to the introduction of sulfonamides in 1936, management of acute otitis media included watchful waiting or, when the suppurative process produced severe clinical signs or complications, use of myringotomy to drain the middle ear abscess. Spread of infection to the mastoid, meninges, and other intracranial foci was a feared complication of otitis media.

After the advent of sulfonamides and later of penicillin and other antibiotics, the frequency of complications of otitis media showed a dramatic decline, from approximately 20 to 5 per cent (Sorensen, 1977). In 1938, the frequency of mastoidectomy was 20 per cent, while in 1948 it was 2.5 per cent (Sorensen, 1977). In some studies it even dropped to zero (Herberts et al., 1971). Mortality from acute otitis media was a concern prior to the advent of usage of antimicrobial agents (Sorensen, 1977).

Most experts agree that all cases of acute otitis media should be treated with antimicrobial agents. This concensus is based on the facts that susceptible organisms, predominantly bacterial pathogens, are isolated from the majority of middle ear effusions of children who have acute otitis media and that there has been a significant decline in the incidence of suppurative intratemporal and intracranial complications of otitis media since the advent of use of antimicrobial agents. On the other hand, some physicians believe that antimicrobial therapy is used too frequently, and should not be instituted for routine episodes of otitis media, but should be reserved for severe cases, for otitis media associated with suppurative complications, for effusions that become chronic, or for treating certain high-risk children (Diamant and Diamant, 1974).

Many children with acute otitis media improve without use of antimicrobial agents. The use of a placebo group in a comparative trial with one or more antimicrobial agents has been studied by many investigators in the past 30 years. Some of these studies yield important information on the course of infection of the middle ear unmodified by an antimicrobial agent (at least, not at onset).* Results from representative studies provide important insights into the value of antimicrobial agents and use of myringotomy alone or in combination with a drug. Only studies that used a method of aspiration of middle ear fluid to define the microbiology of infection will be cited.

1. Rudberg (1954) evaluated 1365 cases of acute, uncomplicated otitis media treated as inpatients or outpatients at the Ear, Nose and Throat Department of Sahlgrensk Sjukhuset, Gothenberg, between January, 1951, and May, 1952. All patients were confined to bed and had daily syringing of the ear as long as discharge was present. If spontaneous perforation did not occur, myringotomy was performed. Four regimens of antimicrobial agents were used: penicillin G tablets or triple

---

*These studies should not be considered to describe the natural course of otitis media, since all include a procedure that drains variable amounts of fluid: tympanocentesis (aspiration); or myringotomy (incision and drainage); in some cases, the procedure was repeated at frequent intervals.

sulfa oral preparation alone or in combination, or an IM injection of a combination of benzathine and procaine penicillin. A fifth group received none of the drug regimens. The criteria for efficacy included the duration of discharge and incidence of complications. Two hundred thirty-six to 333 cases were included in each group. The results were as follows:

Duration of ear discharge was significantly shortened in infections due to the pneumococcus and *H influenzae* by the penicillin or sulfonamide preparations when compared with results of placebo; infections due to *S. aureus* and beta-hemolytic streptococcus were favorably altered by use of penicillin, but the results in the sulfonamide group were not significantly different from placebo. Complications including exacerbation of clinical signs, mastoiditis, and failure of the infection to subside occurred significantly more often in the placebo group than in the groups receiving a penicillin, but the complications in patients receiving a sulfonamide were not significantly different from those in the placebo group. Mastoiditis occurred in 44 of 254 (17 per cent) of patients receiving placebo, in 4 of 267 cases treated with sulfonamides, and in none of 844 cases managed with one of the penicillin regimens. The highest incidence of complications occurred in patients with disease due to beta-hemolytic streptococcus and *H. influenzae*.

2. In 1953 Lahikainen reported a study of children who were managed by use of myringotomy alone or in combination with penicillin G. The duration of discharge was significantly decreased in the group who received the antibiotic. No complications occurred in the penicillin-treated group but 9 of 153 patients who had myringotomy alone developed complications, including seven cases of mastoiditis, one case of meningitis, and one case of sinus thrombosis and brain abscess.

3. Van Dishoeck, Derks, and Voorhorst (1959) reported that 50 per cent of 400 children treated with eardrops alone recovered in 7 to 17 days, but 13 children developed mastoiditis requiring operation.

4. Halstead and colleagues in 1968 identified clinical improvement in a majority of patients with suppurative otitis (almost all

had cultures that were positive for *S. pneumoniae* or *H. influenzae*), but one third of the children (13 of 39) continued to be ill.

5. Howie and Ploussard (1972) evaluated various antimicrobial agents and included a group without antimicrobial therapy. Clinical and microbiologic resolution occurred without use of antibiotics in a small number of cases of otitis media due to *S. pneumoniae* (9 of 45, 20 per cent) and a larger number of cases due to *H. influenzae* (9 of 21, 43 per cent).

6. In a more recent study, Lorentzen and Haugsten (1977) evaluated 505 children; three treatment groups were defined, including myringotomy, a course of penicillin V alone, and penicillin V in combination with myringotomy. Significantly more failures occurred in the myringotomy group (15 per cent) than in the penicillin group (4 per cent) or the penicillin plus myringotomy group (5 per cent). Thus, penicillin V was more efficacious than

myringotomy alone, but myringotomy did not add to the effectiveness of the drug.

These studies suggest that many cases of infection of the middle ear resolve spontaneously or with the assistance of surgical drainage. The cases that resolve spontaneously may improve because the contents of the middle ear infection are discharged through the eustachian tube or after spontaneous perforation of the tympanic membrane. The major advantages of antimicrobial agents as compared with placebo (the latter usually including some drainage procedure) are (1) that the duration of drainage or clinical disease is decreased and (2) that the incidence of complications, although low, is significantly decreased, almost to zero.

RESULTS OF RECENT CLINICAL TRIALS

A summary of results of selected clinical trials of various antimicrobial agents in children with acute otitis media is given in Table 16–29. The reports were published between

Table 16–29   SELECTED TRIALS OF ANTIMICROBIAL AGENTS FOR ACUTE OTITIS MEDIA: CLINICAL RESPONSE TO THERAPY*

Investigator	Drugs	Clinical Efficacy	
		Streptococcus pneumoniae	*Haemophilus influenzae* †
Nilson et al., 1969	Amoxicillin	+	−
	Penicillin V†	+	+
	Trisulfapyrimidines		
	Ampicillin	+	+
Howie and Ploussard, 1972	Placebo	−	−
	Ampicillin	+	+
	Erythromycin estolate (E)	+	−
	Trisulfapyrimidines (S)	−	+
	E & S	+	+
Feigin et al., 1973a	Ampicillin	+	+
	Cephalexin	+	−
Howie, Ploussard, and Sloyer, 1974	Ampicillin	+	+
	Amoxicillin	+	+
Howard et al., 1976	Amoxicillin	+	+
	Penicillin	+	−
	Erythromycin estolate	+	−
	E & S	+	+
Stechenberg et al., 1976	Ampicillin	+	+
	Cephalexin	+	−
Gold et al., 1979	Ampicillin	+	+
	Cyclacillin	+	+
Shurin et al., 1980a	Ampicillin	+	+
	Trimethoprim-sulfamethoxazole	+	+
Mandel et al., 1981	Amoxicillin	+	+
	Cefaclor	+	+

*For purposes of this table clinical results are defined as satisfactory (+) or unsatisfactory (−).

†Cases of otitis media due to *H. influenzae* were almost all due to ampicillin-sensitive strains; cases due to beta-lactamase–producing strains were not evaluated or an insufficient number of such cases was enrolled.

Table 16–30   EFFICACY OF SELECTED ANTIMICROBIAL AGENTS FOR THE
COMMON PATHOGENS IN ACUTE OTITIS MEDIA*

| Antimicrobial Agents | S. pneumoniae | H. influenzae | | S. pyogenes 5–10 | S. aureus 2–10 |
		Non–β-Lactamase	β-Lactamase		
Ampicillin or Amoxicillin	+	+	–	+	+
Penicillin V	+	–	–	+	+
Clindamycin	+	–	–	+	+
Erythromycin	+	–	–	+	+
Sulfonamides	+	+	+	–	–
Erythromycin-sulfisoxazole	+	+	+	+	+
Trimethoprim-sulfamethoxazole	+	+	+	–	–
Cefaclor	+	+	+	+	+

*Based on available data from clinical trials.
+Effective; –Not effective.

1961 and 1981 and the list includes only studies that identified the bacterial etiology by aspiration of middle ear fluid. The clinical results were consistent with the results of *in vitro* studies of the activity of the antimicrobial agents (see Table 16–23) and with data about the concentration of drug achieved in middle ear fluid (see Table 16–25).

Because of the marked susceptibility of the pneumococcus for all drugs tested (with the sole exception of sulfonamides), clinical results of drugs for otitis media due to *S. pneumoniae* were uniformly satisfactory. The efficacy of the drugs for infections due to *H. influenzae* was variable. Ampicillin, amoxicillin, cyclacillin, cefaclor, sulfonamides, and trimethoprim-sulfamethoxazole were effective. Penicillin V, erythromycins, and clindamycin were ineffective. Cephalexin was ineffective in a dosage of 50 mg/kg/day (Stechenberg et al., 1976) for infections due to *H. influenzae* but McLinn noted that improved results occurred when 100 mg/kg/day was used. Cases of acute otitis media due to beta-lactamase–producing *H. influenzae* were either not present (such strains were first identified in 1974), were not identified, or were of insufficient number to effect results.

A small number of cases of otitis media due to *S. aureus* were treated successfully with clindamycin (Feigin et al., 1973a). As had been noted in earlier studies, sulfonamides (in this case trisulfapyrimidines) failed to alter the course of acute otitis media due to group A *Streptococcus* (Howie and Ploussard, 1972).

The efficacy of the antimicrobial agents for the common pathogens in acute otitis media is summarized in Table 16–30.

A Strategy for Management of Otitis Media

At present, antimicrobial agents should be administered to children who have acute otitis media. Since the same bacteria found in acute middle ear effusions have been isolated from the ears of children who lack the classic signs and symptoms of acute otitis media and also from chronic effusions, all children who have otitis media with effusion, regardless of the stage, should receive an antimicrobial agent, if one has not been given during the recent past.

Amoxicillin or ampicillin are the currently preferred drugs for initial treatment of otitis media, since they are active both *in vitro* and *in vivo* against *S. pneumoniae* and *H. influenzae*. Other regimens that are satisfactory include trimethoprim-sulfamethoxazole, cefaclor, and combinations of a sulfonamide with benzathine penicillin G (administered by the intramuscular route as a single injection), oral penicillin G or V, clindamycin, or erythromycin. For the child who is allergic to penicillins, trimethoprim-sulfamethoxazole, cefaclor, or erythromycin or clindamycin combined with a sulfonamide provide equivalent antimicrobial coverage.

Dosage schedules have been determined on the basis of studies of clinical pharmacology and results of clinical trials. Oral ampicillin, 50 to 100 mg/kg/24 hr, in four divided doses for 10 days, is recommended. Amoxicillin, 40 mg/kg/24 hr, is equally effective, can be given in three divided doses, and has fewer side effects, such as diarrhea. Ten days of treatment is recommended. If the child is allergic to the penicillins, then a combination of oral erythromycin, 40 mg/kg/24 hr, and sulfisoxazole, 120 mg/kg/24 hr, in four divided doses, is a suitable alternative. The recent availability of a fixed combination of these two antimicrobial agents (Pediazole) is an even more attractive choice, since patient compliance is improved when only one medication need be given instead of two. If beta-lactamase–producing *H. influenzae* or *S. aureus* are suspected or documented by tympanocentesis, then appropriate choices would be the fixed combination of erythromycin and sulfisoxazole, or the new cephalosporin, cefaclor, 40 mg/kg/24 hr in three divided doses.

Intramuscular benzathine penicillin G is an alternative choice if the child is vomiting, there is difficulty in oral administration, or there is doubt concerning patient compliance with the prescribed regimen. This agent is effective against *S. pneumoniae* and *S. pyogenes* but must be combined with a sulfonamide for coverage of *H. influenzae*.

With appropriate antimicrobial therapy, most children with acute bacterial otitis media are significantly improved within 48 to 72 hours. The physician should be in contact with the patient to ascertain that improvement has occurred. If the patient remains toxic or the condition worsens, he or she must be re-evaluated and a change in antimicrobial therapy, myringotomy for drainage, or needle aspiration should be considered.

The current incidence of strains of ampicillin-resistant *H. influenzae* is low (only 3 to 8 per cent of all cases of acute otitis media) and does not require a change in recommendations for initial therapy (Fig. 16–53). However, if the patient does not respond to initial therapy with ampicillin or amoxicillin, infection with a resistant strain of *H. influenzae* should be considered. Toxicity with persistent or recurrent fever or otalgia, or both, should prompt the clinician to recommend tympanocentesis or myringotomy, or both, to identify the causative organism; a specific antimicrobial agent may then be chosen on the basis of the results of the culture of the middle ear effusion and sensitivity testing. However, if signs persist but the child is not toxic and aspiration to culture the middle ear effusion is not performed, the initial antimicrobial agent should be changed to a regimen to which most uncommon organisms, such as a beta-lactamase–producing *H. influenzae* or *S. aureus*, would be sensitive. If ampicillin or amoxicillin was initially given, then the combination of erythromycin-sulfisoxazole of cefaclor should be administered. Trimethoprim-sulfamethoxazole (8 mg trimethoprim plus 40 mg sulfamethoxazole/kg/24 hr in three divided doses) appears to be effective when ampicillin-resistant *H. influenzae* is present or suspected to be present. However, this combination is apparently not effective when *S. pyogenes* or *S. aureus* is the causative organism and therefore should not be the drug of choice as initial treatment of otitis media with effusion.

Schwartz et al. (1981) studied children whose clinical signs did not resolve after initial therapy of a 10-day course of ampicillin, amoxicillin, or erythromycin-sulfonamide mixture. Middle ear fluid was aspirated and cultured for bacteria: ampicillin-resistant *H. influenzae* was found in

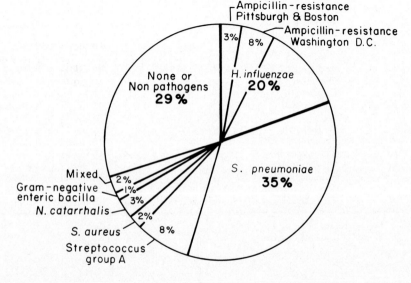

Figure 16–53 Bacteriology of otitis media with effusion and reported incidence of ampicillin-resistant *H. influenzae*.

about one third (31 per cent), ampicillin-susceptible strains of *S. pneumoniae* or *H. influenzae* were identified in about one half (51 per cent), and no bacterial growth was found in the other fluids. Teele et al. (1981b) also studied children who failed to respond to therapy and noted the following results: 19 per cent had organisms resistant to initial therapy, and 57 per cent had no bacteria isolated from the middle ear fluids. Thus, although some children who fail clinically do so because of a bacterial pathogen resistant to initial therapy, many children have bacteria that are susceptible to the drug and some have negative bacterial cultures and presumably have a nonbacterial microorganism as the cause of otitis media or some other reason for the persistent fever.

The bacteriology of middle ear infection in children who have recurrent episodes of acute otitis media is similar to that found in first episodes; the predominant pathogens are *S. pneumoniae* (although of different serotypes) and nontypable strains of *H. influenzae*. Thus, the child with a recurrent episode of otitis media should be treated initially with the same antimicrobial regimens as the child with a first episode of middle ear infection.

DURATION OF THERAPY

Physicians must rely on empirically derived schedules of therapy to plan drug regimens that lead to rapid and complete resolution of disease but minimal risk in terms of clinical or microbiologic failure or drug toxicity. For treatment of otitis media, opinions vary and the data are not easy to interpret. The dosage schedules presented in Table 16–31 appear appropriate for a 10-day course on the basis of currently available data.

For neonates and immunosuppressed children, and whenever an unusual organism is isolated from the middle ear culture, the appropriate antimicrobial agent should be selected according to the results of the sensitivity testing.

Even though the efficacy of antimicrobial agents has not been tested in controlled clinical trials in children with chronic middle ear effusions, the same antimicrobial agents recommended for acute otitis media should be administered for chronic otitis media with effusion. In addition, children who have a persistent middle ear effusion following an initial 10-day course of an antimicrobial agent such as ampicillin (or amoxicillin) may benefit from a therapeutic trial with erythromycin-sulfisoxazole, trimethoprime-sulfamethoxazole, or cefaclor. However, the efficacy of treatment with one of these agents for this stage of the disease has not been subjected to clinical trials.

Selected Aspects of Administration of Antimicrobial Agents

DOSAGE SCHEDULES FOR INFANTS AND CHILDREN

Dosage schedules of antimicrobial agents useful in otitis media are listed for infants (beyond the newborn period) and children in Table 16–31. Oral regimens are used for otitis media due to susceptible organisms in the

Table 16–31 DAILY DOSAGE SCHEDULE FOR ANTIMICROBIAL AGENTS USEFUL IN OTITIS MEDIA

Penicillin G	50,000 μ/kg in 4 doses*
Penicillin G (benzathine salt)†	<30 lbs — 600,000 μ in 1 dose
	>30 lbs — 1,200,000 μ in 1 dose
Penicillin V	50 mg/kg in 4 doses
Ampicillin	50–100 mg/kg in 4 doses*
Amoxicillin	40 mg/kg in 3 doses
Oxacillin	50 mg/kg in 4 doses*
Cloxacillin	50 mg/kg in 4 doses*
Dicloxacillin	25 mg/kg in 4 doses*
Nafcillin	50 mg/kg in 4 doses*
Cephalexin	100 mg/kg in 4 doses*
Cefaclor	40 mg/kg in 3 doses
Erythromycins	40 mg/kg in 4 doses
Clindamycin	25 mg/kg in 4 doses
Sulfisoxazole	120 mg/kg in 4 doses
Trisulfapyrimidine	120 mg/kg in 4 doses
Trimethoprim-sulfamethoxazole (TMP-SMZ)	8 mg TMP; 40 mg SMZ in 2 doses

*Schedule at least one hour before or two hours after meals.
†Route IM; all other PO.

Table 16–32 DAILY DOSAGE SCHEDULES FOR ANTIMICROBIAL AGENTS OF VALUE IN INFANTS (OTHER THAN NEONATES) AND CHILDREN WITH OTITIS MEDIA AND SEPSIS OR SUPPURATIVE COMPLICATIONS

Drug	Route	Dosage/kg/24 hours
Penicillin G	IV, IM	100,000–400,000 μ in 4-6 doses*
Methicillin	IV, IM	200 mg in 4–6 doses
Oxacillin	IV, IM	200 mg in 4–6 doses
Nafcillin	IV, IM	200 mg in 4–6 doses
Ampicillin	IV, IM	200–300 mg in 4–6 doses*
Carbenicillin	IV, IM	400–600 mg in 4–6 doses*
Ticarcillin	IV, IM	200–300 mg in 4–6 doses*
Cephalothin	IV, IM	200 mg in 4–6 doses
Cefazolin	IV, IM	100 mg in 4 doses
Moxalactam	IV, IM	200 mg in 4 doses
Erythromycin	IV	50 mg in 4 doses†
Clindamycin	IM, IV	40 mg in 3–4 doses
Vancomycin	IV	40 mg in 2–4 doses
Chloramphenicol	IV	50–100 mg in 4 doses*
Kanamycin	IV, IM	15 mg in 2–3 doses†
Gentamicin	IV, IM	5–7.5 mg in 3 doses†
Tobramycin	IV, IM	5 mg in 3 doses†
Amikacin	IV, IM	15 mg in 2 doses†
Sulfisoxazole	IV	120 mg in 4 doses

*Use high dosage schedule if meningitis is diagnosed or suspected.

†Administer in a continuous drip or by slow infusion in 30–60 minutes or more.

absence of suppurative complications. Parenteral administration should be considered for severe infections due to less susceptible organisms and when sepsis or suppurative complications are present or imminent (Table 16–32.)

DOSAGE SCHEDULES FOR NEWBORN INFANTS (Table 16–33)

The clinical pharmacology of antimicrobial agents administered to the newborn infant is unique and cannot be extrapolated from the results of studies done in older children or adults. Physiologic and metabolic processes that affect the distribution, metabolism, and excretion of drugs undergo rapid changes during the first few weeks of life. The increased efficiency of kidney function after the first seven days of life requires a decrease in the interval between doses of penicillins and aminoglycosides to maintain high concentrations of drug in blood and tissues. Thus, different dosage schedules are provided for the first week of life and for subsequent weeks of the neonatal period. A recent monograph by McCracken and Nelson (1977) provides detailed information about the clinical pharmacology of antimicrobial agents in the newborn infant.

SHOULD DOSAGES BE DETERMINED BY WEIGHT OR BY SURFACE AREA?

In most standard pediatric texts and in the drug package inserts prepared by manufacturers, dosages of antibiotics for children are usually based on weight. Some investigators suggest that calculation of dosage by surface area may result in more reliable concentrations of drug in serum (Siber, Smith, and Levin, 1979). The latter method may be more reliable for some drugs such as the aminoglycosides that are distributed in extracellular fluid, since body surface area correlates more closely with extracellular fluid volume, and more predictable serum levels have been achieved by using dosages calculated on the basis of surface area than by using those based on weight. For the time being, however, it seems to be important to use calculations based on weight to determine dosage schedules.

USE OF ORAL PREPARATIONS FOR SERIOUS INFECTIONS

Oral preparations of antimicrobial agents vary in their degree of absorption from individual to individual and from dose to dose in the same individual. Because higher and more consistent serum concentrations of drug are achieved after parenteral administration, the latter routes are preferable for serious infections. Recent studies (Nelson, 1978; Nelson et al., 1978; Tetzlaff et al., 1978) of the effectiveness of antibiotics administered by mouth to children with infections of the bones and joints suggest that this mode of administration should be considered for at least a portion of the course of administration for children with severe infectious diseases. For oral use of drugs for serious infections it is recommended that (1) the patient be able to swallow and retain the medication; (2) the dose be sufficiently high to provide adequate bactericidal concentrations of drug at the site of infection; (3) the hospital laboratory be capable of performing tests to determine the concentration of drug in blood and the minimal inhibitory and minimal bactericidal concentrations of the antibiotic.

FOOD INTERFERES WITH THE ABSORPTION OF SOME ORAL ANTIMICROBIAL AGENTS

The absorption of some oral antimicrobial agents is significantly decreased when the drug is taken with food or near mealtime.

Table 16–33 ANTIBACTERIAL DRUGS FOR NEWBORN INFANTS

| Drug (Generic) | Route | Dosage/kg/24 hours | |
		<7 Days of Age	7–28 Days of Age
Penicillin G, crystalline	IV, IM	50,000–100,000 U* in 2 doses	100,000–250,000 U* in 3 doses
Penicillinase-resistant penicillins			
Methicillin	IV, IM	50–100 mg in 2 doses	100–200 in 3 doses
Oxacillin	IV, IM	50–100 mg in 2 doses	100–200 mg in 3 doses
Nafcillin	IM	50–100 mg in 2 doses	100–200 mg in 3 doses
Broad-spectrum penicillins			
Ampicillin	IV, IM	100 mg in 2 doses	200–300 mg* in 3 doses
Carbenicillin	IV, IM	200–300 mg in 2–4 doses	400 mg in 4 doses
Aminoglycosides**			
Kanamycin***	IV,†IM	15 mg in 2 doses	15 mg in 2 doses
Gentamicin	IV,†IM	5 mg in 2 doses	7.5 mg in 3 doses
Tobramycin	IV,†IM	4 mg in 2 doses	6 mg in 3 doses
Amikacin	IV,†IM	15 mg in 2 doses	15 mg in 2 doses
Polymyxins			
Polymyxin B	IM	2.5 mg in 4 doses	2.5 mg in 4 doses
Colistimethate	IV, IM	2.5–5 mg in 2–4 doses	2.5–5 mg in 2–4 doses
Chloramphenicol**	IV	Premature — 25 mg in 2 doses Term—25 mg in 2 doses	Premature—25 mg in 2 doses Term—50 mg in 2 doses
Vancomycin	IV‡	30 mg in 2 doses	45 mg in 3 doses

*The higher dose is recommended in the treatment of meningitis.

**Serum concentrations should be assayed to determine the optimal dose.

***Higher doses have been recommended on the basis of pharmacologic studies by some. However, improved therapeutic efficacy and lack of long-term toxicity for these regimens has not been demonstrated. These doses/kg/24 hrs are as follows:

	<7 Days	7–28 Days
Kanamycin	15–20 mg in 2 doses	20–30 mg in 2 or 3 doses
Amikacin	15 mg in 2 doses	20–30 mg in 2 or 3 doses

†Intravenous administration given in a 20–30 min interval.

‡Intravenous administration given in a 30–60 min interval.

These drugs include unbuffered penicillin G, the penicillinase-resistant penicillins (nafcillin, oxacillin, cloxacillin, and dicloxacillin), ampicillin, and lincomycin. Milk, milk products, and other foods or medications containing calcium or magnesium salts interfere with absorption of the tetracyclines. Absorption of penicillin V, buffered penicillin G, amoxicillin, cefaclor, chloramphenicol, erythromycin, and clindamycin is only slightly affected by food. Antibiotics whose absorption is affected by concurrent administration of food should be taken one or more hours before or two or more hours after meals. A four-times-per-day dosage schedule could call for the drug to be given on arising, one hour before lunch, one hour before supper, and at bedtime.

INTRAVENOUS VS INTRAMUSCULAR ADMINISTRATION

After intravenous administration of an antimicrobial agent, there is a brief period when the concentration of drug in serum is higher than that following intramuscular administration. However, no therapeutic advantage of administering antibiotics intravenously as opposed to intramuscularly has been demonstrated. Intravenous administration should be used if the patient is in shock or suffers from a bleeding diathesis. If prolonged parenteral therapy is anticipated, the pain on injection and the small muscle mass of the young child preclude the intramuscular route and make intravenous therapy preferable. The physician must be alert for thrombophlebitis that may result from prolonged intravenous administration and sterile abscesses that may follow intramuscular administration.

Chloramphenicol, the tetracyclines, and erythromycin should be administered by the intravenous rather than the intramuscular route. Chloramphenicol is poorly absorbed from intramuscular sites. The intramuscular injection of parenteral tetracyclines and erythromycin causes local irritation and pain.

"Push" vs "Continuous" or "Steady Drip" Intravenous Administration

Antimicrobial agents may be administered intravenously by the "push" method, in which the drug is provided over a period of 5 to 15 minutes; by "steady drip" over one to two hours; or by "continuous drip," whereby the drug is given throughout the period of administration. The "push" method results in high levels of antibacterial activity in serum for short periods, whereas the "steady" or "continuous drip" method produces a lower but more sustained level of activity. There are no data that indicate a clinical advantage of one method over the other. Rather, the important criterion of clinical and microbiologic efficacy appears to be maintenance of a sufficient level of antimicrobial activity at the site of infection so that persisting organisms cannot multiply. The permissible period without antibiotic activity may be relatively brief for rapidly growing bacteria, such as gram-positive cocci, and longer for organisms that multiply at a slower rate, such as *Mycobacterium tuberculosis.*

Rapid administration (less than five minutes) of large intravenous doses of penicillin should be avoided because of possible central nervous system effects due to extraordinarily high tissue concentrations. Aminoglycosides given by the intravenous route should be infused over one to two hours. Because high concentrations of drug may cause eighth nerve toxicity, the aminoglycosides should never be given by the "push" method.

Antimicrobial activity may deteriorate if drugs are kept in solution at room temperature for prolonged periods, as might occur with use of the "continuous drip" method. Penicillins lose activity when stored in this fashion over time. Therefore, it is good practice to administer fresh solutions of penicillins every six to eight hours when the "continuous drip" method is used.

Dosage Schedules in Children with Renal Insufficiency

The kidney is the major organ of excretion for most antimicrobial agents, including the penicillins, cephalosporins, aminoglycosides, polymyxins, and tetracyclines (with the exception of doxycycline). Impaired excretion may result in high and possibly toxic concentrations of drug in the blood and tissues. Therefore, alterations in dosage schedules must be considered in children with diminished renal function. Drugs that are eliminated by nonrenal mechanisms and therefore do not require adjustment of dosage schedule in cases of renal impairment include erythromycin, chloramphenicol, and doxycycline. Agents requiring dosage adjustments only when renal failure is severe include most penicillins, cephalosporins, and clindamycin. Agents that require careful adjustment of dosage in renal impairment include carbenicillin and ticarcillin (because of the high dosage schedules used), the aminoglycosides, tetracyclines (with the exception of doxycycline), vancomycin, and the polymyxins.

The dosage schedules may be altered by increasing the interval between doses or decreasing individual doses. In most cases, the first dose can be given in the usual amount and the interval between subsequent doses lengthened. Various "rules of thumb" have been developed to guide the physician (Kunin, 1972). These formulas have been developed from studies of adults with renal impairment, and pediatricians must be cautious in adapting the formulas for use in children. Rather, the degree of antimicrobial activity in serum should be established by bioassay when aminoglycosides and other drugs of potential toxicity are administered to children with renal insufficiency. Serum specimens should be obtained at the time of the anticipated peak and trough levels on the first day, and repeat samples should be obtained on subsequent days to make certain that a safe and effective dosage schedule is used (Hewitt and McHenry, 1978).

Ototopical Use of Antimicrobial Agents

Ototopical antimicrobial agents are used for otitis media when a perforation of the tympanic membrane (or tympanostomy tube) and a discharge are present. Neomycin, polymyxin B, chloramphenicol, and gentamicin are the most commonly used drugs. All of the agents are potentially ototoxic and should be used only when necessary. Sensitization does not appear to be an important problem with topical antibiotics, although some patients with chronic dermatoses may react to certain agents, such as neomycin.

What to Look for When Antimicrobial Therapy Fails

If the patient does not respond appropriately to therapy with antimicrobial agents or subsequently has a relapse or recurrence of infection, the physician must consider factors that may contribute to failure, including those that are infection- or disease-related, host-related, or drug-related (Table 16–34).

Infection or Disease Factors

The use of antimicrobial agents for viral infection or incorrect choice of drugs for

Table 16–34 FACTORS CONTRIBUTING TO FAILURE OF ANTIMICROBIAL AGENTS USED FOR TREATMENT OF OTITIS MEDIA

Infection- or Disease-Related
  Antibiotic inappropriate for infection
  Viral or other nonbacterial infection unaffected by
    antibiotics
  Resistant or unusual organism
  Significant focus of infection at another site

Host-Related
  Defect in immune response to infection
  Anatomic defect
  Foreign body present

Drug-Related
  Inadequate compliance
  Improper dosage schedule — route, dose, or duration
  Inadequate diffusion to site of infection
  Deterioration of drug on storage

bacterial infection results in apparent lack of response. A resistant or uncommon organism must be considered.

A significant focus of infection at another site requiring a different regimen or different dosage schedule may be responsible for failure.

HOST FACTORS

Patients whose normal humoral or cellular defense mechanisms are compromised by congenital or acquired disease or immunosuppressive medications suffer from frequent infections, often of the respiratory tract, including otitis media. Bactericidal antibiotics (penicillins, cephalosporins) are usually necessary in treating infection in these patients, since bacteriostatic agents (erythromycin, sulfonamides) depend on normal phagocytic and immunologic mechanisms to eradicate the infection.

Anatomic defects, congenital or traumatic, e.g., cleft palate, may have previously been undetected and may be a cause of frequent episodes of infection in the middle ear.

A foreign body in the nares may serve as a nidus for a persistent suppurative infection that may be transmitted to the ear.

DRUG FACTORS

The most frequent drug-related factor in failure of antibiotic therapy is inadequate compliance. Physicians overestimate the degree of compliance of their patients. Unacceptable taste or odor of drugs may result in poor compliance. Penicillin V, amoxicillin, and ampicillin are somewhat bitter, but ac-

ceptance is usually not a problem. Erythromycin preparations, alone or in fixed combination with sulfonamide, and cefaclor are well accepted. Trimethoprim-sulfamethoxazole and the oral penicillinase-resistant penicillins have a bitter aftertaste, and compliance problems should be anticipated in instructions to parents (Nelson and McCracken, 1980; Schwartz and Schwartz, 1980).

Mattar et al. (1975) evaluated treatment given at home for children with otitis media. Full compliance with prescribed medications occurred in only 5 of 100 patients. Factors limiting compliance included incorrect dosage schedules (36 per cent), early termination (37 per cent), inadequate dispensing of medication at drugstores (15 per cent), spilled medicine (7 per cent), and a series of other errors by physician, pharmacist, and parent (Table 16–35). Compliance improved to more than half when hospital pharmacy personnel gave patients and parents verbal and written instructions for administration of medications that were dispensed with a calibrated measuring device and a calendar to record doses taken.

Other drug-related factors include inappropriate dosage schedule and inadequate duration of therapy. Some antimicrobial agents deteriorate on prolonged storage. Adherence to expiration dates recommended by

Table 16–35 FACTORS IN FAILURE OF PATIENTS TO COMPLY WITH PRESCRIBED MEDICATION*

Physician Errors
  Action of drugs and possible side effects not explained to parent
  Dosage schedule ambiguous or incorrect
  Instructions absent or incomplete
  Multiple drugs prescribed resulting in confusion
  Expensive trade brand used beyond Medicaid reimbursement rate
Pharmacist Errors
  Misleading or incorrect labels
  Underfilling of prescriptions
Community Factors
  Drug stores not open at time of day when parents sought medication
Parent and Home Factors
  Difficulty in giving medication;
    two people often necessary to administer drug
  Use of household teaspoon unsatisfactory
  Bottles broken or spilled
  Schedule of administration unrealistic for parent;
    baby sitter inadequate to dispense medication

*After Mattar, M. E., Markello, J., and Yaffe, S. J. 1975. Pharmaceutic factors affecting pediatric compliance. Pediatrics, 55:101–108.

the manufacturer safeguards against inadequate potency of the drug.

Antimicrobial Agents for Prophylaxis

Chemoprophylaxis implies use of drugs in anticipation of infection, whereas treatment implies use of drugs after infection has taken place or signs of infectious disease are evident. Although indiscriminate use of antimicrobial agents for prophylaxis is to be avoided, many forms of chemoprophylaxis have been extensively tested and are of proven value. Recent studies suggest that chemoprophylaxis may be effective in children with recurrent episodes of acute otitis media.

An antimicrobial agent of value for prophylaxis should be effective for the bacteria most likely to cause disease, should be of limited toxicity and have few side effects, and should be unlikely to decrease in efficacy with prolonged usage (the bacteria should not develop resistance to the drug). The potential liabilities of chemoprophylaxis include alteration of the patient's microflora, allergic or toxic reactions, and relaxation of the physician's watchfulness for the occurrence of disease in his patient.

Children are at risk for recurrent episodes of acute otitis media during a relatively short period of life: most episodes occur between 6 and 24 months of age. If the child who is susceptible to recurrent otitis media could be protected from infection during this period, the morbidity of middle ear disease might be avoided. Thus, the concept of prophylaxis is a worthy one that deserves careful study by investigators, and it may be helpful when used appropriately by physicians who care for children.

Two double-blind controlled trials of chemoprophylaxis in children with acute otitis media have been reported: Maynard et al. (1972) studied Alaskan Eskimo children, and Perrin and coworkers (1974) studied children in Rochester, New York. In the first study, ampicillin or a placebo was administered for one year to children under seven years of age living in Alaskan Eskimo villages. The children received a daily dose or oral ampicillin — 125 mg for those up to 2½ years of age, and 250 mg for older children. Otitis media was defined as a new episode of otorrhea by history or observation of a research nurse who made monthly visits to the villages. The incidence of otorrhea was reduced by approximately 50 per cent in the 173 children receiving ampicillin compared with the 191 children who received a placebo.

In the study by Perrin et al. (1974), sulfisox-

Table 16–36 EFFECTS OF CHEMOPROPHYLAXIS ON RECURRENCE OF OTITIS MEDIA*

	No. of Children (54)	No. of Episodes	
		None	1 or more
First Trial (12/72–2/73)			
Sulfisoxazole	28	25	3
Placebo	26	14	12
Second Trial (3/73–5/73)			
Sulfisoxazole	26	25	1
Placebo	28	19	9

*From Perrin, J. M., Charney, E., MacWhinney, J. B., Jr., McInerny, T. K., Miller, R. L., and Nazarian, L. F. 1974. Sulfisoxazole as chemoprophylaxis for recurrent otitis media: A double-blind crossover study in pediatric practice. N. Engl. J. Med., 291:664–667.

azole or a placebo was administered to 54 children in Rochester, New York, who were 11 months to 8 years of age and had histories of recurrent episodes of acute otitis media (three or more episodes in the previous 18 months, or more than five episodes total). Children received a placebo or 500 mg of sulfisoxazole twice a day for three months. They were then switched to the alternate regimen for another three month period. No specific criteria for otitis media were used by the participating pediatricians (a four-physician group practice in suburban Rochester). A significant decrease in new episodes of acute otitis media occurred in the group of children receiving the antimicrobial agent. The older children, six to eight years of age, showed minimal or insignificant decrease in incidence of otitis media when on the prophylactic regimen. The results of the study are given in Table 16–36.

Biedel (1978) evaluated the effectiveness of sulfonamides (sulfisoxazole or trisulfapyrimidine in a dosage of 100 to 130 mg/kg/24 hr, or sulfamethoxazole in a dosage of 55 mg/kg/24 hr) used at the onset of signs of infection of the upper respiratory tract. Children were enrolled in the program after recovery from a recent acute episode of otitis media. They were placed alternately into treatment (sulfonamide) or control (decongestant) groups when parents called the physician and reported any sign of a new upper respiratory tract infection. Treatment was prescribed for a minimum of six days and any new episodes of otitis media that occurred during the eight weeks following recovery from the original episode of otitis media were recorded. Otitis media was found to recur with a new upper respiratory infection more frequently in children receiving decongestants than in children receiving sulfonamide.

Although the data from these are persuasive, additional studies of more prolonged courses of antimicrobial prophylaxis are needed. Future studies must determine whether the antimicrobial agents decrease the duration of effusion in the middle ear as well as decrease the signs of otitis media and whether prolonged courses will result in significant side effects or development of resistant bacteria.

Should prophylaxis be prescribed for the young child who has recurrent bouts of acute otitis media? Although the studies are inadequate to provide conclusive evidence of the value of chemoprophylaxis, we are impressed with the results. While we await definitive studies of the value of chemoprophylaxis, we believe it is reasonable for the physician to use a drug such as amoxicillin 20 mg per kg every 24 hrs in one dose (conveniently given at bedtime), or a daily dose of sulfonamide 50 mg/kg, for the child who has repeated episodes of otitis media (arbitrarily we consider "repeated episodes" to be three in six months or five in 12 months); this prophylactic regimen should be continued for about six months. Most important, the physician must examine the child at frequent and regular intervals (every month) to be certain that inapparent middle ear effusion does not occur. If a decrease in signs of acute disease occurs but there is persistence of middle ear effusion, surgical intervention should be considered, such as myringotomy and tympanostomy tube insertion.

Decongestants and Antihistamines

Nasal and oral decongestants, administered either alone or in combination with an antihistamine, are currently among the most popular medications for the treatment of otitis media with effusion. The common concept is that these drugs reduce congestion of the mucosa of the eustachian tube; however, the efficacy of this mode of therapy for otitis media with effusion has not been demonstrated.

A number of investigators have evaluated decongestants with or without antihistamines, but the quality of design of the programs has varied and therefore the results are difficult to interpret.

1. Collipp (1961) evaluated the use of phenylephrine hydrochloride nasal spray in treating acute purulent otitis media with effusion in 180 children aged 2 to 14 years. Half of the children were treated with nasal spray by their parents four times per day; the other half received no decongestant. All subjects were given an initial injection of procaine penicillin G and a 10-day course of acetyl sulfisoxazole, chlorpheniramine maleate, and phenylephrine hydrochloride. No statistical differences were noted in the otologic status of the children who received the nasal spray and those who did not.

2. Rubenstein et al. (1965) treated 462 episodes of otitis media with effusion using several antimicrobial agents and the decongestant pseudoephedrine. While some improvement was noted to be the result of treatment with the antimicrobial agents, the addition of pseudoephedrine to the medication regimen did not appear to improve treatment results significantly.

3. Miller (1970) evaluated the effect of a decongestant mixture containing carbinoxamine maleate and pseudoephedrine hydrochloride on 13 children with tympanostomy tubes which had been inserted to treat recurrent otitis media with effusion using drug or placebo in a limited double-blind cross-over design. The success of the placebo or drug was determined by the results of eustachian tube function tests which measured the ability to equilibrate applied negative middle ear pressures. An almost equal number of patients demonstrated "suggestive" positive response or no response to the drug, while none of the children showed any response to the placebo.

4. Stickler et al. (1967), in a follow-up to Rubenstein's study (1965), evaluated the effects of penicillin and antihistamine (chlorpheniramine maleate), of penicillin alone, and of penicillin with sulfonamides on otitis media with effusion. While sulfonamides did not improve the effects of the penicillin, the addition of the antihistaminic agent to penicillin did produce better results.

5. Olson and coworkers (1978) evaluated the efficacy of pseudoephedrine hydrochloride by studying the response to treatment of 96 children who had had acute otitis media with effusion that had

not responded to treatment for two weeks. Following a double-blind protocol which compared the effects of the drug to those of the placebo, the children were treated for at least four weeks and reexamined by pneumatic otoscopy and tympanometry. No significant differences between the treatment groups were found. Although the findings were not statistically significant, these researchers did note that males and children with an allergic history did worse on the decongestant.

6. Holmquist (1977) reported the effect of a combination of ephedrine and antihistamine compared with that of a placebo in a double-blind study on eustachian tube function in 58 patients (62 ears). The eustachian tube function was evaluated by means of air-pressure equalization and tympanometry. In the 28 ears of patients who received the drug, a "positive effect" was noted in 16 (57 per cent), whereas of the 34 ears of subjects who received the placebo, a "positive effect" was reported in only 6 (18 per cent); the difference was statistically significant at the 95 per cent confidence level.

7. However, Fraser et al. (1977) compared ephedrine nose drops; a combination of brompheniramine maleate, phenylephrine hydrochloride, and phenylpropanolamine hydrochloride; autoinflation; and no treatment in children with otitis media with effusion and found no difference in tympanic membrane compliance, middle ear pressure, or audiometric findings between the treatment groups. In addition to problems associated with documentation of otitis media with effusion, the investigators had eight treatment regimens with only 10 or 11 subjects in each group, which leads one to question the design and statistical analysis of the study.

8. In a double-blind study, Roth and coworkers (1977) showed that pseudoephedrine hydrochloride decreased nasal resistance in adults who had an upper respiratory infection.

Past studies, employing a modified inflation-deflation manometric technique to assess eustachian tube function in children who had had recurrent or chronic otitis media with effusion, showed that the obstruction of the eustachian tube was functional rather than mechanical (Bluestone et al., 1974; Cantekin et al., 1976). However, further studies during periods of upper respiratory infection showed that eustachian tube function was decreased from the baseline measurements at these times (Bluestone et al., 1977a). This decrease was attributed to intrinsic mechanical obstruction superimposed on the functional obstruction.

9. In an attempt to determine the effect of an oral decongestant with or without an antihistamine on the ventilatory function of the eustachian tube, two separate studies were conducted in 50 children who had had chronic or recurrent otitis media with effusion, and in whom tympanostomy tubes had been inserted previously (Cantekin et al., 1980a). The first was a double-blind study that compared the effect of an oral decongestant, pseudoephedrine hydrochloride, with that of a placebo in 22 children who developed an upper respiratory infection during an observation period. Certain measures of eustachian tube function were significantly elevated above baseline values during the upper respiratory infection, which was attributed to intrinsic mechanical obstruction of the eustachian tube. It was found that oral decongestants tended to alter these parameters of eustachian tube function in the direction of the baseline (pre–upper respiratory infection) values. Even though the effect was statistically significant, the favorable changes in measurements of tubal function were only partial and were more prominent on the second day of the trial after the subjects had received four doses of the decongestant. However, the administration of a nasal spray of 1 per cent ephedrine had no effect on eustachian tube function in these children.

The second study was a double-blind cross-over design. In this study of 28 children who did not have an upper respiratory infection, the effect of a decongestant-antihistamine combination (pseudoephedrine hydrochloride and chlorpheniramine maleate) was compared with that of a placebo. When the subjects were given the decongestant-antihistamine medication, there were favorable changes in certain eustachian tube function measures that were not observed when they received the placebo. Again, the response differences between the two groups were statistically significant. Even though these two studies indicated that an oral decongestant appeared to affect favorably the eustachian tube function of children who had an upper respiratory infection, and that the combination of an oral decongestant and antihistamine had a similar effect on tubal function in children without an upper respiratory infection, an evaluation of the efficacy of these commonly employed medications must await the results of controlled clinical trials in children with otitis media with effusion.

10. Lildholdt and coworkers (in press) evaluated the effect of a topical nasal decongestant spray on eustachian tube function in 40 children with tympanostomy tubes. Five parameters of tubal function were assessed, employing a modified inflation test and forced-response test before and after spraying the nose with either oxymetazoline hydrochloride or placebo according to a double-blind study design. The results showed no significant differences between the two treatment groups of the study children who had severe functional tubal disorders, as documented by the constrictions of eustachian tube lumen during swallowing.

The conclusion from these studies is that further investigation of the efficacy of topical or systemic decongestants and antihistamines for otitis media with effusion and related conditions of eustachian tube dysfunction is warranted to justify the widespread use of these medications.

Corticosteroids

The administration of adrenocorticosteroids either as a topical nasal spray or in systemic form has been advocated for treatment of otitis media with effusion for the past two decades. Heisee (1963) reported excellent results with depomethylprednisone in 30 allergic patients who had otitis media with effusion. Oppenheimer (1968, 1975) recommended a short-term trial of corticosteroids in children. Shea (1971) also reported success in treating allergic children who had middle ear effusions by a four-day course of prednisone. Persico et al. (1978) treated one group of 160 children with prednisone and ampicillin and another group of 116 children with ampicillin only. They reported a 53 per cent resolution of the effusion in the group that received the steroid and ampicillin treatment as compared to 13 per cent in the group that was treated only with the antibiotic. However, none of these studies was a randomized, controlled trial.

Schwartz et al. (1980) reported 70 per cent success in treating 41 children with a seven-day course of prednisone in a double-blind, placebo-controlled, cross-over study. The prednisone was administered according to the following dosage schedule: 1 mg/kg/day for two days, 0.75 mg/kg/day for two days, and 5-10 mg/day for three days. The steroid appeared to be equally effective in those children who did and in those who did not have a history of allergy. However, the long-term outcome of the treatment was not reported; it would have been especially interesting to have observed the recurrence rates of the otitis media after such treatment.

Essentially no studies have been reported that have evaluated the effects of administering a topical corticosteroid nasal spray. However, Schwartz et al. (1980) noted that when beclomethasone dipropionate spray was given to 10 children with otitis media with effusion, it was effective in only three.

If, indeed, adrenocorticosteroid therapy is effective in the treatment of otitis media with effusion, the mode of action remains only speculative at this time but may be related to the anti-inflammatory action of the drug. Persico et al. (1978) postulated that the drug altered surface tension forces within the lumen of the eustachian tube. Schwartz et al. (1980) suggested that steroids may shrink the lymphoid tissue around the eustachian tube, acting on mucoproteins to decrease the viscosity of the middle ear effusion by reducing tubal edema or reversing metaplasia of the middle ear mucosa.

From these few studies, all of which have significant flaws in experimental design, it appears that a short course of adrenocorticosteroid therapy may be of some help in alleviating the problems of subacute and chronic otitis media with effusion in some children, but proof of efficacy and specific indications for such therapy must await the results of well-designed, randomized, controlled trials.

Immunization

S. pneumoniae is the most frequent bacterial organism isolated from middle ear fluids of children with acute otitis media (Klein, 1981).

Relatively few serotypes are responsible for most infections; about 90 per cent of isolates of *S. pneumoniae* from middle ear fluids are among the 14 types present in the available pneumococcal vaccine (Pneumovax — Merck, Sharp and Dohme; and Pnu-Immune — Lederle Laboratories) (Klein, 1981). Because of the frequency and morbidity of otitis media in young children, the importance of the pneumococcus as an etiologic agent, and the limited number of serotypes responsible for most disease, investigations of use of pneumococcal vaccines for prevention of recurrent episodes of acute otitis media were initiated in 1975 in Boston, Massachusetts, and Huntsville, Alabama, and in 1977 in Oulu and Tampere, Finland. The investigations were completed in 1980 and the results were recently published (Karma et al., 1980; Makela et al., 1980, 1981; Sloyer et al., 1981; Teele et al., 1981a).

A 14-type pneumococcal polysaccharide vaccine was licensed for use in the United States in 1978. The vaccine contains purified polysaccharide antigens of types associated with otitis media in children. These types include 1, 2, 3, 4, 6(6A), 9(9N), 12(12F), 14, 19(19F), 23(23F), 25, 51(7F), and 56(18C). (The capsular designations are listed by the American system of typing with the Danish types listed in parentheses.) A 0.5-ml dose contains 50 μg of each polysaccharide type dissolved in isotonic saline solution containing 0.25 per cent phenol as a preservative and is administered subcutaneously or intramuscularly. The vaccine is well tolerated. Children who receive the vaccine have some pain, erythema, and induration at the site of injection and a small number have a minimal elevation in temperature. No significant reactions have been noted in children.

Each antigen produces an independent antibody response. In older children (more than two years of age) and adults, antibody develops in about two weeks. Studies in children indicate that as with polysaccharide vaccines prepared from capsular materials of *H. influenzae* type b and *N. meningitidis* group C, children less than two years of age exhibit unsatisfactory serologic responses to a single dose regimen. However, *N. meningitidis* group A (Gold et al., 1978) and *S. pneumoniae* type 3 (Makela et al., 1980) evoke significant antibody responses in infants as young as six months, suggesting that some polysaccharides are adequate immunogens in young infants.

Results of the Pneumococcal Vaccine Trials

Types of *S. pneumoniae* present in the vaccine were isolated less frequently from middle ear fluids of children with acute episodes of otitis media following immunization of children in the vaccine group than from children in the control group in each of the three studies. If the estimates of relative risk for the three studies are combined, the overall risk indicates a significant protective effect in children who receive the vaccine.

The number of episodes of otitis media due to types not present in the vaccine and due to other pathogens (predominantly *H. influenzae*) was similar in the vaccine and control groups. Finnish children two to seven years of age who received pneumococcal vaccines had a degree of protection similar to that of younger children: immunized children had 50 per cent fewer episodes of otitis media due to types present in the vaccine.

In spite of the decrease in middle ear infections due to pneumococcal types present in the vaccine, the clinical experience of children in the vaccine groups was similar to that of children in the control groups. In general, the number of children who had one or more episodes of otitis media and the mean number of episodes of acute otitis media after immunization were similar in the vaccine and control groups. There were differences in some subsets: Huntsville children 6 to 12 months of age in the vaccine group had fewer episodes of otitis media than did children in the control group. The duration of middle ear effusion following an episode of pneumococcal otitis media was similar for the vaccine and the control groups (analyzed only by the Boston group).

Conclusions of the Vaccine Trials

There is both promise and disappointment in the results of the three pneumococcal vaccine trials for prevention of new episodes of acute otitis media. The vaccine *was* effective. Children who received either the 8- or 14-type vaccine had significantly fewer episodes of acute otitis media due to types of *S. pneumoniae* present in the vaccine. The disappointment occurred because the clinical experience with otitis media was not significantly altered; the reduction in pneumococcal type-specific infection in vaccinees was of insufficient magnitude to affect the number of episodes of otitis media after immunization.

The results of these studies do not encourage use of current pneumococcal vaccines for prevention of recurrent episodes of acute otitis media. Although episodes of acute otitis media can be prevented (particularly in children two years of age and older who respond more uniformly to the polysaccharide antigens), the reduction may not be sufficient to significantly alter the experience of these children with infections of the middle ear. Studies are underway of more potent pneumococcal immunogens for infants (by conjugations with proteins or other means of increasing immunogenicity), other schedules (two or more doses), and other study designs (use of the vaccine before the first episode of otitis media). Results of a double-blind trial of several thousand Finnish infants immunized with a 14-type pneumococcal vaccine at seven to nine months of age and prior to the first episode of otitis media will be available in 1982.

Immunotherapy and Allergy Control

Since the precise role of allergy in the etiology of otitis media with effusion has not been documented, and since at times it is difficult to establish or confirm the diagnosis of allergy with certainty, it is not possible at this time to quantify the relative efficacy of allergic management of otitis media with effusion in children. (This topic is discussed further in the section on Allergy and Eustachian Tube Obstruction, p. 398 and 417.) In spite of this dilemma of a lack of information, there are clinicians who advocate allergy management for almost all infants and children who have recurrent or chronic otitis media with effusion. Other physicians doubt that allergy plays any part in the etiology of otitis media with effusion and rarely, if ever, consider directing their treatment of a patient with this problem to a possible underlying allergy. For example, Bluestone and Shurin (1974) and Paradise (1980), in extensive reviews of otitis media in infants and children, did not include control of allergy as a management option. On the other hand, there are those who include allergy in the differential diagnosis if there are one or more of the following: (1) past or present atopy in the child, (2) family history of allergy, and (3) signs of upper respiratory allergy present at the time of the clinical examination. These investigators have employed various regimens in their management of allergies, but all have reported obtaining good results from

such treatment (Fernandez and McGovern, 1965; Whitcomb, 1965; Drapper, 1967, 1974; Rapp and Fahey, 1973; Phillips et al., 1974; Kjellman et al., 1976).

Clemis (1976) considers inhalant allergy easiest to identify and treat and therefore advocates searching for inhalant sensitivities before looking for allergies to food and chemicals. In his experience, house dust is the most frequent inhalant allergen identified. When house dust is identified as the problem, he advises "dust proofing" the child's environment (especially the child's bedroom) and using electrostatic air filters. If environmental control measures are not successful in reducing symptoms, then hyposensitization to house dust may be considered. Mold spores are the second most common aeroallergen responsible for nonpollen allergy; for this allergy too he advocates environmental control, and if unsuccessful, hyposensitization. The treatment of choice when an adverse food reactivity is suspected is total dietary elimination of that food. In Clemis's experience, pollinosis plays a much less dominant role than do dusts, molds, and foods in causing otitis media, but when pollinosis is present he recommends hyposensitization. Pets may be a source of allergy; but in this case, hyposensitization is not as successful as elimination of the offending pet from the house. In Clemis's (1976) view, antihistamines are not of benefit in treating otitis media caused by allergy and he advises against the use of cortisone, in either the systemic or topical intranasal forms, for therapy. Waickman (1979) agrees with Clemis that house dust is the most common allergic offender in patients who have otitis media with effusion that persists for two weeks or longer and has been unresponsive to adequate therapy for infection. Other inhalant antigens are considered to be less common offenders than dust, but for all inhalants the Rinkel (1962, 1963) method of immunotherapy is advocated.

Unfortunately, none of these reports was based on randomized, controlled trials but only on the experiences of the clinicians. Nevertheless, there does appear to be some evidence that chronic and recurrent otitis media with effusion may be associated with upper respiratory tract allergy. Therefore, until our state of knowledge of the etiology, method of diagnosis, and management of allergy in relation to otitis media with effusion increases, when a child has recurrent or chronic middle ear disease and evidence of upper respiratory tract allergy, management of the allergy should be considered as a treatment option. A history of itching of the eyes, nose, or throat; of paroxysms of sneezing; and of chronic or frequently recurrent watery rhinorrhea in the presence or absence of the classic signs of nasal allergy should prompt the clinician to evaluate further the possibility that the child has an upper respiratory tract allergy. However, since no convincing clinical trials of the treatment options have been reported, no single method of treatment can be recommended. The treatment of upper respiratory tract allergy is discussed in detail in Chapter 37. It does not seem favorable at present to treat for an allergy those children who have recurrent or chronic or both types of middle ear effusion, and who lack the signs and symptoms of upper respiratory tract allergy. This could change, however, in the event that convincing data were presented which established that the middle ear is a shock organ.

Inflation of the Eustachian Tube–Middle Ear

Procedures that force air through the eustachian tube into the middle ear and mastoid cavities have been employed for over 100 years in an effort to normalize negative intratympanic pressure and eliminate middle ear effusion. The methods of Valsalva and Politzer are the most commonly used in children (Valsalva, 1949; Politzer, 1909). Catheterization of the eustachian tube has also been utilized but is of limited usefulness in children, since the procedure can be frightening and is technically difficult to perform in young patients. All three of these methods are also crude tests of eustachian tube patency and have been described in detail in the section on Physiology, Pathophysiology, and Pathogenesis, p. 375.

From a physiologic standpoint, inflation of the eustachian tube–middle ear–mastoid has merit. Figure 16–54 shows the flask model of the nasopharynx–eustachian tube–middle ear system: liquid is shown in the body and narrow neck of an inverted flask. Relative negative pressure inside the body of the flask prevents the flow of the liquid out of the flask. This is analogous to an effusion in a middle ear that has abnormally high negative pressure. If the air is insufflated up into the liquid, through the neck and into the body of

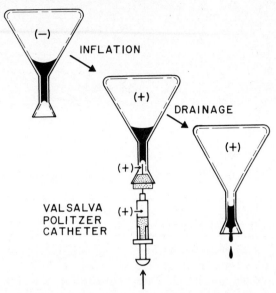

Figure 16–54 Flask model showing the rationale of how inflation of the middle ear promotes draining down the eustachian tube. The eustachian tube–middle ear–mastoid air cell system can be likened to an inverted flask with a long, narrow neck (see text).

the flask, the negative pressure is converted to ambient or positive pressure and the liquid will flow out of the flask. However, if the liquid is of high viscosity, the likelihood of air being forced through the liquid into the body of the flask is remote, especially if the thick liquid completely fills the chamber. Therefore, in the human system a thin, or serous, effusion would be more likely to flow out of the middle ear and down the eustachian tube than a thick, mucoid effusion that fills the middle ear and mastoid cavities.

Theoretically, then, inflation of the eustachian tube–middle ear should be an effective treatment option for children with certain types of otitis media with effusion or atelectasis, or both; however, in reality, there are several problems with this method of management. The self-inflation method of Valsalva is somewhat difficult for children to learn since it is a technique involving forced nasal expiration with the nose and lips closed. Cantekin et al. (1976) tested 66 children between the ages of two and six years who had had chronic or recurrent otitis media with effusion and who had functioning tympanostomy tubes in place. They asked them to try to blow their noses with their glotti closed (Fig. 16–55). None of these children could passively open their eustachian tubes and force air into the middle ear by the Valsalva

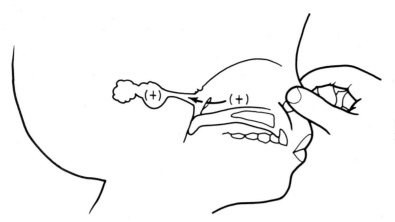

Figure 16–55 Self-inflation of the eustachian tube–middle ear employing the method of Valsalva.

method, even though they developed a maximum nasopharyngeal pressure of 538.8 ± 237.0 mm H_2O. They concluded that the Valsalva method of opening the eustachian tube in this age group was not successful owing to possible tubal compliance problems. Unfortunately, children in this age group have a high incidence of otitis media; for infants, who have the highest incidence of otitis media, the procedure cannot be used at all.

The Politzer method of opening the eustachian tube involves inserting the tip of a rubber air bulb into one nostril while the other nostril is compressed by finger pressure (Fig. 16–56), and then asking the child to swallow while the rubber bulb is compressed. Some children complain of a sudden "pop" in

the ear as the positive pressure is forced up the eustachian tube and have discomfort with the procedure. This method is also extremely difficult to perform in infants.

The major difficulty with both methods is determining whether the middle ear is actually inflated by the procedure. If a child hears a "pop" or has a pressure sensation in the ear, there is only presumptive evidence of passage of air into the middle ear. Auscultation of the ear (listening for the sound of air entering the middle ear during the procedure) is helpful in determining whether or not the procedure is successful, but a sound may be heard even when air does not enter the middle ear. Objective otoscopic evidence that the middle ear is actually inflated would be constituted by the presence of bubbles or a fluid level

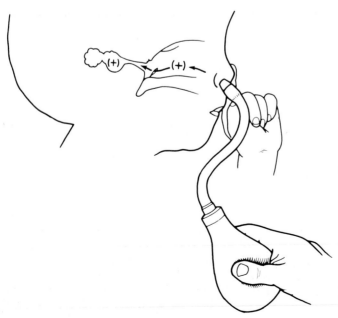

Figure 16–56 Politzer method of inflation of the eustachian tube–middle ear.

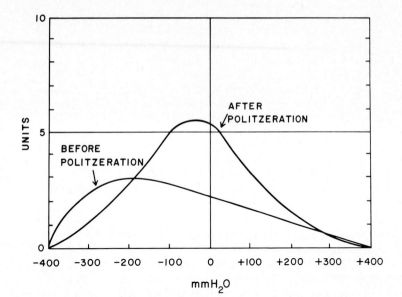

Figure 16–57 Tympanogram demonstrating objective evidence that inflation of the middle ear is successful. Before inflation, the compliance peak is in the negative zone (an effusion pattern), whereas after inflation, the peak is shifted toward the positive pressure zone.

behind the tympanic membrane when these findings were not present prior to inflation. Another excellent method to determine objectively if the inflation is successful is to obtain a tympanogram before and after the procedure: the compliance peak should shift toward or be in the positive pressure zone after inflation (Fig. 16–57). If none of the results of these presumptive or objective methods of determining the success of inflation is definitive, then the clinician cannot be certain that the procedure has been therapeutic. Failure to achieve a successful result may be related to (1) inability of the patient to learn the method; (2) insufficient nasopharyngeal over-pressure to open the eustachian tube passively; (3) eustachian tube abnormality; or (4) a middle ear filled with a very thick mucoid effusion.

Unfortunately, the beneficial effect of the Valsalva and Politzer methods of inflation for treatment of otitis media with effusion or atelectasis has not been subjected to any acceptable randomized, controlled trials. Most of the evidence has been anecdotal. Gottschalk (1966, 1980) described remarkable success with a modification of the Politzer method in over 12,000 patients; the average course of treatment was a minimum of 12 inflations in the office on three separate days. Schwartz and coworkers (1978a) have shown that it is possible to inflate the middle ears of children at home by the Politzer method; they documented the results of the method by tympanometry but did not test its efficacy. The only controlled trial of this method was

reported by Fraser et al. (1977), and they were not able to demonstrate that it was efficacious.

Until well-controlled clinical trials are reported, it would appear reasonable to use the Politzer method of inflating the middle ear for the following conditions. Barotrauma (following flying or swimming) should respond ideally to the Politzer procedure if atelectasis with high negative pressure or an otitis media with effusion or both are present. Inflation of the middle ear should be helpful under these circumstances, since this condition is usually not due to chronic eustachian tube dysfunction, and inflation may resolve the acute, subacute, or chronic disorder rapidly. When a middle ear effusion not due to barotrauma is found in a patient who only occasionally has a problem, and in whom frequently recurrent or chronic disease is not suspected, then the procedure may also be successful, especially if a small amount of serous effusion is visible behind a translucent tympanic membrane. However, it is unlikely that a mucoid or purulent effusion could be evacuated by this technique and if it could be it would probably recur immediately after the procedure. Atelectasis of the tympanic membrane–middle ear, with or without high negative pressure, can also be treated by repeated autoinflation (Valsalva) or the Politzer method, but even if the middle ear is successfully inflated, the benefit is usually only of short duration and the procedure must be repeated frequently. Therefore, it is unlikely that inflation will be successful in alleviating for any length of time frequently recurrent or chronic eustachian tube dysfunction. There is also a remote possibility that bacteria can be forced into the middle ear from the nasopharynx during this procedure.

In conclusion, these procedures may be worthwhile for children with baro-otitis and for children who have an occasional episode of otitis media with effusion or atelectasis, but they are probably not helpful in children who have chronic or frequently recurrent middle ear effusion or atelectasis, or both.

Myringotomy

Myringotomy, or the incision of the tympanic membrane for acute otitis media, was first described by Sir Ashley Cooper in 1802 (Alberti, 1974). This procedure became increasingly popular until the 1940s when antimicrobial agents came into wide use. Nowadays, myringotomy is reserved only for selected cases and performed primarily by otolaryngologists and a handful of primary care physicians; the indications are usually limited to those children who have severe otalgia or suppurative complications, or both. However, facing an apparent recent increase in the prevalence and incidence of acute and chronic otitis media with effusion, considerably more effort, has been made to study the efficacy of myringotomy in the management of otitis media. The potential benefit from more liberal use of the procedure in cases of acute otitis media might be relief of otalgia and a decrease in persistence and recurrence rates. When chronic otitis media with effusion is present, myringotomy may be equally as effective in eliminating the middle ear effusion as when the procedure is followed by the insertion of a tympanostomy tube, with its attendant complications and sequelae, assuming a surgical procedure is indicated at all.

The results of studies conducted in the past to determine the efficacy of myringotomy for acute otitis media are shown in Table 16–37. In the Roddey et al. (1966) study, all 181 children received an antimicrobial agent, and in approximately half of the subjects, myringotomy was performed as well. The only significant difference between the two groups judged by otoscopy at 2, 10, 30, and 60 days, and by audiometry at three to six months, was more rapid pain relief among a small group who had severe otalgia initially. Fewer children who had the myringotomy and antimicrobial therapy. had middle ear effusion at the end of six weeks than those who had received antimicrobials alone, but the difference was not statistically significant. However, if a larger number of children had been involved in the study, the difference might have achieved statistical significance. Herberts et al. (1971) found no difference in the per cent with persistent effusion 10 days after either myringotomy and antimicrobial therapy or antimicrobial therapy alone. Lorentzen and Haugsten (1977) found the "myringotomy only" group to have the same recovery rate (88 per cent) as both the group treated with penicillin V alone and the group that was treated with penicillin V and myringotomy. Puhakka et al. (1979) repeated the same study with 158 children and found that

Table 16–37 PERCENTAGE OF PERSISTENT MIDDLE EAR EFFUSION FOLLOWING INITIAL MYRINGOTOMY AND ANTIMICROBIAL THERAPY COMPARED WITH ANTIMICROBIAL THERAPY ALONE FOR ACUTE OTITIS MEDIA

Investigator	Procedure*	No. of Subjects	Per Cent With Persistent Effusion After: 10–14 Days	4 Weeks	6 Weeks	Statistical Significance Achieved
Roddey, Earle, Haggerty, 1966	AB	121	35	7	2	No
	AB&M	94	24	9	1	
Herberts et al., 1971	AB	81	10	–	–	No
	AB&M	91	18	–	–	
Lorentzen and Haugsten, 1977	AB	190	16	6	–	No
	AB&M	164	20 (Est)	6	–	
Puhakka et al., 1979	AB	90	78	29	–	Yes
	AB&M	68	29	10	–	
Qvarnberg and Palva, 1980	AB	151	50	–	–	Yes
	AB&M	97	28	–	–	
Schwartz and Schwartz, 1980	AB	361	47	–	–	No
	AB&M	415	51	–	–	

*AB – Antibiotic; AB&M – antibiotic and myringotomy.

four weeks after the onset of acute otitis media, 71 per cent of the children who were treated with penicillin V but not myringotomy were cured, whereas 90 per cent of the group that had myringotomy with penicillin V had the same outcome, indicating that "myringotomy clearly accelerates the recovery rate from acute otitis media." Qvarnberg and Palva (1980) reported results of their study of 248 children in which they compared the efficacy of penicillin V and myringotomy, penicillin V alone, and amoxicillin, and concluded that if the first attack of acute otitis media is treated with myringotomy and antibiotics (penicillin V or amoxicillin), cure is the rule; if, however, antibiotics alone (either one) are used, 10 per cent of the patients will run a prolonged course. Schwartz et al. (1981) treated 776 children with a variety of antimicrobial agents, half of whom also had a myringotomy (without aspiration), and found no difference in the relief of pain or in the per cent with persistent effusion 10 days after myringotomy therapy.

Unfortunately, all of these studies had design and methodologic flaws that make interpretation of their results difficult; the question of the value of myringotomy for acute otitis media therefore remains unanswered. For example, in the study conducted by Puhakka and coworkers (1979), myringotomy was performed along with aspiration of the middle ear effusion, but it was a nonrandomized trial. However, children who received a myringotomy had a significantly shorter course of their disease than those who did not have a myringotomy. On the other hand, Schwartz et al. (1981) failed to find a difference between those children who did and did not receive a myringotomy. However, there was no attempt to aspirate the middle ear effusion, and the children were not randomly assigned to the two treatment groups.

Indications

In spite of the lack of convincing evidence to support the routine use of myringotomy for *all* children with acute otitis media, there are certain indications for which there is general consensus at present.

SUPPURATIVE COMPLICATIONS

Whenever a child has acute mastoiditis, labyrinthitis, facial paralysis, or one or more of the intracranial suppurative complications such as meningitis, myringotomy and aspiration should be performed as an emergency procedure. Tympanocentesis should precede the myringotomy to identify the causative organisms. In addition, in such cases the insertion of a tympanostomy tube should be attempted to provide prolonged drainage.

SEVERE OTALGIA REQUIRING IMMEDIATE RELIEF

Even though some studies have failed to show that myringotomy alleviated earache (Schwartz et al., 1981), Roddey and coworkers (1966) did show that acute pain was relieved in those children who received myringotomy. Culture of the effusion is reasonable, since the middle ear is being opened but is not absolutely necessary if there is no reason to suspect an unusual organism.

MICROBIOLOGIC DIAGNOSIS

When severe otalgia or suppurative complications are present in a child with acute otitis media, myringotomy is clearly indicated, since drainage of the middle ear–mastoid air cell system is provided. Although not as compelling as the above indications, whenever a diagnostic tympanocentesis is indicated, a myringotomy for drainage may follow the needle aspiration, especially when a copious amount of middle ear effusion is identified by the tympanocentesis. Myringotomy may then reasonably follow a tympanocentesis when acute otitis media is present and (a) the child is critically ill; (b) there is persistent or recurrent otalgia or fever or both in spite of adequate and appropriate antimicrobial therapy; (c) acute otitis media occurs during the course of antimicrobial therapy given for another infection and the agent should be effective against the most common organisms causing otitis, for example, amoxicillin or ampicillin; (d) the patient is a neonate; or (e) the patient is immunologically compromised. (The specific indications and techniques for tympanocentesis are thoroughly discussed in the section on Diagnosis in this chapter, p. 423.)

The benefit of performing myringotomy on all infants and children with acute otitis media is uncertain at present but is a reasonable procedure, especially if otalgia is present. If a middle ear effusion persists after 10 to 14 days of antimicrobial therapy, myringotomy may also be reasonable if the child is still symptomatic; however, if the child is relatively asymptomatic, the indications for the procedure would be less urgent, since most effusions at this stage would be expected to clear spontaneously during the next several weeks. If the middle ear effusion persists for longer than three months, then surgical drainage would appear to be reasonable. If the procedure can be performed without the need of a general anesthetic, then a myringotomy alone would seem reasonable, reserving the insertion of a tympanostomy tube for those cases in which the effusion recurs soon after the myringotomy incision heals. However, if a general anesthetic is required to perform the surgical drainage of a chronic otitis media with effusion, a myringotomy and tympanostomy tube insertion would seem a reasonable option at present. Unfortunately, convincing controlled trials addressing the efficacy of myringotomy for subacute or chronic otitis media with effusion have not been reported, and until such trials are completed and reported, the above method of management would appear to be appropriate.

Technique of Myringotomy

Tympanocentesis is a needle aspiration of the middle ear contents for diagnostic purposes, but a myringotomy is a procedure in which an incision of the tympanic membrane by a myringotomy knife is made to provide adequate drainage. To accomplish this goal, the incision should be large enough to provide not only adequate and prolonged drainage into the external auditory canal but also aeration of the middle ear to enhance drainage down the eustachian tube. When acute otitis media is present in the infant or young child, adequate restraint employing a sheet or board especially designed for restraining children may be all that is needed, sedation not being necessary. However, for older children, sedation or even general anesthesia may be required. Iontophoresis does not effectively provide anesthesia of the tympanic membrane when acute otitis media is present. However, when a myringotomy is to be performed for a middle ear effusion when acute disease is not present, iontophoresis may be a satisfactory method. The use of a topical solution of phenol gently applied to the exact spot on the tympanic membrane to be opened may be all that is necessary in older children and teenagers. The myringotomy incision should be a wide circumferential incision to encompass both inferior quadrants of the tympanic membrane in order to provide adequate drainage, and an attempt should be made to aspirate as much of the middle ear effusion as possible. Frequently, insertion of the suction tip through the incision on the tympanic membrane will enhance removal of the effusion and provide a larger opening that will, it is hoped, remain open longer than just an incision alone.

The procedure can be performed through an otoscope with a surgical head attached, or, for better magnification and binocular vision, the otomicroscope is more desirable. However, for the routine case, the otoscope is quite adequate, making the procedure readily available to the clinician in settings other than an operating room or otologic outpatient area, where an otomicroscope would be available. By becoming proficient with the otoscope in performing myringotomy, the physician can perform the procedure in neonatal intensive care units, emergency rooms, inpatient pediatric floors, at the child's home, or in any other setting in which a child is examined and is in need of the procedure.

In almost all conditions in which a myringotomy is performed, a diagnostic tympanocentesis may precede the myringotomy. In such instances, the procedure should be performed as described in the section on Diagnosis in this chapter.

Complications and Sequelae of Myrinogotomy

The complications of performing a myringotomy properly are minimal. The persistent otorrhea that follows the procedure and is the most common finding after a myringotomy can hardly be considered a complication, since it is the desired outcome; however, the discharge may become profuse and cause an eczematoid external otitis. If this occurs, meticulous cleaning of the external auditory canal with a cotton-tipped applicator; instillation of otic drops containing hydrocortisone, neomycin, and polymyxin; and insertion of a small piece of cotton in the outer canal which should be changed frequently will usually eliminate the problem. Dislocation of the incudostapedial joint, severing the facial nerve, or puncturing an exposed jugular bulb are dreaded complications but are so rare in experienced hands that they should not deter the trained practitioner from employing the procedure when indicated. The most common sequelae of the procedure are persistent perforation, atrophic scar, or tympanocentesis at the site of the incision. Even though the incidence of these conditions has not been systematically studied in a prospective manner, the risk of any or all occurring do not outweigh the benefits of the myringotomy when indicated. The incidence of these sequelae occurring would rise in children who require repeated myringotomy, and in these patients, a tympanostomy tube should be considered even though its use is not without complications and sequelae.

Tympanostomy Tubes

Myringotomy with insertion of tympanostomy tubes is currently the most common surgical procedure that requires general anesthesia performed in children. The use of tympanostomy tubes was first suggested by Politzer over 100 years ago (1869), but they did not become readily available until they were reintroduced by Armstrong in 1954. Since then they have become increasingly popular. It has been estimated that in 1976 two million tubes were manufactured and, presumably, inserted through the tympanic membranes of probably more than one million patients (Paradise, 1977).

The financial costs of tympanostomy tube surgery have not been formally studied but may be estimated. Physicians' fees for tube insertion average $90 to $125. When they are inserted under general anesthesia, as they invariably are in children, operating room and anesthesia charges are approximately $300 to $500 per procedure. If tympanostomy tubes were inserted in the ears of one million children per year, it would cost approximately $500,000,000 annually. The indirect costs of myringotomy with insertion of tympanostomy tubes — in time lost from school and in lost income to parents as a result of providing support to their children during surgery and afterward — have also not been assessed but may be imagined to be considerable.

There are "costs" of tympanostomy tube insertion which are not financial. For instance, children with tympanostomy tubes usually are restricted from certain activities, such as swimming. However, despite the popularity of tympanostomy tubes (or perhaps because of it), few controlled clinical trials of the efficacy of this method of treatment have been conducted.

Clinical Trials

Several studies have addressed the question of the efficacy of myringotomy and the insertion of tympanostomy tubes for the treatment of otitis media with effusion.

1. Shah (1971) performed a myringotomy and aspiration in one ear, and a myringotomy and aspiration with tympanostomy tube insertion in the opposite ear, on children with bilateral mucoid otitis media with effusion. Adenoidectomies were performed on all of these children at the time that ear surgery was performed. Shah found that the hearing in the ears into which the tympanostomy tubes had been inserted was better than the hearing in the other ears 6 to 12 months after the procedures.

2. Kilby et al. (1972) also performed bilateral myringotomies, inserting a tympanostomy tube into only one ear in a series of children, but they did not perform an adenoidectomy at the same time. These investigators found no difference in the hearing in the two ears two years after surgery when all the tubes had been extruded.

3. Kokko (1974) compared findings in the ears of children who had undergone adenoidectomy, myringotomy, and tympanostomy tube insertion with the findings in the ears of those who had undergone adenoidectomy and myringotomy without insertion of tubes. He found no differences in the pathology present in the tympanic membranes or in the degree of hearing loss present in the two groups four and a half years after the procedures.

4. Yagi (1977) compared 100 children who underwent an adenoidectomy, myringotomy, and tympanostomy tube insertion with 100 children who underwent only adenoidectomy. There were no significant differences between the two groups in (1) the number of children whose hearing problems were "cured" without further surgery; (2) the number of those requiring insertion of tubes owing to recurrence of problems after initial treatment; (3) the number of patients having abnormal tympanic membranes; or (4) the number of patients with more than 20 dB hearing loss 18 months after treatment.

5. Mawson and Fagan (1972) performed adenoidectomy, myringotomy, and tympanostomy tube insertion on a number of children and found that the degree of hearing loss and the number of tympanic membrane abnormalities (such as tympanosclerosis) noted increased the longer the children were followed. They reported that 76 per cent of the children in their study required insertion of another tympanostomy tube within four years of initial treatment.

6. Tos and Poulsen (1976) performed adenoidectomy, myringotomy, and tympanostomy tube insertion in 108 children. During a five- to eight-year follow-up period, they reported that only 2.5 per cent of the children into whose ear tympanostomy tubes had been placed had hearing losses, but that scarring was a frequently observed abnormality.

7. Marshak and Neriah (1981) did a retrospective study on 58 children, half of whom had undergone adenoidectomy and myringotomy for chronic otitis media with effusion and the other half of whom had only had tympanostomy tubes inserted. Only 20.7 per cent of the adenoidectomized children had normal hearing and aerated middle ears during a two-year follow-up, whereas 59 per cent of the children who had had tympanostomy tubes inserted had normal hearing and aerated middle ears during the same period.

These studies demonstrate the problems with myringotomy and tympanostomy tube insertion. *No* randomized clinical trial of the efficacy of myringotomy with tympanostomy tube insertion has been reported, but there appears to be some evidence that tympanostomy tubes allow for normal hearing while they are in place. There is little evidence that tubes prevent recurrence of otitis media with effusion or hearing loss after the tubes are out, and there appears to be some evidence that pathologic changes may occur in the tympanic membrane after the insertion of a tympanostomy tube. However, the use of such tubes may prevent the complications and sequelae of otitis media with effusion or severe atelectasis, or both. It is important to know if the beneficial effects of tympanostomy tube insertion outweigh these potential complications and sequelae.

Need for Randomized Clinical Trials of Tympanostomy Tubes

It is evident from the review of the existing literature that the widespread use of tympanostomy tubes has not been based on any controlled clinical trial. Rather, the popularity of the tubes has been based empirically on their apparent success in restoring hearing and preventing recurrence of otitis media with effusion. However, randomized clinical trials are urgently needed to confirm this apparent success. Such a study is now in progress. In 1979, the Departments of Oto-laryngology and Pediatrics at Children's Hospital of Pittsburgh initiated a clinical study of the efficacy of tympanostomy tubes in infants and children who have chronic otitis media with effusion that has been unresponsive to a standardized medical treatment. Also, a randomized, controlled clinical trial for the prevention of otitis media in infants and children who have frequent recurrent episodes of the disease is also being studied.

In addition, children and adults who have atelectasis of the tympanic membrane–middle ear, especially those with deep retraction pockets in the pars flaccida or the posterosuperior quadrant of the tympanic membrane, should be studied in a controlled clinical trial to determine whether or not the use of tympanostomy tubes prevents progressive changes such as erosion of the incus or cholesteatoma formation, or both, from occurring. Until such studies are completed and reported, the indications for the insertion of tympanostomy tubes must remain empiric.

Rationale for the Use of Tympanostomy Tubes

Even though the procedure has not been tested in controlled clinical trials, tympanostomy tube insertion would appear to be beneficial, since hearing is restored and permanent structural changes within the middle ear may be prevented. The rationale for the procedure may be found in certain aspects of the physiology and pathophysiology of the nasopharynx–eustachian tube–middle ear–mastoid air cell system related to the pathogenesis of otitis media. The eustachian tube has three important physiologic functions in relation to the middle ear: (1) middle ear pressure regulation (Fig. 16–58A), (2) drainage of secretions down the eustachian tube (Fig. 16–58B), and (3) protection of the middle ear from the entrance of unwanted nasopharyngeal secretions (Fig. 16–58C) (Bluestone and Beery, 1976).

Pressure regulation of the middle ear is achieved by contraction of the tensor veli palatini muscle, which actively dilates (opens) the eustachian tube (Cantekin et al., 1980b). Dysfunction of the eustachian tube may be due either to abnormal patency or to obstruction. A patulous eustachian tube (one that is open even at rest) is not as common as one that is semipatulous (i.e., one that has low resistance). Obstruction can be either functional or mechanical. Functional obstruction is due either to increased compliance (decreased stiffness) or to an abnormal opening

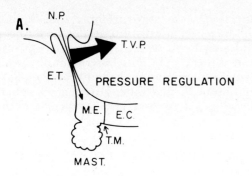

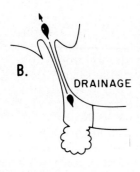

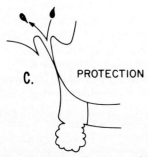

Figure 16–58 Physiologic functions of the eustachian tube related to the middle ear. N.P., nasopharynx; T.V.P., tensor veli palatini muscle; E.T., eustachian tube; M.E., middle ear; T.M., tympanic membrane; E.C., external auditory canal; MAST, mastoid (see text).

mechanism (i.e., tensor veli palatini contraction), or to both. Mechanical obstruction may be due to intrinsic inflammation, infection or allergy, or both (Bluestone et al., 1977a; Bluestone, 1978). Mechanical obstruction could also be the result of extrinsic compression by adenoids (Bluestone et al., 1972c, 1975a), or, more rarely, by a tumor. Nasopharyngeal secretions possibly containing pathogenic bacteria can enter the middle ear–mastoid air cell system by *reflux, insufflation,* or *aspiration,* and can result in otitis media. Severe functional or mechanical eustachian tube obstruction can result in *atelectasis* of the tympanic membrane, or a sterile

middle ear effusion, or both (Bluestone and Beery, 1976).

A functioning tympanostomy tube would maintain ambient pressure within the middle ear and mastoid (Fig. 16–59*A*) and provide adequate drainage both down the eustachian tube and through the tympanostomy tube (Fig. 16–59*B*). Therefore, two physiologic functions of the eustachian tube are fulfilled by the tympanostomy tube. However, the protective function of the eustachian tube may be impaired by tympanostomy tube insertion, since all of the conventional tympanostomy tubes used leave an opening in the

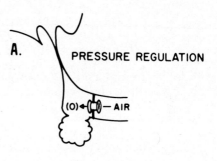

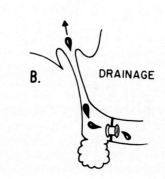

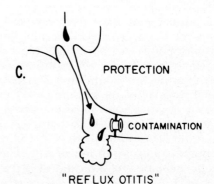

Figure 16–59 Tympanostomy tubes restore pressure regulation (*A*) and drainage (*B*) functions of the eustachian tube but may interfere with its protective function (*C*) owing to loss of the middle ear–mastoid air cushion, which can result in "reflux otitis media" (see text).

tympanic membrane, and the physiologic middle ear cushion is not present if the tympanic membrane is open (Fig. 16–59C). Therefore, reflux of nasopharyngeal secretions into the middle ear may be enhanced when a tympanostomy tube eliminates the middle ear air cushion, a situation that can result in "reflux otitis media" and otorrhea.

The ideal eustachian tube prosthesis would be a transtympanic tube that fulfilled all three of the important physiologic functions of the eustachian tube: pressure regulation, drainage, and protection. In an attempt to develop such a prosthesis, a tube with a semipermeable membrane covering one end of the artificial tube has been developed and is currently being evaluated in a clinical trial (Cantekin and Bluestone, 1976). Such a tube may also be beneficial in preventing contamination of the middle ear by water in the external ear canal during bathing and swimming.

Recommended Indications for Insertion of Tympanostomy Tubes

Even though the efficacy of tympanostomy tubes has not been established, current indications for their use seem reasonable in selected cases until such controlled studies are reported.

CHRONIC OTITIS MEDIA WITH EFFUSION

Patients who have had otitis media with effusion that has been unresponsive to other methods of management for at least three months would appear to be reasonable candidates for the insertion of tympanostomy tubes. Although there are no results available from studies of appropriate design, the most rational of these other treatments for chronic effusions is probably administration of a trial course of antimicrobial drugs. The use of antimicrobial agents is based on results of several studies that have demonstrated the presence of bacteria in chronic middle ear effusions (Senturia et al., 1958; Liu et al., 1975; Healy and Teele, 1977; Riding et al., 1978a). If antimicrobial therapy is unsuccessful, then removal of the middle ear effusion through a myringotomy incision would appear to be warranted. Persistence of otitis media with effusion immediately following myringotomy and aspiration of the effusion would be a compelling indication for the use of a tympanostomy tube. Until controlled studies of the efficacy of myringotomy with tube insertion as compared with myringotomy alone are reported, it would seem reasonable to attempt a myringotomy and aspiration of the middle ear effusion prior to

insertion of a tympanostomy tube in both children and adults who do not require general anesthesia. Presence of a mucoid effusion at the time of initial myringotomy would prompt many clinicians to insert a tympanostomy tube at that time. However, if general anesthesia is necessary to perform a myringotomy, insertion of a tympanostomy tube at the same time, regardless of the type of effusion present, would appear to be reasonable.

Removal of a middle ear effusion that is asymptomatic, especially when significant hearing loss is not present, is questionable. If air is visualized behind a translucent tympanic membrane (i.e., bubbles or a fluid level are visible), the condition would appear to be less severe. However, most children with effusion have some degree of conductive hearing loss and the short- or long-term effects of even modest degrees of hearing loss on the development of a child have not been measured adequately (Hanson and Ulvestad, 1979). In addition, it is not known what chronic irreversible changes, such as adhesive otitis media, tympanosclerosis, ossicular discontinuity, or cholesteatoma, might occur in the middle ear space if such an effusion is not treated. Therefore, the ultimate decision for use of tympanostomy tubes for chronic otitis media with effusion must be based on many factors, most of which remain arbitrary. At present, however, it seems to be reasonable to insert tympanostomy tubes to restore hearing and prevent possible complications and sequelae of recurrent and chronic otitis media with effusion.

RECURRENT OTITIS MEDIA WITH EFFUSION

Many children, especially infants, have recurrent episodes of acute otitis media with effusion that respond to medical therapy or resolve spontaneously; in these patients the middle ear effusion does not become chronic. However, it would still be desirable to prevent these episodes when they occur frequently over a relatively short period of time, since hearing is affected when the middle ear effusion is present and the child may be uncomfortable owing to accompanying otalgia and fever. At present, there are three popular treatments for such episodes: (1) antimicrobial prophylaxis, (2) adenoidectomy with or without tonsillectomy, and (3) myringotomy with insertion of tympanostomy tubes. Unfortunately, none of these methods of management has been satisfactorily tested in a randomized clinical trial.

In spite of the relative lack of proof of their efficacy, tympanostomy tubes may reasonably be assumed to prevent otitis media with effusion. Presumably, the tube would prevent aspiration of infected nasopharyngeal secretions into the middle ear, since ambient rather than negative middle ear pressure would be present. Absence of negative middle ear pressure could also prevent accumulation of a noninfected middle ear effusion. In addition, a nonintact tympanic membrane would allow for excellent drainage down the eustachian tube of any secretions entering the middle ear. However, in children with semipatulous eustachian tubes, reflux of nasopharyngeal secretions could be enhanced when the tympanic membrane is not intact, resulting in otorrhea secondary to reflux otitis media. Studies of appropriate design to test these hypotheses are lacking. Although data are not available, myringotomy with insertion of a tympanostomy tube appears to the authors to be helpful for children who suffer frequent recurrent attacks of acute otitis media. Three or more episodes during the preceding six months, or at least four episodes during the preceding year with the last episode occurring during the preceding six months, would be indications for performing this procedure. However, for such children a trial of antimicrobial prophylaxis would be an acceptable alternative management option, reserving myringotomy with insertion of tympanostomy tubes for those children in whom chemoprophylaxis has failed. Antimicrobial prophylaxis should be considered only in those children who have no evidence of a middle ear effusion between the acute attacks. For those children who have recurrent acute episodes superimposed on a chronic otitis media with effusion, tympanostomy tubes should be inserted.

Eustachian Tube Dysfunction and Atelectasis of the Tympanic Membrane

Tympanostomy tubes may restore normal middle ear pressure in patients who have eustachian tube dysfunction but who do *not* have a middle ear effusion when one or more of the following conditions is present: (1) otalgia, (2) significant and symptomatic conductive hearing loss, (3) vertigo, and (4) tinnitus. If these signs and symptoms are believed to be due to eustachian tube obstruction and not related to a condition that can be improved by medical treatment (e.g., sinusitis), then tympanostomy tubes often provide relief. This is not usually the case in patients with a patulous or semipatulous eustachian tube. When an abnormally patent eustachian tube is suspected, a trial with just a myringotomy should first be attempted. If the patient is symptom-free when the tympanic membrane is not intact, a tympanostomy tube can then be inserted. However, if the symptoms are not eliminated or become worse, a tympanostomy tube should not be inserted. While the tympanic membrane is open, a test of eustachian tube function should be performed in an effort to determine the specific type of dysfunction present. If the function of the eustachian tube is normal, another cause of the symptoms (e.g., inner ear pathology) should be sought.

Atelectasis of the middle ear may be the result either of passive collapse of the tympanic membrane due to lack of stiffness of the drum or of active retraction of the tympanic membrane secondary to high negative middle ear pressure. Atelectasis may be either generalized or localized or both and may be accompanied by a retraction pocket in the pars flaccida or posterosuperior portion of the tympanic membrane. These two portions of the tympanic membrane are the most compliant areas of the drum (Khanna and Tonndorf, 1972). A severe retraction pocket in the posterosuperior portion of the tympanic membrane may cause irreversible destruction of the incus, with resultant conductive hearing loss. Progression of such a retraction pocket may also result in a cholesteatoma. This sequence of events has been shown to be associated with eustachian tube dysfunction (Bluestone et al., 1977b) and may be reversed by insertion of a tympanostomy tube. However, if the retraction pocket is associated with adhesive otitis media, in which the tympanic membrane is adherent to the incudostapedial joint and the surrounding area, restoration of normal intratympanic pressure with a tympanostomy tube may not be successful in returning the tympanic membrane to its neutral position. Following tympanostomy tube insertion, persistence of such a retraction pocket in the attic or the posterosuperior quadrant or both may require a tympanoplastic procedure in an effort to prevent progressive disease. However, when a tympanoplasty procedure is performed in such ears and eustachian tube function is abnormal, a tympanostomy tube should be considered postoperatively to maintain normal middle ear regulation of pressure, which should prevent recurrence of the retraction

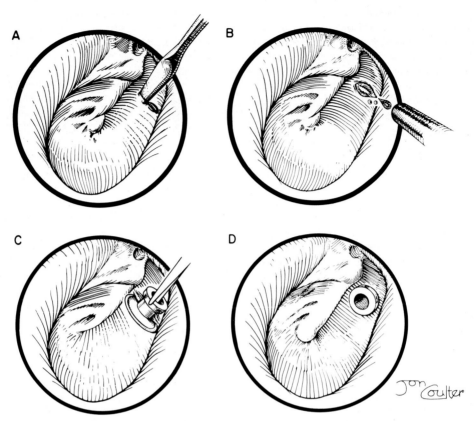

Figure 16–60 Method of insertion of a tympanostomy tube. *A*, Radial incision in the tympanic membrane; *B*, Middle ear effusion aspirated; *C*, Short, biflanged tympanostomy tube (Armstrong type) inserted using alligator forceps; *D*, Tube position in anterosuperior portion of tympanic membrane.

pocket and possibly the development of a cholesteatoma (Bluestone et al., 1978, 1979a).

Surgical Technique and Type of Tube Employed

Insertion of a tympanostomy tube into the posterosuperior quadrant of the tympanic membrane is not advised, since this is the most compliant part of the pars tensa and may result in a permanent perforation or an atrophic scar with subsequent retraction pocket. A retraction pocket could lead to necrosis of the incus or formation of a cholesteatoma or both. Insertion of a tympanostomy tube under the annulus also may result in a cholesteatoma. It seems more appropriate to insert the tube into the anterior portion of the pars tensa. In fact, when there is severe generalized atelectasis, the anterosuperior portion may be the only area into which a tympanostomy tube can be inserted (Fig. 16–60).

The type of tube employed varies with the surgeon. The short, biflanged tubes appear to provide adequate middle ear aeration without a high incidence of obstruction of the lumen by mucus or cerumen, but water can more readily enter the ear through a short tube. However, when the longer type of tube is used there is a greater chance of obstruction of the lumen. The size of the lumen of the tube is quite variable, but if the lumen is too small obstruction is a problem, and if the lumen is too large removal or spontaneous extrusion of the tube could result in a persistent perforation. Tubes are made of various materials, but no data are available to show the superiority of one type of biocompatible material over another.

Much controversy exists concerning the indications for insertion of tympanostomy tubes that are more or less "permanent." Insertion of such tubes may be warranted in selected patients: those in whom tympanostomy tubes have frequently been tried and in whom eustachian tube dysfunction appears to be not only chronic but also not likely to improve in the near future. "Permanent" tubes may also be used in adults with long-standing chronic otitis media with effusion or severe atelectasis. However, these tubes should not be used in children, since the incidence of otitis media with effusion and atelectasis of the tympanic membrane progressively decreases with advancing age during childhood. This is true even for children with cleft palates who have had repeated myringotomies. On the infrequent occasions when permanent tympanostomy tubes are used in children, the function of the eustachian tube should be tested periodically to determine when and if there is evidence of improvement so that the tube may be removed.

Even though many ways to assess eustachian tube function have been tried, there is currently no known method that surpasses observation of the middle ear when the tympanic membrane is intact. Therefore, the best way to determine if a patient needs another tympanostomy tube after the tube extrudes spontaneously is to examine the ears frequently.

When Should Tympanostomy Tubes Be Removed?

In general, once tubes have been inserted, they should be permitted to extrude spontaneously into the external auditory canal and not be removed surgically. The rationale for such managment is based on experience surgically. The rationale for such management is based on experience rather than on any controlled clinical trials: in children with the tympanostomy tube in place, when eustachian tube function is assessed it has not been shown to change significantly, even after several years (Beery et al., 1979).

There are, however, some exceptions to this generalization. Serial eustachian tube function tests should be carried out and if significant improvement does occur, then the tympanostomy tube may be removed.

Most tympanostomy tubes remain in the tympanic membrane for 6 to 12 months, although some have been known to remain in place for years. In children in whom tympanostomy tubes were inserted bilaterally and one tube subsequently extrudes but the other remains in place for a prolonged period, the remaining tube can usually be removed if the opposite middle ear remains free of high negative middle ear pressure or middle ear effusion or both for at least one year after the spontaneous extrusion of the opposite tube. This method of management is based on the observation that eustachian tube function is usually about the same in both ears in children. If high negative middle ear pressure, or otitis media with effusion, or both, occur during the observation period, the tube in the opposite ear should not be removed. Unfortunately, this method of management cannot be employed in adults, since eustachian tube function may not be symmetrical.

Complications and Sequelae

Complications of insertion of tympanostomy tubes include scarring of the tympanic membrane (tympanosclerosis) and localized or diffuse membrane atrophy, with or without retraction pockets, or atelectasis, or both (Mawson and Fagan, 1972; Kokko, 1974; Muenker, 1980). Much less commonly, a perforation may remain at the insertion site following extrusion of the tube, or a cholesteatoma may develop. Other complications include secondary infection accompanied by otorrhea through the tube, and dislocation of the tube into the middle ear cavity.

The most common complication of tympanostomy tube insertion is otorrhea through the lumen of the tube. This is usually the result of reflux of nasopharyngeal secretions into the middle ear. Otorrhea occurred in two thirds of infants with unrepaired cleft palates who had had tympanostomy tubes inserted to treat chronic otitis media with effusion and who were followed during the first two years of life (Paradise and Bluestone, 1974). However, otorrhea may also occur in children without cleft palates in whom tubes have been inserted. When this occurs, a culture should be obtained from the middle ear by obtaining an aspirate through the tympanostomy tube. A preliminary culture of the ear canal and meticulous cleaning of the ear canal should precede the aspiration of the middle ear. Oral systemic antimicrobial therapy should be guided by the results of the middle ear culture and sensitivity studies. Topical antimicrobials and irrigation of the middle ear with a variety of agents have been advocated, but the ototoxic effect of these medications must be considered.

If oral systemic and topical antimicrobial therapy fails, usually after several weeks of treatment the patient should have the middle ear aspirated with the aid of an otomicroscope and a topical hydrocortisone, and an antimicrobial agent should be instilled directly into the middle ear through the tympanostomy tube. Again, the choice of a topical antimicrobial drug would depend on the results of the middle ear culture. The instillation of topical drops should be repeated daily until the middle ear is free of discharge. The organism which most frequently causes persistent otorrhea that is unresponsive to this type of management is *P. aeruginosa*. In the occasional case in which daily instillation of a topical antimicrobial drug fails, intravenous administration of an antimicrobial agent that is effective against *P. aeruginosa* may be necessary. Removal of the tube after such treatment may be attempted, but this usually results in recurrence of the effusion. Removal of the tube in an effort to eliminate the discharge also frequently results in recurrence of effusion.

When frequently recurrent episodes of acute otitis media occur despite the presence of a functioning tympanostomy tube, antimicrobial prophylaxis should be given to prevent the recurrent middle ear infection and otorrhea. The selection of antibiotic and dose would be the same as recommended for antimicrobial prophylaxis alone. The results of cultures from the previous ear discharge would aid in the selection of the most appropriate antimicrobial agent.

Protection of the Ear When Tubes Are in Place

Water from bathing or swimming should not be allowed to enter the middle ear through the tympanostomy tube, since contamination usually results in otitis media and discharge. During bathing or hair washing a wad of either lamb's wool or petroleum jelly over cotton should be inserted into the external auditory meatus. A custom-made ear mold is usually effective in protecting the middle ear and may be used to permit the patient to swim.

Conclusions

It is extremely important to determine the efficacy of insertion of tympanostomy tubes in patients with recurrent or chronic otitis media with effusion, as well as with certain related conditions such as atelectasis of the tympanic membrane–middle ear. However, the apparent beneficial results obtained by this technique warrant its continued use until such time as randomized clinical studies of this procedure are able to show that the disadvantages outweigh the benefits.

It does not seem that the use of tympanostomy tubes is a modern fad that will become obsolete in the near future. Recurrent and chronic otitis media with effusion is extremely prevalent in infants and young children,

but it is a condition that is highly age-related. Since hearing loss secondary to otitis media during infancy and early childhood may impair language or cognitive development, and since insertion of tympanostomy tubes permits hearing preservation and probably prevents many of the complications and sequelae of otitis media while the tubes are in place, their use is advocated despite the fact that otitis media usually improves with increasing age.

Until randomized clinical trials are conducted, tympanostomy tubes are indicated in the following types of cases: (1) chronic otitis media with effusion that has been present for at least three months and is unresponsive to or not improving progressively with other methods of management, e.g., antimicrobial therapy (such a couse should either be documented or be evident from the history); (2) recurrent otitis media with effusion, at least three episodes within the preceding six months, the frequency being documented or evident from the history; (3) eustachian tube dysfunction resulting in one or more of the following: significant and symptomatic hearing loss, otalgia, vertigo, tinnitus, and severe atelectasis, especially in those ears in which a deep retraction pocket is present in the posterosuperior quadrant or pars flaccida or both; and (4) following tympanoplasty, when eustachian tube function is known to be poor; and (5) presence of a suppurative complication.

Tonsillectomy and Adenoidectomy

Adenoidectomy performed either separately or in combination with tonsillectomy is the most common major surgical procedure employed to prevent otitis media; myringotomy with tympanostomy tube insertion is the most common minor surgical procedure for otitis media with effusion (Paradise, 1977).

Tonsil and adenoid surgery are the most common major operations performed in the United States; approximately one fourth of all children are subjected to tonsillectomy and adenoidectomy during childhood. Such operations account for about one half of all major surgical operations performed on children, one fourth of all hospital admissions of children, and 10 per cent of hospital bed-days utilized by children. In 1979, about 634,000 procedures on the tonsils and adenoids were performed in the United States (Ament, 1980), which, as shown in Figure 16–61,

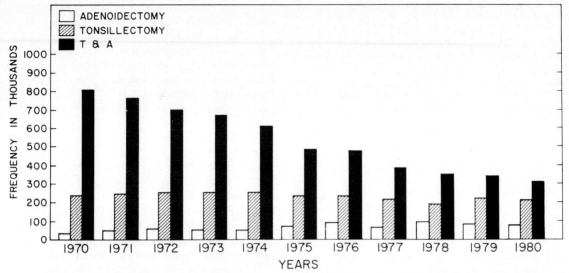

Figure 16–61 Frequency of tonsillectomies and adenoidectomies in all United States nonfederal, short-term hospitals (estimated in the Hospital Record Study, 1980).

represents a significant reduction from the over one million such operations performed 10 years earlier.

However, this decrease in the total number of tonsil and adenoid operations may be related to a change in demography, since the total reduction during the same period in the number of children in the age group concerned was approximately 20 per cent. Although the number of adenoidectomies without tonsillectomy remained relatively small in comparison to the number of tonsillectomies either performed separately or in combination with adenoidectomy, there was more than a twofold increase in the performance of adenoidectomy without tonsillectomy. Also, there appears to be a wide variation in the rate of performance of these operations by region of the country; the rates for adenoidectomy vary the most widely (National Center for Health Statistics, 1974). However, there are no data available related to the indications for which these operations were performed. Certainly, for many, otitis media was one of the indications and in many instances the only indication for adenoidectomy either with or without tonsillectomy.

Previous Clinical Trials

Despite the high frequency of their performance, it has never been established through controlled scientific studies that the benefits of tonsil and adenoid surgery for otitis media outweigh their cost in any age group of children. In the past, there have been only a few prospective clinical trials of tonsillectomy and adenoidectomy. The fol-

lowing is a summary of the results of these studies as they relate to the efficacy of the surgical procedures for prevention of otitis media. In 1930, Kaiser reported the results of following 4400 children, on one half of whom tonsillectomy and adenoidectomy were performed (the indications for surgery were not reported). Table 16–38 shows the results of his retrospective analysis of the prevalence of purulent otorrhea 10 years after surgery. Even though there was no difference in incidence of purulent otorrhea in the operated and unoperated children, the study cannot be considered to indicate conclusively the lack of efficacy of tonsillectomy and adenoidectomy in preventing otitis media, since (1) the two groups may not have been similar at the outset, (2) they were not ran-

Table 16–38 PREVALENCE OF PURULENT OTORRHEA IN 2200 CHILDREN WHO RECEIVED TONSILLECTOMY WITH ADENOIDECTOMY (T&A) AND 2200 "COMPARABLE" CHILDREN WHO DID NOT*

	T&A (%)	NO T&A (%)
Before operation	15	12
10 years after operation	5	6

*From Kaiser, A. D. 1930. Results of tonsillectomy: A comparative study of 2,200 tonsillectomized children with an equal number of controls three and ten years after operation. JAMA, 95:837–842.

Table 16–39 MEAN INCIDENCE OF OTITIS MEDIA IN CHILDREN AGED 2–15 YEARS RECEIVING TONSILLECTOMY WITH ADENOIDECTOMY (T&A) COMPARED WITH CONTROL GROUP*

	Control (No.)	T&A (No.)	t
First year	0.33 (154)	0.17 (222)	2.52†
Second year	0.17 (139)	0.14 (213)	0.54

*From McKee, W. J. 1963. A controlled study of the effects of tonsillectomy and adenoidectomy in children. Br. J. Prev. Soc. Med., 17:46–49.
†Significant change $P<0.01$

domized, (3) the analysis was retrospective, and (4) only purulent otorrhea was considered in the measurement of the effectiveness of tonsillectomy and adenoidectomy.

The first truly prospective clinical trial of tonsillectomy and adenoidectomy was reported by McKee (1963a). The criterion for entry into the study was a history of at least three episodes of "throat infection" or of acute upper respiratory tract infection with cervical adenitis during the preceding year. Table 16–39 shows the mean incidence of otitis media one and two years following treatment, in those (randomly chosen) children who underwent tonsillectomy and adenoidectomy compared with those who did not.

The mean incidence of otitis media among control subjects was twice as high as among children having the tonsillectomy and adenoidectomy during the first year of the trial, but during the second year there was no difference in incidence of otitis media in the operated and control groups. However, this study was based on the occurrence of sore throats, and not on the presence of middle ear disease in the year preceding the study. In fact, subjects were initially excluded from the study if they had "marked deafness, or recurrent or chronic otitis media." In addition, the follow-up evaluation was based solely on interview data, with no objective examinations being made, and no attempt was made to detect asymptomatic otitis media with effusion or impairment of hearing.

In a second study, McKee (1963b) attempted to distinguish the effects of tonsillectomy from those of adenoidectomy. The criterion for entry into the study was the same as in the first study, and, again, children with deafness and otitis media were excluded. Two hundred children were randomly assigned to undergo either tonsillectomy and adenoidectomy, or adenoidectomy only. Table 16–40 shows that the mean incidence of otitis media in each of the two surgical groups was approximately the same.

Therefore, McKee concluded from the two studies that otitis media was infrequent after adenoidectomy or tonsillectomy and adenoidectomy, and that the combined operation did not offer any particular advantages in the prevention of the disease. Even though the studies did not select children with a high morbidity of otitis media, McKee stated that it was reasonable to infer that adenoidectomy without tonsillectomy was indicated for the prevention of otitis media with effusion.

In 1967, Mawson and coworkers reported their prospective study of tonsillectomy and adenoidectomy. The design of their experiment was similar to that of the first McKee study in that an unspecified number of children who were severely affected were excluded and operated upon. Minimal criteria for entry were not described. Table 16–41 shows the relative incidence of earache and otitis media before, and one and two years after, randomization of 404 children into either the tonsillectomy and adenoidectomy or control group.

There was no apparent difference at any age between the two groups. However, as can be seen from Table 16–41, over one half of the children apparently did not have otitis media prior to entry, and the occurrence of asymptomatic otitis media with effusion or the incidence of hearing loss was not reported.

Table 16–40 INCIDENCE AND DURATION OF OTITIS MEDIA IN CHILDREN AGED 2–5 RECEIVING TONSILLECTOMY WITH ADENOIDECTOMY (T&A) OR ADENOIDECTOMY (A) ONLY*

Operation	A	T&A	t
No. of children	97	98	
No. of episodes (per year)	0.16	0.22	0.84
Mean duration (days per year)	0.55	0.74	0.61

*From McKee, W. J. 1963. The part played by adenoidectomy in the combined operation of tonsillectomy with adenoidectomy: Second part of a controlled study in children. Br. J. Prev. Soc. Med., 17:133–140.

Table 16–41 RELATIVE FREQUENCY INCIDENCE OF EARACHE AND OTITIS MEDIA IN 404 CHILDREN RECEIVING TONSILLECTOMY WITH ADENOIDECTOMY (T&A) COMPARED WITH CONTROL GROUP*

Number of Episodes	Relative Frequency					
	Year Prior to Trial		1st Year of Trial		2nd Year of Trial	
	T&A (%)	Control (%)	T&A (%)	Control (%)	T&A (%)	Control (%)
0	63	65	59	57	58.5	57.5
1	5	4.5	7.5	15	7	9.5
2–3	19	22.5	15.5	18	9	11
4–6	6	3	3.5	2	1	1.5
>7	5	4	–	2.5	–	1

*From Mawson, S. R., Adlington, R., and Evans, M. 1967. A controlled study evaluation of adeno-tonsillectomy in children. J. Laryngol. Otol., 81:777–790.

In a study from New Zealand, using an experimental design similar to McKee's, Roydhouse reported his findings in 1970. In addition to the group of children who were referred for tonsillectomy and adenoidectomy and who were randomized into surgery and no-surgery groups, a third matched group of children who were presumably normal were followed during the trial. Table 16–42 shows the mean incidence of otitis media in the three groups: tonsillectomy and adenoidectomy, tonsillectomy and adenoidectomy withheld, and controls. The results were similar to those reported by McKee, in that there was a reduction in the incidence of otitis media in the first year after tonsillectomy and adenoidectomy, but this difference was not maintained into the second year. However, in the second year of the trial, the total duration of otitis media in the tonsillectomy and adenoidectomy group was less than 60 per cent as long as it had been before surgery. Roydhouse concluded that the operation not only reduced the incidence of otitis media quickly in the first year, but also reduced the severity in both years. However, as in the previous studies, patients whose main symptoms were aural were excluded and there was no attempt to detect asymptomatic otitis media with effusion or impairment in hearing. In a second clinical trial, Roydhouse (1980) randomly divided 100 children with persistent otitis media into two groups: adenoidectomy with tympanostomy tube insertion and tympanostomy tube insertion alone. All had failed a nonsurgical treatment regimen. He compared these two groups to a third group of 69 other children who had had otitis media but had all been found to be free of middle ear effusion following the nonsurgical management and received no surgical treatment.

The cure rate was similar in each of the operative groups, with a greater relapse rate in the nonadenoidectomy group, which required 9 per cent more tympanostomy tube insertions. An estimation from radiographs of the size of the adenoids showed that the group cured without surgery had somewhat smaller adenoids. The relapse rate in the nonadenoidectomy surgical group was independent of the size of the adenoids. The study failed to show a favorable outcome following adenoidectomy.

Unfortunately, all of these prospective controlled studies had one or more of the following limitations in experimental design: (1) entry into the study was based on the occurrence of a sore throat and not on the presence of otitis media; (2) objective evidence of otitis media was not documented by tympanometry or audiometry; (3) no other surgical procedures that may have been performed (myringotomy or tympanostomy tube inser-

Table 16–42 MEAN INCIDENCE PER YEAR OF OTITIS MEDIA IN CHILDREN RECEIVING TONSILLECTOMY WITH ADENOIDECTOMY (T&A) COMPARED WITH TWO CONTROL GROUPS*

	T&A (No.)	T&A Withheld (No.)	Control (No.)
1st Year of Trial	0.19 (251)	0.29 (175)	0.12 (173)
2nd Year of Trial	0.09 (204)	0.07 (122)	0.08 (173)

*From Roydhouse, N. 1970. A controlled study of adenotonsillectomy. Arch. Otolaryngol., 92:611–616.

tions, for example) were reported; (4) the technique of adenoidectomy — e.g., "midline sweep" or thorough removal of adenoid tissue from the fossa of Rosenmüller — was not described, nor was evidence of complete removal of the adenoids documented; and (5) nasal and eustachian tube functions were not assessed objectively.

Children's Hospital of Pittsburgh Study

At the Children's Hospital of Pittsburgh a randomized, controlled trial is currently in progress to determine the efficacy of tonsillectomy and adenoidectomy (see Chapter 48). The effect of adenoidectomy on otitis media with effusion is one of the primary research questions, and an attempt is being made to document and control those factors cited as lacking in the previous studies cited above. The criterion for entry into the study (to deal with the adenoidectomy-for-otitis media-with-effusion problem) is documented episodes of recurrent or persistent otitis media with effusion in a child who had had a myringotomy and insertion of a tympanostomy tube at least once previously. Applying stringent surgical indications, of course, requires careful evaluation. After initial examination, each patient is examined every six weeks and at the time of any respiratory illness. Pneumatic otoscopy is always performed at every visit. A trained interviewer telephones each home every two weeks to determine whether there had been apparent or suspected illness, to make sure that any ill child is brought in promptly for examination, and to obtain routine information on school attendance, medication usage, and a number of minor symptoms.

Basic allergy screening is part of every child's work-up. A nasal smear is examined for eosinophiles, and a battery of skin tests using common inhalant allergens is applied. Other regularly performed studies include lateral soft tissue radiographs of the nasopharynx to assess adenoid size; sinus radiographs when sinusitis is suspected; and audiometry and tympanometry to evaluate hearing and middle ear status and tympanic membrane compliance.

The degree of middle ear disease developing respectively in the adenoidectomy and nonadenoidectomy groups is measured on the basis of three main parameters: (1) number of episodes per year of otitis media with effusion, (2) months of middle ear effusion, and (3) frequency with which myringotomy is carried out subsequent to entering the clinical trial.

Data concerning subjects assigned randomly either to receive adenoidectomy or to enter the nonadenoidectomy control group are maintained separately from data concerning subjects whose parents decline randomization and opt for or against adenoidectomy. However, the two groups of data appear similar.

Preliminary analyses of data currently available may be summarized by stating that, in study subjects, (1) adenoidectomy by no means eliminates the problem of recurrent otitis media, and (2) it remains at the present time uncertain whether or not adenoidectomy somewhat reduces the rate, severity, or duration of recurrent episodes (Paradise et al., 1980). The following variables are being examined as potentially important in affecting the outcome of adenoidectomy for otitis media with effusion: age, sex, race, allergy, adenoid size, and eustachian tube function.

This study does not address the question of whether tonsillectomy and adenoidectomy are more effective in the prevention of otitis media with effusion than adenoidectomy alone, nor will it answer the question of the relative value of adenoidectomy with or without tonsillectomy for children who have not received myringotomy and insertion of tympanostomy tubes in the past. These questions are being addressed at present in a randomized clinical trial currently being conducted at the same institution.

Effect of Adenoidectomy on Eustachian Tube Function

In an attempt to improve criteria for the preoperative selection of patients for adenoidectomy, radiographic studies of the nasopharynx and eustachian tube prior to surgery and after adenoidectomy were reported (Bluestone et al., 1972c). Of 27 patients who had preoperative obstruction of the nasopharyngeal end of the eustachian tube, adenoidectomy appeared to be helpful in 19 (70 per cent). Results appeared to be quite poor in children with nasal allergy: only 2 out of 10 had good results. Furthermore, children who preoperatively showed reflux of contrast medium from the nasopharynx into the middle ear did not benefit from adenoidectomy. In this study, 20 of 33 children (60 per cent) seemed to have a favorable response to adenoidectomy, but eight had worse middle ear disease after the operation than before. For example, a few of the children who had asymptomatic otitis media with effusion prior to adenoidectomy developed recurrent acute symptomatic otitis media with effusion following the procedure. Figure 16–62 shows an

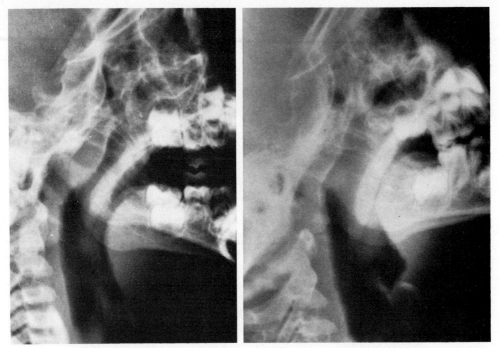

Figure 16–62   Lateral roentgenograms of the soft tissues of the head and neck of a child with chronic otitis media with effusion. Prior to adenoidectomy, the adenoids were considered to be of only moderate size (left). On the postadenoidectomy roentgenogram, they appeared slightly smaller (right).

example of a lateral roentgenographic study of a child with chronic secretory otitis media who received an adenoidectomy. Before surgery the adenoids were adjudged to be of only moderate size. Eight weeks following the adenoidectomy the adenoid size appeared only somewhat smaller. However, when the pre- and postadenoidectomy submental-vertex views were compared in the same child, the function of the eustachian tube at the nasopharyngeal end appeared obstructed before the operation and normal following the operation (Fig. 16–63). This example demonstrates that lateral roentgenographic views alone may not be sufficient to assess the effect of the adenoids on the nasopharyngeal end of the eustachian tube.

The ventilatory function of the eustachian tube has been studied using the inflation-deflation manometric technique both before and after adenoidectomy in a group of children with otitis media with effusion in whom a tympanostomy tube had been inserted (Bluestone et al., 1975a). Inflation-deflation studies of the eustachian tube were obtained in ears that remained intubated, aerated, and dry both before and eight weeks after adenoidectomy. Nasal pressures during swallowing were also determined in some. The re-

sults of this study indicated that, following adenoidectomy, eustachian tube ventilatory function improved in some and remained the same in others, and in a few children the function appears to have been made worse. Improvement was related to a reduction of extrinsic mechanical obstruction of the eustachian tube (Fig. 16–64), or to nasal obstruction due to the adenoids (see Fig. 16–12), while in those in whom the function was adjudged worse the tube was considered to be more pliant after the adenoidectomy than before. This increase in compliance was attributed to loss of adenoid support of the eustachian tube in the fossa of Rosenmüller (Fig. 16–65). A comparable situation was described in the radiographic study in which several of the children demonstrated reflux of radiopaque liquid medium from the nasopharynx into the middle ear after the adenoidectomy but not before (Fig. 16–66).

However, neither of these studies included control subjects. In the current study of tonsillectomy and adenoidectomy being conducted at the Children's Hospital of Pittsburgh, eustachian tube ventilatory function studies employing the inflation-deflation manometric technique are performed prior to and after randomized selection of children for the

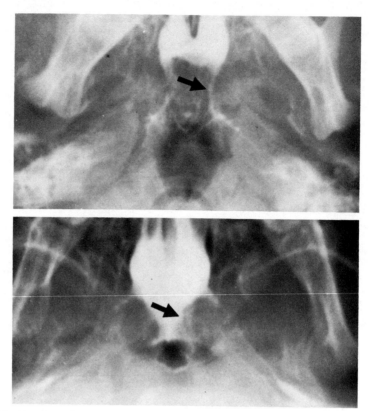

Figure 16–63 Preadenoidectomy submental-vertex roentgenogram (top) demonstrating extrinsic compression of the nasopharyngeal end of the eustachian tube (arrow) in the same child described in Figure 16–62. Following adenoidectomy (bottom), contrast material entered the mouth of the eustachian tube, and the torus tubarius (arrow) was not obstructed by the adenoids.

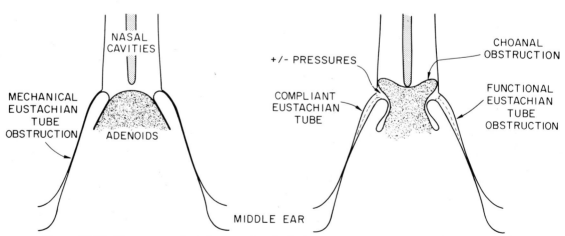

Figure 16–64 Two proposed mechanisms by which obstructive adenoids could alter eustachian tube function. The adenoids can cause extrinsic mechanical compression of the eustachian tube in the fossa of Rosenmüller (left). Obstruction of the posterior nasal choanae may result in abnormal nasopharyngeal pressures that develop during swallowing (Toynbee phenomenon) and result in insufflation into the middle ear of nasopharyngeal secretions or prevent the tube from opening, or both (right).

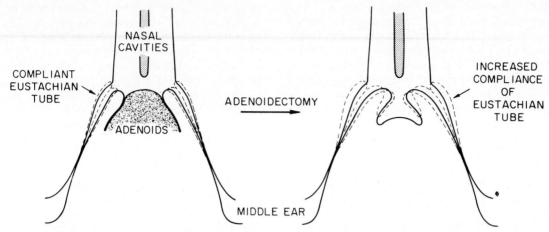

Figure 16–65 Proposed mechanism by which removal of adenoids can result in a more pliant eustachian tube after surgery than before. The increase in compliance following the surgery may be due to decrease in tubal support as a result of the adenoids being removed from the fossa of Rosenmüller.

study and at any time an upper respiratory tract infection supervenes. Since eustachian tube ventilatory function has been shown to be affected adversely by an upper respiratory tract infection (Bluestone 1977a), it is important to assess this function when an upper respiratory tract infection is present as well as when infection is absent in children both before and after randomization into either the adenoidectomy or control group. The goal of this study is to determine if adenoidectomy is efficacious in preventing otitis media with effusion in children, and, if so, whether or not a simple eustachian tube function test may be helpful in determining who may be helped by the procedure. An

additional question would be which type of adenoidectomy ("mid-line sweep" alone or additional removal of the adenoids from the fossa of Rosenmüller) is indicated for the individual child. It is hoped that some or all of these questions will be answered by the current studies.

Conclusions

The previous prospective studies to determine the efficacy of tonsillectomy and adenoidectomy or adenoidectomy for otitis media have shown a modest reduction in the incidence of ear disease in some studies (McKee, 1963a, 1963b; Roydhouse, 1970) but no reduction in others (Kaiser, 1930; Mawson et al., 1967; Roydhouse, 1980) following sur-

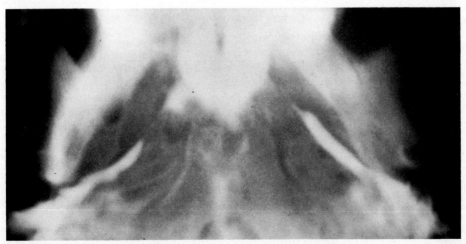

Figure 16–66 Postadenoidectomy roentgenogram of a child who demonstrated reflux of radiopaque media from the nasopharynx into the middle ear. This did not occur during the preadenoidectomy roentgenographic study.

gery. However, all of these studies, unfortunately, suffered from shortcomings in design and method. The current studies of tonsillectomy and adenoidectomy being conducted in Pittsburgh are attempting to eliminate the problems of the earlier studies and to answer the question of whether adenoidectomy is helpful in decreasing otitis media, so that children who stand to benefit can be helped while those who may not can be spared the cost, discomfort, and risks of surgery.

Tympanoplasty for Atelectasis of the Tympanic Membrane–Middle Ear

In selected cases in which a perforation of the tympanic membrane is absent but severe atelectasis is present, a tympanoplasty procedure may be indicated. (When a perforation of the tympanic membrane is present, a tympanoplasty may also be indicated, which is discussed in Chapter 17 — Intratemporal Complications and Sequelae of Otitis Media). The most compelling indication for such a procedure would be the presence of a deep retraction pocket in the posterosuperior portion of the pars tensa which is unresponsive to nonsurgical and other surgical methods of management previously described for this defect. For example, if a tympanostomy tube had been inserted previously, but the retraction pocket did not return to the neutral position after several months of equalization of the intratympanic pressure, a tympanoplasty should be considered, since adhesive otitis media is most likely binding the drum to the ossicles and surrounding structures within the middle ear. Even though the natural history of such deep retraction pockets has not been formally studied, the risk of erosion necrosis of the incus or formation of a cholesteatoma, or both, appears to be quite high. It is frequently difficult to determine if there is only a retraction pocket present or a cholesteatoma has already developed; therefore, a very thorough examination of the entire external canal and tympanic membrane should be performed using the otomicroscope. An examination under general anesthesia will be required for all infants and children in whom the examination is unsatisfactory without general anesthesia. At the time of the examination under anesthesia, a thorough examination of the retraction pocket employing a curved, blunt probe should be performed to determine the extent of the pocket. In addition, the continuity of the incus and stapes should be assessed, since

erosion of the long process of the incus may require surgical correction. Frequently, when nitrous oxide is employed as one of the anesthetic agents, the retraction pocket can be seen to balloon laterally, as visualized through the otomicroscope. When this occurs, insertion of the tympanostomy tube will usually be sufficient to eliminate the retraction pocket. However, reinsertion of the tube may be needed if a retraction pocket recurs after spontaneous extubation.

There are many techniques advocated for repair of a severely atelectatic tympanic membrane, many of which have been shown to be quite successful (Sheehy, 1977; Goodhill, 1979). However, the surgeon should be cautioned that even though the graft "takes," the child will most likely have persistent eustachian tube dysfunction with sustained fluctuating or negative intratympanic pressure after the procedure, which could result in recurrence of the retraction pocket months or years later. Therefore, a tympanostomy tube should be inserted at the time of the tympanoplasty surgery and reinserted if atelectasis begins to recur after the tympanostomy tube is spontaneously extruded. Some surgeons prefer to use tragal cartilage attached to its perichondrium to cover the area of the retraction pocket to prevent recurrence of an attic or posterosuperior retraction pocket (Heermann et al., 1970).

All children who require a tympanoplasty for severe atelectasis must be followed at relatively frequent intervals for the first year after the procedure and at appropriate intervals for several succeeding years, since recurrence of the atelectasis should always be anticipated.

Mastoidectomy and Middle Ear Surgery for Chronic Otitis Media with Effusion

On very rare occasions a child will require a mastoidectomy and middle ear surgery to eliminate chronic otitis media with effusion when all other nonsurgical and surgical methods of management have failed. The operation, which has been advocated by Proctor (1971) and Paparella (1973) and described in detail by Proud and Duff (1976) should be reserved only for those children in whom a thorough search for an underlying cause of the chronic middle ear effusion has failed to uncover a cause, or, if a cause was found, appropriate management has failed to alleviate the problem (for example, the repair of a cleft palate). In addition, all attempts should have been made to maintain an aerated middle ear space by means of a myringotomy and insertion of a tympanostomy tube, even though the procedure may have to be repeated many times for years. If, however, the myringotomy and thorough aspiration of the middle ear fluid is unsuccessful in eliminating the effusion and the insertion of a tympanostomy tube fails to provide an aerated middle ear space, the child may be considered a candidate for a mastoidectomy. Examination of the mastoid and middle ear space at the time of surgery may reveal a previously unsuspected mastoid osteitis, cholesterol granuloma, or cholesteatoma (see Chapter 17 — Intratemporal Complications and Sequelae of Otitis Media). However, even when these conditions are not present, the usual findings will be a cellular mastoid containing edematous, hyperplastic mucosa, with granulomatous tissue, polypoid tissue, and a very thick mucoid effusion. The condition is usually reversible with mastoid–middle ear surgery, but an aerated middle ear–mastoid air cell system should be maintained by the insertion of a tympanostomy tube at the time of the mastoid surgery; the tube should be reinserted if the otitis media with effusion or atelectasis or both recur.

It should be stressed that mastoidectomy and middle ear surgery are *rarely* indicated and should be performed only in those few children for whom other appropriate methods have been unsuccessful.

Hearing Aids

A management option recommended by some clinicians as an alternative to surgical intervention is the fitting of a hearing aid on a child who has a conductive hearing loss due to chronic otitis media with effusion or chronic atelectasis of the tympanic membrane, or both. The rationale for this approach is that it is the hearing loss that may interfere with normal development of speech, language, and learning and that the middle ear condition is self-limited and should improve as the child grows older. The fallacy in this argument is that we just don't know the natural history of chronic middle ear effusions and atelectasis. In some cases, these conditions can lead to middle ear damage. An excellent example is the cleft palate population in which cholesteatoma formation is a frequent sequela in spite of what apparently is aggressive medical, and even sur-

gical, management of the ever-present chronic middle ear effusions and atelectasis. Therefore, the fitting of a hearing aid on such individuals could obscure the pathologic complications and sequelae of otitis media in an effort to promote adequate hearing.

On the other hand, fitting a hearing aid on selected children should be considered and attempted when the hearing loss is interfering with the child's development and the middle ear disease cannot be reversed by medical or surgical methods. Insertion of tympanostomy tubes usually restores the hearing to adequate levels when a chronic otitis media with effusion is present. In some ears, especially with severe atelectasis of the tympanic membrane, a tympanostomy tube is either difficult to insert or remains in place for only a short period. Fluctuating hearing loss in such children could be detrimental and amplification of the hearing may be beneficial. Likewise, a child who already has damage to the ossicular chain and for whom reconstructive middle ear surgery is withheld until the child is older may also be a good candidate for a hearing aid.

Therefore, the fitting of hearing aids should be considered in selected children, but close medical monitoring of such children is mandatory so that the possible development of the complications and sequelae of otitis media and atelectasis are not masked.

Management of Special Populations

There are certain types of children who are known to be at high risk for developing otitis media and in whom continuing surveillance and more attentive management is necessary to prevent the complications and sequelae of the disease. In addition, children who have handicaps otherwise unrelated to middle ear disease may deserve special attention, since the occurrence of otitis media with its attendant conductive hearing loss may further compromise the pre-existing handicap and possibly interfere with the educational and social development of the child.

Infants and Children with Cleft Palate

Since otitis media with effusion is a universal finding in infants with an unrepaired cleft palate (Stool and Randall, 1967; Paradise et al., 1969), it seems reasonable to attempt to maintain these children's middle ears free of effusion and with normal pressures. Since there is always a conductive hearing loss and usually discomfort associated with a middle ear effusion, elimination of the otitis media as early in life as possible should be the goal of management. Medical treatment, such as a trial of antimicrobial therapy in young infants with an unrepaired cleft palate, has not been systematically tested; however, in older infants and children, the nonsurgical methods of management have usually been unsuccessful in the elimination of the middle ear effusion and restoration of hearing. Therefore, the most reasonable method of management for young infants with an unrepaired cleft palate would be the insertion of a tympanostomy tube as early in life as feasible (Bluestone, 1971; Paradise and Bluestone, 1974). If a repair of a cleft lip is performed at two or three months of age, the tympanostomy tubes can be inserted at this time. In any event, a tympanostomy tube should probably be inserted sometime during the first six months of life. The overall reduction in middle ear disease which follows palate repair would appear to constitute a basis for consideration of earlier repair than might otherwise be undertaken (Paradise and Bluestone, 1974). Paradise et al. (1969) pointed out that the middle ear damage and hearing loss prevalent during later life in patients who had cleft palates probably originated with chronic middle ear effusion in infancy; they further suggest that the restrictions in language skill (McWilliams, 1966) and the psychological problems that also seem to be prevalent in these patients later in life may have the same origin, since the persistent middle ear effusion of infants with cleft palates is probably accompanied by variable degrees of hearing loss. When spontaneous extubation occurs in these children, the tubes should be reinserted if otitis media with effusion recurs.

Patients with a cleft palate and otitis media should not be considered candidates for adenoidectomy, since there is a distinct possibility that the operation may worsen velopharyngeal function. In a retrospective study by Severeid (1972), adenoidectomy was not found to be effective in relieving otitis media in children with cleft palates.

Other Craniofacial Malformations

All children with a craniofacial malformation who have an associated cleft palate will have a high incidence of otitis media early in life. Otitis media in these children should be managed as previously outlined for children with only cleft palates. Children in this category include those with Pierre-Robin anomalad (glossoptosis, micrognathia, and cleft of the soft palate) and those with trisomy 21 (Down syndrome). The latter have an extremely high incidence of otitis media with effusion. Balkany et al. (1978, 1979) have reported that over 50 per cent of such children will have a middle ear effusion and that more than three fourths have a conductive hearing loss. Antimicrobial therapy is usually not successful in eliminating the effusion, and most will require a myringotomy and tympanostomy tube insertion to restore the hearing to normal. If a conductive hearing loss persists after successful placement of a tympanostomy tube (the middle ear appears to be aerated), then an ossicular malformation should be suspected, since this congenital anomaly is commonly found in association with these syndromes.

Even though the incidence of otitis media with effusion in many of the infants and children with craniofacial malformations has not been formally studied, children with some of the following malformations are considered to be at high risk for developing middle ear effusions: mandibulofacial dysostosis (Treacher-Collins syndrome), craniofacial dysostosis (Crouzon disease), gonadal dysgenesis (Turner syndrome), and mucopolysaccharidosis (Hunter-Hurler syndrome) (Table 16–43). However, any child with a congenital craniofacial malformation should be followed to detect the development of otitis media with effusion; should he acquire this problem he might most reasonably be managed by myringotomy with insertion of a tympanostomy tube.

Table 16–43 CRANIOFACIAL MALFORMATIONS AND SYNDROMES ASSOCIATED WITH HIGH INCIDENCE OF OTITIS MEDIA WITH EFFUSION

Cleft palate, micrognathia, glossoptosis (Pierre-Robin anomalad)
Trisomy-21 (Down syndrome)
Trisomy-13-15 (Patau syndrome)
Mandibulofacial dysostosis (Treacher-Collins syndrome)
Oculoauricular vertebral dysplasia (Goldenhar syndrome)
Acrocephalosyndactyly (Apert syndrome)
Gonadal dysgenesis (Turner syndrome)
Craniometaphyseal dysplasia (Pyle syndrome)
Osteopetrosis (Albers-Schonberg disease)
Achondroplasia (Parrot disease)
Mucopolysaccharidoses (Hunter-Hurler syndrome)
Orofacial-digital syndrome (Mohr syndrome)

Racial Groups

Certain racial groups are believed to have a high incidence of otitis media with effusion: American natives (Indians and Eskimos), the Maori of New Zealand, natives of Guam, Greenland Eskimos, Australian aborigines, and Lapplanders. The prevalence and incidence of otitis media have not been systematically studied in these populations (or in other racial groups not listed which might also show such trends). However, early in life the children of these populations appear to develop recurrent acute otitis media, perforation of the tympanic membrane, otorrhea, and a propensity for chronic otitis media with discharge as a later sequelae. When infants in these racial groups contract upper respiratory tract infections, which are so frequently associated with the ear disease, they should be aggressively treated by medical means, and antimicrobial therapy should be instituted for the otitis media as early as possible. If a perforation occurs, which appears to be part of the natural history of the ear disease in these children, then meticulous cleansing of the purulent material from the canal (aural toilet) should be performed frequently. In addition, an appropriate topical aural antibiotic, selected on the basis of the results of the culture, should be instilled. Animicrobial prophylaxis is a reasonable treatment option for such children. Ensign et al. (1960) demonstrated a decreased incidence of otitis media in American Indians when prophylactic doses of a sulfonamide were administered. In a later study, Maynard and coworkers (1972) were able to decrease the incidence of otorrhea in about 50 per cent of Alaskan Eskimos who were given a prophylactic daily dose of ampicillin over a one-year period. For those children in whom compliance was considered best, there was a two-thirds reduction in the incidence of ear discharge.

The insertion of tympanostomy tubes into the ears of such children has not been as successful in alleviating the recurrent otitis media as it has in children with cleft palates. This may be due to the basic differences in the etiology and pathogenesis of the disease in these two groups of children: children with cleft palates usually have otitis media with effusion, while American natives more commonly have recurrent otitis media, followed by perforation and discharge.

If a perforation persists in infants and children who have a racial predilection for developing otitis media, and a tympanoplasty is not performed, a hearing aid should be fitted to rehabilitate the child's hearing.

Compromised Host

Infants and children who have congenital, acquired, or drug-induced compromise of their immune system require special consideration when an otitis media is present (Table 16–44). Children with a congenital condition that compromises their defense system are more susceptible to infections in general and may be more susceptible to otitis media in specific. When an otitis media is present in patients with immune deficiency, the possibility of an unusual organism should be considered (Table 16–45). Medications such as corticosteroids, antibiotics, and cytotoxic drugs may compromise the immune system. Lymphoproliferative disease states such as lymphoma or leukemia may also compromise the host.

For such children, the occurrence of acute signs and symptoms of otitis media warrants identification of the causative organism employing tympanocentesis and possibly drainage, i.e., myringotomy. Culture and sensitivity testing of the middle ear aspirate will be helpful in selecting the appropriate antimicrobial agent effective against the causative organism. In certain children who are immunocompromised, frequently recurrent and chronic otitis media are potentially life-threatening, and more permanent drainage may be required; therefore a myringotomy and insertion of tympanostomy tube should be considered to eliminate the middle ear effusion and prevent recurrence of suppurative disease, so as to prevent intracranial and intratemporal complications such as labyrinthitis or meningitis.

Immotile Cilia Syndrome

Infants and children with chronic otitis media with effusion, paranasal sinusitis, and bronchitis (and bronchiectasis) should be suspect of having a chronic respiratory tract infection secondary to abnormal cilia that will significantly interfere with the mucociliary transport system (Eliasson et al., 1977). It is now appreciated that Kartagener syndrome (dextrocardia with situs inversus, bronchiectasis, sinusitis, or agenesis of the frontal sinuses) is associated with the immotile cilia syndrome. Patients with this condition should have a bilateral myringotomy and tympanostomy tube insertion to eliminate the middle

Table 16–44 CLASSIFICATION OF CONDITIONS THAT RESULTED IN INCREASED SUSCEPTIBILITY TO INFECTIONS INCLUDING OTITIS MEDIA IN WHICH AN UNUSUAL ORGANISM SHOULD BE SUSPECT

Congenital	Acquired	Drug-induced
B-cell Deficiency	Neoplasms	Anti-inflammatory
Hypogammaglobulinemia	Acute and chronic leukemia	Aspirin
X-linked agammaglobulinemia	Hodgkin disease	Corticosteroid
IgA deficiency	Non-Hodgkin lymphoma	Indomethacin
Common variable deficiency	Sarcoma	Phenylbutazone
T-cell Deficiency	Carcinoma	Gold salts
DiGeorge syndrome	Weber-Christian disease	Antimicrobials
Nucleoside phosphorylase deficiency	Inflammatory	Chloramphenicol
Thymic dysplasia	Acute infection	Tetracycline
Chronic mucocutaneous candidiasis	Neonatal infections	Penicillin derivatives
T- and B-cell Deficiencies	Lepromatous leprosy	Sulfonamides
Cartilage-hair hypoplasia	Felty syndrome	Streptomycin
Ataxia telangiectasia	Rheumatoid arthritis	Gentamicin
Wiskott-Aldrich syndrome	Metabolic	Amphotericin
Reticular dysgenesis	Diabetes mellitus	Antiparasitics
Nezelof syndrome	Renal disease	Levamisole
Phagocyte Defects	Hepatic cirrhosis	Niridazole
Neutropenia	Hyperosmolar states	Suramin
Chronic granulomatous disease	Protein-calorie malnutrition	Cytotoxic
Chediak-Higashi syndrome	Storage diseases	Cyclophosphamide
Lazy leukocyte syndrome	Anemias	Azathioprine
Myeloperoxidase deficiency	Neutropenia	Methotrexate
Hyper IgE syndrome	Chronic hemolytic anemia	6-Mercaptopurine
Others	Sickle cell disease	5-Fluorouracil
Down syndrome	Others	Phenothiazines
Complement deficiencies	Alcoholism	Chlorpromazine
Glucose-6-phosphate dehydrogenase deficiency	Malakoplakia	Mepazine
Hyper IgE syndrome (with normal phagocytes)	Burn	Diuretics
	Systemic lupus erythematosus	Thiazides
		Ethacrynic acid
		Mercurial diuretics
		Antithyroid
		Thiouracil derivatives
		Methimazole
		Antiarrhythmics
		Quinidine
		Procainamide
		Propranolol
		Anticonvulsants
		Phenytoin
		Phenobarbital
		Other
		Anesthesia

ear effusion, restore the hearing, and prevent the complications and sequelae of otitis media with effusion. Nonsurgical methods of management may be effective, such as antimicrobial agents, but when a persistent effusion is present, myringotomy with insertion of a tympanostomy tube is indicated.

Concurrent Permanent Hearing Loss

Infants and children with preexisting hearing losses who subsequently develop otitis media with effusion or abnormal negative middle ear pressure (atelectasis) or both are at higher risk for impairment of language acquisition and learning than are those children whose hearing loss is due to the middle ear effusion–negative pressure alone. Therefore, the former children should be observed at more frequent intervals than children without a concurrent permanent hearing loss and may require more aggressive management for the superimposed conductive hearing loss, since it is amenable to treatment. The preexisting hearing loss may be conductive, sensorineural, or mixed. The child with a congenital malformation of the middle ear ossicles with a conductive hearing loss may develop persistent or recurrent otitis media with effusion or high negative pressure,

Table 16–45 UNUSUAL MICROBIAL AGENTS THAT MAY BE FOUND IN OTITIS MEDIA OF A COMPROMISED HOST

Bacteria	Fungi
Aerobic and/or Facultative Anaerobic	Candida species
Gram-negative bacilli	Aspergillus species
Haemophilus (penicillin-resistant)	
Pseudomonas species	
Proteus species	
Klebsiella species	
Escherichia coli	
Enterobacter species	
Serratia species	
Gram-negative cocci or coccobacilli	
Branhamella catarrhalis	
Moraxella lacunata	
Gram-positive cocci	
Pneumococcus (resistant)	
Streptococcus species	
Staphylococcus species	
Enterococcus species	
Non-Enterococcus species	
Gram-positive bacilli	
Bacillus species	
Corynebacterium species	
Listeria monocytogenes	
Anaerobic	
Peptococcus	
Bacteroides species	
Higher Bacteria	
Actinomyces israelii	
Mycobacterium species	
Nocardia species	

which would increase his hearing handicap. Likewise, children who have a preexisting sensorineural hearing loss of some degree are often severely handicapped socially and educationally if they then acquire a middle ear effusion. These children should be managed in the same way as those without a concurrent hearing loss from another etiology, but it is even more important to eliminate the middle ear effusion in these children rapidly and to prevent the development of any further hearing loss, if possible. If medical treatment does not eliminate the superimposed conductive hearing loss within a relatively short time, a myringotomy and insertion of a tympanostomy tube should be considered at an earlier time than for children without a concurrent hearing loss. Middle ear effusion is common in all children but appears to have an even higher incidence in some children with a congenital middle ear malformation (e.g., Down syndrome) and those who have a sensorineural loss. For this reason, surgical intervention should be considered earlier in children who have recurrent middle ear effusion and persistent or fluctuating conductive hearing loss to prevent further impairment of hearing and, consequently, of development.

Today many children with moderate to severe permanent hearing losses attend regular schools ("mainstreaming") and some may not even require a hearing aid. Regardless of their functional level of hearing, however, any child who has such a hearing loss should be evaluated more frequently for possible occurrence of otitis media with effusion than should the child without a permanent hearing loss. Children of all ages are at high risk but infants, preschoolers, and young school-age children are at particular risk, since the incidence of otitis media is higher in these age groups. Examination of such infants and children twice a year would appear to be a reasonable goal if the child had no past history or evidence of the disease, but more frequent evaluation (three or four times per year) is desirable for those children who have had recurrent middle ear effusions. Since all infants and young children are at high risk for developing otitis media with effusion and high negative pressure, all infants identified as having a sensorineural hearing loss early in life should be more frequently examined for possible recurrence of otitis media. Even if such children show no objective evidence of middle ear effusion by otoscopy or tympanometry, or both, if there is a history of fluctuating hearing loss the child should be actively treated, since the presence of even transient high negative pressure may lead to a compounding of the educational handicap.

Schools or Programs for the Deaf

Children with severe to profound deafness who are enrolled in schools for the deaf or in special programs in regular schools ("mainstreamed") are at high risk for compounding their handicaps if they develop an added conductive hearing loss secondary to otitis media with effusion or high negative pressure, or both. Since the incidence of intercurrent middle ear problems appears to be high in such children, early identification employing a formal screening program such as the one proposed earlier (see Diagnosis of Otitis Media) is mandatory. Some children develop troublesome cerumen that obstructs the ear canal and may interfere with the function of a hearing aid. Such children should be examined frequently and the cerumen periodically removed. As suggested earlier, otitis media with effusion or high negative pressure or both should be suspected during periods of upper respiratory tract infection when the children have signs and symptoms of otologic disease such as otorrhea and otalgia, or when there has been a noticeable loss of hearing reported by the parents or teachers. Regular periodic screening employing otoscopy or tympanometry or both will identify those children with middle ear problems who might otherwise be overlooked, since obvious signs and symptoms associated with hearing loss may be absent.

Treatment of such children would depend upon the type, severity, frequency, and duration of the middle ear problem. However, more aggressive treatment is indicated for this special population. Myringotomy and tympanostomy tube insertion should be considered earlier in such children when otitis media with effusion is frequently recurrent or chronic. Since sustained or transient high negative middle ear pressure without a middle ear effusion can cause a persistent or fluctuating conductive hearing loss, the insertion of tympanostomy tubes should also be considered at an earlier time than in nondeaf children. The presence of a hearing aid will not interfere with the function of tympanostomy tubes, since a small bore hole can be placed in the ear mold to provide ventilation. It is important when tympanostomy tubes are inserted in such children that a short tube be used so that the ear mold may be inserted.

Early identification and appropriate management of middle ear disease in a child with severe to profound deafness, especially those who utilize their residual hearing, is imperative so that maximum habilitation may be accomplished.

Acknowledgment

The authors want to thank Ms. Sandra Arjona for her patient, diligent, and painstaking work during the preparation of this chapter and Chapters 17 and 18. They would also like to thank Mr. Jon Coulter for design and preparation of the artwork, Ms. Diana Mathis for copy editing these three chapters and Bruce Johnston for verifying the references for Chapters 16 to 18.

SELECTED REFERENCES

Paradise, J.L. 1980. Otitis media in infants and children: Review article. Pediatrics, 65:917-943.

In this well-written article, the author not only provides a comprehensive review of the literature on otitis media with effusion, but also gives the pediatrician's viewpoint.

Proceedings of the Second National Conference on Otitis Media. 1979. Wiet, R.J., and Coulthard, S. (Eds.) Columbus, Ohio, Ross Laboratories.

This monograph contains concise, well-written papers on the epidemiology, etiology, pathogenesis, diagnosis, management, complications, and sequelae of otitis media.

Lim, D.J., Bluestone, C.D., and Senturia, B.H. (Eds.) 1976. Recent Advances in Middle Ear Effusions. Ann. Otol. Rhinol. Laryngol., 85(25).

This supplement consists of the papers that were presented at the First International Symposium on Otitis Media in Columbus, Ohio, 1975, and contains information that is still excellent.

Senturia, B.H., Bluestone, C.D., and Lim, D.J. (Eds.) 1980. Recent advances in otitis media with effusion. Ann. Otol. Rhinol. Laryngol., 89(68).

Contained within this supplement is the current state of our knowledge concerning otitis media with effusion.

Schuknecht, H.F. 1974. Pathology of the ear. Cambridge, Mass., Harvard University Press, pp. 23–40, 97–105, 215–224.

This text has the best description of the pathology of otitis media and certain related conditions.

REFERENCES

Alberti, P. W. 1974. Myringotomy and ventilating tubes in the 19th century. Laryngoscope, 84:805–815.

Alberti, P. W., and Kristensen, R. 1970. The clinical application of impedance audiometry: A preliminary appraisal of an electro-acoustic impedance bridge. *Laryngoscope*, 80:735–746.

Alt, A. 1878, 1879. Heilunger taubstummheit erzielte durch beseitigung einer otorrhoe und einer angebornen gaumenspalate. Arch. Augen Ohrenh, 7:211, and Schmidt's Jahrbuecher, 183:277.

Ament, R. P. 1980. Hospital Record Study, Professional Activity Study. Ann Arbor, MI, Commission on Professional and Hospital Activities.

American Academy of Pediatrics. 1977. Otitis Media. Evanston, IL, Committee on Infectious Diseases, pp. 160–163.

Applebaum, P. C., Bhamjee, A., Scragg, J. N., Hallett, A. F., Brown, A. J., and Cooper, R. C. 1977. *Streptococcus pneumoniae* resistant to penicillin and chloramphenicol. Lancet, 2:995–997.

Armstrong, B. W. 1954. A new treatment for chronic secretory otitis media. Arch. Otolaryngol., 59:653–654.

Aschan, G. K. 1952. Observations on the Eustachian tube. Acta Soc. Med. Upsalien, 57:1–13.

Aschan, G. K. 1955. The anatomy of the Eustachian tube with regard to its function. Acta Soc. Med. Upsalien, 60:131–149.

Aschan, G. K. 1966. Hearing and nasal function correlated to postoperative speech in cleft palate patients with velopharyngoplasty. Acta Otolaryngol. (Stockh.), 61:371–379.

Auritt, W. A., Hervada, A. R., and Fendrick, G. 1978. Fatal pseudomembranous enterocolitis following oral ampicillin therapy. J. Pediatr., 93:882–883.

Austrian, R., Howie, V. M., and Ploussard, J. H. 1977. The bacteriology of pneumococcal otitis media. Johns Hopkins Med. J., 141:104–111.

Bakwin, H., and Jacobinzer, H. 1939. Prevention of purulent otitis media in infants. J. Pediatr., 14:730–736.

Balkany, T. J., Berman, S. A., Simmons, M. A., and

Jafek, B. W. 1978. Middle ear effusions in neonates. Laryngoscope, 88:398–405.

Balkany, T. J., Downs, M. P., Jafek, B. W., and Krajicek, M. J. 1979. Hearing loss in Down's syndrome. A treatable handicap more common than generally recognized. Clin. Pediatr., 18(2):116–118.

Barza, M. 1978. The nephrotoxicity of cephalosporins: An overview. J. Infect. Dis., 137:S60–S73.

Bass, J. W., Steele, R. W., Wiebe, R. A., and Dierdorff, E. P. 1971. Erythromycin concentrations in middle ear exudates. Pediatrics, 48:417–422.

Bauer, F. 1975. Tubal function in the glue ear: Urea for glue ears. J. Laryngol. Otol., 89:63–71.

Bauer, A. W., Kirby, W. M., Sherris, J. C., and Turck, M. 1966. Antibiotic susceptibility testing by a standardized single disk method. Am. J. Clin. Pathol., 45:493–496.

Beatty, H. G. 1936. The care of cleft palate patients. Laryngoscope, 46:203–206, 1936.

Beery, Q. C., Bluestone, C. D., and Cantekin, E. I. 1975. Otologic history, audiometry and tympanometry as a case finding procedure for school screening. Laryngoscope, 85:1976–1985.

Beery, Q. C., Doyle, W. J., Cantekin, E. I., and Bluestone, C. D. 1979. Longitudinal assessment of Eustachian tube function in children. Laryngoscope, 89:1446–1456.

Beery, Q. C., Doyle, W. J., Cantekin, E. I., Bluestone, C. D., and Wiet, R. J., 1980. Eustachian tube function in an American Indian population. Ann. Otol. Rhinol. Laryngol., 89(68):28–33.

Bennett, M. 1972. The older cleft palate patient: A clinical otologic-audiologic study. Laryngoscope, 82:1217–1225.

Bennett, M., Ward, R. H., and Tait, C. A. 1968. Otologic-audiologic study of cleft palate children. Laryngoscope, 78:1011–1019.

Berdal, P., Brandtzaeg, P., Froland, S., Henriksen, S., and Skrede, S. 1976. Immunodeficiency syndromes with otorhinolaryngological manifestations. Acta Otolaryngol. (Stockh.), 82:185–192.

Bergman, A. B., and Haggerty, R. J. 1962. The emergency clinic: A study of its role in a teaching hospital. Am. J. Dis. Child., 104:36–44.

Bergstrom, L. 1978. Congenital and acquired deafness in clefting and craniofacial syndromes. Cleft Palate J., 15(3):254–261.

Berman, S. A., Balkany, T. J., and Simmons, M. A. 1978. Otitis media in the neonatal intensive care unit. Pediatrics, 62:198–201.

Bernstein, J. M. 1976. Biological mediators of inflammation in middle ear effusions. Ann. Otol. Rhinol. Laryngol., 85(25):90–96.

Bernstein, J. M. 1980. Immunological reactivity in otitis media with effusion. In Oehling, A., Mathov, E., Glazer, I., and Arbesman, C. (Eds.): Advances in Allergology and Immunology. Oxford, Pergamon Press, pp. 139–146.

Bernstein, J. M., Hayes, E. R., Ishikawa, T., Tomasi, T. B., and Herd, J. K. 1972. Secretory otitis media: A histopathologic and immunochemical report. TAAOO, 76:1305–1318.

Bernstein, J. M., and Reisman, R. 1974. The role of acute hypersensitivity in secretory otitis media. TAAOO, 78:ORL 120–ORL 127.

Bernstein, J. M., Okazaki, T., and Reisman, R. E. 1976. Prostaglandins in middle ear effusions. Arch. Otolaryngol., 102:257–258.

Bernstein, J. M., Schenkein, H. A., Genco, R. J., and

Bartholomew, W. 1978. Complement activity in middle ear effusions. Clin. Exp. Immunol., 33:340–346.

Bernstein, J. M., Myers, D., Kosinski, D., Nisengard, R., and Wicher, K. 1980. Antibody coated bacteria in otitis media with effusions. Ann. Otol. Rhinol. Laryngol., 89(68):104–109.

Bernstein, J. M., and Ogra, P. L. 1980. Mucosal immune system: Implications in otitis media with effusion. Ann. Otol. Rhinol. Laryngol., 89(68):326–332.

Berry, M. F., and Eisenson, J. 1956. Speech Disorders: Principles and Practices of Therapy. New York, Appleton-Century-Crofts, Inc..

Bess, F. H., Lewis, H. D., and Cieliczka, B. T. 1975. Acoustic impedance measurements in cleft palate children. J. Speech Hear. Res., 40(1):13–24.

Biedel, C. W. 1978. Modification of recurrent otitis media by short-term sulfonamide therapy. Am. J. Dis. Child., 132:681–683.

Bjuggren, G., and Tunevall, G. 1952. Otitis in childhood: A clinical and serobacteriological study with special reference to the significance of Haemophilus influenzae in relapses. Acta Otolaryngol., 42:311–328.

Bland, R. D. 1972. Otitis media in the first six weeks of life: Diagnosis, bacteriology, and management. Pediatrics, 49:187–197.

Bluestone, C. D. 1971. Eustachian tube obstruction in the infant with cleft palate. Ann. Otol. Rhinol. Laryngol., 80(2):1–30.

Bluestone, C. D. 1975. Assessment of Eustachian tube function. In Jerger, J. (Ed.): Handbook of Clinical Impedance Audiometry. New York, American Electromedics Corp., pp. 127–148.

Bluestone, C. D. 1978. Eustachian tube function and allergy in otitis media. Pediatrics, 61:753–760.

Bluestone, C. D. 1979. Eustachian tube dysfunction. In Wiet, R. J., and Coulthard, S. W. (Eds.): Proceedings of the Second National Conference on Otitis Media. Columbus, OH, Ross Laboratories, pp. 50–58.

Bluestone, C. D. 1980. Assessment of Eustachian tube function. In Jerger, J., and Northern, J. (Eds.): Clinical Impedance Audiometry. Acton, MA, American Electromedics Corp., pp. 83–108.

Bluestone, C. D., Paradise, J. L., and Beery, Q. C. 1972a. Physiology of the Eustachian tube in the pathogenesis and management of middle ear effusions. Laryngoscope, 82:1654–1670.

Bluestone, C. D., Paradise, J. L., Beery, Q. C., and Wittel, R. 1972b. Certain effects of cleft palate repair on Eustachian tube function. Cleft Palate J., 9:183–193.

Bluestone, C. D., Wittel, R. A., Paradise, J. L., and Felder, H. 1972c. Eustachian tube function as related to adenoidectomy for otitis media. TAAOO, 76:1325–1339.

Bluestone, C. D., Wittel, R. A., and Paradise, J. L. 1972d. Roentgenographic evaluation of Eustachian tube function in infants with cleft and normal palates. Cleft Palate J., 9:93–100.

Bluestone, C. D., Beery, Q. C., and Paradise, J. L. 1973. Audiometry and tympanometry in relation to middle ear effusions in children. Laryngoscope, 83:594–604.

Bluestone, C. D., Beery, Q. C., and Andrus, W. S. 1974. Mechanics of the Eustachian tube as it influences susceptibility to and persistence of middle ear effusions in children. Ann. Otol. Rhinol. Laryngol., 83(11):27–34.

Bluestone, C. D., and Shurin, P. A. 1974. Middle ear

diseases in children: Pathogenesis, diagnosis, and management. Pediatr. Clin. North Am., *21*:379–400.

Bluestone, C. D., Cantekin, E. I., and Beery, Q. C. 1975a. Certain effects of adenoidectomy on Eustachian tube ventilatory function. Laryngoscope. *85*:113–127.

Bluestone, C. D., Cantekin, E. I., Beery, Q. C., and Paradise, J. L. 1975b. Eustachian tube ventilatory function in relation to cleft palate. Ann. Otol. Rhinol. Laryngol., *84*:333–338.

Bluestone, C. D., and Beery, Q. C. 1976. Concepts on the pathogenesis of middle ear effusions. Ann. Otol. Rhinol. Laryngol. *85*(25):182–186.

Bluestone, C. D., Cantekin, E. I., and Beery, Q. C. 1977a. Effect of inflammation on the ventilatory function of the Eustachian tube. Laryngoscope, *87*:493–507.

Bluestone, C. D., Cantekin, E. I., Beery, Q. C., Douglas, G. S., Stool, S. E., and Doyle, W. J. 1977b. Functional Eustachian tube obstruction in acquired cholesteatoma and related conditions. *In* McCabe, B. F., Sade, J., and Abramson, M. (Eds.): Cholesteatoma: First International Congress. Birmingham, Aesculapius Pub. Co., pp. 325–335.

Bluestone, C. D., Cantekin, E. I., Beery, Q. C., and Stool, S. E. 1978. Function of the Eustachian tube related to surgical management of acquired aural cholesteatoma in children. Laryngoscope, *88*:1155–1163.

Bluestone, C. D., Cantekin, E. I., and Douglas, G. S. 1979a. Eustachian tube function related to the results of tympanoplasty in children. Laryngoscope, *89*:450–458.

Bluestone, C. D., Michaels, R. H., Stool, S. E., Wright, C. M., Beery, Q. C., Zanotti, M. L., Grundfast, K. M., and Mandel, E. M. 1979b. Cefaclor compared with amoxycillin in acute otitis media with effusion: A preliminary report. Postgrad. Med. J., *55*(4):42–49.

Bordley, J. E., and Kapur, Y. P. 1972. The histopathological changes in the temporal bone resulting from acute smallpox and chickenpox infection. Laryngoscope, *82*:1477–1490.

Braun, P. 1969. Hepatotoxicity of erythromycin. J. Infect. Dis., *119*:300–306.

Brook, I. 1979. Bacteriology and treatment of chronic otitis media. Laryngoscope, *89*:1129–1134.

Brook, I., Anthony, B. F., and Finegold, S. M. 1978. aerobic and anaerobic bacteriology of acute otitis media in children. J. Pediatr., *92*:13–15.

Brook, I., and Schwartz, R. 1981. Anaerobic bacteria in acute otitis media. Acta Otolaryngol., *91*:111–114.

Brooks, D. 1968. An objective method of detecting fluid in the middle ear. Int. Audiol., *7*:280–286.

Brooks, D. 1969. The use of the electroacoustic impedance bridge in the assessment of middle ear function. Int. Audiol., *8*:563–569.

Brooks, D. 1971. Electroacoustic impedance bridge studies on normal ears of children. J. Speech Hear. Res., *14*:247–253.

Brooks, D. 1974. Impedance bridge studies on normal and hearing impaired children. Acta Otorhinolaryngol. Belg., *28*:140–145.

Brunck, W. 1906. Die Systematische Untersuchung des Sprachorganes bei Angeborenen Gaumendefekte in Ihrer Beziehung zur Prognose und Therapie. B. Angestein, Leipzig.

Bush, P. J., and Rabin, D. L. 1980. Racial differences in encounter rates for otitis media. Pediatr. Res., *14*:1115–1117.

Bylander, A. 1980. Comparison of Eustachian tube function in children and adults with normal ears. Ann. Otol. Rhinol. Laryngol., *89*(68):20–24.

Cambon, K., Galbraith, J. D., and Kong, G., 1965. Middle ear diseases in Indians of the Mount Currie reservation, British Columbia. Can. Med. Assoc. J., *93*:1301–1305.

Cantekin, E. I., and Bluestone, C. D. 1976. A membrane ventilating tube for the middle ear. Ann. Otol. Rhinol. Laryngol., *85*(25):270–276.

Cantekin, E. I., Bluestone, C. D., and Parkin, L. P. 1976. Eustachian tube ventilatory function in children. Ann. Otol. Rhinol. Laryngol., *85*(25):171–177.

Cantekin, E. I., Bluestone, C. D., Saez, C. A., Doyle, W. J., and Phillips, D. 1977. Normal and abnormal middle ear ventilation. Ann. Otol. Rhinol. Laryngol., *86*(41):1–15.

Cantekin, E. I., Doyle, W. J., Reichert, T. J., Phillips, D. C., and Bluestone, C. D. 1979a. Dilation of the Eustachian tube by electrical stimulation of the mandibular nerve. Ann. Otol. Rhinol. Laryngol., *88*:40–51.

Cantekin, E. I., Saez, C. A., Bluestone, C. D., and Bern, S. A. 1979b. Airflow through the Eustachian tube. Ann. Otol. Rhinol. Laryngol., *88*:603–612.

Cantekin, E. I., Bluestone, C. D., Rockette, H. E., and Beery, Q. C. 1980a. Effect of decongestant with or without antihistamine on Eustachian tube function. Ann. Otol. Rhinol. Laryngol., *89*(68):290–295.

Cantekin, E. I., Phillips, C. D., Doyle, W. J., Bluestone, C. D., and Kimes, K. K. 1980b. Effect of surgical alterations of the tensor veli palatini muscle on Eustachian tube function. Ann. Otol. Rhinol. Laryngol., *89*(68):47–53.

Cates, K. L., Gerrard, J. M., Giebink, G. S., Lund, M. E., Bleeker, E. Z., O'Leary, M. C., Krivit, W., and Quie, P. G. 1978. A penicillin-resistant pneumococcus. J. Pediatr., *93*:624–626.

Chandra, R. K. 1979. Prospective studies of the effect of breast feeding on incidence of infection and allergy. Acta Paediatr. Scand., *68*:691–694.

Chaudhuri, P. K., and Bowen-Jones, E. 1978. An otorhinolaryngological study of children with cleft palates. J. Laryngol. Otol., *92*(1):29–40.

Clarke, T. A. 1962. Deafness in children: Otitis media and other causes; a selective survey of prevention and treatment and of educational problems. Proc. R. Soc. Med., *55*:61–70.

Clements, D. A. 1978. Otitis media and hearing loss in a small aboriginal community. Med. J. Aust., *1*:665–667.

Clemis, J. D. 1976. Allergic factors in management of middle ear effusions. Ann. Otol. Rhinol. Laryngol., *85*(25):259–262.

Coffey, J. D. Jr. 1966. Otitis media in the practice of pediatrics: Bacteriological and clinical observations. Pediatrics, *38*:25–32.

Coffey, J. D., Jr. 1968. Concentration of ampicillin in exudate from acute otitis media. J. Pediatr., *72*:693–695.

Coffey, J. D., Jr., Martin, A. D., and Booth, H. N. 1967. *Neisseria catarrhalis* in exudative otitis media. Arch. Otolaryngol., *86*:403–406.

Collipp, P. J. 1961. Evaluation of nose drops for otitis media in children. Northwest Med., *60*:999–1000.

Compere, W. E., Jr. 1960. The radiologic evaluation of Eustachian tube function. Arch. Otolaryngol., *71*:386–389.

Compere, W. E., Jr.: Radiologic evaluation of the Eustachian tube. Otolaryngol. Clin. North Am., *3*:45–49, 1970.

Craig, H. B., Stool, S. E., and Laird, M. A. 1979. Project "Ears": Otologic maintenance in a school for the deaf. Am. Ann. Deaf, *124*:458–467.

Crysdale, W. S. 1976. Rational management of middle ear effusions in cleft palate patients. J. Otolaryngol., *5*(6):463–467.

Cunningham, A. S., 1977. Morbidity in breast-fed and artificially fed infants. J. Pediatr., *90*:726–729.

Danon, J. 1980. Cefotaxime concentrations in otitis media effusion. J. Antimicrob. Chemother., *6*(Suppl. A):131–132.

Dawson, C., Wood, T. R., Rose, L., and Hanna, L. 1967. Experimental inclusion conjunctivitis in man. Keratitis and other complications Arch. Ophthalmol., *78*:341–349.

Deinard, A. S., Dassenko, D., Kloster, B., Welle, P., and Zavoral, J. 1980. Otogenous tetanus. J.A.M.A., *243*:2156.

Diamant, M., and Diamant, B. 1974. Abuse and timing of use of antibiotics in acute otitis media. Arch. Otolaryngol., *100*:226–232.

Domagk, G. 1935. Ein beitrag zur Chemotherapie der bakteriellen Infektionen. Dtsch. Med. Wochenschr., *61*:250–253.

Domart, A., Hazard, J., and Husson, R. 1961. Fatal bone marrow aplasia after intramuscular chloramphenicol administration in two adults. Sem. Hop. Paris, *37*:2256–2258.

Downes, J. J. 1959. Primary diphtheritic otitis media. Arch. Otolaryngol., *70*:27–31.

Downs, M. P. 1980. Identification of children at risk for middle ear effusion problems. Ann. Otol. Rhinol. Laryngol., *89*(68):168–171.

Doyle, W. J. 1977. A functiono-anatomic description of Eustachian tube vector relations in four ethnic populations — an osteologic study. Ph.D. Dissertation.

Doyle, W. J. 1979. Boston genetic study. Personal Communication.

Doyle, W. J., Cantekin, E. I., and Bluestone, C. D. 1980a. Eustachian tube function in cleft palate children. Ann. Otol. Rhinol. Laryngol., *89*(68):34–40.

Doyle, W. J., Cantekin, E. I., Bluestone, C. D., Phillips, D. C., Kimes, K. K., and Siegel, M. I. 1980b. Nonhuman primate model of cleft palate and its implications for middle ear pathology. Ann. Otol. Rhinol. Laryngol., *89*(68):41–46.

Draper, W. L. 1967. Secretory otitis media in children: A study of 540 children. Laryngoscope, *77*:636–653.

Draper, W. L. 1974. Allergy in relationship to the Eustachian tube and middle ear. Otolaryngol. Clin. North Am., *7*:749–755.

Drettner, B. 1960. The nasal airway and hearing in patients with cleft palate. Acta Otolaryngol. (Stockh.), *52*:131–142.

Drury, D. W. 1925. Diphtheria of the ear. Arch. Otolaryngol., *1*:221–230.

Dugdale, A. E., Canty, A., Lewis, A. N., and Lovell, S. 1978. The natural history of chronic middle ear disease in Australian aboriginals: A cross-sectional study. Med. J. Aust., Spec. Suppl., *1*:6–8.

Eguchi, S. 1975. A new acoustical measurement of tubal opening. Otologia (Fukuoka), *21*:154–157.

Eliasson, R., Mossberg, B., Camner, P., and Afzelius, B. A. 1977. The immotile cilia syndrome: A congenital ciliary abnormality as an etiologic factor in chronic airway infections and male sterility. N. Engl. J. Med., *297*:1–6.

Elbrnd, O., and Larsen, E. 1976. Mucociliary function of the Eustachian tube. Arch. Otolaryngol., *102*:539–541.

Elner, A. 1972. Indirect determination of gas absorption from the middle ear. Acta Otolaryngol. (Stockh.), *74*:191–196.

Elner, A. 1977. Quantitative studies of gas absorption from the normal middle ear. Acta Otolaryngol. (Stockh.), *83*:25–28.

Elner, A., Ingelstedt, S., and Ivarsson, A. 1971a. A method for studies of middle ear mechanics. Acta Otolaryngol. (Stockh.), *72*:191–200.

Elner, A., Ingelstedt, S., and Ivarsson, A. 1971b. Indirect determination of the middle ear pressure. Acta Otolaryngol. (Stockh.), *72*:255–261.

Elner, A., Ingelstedt, S., and Ivarrson, A. 1971c. The elastic properties of the tympanic membrane system. Acta Otolaryngol. (Stockh.), *72*:397–403.

Elner, A., Ingelstedt, S., and Ivarsson, A. 1971d. The normal function of the Eustachian tube: A study of 102 cases. Acta Otolaryngol. (Stockh.), *72*:320–328.

Elpern, B. S., Naunton, R. F., and Perlman, H. B. 1964. Objective measurement of middle ear function: The Eustachian tube. Laryngoscope, *74*:359–371.

Ensign, P. R., Ubanich, E. M., and Moran, M. 1960. Prophylaxis for otitis media in an Indian population. Am. J. Public Health, *50*:195–199.

Evans, W. E., Feldman, S., Barker, L. F., Ossi, M., and Chaudhary, S. 1978. Use of gentamicin serum levels to individualize therapy in children. J. Pediatr., *93*:133–137.

Feigin, R. D., Kenney, R. E., Nusrala, J., Shackelford, P. G., and Lins, R. D. 1973a. Efficacy of clindamycin therapy for otitis media. Arch. Otolaryngol., *98*:27–31.

Feigin, R. D., Shackelford, P. G., Campbell, J., Lyles, T. O., Schechter, M., and Lins, R. S. 1973b. Assessment of the role of *Staphylococcus epidermidis* as a cause of otitis media. Pediatrics, *52*:569–575.

Feingold, M., Klein, J. O., Haslam, G. E., Tilles, J. G., Finland, M., and Gellis, S. S. 1966. Acute otitis media in children: Bacteriological findings in middle ear fluid obtained by needle aspiration. Am. J. Dis. Child., *111*:361–365.

Ferber, A., and Holmquist, J. 1973. Roentgenographic demonstration of the Eustachian tube in chronic otitis media. Acta Radiol. (Diagn.) (Stockh.), *14*:667–672.

Fernandez, A. A., and McGovern, J. P. 1965. Secretory otitis media in allergic infants and children. South. Med. J., *58*:581–586.

Findlay, R. C., Stool, S. E., and Svitko, C. A. 1977. Tympanometric and otoscopic evaluations of a school-age deaf population: A longitudinal study. Am. Ann. Deaf, *122*:407–413.

Finegold, S. M. 1981. Anerobic infections in otolaryngology. Ann. Otol. Rhinol. Laryngol., *90*(84):13–16.

Finland, M., and Hewitt, W. L. (Guest Eds.) 1971. Second international symposium on gentamicin, an aminoglycoside antibiotic. J. Infect. Dis., *124*:S1–S300.

Finland, M., Brumfitt, W., and Kass, E. H. (Guest Eds.) 1976. Advances in aminoglycoside therapy: Amikacin. J. Infect. Dis., *134*:S235–S460.

Finland, M., and Neu, H. C. (Guest Eds.) 1976. Tobramycin. Symposium of the ninth international congress of chemotherapy in London, England. J. Infect. Dis., *134*:S1–S234.

Fischer, G. W., Sunakorn, P., and Duangman, C. 1977. Otogenous tetanus: A sequela of chronic ear infections. Am. J. Dis. Child., *131*:445–446.

Fischer, J. J., McAdams, J. A., Entis, G. N., Cotton, R., Ghory, J. E., and Ausdenmoore, R. W. 1978. Middle ear ciliary defect in Kartagener's syndrome. Pediatrics, *62*:443–445.

Flisberg, K. 1966. Ventilatory studies on the Eustachian tube: A clinical investigation of cases with perforated eardrums. Acta Otolaryngol. (Stockh.), Suppl. 219.

Fraser, J. G., Mehta, M., and Fraser, P. M. 1977. The medical treatment of secretory otitis media: A clinical trial of three commonly used regimens. J. Laryngol. Otol., *91*:757–765.

Fuchs, P. C., Gavan, T. L., Gerlach, E. H., Jones, R. N., Barry, A. L., and Thornsberry, C. 1977. Ticarcillin: A collaborative *in vitro* comparison with carbenicillin against over 9,000 clinical bacterial isolates. Am. J. Med. Sci., *274*:255–263.

Giebink, G. S., and Quie, P. G. 1978. Otitis media: The spectrum of middle ear inflammation. Ann. Rev. Med., *29*:285–306.

Giebink, G. S., Mills, E. L., Huff, J. S., Edelman, C. K., Weber, M. L., Juhn, S. K., and Quie, P. G. 1979. The microbiology of serous and mucoid otitis media. Pediatrics, *63*:915–919.

Giebink, G. S., Berzins, I. K., Cates, K. L., Huff, J. S., and Quie, P. G. 1980. Polymorphonuclear leukocyte function during otitis media. Ann. Otol. Rhinol. Laryngol., *89*(68):138–142.

Ginsburg, C. M., McCracken, G. H., and Nelson, J. D. 1981. Pharmacology of oral antibiotics used for treatment of otitis media and tonsillopharyngitis in infants and children. Ann. Otol. Rhinol. Laryngol., *90*:37–43.

Goetzinger, C. P., Embrey, J. E., Brooks, R., and Proud, G. O. 1960. Auditory assessment of cleft palate adults. Acta Otolaryngol. (Stockh.), *52*:551–557.

Gold, J. A., Hegarty, C. P., Deitch, M. W., and Walker, B. R. 1979. Double-blind clinical trials of oral cyclacillin and ampicillin. Antimicrob. Agents Chemother., *15*:55–58.

Gold, R., Lepow, M. L., Goldschneider, I., Draper, T. S., and Gotschlick, E. C. 1978. Antibody responses of human infants to three doses of Group A *Neisseria meningitidis* polysaccharide vaccine administered at two, four, and six months of age. J. Infect. Dis., *138*:731–735.

Goodhill, V. 1979. Ear Diseases, Deafness, and Dizziness. Hagerstown, Md., Harper and Row Pub., pp. 356–379.

Gorbach, S. L., and Bartlett, J. G. 1977. Pseudomembranous enterocolitis: A review of its diverse forms. J. Infect. Dis., *135*:S89–S94.

Gottschalk, G. H. 1966. Further experience with controlled middle ear inflation in treatment of serous otitis. EENT Monthly, *45*:49–51.

Gottschalk, G. H. 1980. Nonsurgical management of otitis media with effusion. Ann. Otol. Rhinol. Laryngol., *89*(68):301–302.

Graham, M. D. 1963. A longitudinal study of ear disease and hearing loss in patients with cleft lips and palates. TAAOO, *67*:213–222.

Graham, M. D., and Lierle, D. M. 1962. Posterior

pharyngeal flap palatoplasty and its relation to ear disease and hearing loss: A preliminary report. Laryngoscope, *72*:1750–1755.

Gray, B. M., Converse, G. M., and Dillon, H. C., Jr. 1979. Serotypes of *Streptococcus pneumoniae* causing disease. J. Infect. Dis., *140*:979–983.

Green, G. R., Rosenblum, A. H., and Sweet, L. C. 1977. Evaluation of penicillin hypersensitivity: Value of clinical history and skin testing with penicilloylpolysine and penicillin G. A cooperative prospective study of the penicillin study group of the American Academy of Allergy. J. Allergy Clin. Immunol., *60*:339–345.

Grilliat, J. P., Streiff, F., and Hua, G. 1966. Fatal cytopenia after chloramphenicol hemisuccinate therapy. Ann. Med. (Nancy), *5*:754–762.

Gronroos, J. A., Kortekangas, A. E., Ojala, L., and Vuori, M. 1964. The aetiology of acute middle ear infection. Acta Otolaryngol. (Stockh.), *58*:149–158.

Guillerm, R., Riu, R., Badre, R., LeDen, R., and LeMouel, C. 1966. Une nouvelle technique d'exploration fonctionelle de la trompe d'Eustache: la sonomanometrie tubaire. Ann. Otolaryngol. Chir. Cervicofac., *83*:523–543.

Gutzmann, H. 1893. Zur Prognose und Behandlung der angeborenen Gaumendefekte. Mschr. Sprachheilk.

Gyergyay, A. 1932. Neue Wege zur Erkennung der Physiologie und Pathologie der Ohrtrompete. Monatsschr. Ohrenheilkd. Laryngorhinol., *66*:769.

Halfond, M. M., and Ballenger, J. J. 1956. An audiologic and otorhinologic study of cleft lip and cleft palate cases. Arch. Otolaryngol., *64*:58–62.

Halstead, C., Lepow, M. L., Balassanian, N., Emmerich, J., and Wolinsky, E. 1968. Otitis media: Clinical observations, microbiology and evaluation of therapy. Am. J. Dis. Child., *115*:542–551.

Hanson, D. G., and Ulvestad, R. F. (Eds.) 1979. Otitis media and child development: Speech, language, and education. Ann. Otol. Rhinol. Laryngol., *88*(60):1–111.

Harding, A. L., Anderson, P., Howie, V. M., Ploussard, J. H., and Smith, D. H. 1973. *Haemophilus influenzae* isolated from children with otitis media. *In* Sell, S. H. W., and Kargon, D. T. (Eds.): Haemophilus Influenzae. Nashville, Vanderbilt University Press, pp. 21–28.

Harford, E. R., Bess, F. H., Bluestone, C. D., and Klein, J. O. (Eds.) 1978. Impedance Screening for Middle Ear Disease in Children. New York, Grune and Stratton.

Harrison, R. J., and Phillips, B. J. 1971. Observations on hearing losses of preschool cleft palate children. J. Speech Hear. Disord. *36*(2):252–256.

Healy, G. B., and Telle, D. W. 1977. The microbiology of chronic middle ear effusions in young children. Laryngoscope, *87*:1472–1478.

Heermann, J., Jr., Heermann, H., and Kopstein, E. 1970. Fascia and cartilage palisade tympanoplasty: Nine years experience. Arch. Otolaryngol., *91*:228–241.

Heisee, J. W., Jr. 1963. Secretory otitis media: Treatment with depomethylprednisone. Laryngoscope, *73*:54–59.

Heller, J. C., Hochberg, L., and Milano, G. 1970. Audiologic and otologic evaluation of cleft palate children. Cleft Palate J., *7*:774–783.

Henderson, F. W., Collier, A. M., Clyde, W. A., Jr., et al.

1977. The epidemiology of acute otitis media in childhood. Abstract, Interscience Conference on Antimicrobial Agents and Chemotherapeutics.

Herberts, G., Jeppson, P. H., Nylen, O., and Branefors-Helander, P. 1971. Acute otitis media: Etiological and therapeutical aspects of acute otitis media. Prac. Otol. Rhinol. Laryngol., *33*:191–202.

Hewitt, W. L., and McHenry, M. C. 1978. Blood level determinations of antimicrobial drugs. Some clinical considerations. Med. Clin. North Am., *62*:1119–1140.

Hill, H. R., Book, L. S., Hemming, V. G., and Herbst, J. J. 1977. Defective neutrophil chemotactic responses in patients with recurrent episodes of otitis media and chronic diarrhea. Am. J. Dis. Child., *131*:433–436.

Hoekelman, R. A. 1977. Infectious illness during the first year of life. Pediatrics, *59*:119–121.

Holborow, C. 1970. Eustachian tube function: Changes in anatomy and function with age and the relationship of these changes with aural pathology. Arch. Otolaryngol., *92*:624–626.

Holmes, E. M., and Reed, G. F. 1955. Hearing and deafness in cleft palate patients. Arch. Otolaryngol., *62*:620–624.

Holmquist, J. 1969a. Eustachian tube function in patients with eardrum perforations following chronic otitis media. Acta Otolaryngol. (Stockh.), *68*:391–401.

Holmquist, J. 1969b. Eustachian tube function assessed with tympanometry. Acta Otolaryngol. (Stockh.), *68*:501–508.

Holmquist, J. 1970. Middle ear ventilation in chronic otitis media. Arch. Otolaryngol., *92*:617–623.

Holmquist, J. 1972. Tympanometry in testing auditory tubal function. Audiology, *11*:209–212.

Holmquist, J. 1977. Medical treatment in ears with Eustachian tube dysfunction. Presented at the Symposium on Physiology and Pathophysiology of the Eustachian Tube and Middle Ear, Freiburg, West Germany.

Honjo, I., Okazaki, N., and Kumazawa, T. 1979. Experimental study of the Eustachian tube function with regard to its related muscles. Acta Otolaryngol. (Stockh.), *87*:84–89.

Howard, J. E., Nelson, J. D., Clashen, J., and Jackson, L. H. 1976. Otitis media of infancy and early childhood: A double-blind study of four treatment regimens. Am. J. Dis. Child, *130*:965–970.

Howie, V. M. 1975. Natural history of otitis media. Ann. Otol. Rhinol. Laryngol., *84*(Suppl. 19):67–72.

Howie, V. M., and Ploussard, J. H. 1969. The *"in vivo* sensitivity test"*: Bacteriology of middle ear exudate during antimicrobial therapy in otitis media. Pediatrics, *44*:940–944.

Howie, V. M., Ploussard, J. H., and Lester, R. L. 1970. Otitis media: A clinical and bacteriological correlation. Pediatrics, *45*:29–35.

Howie, V. M., and Ploussard, J. H. 1972. Efficacy of fixed combination antibiotics versus separate components in otitis media. Clin. Pediatr. (Phila.), *11*:205–214.

Howie, V. M., Ploussard, J. H., Sloyer, J. L., and Johnston, R. B., Jr. 1973. Immunoglobulins of the middle ear fluid in acute otitis media: Relationship to serum immunoglobulin concentrations and bacterial cultures. Infect. Immun., *7*:589–593.

Howie, V. M., Ploussard, J. H., and Sloyer, J. 1974. Comparison of ampicillin and amoxicillin in the treatment of otitis media in children. J. Infect. Dis., *129*:S181–S184.

Howie, V. M., Ploussard, J. H., and Sloyer, J. 1975. The "otitis prone" condition. Am. J. Dis. Child., *129*:676–678.

Ingelstedt, S., and Ortegren, U. 1963. Qualitative testing of the Eustachian tube function. Acta Otolaryngol. (Stockh.), Suppl. 182:7–23.

Ingelstedt, S., Ivarsson, A., and Jonson, B. 1967a. Mechanics of the human middle ear; Pressure regulation in aviation and diving: A nontraumatic method. Acta Otolaryngol. (Stockh.), Suppl. 228.

Ingelstedt, S., Ivarsson, A., and Jonson, B. 1967b. Quantitative determination of tubal ventilation during changes in ambient pressure as during ascent and descent in aviation. Acta Otolaryngol. (Stockh.), Suppl. 228:31–34.

Ingelstedt, S., and Bylander, A. 1978. A comparison of the Eustachian tube function in fifty children and fifty adults with normal ears. Presented at the Association for Research in Otolaryngology Meeting, St. Petersburg, Florida.

Jacobs, M. R., Koornhof, H. J., Robins-Browne, R. M., Stevenson, C. M., Vermaak, Z. A., Freiman, I., Miller, G. B., Witcomb, M. A., Isaacson, M., Ward, J. I., and Austrian, R. 1978. Emergence of multiply resistant pneumococci. N. Engl. J. Med., *299*:735–740.

Jaffe, B. F., Hurtado, F., and Hurtado, E. 1970. Tympanic membrane mobility in the newborn with seven months follow-up. Laryngoscope, *80*:36–48.

Jerger, J. 1970. Clinical experience with impedance audiometry. Arch. Otolaryngol., *92*:311–324.

Jonson, B., and Rundcrantz, H. 1969. Posture and pressure within the internal jugular vein. Acta Otolaryngol. (Stockh.), *68*:271–275.

Juhn, S. K., and Huff, J. S. 1976. Biochemical characteristics of middle ear effusions. Ann. Otol. Rhinol. Laryngol., *85*(25):110–116.

Kaiser, A. D. 1930. Results of tonsillectomy: A comparative study of 2,200 tonsillectomized children with an equal number of controls three and ten years after operation. J.A.M.A., *95*:837–842.

Kamme, C. 1970. Evaluation of the *in vitro* sensitivity of *Neisseria catarrhalis* to antibiotics with respect to acute otitis media. Scand. J. Infect. Dis., *2*:117–120.

Kamme, C. 1980. Penicillin-resistant *Branhamella catarrhalis*. Lakartidningen, *77*:4858–4859.

Kamme, C., Lundgren, K., and Rundcrantz, H. 1969. The concentration of penicillin V in serum and middle ear exudate in acute otitis media in children. Scand. J. Infect. Dis., *1*:77–83.

Kamme, C., Ageberg, M., and Lundgren, K. 1970. Distribution of *Diplococcus pneumoniae* types in acute otitis media in children and influence of the types on the clinical course in penicillin V therapy. Scand. J. Infect. Dis., *2*:183–190.

Kaplan, G. J., Fleshman, J. K., Bender, T. R., Baum, C., and Clark, P. S. 1973. Long-term effects of otitis media: A ten-year cohort study of Alaskan Eskimo children. Pediatrics, *52*:577–585.

Karma, P., Palva, A., and Kokko, E. 1976. Immunological defects in children with chronic otitis media. Acta Otolaryngol. (Stockh.), *82*:193–195.

Karma, P., Luotonen, J., Timonen, M., Pontynen, S., et al.

1980. Efficacy of pneumococcal vaccination against recurrent otitis media. Preliminary results of a field trial in Finland. Ann. Otol. Rhinol. Laryngol., 89(68):357–362.

Kass, E. H., and Evans, D. A. (Guest Eds.) 1979. Future prospects and past problems in antimicrobial therapy: The role of cefoxitin. Rev. Infect. Dis., 1:1–244.

Kaufman, R. S. 1970. Hearing loss in children with cleft palates. N.Y. State J. Med., 70(20):2555–2558.

Kessner, D. M., Snow, C. K., and Singer, J. 1974. Assessment of Medical Care for Children, Vol. 3. Washington, D. C., Institute of Medicine, National Academy of Sciences.

Khanna, S. M., and Tonndorf, J. 1972. Tympanic membrane vibrations in cats studied by time-averaged holography. J. Acoust. Soc. Am., 51:1904–1920.

Kilby, D., Richards, S. H., and Hart, G. 1972. Grommets and glue ears. Two year results. J. Laryngol. Otol., 86:881–888.

Kinmonth, A. L., Storrs, C. N., and Mitchell, R. G. 1978. Meningitis due to chloramphenicol-resistant *Haemophilus influenzae* type b. Br. Med. J., 1:694.

Kirby, W. M. M. (Chrmn.) 1970. Symposium on carbenicillin. A clinical profile. J. Infect. Dis., 122:S1–S116.

Kjellman, N. I., Synnerstad, B., and Hansson, L. O. 1976. Atopic allergy and immunoglobulins in children with adenoids and recurrent otitis media. Acta Paediatr. Scand., 65:593–600.

Klein, J. O. 1976. Otitis media in the newborn infant. *In* Remington, J. S., and Klein, J. O. (Eds.): Infectious Diseases of the Fetus and Newborn Infant. Philadelphia, W. B. Saunders Co., p. 807.

Klein, J. O. 1981. Epidemiology of pneumococcal disorders in infants and children. Rev. Infect. Dis., 3:246–253.

Klein, J. O., and Bratton, L. 1973. Unpublished data.

Klein, J. O., and Teele, D. W. 1976. Isolation of viruses and mycoplasmas from middle ear effusions: A review. Ann. Otol. Rhinol. Laryngol. 85 (Suppl. 25):140–144.

Klein, B. S., Dollete, F. R., and Yolken, R. H. 1982. The role of respiratory syncytial virus and other viral pathogens in acute otitis media. J. Pediatr. 101:16–20.

Klimek, J. J., Nightingale, C., Lehmann, W. B., and Quintiliani, R. 1977. Comparison of concentrations of amoxicillin and ampicillin in serum and middle ear fluid of children with chronic otitis media. J. Infect. Dis., 135:999–1002.

Klimek, J. J., Bates, T. R., Nightingale, C., Lehmann, W. B. Ziemniak, J. A., and Quintiliani, R. 1980. Penetration characteristics of trimethoprim-sulfamethoxazole in middle ear fluid of patients with chronic serous otitis media. J. Pediatr., 96:1087–1089.

Koch, H., and Dennison, N. J. 1974. Office visits to pediatricians. National Ambulatory Medical Care Service, National Center for Health Statistics. Hyattsville. Md.

Kokko, E. 1974. Chronic secretory otitis media in children: A clinical study. Acta Otolaryngol. (Stockh.), Suppl. 327:7–44.

Korsan-Bengstein, M., and Nylen, O. 1974. A follow-up study of cleft children treated with primary bone grafting. Scand. J. Plast. Reconstr. Surg., 8:161–163.

Kunin, C. M. 1972. Antibiotic usage in patients with renal impairment. Hosp. Pract., 7:141–149.

LaFaye, M., Gaillard de Collogny, L., Jourde, H., Plagne, R., Callier, J., and Meyniel, G. 1974. Étude de la permeabilité de la trompe d'Eustache par les radioisotopes. Ann. Otolaryngol. Chir. Cervicofac., 91:665–680.

Lahikainen, E. A. 1953. Clinico-bacteriologic studies on acute otitis media: Aspiration of tympanum as diagnostic and therapeutic method. Acta Otolaryngol. (Suppl.) (Stockh.) 107:1–82.

Lahikainen, E. A. 1970. Penicillin concentration in middle ear secretion in otitis. Acta Otolaryngol. (Stockh.), 70:358–362.

Lahikainen, E. A., Vuori, M., and Virtanen, S. 1977. Azidocillin and ampicillin concentrations in middle ear effusion. Acta Otolaryngol. (Stockh.), 84:227–232.

Lang, R. W., Liu, Y. S., Lim, D. J., and Birck, H. G. 1976. Antimicrobial factors and bacterial correlation in chronic otitis media with effusion. Ann. Otol. Rhinol. Laryngol., 85(25):145–151.

Lannois, M. 1901. De l'état de l'oreille moyenne dans les fissures congenitales du palais. Rev. Hebd. Laryngol., 21:177–184.

Levine, B. B. 1966. Immunologic mechanisms of penicillin allergy. A haptenic model system for the study of allergic diseases of man. N. Engl. J. Med., 275:1115–1125.

Levine, B. B., Redmond, A. P., Fellner, M. J., Voss, H. E., and Levytska, V. 1966. Penicillin allergy and the heterogeneous immune responses of man to benzylpenicillin. J. Clin. Invest., 45:1895–1906.

Lewis, D. M., Schram, J. L., Lim, D. J., Birck, H. G., and Gleich, G. 1978. Immunoglobulin E in chronic middle ear effusions: Comparison of RIST, PRIST, and RIA techniques. Ann. Otol. Rhinol. Laryngol. 87:197–201.

Lewis, D. M., Schram, J. L., Birck, H. G., and Lim, D. J. 1979. Antibody activity in otitis media with effusion. Ann. Otol. Rhinol. Laryngol. 88:392–396.

Lildholdt, T., Cantekin, E. I., Marshak, G., Bluestone, C. D., Rohn, D. C., and Schuit, K. E. 1981. Pharmacokinetics of cefaclor in chronic middle ear effusions. Ann. Otol. Rhinol. Laryngol. 90(84):44–47.

Lilholdt, T., Cantekin, E. I., Bluestone, C. D., and Rockette, H. E. 1982. Effect of nasal decongestant on Eustachian tube function in children with tympanostomy tubes. Acta Otolaryngol. (Stockh.), in press.

Lindsay, W. K., LeMeusurier, A. B., and Farmer, A. W. 1962. A study of the speech results of a large series of cleft palate patients. Plast. Reconstr. Surg., 29:273–288.

Ling, D., McCoy, R. H., and Levinson, E. D. 1969. The incidence of middle ear disease and its educational implications among Baffin Island Eskimo children. Can. J. Public Health, 60:385–390.

Linthicum, F. H., Body, H., and Keaster, J. 1959. Incidence of middle ear disease in children with cleft palate. Cleft Palate Bull., 9:23–25.

Liu, Y. S., Lim, D. J., Lang, R. W., and Birck, H. G. 1975. Chronic middle ear effusions: Immunochemical and bacteriological investigations. Arch. Otolaryngol., 101:278–286.

Liu, Y. S., Lim, D. J., Lang, R., and Birck, H. G. 1976. Micro-organisms in chronic otitis media with effusion. Ann. Otol. Rhinol. Laryngol., 85(25):245–249.

Loeb, W. J. 1964. Speech, hearing and the cleft palate. Arch. Otolaryngol., 79:1–14.

Lorentzen, P., and Haugsten, P. 1977. Treatment of acute

suppurative otitis media. J. Laryngol. Otol., *91*:331–340.

Lous, J., and Fiellau-Nikolajsen, M. 1981. Epidemiology of middle ear effusion and tubal dysfunction: A one year prospective study comprising monthly tympanometry in 387 nonselected seven year old children. Int. J. Pediatr. Otorhinolaryngol., *3*:303–317.

Lundgren, K., Ingvarsson, L., and Rundcrantz, H. 1979. The concentration of penicillin V in middle ear exudate. Int. J. Pediatr. Otorhinolaryngol., *1*:93–96.

Luotonen, J., Herva, E., Karma, P., Timonen, M., Leinonen, M., and Makela, P. H. 1981. The bacteriology of acute otitis media in children with special reference to *Streptococcus pneumoniae* as studied by bacteriological and antigen detection methods. Scand. J. Infect. Dis., *13*:177–183.

Lynn, G. E., and Benitez, J. T. 1974. Temporal bone preservation in a 2600 year old Egyptian mummy. Science, *183*:200–202.

MacAdam, A. M., and Rubio, T. 1977. Tuberculous otomastoiditis in children. Am. J. Dis. Child., *131*:152–156.

Mace, J. W., Janik, D. S., Sauer, R. L., and Quilligan, J. J. 1977. Penicillin-resistant pneumococcal meningitis in an immunocompromised infant. J. Pediatr., *91*:506–507.

Mach, E., and Kessel, J. 1872. Die Function der Trommelhohle und der Tuber Eustachii sitzungsber. Weiner Akad. Math. Natur. Wiss., *66*:329.

Magnus, A. 1864. Werhalten des Gehor-organs in konprimirter Luft. Arch. Ohren., *1*:269.

Makela, P. H., Sibakov, M., Herva, E., and Henricksen, J. 1980. Pneumococcal vaccine and otitis media. Lancet, *2*:547–551.

Makela, P. H., Leinonen, M., Tukander, J., and Karma, P. 1981. A study of the polyvaccine in prevention of clinically acute attacks of recurrent otitis media. Rev. Infect. Dis., *3*:S124–S130.

Mandel, E. M., Bluestone, C. D., Cantekin, E. I., Ghorbanian, N. S., and Rockette, H. 1981. Comparison of cefaclor and amoxicillin for acute otitis media with effusion. Ann. Otol. Rhinol. Laryngol., *90*:48–52.

Marshak, G., and Neriah, Z. B. 1981. Adenoidectomy versus tympanostomy in chronic secretory otitis media. Ann. Otol. Rhinol. Laryngol., *89*(68):316–318.

Masters, F. W., Bingham, H. G., and Robinson, D. W. 1960. The prevention and treatment of hearing loss in the cleft palate child. Plast. Reconstr. Surg., *25*:503–509.

Mattar, M. E., Markello, J., and Yaffe, S. J. 1975. Pharmaceutic factors affecting pediatric compliance. Pediatrics, *55*:101–108.

Mawson, S. R. 1974. The Eustachian tube. *In* Mawson, S. R.: Diseases of the Ear. Baltimore, The Williams and Wilkins Co.

Mawson, S. R., Adlington, R., and Evans, M. 1967. A controlled study evaluation of adeno-tonsillectomy in children. J. Laryngol. Otol. *81*:77–790.

Mawson, S. R., and Fagan, P. 1972. Tympanic effusions in children: Long-term results of treatment by myringotomy, aspiration, and indwelling tubes (grommets). J. Laryngol. Otol. *86*:105–119.

Maynard, J. E., Fleshman, J. K., and Tschopp, C. F. 1972. Otitis media in Alaskan Eskimo children: Prospective evaluation of chemoprophylaxis. J.A.M.A., *219*:597–599.

McCracken, G. H., Jr., and Nelson, J. D. 1977. Antimicrobial Therapy for Newborns. Practical Application of Pharmacology to Clinical Usage. New York, Grune and Stratton.

McKee, W. J. 1963a. A controlled study of the effects of tonsillectomy and adenoidectomy in children. Br. J. Prev. Soc. Med., *17*:46–49.

McKee, W. J. 1963b. The part played by adenoidectomy in the combined operation of tonsillectomy with adenoidectomy: Second part of a controlled study in children. Br. J. Prev. Soc. Med., *17*:133–140.

McLinn, S. E. 1976. Letter: Cephalosporins in otitis media. Can. Med. Assoc. J., *114*:13–14.

McNicoll, W. D., and Scanlon, S. G. 1979. Submucous resection: The treatment of choice in the nose-ear distress syndrome. J. Laryngol. Otol., *93*:357–367.

McWilliams, B. J. 1966. Speech and hearing problems in children with cleft palate. J. Am. Med. Wom. Assoc. *21*:1005.

Means, B. J., and Irwin, J. V. 1954. An analysis of certain measures of intelligence and hearing loss in a sample of Wisconsin cleft palate population. Cleft Palate Bull., *4*:4.

Mehta, D., and Erlich, M. 1978. Serous otitis media in school for the deaf. Volta Rev., *80*:75–80.

Meissner, K. 1939. Ohrenerkrankungen bei Gaumenspalten. Hals-Nasen-und Ohrenarzt, *30*:6–20.

Metz, O. 1946. The acoustic impedance measured in normal and pathological ears. Acta Otolaryngol. (Stockh.), Suppl. 63.

Miller, G. F., Jr. 1965. Eustachian tube function in normal and diseased ears. Arch. Otolaryngol., *81*:41–48.

Miller, G. F. 1970. Influence of an oral decongestant on Eustachian tube function in children. J. Allergy, *45*:187–193.

Miller, M. H. 1956. Hearing losses in cleft palate cases: The incidence, type, and significance. Laryngoscope, *66*:1492–1496.

Moellering, R. C., Jr. (Guest Ed.). 1978. Symposium on cefamandole. J. Infect. Dis., *137* (Suppl):S1–S194.

Moellering, R. C., Jr., and Swartz, M. N. 1976. Drug therapy. The newer cephalosporins. N. Engl. J. Med., *294*:24–28.

Mogi, G., Yoshida, T., Honjo, S., and Maeda, S. 1973. Middle ear effusions: Quantitative analysis of immunoglobulins. Ann. Otol. Rhinol. Laryngol., *82*:196–202.

Mogi, G., Honjo, S., Maeda, S., Yoshida, T., and Watanabe, N. 1974. Immunoglobulin E (IgE) in middle ear effusions. Ann. Otol. Rhinol. Laryngol., *83*:393–398.

Mogi, G., Maeda, S., Yoshida, T., and Watanabe, N. 1976. Immunochemistry of otitis media with effusion. J. Infect. Dis., *133*:126–136.

Mortimer, E. A., Jr., and Watterson, R. L., Jr. 1956. A bacteriologic investigation of otitis media in infancy. Pediatrics, *17*:359–366.

Muenker, G. 1980. Results after treatment of otitis media with effusion. Ann. Otol. Rhinol. Laryngol., *89*(68):308–311.

Murrary, D. L., Singer, D. A., and Singer, A. B. 1980. Cefaclor: A cluster of adverse reactions. N. Engl. J. Med., *303*:1003.

Murti, K. G., Stern, R. M., Cantekin, E. I., and Bluestone, C. D. 1980. Sonometric evaluation of Eustachian tube function using broadband stimuli. Ann. Otol. Rhinol. Laryngol., *89*(68):178–184.

Naiditch, M. J., and Bower, A. G. 1954. Diphtheria: A study of 1,433 cases observed during a ten-year period at Los Angeles County Hospital. Am. J. Med., *17*:229–245.

National Center for Health Statistics. 1974. Surgical Operations in Short-Stay Hospitals: United States — 1971. DHEW Publication No. HRA-75-1769. Rockville, Md., United States Department of Health, Education, and Welfare.

Naunton, R. F., and Galluser, J. 1967. Measurements of Eustachian tube function. Ann. Otol. Rhinol. Laryngol., *76*:455–471.

NDTI Review. 1970. Leading diagnoses and reasons for patient visits. *1*:18–23.

Nelson, J. D. 1978. Oral antibiotic therapy for serious infections in hospitalized patients. J. Pediatr., *92*:175–176.

Nelson, J. D., Howard, J. B., and Shelton, S. 1978. Oral antibiotic therapy for skeletal infections of children. J. Pediatr., *92*:131–134.

Nelson, J. D., and McCracken, G. H. 1980. The drug of choice for otitis media? J. Pediatr. Infect. Dis., *6*:5.

Nelson, J. D., Ginsburg, C. M., McLeland, O., Clahsen, J., Culbertson, M. C., Jr., and Carder, H.: Concentrations of antimicrobial agents in middle ear fluid, saliva and tears. Int. J. Pediatr. Otorhinolaryngol., *3*:327–334.

Neu, H. C. 1978. A symposium on the tetracyclines: A major appraisal. Introduction. Bull. N. Y. Acad. Med., *54*:141–155.

Nilson, B. W., Poland, R. L., Thompson, R. S., Morehead, D., Baghdassarian, A., and Carver, D. H. 1969. Acute otitis media: Treatment results in relation to bacterial etiology. Pediatrics, *43*:351–358.

Noone, R. B., Randall, P., Stool, S. E., Hamilton, R., and Winchester, R. A. 1973. The effect on middle ear disease of fracture of the pterygoid hamulus during palatoplasty. Cleft Palate J., *10*:23–33.

Odoi, H., Proud, G. O., and Toledo, P. S. 1971. Effects of pterygoid hamulotomy upon Eustachian tube function. Laryngoscope, *81*:1242–1244.

Ogawa, S., Satoh, I., and Tanaka, H. 1976. Patulous Eustachian tube. A new treatment with infusion of absorbable gelatin sponge solution. Arch. Otolaryngol., *102*:276–280.

Olson, A. L., Klein, S. W., Charney, E., MacWhinney, J. B., McInerny, T. K., Miller, R. L., Nazarian, L. F., and Cunningham, D. 1978. Prevention and therapy of serous otitis media by oral decongestant: A double-blind study in pediatric practice. Pediatrics *61*:679–684.

Oppenheimer, P. 1968. Short-term steroid therapy — treatment of serous otitis media in children. Arch. Otolaryngol., *88*:138–140.

Oppenheimer, R. P. 1975. Serous otitis: Review of 992 patients. EENT Monthly, *54*:316–318.

Ostfeld, E., and Altmann, G. L. 1980. Evaluation of countercurrent immunoelectrophoresis as a diagnostic tool in bacterial otitis media. Ann. Otol. Rhinol. Laryngol., *89*(68):110–114.

Ostfeld, E., and Rubinstein, E. 1980. Acute gram-negative bacillary infections of middle ear and mastoid. Ann. Otol. Rhinol. Laryngol., *89*:33–36.

Page, J. R. 1935. Report of acute infections of middle ear and mastoid process at Manhattan Eye, Ear, and Throat Hospital during 1934: Their prevalence and virulence. Laryngoscope, *45*:839–843.

Palva, T., Holopainen, E., and Karma, P. 1976. Protein and cellular protein of glue ear secretions. Ann. Otol. Rhinol. Laryngol., *85*(25):103–109.

Palva, T., Hayry, P., and Ylikoski, J. 1980. Lymphocyte morphology in middle ear effusions. Ann. Otol. Rhinol. Laryngol., *89*(68):143–146.

Pannbacker, M. 1969. Hearing loss and cleft palate. Cleft Palate J., *6*:50–56.

Paparella, M. M. 1973. The middle ear effusions. *In* Paparella, M. M., and Shumrick, D. A. (Eds.): Otolaryngology, Vol. I. Philadelphia, W. B. Saunders Co., pp. 93–112.

Paparella, M. M., and Dickson, R. I. 1969. The recurrent middle ear effusions. Otolaryngol. Clin. North Am., *2*:53–70.

Paparella, M., Hiraide, F., Juhn, S. K., and Kaneko, Y. 1970. Cellular events involved in middle ear fluid production. Ann. Otol. Rhinol. Laryngol., *79*:766–779.

Paparella, M. M., Oda, M., Hiraide, F., and Brady, D. 1972. Pathology of sensorineural hearing loss in otitis media. Ann. Otol. Rhinol. Laryngol., *81*:632–647.

Paradise, J. L. 1977. On tympanostomy tubes: Rationale, results, reservations, and recommendations. Pediatrics, *60*:86–90.

Paradise, J. L. 1980. Otitis media in infants and children. Pediatrics, *65*:917–943.

Paradise, J. L., Bluestone, C. D., and Felder, H. 1969. The universality of otitis media in fifty infants with cleft palate. Pediatrics, *44*:35–42.

Paradise, J. L., and Bluestone, C. D. 1974. Early treatment of the universal otitis media of infants with cleft palate. Pediatrics, *53*:48–54.

Paradise, J. L., Bluestone, C. D., Rogers, K. D., and Taylor, F. H. 1980. Efficacy of adenoidectomy in recurrent otitis media: Historical overview and preliminary results from a randomized, controlled trial. Ann. Otol. Rhinol. Laryngol., *89*(68):319–321.

Paredes, A., Taber, L. H., Yow, M. D., Clark, D., and Nathan, W. 1976. Prolonged pneumococcal meningitis due to an organism with increased resistance to penicillin. Pediatrics, *58*:378–381.

Parisier, S. C., and Khilnani, M. T. 1970. The roentgenographic evaluation of Eustachian tubal function. Laryngoscope, *80*:1201–1211.

Parker, C. W. 1972. Allergic drug responses — mechanisms and unsolved problems. CRC Crit. Rev. Toxicol., *1*:261–281.

Pelton, S. I., Shurin, P. A., and Klein, J. O. 1977. Persistence of middle ear effusion after otitis media. Pediatr. Res., *11*:504.

Pelton, S. I., Teele, D. W., Shurin, P. A., and Klein, J. O. 1980. Disparate cultures of middle ear fluids. Am. J. Dis. Child., *134*:951–953.

Perlman, H. B. 1939. The Eustachian tube: Abnormal patency and normal physiologic state. Arch. Otolaryngol., *30*:212–238.

Perlman, H. B. 1951. Observations on the Eustachian tube. Arch. Otolaryngol., *53*:370–385.

Perrin, J. M., Charney, E., MacWhinney, J. B., Jr., McInerny, T. K., Miller, R. L., and Nazarian, L. F. 1974. Sulfisoxazole as chemoprophylaxis for recurrent otitis media: A double-blind crossover study in pediatric practice. N. Engl. J. Med., *291*:664–667.

Persico, M., Podoshin, L., and Fradis, M. 1978. Otitis media with effusion: A steroid and antibiotic therapeutic trial before surgery. Ann. Otol. Rhinol. Laryngol., *87*:191–196.

Petz, L. D. 1978. Immunologic cross-reactivity between penicillins and cephalosporins: A review. J. Infect. Dis., *137*:S74–S79.

Petz, L. D., and Fudenberg, H. H. 1966. Coombs-positive hemolytic anemia caused by penicillin administration. N. Engl. J. Med., *274*:171–181.

Pfisterer, H. 1958. Recent knowledge concerning impairment of hearing in patients with palatal fissure. HNO (Berl.), *6*:307–309.

Phillips, M. J., Knight, N. J., Manning, H., Abbott, A. L., and Tripp, W. G. 1974. IgE and secretory otitis media. Lancet, 2:1176–1178.

Pieraggi, J. 1974. Interet de la sonomanometrie dans le prognostic de la microchirurgie auriculaire. Rev. Laryngol. Otol. Rhinol. (Bord.), 95:319–324.

Politzer, A. 1862. Ueber die willkurlichen bewegungen des trommelfells. Weiner Med. Halle. Nr., 18:103.

Politzer, A. 1865, 1869. Lehrbuch der Ohrenheilkunde. 5. Auflage Vol. I, Stuttgart, F. Enke.

Politzer, A. 1883. Diseases of the Ear. Cassells, J. P. (Trans.-Ed.) Philadelphia, Henry C. Lea's Son and Co., pp. 375–377.

Politzer, A. 1909. Diseases of the Ear. Philadelphia, Lea and Febiger.

Porter, T. A. 1974. Otoadmittance measurements in a residential deaf population. Am. Ann. Deaf, 119:47–52.

Potsic, W. P., Cohen, M., Randall, P., and Winchester, R. 1979. A retrospective study of hearing impairment in three groups of cleft palate patients. Cleft Palate J., 16(1):56–58.

Prellner, K., Nilsson, N. I., Johnson, U., and Laurell, A. B. 1980. Complement and Clq binding substances in otitis media. Ann. Otol. Rhinol. Laryngol., 89(68):129–132.

Proctor, B. 1967. Embryology and anatomy of the Eustachian tube. Arch. Otolaryngol., 86:503–514.

Proctor, B. 1971. Attic-aditus block and the tympanic diaphragm. Ann. Otol. Rhinol. Laryngol., 80:371–375.

Proud, G. O., and Duff, W. E. 1976. Mastoidectomy and epitympanotomy. Ann. Otol. Rhinol. Laryngol., 85(25):289–292.

Puhakka, H., Virolainen, E., Aantaa, E., Tuohimaa, P., Eskola, J., and Ruuskanen, O. 1979. Myringotomy in the treatment of acute otitis media in children. Acta Otolaryngol. (Stockh.), 88:122–126.

Pulec, J. L. 1967. Abnormally patent Eustachian tubes: Treatment with injection of polytetrafluoroethylene (Teflon) paste. Laryngoscope, 77:1543–1554.

Qvarnberg, Y., and Palva, T. 1980. Active and conservative treatment of acute otitis media: Prospective studies. Ann. Otol. Rhinol. Laryngol., 89(68):269–270.

Raikundalia, K. B. 1975. Analysis of suppurative otitis media in children: Aetiology of non-suppurative otitis media. Med. J. Aust., 1:749–750.

Rapp, D. J., and Fahey, D. 1973. Review of chronic secretory otitis and allergy. J. Asthma Res., 10:193–218.

Rathbun, T. A., and Mallin, R. 1977. Middle ear disease in a prehistoric Iranian population. Bull. N. Y. Acad. Med., 53:901–905.

Reed, D., Struve, S., and Maynard, J. E. 1967. Otitis media and hearing deficiency among Eskimo children: A cohort study. Am. J. Public Health, 57:1657–1662.

Restrepo, M. A., and Zambrano, F. 1968. II. Late onset aplastic anemia secondary to chloramphenicol. Report of ten cases. Antioquia Medica, 18:593–606.

Rich, A. R. 1920. A physiological study of the Eustachian tube and its related muscles. Bull. Johns Hopkins Hosp., 31:206–214.

Riding, K. H., Bluestone, C. D., Michaels, R. H., Cantekin, E. I., Doyle, W. J., and Poziviak, C. 1978a. Microbiology of recurrent and chronic otitis media with effusion. J. Pediatr., 93:739–743.

Riding, K. H., Reichert, T. J., Findlay, R. C., and Stool, S. E. 1978b. Tympanometric and otologic evaluation of students in a school for the deaf. In Harford, E. R.,

Bess, F. H., Bluestone, C. D., and Klein, J. O. (Eds.): Impedance Screening for Middle Ear Disease in Children. New York, Grune and Stratton, pp. 279–291.

Rifkind, D. R., Chanock, R. M., Kravetz, H., Johnson, K., and Knight, V. 1962. Ear involvement (myringitis) and primary atypical pneumonia following inoculation of volunteers with Eaton agent. Am. Rev. Respir. Dis., 85:479–489.

Rinkel, H. J. 1962, 1963. The management of clinical allergy. Arch. Otolaryngol., Part I — 76:491–508, 1962; Part II — 77:42–75, 1963; Part III –77:205–225, 1963; Part IV — 77:302–326, 1963.

Riu, R., Flottes, L., Bouche, J., and LeDen, R. 1966. La physiologie de la trompe d'Eustache. Paris, Librarie Anette.

Roddey, O. F., Jr., Earle, R., Jr., and Haggerty, R. 1966. Myringotomy in acute otitis media: A controlled study. J.A.M.A., 197:849–853.

Rogers, R. L., Kirchner, F. R., and Proud, G. O. 1962. The evaluation of Eustachian tubal function by fluorescent dye studies. Laryngoscope, 72:456–467.

Rood, S. R., and Doyle, W. J. 1978. Morphology of tensor veli palatini, tensor tympani, and dilatator tubae muscles. Ann. Otol. Rhinol. Laryngol., 87:202–210.

Roth, R. P., Cantekin, E. I., Bluestone, C. D., Welch, R. M., and Cho, Y. W. 1977. Nasal decongestant activity of pseudoephedrine. Ann. Otol. Rhinol. Laryngol., 86:235–242.

Roydhouse, N. 1970. A controlled study of adenotonsillectomy. Arch. Otolaryngol., 92:611–616.

Roydhouse, N. 1980. Adenoidectomy for otitis media with mucoid effusion. Ann. Otol. Rhinol. Laryngol., 89(68):312–315.

Ruben, R. J., and Math, R. 1978. Serous otitis media associated with sensorineural hearing loss in children. Laryngoscope, 88:1139–1154.

Rubenstein, M. M., McBean, J. B., Hedgecock, L. D., and Stickler, G. B. 1965. The treatment of acute otitis media in children: A third clinical trial. Am. J. Dis. Child., 109:308–313.

Rubin, M. 1978. Serous otitis media in severely to profoundly hearing impaired children, ages 0 to 6. Volta Rev., 80:81–85.

Rudberg, R. D. 1954. Acute otitis media: Comparative therapeutic results of sulfonamide and penicillin administered in various forms. Acta Otolaryngol., 113:1–79.

Sade, J. 1966. Pathology and pathogenesis of serous otitis media. Arch. Otolaryngol., 84:297–305.

Sataloff, J., and Fraser, M. 1952. Hearing loss in children with cleft palates. Arch. Otolaryngol., 5561–64.

Satoh, I., Watanabe, I., and Saindo, T. 1970. Measurement of Eustachian tube function. Arch. Otolaryngol., 92:329–334.

Schachter, J., Grossman, M., Holt, J., Sweet, R., Goodner, E, and Mills, J. 1979. Prospective study of chlamydial infection in neonates. Lancet, 2:377–379.

Schaefer, O. 1971. Otitis media and bottle-feeding. An epidemiological study of infant feeding habits and incidence of recurrent and chronic middle ear disease in Canadian Eskimos. Can. J. Public Health, 62:478–489.

Schwartz, D. M., Schwartz, R. H., and Redfield, N. P. 1978a. Treatment of negative middle ear pressure and serous otitis media with Politzer's technique: An old procedure revised. Arch. Otolaryngol., 104:487–490.

Schwartz, R. H. 1981. Bacteriology of otitis media: A

review. Otolaryngol. Head Neck Surg., *89*:444–450.

Schwartz, R. H., Rodriguez, W. J., Khan, W. N., and Ross, S. 1977. Acute purulent otitis media in children older than five years: Incidence of Haemophilus as a causative organism. J.A.M.A., *238*:1032–1033.

Schwartz, R., Barsanti, R. G., and Rodriguez, W. J.: Private practice view of otitis media. Pediatrics, *61*:937–938.

Schwartz, R., Rodriguez, W. J., Mann, R., Khan, W., and Ross, S. 1979. The nasopharyngeal culture in acute otitis media: A reappraisal of its usefulness. J.A.M.A., *241*:2170–2173.

Schwartz, R.H., Puglese, J., and Schwartz, D.M. 1980. Use of a short course of prednisone for treating middle ear effusion: A double-blind crossover study. Ann. Otol. Rhinol. Laryngol., *89*(68):296-300.

Schwartz, R.H., and Schwartz, D.M. 1980. Acute otitis media: Diagnosis and drug therapy. Drugs, *19*:107-118.

Schwartz, R.H., and Rodriguez, W.J. 1981. Acute otitis media in children eight years old and older: A reappraisal of the role of *Haemophilus influenzae*. Am. J. Otolaryngol., *2*:19-21.

Schwartz, R.H., Rodriguez, W.J., and Schwartz, D.M. 1981. Office myringotomy for acute otitis media: Its value in preventing middle ear effusion. Laryngoscope, *91*:616–619.

Scott, J. L., Finegold, S.M., Belkin, G.A., and Lawrence, J.S. 1965. A controlled double-blind study of the hematologic toxicity of chloramphenicol. N. Engl. J. Med., *272*:1137-1142.

Sellars, S.L., and Seid, A.B. 1973. Aural tuberculosis in childhood. S. Afr. Med. J., *47*:216-218.

Senturia, B.H., Gessert, C.F., Carr, C.D., and Bauman, E.S.: Studies concerned with tubotympanitis. Ann. Otol. Rhinol. Laryngol., *67*:440-467.

Senturia, B.H., Bluestone, C.D., Klein, J.O., Lim, D.J., and Paradise, J.L. 1980a. Report of the ad hoc committee on definition and classification of otitis media with effusion. Ann. Otol. Rhinol. Laryngol., *89*(68):3-4.

Senturia, B.H., Marcus, M.D., and Lucente, F.E. 1980b. Diseases of the External Ear: An Otologic-Dermatologic Manual, 2nd ed. New York, Grune and Stratton.

Severeid, L.R. 1972. A longitudinal study of the efficacy of adenoidectomy in children with cleft palate and secondary otitis media. TAAOO, *76*:1319-1324.

Shah, N. 1971. Use of grommets in "glue" ears. J. Laryngol. Otol., *85*:283-287.

Shah, K.N., and Desai, M.P. 1969. *Ascaris lumbridoides* from the right ear. Indian Pediatr., *6*:92-93.

Shaw, J.R., Todd, N.W., Goodwin, M.H., and King, G.H. 1979. Observations on otitis media among four Indian populations in Arizona. *In* Wiet, R.J., and Coulthard, S. (Eds.): Proceedings of the Second National Conference on Otitis Media. Columbus, Ohio, Ross Laboratories, 1979.

Shea, J.J. 1971. Autoinflation treatment of serous otitis media in children. J. Laryngol. Otol., *85*:1254-1258.

Sheehy, J.L. 1977. Surgery of chronic otitis media. *In* English, G. (Ed.): Otolaryngology, Vol. I. Hagerstown, Md., Harper and Row, Pub.

Shurin, P.A., Pelton, S.S., and Klein, J.O. 1976. Otitis media in the newborn infant. Ann. Otol. Rhinol. Laryngol., *85*(25):216-222.

Shurin, P.A., Howie, V.M., Pelton, S.I., Ploussard, J.H., and Klein, J.O. 1978. Bacterial etiology of otitis media during the first six weeks of life. J. Pediatr., *92*:893-896.

Shurin, P.A., Pelton, S.I., Donner, A., Finkelstein, J., and Klein, J.O. 1980a. Trimethoprim-sulfamethoxazole compared with ampicillin in the treatment of acute otitis media. J. Pediatr., *96*:1081-1087.

Shurin, P.A., Pelton, S.I., Tager, I.B., and Kasper, D.L. 1980b. Bactericidal antibody and susceptibility to otitis media caused by non-typable strains of *Haemophilus influenzae*. J. Pediatr., *97*:364-369.

Siber, G.R., Smith, A.L., and Levin, M.J. 1979. Predictability of peak serum gentamicin concentration with dosage based on body surface area. J. Pediatr., *94*:135-138.

Siedentop, K.H., Loewy, A., Corrigan, R.A., and Osenar, S.B. 1978. Eustachian tube function assessed with tympanometry. Ann. Otol. Rhinol. Laryngol., *87*:163-169.

Siegel, S. C. 1979. Allergy as it relates to otitis media. *In* Wiet, R.J., and Coulthard, S.W. (Eds.): Proceedings of the Second National Conference on Otitis Media. Columbus, Ohio, Ross Laboratories, pp. 25-29.

Siirala, U., and Lahikainen, E.A. 1952. Some observations on the bacteriostatic effect of the exudate in otitis media. Acta Otolaryngol. (Stockh.), Suppl. 100:20-25.

Siirala, U., Tarpila, S., and Halonen, P. 1961. Inhibitory effect of sterile otitis media exudates on the cytopathogenicity of herpes simplex, poliomyelitis, and adenoviruses in HeLa cells. Acta Otolaryngol. (Stockh.), *53*:230-236.

Silverstein, H., Bernstein, J.M., and Lerner, P.I. 1966. Antibiotic concentrations in middle ear effusion. Pediatrics, *38*:33-39.

Skolnick, E.M. 1958. Otologic evaluation in cleft palate patients. Laryngoscope, *68*:1908-1949.

Sloyer, J.L., Jr., Howie, V.M., Ploussard, J.H., Amman, A.J, Austrian, R., and Johnston, R.B. 1974. Immune response to acute otitis media in children. I. Serotypes isolated in serum and middle ear fluid antibody in pneumococcal otitis media. Infect. Immun., *9*:1028-1032.

Sloyer, J.L., Jr., Cate, C.C., Howie, V.M., Ploussard, J.H., and Johnston, R.B. 1975. The immune response to acute otitis media in children. II. Serum and middle ear antibody in otitis media due to *Haemophilus influenzae*. J. Infect. Dis., *132*:685-688.

Sloyer, J.L., Howie, V.M., Ploussard, J.H., Schiffman, G.D., and Johnston, R.B. 1976. Immune response to acute otitis media: Association between middle ear antibody and the clearing of clinical infection. J. Clin. Microbiol., *4*:306-308.

Sloyer, J.L., Jr., Howie, V.M., Ploussard, J.H., Bradoc, J., Hatercorn, M., and Ogra, P.L. 1977. Immune response to acute otitis media in children. II. Implications of viral antibody in middle ear fluid. J. Immunol., *118*:248-250.

Sloyer, J.L., Jr., Ploussard, J.H., and Howie, V.M. 1981. Efficacy of polysaccharide vaccine in preventing acute otitis media in infants in Huntsville, Alabama. Rev. Infect. Dis., *3*:S119-S123.

Sly, R.M., Zambie, M.F., Fernandes, D.A., and Fraser, M. 1980. Tympanometry in kindergarten children. Ann. Allergy. *44*:1-7.

Sobeslavsky, O., Syrucek, L., Bruckoya, M., and Abrahamovic, M. 1965. The etiological role of *Mycoplasma pneumoniae* in otitis media in children. Pediatrics, 35:652–657.

Solomon, N.E., and Harris, L.J. 1976. Otitis Media in Children. Assessing the Quality of Medical Care Using Short-Term Outcome Measures. Quality of Medical Care Assessment Using Outcome Measures: Eight Disease-Specific Applications. Santa Monica, CA, Rand Corp.

Sorensen, H. 1977. Antibiotic in suppurative otitis media. Otolaryngol. Clin. North Am., 10:45-50.

Spivey, G.H., and Hirschhorn, N. 1977. A migrant study of adopted Apache children. Johns Hopkins Med. J., 140:43-46.

Spriesterbach, D.C., Lierle, D.M., Moll, K.L., and Prather, W.F. 1962. Hearing loss in children with cleft palates. Plast. Reconstr. Surg., 30:336-347.

Stanievich, J.F., Bluestone, C.D., Lima, J.A., Michaels, R.H., Rohn, D., and Effron, M. Z. 1981. Microbiology of chronic and recurrent otitis media with effusion in young infants. Int. J. Pediatr. Otorhinolaryngol., 3:137-143.

Stechenberg, B.W., Anderson, D., Chang, M.J., Dunkle, L., Wong, M., vanReken, D., Pickering, L.K., and Feigin, R.D. 1976. Cephalexin compared to ampicillin treatment of otitis media. Pediatrics, 58:532-536.

Steinberg, E.A., Overturf, G.D., Wilkins, J., Baraff, L.J., Streng, J.M., and Leedom, J.M. 1978. Failure of cefamandole in treatment of meningitis due to *Haemophilus influenzae* type b. J. Infect. Dis., 137:S180-S186.

Stickler, G.B., and McBean, J.B. 1964. The treatment of acute otitis media in children: A second clinical trial. J.A.M.A., 187:85-89.

Stickler, G.B., Rubenstein, M.M., McBean, J.B., Hedgecock, L.D., Hugstad, B.A., and Griffing, T. 1967. Treatment of acute otitis media in children: A fourth clinical trial. Am. J. Dis. Child., 114:123-130.

Stool, S.E., and Randall, P. 1967. Unexpected ear disease in infants with cleft palate. Cleft Palate J., 4:99-103.

Stool, S.E., Craig, H.B., and Laird, M.A. 1980. Screening for middle ear disease in a school for the deaf. Ann. Otol. Rhinol. Laryngol., 89(68):172-177.

Stroud, M.H., Spector, G.J., and Maisel, R.H. 1974. Patulous Eustachian tube syndrome: Preliminary report of the use of the tensor veli palatini transposition procedure. Arch. Otolaryngol., 99:419-421.

Suehs, O.W. 1952. Secretory otitis media. Laryngoscope, 62:998-1027.

Taylor, G.D. 1972. The bifid uvula. Laryngoscope, 82:771-778.

Teele, D.W., and Klein, J.O.: Unpublished data.

Teele, D.W., Norton, C.C., and Klein, J.O.: Unpublished data.

Teele, D.W., Healy, G.B., and Tally, F.P. 1980a. Persistent effusions of the middle ear: Cultures for anaerobic bacteria. Ann. Otol. Rhinol. Laryngol., 89(68):102-103.

Teele, D.W., Klein, J.O., and Rosner, B.A. 1980b. Epidemiology of otitis media in children. Ann. Otol. Rhinol. Laryngol., 89(68):5-6.

Teele, D.W., Klein, J.O., and the Greater Boston Collaborative Otitis Media Program. 1980c. Beneficial effects of breastfeeding on the duration of middle ear effusion after the first episode of acute otitis media. Pediatr. Res., 14:494.

Teele, D.W., Klein, J.O., and the Greater Boston Colla-

borative Otitis Media Study Group. 1981a. Use of polyvaccine for prevention of recurrent acute otitis media in infants in Boston. Rev. Infect. Dis.,3:S113-S118.

Teele, D.W., Pelton, S.I., and Klein, J.O. 1981b. Bacteriology of acute otitis media unresponsive to initial antimicrobial therapy. J. Pediatr., 98:537–539.

Tetzlaff, T.R., Ashworth, C., and Nelson, J.D. 1977. Otitis media in children less than 12 weeks of age. Pediatrics, 59:827-832.

Tetzlaff, T.R., McCracken, G.H., Jr., and Nelson, J.D. 1978. Oral antibiotic therapy for skeletal infections of children. II. Therapy of osteomyelitis and suppurative arthritis. J. Pediatr., 92:485–490.

Thomsen, J., Meistrup-Larson, K.I., Sorensen, H., Larsen, P.K., and Mygind, N. 1980. Penicillin and acute otitis: Short and long term results. Ann. Otol. Rhinol. Laryngol., 89(68):271-274.

Thomsen, K.A. 1958a. Investigations on the tubal function and measurement of the middle ear pressure in pressure chamber. Acta Otolaryngol. (Stockh.), Suppl. 140:269-278.

Thomsen, K.A. 1958b. Investigations on Toynbee's experiment in normal individuals. Acta Otolaryngol. (Stockh.), Suppl. 140:263-268.

Thorington, J. 1892. Almost total destruction of the velum palati corrected by an artificial soft palate, producing not only greatly improved speech, but an immediate increase of audition. Med. News,61:269, and Ann. Mal l'Oreille Larynx, p. 694.

Timmermans, F.J., and Gerson, S. 1980. Chronic granulomatous otitis media in bottle-fed Inuit children. Can. Med. Assoc. J., 122:545-547.

Tipple, M.A., Beem, M.O., and Saxon, E.M. 1979. Clinical characteristics of the afebrile pneumonia associated with chlamydia trachomatis infection in infants less than six months of age. Pediatrics, 63:192-197.

Tos, M., and Polusen, G. 1976. Secretory otitis media: Late results of treatment with grommets. Arch. Otolaryngol., 102:672–675.

Turner, A.L., and Fraser, J.S. 1915. Tuberculosis of the middle ear cleft in children: A clinical and pathological study. J. Laryngol. Rhinol. Otol., 30:209-247.

Valsalva, A. 1949. Trachus de aure humana. *In* Stevenson, R.S., and Guthrie, D. (Eds.): A History of Otolaryngology. Edinburgh, E. and S. Livingstone, Ltd.

Van Dishoeck, H.A.E., Derks, A.C.W., and Voorhorst, R. 1959. Bacteriology and treatment of acute otitis media in children. Acta Otolaryngol. (Stockh.), 50:250-262.

Variot, G. 1904. Écoulement de lait par l'oreille d'un mourisson atteint de division congenitale du voile du palais. Bull. Soc. Pediatr. Paris, 6:387.

Veltri, R.W., and Sprinkle, P.M. 1973. Serous otitis media: Immunoglobulin and lysozyme levels in middle ear fluids and serum. Ann. Otol. Rhinol. Laryngol., 82:297-301.

Venker, H. 1973. Sonomanometric investigation of the Eustachian tube function and tympanoplasty. ORL, 35:233-236.

Virolainen, E., Puhakka, H., Aantaa, E., Tuohimaa, P., Ruuskanen, O., and Meurman, O.H. 1980. Prevalence of secretory otitis media in seven to eight year old school children. Ann. Otol. Rhinol. Laryngol., 89(68):7-10.

Virtanen, H. 1977. Eustachian Tube Sound Conduction — Sonotubometry, An Acoustical Method for

Objective Measurement of Auditory Tubal Opening. Thesis, Department of Otolaryngology, University of Helsinki, Finland.

Virtanen, H. 1978. Sonotubometry: An acoustical method for objective measurement of auditory tubal opening. Acta Otolaryngol. (Stockh.), 86:93-103.

Virtanen, S., and Lahikainen, E.A. 1979. Ampicillin concentrations in middle ear effusions in acute otitis media after administration of bacampicillin. Infection, 7(5):472-474.

Waickman, F.G. 1979. Allergic management of otitis media. Transactions of the Second National Conference on Otitis Media. Columbus, Ohio, Ross Laboratories, pp. 109-114.

Wallerstein, R.O., Condit, P.K., Kasper, C.K., Brown, J.W., and Morrison, F.R. 1969. Statewide study of chloramphenicol therapy and fatal aplastic anemia. J.A.M.A., 208:2045-2050.

Walton, W.K. 1973. Audiometrically "normal" conductive hearing losses among the cleft palate. Cleft Palate J., 10:99-103.

Ward, J. 1981. Antibiotic-resistant Streptococcus pneumoniae: Clinical and epidemiological aspects. Rev. Infect. Dis., 3:254-266.

Ward, J.I., Tsai, T.F., Filice, G.A., and Fraser, D.W. 1978. Prevalence of ampicillin- and chloramphenicol-resistant strains of Haemophilus influenzae causing meningitis and bacteremia: National survey of hospital laboratories. J. Infect. Dis., 138:421–424.

Ward, P. A., and McClean, R. 1978. Complement activity. In Bellanti, J.A. (Ed.): Immunology II. Philadelphia, W.B. Saunders Co. pp. 138-150.

Warren, W.S., and Stool, S.E. 1971. Otitis media in low-birth-weight infants. J. Pediatr., 79:740-743.

Webster, J.C. 1980. Middle ear function in the cleft palate patient. J. Laryngol. Otol., 94(1):31-37.

Welin, S. 1947. On the radiologic examination of the Eustachian tube in cases of chronic otitis. Acta Radiol. (Stockh.), 28:95-103.

Whaley, J.B. 1957. Otolaryngologist's role in the care of cleft palate patients. J. Can. Dent. Assoc., 23:574-575.

Whitcomb, N.J. 1965. Allergy therapy in serous otitis media associated with allergic rhinitis. Clin. Allergy, 23:232-236.

Wittenborg, M.H., and Neuhauser, E.B. 1963. Simple roentgenographic demonstration of Eustachian tubes and abnormalities. Am. J. Roentgenol. Rad. Ther. Nucl. Med., 89:1194-1200.

Wong, D.T., and Ogra, P.L. 1980. Immunology of tonsils and adenoids — an update. Int. J. Pediatr. Otorhinolaryngol., 2:181-191.

Yaffe, S.J. 1975. Requiem for tetracyclines. Pediatrics. 55:142-143.

Yagi, H.A. 1977. The surgical treatment of secretory otitis media in children. J. Laryngol. Otol., 91:267-270.

Yules, R.B. 1970. Hearing in cleft palate patients. Arch. Otolaryngol., 91:319-323.

Zollner, R. 1942. Anatomie, Physiologie und Klinik der Ohrtrompete. Berlin, Springer Verlag.

Zonis, R.D. 1968. Chronic otitis media in the Southwestern American Indian. Arch. Otolaryngol., 88: 360–365.

INTRATEMPORAL COMPLICATIONS AND SEQUELAE OF OTITIS MEDIA

Charles D. Bluestone, M.D.

Jerome O. Klein, M.D.

The intracranial suppurative complications of otitis media are relatively uncommon today except in neglected cases. However, those that occur within the aural cavity and adjacent structures of the temporal bone are more common, and awareness of them is essential in management of children with otitis media, for even though many of the less serious conditions are not life-threatening, the quality of life may be severely affected. The aural and intratemporal complications and sequelae of otitis media are hearing loss, perforation of the tympanic membrane, chronic suppurative otitis media, retraction pocket, acquired cholesteatoma, mastoiditis, petrositis, labyrinthitis, adhesive otitis media, tympanosclerosis, ossicular discontinuity and fixation, facial paralysis, cholesterol granuloma, infectious eczematoid dermatitis, and necrotizing ("malignant") external otitis (Fig. 17–1). For many of these disorders, surgery is indicated, but the emphasis in this chapter has been on concepts of surgical management as they relate to infants and children, rather than on explicit descriptions of surgical techniques. For details of the surgical techniques, the reader is referred to current texts and atlases (see Selected References).

HEARING LOSS

Hearing loss is by far the most prevalent complication and morbid outcome of otitis media with effusion and may be caused by one or more of the intra-aural complications or sequelae. To a varying degree, fluctuating or persistent loss of hearing is always associated with acute or chronic otitis media with effusion. The presence of high negative pressure within the middle ear (atelectasis) in the absence of an effusion can also be associated with a significant hearing loss. The prevalence of hearing loss in children roughly corresponds to the prevalence of otitis media in the same population (Solomon and Harris, 1976). The audiogram usually reveals a mild to moderate conductive loss. However, there may be a sensorineural component, generally attributed to the effect of increased tension and stiffness of the round window membrane. This hearing loss is usually reversible with resolution of the effusion, but permanent conductive hearing loss can result from irreversible changes secondary to recurrent acute or chronic inflammation, such as adhesive otitis media or ossicular discontinuity. Irreparable sensorineural loss may also occur, presumably as the result of chronic spread of infection through the round window membrane (Paparella et al., 1972). Although uncommon today, suppurative labyrinthitis secondary to otitis media may cause sensorineural hearing loss (with or without vertigo). More commonly, a perilymphatic fistula in the oval or round window, or both, may be present when otitis media results in sensorineural hearing loss (Grundfast and Bluestone, 1978). Audiometry can give reliable results when performed in children over

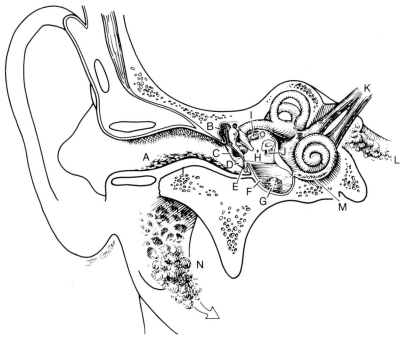

Figure 17-1   Intratemporal complications and sequelae of otitis media include *A*, Infectious eczematoid dermatitis; *B*, Cholesteatoma; *C*, Retraction pocket of the tympanic membrane; *D*, Tympanosclerosis; *E*, Perforation of the tympanic membrane; *F*, Chronic suppurative otitis media; *G*, Cholesterol granuloma; *H*, Ossicular discontinuity; *I*, Facial paralysis; *J*, Adhesive otitis media with fixation of the ossicles; *K*, Hearing loss; *L*, Petrositis; *M*, Labyrinthitis; *N*, Mastoiditis with extension into the neck (Bezold abscess).

two years of age, but children under two years are the group at highest risk for effusions and associated hearing loss, and in these patients, standard audiometric assessment is difficult to perform reliably. However, an attempt should be made to assess the hearing in all infants and children who have recurrent or chronic otitis media.

Most investigators have found a substantial incidence of hearing loss in children who have apparently recovered from acute otitis media. In the study by Fry et al. (1969), a loss of 20 dB or more was found in 17 per cent of children who had had an episode of otitis media 5 to 10 years previously, as compared to 4.5 per cent in matched controls. Reed et al. (1967), in a longitudinal study, showed a statistically significant association between the frequency of episodes of otitis media and a hearing loss of greater than 26 dB (International Standards Organization, ISO). Of children who had an average of less than one episode of otitis media per year, 35 per cent had hearing loss, and among children who had one or more attacks, 49 per cent had loss of hearing, whereas in children with no diag-

nosed episodes, only 15 per cent had hearing loss. Other studies with somewhat differing criteria have found the incidence of hearing loss associated with acute otitis media to vary between 6 and 30 per cent (Lowe et al., 1963; Neil et al., 1966).

Olmstead and coworkers (1964) studied children 2½ to 12 years of age seen in the outpatient department of St. Christopher's Hospital in Philadelphia with a diagnosis of acute otitis media. Of 82 children included in the study, 33 per cent had no loss of hearing on the initial audiometric test following acute infection; 40 per cent had loss of hearing (15 dB) initially, which disappeared in one to six months; 12 per cent had loss of hearing throughout the six month period of observation; and 15 per cent had loss of hearing initially but were lost to the study between one and four months after the acute episode of otitis media. The children in the study had no prior history of hearing difficulty or chronic ear infection. Otoscopic examinations were not performed after the initial diagnosis, and data were not presented about the duration of fluid in the middle ear. These data indicate that after a single episode of acute otitis media, many children have prolonged impairment of hearing.

Kessner et al. (1974), in a large-scale community survey of children in Washington, D.C., found that approximately 19 per cent had hearing loss of 15 dB or greater. Of the 108 children with hearing loss, only two had a sensorineural loss, the rest having the conductive type. Only half of all those with hearing loss had otoscopic evidence of tympanic membrane–middle ear pathology. Most likely, the others without otoscopic evidence of effusion had high negative pressure or inflammatory changes within the middle ear, or both, which was not evident on routine otoscopic examination. Downs (1975) reported that the prevalence of hearing loss greater than 15 dB in preschool children was between 10 and 15 per cent. Bluestone et al. (1973) reported that most children with effusions (subsequently documented at the time of surgery) had significant impairment of hearing. Therefore, whenever an otitis media with effusion is diagnosed by otoscopy or by tympanometry, there is a usually concurrent hearing loss.

Effects on Learning Processes

Do children suffer long-term sequelae either of recurrent episodes of acute otitis media (fluid in the middle ear plus signs of acute illness) or of persistent effusions of the middle ear (fluid in the middle ear with minimal or no signs or symptoms)? Such sequelae might include depressed scores on intelligence tests, impaired hearing, impaired speech and language, and poor performance in school.

The relation between sensorineural hearing loss and impairment in the cognitive, language, and emotional development of children has been studied. Young and McConnell (1957) compared children who had 30 dB or more hearing losses with children with normal hearing and found the hearing-handicapped children to be significantly retarded in development of vocabulary. In another study, Kodman (1963) showed that children with significant hearing losses were placed below their expected grade levels in school. Goetzinger et al. (1964) found that children who either had a congenital hearing loss or had acquired a hearing

loss in the first year of life had poorer articulation and auditory discriminatory abilities than those who had not. Fisher (1966) reported a high rate of maladjusted behavior patterns in children who had hearing losses of 20 to 64 dB. Peckham et al. (1972) also related hearing impairment to disturbances in psychosocial adjustment.

The association between developmental problems and persistent or fluctuant hearing loss associated with otitis media has also been studied. The following investigators have examined this association.

1. Wishik et al. (1958) defined intermittent hearing loss (presumably due to otitis media) as failure to pass one audiometric test during an eight-year study period. Children who had intermittent hearing losses according to this criterion were found to have been delayed in grade placement when compared to children with normal hearing.

2. Holm and Kunze (1969) studied the effect of chronic otitis media on language and speech development. Children aged five to nine years with a history of chronic otitis media and with hearing fluctuations documented by audiograms were compared to a control group matched for age, sex, and socioeconomic background. Language skills were compared by means of the Illinois Test of Psycholinguistic Abilities (ITPA), the Peabody Picture Vocabulary Test, the Templin-Darley Picture Articulation Screening Test, and the Meechan Verbal Language Development Scale. Children with a history of chronic otitis media were delayed in all language skills requiring the receiving or processing of auditory stimuli, but the groups were not different in tests measuring visual and motor skills.

   The disease cohort was selected from children referred to an ear, nose, and throat clinic. Diagnosis of otitis media was made by history alone; examinations of the middle ear were not performed during the study. The sample size was small; there were 16 children in the diseased group and 16 in the control group.

3. Kaplan et al. (1973) studied the effects of recurrent episodes of acute otitis media (defined as the presence of a draining ear) on Eskimo children. They followed the children prospectively during their

first four years of life and then tested them at age 10 years for morbidity. They administered tests to assess hearing, intelligence, and school performance. Children with recurrent episodes of otitis media during the first two years of life and with loss of hearing of 26 dB had lower scores in tests of reading, mathematics, and language than did children in a control group.

American Eskimo children have exceptionally high rates of middle ear disease. Because otorrhea was the sole criterion by which these investigators defined history of otitis media, they presented no data concerning the presence or duration of middle ear effusions or episodes of acute otitis media that did not result in otorrhea.

4. Lewis (1976) studied children from the schools of a community of aborigines near Brisbane, Australia. Children aged seven to nine years who had been noted to have hearing deficits measured on audiometric or tympanometric tests over a four-year period were compared with age-matched control children who had consistently passed the audiometric tests and who were presumed to be disease-free. "Speech hearing" tests, the Wepman Auditory Discrimination Test, and a test of phonemic synthesis similar to subtests of the ITPA were performed. The results of these tests indicated that the children with chronic middle ear disease had mean scores for speech and language development that were significantly lower than those of the children without a history of ear disease. The sample size was small (32 children).

5. Needleman (1977) evaluated 20 children with a history of recurrent otitis media with fluctuations in hearing as documented by audiograms and 20 control subjects matched for age, grade, and socioeconomic status but with no history of problems with hearing or recurrent ear infections. The children were tested to evaluate their phonologic development. Tests of phonologic skills included the Templin-Darley Screening Test of Articulation, the Goldman-Fristoe-Woodcock Test for Auditory Discrimination, selected subtests of the ITPA, and ability to repeat sentences. Children with a history of chronic otitis media had poorer phonologic abilities than did matched normal children. The authors note that these phonologic skills are a prerequisite for learning to read and that phonologic difficulties may result in educational retardation. This study was retrospective and was based on history alone. The criteria did not include documentation of past or present middle ear disease.

6. Zinkus et al. (1978) studied 40 children aged 6 to 11 years of age who had been referred for evaluation of suspected learning disability. One group of 18 children had histories of multiple episodes of otitis media during the first three years of life. Thirteen of these children had a measurable loss of hearing when they were evaluated. The second group of 22 children had a history of few episodes of otitis media, and all but two had normal hearing. Children with a history of chronic otitis media showed significant delays in speech and language development and did poorly on measurements of intelligence that involved auditory skills, although they performed normally on tests that depended on visual skills.

This study was retrospective and depended on the history of past episodes of otitis media. No documentation of the presence or absence of disease of the middle ear was included.

These reports are disturbing, but each is flawed in design or of uncertain relevance to most children because of one or more of the following features: (1) reliance on retrospective history of acute otitis media, (2) uncertain validity of diagnosis of otitis media, (3) lack of information about middle ear effusion, (4) presence of significant hearing impairment in subjects at the time of tests of speech and language, (5) small numbers of subjects, (6) special populations tested (Australian aborigines or Alaskan Eskimos, for example), and (7) inadequate criteria for selection of children without disease used for comparison. These inadequacies prevent application of these results to planning care for young children, but they do not prevent concern that many children may suffer from such morbidity.

Conclusions

Hearing loss, to some degree, is present when there is an effusion within the middle ear. When the hearing loss is due to otitis media, it is usually of the conductive type; when the effusion resolves, the hearing in most children returns to normal. However, in some children who have one or more of the complications or sequelae of otitis media, the loss of hearing may be permanent, with the loss being conductive or sensorineural or both. Severe hearing loss can cause language, speech, and developmental impairments, and moderate loss of hearing appears to delay or impair language skills in children. However, for children who have only a conductive hearing loss when an effusion or high negative pressure or both are present within the middle ear, the proof of later language or developmental impairment is not yet established. Nevertheless, prevention of otitis media and its related conditions and of the possible structural changes that they may cause within the middle ear is desirable, since recurrent episodes of acute otitis media or persistent middle ear effusion have been shown to be detrimental to hearing.

PERFORATION OF THE TYMPANIC MEMBRANE

A perforation of the tympanic membrane that is secondary to otitis media (and certain related conditions, such as atelectasis of the tympanic membrane) can be classified according to its duration, the area of the eardrum involved, its size, and the presence or absence of associated conditions, such as otitis media or cholesteatoma. In addition, the perforation may not be spontaneous (a result of a middle ear infection) but may be a complication of a surgical procedure to manage otitis media, such as a myringotomy and tympanostomy tube insertion. An acute perforation is most frequently secondary to an espisode of acute otitis media, whereas if it persists for two or three months, it is considered chronic. These perforations occur in the pars tensa and involve one or more of the following quadrants: anterosuperior, anteroinferior, posterosuperior, or posteroinferior. The defect may involve almost the entire pars tensa or may be so small as to be detectable only when visualized with the otomicroscope or when the electroacoustic impedance bridge measures a volume larger than the expected ear canal volume. Otitis media (with or without discharge) may be present or absent; when chronic otitis media with discharge is

present, the condition is called chronic suppurative otitis media, which is described in detail in the next section. Likewise, a perforation may be associated with some of the other complications and sequelae described in this chapter.

In the past, perforations have been classified into "central" and "marginal" types. Regardless of size, if there is a rim of tympanic membrane remaining at all borders, the perforation has been classified as being of the "central" type, whereas when any part of the perforation extends to the annulus, it has been termed a "marginal perforation." Similarly, a defect in the pars flaccida has been commonly called an "attic perforation." However, the so-called "marginal perforation" of the pars tensa, which usually occurs in the posterosuperior portion, and the "attic perforation" are in reality either a deep retraction pocket or a cholesteatoma (Fig. 17–2). There is usually no continuity between the *defect* in the membrane and the middle ear until late in the disease process, when infection destroys the membrane of the pocket or the matrix of the cholesteatoma. Therefore, the terms "marginal perforation" and "attic perforation" are misnomers; they were applied on the basis of observations made prior to the availability of the otomicroscope, modern middle ear surgery, advances in temporal bone histopathology, the use of the electroacoustic impedance bridge, and a better understanding of the pathogenesis of a retraction pocket and cholesteatoma (both of which are described in a separate section in this chapter). In this section, only acute and chronic perforations (with and without acute otitis media) will be discussed.

Acute Perforation

Etiology

An acute perforation (not due to trauma) is usually secondary to acute otitis media but may also occur during the course of chronic otitis media with effusion. Since a spontaneous perforation commonly accompanies an episode of acute middle ear infection, it may be part of the natural history of the disease process rather than a complication. Because such a perforation allows pus to drain into the external canal and enhances drainage of pus down the eustachian tube (see Chap. 16, p. 375), a perforation of the eardrum that

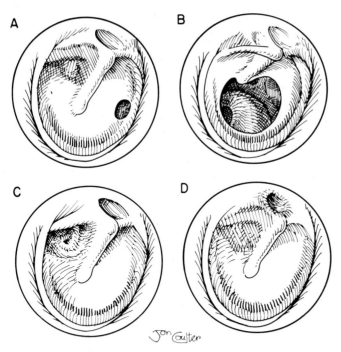

Figure 17–2 Examples of defects in the tympanic membrane. *A,* A small "central" perforation in the anteroinferior portion of the pars tensa of the tympanic membrane. *B,* A "central" perforation that involves approximately half of the pars tensa. *C,* A deep retraction pocket in the posterosuperior portion of the pars tensa that has been incorrectly called a "marginal perforation." *D,* A deep retraction pocket in the pars flaccida that has been inappropriately called an "attic perforation."

adequately drains the middle ear may prevent further spread of infection within the temporal bone or, more importantly, into the intracranial cavity. Infants and children of certain racial groups, such as Alaskan natives (Eskimos) and American Indians, have a high incidence of spontaneous perforation with discharge; the eardrum is perforated spontaneously with almost every episode of acute otitis media. The disease runs a similar course in certain other children not belonging to these high-risk populations. The perforation may occur in these individuals because of the presence of a semipatulous eustachian tube (Beery et al., 1980). A eustachian tube with low resistance would permit a larger bolus of bacteria-laden purulent material from the nasopharynx to enter the middle ear, causing a more fulminating infection than would occur if the eustachian tube had either normal or high resistance. An alternative explanation of why some children seem to suffer a perforated eardrum with each episode of acute otitis media while others do not could be that there are differences in the virulence of the bacteria or resistance of the host. It has been postulated that certain bacteria that cause acute otitis media are more virulent than others, such as the type 3 pneumococcus. Even a mild middle ear infection in a compromised host could result in a spontaneous tympanic membrane perforation and profuse aural discharge.

Management

The organisms that are most frequently cultured from an aural discharge when acute otitis media is present are the same as those that have been cultured from acute middle ear effusions when a tympanocentesis has been performed, that is, *Streptococcus pneumoniae* and *Haemophilus influenzae*. Therefore, antimicrobial therapy for children with perforated eardrums should be the same as that recommended for those with acute otitis media when a perforation is not present (see Chap. 16, p. 460). However, when an aural discharge is present, it may be desirable to culture the drainage. The indications for obtaining a culture in such cases would be similar to those for performing a tympanocentesis when acute otitis media (without a perforation) is present: (1) the child is critically ill or toxic; (2) there is an unsatisfactory clinical response to antimicrobial therapy, such as persistence or recurrence of fever or otalgia, or both; (3) a suppurative complication, such as acute mastoiditis with periostitis, is present or impending; (4) a discharge is occurring in the neonate, the very young infant, or the immunologically deficient patient, in each of whom an unusual organism may be present; and (5) the purulent otorrhea persists in spite of a full course of antimicrobial therapy. The antimicrobial agent(s) can then be adjusted according to the results of the smear, culture, and sensitivity testing. The most effective method to obtain a sample of the discharge is to remove as much as possible of the purulent material from the external canal by suction or cotton-tipped applicator and then to aspirate pus directly at or through the perforation, using a spinal needle attached to a tuberculin syringe or an Alden-Senturia trap (Storz Instrument Co., St. Louis) and suction.

Even though some experts would argue against the use of ototopical medication when a perforation is present because of the potential danger of ototoxicity, some children should have otic drops instilled into the external canal. In particular, ototopical medication will usually be beneficial when infectious eczematoid external otitis complicates the picture (see Infectious Eczematoid Dermatitis, p. 560). The application of an antibiotic-cortisone otic medication whenever a discharge is present has been advocated by many clinicians despite the possibility of ototoxicity, since the topical medication may prevent an external canal infection from occurring and hasten the resolution of the middle ear infection.

In any event, the discharge, especially when profuse, should be prevented from draining onto the pinna and adjacent areas, since this usually results in dermatitis. The parent should be instructed to keep cotton in the external auditory meatus and change it as often as necessary to keep the canal as dry as possible. Cotton-tipped applicators should not be used by the child or the parent.

Healing of the tympanic membrane frequently follows cessation of the suppurative process. The defect usually closes within a week of the onset of the infection; however, when persistent discharge lasts longer than the initial 10 day course of antibiotic treatment, the child requires more intensive evaluation and aggressive management. In addition to obtaining a culture of the purulent material from the middle ear and adjusting the antimicrobial agent(s), frequent cleaning of the canal followed by instillation of ototopical drops may also be required. The presence of acute mastoiditis with periosteitis or acute mastoid osteitis should be suspected if the child has persistent otalgia, tenderness of the ear to touch, erythema, and swelling in the postauricular area. Roentgenograms of the mastoids may be helpful but are not always diagnostic of mastoid osteitis (see Mastoiditis, p. 546). Spread of the infection outside the middle ear and mastoid may be diagnosed on computerized tomograms. Even if an intratemporal (or intracranial) complication is not readily apparent, if the aural discharge persists for two or three weeks after the onset of the acute otitis media, the child should be hospitalized if appropriately administered oral antibiotics (selected on the basis of the culture results) have failed to resolve the infection. The child should also be evaluated again thoroughly to search for an underlying illness that would interfere with the resolution of the infection. The otologic assessment should include an examination of the entire external canal and tympanic membrane, using the otomicroscope to determine if another otologic condition is present, such as a cholesteatoma or neoplasm. If an adequate examination cannot be performed with the child awake, it should be carried out under general anesthesia, at which time a culture directly from the middle ear (or biopsy) can be obtained. If no other condition besides the perforation and subacute otitis media is found, parenteral antimicrobial agents should be administered, and appropriate ototopical drops should be directly instilled once or twice a day (using a needle attached to a syringe) into the middle ear through the perforation, with the aid of the otomicroscope. The selection of both the systemic and topical antimicrobial agents should be based on the results of the culture (see Tables 16–32 and 17–1). Frequently, a gram-negative organism (such as *Pseudomonas aeruginosa)* is present at this stage, and management is essentially as recommended under Chronic Suppurative Otitis Media.

With this method of management, the infection will usually subside; however, if the discharge persists, an exploratory tympanotomy and complete simple mastoidectomy are indicated, even if there are no signs and symptoms of mastoid osteitis present and if the roentgenograms fail to show osteitis, that is, "coalescence." During the surgery on the middle ear and mastoid, a thorough search for another cause of the persistent infection must be made. On occasion, a cholesteatoma or neoplasm that could not be visualized through the otomicroscope will be found. Resolution of the infection in the middle ear and mastoid will invariably follow the surgery, since mastoid osteitis is the usual cause of this complication of acute otitis media.

Fortunately, nowadays, the occurrence of such cases is uncommon, and the perforation

Table 17–1 TOPICAL ANTIBIOTIC THERAPY FOR CHRONIC OTITIS MEDIA

Polymyxin B
Colistin (polymyxin E)
  Sensitive organisms
    Pseudomonas aeruginosa
    Escherichia coli
    Klebsiella sp
    Enterobacter sp
  Resistant organisms
    Proteus sp
    Bacteroides fragilis
  Gram-positive cocci

Neomycin
  Sensitive organisms
    Many gram-positive and gram-negative organisms,
    e.g., *S. aureus*, Proteus sp.
  Resistant organisms
    Many *Pseudomonas* sp, all anaerobes

Chloramphenicol
  Sensitive organisms
    Staphylococcus, coagulase-positive
    Staphylococcus, coagulase-negative
    Group A *Streptococcus*
    Escherichia coli
    Proteus mirabilis
    Klebsiella
    Enterobacter

(Adapted from Fairbanks, D. N. 1981. Antimicrobial therapy for chronic suppurative otitis media. Ann. Otol. Rhinol. Laryngol., 90(84):58.)

usually heals rapidly; however, not infrequently, the defect will remain open without evidence of otitis media (with or without discharge). If the perforation remains free of infection, it will frequently close in a few months. At this stage, no attempt at surgical closure of an uncomplicated perforation, even though there are no signs of otitis media, is indicated. If there is no sign of progressive healing after three or more months, management should be as described next for a chronic perforation of the tympanic membrane.

Chronic Perforation

It is not uncommon for a perforation of the tympanic membrane to remain open after an episode of acute otitis media or following spontaneous extrusion (or removal) of a tympanostomy tube. When the perforation is present with no signs of healing and there are no signs of otitis media for several months, the perforation is considered to be chronic and possibly "permanent." If chronic suppurative otitis media is present, the perforation may close spontaneously following appropriate treatment (see Chronic Suppurative Otitis Media in this chapter). The healing of the perforation is most likely being prevented by the presence of squamous epithelium at the edges of the perforation. The effect on hearing of a small chronic perforation, regardless of its location and in the absence of other middle ear abnormalities, is not significant. However, a large perforation can be associated with an appreciable conductive hearing loss, for example, 20 to 30 dB.

Even though the incidence of chronic perforations in the pediatric population has not been formally studied, the rate is high. The incidence of tympanoplasties performed in children would not accurately reflect the true incidence of chronic perforation, since many physicians elect to withhold surgery until later in life. However, next to myringotomy, with or without tympanostomy tube insertion, tympanoplasty is the most common ear operation performed in children and is the most common of all major surgical procedures performed on the ears of children (Avery et al., 1976).

Chronic perforations as complications of otitis media are more prevalent in the racial groups that also have a high prevalence and incidence of acute perforations associated with acute middle ear infection. In 1970, new cases of chronic perforation (with or without chronic suppurative otitis media) were reported in 8 per cent of the native population of Alaska, although this rate appears to be dropping more recently (Wiet et al., 1980). Similar rates are found in American Indian populations. Between 1971 and 1974, there were 114 Alaskan native children aged 6 to 10 years who had tympanoplasty procedures performed for chronic perforations (apparently without suppurative otitis media). As a complication of tympanostomy tube insertion, chronic perforations appear to be quite high in some centers. Of 1062 ears of children who received tympanostomy tubes in one study reported from West Germany, 26 ears (2.5 per cent) had a persistent perforation (Muenker, 1980). However, this figure is dependent on the site of the tube placement and the type of tube used (see Chapter 16, Tympanostomy Tubes).

Management

The management of so-called "dry" chronic perforations in children is both difficult and controversial. On the one hand, the perforation provides ventilation and drainage of the middle ear, but on the other hand, the physiologic protective function of the eustachian tube–middle ear system is impaired. The middle ear and mastoid air cells no longer have an air cushion to prevent nasopharyngeal secretions from entering the ear, which can result in "reflux otitis media" (Fig. 17–3). In addition, the open tympanic membrane can permit contaminated water to enter the middle ear during bathing and swimming. Therefore, the dilemma of when to close such a perforation is comparable to that regarding the most appropriate time to remove a tympanostomy tube; a small, uncomplicated chronic perforation and a tympanostomy tube have similar benefits and risks. Like a tympanostomy tube, a perforation may be beneficial for a child who had had recurrent or chronic otitis media with effusion prior to the development of the perforation, but recurrent acute "reflux otitis media" with discharge may become a prob-

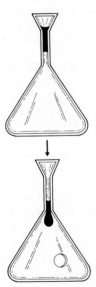

Figure 17–3 Flask model showing how a perforation of the tympanic membrane may result in reflux of nasopharyngeal secretions into the middle ear. The nasopharynx–eustachian tube–middle ear–mastoid air cell system is likened to a flask with a narrow neck. When the system is intact, liquid is prevented from entering the body of the flask, but when the body of the flask is not intact, i.e., when a perforation is present, liquid can readily flow through the system.

lem, making closure of the eardrum defect a consideration. However, recurrent acute otitis media that results in otorrhea through a chronic perforation can be effectively treated and even prevented without repair of the tympanic membrane. When the episodes are infrequent, the treatment of each bout should be the same as recommended for an acute perforation that is associated with acute otitis media. However, if the episodes of acute infection are frequent and the interval between bouts short, then a prolonged course of a prophylactic antimicrobial agent will usually prevent the recurrent middle ear infection and discharge. The selection of the agent should be based on the results of the cultures obtained from the previous episodes of discharge. Dosage and duration of the treatment should be the same as recommended for children who have had frequently recurrent acute otitis media without a perforation (Chap. 16, Antimicrobial Agents for Prophylaxis, p. 468). Children in whom an attack of acute middle ear infection and discharge persists despite adequate medical treatment and in whom the infection is thought to be chronic should be evaluated and managed as described in the section on Chronic Suppurative Otitis Media. Fortunately, most children who have a defect in the eardrum that is thought to be preventing otitis media can be watched until the risk of recurrence of infection is low enough to consider surgical closure of the perforation. Since the perforation, like a tympanostomy tube, may be preventing the development of a retraction pocket and, subsequently, of a cholesteatoma if the function of the eustachian tube is poor, it is desirable to delay such surgery as long as possible in order to prevent such complications. On the other hand, surgery for a chronic perforation should not necessarily be withheld in children because of recurrent episodes of otitis media and discharge, since the perforation may be causing the middle ear infection (owing to reflux from the nasopharynx), rather than preventing disease.

Indications for Repair of the Perforation. Indications for repair of a chronic perforation in adults have been defined by many surgeons, but most have emphasized that the results of this type of surgery are not as successful in children (Armstrong, 1965; Goodey and Smyth, 1972; Mawson and Ludman, 1979). Some have commented upon this in the literature, attributing their findings to the higher incidence of upper respiratory tract infection leading to otitis media in children and the unpredictability of their eustachian tube function. Optimal ages at which to perform tympanoplastic surgery have variously been stated to be from three years to puberty (Mawson and Ludman, 1979; Bailey, 1976; Glasscock, 1976; Storrs, 1976). Paparella (1977) states that tympanoplasty can be performed in children of almost any age. However, Sheehy and Anderson (1980) do not recommend elective tympanic membrane grafting on children who are younger than seven years of age because of the possibility of postoperative otitis media.

Studying eustachian tube function before the patient with a chronic perforation of the tympanic membrane is operated upon may be helpful in determining the potential results of tympanoplasty surgery. Holmquist (1968) studied eustachian tube function in adults before and after tympanoplasty and reported that the operation had a high rate of success in patients with good eustachian tube function (that is, those who could equilibrate applied negative pressure) but that in patients without good tubal function, surgery frequently failed to close the perforation. Miller and Bilodeau (1967) and Siedentop (1968) reported similar findings, but Ekvall (1970), Lee and Schuknecht (1971), Andreasson and Harris (1979), Cohn et al. (1979), and Virtanen et al. (1980) found no correlation between the results of the inflation-deflation tests and success or failure of tympanoplasty. Most of these studies failed to define the criteria for "success," and the postoperative follow-up period was too short. Bluestone et al. (1979) assessed children prior to tympanoplasty and found that of 51 ears of 45 children, 8 ears could equilibrate an applied negative pressure (-200 mm H_2O) to some degree, and in 7 of these ears the graft took, no middle ear effusion occurred, and no other perforation developed during a follow-up period of between one and two years. However, as was found in studies in adults, failure to equilibrate an applied negative pressure did not predict failure of the tympanoplasty (see Chap. 16, Tests of Ventilatory Function, p. 378).

The conclusion to be drawn from these studies is that if the patient is able to equilibrate an applied negative pressure, regardless of age, the success of tympanoplasty is likely, but failure to pass this difficult test will not help the clinician in deciding not to operate. However, the value of testing a patient's ability to equilibrate negative pressure lies in the possibility of determining from the test results if a young child is a candidate for tympanoplasty when one might decide on the basis of other findings alone to withhold surgery until the child is older. These tests are also of value in the diagnosis of severe or total mechanical obstruction, conditions that contraindicate the performance of a simple myringoplasty rather than a tympanoplasty; further evaluation and medical or surgical management of such patients may be indicated depending upon the condition of the ear. The child should be examined for the possible presence of a nasopharyngeal tumor, and if none is found, the cause of obstruction could be mucosal swelling of the middle ear end of the eustachian tube, which may respond to medical treatment, such as ototopical medication. If the obstruction persists despite medical treatment and if a repair of the perforation is to be performed, an exploration of the middle ear and bony (protympanic) portion of the eustachian tube should be part of the examination. It is possible that an unsuspected cholesteatoma will be found to be the cause of the obstruction.

In addition to inflation-deflation studies in the ear with a perforation, otoscopic and tympanometric assessment of the contralateral ear with an intact tympanic membrane may be helpful in predicting the success of surgery. Since the best indication of eustachian tube function is obtained by observing the status of the middle ear over a period of at least one year, that is, four seasons, and since eustachian tube function is usually the same bilaterally in children, the status of the contralateral ear with an intact tympanic membrane may be a good indicator of the expected functioning of the middle ear with a perforated eardrum following repair of the eardrum. If recurrent or persistent high negative pressure or effusion or both are present within the middle ear or if there is a retraction pocket in the posterosuperior quadrant of the pars tensa or in the pars flaccida, or a cholesteatoma, tympanoplasty is usually unsuccessful. Figure 17–4 shows an example of test results of an ideal case for tympanoplasty, whereas Figure 17–5 is an example of results that would indicate that the child is an uncertain candidate for surgical repair of the tympanic membrane.

If a child has a unilateral perforation and if insertion of a tympanostomy tube is indicated in the opposite, intact side to prevent recurrent otitis media with effusion, or to eliminate

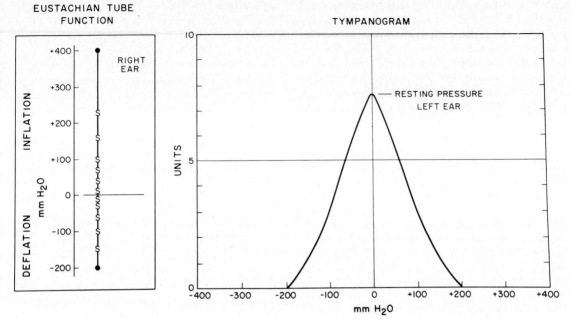

Figure 17–4 Pretympanoplasty evaluation of a child who had normal results on the inflation-deflation eustachian tube function test in the perforated ear and normal resting pressure in the contralateral ear with an intact tympanic membrane. S–swallow.

a chronic middle ear effusion, or to ventilate a severely atelectic tympanic membrane (with or without a retraction pocket), tympanoplasty for an uncomplicated chronic perforation would be contraindicated until these conditions are absent and a tympanostomy tube is no longer required. Again, an observation period of at least one year will be required.

There is no available evidence to support

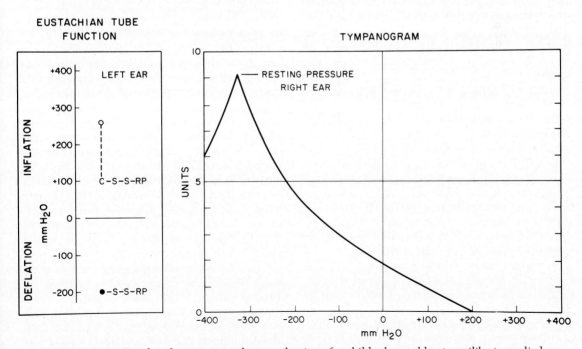

Figure 17–5 Results of pretympanoplasty evaluation of a child who could not equilibrate applied positive or negative pressure during the inflation-deflation eustachian tube test in the ear with the perforation. A tympanogram of the contralateral ear with an intact tympanic membrane revealed high negative pressure. O–opening pressure, C–closing pressure, S–swallow, RP–residual pressure.

the belief that removal of the adenoids (and tonsils) improves the success rate of tympanoplasty, and until such studies are available, surgical removal of these structures for the ear condition alone should be considered of uncertain benefit. Two retrospective studies in children failed to show that adenoidectomy had any effect on the outcome of tympanoplasty (Bluestone et al., 1979; Buchwach and Birck, 1980). Most surgeons agree that there should be no signs of otitis media in the ear prior to a tympanoplasty; that is, the ear should be "dry," since the presence of discharge is associated with failure of the tympanoplasty (Armstrong, 1965). When an acquired cholesteatoma is found in the operated ear, tympanoplasty will most likely be less than optimally successful (Bluestone et al., 1979). When a tympanoplasty is withheld in a child who has significant hearing loss, a hearing aid should be considered until such time as the procedure is performed and hearing improvement is achieved.

In children who have bilateral perforations and in whom eustachian tube function tests show no active function when negative pressure is applied, it is uncertain whether or not tympanoplasty would be successful. A better test of tubal function must be devised and the results correlated with the results of the surgery before it will be possible to determine the probable degree of success to be expected from tympanoplasty in these cases. When a tympanoplasty must be performed and the function of the eustachian tube is thought to be poor, a tympanostomy tube should be inserted.

Surgical Techniques. Once the decision is made to close a chronic perforation of the tympanic membrane of a "dry" ear surgically, a technique should be chosen that will have the greatest chance of success with the least risk to the child. To perform most surgical procedures to repair a perforation in children, a general anesthetic will be required, whereas in adults, especially when the perforation is small, local anesthesia is adequate. Therefore, the benefits of surgery in a child must outweigh the risks of general anesthesia.

When no other middle ear abnormalities are present, a small perforation may heal if the epithelium is removed from its edges and if the circumference of the perforation is cauterized with trichloroacetic acid. A rayon, silk, or plastic wrap (for example, Saran Wrap) patch can then be placed over the defect. This simple technique can be done as an outpatient procedure, with local anesthesia in older children and adolescents, but general anesthesia may be necessary in young children. The procedure should be performed only if the hearing is normal or only slightly impaired and if the remaining portion of the tympanic membrane is translucent; these two criteria must be met in order to avoid the possibility that the ossicles may be involved or that a tympanic membrane–middle ear cholesteatoma, that is, migration of squamous epithelium through the perforation into the middle ear, may be present. These same criteria also apply to the next, somewhat more involved, type of repair, a myringoplasty. This procedure is similar to the simple closure, except that cautery is usually not used, a larger defect can be repaired, and a fresh autograft should be employed, such as temporalis fascia, tragal perichondrium, or earlobe fat. However, neither procedure involves exploration of the middle ear; therefore, in most children, the middle ear (including the medial side of the tympanic membrane remnant) must be inspected during tympanoplasty to rule out the possible presence of another pathologic condition that may require more extensive surgery. In one large study reported by Sheehy and Anderson (1980), the 472 myringoplasties performed during the years 1967 to 1977 represented only 10 per cent of all the primary operations performed at their center, and of these, 88 per cent were performed in patients 16 years of age or older.

Of all the techniques of tympanoplasty that are currently advocated (see Selected References), none is specifically designed for children. In general, the surgical techniques are the same for children as for adults; however, certain considerations should be kept in mind when performing a tympanoplasty in a child. Since the external canal is frequently smaller in children than in adults, a postauricular (or endaural) approach may be required to achieve adequate visualization of the tympanic membrane and middle ear. A transcanal approach should be reserved for only those children whose ear canals are large enough to provide proper exposure of the entire operative field. Autografts are preferred over homografts and heterografts, since we have inadequate information at present to determine the long-term effects of using the latter grafts. For the same reason, when an ossicular chain abnormality is present, a type II or III tympanoplasty (Fig. 17–6), or an autograft ossicle, should be used for the ossiculoplasty rather

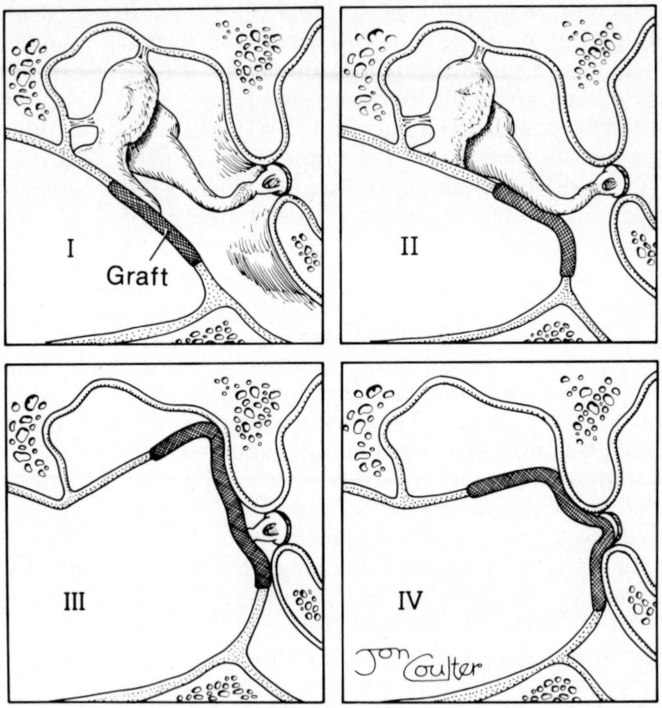

Figure 17–6 Tympanoplasty surgical procedures. Type I, ossicular chain intact; Type II, graft lies on incus; Type III, graft is on stapes superstructure; Type IV, graft is on stapes footplate.

than inert material (see Ossicular Discontinuity and Fixation). A type IV tympanoplasty is invariably unsuccessful in children. The preference for a technique that involves placing the graft lateral to the tympanic membrane has some merit, since laterally placed grafts have been shown to have a higher initial "take rate" in children (Bluestone et al., 1979). The failure of medially placed grafts may be related to the fluctuating negative pressure that is so commonly present in the middle ears of children and that could conceivably enhance the take of a lateral graft but tend to pull a medial graft away from the tympanic membrane. For smaller perforations, a medial graft may be satisfactory, but for a large perforation, the laterally placed fascia graft appears to give better results and, when performed properly, should not lead to the postoperative complication of "blunting" in the anterior sulcus or lateral healing of the graft (Sheehy and Anderson, 1980).

The routine addition of an extensive simple mastoidectomy to a tympanoplasty procedure in children who show no evidence of disease in the mastoid is not justified. The risk of prolonging the general anesthesia does not outweigh the remote possibility of finding occult disease, nor is the risk justified by increasing the middle ear–mastoid air volume, which has been purported to enhance the success rate of

tympanoplasty. In addition, obtaining routine preoperative roentgenograms of the mastoid without any evidence of disease in the area also does not appear to be justified owing to the potential hazards of radiation.

The problems associated with postoperative care of the patient are greater when the patient is a child than an adult, especially if the patient is a young child. These problems must be considered before deciding to perform elective tympanic grafting.

Outcome

Unfortunately, regardless of the technique and despite adequate follow-up, tympanoplasty is not as successful in children as it is in adults, which is probably the reason why many surgeons wait until a child grows older to do the procedure. In children, the criteria that must be met for a tympanoplasty done to repair an uncomplicated perforation to be successful are take of the initial graft (the tympanic membrane remains intact) and absence of high negative middle ear pressure, atelectasis, retraction pocket, otitis media with effusion, or cholesteatoma for a follow-up period of at least two years. Improvement in hearing is also an important goal. In a study of 45 children (51 ears) in which the preceding criteria were used to evaluate the outcome of tympanoplasty, less than half of the tympanoplasties followed for one to two years were successful (Bluestone et al., 1979). However, some of the cases initially had cholesteatoma. Buchwach and Birck (1980) reported an overall success rate of 66 per cent for type I tympanoplasties in 74 children (80 ears). In their retrospective study, the age of the child was not related to the outcome.

Conclusions

Children are uncertain candidates for tympanoplastic surgery, since as a group their eustachian tube function is not as good as that of adults. However, in selected cases, the procedure may be successful. For some children, tympanoplasty appears to be contraindicated, whereas in others, the outcome of the operation is less certain. The problem for the clinician is deciding which child should have the perforation repaired. The development of an improved method of testing the eustachian tube, a method that is more indicative of the actual function available for clinical use, could possibly help in this decision-making process. A controlled study of the indications for tympanoplasty in a large group of children is needed.

CHRONIC SUPPURATIVE OTITIS MEDIA
(Chronic Suppurative Otitis Media and Mastoiditis, Chronic Otitis Media with Perforation and Discharge, Chronic Otitis Media)

Chronic suppurative otitis media is a stage of ear disease in which there is chronic inflammation of the middle ear and mastoid and in which a "central" perforation of the tympanic membrane and discharge (otorrhea) are present. Mastoiditis is invariably a part of the pathologic process. The condition has been called simply chronic otitis media, but this term can be confused with chronic otitis media with effusion, in which no perforation is present. It is also called chronic suppurative otitis media and mastoiditis, chronic purulent otitis media, and chronic otomastoiditis. The most descriptive term is chronic otitis media with perforation, discharge, and mastoiditis (Senturia et al., 1980a), but this is not common usage. When a cholesteatoma is also present, the term chron-

ic suppurative otitis media with cholesteatoma is used; however, because an acquired aural cholesteatoma does not have to be associated with chronic suppurative otitis media, cholesteatoma is not part of the pathology of the type of ear disease described in this section but is presented as a separate entity in the following section.

Epidemiology

Most studies that have reported the prevalence of chronic suppurative otitis media in children include children who also have cholesteatoma, so that accurate data on the incidence of chronic suppurative otitis media alone are not available. In a study conducted by the School Health Service in Great Britain, the number of children found to have chronic otitis media at the periodic medical inspections was about 9 in 1000 (Mawson and Ludman, 1979).

This type of chronic ear disease has a high prevalence in children of certain racial groups. The studies of American Indians (Cambon et al., 1965; Zonis, 1970; DeBlanc, 1975; Wiet et al., 1980), Canadian and Alaskan (Eskimo) natives (Maynard, 1969; Baxter and Ling, 1974), Australian aboriginal children (McCafferty et al., 1977), and others, such as the Maoris of New Zealand, have shown an extremely high prevalence and incidence of chronic suppurative otitis media among these populations. In addition, the prevalence of chronic suppurative otitis media is higher in children in these racial groups than in the Caucasian population living in the same area (Ratnesar, 1977). Cholesteatoma is not commonly associated with the chronic ear disease found in these populations. In a study of 4193 Alaskan native school children conducted in 1971, 1274 (30 per cent) had perforated tympanic membranes, but in only 144 (3 per cent) was a cholesteatoma also diagnosed (Tschopp, 1977). Ratnesar (1977) reported similar findings in a study of Canadian Eskimos and Indians but also found a higher incidence of cholesteatoma in the Caucasians living in the same area. Similarly, McCafferty and coworkers (1977) studied 3663 Australian aboriginal children and found that 70 per cent of their ears were abnormal; 12 per cent had chronic otitis media, but less than 1 per cent had a cholesteatoma. Ear disease has an early onset in these children; Maynard (1969) reported that most Eskimo children had chronic otitis media before the age of two years.

These epidemiologic studies appear to be describing the etiology and pathogenesis of chronic suppurative otitis media that is *not* associated with cholesteatoma. By studying the natural history of the ear disease in these population groups, the pathogenesis of this type of ear disease can be better understood.

Pathogenesis, Etiology, and Pathology

Even though the pathogenesis of chronic suppurative otitis media is not completely known, it is considered to be the chronic stage that follows an attack of acute otitis media in which a perforation has developed followed by discharge. However, the sequence of events does not have to progress directly from the acute to the chronic form. A perforation secondary to an acute otitis media can become chronic without any evidence of middle ear inflammation, that is, a "dry" perforation. Some authors consider this stage to be an "inactive" stage of chronic otitis media, since a middle ear (and mastoid) infection with discharge through the perforation may occur at any time. However, some children have a perforation that rarely, if ever, occurs with a discharge after the initial acute episode in which the perforation developed, and the middle ear mucous membrane remains normal. Therefore, only a chronic perforation that is associated with chronic inflammation of the middle ear–mastoid should be considered to be chronic suppurative otitis media (see Perforation of the Tympanic Membrane, p. 517). However, the pathogenesis may be the same for acute or chronic perforations with or without otitis media.

Doyle (1977), in studies of the bony craniofacial structures of Eskimo, American Indian, Caucasian, and Negro individuals, found that there were anatomic differences in the structures of the eustachian tube among these groups. Beery et al. (1980) studied 25 White Mountain Apache Indians ranging in age from 3 to 36 years and found that their eustachian tubes were semipatulous (of low resistance) in comparison to those of a group of Caucasians. In this study, the function of the eustachian tube was assessed directly through chronic perforations of the eardrum, employing the inflation-deflation and forced-response tests. These studies would appear to indicate that these racial groups and the segment of the Caucasian population that has chronic suppurative otitis media have eustachian tubes that permit reflux of nasopharyngeal secretions into the middle ear; reflux acute otitis media develops, and the tympanic membrane perforates. In some individuals, the reflux of nasopharyngeal secretions continues after the initial episode, while in others, the process recurs with each upper respiratory tract infection. The perforation enhances the reflux of the secretions from the nasopharynx, since the middle ear–mastoid air cushion is abolished (see Chap. 16, Physiology, Pathophysiology, and Pathogenesis, p. 373).

However, these individuals rarely have a cholesteatoma in the posterosuperior quadrant of the pars tensa or in the pars flaccida, and if a cholesteatoma is present, it is usually due to migration of epithelium through the "central" perforation, which is uncommon; an even more rare and unproved pathogenesis of cholesteatoma is that which is secondary to metaplasia of the middle ear mucous membrane. Since most cholesteatomas are the final step in a sequence of events that begins with negative middle ear pressure, progresses to atelectasis, and then leads to a retraction pocket, the development of a cholesteatoma should be rare when a "central" perforation is present, since the middle ear pressure is always ambient (see Cholesteatoma and Retraction Pocket, p. 530). Therefore, even though children who have chronic suppurative otitis media have a morbid process, they appear to be protected from developing an attic or posterosuperior type of cholesteatoma. It is important to keep these facts in mind when considering the surgical management of the perforation after elimination of the chronic middle ear and mastoid infection.

Chronic suppurative otitis media develops from a chronic bacterial infection. However, the bacteria that caused the initial episode of acute otitis media with perforation are usually not those that are isolated from the chronic discharge when there is a chronic infection in the middle ear and mastoid. Thus, the antimicrobial therapy recommended for acute otitis media will not be effective for most cases of chronic suppurative otitis media. The most common organisms are the gram-negative bacilli, *P. aeruginosa* and *Proteus* sp; however, *Staphylococcus aureus* has also been cultured (Friedman, 1957), as have anaerobes from ears with chronic otitis media. It is probable that these organisms are present in the ear canal and enter the chronically infected middle ear through the perforation.

It is important to understand the pathology of chronic otitis media, since the decision for or against surgical intervention may depend on the pathologic changes in the middle ear and mastoid. These include edema, submucosal fibrosis, and infiltration with chronic inflammatory cells, which together cause thickening of the mucous membrane (Schuknecht, 1974). Polyps may result from excessive mucosal edema; in the more advanced stage, not only are polypoid tissue and granulation tissue present, but also osteitis of the mastoid bone, ossicles, and labyrinth may be observed. Adhesive otitis media and sclerosis of bone may occur with healing. Tympanosclerosis may also be present and is commonly associated with this disease in Alaskan (Eskimo) natives (Wiet et al., 1980). If intensive medical treatment is instituted early, these pathologic changes may be reversible without surgery. However, when longstanding chronic disease has led to irreversible changes, middle ear and mastoid surgery is usually indicated to eradicate the infection.

Diagnosis

A purulent, mucoid, or serous discharge coming through a "central" perforation of the tympanic membrane for at least two or three months is evidence of chronic suppurative otitis media. Frequently, a polyp will be seen coming through the perforation (Fig. 17–7). The size of the perforation has no relation to the duration or severity of the disease, but frequently the defect involves most of the pars tensa. There is no otalgia, tenderness to touch in the mastoid area or pinna, vertigo, or fever. When any of these signs or symptoms is present, the examiner should look for a possible suppurative intratemporal or intracranial complication. A search for the underlying cause of the infection may reveal the presence of paranasal sinusitis, which must be actively treated, since the ear infection may not respond to medical treatment until the sinusitis resolves. An upper respiratory tract allergy or a nasopharyngeal tumor may also be contributing to the pathogenesis of chronic otitis media and will need to be managed appropriately (see Chap. 16, p. 393).

The diagnostic evaluation must include a smear, culture, and sensitivity testing of the discharge. This should be done as described in the section on perforation of the tympanic membrane in this chapter.

However, one of the most important parts of the evaluation is a complete examination, with the aid of the otomicroscope, of the ear canal, tympanic membrane, and, if the perforation is large enough, the middle ear. If a satisfactory examination cannot be performed with the child awake, then an exami-

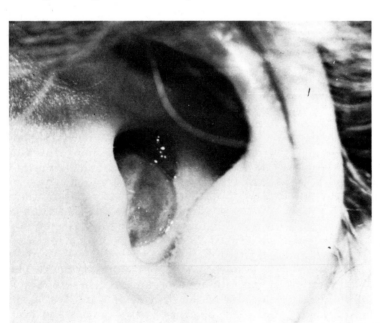

Figure 17–7 Aural polyp in external auditory meatus. The polyp came through a large perforation of an ear with chronic suppurative otitis media.

nation under general anesthesia will be necessary. At this time, the discharge can be aspirated, and a culture from the middle ear can be obtained; in addition, a search for a polyp or unsuspected cholesteatoma or neoplasm should be conducted.

A conductive hearing loss usually accompanies chronic otitis media. If greater than a 20 to 30 dB hearing loss is found, the ossicles may be involved; however, the patient may also have a sensorineural component, which is most likely due to a serous labyrinthitis (Paparella et al., 1972). Impedance testing may be helpful if purulent material in the ear canal prevents visualization of the eardrum adequate to identify a possible perforation. If a perforation is present, the measured volume of the external canal will be larger than expected; however, the tympanometric pattern may be flat despite the presence of a perforation if the volume of air in the middle ear and mastoid is small. When this is suspected, the pressure on the pump-manometer of the impedance bridge can be increased in an attempt to force open the eustachian tube; if the tube can be opened with positive air pressure from the pump-manometer, a perforation must be present.

Roentgenograms of the mastoid should be obtained in every case; if tomograms can be obtained as well, they will be the most informative. In the typical case, the sclerotic or undeveloped mastoid will appear "cloudy." However, if a defect in the bone due to osteitis is present, the area will appear on the roentgenogram. Discontinuity of the ossicular chain, if present, may be visualized if tomography is used.

Unusual causes of a chronic draining ear include neoplasm, eosinophilic granuloma, or an unusual bacterial infection. These must be considered in the differential diagnosis of chronic suppurative otitis media.

Management

Medical management of chronic otitis media is directed toward eliminating the infection from the middle ear and mastoid. Since the bacteria most frequently cultured are gram-negative, antimicrobial agents should be selected to be effective against these organisms. Various topical preparations are available, including hydrocortisone and antibiotics such as polymyxins B or E, neomycin, and gramicidin (Table 17–1). The purulent material should be prevented from spreading onto the adjacent area of the pinna and neck by keeping cotton in the external meatus. Orally administered antibiotics are usually not effective unless an organism is seen on the Gram stain or is cultured from the discharge, such as *S. aureus,* a beta-lactamase–producing *H. influenzae,* or *Branhamella catarrhalis.* Oral antibiotics are also effective against the organisms that commonly cause acute otitis media, such as Pneumococcus.

If the discharge fails to resolve rapidly with antibiotic medication, then more aggressive medical management will be required. Topical gentamicin (Genoptic) should be used, since the most common causative organism is *P. aeruginosa.* This medication can be used at home, but the best method is for the child to return to the outpatient facility daily so that the discharge can be thoroughly aspirated and the ototopical gentamicin can be directly instilled into the middle ear through the perforation, employing the otomicroscope. Frequently, the discharge will rapidly improve with this type of treatment within a week, after which the eardrops may be administered at home until there is complete resolution of the middle ear–mastoid inflammation.

If it is not feasible for the child to be treated on an ambulatory basis or if the suppurative process continues despite the method of management just described, then the patient should be hospitalized, and parenteral carbenicillin (effective against *P. aeruginosa)* should be administered in adequate doses (see Table 16–32). Using the otomicroscope and following aspiration and débridement of the discharge from the ear canal and middle ear, if the smear shows gram-negative bacilli, an appropriate topical agent such as gentamicin should be directly instilled into the middle ear through the perforation twice daily. In almost all children, the middle ear will be free of discharge, and the signs of otitis media will be greatly improved or absent within 7 to 10 days after initiating this method of management. If resolution does in fact occur, the child should be discharged and followed on an ambulatory basis at periodic intervals to watch for signs of spontaneous closure of the perforation, which frequently happens after the middle ear and mastoid are no longer infected. However, if the perforation persists or if another abnormality requiring surgery is present, such as an ossicular chain disarticulation, tympanoplastic surgery should be considered. When a chronic ("dry") perforation is present, the indications for repair of the tympanic membrane would be similar to those outlined in the previous section (see Perforation of the Tympanic Membrane, p. 521). However, frequent episodes of acute and chronic infection would be a possible indication to explore the middle ear (and possibly the mastoid) and to perform a tympanoplasty. The decision to do a mastoidectomy should depend on the roentgenographic findings and the preference of the surgeon, but routine mastoidectomy is not necessary if the perforation is not associated with another abnormality that would warrant an exploration of the mastoid. In most children who have had complete resolution of the infection in the middle ear and mastoid but who have a persistent, chronic ("dry") perforation and in whom a tympanoplasty is performed, the addition of a mastoidectomy is of limited value for either diagnosis or management. In such cases, the mastoid was most likely converted to a more normal state if the discharge was absent for several months.

When the discharge fails to respond to the intensive medical therapy described earlier, surgery on the middle ear and mastoid is indicated. For most children, a complete simple mastoidectomy combined with a transcanal tympanotomy with removal of the infected mucous membrane and bone will usually result in resolution of the chronic suppurative middle ear infection and the chronic irreversible mastoid osteitis. No attempt should be made to perform reconstructive middle ear surgery, such as a tympanoplasty or an ossiculoplasty. These procedures should be performed as a planned second-stage operation or later in life, depending upon the status of the ear during the postoperative period.

It is not uncommon that a cholesteatoma is present when an ear with chronic suppurative otitis media fails to respond to intensive medical treatment, even though no preoperative evidence for the presence of cholesteatoma was identified by otomicroscopy or roentgenography. The cholesteatoma usually is found in the middle ear (and mastoid) following migration of the squamous epithelium through the perforation in the tympanic membrane. When a cholesteatoma is found, surgical removal as outlined in the next section is indicated. With the possible exception of finding a cholesteatoma, there is seldom a reason to perform a modified radical or radi-

cal mastoidectomy for chronic suppurative otitis media, since it is a disease of the mucous membrane and mastoid bone, and adequate control can be achieved without "taking the canal down."

Conclusions

Most children who have chronic suppurative otitis media that is refractory to ototopical medication and orally administered antimicrobial agents will require (1) a thorough examination of the external canal and tympanic membrane with the otomicroscope (usually under general anesthesia); (2) a culture obtained directly from the middle ear; (3) direct instillation of the appropriate ototopical medication into the middle ear once or twice a day using the otomicroscope to visualize the middle ear; and, if the suppurative process is severe, (4) hospitalization and the parenteral administration of an antimicrobial agent. The ototopical medication and the systemic antimicrobial therapy should be selected following microbiologic assessment of the discharge. Middle ear and mastoid surgery should be reserved for those children who fail to respond to intensive medical therapy.

CHOLESTEATOMA AND RETRACTION POCKET

Keratinizing stratified squamous epithelium and an accumulation of desquamating epithelium of keratin within the middle ear or other pneumatized portions of the temporal bone is called a keratoma or, more commonly, a cholesteatoma. Aural cholesteatomas can be classified into two types: "congenital" and acquired. A "congenital" cholesteatoma has been defined as a congenital rest of epithelial tissue and appears as a white, cyst-like structure within the middle ear (intratympanic) or temporal bone. The tympanic membrane is intact, and it is apparently not a sequela of otitis media or eustachian tube dysfunction (Cawthorne and Griffith, 1961; Derlacki and Clemis, 1965) (see Chap. 14). Acquired cholesteatoma may be secondary to implantation or may be a sequela of otitis media or a retraction pocket or both. Implantation cholesteatoma may develop either from epithelium that has migrated through a traumatic perforation of the tympanic membrane or from epithelium that has been inadvertently overlooked in the middle ear or mastoid during surgery of the ear (iatrogenic) (Brandow, 1977).

However, the most common cholesteatoma is the acquired type, which is secondary to middle ear disease. In a study of 1024 patients (adults as well as children), a cholesteatoma was found in the attic in 42 per cent, in the posterosuperior quadrant in 31 per cent, in 18 per cent when there was a "total" perforation, in 6 per cent when there was a "central" perforation, and in 3 per cent when there was no perforation (Sheehy et al., 1977). However, it is possible that the patients in whom the cholesteatoma was associated with a "total" perforation originally had involvement of the posterosuperior portion of the pars tensa. In children, the most common defect in the tympanic membrane begins developing in the posterosuperior quadrant of the pars tensa or, somewhat less commonly, in the pars flaccida. The term "marginal perforation" has been used to describe the defect in the posterosuperior quadrant, and the defect in the pars flaccida has been called an "attic perforation," but in reality, these are not perforations but are either retraction pockets or cholesteatomas that appear otoscopically to be perforations (Fig. 17–2). No continuity between the defect and the middle ear occurs until later in the disease process (see Perforation of the Tympanic Membrane, p. 517). Retraction pockets of the tympanic membrane are also described in Chapter 16 on p. 438.

Epidemiology, Natural History, and Complications

Harker and Koontz (1977), in a study of the general population in Iowa, reported the overall incidence of cholesteatoma to be 6 per 100,000; in children up to 9 years of age, the incidence was 4.7 per 100,000, while in children 10 to 19 years old, the incidence of 9.2 per 100,000 was the highest for all age groups. Cholesteatoma is a common sequela in children with cleft palate. Severeid (1977) reviewed the records of 160 children and young adults with cleft palates (70 per cent were 10 to 16 years of age), all of whom had had a history of ear disease, and found the incidence of cholesteatoma to be 7.1 per cent; the posterosuperior portion of the pars tensa was the most common site. In contrast to this

high incidence of cholesteatoma in the cleft palate population is the rare occurrence of cholesteatoma in Alaskan (Eskimo) natives, American Indians (Hinchcliffe, 1977), and Australian aboriginal children (McCafferty et al., 1977), in whom other middle ear disease is very common. This remarkable difference in the incidence of cholesteatoma in children with cleft palates and in certain racial groups, both of which have a high prevalence and incidence of otitis media, is most likely related to differences in the pathogenesis and natural history of the respective middle ear disease processes.

Cholesteatoma in children is considered to be a more aggressive disease than that occurring in adults (Baron, 1969; Derlacki, 1973; Schuknecht, 1974) for two reasons: (1) Very extensive disease is found at the time of surgery more frequently in children than in adults, and (2) higher rates of residual (persistent) and recurrent cholesteatoma following surgery have been found in children compared to the rates in adults (Abramson et al., 1977). Palva et al. (1977) compared 65 children with cholesteatomas with 65 adults with the same disease and found that whereas 22 per cent of the children had extensive disease that filled the middle ear and mastoid, only 6 per cent of adults had such extensive disease. However, despite the finding that cholesteatomas in children tend to be more extensive than those occurring in adults, childhood cholesteatoma may still be confined to the mesotympanum or epitympanum.

Ritter (1977) compared an epidemiologic study in Michigan of 152 cases of cholesteatoma identified during the period from 1965 to 1970 to a similar study from Massachusetts of 303 cases that were identified during a period prior to the use of antimicrobial agents (1925 to 1936). He found in both series that about 45 per cent of cases of cholesteatoma were operated on before the patient was 20 years of age, that in approximately 65 per cent of the patients, the aural discharge had begun by 11 years of age, and that the distribution of sites on the tympanic membrane where the defect was located were about the same. He concluded that antimicrobial agents have not altered the incidence and natural history of cholesteatoma during the 40 years between the two studies.

However, prior to the advent of the widespread use of antimicrobial agents and modern otologic surgery, complications of cholesteatoma were common, and for many children when infection involved the intracranial cavity, the result was death. Nowadays, serious complications of cholesteatoma in children are uncommon. In a study of 181 children who had cholesteatoma, 8 (4.4 per cent) developed a labyrinthine fistula, and one suffered facial paralysis, but none had intracranial complications (Sheehy et al., 1977). However, in the same study, which also included 843 adults, the incidence of both intratemporal and intracranial complications increased the longer the cholesteatoma was present. Because most of the adults could date the onset of their disease to childhood and because diagnosis and surgery for cholesteatoma is the best way to prevent serious complications, physicians dealing with ear problems in children should treat suspected cholesteatoma early and aggressively.

The incidence of retraction pockets has not been formally studied, but a retraction pocket is a common sequela of atelectasis of the tympanic membrane with or without otitis medial with effusion. The incidence in individuals with cleft palates must be greater than that of cholesteatoma in this population (7.1 per cent), since a retraction pocket precedes the development of a cholesteatoma in children with cleft palate (Bluestone et al., 1982).

Pathogenesis

Many hypotheses regarding the pathogenesis of cholesteatoma have been proposed; the following are the most popular: (1) metaplasia of the middle ear and attic due to infection (Wendt, 1873; Tumarkin, 1938); (2) invasive hyperplasia of the basal layers of the meatal skin adjoining the upper margin of the tympanic membrane (Nager, 1925; Hellman, 1925; Lange, 1932; Ojala and Saxen, 1952; Ruedi, 1958); (3) invasive hyperkeratosis of the deep external auditory canal (McGuckin, 1961); and (4) retraction or collapse of the tympanic membrane with invagination secondary to eustachian tube dysfunction (Habermann, 1888; Bezold, 1889; Wittmaack, 1933). In addition, there are those who consider the condition not to be acquired at all but to be an embryonic epidermal rest occurring in the attic (McKenzie, 1931; Teed, 1936; Diamant, 1952).

Bluestone et al. (1977) reported preliminary findings of varying degrees of function-

al rather than mechanical (anatomic) obstruction of the eustachian tube in 13 children and adults who had a retraction pocket or an acquired cholesteatoma. Subsequently, the findings in 12 children with acquired cholesteatoma, all of whom had functional obstruction of the eustachian tube, were also reported by the same group (Bluestone et al., 1978). Children were specifically studied, since the development of an acquired cholesteatoma with its attendant irreversible changes was thought to occur early in life and since the function of the eustachian tube might improve with growth and development. In these children, the function of the eustachian tube was assessed by the modified inflation-deflation technique (after Ingelstedt et al., 1963). Another study was undertaken by Bluestone and coworkers (1982) to clarify further the cause of this functional obstruction by employing a new test of eustachian tube function, the forced-response test (Cantekin et al., 1979), and to evaluate a larger group of children who had either a cholesteatoma or a retraction pocket. In addition, children with an apparently "congenital" cholesteatoma were also studied, and the results obtained in both groups were then compared to the results of testing children who had traumatic perforation of the tympanic membrane but who otherwise were considered to be otologically "normal." Another goal of the study was to determine if there were any differences in eustachian tube function between ears that had a posterosuperior or pars flaccida retraction pocket or cholesteatoma, a central perforation and a cholesteatoma, and ears with "congenital" cholesteatoma.

From these studies, it appears that the basic problem in children with acquired cholesteatoma is functional obstruction of the eustachian tube due to constriction rather than dilation of the tube during swallowing. (This type of functional obstruction of the eustachian tube was present in subjects with a retraction pocket or cholesteatoma regardless of the site.) Abnormal functioning of the tube then results in impaired ventilation of the middle ear–mastoid air cell system, which in turn results in fluctuating or sustained high negative middle ear pressure. Periodic, rather than regular, ventilation could result in wide variations in middle ear pressures that would produce greater than normal excursions of the tympanic membrane. The membrane would then lose elasticity and would become flaccid and, eventually, atelectatic. The most flaccid parts of the tympanic membrane are the posterosuperior and pars flaccida areas (Khanna and Tonndorf, 1972). When the atelectasis becomes severe and localized in these sites, a retraction pocket forms. Inflammation between the medial portion of the retracted or collapsed tympanic membrane could then result in adhesive changes and could fix the pocket to the ossicles or surrounding structures, or both. The next stage in this series of events would be discontinuity of the ossicles or cholesteatoma formation, or both. Figures 17–8 and 17–9 show the progression from the stage of a retraction pocket with atelectasis to adhesive otitis and finally to cholesteatoma.

The distinction between a deep retraction pocket and a cholesteatoma in either the posterosuperior quadrant of the pars tensa or the pars flaccida can be difficult even with the aid of the otomicroscope. The transition between the two conditions usually follows a progressive change from a retraction pocket to cholesteatoma; however, the factors involved in this transition remain obscure at present, although infection within the retraction pocket–sac appears to be important in the process.

Children who have a central perforation and cholesteatoma are of particular interest. The cholesteatoma in these cases most likely develops as a result of migration of epithelium from the tympanic membrane through the perforation and into the middle ear. However, it must be stressed that in children this type of acquired cholesteatoma is less common compared to the posterosuperior or attic type.

It is uncertain that "congenital" cholesteatomas are truly congenital in origin. Children who have an intratympanic cholesteatoma may have had otitis media with effusion. It could be argued, on the one hand, that intratympanic cholesteatoma is the result of metaplasia secondary to middle ear inflammation and that it is not "congenital" (Sade, 1977); on the other hand, otitis media with effusion, when present, may be unrelated to a congenital rest. The fact that children who have "congenital" cholesteatomas tend to be younger than those who present with a retraction pocket or acquired cholesteatoma would support the origin of a cholesteatoma medial to an intact tympanic membrane as being congenital. In any event, most acquired cholesteatomas not due to implantation are secondary to otitis media or a retraction pock-

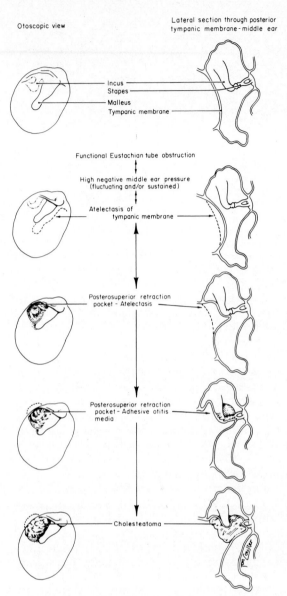

Figure 17–8 Chain of events in the pathogenesis of acquired aural cholesteatoma in the posterosuperior portion of the pars tensa or the tympanic membrane.

et, or both, and some children who have an apparently "congenital" cholesteatoma may have developed the disease in the same way (Sobol et al., 1980).

It has been shown that all infants with an unrepaired cleft palate have otitis media with effusion (Stool and Randall, 1967; Paradise et al., 1969) and that they have functional obstruction of the eustachian tube due to impairment of the tubal opening mechanism (Bluestone, 1971; Bluestone et al., 1972, 1975). Recent studies of infants, children, and adolescents with cleft palate demonstrate

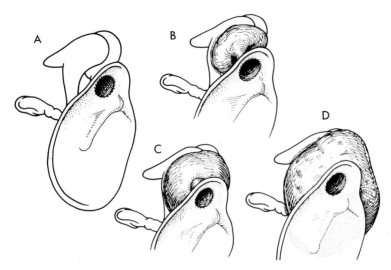

Figure 17–9 Evolution of acquired attic cholesteatoma. *A*, Attic retraction pocket that appears on otoscopic examination to be a "perforation." *B*, A narrow neck sac developing. *C*, Enlargement of the sac with erosion of the ossicles. *D*, A large cholesteatoma sac, a portion of which can be seen through the eardrum.

constriction of the eustachian tube during the forced-response test (Doyle et al., 1980). Cholesteatoma is a common sequela of middle ear disease in patients with cleft palate (Severeid, 1977). The cleft palate child, therefore, represents an *in vivo* model of the type of functional eustachian tube obstruction that can result in an acquired cholesteatoma. Because this type of dysfunction also occurs commonly in Caucasians who have otitis media or atelectasis but who do not have cleft palate (Cantekin et al., 1979), they are also at risk for developing cholesteatoma.

On the other hand, cholesteatoma has rarely been identified in American Indian populations (Wiet et al., 1980). Jaffe (1969) reported that attic "perforations" are rarely found in Navajo children; in over 200 tympanoplasties performed to repair central perforations, no cholesteatoma was found. Wiet (1979), in a study of 600 White Mountain Apache Indians, also reported a low incidence of cholesteatoma; the few cases he found were mostly of the attic type. In a subsequent study by Beery et al. (1980), otoscopic examination of 25 Apache Indians revealed no cholesteatomas. The eustachian tube function was tested in these Indians employing the inflation-deflation and forced-response tests, which revealed the presence of a eustachian tube that had low resistance to airflow (was semipatulous) but had active muscle function. This type of tube would probably preclude the development of high negative middle ear pressure, a retraction pocket, or cholesteatoma. The Apache Indian appears to have a eustachian tube that allows for easier passage of gas and liquid than does the Caucasian

with or without cleft palate. The middle ear of the Apache individual is very easily ventilated and, consequently, is not protected from unwanted secretions from the nasopharynx. It appears that the structure of the eustachian tube of the Apache Indian of the White Mountain Reservation is conducive to the development of "reflux" otitis media, perforation, and discharge.

Therefore, some American Indian tribes would appear to be *in vivo* models of the semipatulous eustachian tube that actively dilates during swallowing. Cholesteatoma formation is rarely seen in such ears, since the middle ear is aerated either by the eustachian tube or by a central perforation, or both. By studying these *in vivo* models, we can gain a clearer perspective of the whole spectrum of eustachian tube dysfunction (see Chapter 16, p. 393).

Microbiology

When a cholesteatoma is infected, the organisms cultured from the discharge are similar to those identified from ears with chronic suppurative otitis media: *P. aeruginosa* and *Proteus* sp are the most commonly identified aerobic bacteria, and *Bacteroides* and *Peptococcus-Peptostreptococcus* are the most commonly seen anaerobic organisms. Multiple bacteria were cultured from the discharges of over half of 30 patients with cholesteatomas studied by Harker and Koontz (1977; Table 17–2). Karma and coworkers (1978) reported that when they cultured 18 infected cholesteatomas, in half of the cul-

Table 17–2 BACTERIOLOGY OF INFECTED CHOLESTEATOMAS IN 30 CHILDREN AND ADULTS

Organism	No. Cases Present
Aerobes	
Pseudomonas aeruginosa	11
Pseudomonas fluorescens	2
Proteus sp	4
Escherichia coli	4
Klebsiella-Enterobacter-Serratia sp	4
Streptococcus sp	8
Alcaligenes-Achromobacter sp	3
Staphylococcus aureus	1
Staphylococcus epidermidis	2
CBC Group F	2
Anaerobes	
Bacteroides	13
Peptococcus-Peptostreptococcus sp	11
Propionibacterium acnes	8
Fusobacterium sp	4
Bifidobacterium sp	3
Clostridium sp	3
Eubacterium sp	2

(Adapted from Harker, L. A., and Koontz, F. P. 1977. The bacteriology of cholesteatoma. *In* McCabe, B. F., Sade, J., and Abramson, M. (Eds.). Cholesteatoma: First International Conference. New York, Aesculapius Pub., pp. 264–267.)

tures, both aerobic and anaerobic bacteria were found. From the results of the preceding studies, it seems that the most appropriate ototopical medication and systemic antimicrobial therapy for patients who have an infected cholesteatoma would be agents that are effective against gram-negative organisms and anaerobic bacteria; however, the results of culturing the discharge will aid in selecting the proper antimicrobial therapy. These considerations may be life-saving when an intratemporal or intracranial complication of cholesteatoma is present. In addition, preoperative and postoperative antimicrobial therapy for patients with profuse otorrhea may also be necessary to prevent development of a postoperative infection.

Pathology

The pathology of a cholesteatoma is characterized by the presence of keratinizing stratified squamous epithelium, with accumulation of desquamating epithelium or keratin within the middle ear cleft or other pneumatized portions of the temporal bone. Usually a cyst-like structure is produced by the keratin-izing squamous epithelium. Laminated keratin from its inverted surface accumulates within the cavity, which may also contain necrotic tissue and purulent material (Fig. 17–10). If the pocket is dry, the rate of exfoliation may be slow (Schuknecht, 1974). A cholesteatoma may or may not be infected or associated with chronic suppurative otitis media. Sheehy and coworkers (1977) reported that of 1024 children and adults with cholesteatoma, 26 per cent had no history of an aural discharge in the past, in 53 per cent it had been intermittent, and in only 21 per cent of the patients was discharge reported as being continuous. When these patients had surgery, almost half had no evidence of discharge.

The cholesteatoma usually causes bone resorption, which is thought to be secondary to pressure erosion as the mass enlarges or possibly due to the activity of collagenase (Abramson, 1969). Erosion of bone can occur anywhere in the temporal bone, although the ossicles are commonly involved. Ossicular erosion can result in discontinuity (usually erosion of the long process of the incus) and a conductive hearing loss or fistulization of the labyrinth. (The lateral semicircular canal is a common site of erosion.)

Alternately, the epidermis may invade the aerated space of the temporal bone and form an incomplete surface lining into which the desquamated keratin debris overflows. This process may give the impression that the mucous membrane is converted by metaplasia to keratinizing squamous epithelium (Sade, 1977); however, there apparently is no histopathologic support for this hypothesis (Schuknecht, 1974).

Cholesteatoma in children, in contrast to adults, will frequently extend into the cell tracts of the temporal bone, since pneumatization is usually more extensive in children than in adults (Schuknecht, 1974). This finding may explain the commonly held belief that cholesteatoma in children is more invasive than in adults and, therefore, that it is more difficult to cure surgically in younger patients.

Diagnosis

The signs and symptoms of cholesteatoma are such that the disease may go undetected for many years in all age groups, but in children this is an even greater problem.

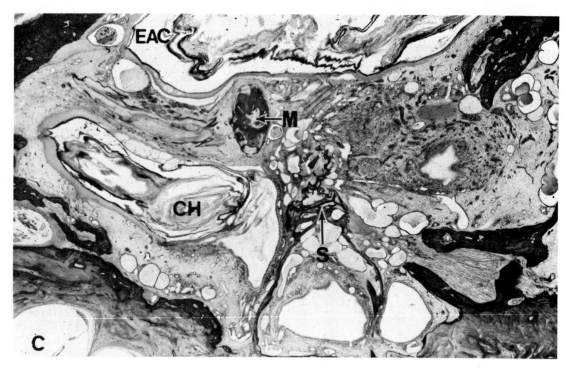

Figure 17–10 Cholesteatoma (H and E stain × 16). CH, cholesteatoma; EAC, external auditory canal; M, malleus; S, stapes; C, cochlea. (Courtesy of I. Sando, M.D.)

Most adults have a history of hearing loss, which is usually progressive and associated with recurrent ear discharge. However, children rarely complain of hearing loss, especially if the disease is unilateral, frequently there is no discharge, and otalgia may be absent in most children and adults. In addition, children are usually unaware of the more subtle symptoms associated with the disease, such as fullness in the ear, tinnitus, mild vertigo, and the foul smell of the discharge, when present. Fever is not a symptom of cholesteatoma; when it accompanies this disease, and especially when otalgia is also present, a search for an intratemporal or intracranial complication must be made. Other signs and symptoms, such as facial paralysis, severe vertigo, vomiting, and headache, should also alert the physician to the presence of a suppurative complication. In children, the attic type of cholesteatoma appears to be less symptomatic than a cholesteatoma in the posterosuperior quadrant, since the latter type is frequently preceded by symptomatic recurrent or chronic otitis media with effusion and an early onset of ossicular discontinuity with a significant hearing loss. However, in both types, the preceding atelectasis and retraction pocket may not

be associated with significant symptomatology in children. The intratympanic "congenital" cholesteatoma, which may be secondary to otitis media, is even more obscure, since hearing loss may be a late sequela and discharge is not present.

Examination of the ear with an otoscope or, more accurately, with the otomicroscope, is the most effective way to diagnose cholesteatoma. Usually white, shiny, greasy flakes of debris, which may or may not be associated with a foul-smelling discharge, will be seen in a defect in the posterosuperior portion of the pars tensa or the attic or through a large perforation. A polyp may be seen coming through the defect, which, like a crust, can prevent adequate visualization of the tympanic membrane. A crust overlying the area of the posterosuperior quadrant or the pars flaccida must be removed, since a retraction pocket or cholesteatoma may be present. The size of the defect in the tympanic membrane may not be indicative of the extent of the cholesteatoma, since a small defect, especially in the attic, may be associated with extensive cholesteatoma. On the other hand, the cholesteatoma may be confined only to the attic or middle ear despite the presence of a large defect. If an adequate examination of the child's ear is not possible with the child awake, then an examination under anesthesia is indicated. Every child who must be given a general anesthetic for myringotomy (with or without the insertion of a typanostomy tube) should have an examination of the entire tympanic membrane in order to identify a possible cholesteatoma or its precursor, a retraction pocket. In addition, an intratympanic cholesteatoma may be visualized through the tympanic membrane or through the incision following a myringotomy.

It is not always possible to determine if the defect is a retraction pocket or a "dry" cholesteatoma; however, even though this distinction cannot be made, the management of the defect will usually be the same.

There is no tympanometric pattern that is diagnostic of a cholesteatoma. An abnormal tympanogram should alert the clinician to the presence of middle ear disease, but the tympanogram may be normal even when a cholesteatoma is present. Impedance testing may reveal a perforation of the tympanic membrane, but in children this occurs less commonly than in adults. Likewise, audiometric testing may reveal a conductive hearing impairment or possibly a mixed conductive and sensorineural deficit, but a cholesteatoma may be present without the presence of a loss of hearing. A sensorineural hearing loss is presumably due to serous labyrinthitis (Paparella et al., 1972) or possibly to a labyrinthine fistula.

Roentgenograms of the temporal bone should be obtained when a cholesteatoma is suspected; polytomography is even more helpful. The roentgenograms should be studied carefully to identify the extent of the cholesteatoma, possible ossicular involvement, and any complication that might be present, such as a labyrinthine fistula. The radiographs should be restudied preoperatively when planning the surgical procedure.

When aural discharge accompanying cholesteatoma is profuse, microbiologic assessment of the discharge is indicated so that the infection can be controlled preoperatively by administering the most appropriate antimicrobial agent(s) (p. 463, Table 16–32).

Prevention and Management

Rational management of children with cholesteatoma and conditions that may be cau-
sally related to this disease should be based upon an understanding of its pathogenesis. The presence of a deep retraction pocket in the posterosuperior or pars flaccida area of the tympanic membrane, if persistent, must be managed promptly by insertion of a tympanostomy tube in an effort to return the tympanic membrane to the neutral position and to prevent formation of adhesions between the tympanic membrane and the middle ear structures (Fig. 16–51, upper panel). In children, the retraction pocket may be seen to distend during inhalation anesthesia (while looking through the otomicroscope); this is a good sign that the tympanic membrane will return to the normal position following the insertion of a tympanostomy tube. On the other hand, if the retraction pocket does not distend during anesthesia, then the surgeon should carefully examine the depth and extent of the pocket, probing gently with a blunt right-angled hook. Mirrors may also help to visualize the extent of the pocket, or the 90 degree needle telescope (Olympus Co.) may be used to determine the exact borders of the pocket. A retraction pocket can extend into any area of the middle ear, but most frequently it is found extending into the epitympanum and sinus tympani. If the retraction pocket persists after the middle ear has been ventilated by a tympanostomy tube that has been in place for several weeks or months (Fig. 16–51, lower panel), then the surgeon should consider performing a tympanoplasty procedure to prevent ossicular discontinuity or the development of a cholesteatoma, or both. Heermann et al. (1970) advocate the use of cartilage to support the tympanic membrane graft to prevent recurrence of the retraction pocket. Especially in children, a tympanostomy tube should probably be inserted into the tympanic membrane remnant, since eustachian tube function will most likely remain poor postoperatively.

If a cholesteatoma is found in the posterosuperior or attic area during the examination of a child, an attempt should be made to remove the cholesteatoma debris. If most or all of this material can be removed and if the extent of the sac can be visualized adequately, then a tympanostomy tube should be inserted. A few children have been found to have normal tympanic membranes within one month following such "débridement" and tympanostomy tube insertion. However, when this uncommon event occurs, long-term follow-up of these children must include reinsertion of a tympanostomy tube if the retraction pocket recurs.

Surgical Procedure

When a cholesteatoma is present, surgical intervention is indicated. The only exceptions to this form of management would be unusual cases (just described) in which simple "débridement" and insertion of a tympanostomy tube are successful, or the presence of a concomitant disease that would make surgery under general anesthesia a hazard to the child's health. The surgical procedures that are currently employed to eradicate a cholesteatoma are briefly described next. These procedures may also be performed for other conditions described in this chapter, but for detailed descriptions of the surgical techniques, the reader is referred to the Selected References at the end of this chapter.

The procedures can be divided into those that provide exposure and removal of disease from the middle ear and mastoid and those that are designed to reconstruct the middle ear to preserve or restore hearing. A *tympanotomy* is a surgical procedure that opens the middle ear space. In an *exploratory tympanotomy,* a tympanomeatal flap is elevated so that the middle ear and its structures can be viewed directly. Exploratory tympanotomy is indicated when it is suspected that there is an abnormality, such as intratympanic cholesteatoma or ossicular chain abnormality, or as a planned second-stage procedure after a tympanoplasty with or without a mastoidectomy has been performed to manage cholesteatoma.

A *myringoplasty* is the surgical repair of a defect in the tympanic membrane with no attempt made to explore the middle ear. A perforation (or retraction pocket) is commonly repaired by utilizing autogenous connective tissue graft (temporalis fascia or compressed adipose tissue from the earlobe) as a lattice onto which epithelial cells can migrate from the edges of the existing perforation. The procedure is employed to manage a simple uncomplicated tympanic membrane perforation without cholesteatoma. *Tympanoplasty* is the surgical reconstruction of the tympanic membrane–ossicle transformer mechanism. If a perforation is present, it is repaired with a connective tissue graft, but unlike a myringoplasty, the middle ear is explored. Ossicles can be repositioned (ossiculoplasty) to restore ossicular chain continuity. Traditionally, tympanoplasty operations

are characterized according to the degree to which the reconstructed ossicular chain approximates the anatomic juxtaposition of ossicles in the normal middle ear (see Perforation of the Tympanic Membrane, p. 517; and Ossicular Chain Discontinuity and Fixation, p. 544).

Mastoidectomy involves the surgical exposure and removal of mastoid air cells. There are several types of mastoidectomy (Fig. 17–11). In a *complete simple "cortical" mastoidectomy* (Fig. 17–11A), the mastoid air cell system is exenterated, including the epitympanum, but the canal wall is left intact. The operation is performed when acute or chronic mastoid osteitis is present and is freqently part of the surgical procedure advocated by some surgeons for cholesteatoma. A *posterior tympanotomy* or *facial recess tympanotomy* (Fig. 17–11B) involves exenteration of mastoid air cells followed by formation of an opening between the mastoid and middle ear created in the posterior wall of the middle ear lateral to the facial nerve and medial to the chorda tympani. This procedure is an extension of the complete simple mastoidectomy that allows better visualization of the facial recess without removing the canal wall and is primarily advocated for ears in which a cholesteatoma is present. A *modified radical mastoidectomy* (Fig. 17–11C) is an operation in which a portion of the posterior ear canal wall is removed and a permanent mastoidectomy cavity is created, but the tympanic membrane and some or all of the ossicles are left. The procedure is usually performed when a cholesteatoma cannot be removed without removing the canal wall; some function may be preserved. *Radical mastoidectomy* (Fig. 17–11D) involves exenteration of all mastoid air cells, opening of the epitympanum, and removal of the posterior ear canal wall along with the tympanic membrane, the malleus, and the incus. Only the stapes, or the footplate of the stapes, remains. No attempt is made to preserve or improve function. By removing the posterior ear canal wall, the exenterated mastoid cellular area, middle ear, and external auditory canal communicate, forming a common single cavity. The procedure is indicated when there is extensive cholesteatoma present in the middle ear and mastoid that cannot be removed by a less radical procedure. In addition, the operation may be indicated when a suppurative complication of otitis media is present.

When a tympanoplasty operation is done in conjunction with mastoidectomy, the com-

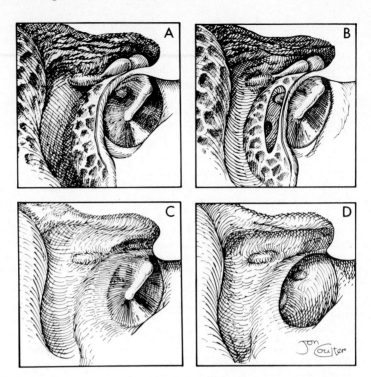

Figure 17–11 Examples of four types of mastoid surgery. *A,* Complete simple ("cortical") mastoidectomy in which the canal wall has been left intact. However, the exposure of the epitympanum is an important part of the surgical procedure. *B,* A posterior tympanotomy–facial recess access to the middle ear has been added to the complete simple mastoidectomy. *C,* Modified radical mastoidectomy. *D,* Radical mastoidectomy.

bined procedure is termed mastoidectomy-tympanoplasty. Mastoidectomy operations that leave the posterior ear canal wall intact are termed "closed cavity," "canal wall up," or "intact canal wall" procedures, whereas those in which the posterior canal is partially removed are called "open cavity" or "canal wall down" procedures.

Type of Surgical Procedure Related to Outcome

There has been a great deal of controversy concerning the best surgical methods to eradicate cholesteatoma from the middle ear and mastoid in all age groups. Some surgeons prefer to perform mastoidectomy and middle ear surgery or "canal wall up" procedures, in which the cholesteatoma is removed without leaving a mastoid cavity and in which function is preserved or restored by performing a tympanoplasty (with or without an ossiculoplasty) (Jansen, 1963; Sheehy and Patterson, 1967; Smyth, 1972; Austin, 1976; Glasscock, 1977). Most of the surgeons who advocate the "intact canal wall" procedure perform a "planned second stage" exploratory tympanotomy, at which time cholesteatoma can be removed that had been left either purposefully in a critical area, such as over a labyrinthine fistula, or inadvertently. However, opponents to this approach prefer to perform either a modified radical mastoidectomy or, when the cholesteatoma is extensive, a radical mastoidectomy, since they consider the rate of persistence (residual) or recurrence, or both, of cholesteatoma following the "intact canal wall" procedures to be unacceptably high (Abramson et al., 1977). The advocates of the "canal wall down" approach would rather sacrifice the potential preservation or restoration of function (in some procedures leaving the patient with a "mastoid bowl") for a better chance at total removal of the cholesteatoma, that is, a low rate of residual and recurrent disease. Palva et al. (1977) advocate performing a modified radical mastoidectomy in which the mastoidectomy cavity is obliterated with subcutaneous tissue, that is, a Palva flap, to eliminate the "mastoid bowl," and an attempt is made to improve or preserve the hearing. However, when he compared 65 children and 65 adults who underwent the procedure to remove cholesteatoma, the three patients in whom a postoperative residual cholesteatoma occurred were children.

Unfortunately, at present there have been no randomized controlled trials of these two approaches to determine the best method. Therefore, both are currently acceptable in adults, but when a cholesteatoma is present in the ear of a child, the evidence currently available would appear to direct the surgeon toward the "canal wall down" procedures. This approach in children is based on several factors, of which two have already been described: The first is that cholesteatoma is more invasive in children compared to adults, and the second is that several studies have shown that there is a higher rate of residual and recurrent cholesteatoma following intact canal wall mastoidectomy-tympanoplasty procedures in children than in adults (Smyth, 1977). Sheehy (1978) reported that residual cholesteatoma was either purposely left or found at the second-stage procedure in 51 per cent of children, compared to only 30 per cent of adults. Abramson et al. (1977) found that children below the age of nine years had a significantly greater rate of postoperative cholesteatoma than adults following either an "intact canal wall" or a "canal wall down" procedure but that the rate in children who had "intact canal wall" mastoidectomy was more than twice as high as that in children who underwent modified radical mastoidectomy ("canal wall down").

Another factor that influences the type of procedure selected for children is that almost all children with cholesteatoma have poor eustachian tube function, which would make them at risk for developing recurrent or chronic middle ear effusion following tympanoplasty (with or without mastoidectomy). Still another, more important, factor is that the same sequence of events that led to development of the initial cholesteatoma can recur, particularly in the posterosuperior or pars flaccida area.

Current Recommendations

At either end of the spectrum of the disease, the decision as to the most appropriate surgical management of cholesteatoma is relatively straightforward. For children who have a small cyst-like cholesteatoma that is localized to the mesotympanum or epitympanum and that can be removed easily, a tympanoplasty can be successful. Performance of a second-stage exploratory tympanotomy should be considered six months after the initial procedure to uncover residual or recurrent disease. This time interval is somewhat shorter than that advocated for adults, but residual cholesteatoma grows more rapidly in children than in adults. However, this may not be necessary if the tympanic membrane is translucent without evidence of progressive disease medial to the drum and if the hearing is stable during the postoperative

follow-up period (and no second-stage ossiculoplasty is planned). In these cases, the child may be observed. However, a "second look" should be performed if the tympanic membrane is opaque or if a progressive loss of hearing develops. If residual cholesteatoma is found during this second procedure and if it is extensive, a "canal wall down" procedure should be performed, that is, a modified radical mastoidectomy or radical mastoidectomy. On rare occasions, only a small remnant of the original cholesteatoma will be found to be present at this second exploration (with no other apparent spread of cholesteatoma); this remnant should be removed, and a third-stage procedure should be planned. On the other hand, if no cholesteatoma is found at the planned second-stage procedure, the child is most likely free of the original cholesteatoma. These children must nevertheless be followed by periodic examination for years: If severe atelectasis or a retraction pocket develops, prompt myringotomy and insertion of a tympanostomy tube are indicated. An alternative approach for a small attic cholesteatoma would be *atticotomy*, that is, exteriorization, especially when a second-stage procedure is not feasible.

At the other end of the spectrum is the extensive cholesteatoma that involves all or most of the middle ear and mastoid, in which the disease has left only remnants of the ossicles. For this condition, a radical mastoidectomy would be indicated. However, the problem for the surgeon is deciding how to manage the majority of cholesteatomas in children that are neither small and easily removed nor so extensive that only radical surgery is indicated. The recommendation at this time is to select the operative procedure that most likely will give the best outcome for that individual child.

A modified mastoidectomy and, when possible, a tympanoplasty would appear to be the most appropriate procedures. All children do not have to have a "routine" planned second-stage exploratory operation, but if extensive disease was found at the initial procedure, an exploratory tympanotomy six months after the original surgery should be seriously considered, since there has been a high rate of residual cholesteatoma found in children, even after a "canal wall down" procedure. As advocated by Shambaugh (Shambaugh and Glasscock, 1980), a Bondy modified radical mastoidectomy using the endaural approach is still an excellent choice when an attic cholesteatoma is present. This procedure is especially appropriate for children in whom the cholesteatoma is lateral to the ossicles in the epitympanum and has spread into the mastoid but does not involve the mesotympanum.

When a modified radical or radical mastoidectomy has been performed, the open mastoid cavity should probably not be obliterated with a connective tissue flap, bone pate, or plastic material, since residual cholesteatoma may occur in the mastoid cavity and since the long-term outcome of these procedures in large groups of children has yet to be reported.

When tympanoplasty is performed in children at the same time that a mastoidectomy is performed to eradicate a cholesteatoma, the results of the tympanoplasty have been poor (Bluestone et al., 1979). Failure of the tympanoplasty is associated with one or more of the following conditions: sloughing of the graft, recurrence of high negative middle ear pressure and a retraction pocket, recurrent or chronic otitis media with effusion, or recurrence of cholesteatoma. Other studies of large numbers of adults and children who underwent tympanoplasties at the time of surgery to remove cholesteatoma have also shown that tympanoplasties in such patients are not successful (Cody, 1977). When chronic suppurative otitis media is present in addition to the cholesteatoma, a tympanoplasty should be withheld or performed as a second-stage procedure (see Chronic Suppurative Otitis Media, p. 526). In addition, when a cholesteatoma is infected, with or without the presence of chronic suppurative otitis media (and mastoiditis), preoperative control of the infection with antimicrobial agents is desirable, since the presence of infection may affect the outcome of the tympanoplasty as well as increase the risk of developing a postoperative wound infection. When a tympanoplasty for cholesteatoma is performed, then artificial ventilation of the middle ear must also be provided by a tympanostomy tube. However, in older children, eustachian tube function may be adequate to ventilate the middle ear, and tympanoplasty can be performed without tympanostomy tube insertion. When tympanoplasty is performed in children, cartilage should be placed to support the tympanic membrane defect and thus prevent recurrence of cholesteatoma.

When the cholesteatoma is extensive and a radical mastoidectomy is necessary to control the disease, then the middle ear end of the poorly functioning eustachian tube should be closed surgically, since the middle ear–mastoidectomy cavity is then an open system (Bluestone et al., 1978). Otherwise, nasopharyngeal secretions could reflux into the middle ear–mastoidectomy cavity, resulting in inflammation and otorrhea (Fig. 17–12). The most effective way to obliterate the bony portion of the eustachian tube is with bone

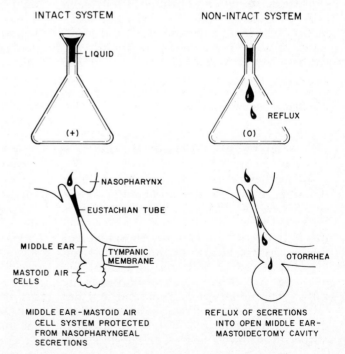

Figure 17–12 Liquid flow through a flask is compared with the nasopharynx–eustachian tube–middle ear–mastoid air cell system. When the system is intact, liquid is prevented from flowing into the body of the flask (middle ear–mastoid air cells). By contrast, the nonintact system permits liquid to reflux into the flask. This condition is analogous to a perforation of the tympanic membrane in which reflux of nasopharyngeal secretions could occur, since the middle ear–mastoid air cushion is lost. Similarly, following a radical mastoidectomy, the presence of a patent eustachian tube could cause troublesome otorrhea (see text).

pate. Closure of the eustachian tube at the time of radical mastoidectomy, although not universally performed by modern otologic surgeons, is not a new addition to the procedure but has been advocated for many years. Closure of the middle ear portion of the tube is also indicated for patients who have had a radical mastoidectomy performed in the past and who have intermittent or persistent postoperative aural discharge. Eustachian tube function tests should be performed, and if the tube is found to be patent, revision middle ear–mastoid surgery should be performed, and surgical closure of the eustachian tube should be done if a tympanoplasty is not going to be performed at the time of the revision surgery or planned in the future.

Conclusions

In children with a retraction pocket or acquired cholesteatoma in the posterosuperior or pars flaccida portion of the tympanic membrane, active function of the eustachian tube is abnormal; constriction, rather than dilatation, of the eustachian tube occurs during swallowing. Acquired cholesteatoma not secondary to implantation is a sequela of otitis media or a retraction pocket, or both. The type of surgery chosen to manage these conditions in children should be selected on the basis not only of the site and extent of the cholesteatoma but also of other factors, such as patient age, presence or absence of otitis media, eustachian tube function, and availability of health care. The operation must be tailored for each child. Prevention of the pathologic conditions that predispose to this type of cholesteatoma is the most effective method of management.

ADHESIVE OTITIS MEDIA

Adhesive otitis media is a result of healing following chronic inflammation of the middle ear and mastoid. The mucous membrane is thickened by proliferation of fibrous tissue, which frequently impairs the movement of the ossicles, resulting in a conductive hearing loss. Schuknecht (1974) has described the pathology as a proliferation of fibrous tissue within the middle ear and mastoid and has termed the condition fibrous sclerosis. When there are cystic spaces present, it is called fibrocystic sclerosis, and when there is new

bone growth in the mastoid, he has classified it as fibro-osseous sclerosis.

There are no data available on the prevalence of adhesive otitis media in children, but the condition is common in those who have had recurrent acute or chronic otitis media with effusion or atelectasis of the tympanic membrane–middle ear, or both. Unfortunately, we have no data from which to establish the probability with which a child who has a middle ear effusion or atelectasis might develop adhesive otitis media. However, the possibility of adhesive changes occurring when inflammation is present in the middle ear and mastoid must be seriously considered when selecting the most appropriate medical or surgical treatment of children who have recurrent acute and chronic otitis media with effusion or atelectasis. In addition to fixation of the ossicles, adhesive otitis media may result in ossicular discontinuity and conductive hearing loss due to rarefying osteitis, especially of the long process of the incus. When there is severe localized atelectasis (a retraction pocket) in the posterosuperior portion of the pars tensa of the tympanic membrane, adhesive changes may bind the eardrum to the incus, stapes, and other surrounding middle ear structures and cause resorption of the ossicles. Once adhesive changes bind the tympanic membrane in this area, the development of a cholesteatoma is also possible (Fig. 17–13). Timely ventilation of the middle ear and mastoid prior to the adhesive changes may return the tympanic membrane to the normal position, thus preventing ossicular damage. If medical treatment fails, then a myringotomy should be performed, and a tympanostomy tube should be inserted in an attempt to reverse the potentially progressive pathologic condition. However, if the tympanic membrane is still attached to the ossicles in spite of tympanostomy tube insertion, then adhesive otitis media is present, and in children, tympanoplasty should be considered to prevent further structural damage, since the process may progress owing to persistent eustachian tube obstruction.

When ossicular discontinuity or fixation has occurred, an ossiculoplasty may be performed to restore function but is not always successful. When the middle ear and mastoid are bound by adhesive otitis media, the results of ossiculoplasty frequently are not permanent owing to recurrence of the adhesive process. However, surgery should be consid-

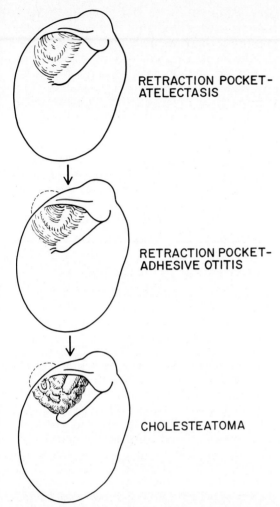

RETRACTION POCKET-
ATELECTASIS

RETRACTION POCKET-
ADHESIVE OTITIS

CHOLESTEATOMA

Figure 17–13 Sequence of events leading from a localized area of atelectasis (retraction pocket) in the posterosuperior portion of the pars tensa of the tympanic membrane to a cholesteatoma and ossicular discontinuity. Adhesive otitis media in this area is shown as the stage between atelectasis and the development of a cholesteatoma.

ered (Shambaugh and Glasscock, 1980). The best method to manage adhesive otitis media is prevention, which involves the treating of its precursors, acute and chronic otitis media with effusion and atelectasis (see Chap. 16).

TYMPANOSCLEROSIS

Tympanosclerosis may be a sequela of chronic middle ear inflammation or the result of trauma. It is characterized by the presence of whitish plaques in the tympanic membrane and nodular deposits in the submucosal layers of the middle ear (Igarashi et al.,

1970). The pathology in the tympanic membrane occurs in the lamina propria, while within the middle ear the pathology is in the basement membrane; in both sites, there is hyalinization followed by deposition of calcium and phosphate crystals. Conductive hearing loss may occur if the ossicles become imbedded in the deposits.

The condition was first described by von Troltsch (1869), who called it "sclerosis," but it was Zollner (1956) who called the disorder tympanosclerosis and differentiated it from otosclerosis. Schuknecht (1974) prefers the term "hyalinization" rather than tynpanosclerosis, since the histopathologic condition is that of hyalin degeneration, which is the result of a healing reaction characterized by fibroblastic invasion of the submucosa, followed by thickening and fusion of collagenous fibers into a homogeneous mass. He also described the hyalinized collagen around the ossicles.

Even though no reliable data are available tympanosclerosis of the tympanic membrane is a very common sequela in children who have or have had recurrent or chronic otitis media with effusion and also is common at the site of a healed, spontaneous perforation or following myringotomy, especially if a tympanostomy tube had been inserted. It would appear that the chalky patch seen in the tympanic membrane of children may be due to inflammation or trauma, or both. However, in the pediatric age group as a whole, the condition is not common in the middle ear, especially in infants and young children. In particular, ossicular involvement is rare in very young children. Of 311 cases of tympanosclerosis studied by Kinney (1978), only 20 per cent occurred in individuals 30 years of age or younger. This would imply that the condition in the middle ear may take many years to develop. However, Schiff et al. (1980) propose the hypothesis that tympanosclerosis has an immune component that occurs in the middle ear following an insult or mucosal disruption and that there is also a genetic component, which would explain the low incidence of the condition in children who have such a high prevalence and incidence of middle ear inflammation.

The preceding hypothesis may be the explanation for the relatively high rate of tympanosclerosis among children who are Alaskan natives (Eskimos) and American Indians (Wiet, 1979; Jaffe, 1969; DeBlanc, 1975). However, other factors may predispose these children to the disease, such as differences in eustachian tube function. Weider (Wiet et al., 1980) reported that tympanosclerosis affected a higher percentage of Alaskan native children than children of a similar age in his New Hampshire private practice; tympanosclerosis of the tympanic membrane or the ossicles or both was found in 78 (68 per cent) of 114 Alaskan native children who had tympanoplasty surgery, while only seven such cases were diagnosed in 377 consecutive tympanoplasties performed on children in his practice. In addition, he also found that far advanced tympanosclerosis that resulted in fixation of the ossicular chain occurred at an early age in the Alaskan native children but not in children in his practice.

No surgical correction, such as tympanoplasty, is indicated when tympanosclerosis of the tympanic membrane, even though extensive, is the only abnormality of the middle ear. If a middle ear effusion is present and a myringotomy, with or without a tympanostomy tube insertion, is indicated, the incision should be placed, if possible, in an area without involvement, leaving the affected area untouched. Removal of large tympanosclerotic plaques may result in a permanent perforation of the tympanic membrane. When an incision must be made in an area of tympanosclerosis, then only that amount necessary to perform the procedure should be removed. When a tympanoplasty is being performed to repair a perforation of the tympanic membrane and tympanosclerosis is present in the drum remnant, removal of the plaque is optional: the plaque may remain if the area of tympanosclerosis does not interfere with the surgical procedure and is not impeding function. When tympanosclerosis is the cause of ossicular fixation and a tympanoplasty procedure is elected, the methods of removal of the plaques and ossiculoplasty described by Shambaugh and Glasscock (1980) are appropriate for the rare child with this advanced stage of tympanosclerosis. However, refixation of the ossicles is not uncommon even after apparently adequate surgical removal of the plaques and ossiculoplasty. If surgery is not performed or is not successful in restoring the hearing loss, then a hearing aid should be considered.

Even though the pathogenesis of tympanosclerosis is not understood, it seems most likely that appropriate management of recurrent and chronic middle ear inflammation in infants and children is the best method of prevention. Since it also occurs following trauma to the tympanic membrane, myringotomy with tympanostomy tube placement should be performed with tympanosclerosis as one of the potential complications and sequelae in mind. However, in general, tympanosclerosis involving the tympanic membrane does not appreciably affect function, although when the ossicles are involved, the patient may have a significant conductive hearing loss. Thus, tympanostomy tubes may, on the one hand, increase the incidence of tympanosclerosis of the tympanic membrane, but on the other hand, their placement may decrease the frequency of ossicular fixation due to this disease later in life.

OSSICULAR DISCONTINUITY AND FIXATION

Ossicular interruption is the result of rarefying osteitis secondary to chronic middle ear inflammation. A retraction pocket or cholesteatoma may also cause resorption of the ossicles. The long process of the incus is most commonly involved, which results in incudostapedial disarticulation. The commonly accepted reason given for this portion of the incus being eroded is its poor blood supply; however, since the tympanic membrane frequently becomes attached to this part of the incus when a posterosuperior retraction pocket is present, adhesive otitis media may be the cause of the osteitis and subsequent erosion. Also, cholesteatoma is commonly found in the same area (Bluestone et al., 1977). The stapes, or more specifically its crural arches, is the second most commonly involved ossicle. The etiology of stapes fixation is more likely to be associated with presence of a retraction pocket or cholesteatoma rather than with decreased vascular supply. Less commonly, the body of the incus and manubrium of the malleus may also be eroded. The ossicles may become fixed by fibrous tissue secondary to adhesive otitis media or, more rarely in children, secondary to tympanosclerosis. Neither the incidence of ossicular discontinuity and fixation nor the natural history of the pathologic conditions that precede these abnormalities has been formally studied in children. However, ossicular discontinuity is commonly associated with a deep retraction pocket or cholesteatoma in the posterosuperior portion of the tympanic membrane. Disarticulation or fixation of the ossicles may also occur when there is a central perforation of the tympanic membrane with or without the presence of chronic suppurative otitis media and, more rarely, when the tympanic membrane is intact.

The hearing loss is conductive when the ossicular chain is affected, and the degree is dependent upon the site and degree of involvement of the ossicle(s) as well as upon the presence or absence of associated conditions such as a perforation of the tympanic membrane. When there is a discontinuity of the incudostapedial joint and the tympanic membrane is intact, a maximal conductive hearing loss may be present, that is, 50 to 60 dB. However, when the same ossicular pathologic condition is present and a perforation is also present, the hearing loss may be less severe. Erosion of the manubrium of the malleus is usually associated with a perforation of the tympanic membrane but does not contribute to the hearing loss.

Diagnosis

The diagnosis of the ossicular chain abnormalities that are secondary to otitis media and its related conditions can frequently be made by visualization of the defect through the otoscope or, more accurately, with the otomicroscope. Erosion of the long process of the incus can usually be seen when a deep posterosuperior retraction pocket is present. The presence of a significant conductive hearing loss, for example, greater than 30 dB, when a perforation of the tympanic membrane is present would be presumptive evidence of ossicular involvement. However, when the tympanic membrane is normal, a significant conductive loss may be due to inflammatory ossicular involvement that has occurred in the past, but congenital ossicular abnormalities and otosclerosis must be part of the differential diagnosis. In addition to the history, otoscopic examination, and conventional audiometric testing, impedance audiometry may aid in the diagnosis. A tympanogram showing high compliance would be presumptive evidence of ossicular chain discontinuity when there is a significant conductive hearing loss present. If the compliance is low, ossicular fixation would be more likely. However, the accuracy with which tympanometry can differentiate between ossicular discontinuity and fixation is not high, since several other parameters in the middle ear, such as mobility of the tympanic membrane, affect the shape of the tympanogram. Polytomography may also aid in identifying ossicular discontinuity but usually is of diagnostic benefit only when a large defect is present. The most accurate way to diagnose these defects is exploration of the middle ear, either during exploratory tympanotomy, when the tympanic membrane is intact, or by inspection of the entire ossicular chain when middle ear and mastoid surgery, such as tympanoplasty, is indicated.

Management

Management of ossicular deformities in children is similar to that described for adults, with some notable exceptions. Most adults who have ossicular discontinuity or fixation no longer are at risk of developing otitis media with effusion or high negative pressure within the middle ear due to eustachian tube dysfunction, but many children still have or will have these conditions, which could interfere with the success of reconstructive middle ear surgery generally and ossiculoplasty specifically. Therefore, the indications for timing and the type of middle ear surgery may be different for children. When an ossicular deformity is suspected and the tympanic membrane is intact without evidence of otitis media or any of its other complications or sequelae, such as retraction pocket or cholesteatoma, then the decision to perform an exploratory tympanotomy to diagnose and possibly repair the ossicular deformity would depend on several considerations. First, and most important, is the child still at risk of developing a middle ear effusion or atelectasis (retraction pocket), or both? As a general rule, if neither condition has occurred in either ear for a year or longer, the risk is low; however, the younger the child, the higher the risk. If further middle ear disease may still occur, the operation should be delayed. The second consideration is the degree of hearing loss and whether or not the defect is unilateral or bilateral. A child who has a maximum conductive hearing loss in both ears would be a very likely candidate for surgical intervention, while the child who only has a unilateral mild conductive loss should not be operated upon. Another important consideration is the need for general anesthesia to perform the surgery in all children. The benefit of surgery must be weighed against the risk of general anesthesia. For the child who has a bilateral maximum conductive hearing loss, the benefit of hearing improvement may outweigh the risk of general anesthesia, whereas the risk of anesthesia may not override the potential chance of improving the hearing in a child with only a unilateral loss of hearing. Withholding the reconstructive surgery until the child is able to tolerate a local anesthetic (adolescence) is a preferred option when the hearing loss is unilateral and especially when it is only mild to moderate in degree. Whenever the decision to operate is delayed until the child is older, a hearing aid should be considered, even when the hearing loss is unilateral.

When middle ear surgery is indicated owing to the presence of a perforation of the tympanic membrane with or without chronic suppurative otitis media, a cholesteatoma, or a retraction pocket, the very fact that the patient is a child still affects the decision as to whether or not to perform an ossiculoplasty. This is because children are at increased risk of suffering future episodes of otitis media and of developing atelectasis or adhesive otitis media. When these conditions are a possiblity, the surgeon should consider staging the surgery and performing the ossiculoplasty when the child is older.

The various ways in which ossicles that are either eroded or fixed may be reconstructed have been adequately described elsewhere. However, it is important to reiterate that the type of ossiculoplasty chosen for a child may be different than that performed in an adult. We feel, and most experts agree, that in general, middle ear ossicular implants should not be used in children unless absolutely necessary, as neither the safety nor the efficacy of these prostheses has been proved over a long enough period of time to warrant insertion in the middle ear of a child. However, some surgeons advocate the use of homograft ossicles in children. Whenever possible, only the child's own tissue should be used to reconstruct the ossicular chain. For the most common discontinuity encountered, that of the incudostapedial joint, an incus transposition or insertion of a fitted incus is the ideal procedure (Fig. 17–14). When the stapes crura are missing, the shaped incus can usually be inserted between the mobile footplate of the stapes and the malleus handle. For all age groups, whenever the stapes is fixed, a stapedectomy should not be performed unless the tympanic

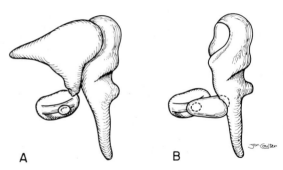

Figure 17–14   The most common ossicular discontinuity present in children is at the incudostapedial joint and is due to erosion of the long process of the incus (*A*). An autograft fitted incus is the recommended procedure for children (*B*).

membrane is intact, and in children who have had otitis media, stapedectomy should rarely, if ever, be performed, even when the tympanic membrane is intact, since a recurrence of otitis media with suppurative labyrinthitis as a complication would be an ever-present risk. Freeing of other fixed ossicles can be attempted in children, but refixation often occurs, as adhesive otitis media, which is the most frequent cause of fixation, commonly leads to further fibrosis.

The most effective method of managing ossicular discontinuity and fixation is prevention of the diseases that cause these ossicular abnormalities. Of special note is the early diagnosis and management, usually by insertion of a tympanostomy tube, of a posterosuperior retraction pocket in which the tympanic membrane is lying on the incus and stapes (see Chap. 16, Atelectasis of the Tympanic Membrane–Middle Ear and High Negative Middle Ear Pressure p. 438).

MASTOIDITIS

The proximity of the mastoid to the middle ear cleft suggests that most cases of suppurative otitis media are associated with inflammation of the mastoid air cells. The incidence of clinically significant mastoiditis, however, is low since the introduction of antimicrobial agents. Nevertheless, acute and chronic disease still occurs and may be responsible for significant morbidity and life-threatening disease.

At birth, the mastoid consists of a single cell, the antrum, connected to the middle ear by a small channel, the aditus ad antrum (Fig. 17–15). Pneumatization of the mastoid bone takes place soon after birth and is usually

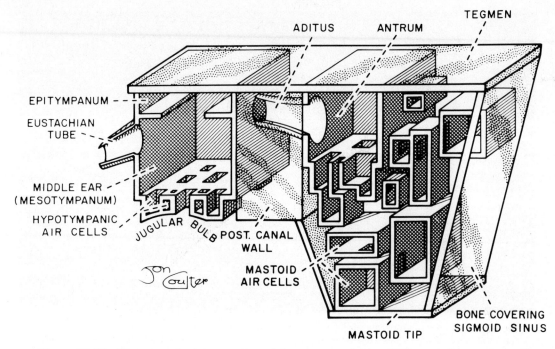

Figure 17–15 Diagrammatic representation of the anatomy of the middle ear and mastoid air cell system, showing the narrow connection (aditus ad antrum) between the two, which is sometimes referred to as the "bottle-neck" when acute infection cannot drain from the mastoid into the middle ear.

extensive by two years of age. The process may continue throughout life. The clinical importance of the mastoid is related to contiguous structures, including the posterior cranial fossa, the middle cranial fossa, the sigmoid and lateral sinuses, the canal of the facial nerve, the semicircular canals, and the petrous tip of the temporal bone. The mastoid air cells are lined with modified respiratory mucosa, and all are interconnected with the antrum.

Infection in the mastoid proceeds after middle ear infection through the following stages: (1) Hyperemia and edema of the mucosal lining of the pneumatized cells, (2) accumulation of serous and then purulent exudates in the cells, (3) demineralization of the cellular walls and necrosis of bone due to pressure of the purulent exudate on the thin bony septa and ischemia of the septa caused by decrease in blood flow, (4) formation of abscess cavities due to the coalescence of adjacent cells following destruction of the cell walls, and (5) escape of pus into contiguous areas.

This process may halt at any stage with subsequent resolution. When infection persists for more than a week or 10 days, however, inflammatory granulation tissue forms in the pneumatic cavity. A hypertrophic osteitis

develops, which results in thickening and sclerosis of the cellular walls and reduction in size of the cellular space. There may be repeated cycles of absorption and deposition of bone. If the infection remains chronic but low-grade, there is thickening of the mucosa caused by a fibrinous exudate, which may become organized and may lead to permanent adhesions. Columnar metaplasia with new gland formation may lead to extensive production of mucus in the former cells.

Mastoiditis can be classified into acute and chronic. Acute mastoiditis is further subdivided according to the pathologic stage present, which has clinical significance, since management is dependent upon the stage of the disease. Unfortunately, because of failure to appreciate the natural history and pathologic process of acute mastoiditis, there is a great deal of confusion in the minds of clinicians, as well as in the current literature, regarding the most appropriate management of each stage.

Acute Mastoiditis

In almost every child who has acute otitis media, the mastoid air cells are also inflamed; thus, acute mastoiditis is a natural extension

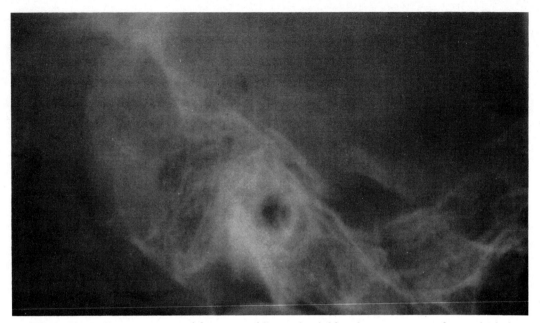

Figure 17–16 Roentgenogram of the temporal bone of a child with acute otitis media in which the mastoid air cells show signs of inflammation without osteitis. The diagnosis was acute mastoiditis, which is usually present during episodes of acute middle ear infection and is most frequently self-limited.

and part of the pathologic process of the acute middle ear infection. No specific signs or symptoms of the mastoid infection are present in this most common stage of mastoiditis. The hearing loss, otalgia, and fever are due primarily to the acute infection within the middle ear. Roentgenograms of the mastoid area are usually read as "cloudy mastoids," which is, in reality, indicative of inflammation. No mastoid osteitis is evident on the roentgenograms (Fig. 17–16). The process is usually reversible, as the middle ear–mastoid effusion resolves, either as a natural process or as a result of treatment of the acute infection. If resolution of the infection does not occur at this stage, one or more of the following conditions can develop: (1) acute mastoiditis with periosteitis, (2) acute mastoid osteitis (with or without a subperiosteal abscess), or (3) chronic mastoiditis.

A condition called "masked mastoiditis" has been described for which a complete simple mastoidectomy has been advocated (Mawson and Ludman, 1979). The disease appears to be a subacute stage of otitis media and mastoiditis (without osteitis) that is characterized by the same signs and symptoms as acute otitis media, except that they are persistent and less severe. The progression to this stage is attributed to failure of the initial antimicrobial agent to resolve the middle ear

infection within a short period. Persistent otalgia and fever while on an antimicrobial agent are indications for a tympanocentesis-myringotomy to identify the causative organism and to promote drainage. In selected children, especially for those patients who have had frequently recurrent episodes of acute otitis in the past, the insertion of a tympanostomy tube (in addition to the appropriate antimicrobial therapy) will resolve the problem. No mastoid surgery is indicated unless mastoid osteitis is present.

Acute Mastoiditis with Periosteitis

At this stage, the infection within the mastoid air cells spreads to the periosteum covering the mastoid process, causing periosteitis (Fig. 17–17). The route of infection from the mastoid cells to the periosteum is by venous channels, usually the mastoid emissary vein. The condition should not be confused with the presence of a subperiosteal abscess, since the management of the latter condition requires incision and drainage of the abscess and a complete simple (cortical) mastoidectomy, while the former usually responds to immediate but less aggressive surgical intervention.

When acute mastoiditis with periosteitis

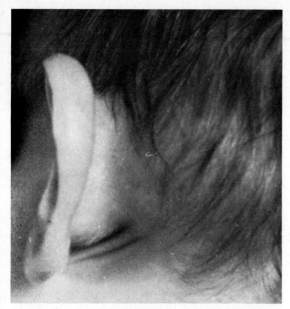

Figure 17–17 An example of postauricular periosteitis. This two year old boy had acute otitis media and mastoiditis. In addition to fever and otalgia, there was postauricular swelling, erythema, tenderness to touch, and loss of the postauricular crease but no evidence of a subperiosteal abscess or roentgenographic evidence of mastoid osteitis. Management consisted of tympanocentesis-myringotomy (and tympanostomy tube insertion) and parenteral antimicrobial therapy, which resulted in complete resolution of the postauricular involvement 24 hours after the beginning of treatment.

occurs in the absence of roentgenographic evidence of osteitis of the mastoid, management should consist of hospitalization, immediate tympanocentesis (for aspiration and microbiologic assessment of the middle ear–mastoid effusion), and myringotomy for drainage of the system. The insertion of a tympanostomy tube is desirable and will enhance drainage over a longer period of time than myringotomy alone. Parenteral antimicrobial agents should be administered as described under Acute Mastoid Osteitis.

Resolution of the periosteal involvement should occur within 24 to 48 hours after the tympanic membrane has been opened for drainage and adequate and appropriate antimicrobial therapy has begun. Surgical drainage of the mastoid, that is, complete simple mastoidectomy, should be performed if the symptoms of the acute infection, such as fever and otalgia, persist, if the postauricular involvement does not progressively improve, or if a subperiosteal abscess develops.

Failure to institute immediate treatment at

this stage may result in the development of acute mastoid osteitis with or without a subperiosteal abscess or, more dangerous to the child, a suppurative intratemporal or intracranial complication such as lateral sinus thrombosis, extradural abscess, or meningitis.

Acute Mastoid Osteitis (Acute "Coalescent" Mastoiditis, Acute Surgical Mastoiditis)

If the infection within the mastoid progresses, rarefying osteitis can cause destruction of the bony trabeculae that separate the mastoid cells so that there is a "coalescence" of the cells. At this stage, a mastoid empyema is present. The pus may spread in one or more of the following directions: (1) anterior to the middle ear through the aditus ad antrum, in which case spontaneous resolution usually occurs; (2) lateral to the surface of the mastoid process, resulting in a subperiosteal abscess (Fig. 17–18); (3) anteriorly, burrowing beneath the skin to form a soft tissue abscess below the pinna or behind the attachment of the sternocleidomastoid muscle in

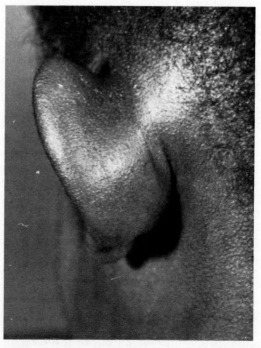

Figure 17–18 An example of a subperiosteal abscess in a child who had acute mastoid osteitis. Note that the pinna is displaced inferiorly and anteriorly, with obliteration of the postauricular crease due to the abscess.

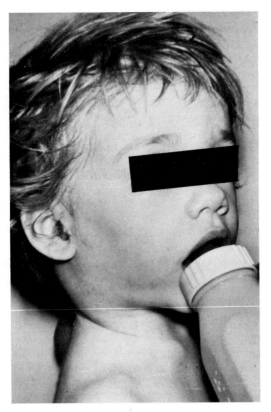

Figure 17–19 An abscess in the neck (Bezold abscess) can be seen in this child who has a draining ear due to acute otitis media. The pus has extended from acute mastoid osteitis and empyema into the neck.

membrane. A fluctuant subperiosteal abscess may be present or even a draining fistula from the mastoid to the postauricular area (Fig. 17–21). The patient may be toxic and febrile with systemic signs of acute illness. In the subacute disease, fever may be prolonged and low-grade with occasional temperature spikes.

Conversely, the tympanic membrane and middle ear may appear almost normal when mastoid osteitis is present. In such cases, the acute middle ear effusion drains through the eustachian tube, in which case there is resolution of the otitis media, but if an obstruction between the middle ear and mastoid is present, then infection in the mastoid becomes trapped and can cause osteitis. The obstruction is usually due to the presence of mucosal swelling or granulation tissue at the aditus ad antrum, or the "bottleneck" of the middle ear–mastoid system. In these cases, the condition of the tympanic membrane and middle ear may not be a reliable indication of mastoid infection. When no external stigmas of extension of pus from the mastoid, such as a subperiosteal abscess, are evident, roentgenograms of the mastoids must be obtained to rule out the presence of an acute mastoid

the neck, which is known as a Bezold abscess (Fig. 17–19); (4) medial to the petrous air cells, resulting in petrositis; or (5) posterior to the occipital bone, which can result in osteomyelitis of the calvarium or a Citelli abscess. Infection may also spread to the labyrinth and facial nerve or into the intracranial cavity, causing one or more suppurative complications, such as an extradural abscess or meningitis.

Clinically, the major signs of mastoid osteitis are a reflection of the underlying inflammatory process and include swelling, redness, and tenderness to touch over the mastoid bone. The pinna is displaced outward and downward (Fig. 17–20), and swelling or sagging of the posterosuperior canal wall may also be present. A purulent discharge may issue through a perforation in the tympanic membrane. Ear drainage may be persistent, and the ear canal is filled with pus and debris, or there may be a nipple-like protrusion at the site of the perforation of the tympanic

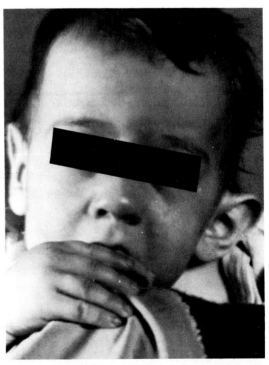

Figure 17–20 Acute mastoid osteitis in an infant showing the outward displacement of the pinna.

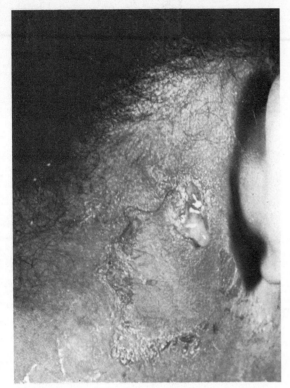

Figure 17–21   An example of a postauricular fistula with purulent discharge in a child who had acute mastoid osteitis.

osteitis when otitis media is not obvious. Any child with a fever of unknown origin should have, as part of the search for the cause of the fever, roentgenograms of the mastoids to rule out the possibility that the fever is caused by acute mastoid osteitis (without otitis media).

Incidence

Before antimicrobial agents were widely used, acute mastoid osteitis was the most common suppurative complication of acute otitis media and frequently resulted in death. The frequency of mastoidectomy for this condition in 1938 was 20 per cent, whereas it was 2.8 per cent in 1948, with an almost 90 per cent reduction in the mortality rate during that period (Sorensen, 1977). A more recent study from Finland found that 29 cases of acute mastoiditis were reported during the period from 1956 to 1971 (Juselius and Kaltiokallio, 1972). It would appear that the frequency of this complication has significantly dropped, but it is still present, even in this, the age of antibiotics.

Bacteriology

Acute mastoiditis may be caused by the same organisms responsible for acute otitis media, *Streptococcus pneumoniae* and *Haemophilus influenzae*. In subacute or chronic cases, *Staphylococcus aureus* and gram-negative enteric bacilli, including *Escherichia coli,* Proteus species, and *Pseudomonas aeruginosa,* may be present and are responsible for a persistent and indolent discharge.

Diagnosis

The diagnosis should be suspected on the basis of clinical signs. Roentgenograms of the mastoid area may show one or more of the following signs: (1) haziness, distortion, or destruction of the mastoid outline; (2) loss of sharpness of the shadows of cellular walls due to demineralization, atrophy, and ischemia of the bony septa (Fig. 17–22); (3) decrease in the density and cloudiness of the areas of pneumatization due to inflammatory swelling of the air cells; (4) in long-standing cases, there is a chronic osteoblastic inflammatory reaction that may obliterate the cellular structure. Small abscess cavities in sclerotic bone may be confused with pneumatic cells.

Cultures for bacteria from ear drainage must be taken with care and concern for discriminating fresh drainage from the debris in the external canal. The canal must be initially cleaned, and if fresh pus is exuding through a perforation in the tympanic membrane, the discharge is cultured at the point of exit from the tympanic membrane with a cotton-tipped wire swab or, preferably, a needle and syringe under direct view. A Gram stain of the pus provides immediate information about the responsible organisms.

Management

Antimicrobial agents are the mainstay of treatment of acute disease. If the case is otherwise uncomplicated (that is, there was no prior infection), it is likely that *S. pneumoniae* or *H. influenzae* is responsible, and ampicillin in a dosage schedule for severe disease is suitable (see Table 16–32). If the disease has persisted for weeks or longer, coverage for *S. aureus* and gram-negative organisms must be provided. It is of the utmost importance to obtain cultures from the site of infection to guide therapy, but initial treatment may begin with a penicillinase-resistant penicillin (nafcillin, oxacillin, or methicillin)

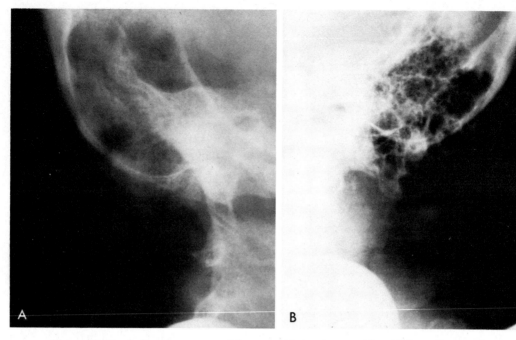

Figure 17-22 *A*, Roentgenogram of the mastoid showing osteitis with loss of septae between the mastoid air cells, which has been termed "coalescent" mastoiditis. *B*, A normal mastoid.

and an aminoglycoside (gentamicin or tobramycin). This regimen may be altered by the findings from a Gram stain of purulent material or by the results of cultures and sensitivity tests.

A complete simple ("cortical") mastoidectomy must be performed when there is evidence of acute mastoid osteitis, especially when the mastoid empyema has extended outside the mastoid bone. The procedure should be considered an emergency, but the timing of the operation must be dependent upon the status of the child. Ideally, sepsis should be under control, and the patient must be able to tolerate a general anesthetic. The procedure is described in detail in current texts (Shambaugh and Glasscock, 1980) (see Fig. 17-11*A*), but in general, the goal is to clean out the mastoid infection and drain the mastoid air cell system into the middle ear by eliminating any obstruction that is caused by edema or granulation tissue in the aditus ad antrum and to provide external drainage. Drains should be inserted into the mastoid cavity and into any abscess that has developed adjacent to the mastoid cavity. To drain and ventilate the middle ear, a tympanostomy tube should be inserted, if not already in place. If a suppurative intratemporal or intracranial complication is also present, surgical intervention for these conditions may also be required (see Chap. 18).

Failure to control the infection in the acute stage of mastoid osteitis may lead to a chronic infection within the mastoid bone or to one of the suppurative complications.

Chronic Mastoiditis

Chronic mastoiditis is invariably associated with chronic suppurative otitis media. The mastoid may be poorly pneumatized or sclerotic. The chronic infection at this stage may be brought under control by medical treatment, but when there are extensive granulation tissue and osteitis in the mastoid, mastoidectomy is usually necessary to eliminate the chronic mastoid osteitis, especially if a cholesteatoma is present (see Chronic Suppurative Otitis Media, p. 526, and Cholesteatoma and Retraction Pocket, p. 530).

PETROSITIS

Petrositis is a rare suppurative complication that is secondary to an extension of infection from the middle ear and mastoid into the petrous portion of the temporal bone. All the inflammatory and cellular changes described as occurring in the mastoid can also occur in the pneumatized petrous pyramid. Only about 30 per cent of the individuals have well-pneumatized petrous bones (Ranier, 1938), but in these individuals, infection of the temporal petrosa may be more frequent than appreciated by clinical and roentgenographic signs, since there is communication of the petrosal air cells with the mastoid–middle ear. Pneumatization usually does not occur before three years of age.

Petrositis may be either acute or chronic. In the acute form, there is extension of acute otitis media and mastoiditis into the pneumatized petrous air cells. The condition, like acute mastoiditis, usually is self-limited with resolution of the acute middle ear and mastoid infection, but on occasion the infection in the petrous portion of the temporal bone does not drain owing to mucosal swelling or because granulation is obstructing the passage from the petrous air cells to the mastoid and middle ear, which results in acute petrous osteomyelitis. Nowadays, the widespread use of antimicrobial agents has made this an extremely rare complication. However, chronic petrous osteomyelitis can be a complication of chronic suppurative otitis media or cholesteatoma, or both, and is much more common than the acute type. Pneumatization of the petrous portion of the temporal bone does not have to be present, since the infection can invade the area by thrombophlebitis, osteitis, or along fascial planes (Allam and Schuknecht, 1968). The infection may persist for months or years, with mild and intermittent signs and symptoms, or may spread to the intracranial cavity and result in one or more of the suppurative complications of ear disease, such as an extradural abscess or meningitis.

The organisms that cause acute petrositis are the same as those that cause acute mastoid osteitis: *S. pneumoniae* and *H. influenzae.* However, chronic petrous osteomyelitis may be caused by the bacteria found in association with chronic suppurative otitis media and cholesteatoma, such as *P. aeruginosa* or Proteus species.

The disease is characterized by pain behind the eye, deep ear pain, persistent ear discharge, and sixth nerve palsy. Eye pain is due to irritation of the ophthalmic branch of the fifth cranial nerve. On occasion, the maxillary and mandibular divisions of the fifth nerve will be involved, and pain will occur in the teeth and jaw. A discharge from the ear is common with acute petrositis but may not be present with chronic disease. Paralysis of the sixth cranial nerve leading to diplopia is a late

complication (Glasscock, 1972). Acute petrous osteomyelitis should be suspected when persistent purulent discharge follows a complete simple mastoidectomy for mastoid osteitis. The triad of pain behind the eye, aural discharge, and sixth nerve palsy is known as Gradenigo syndrome.

Diagnosis

The diagnosis of acute petrous osteomyelitis is suggested by its unique clinical signs. Standard roentgenograms of the temporal bones may show clouding with loss of trabeculation of the petrous bone. The visualization is uncertain, however, because of normal variation in pneumatization (including asymmetry) and the obscuring of the petrous pyramids by superimposed shadows of other portions of the skull. However, polytomograms of the temporal bones can be diagnostic, and computerized tomography should always be performed to rule out the possibility of an extension of the infection into the cranial cavity.

Treatment

Management of acute petrositis is similar to that described for acute mastoiditis, since at this stage it can be considered as further spread of infection within the pneumatized petrous portion of the temporal bone. However, when acute petrous osteomyelitis and acute mastoid osteitis are present together, a more aggressive surgical approach to management will be required than when only the mastoid is involved. As described for patients with acute mastoid osteitis, tympanocentesis-myringotomy (for smear and culture and for drainage) should be performed immediately, and adequate doses of antimicrobial agents should be administered. A complete simple mastoidectomy must also be performed to remove the irreversible mucosal and bone infection, but when the petrous part of the temporal bone is involved, wide exploration of the cell tracts from the mastoid to the petrous portion of the temporal bone should also be part of the surgical procedure to provide adequate drainage. A tympanostomy tube should be inserted into the tympanic membrane if one is not already present. When a large perforation of the tympanic membrane is present, no attempt at reconstruction should be made, since, like the tympanostomy tube, drainage of the middle ear is an important part of management. This approach will usually be adequate for resolution of the petrous infection; however, if drainage of the middle ear, mastoid, and petrosa cannot be achieved by performing a complete simple mastoidectomy, then a modified radical mastoidectomy or, more appropriately, a radical mastoidectomy, may be necessary. However, in children in whom an "extensive" complete simple mastoidectomy (or radical mastoidectomy) fails to resolve the persistent profuse discharge from the mastoid wound and middle ear and for most cases of chronic petrous osteomyelitis, more extensive temporal bone surgery is indicated. The various surgical approaches to the deep petrosal cells have been adequately described by Shambaugh and Glasscock (1980), including the approach through the middle cranial fossa, which usually can preserve the labyrinth, carotid artery, and facial nerve (Glasscock, 1969).

LABYRINTHITIS

This complication of otitis media occurs when infection spreads into the cochlear and vestibular apparatus. The usual portals of entry are the round window and, less commonly, the oval window, but invasion may take place from an infectious focus in an adjacent area, such as the mastoid antrum, the petrous bone, and the meninges, or as a result of bacteremia. Schuknecht (1974) has classified labyrinthitis into four types: (1) acute serous (toxic) labyrinthitis, in which there may be bacterial toxins or biochemical involvement, but no bacteria are present; (2) acute suppurative (purulent) labyrinthitis, in which bacteria have invaded the otic capsule; (3) chronic labyrinthitis, which is secondary to soft tissue invasions, usually by cholesteatoma and granulation tissue or fibrous tissue; and (4) labyrinthine sclerosis, in which there is replacement of the normal labyrinthine structures by fibrous tissue and bone. Labyrinthitis has also been classified into localized (circumscribed) and generalized types.

Acute Serous (Toxic) Labyrinthitis (with or without Perilymphatic Fistula)

The acute serous type of labyrinthitis is considered to be one of the most common suppurative complications of otitis media. Paparella et al. (1972) described the histopathologic evidence of serous labyrinthitis in most of the temporal bone specimens from patients who had otitis media. Bacterial toxins from the infection in the middle ear may enter the inner ear, primarily through an intact round window or through a congenital defect. The portal of entry may also be through an acquired defect of the labyrinth, such as from head trauma or previous middle ear or mastoid surgery. Biochemical changes within the labyrinth have also been found. The cochlea is usually more severely involved than the vestibular system. Paparella et al. (1980) reviewed the audiograms of 232 patients who had surgery for chronic otitis media and found a significant degree of bone conduction loss in the younger age groups. In addition, there was a marked difference in the presence and degree of sensorineural hearing loss in the affected ear, as compared to the normal ear, in patients of all age groups who had unilateral disease. They postulated that the high-frequency sensorineural hearing loss that frequently accompanies this disease is due to a pathologic insult to the basal turn of the cochlea. Fluctuating sensorineural hearing loss has been described in patients with otitis media and has been thought to be due to either endolymphatic hydrops (Paparella et al., 1979) or to a perilymphatic fistula (Grundfast and Bluestone, 1978).

The signs and symptoms of serous labyrinthitis (especially when a perilymphatic fistula is present) are a sudden, progressive, or fluctuating sensorineural hearing loss or vertigo, or both, in association with otitis media or one or more of its complications or sequelae, such as mastoid osteitis. The loss of hearing is usually mixed, that is, there are both conductive and sensorineural components, when serous labyrinthitis is a complication of otitis media. However, in some children who have recurrent middle ear infection, the hearing may be normal between episodes, while in other children, a mild or moderate sensorineural hearing loss only will be present at all times. The presence of vertigo may not be obvious in children, especially infants. Older children may describe a feeling of spinning or turning, while younger children may not be able to verbalize concerning the symptoms but manifest the dysequilibrium by falling, stumbling, or "clumsiness." The vertigo may be mild and

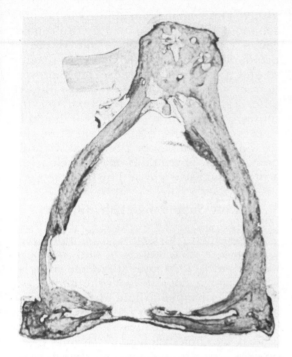

Figure 17–23 Congenital defect in the footplate of the stapes removed from an infant who had a Mondini malformation.

momentary, and it may tend to recur over months or years. Spontaneous nystagmus may also be present, but the signs and symptoms of acute suppurative labyrinthitis, such as nausea, vomiting, and deep-seated pain, are usually absent. Fever, if present, is usually due to a concurrent upper respiratory tract infection or acute otitis media.

The presence of a labyrinthine fistula may be identified by performing a fistula test employing a Siegle pneumatic otoscope or by applying positive and negative external canal pressure using the pump-manometer system of an impedance bridge. The fistula test is considered positive if nystagmus or vertigo is produced by the application of the pressures. Electronystagmography is an objective way of documenting the presence or absence of the nystagmus, but the findings of the fistula test may be misleading, since there can be false-positive and false-negative results. The test can be done in the presence of a perforation of the tympanic membrane or tympanostomy tube. Fistulas are frequently associated with congenital or acquired defects in the temporal bone, such as the Mondini malformation (Fig. 17–23). Polytomography may be helpful in identifying such defects (Fig. 17–24).

When otitis media with effusion is present, a tympanocentesis and myringotomy should be performed for microbiologic assessment of the middle ear effusion and drainage. If possible, a tympanostomy tube should also be inserted for more prolonged drainage and in an attempt to ventilate the middle ear. Antimicrobial agents should be administered. Following resolution of the otitis media with

Figure 17–24 Polytomogram of the temporal bone of a nine month old girl, showing a dilated vestibule (V) and cochlea (C). The child had a fluctuating sensorineural hearing loss documented by auditory brain stem response audiometry when otitis media with effusion was present. Bilateral tympanotomy revealed a congenital defect of the oval window with a perilymphatic fistula. Following repair of the oval window defect, the hearing remained normal.

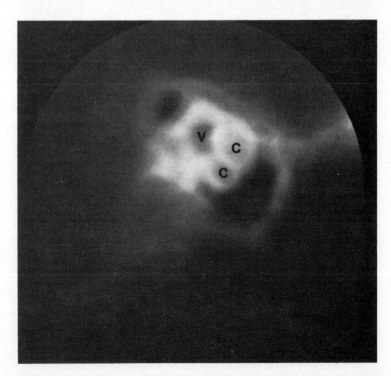

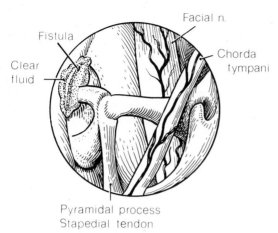

Figure 17–25 Abnormal stapes seen in the left ear. The anterior crus is straight rather than being curved, and it joins the central portion rather than the anterior edge of the footplate.

effusion, the signs and symptoms of the labyrinthitis should rapidly disappear; however, sensorineural hearing loss may persist. If the diagnostic assessment is indicative of a possible congenital or acquired defect of the labyrinth, an exploratory tympanotomy should be performed as soon as the middle ear is free of infection. If a perilymphatic fistula is found, it should be repaired employing either adipose tissue from the earlobe, temporalis fascia, or tragal perichondrium. Even when no defect of the oval or round window is identified, but a fistula is still suspected, the stapes footplate and round window should be covered with connective tissue, since a leak may not be present at the time of the tympanotomy but may recur (Grundfast and Bluestone, 1978). A tympanostomy tube should be reinserted if recurrent otitis media persists (Fig. 17–25).

When acute mastoid osteitis, chronic suppurative otitis media, or cholesteatoma is present, definitive medical and surgical management of these conditions is essential in eliminating the labyrinthine involvement. A careful search for a labyrinthine fistula must be performed when mastoid surgery is indicated. However, a labyrinthectomy is not indicated for serous labyrinthitis.

Any child with sensorineural hearing loss (with or without vertigo) who also has recurrent acute or chronic otitis media with effusion should be carefully evaluated for the possible existence of serous labyrinthitis, which can be secondary to a perilymphatic fistula. This combination appears to be quite common, and failure to identify this complication can result in irreversible severe to profound hearing loss, making early diagnosis and prevention imperative. Since prevention of sensorineural hearing loss due to other causes (such as congenital or viral causes) is not yet possible, our goal should be to prevent this loss of function in those children in whom it can be prevented. In addition, serous labyrinthitis may develop into acute suppurative labyrinthitis.

Acute Suppurative Labyrinthitis

Suppurative (purulent) labyrinthitis may develop as a complication of otitis media or may be one of its complications and sequelae when bacteria migrate from the middle ear into the perilymphatic fluid through the oval or round window, a preexisting temporal bone fracture, an area where bone has been eroded by cholesteatoma or chronic infection, or through a congenital defect. (The most common way that bacteria enter the labyrinth is from the meninges, but migration by this route is usually not a complication of otitis media.)

The incidence of suppurative labyrinthitis as a complication of otitis media is unknown, but it is rare since the widespread use of antibiotics. In a series of 96 cases of suppurative intratemporal and intracranial complications of acute and chronic otitis media that were treated during the period from 1956 to 1971, there were only five cases of suppurative labyrinthitis, all of which were secondary to cholesteatoma that had caused a labyrinthine fistula (Juselius and Kaltiokallio, 1972).

The sudden onset of vertigo, dysequilibrium, deep-seated pain, nausea and vomiting, and sensorineural hearing loss during an episode of acute otitis media or an exacerbation of chronic suppurative otitis media indicates that labyrinthitis had developed. The hearing loss is severe, and there is loss of the child's ability to repeat words shouted in the affected ear with masking of sound in the opposite ear. Often, spontaneous nystagmus and past pointing can be observed. Initially, the quick component of the nystagmus is toward the involved ear, and there is a tendency to fall toward the opposite side. However, when there is complete loss of vestibular function, the quick component will be toward the normal ear. Laboratory and radiographic studies are not of much diagnostic value. In the absence of associated meningitis, the cerebrospinal fluid pressure and cell count are normal.

Frequently, the onset of suppurative labyrinthitis may be followed by facial paralysis, meningitis, or both. In later stages, cerebellar abscess can develop. Thus, suppurative labyrinthitis is a serious complication of otitis media. The development of purulent labyrinthitis means that infection has spread to the inner ear fluid, and infection can then spread to the subarachnoid space through the cochlear aqueduct, the vestibular aqueduct, or the internal auditory canal.

The treatment of suppurative labyrinthitis in the absence of meningitis consists of otologic surgery combined with intensive antimicrobial therapy. If this complication is due to acute otitis media, immediate tympanocentesis and myringotomy with tympanostomy tube insertion are indicated, as described when serous labyrinthitis is present. If acute mastoid osteitis is present, a complete simple mastoidectomy should be performed; however, because this complication is usually secondary to cholesteatoma, a radical mastoidectomy is required. A radical or modified radical mastoidectomy is required. A radical or modified radical mastoidectomy is also appropriate when chronic suppurative otitis media is present without cholesteatoma. If meningitis has also occurred in association with suppurative labyrinthitis, then otologic surgery other than a diagnostic and therapeutic tympanocentesis-myringotomy should be delayed until the meningitis is under control. A labyrinthectomy should be performed only if there is complete loss of labyrinthine function or if the infection spreads to the meninges in spite of adequate antimicrobial therapy. Initially, parenteral antimicrobial agents appropriate to manage the primary middle ear and mastoid disease present should be administered, but since cholesteatoma and chronic suppurative otitis media are the most frequent causes of suppurative labyrinthitis, antimicrobials effective for the gram-negative organisms (*P. aerurinosa* and *Proteus*) are frequently required (see Table 16–32). However, the results of culturing the middle ear effusion, purulent discharge, or the cerebrospinal fluid may alter the selection of the antibiotics.

Chronic Labyrinthitis

The most common cause of chronic labyrinthitis as a complication of middle ear disease is a cholesteatoma that has eroded the labyrinth, resulting in a fistula. Osteitis may also cause bone erosion of the otic capsule. The fistula most commonly occurs in the lateral semicircular canal and is filled by squamous epithelium of a cholesteatoma, granulation tissue, or fibrous tissue entering the labyrinth. The middle ear and mastoid are usually separated at the site of the fistula from the inner ear by the soft tissue, but when there is continuity, acute suppurative labyrinthitis may develop.

The signs and symptoms of chronic labyrinthitis are similar to those of the acute forms of the disease (for example, sensorineural hearing loss and vertigo) except that their onset is more subtle rather than more sudden. The disease is characterized by slowly progressive loss of cochlear and vestibular function over a prolonged period of time. The fistula test may be helpful in making the diagnosis of a labyrinthine fistula, and polytomography may reveal a defect. When there is complete loss of function, no signs or symptoms of labyrinthine dysfunction may be present.

Since a cholesteatoma is the most common cause of this type of labyrinthitis, middle ear and mastoid surgery must be performed. For children with a labyrinthine fistula due to a cholesteatoma, a modified radical or radical mastoidectomy is the procedure of choice. When labyrinthine function is still present, the cholesteatoma matrix overlying the fistula should be left undisturbed, since removal can result in total loss of function. Even though there are advocates of performing an intact canal wall procedure and also surgeons who prefer to remove the cholesteatoma matrix, either at the time of the initial surgery or in a second-stage procedure, the most conservative approach is recommended when a cholesteatoma has caused a labyrinthine fistula in a child.

Failure to make the diagnosis of this complication and to perform the surgery as soon as possible may result in complete loss of cochlear and vestibular function with possible development of labyrinthine sclerosis or an acute suppurative labyrinthitis, which can cause a life-threatening intracranial complication, such as meningitis.

Labyrinthine Sclerosis

Labyrinthine sclerosis is caused by fibrous replacement or new bone formation (labyrinthitis ossificans) in part or all of the labyrinth, with resulting loss of labyrinthine function. Because this condition is the end stage of healing after acute or chronic labyrinthitis, prevention of middle ear disease is the most effective way to prevent labyrinthine sclerosis.

FACIAL PARALYSIS

Facial paralysis may occur during an episode of acute otitis media because of exposure of the facial nerve from a congenital bony dehiscence within the middle ear (Figs. 17–26 and 17–27). Facial paralysis is a relatively frequent complication of acute otitis media in infants and children, and when it occurs as an isolated complication, tympanocentesis and a myringotomy should be performed, and parenteral antibiotics should be administered. The paralysis will usually improve rapidly without requiring further surgery (facial nerve decompression). Mastoidectomy is not indicated unless acute mastoid osteitis (acute "coalescent" mastoiditis) is present. However, if there is complete loss of facial function and if electrophysiologic testing indicates the presence of degeneration or

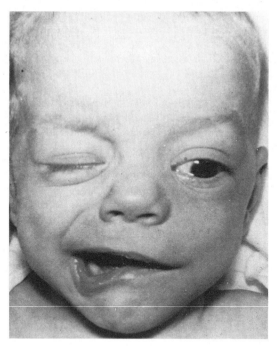

Figure 17–27 An infant in whom left facial paralysis developed a day after the onset of acute otitis media.

progressive deterioration of the nerve, then facial nerve decompression may be necessary to achieve complete return of function.

During the period from 1960 to 1980, there were 35 cases of facial paralysis associated with acute otitis media at the Children's

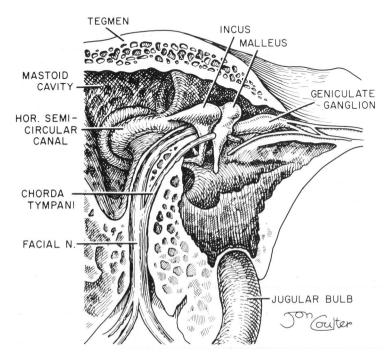

Figure 17–26 The course of the facial nerve shown in the middle ear and mastoid. The nerve can be involved by infection in these areas and can result in facial paralysis.

Hospital of Pittsburgh and The Eye and Ear Hospital of Pittsburgh. The paralysis was partial in 22 (63 per cent) and complete in 13 (37 per cent). In most instances, initial treatment consisted of antimicrobial therapy and myringotomy. However, of these 35 individuals, seven (20 per cent) had further surgery; five underwent facial nerve decompression, and two had simple mastoidectomies (all seven of these children had complete facial paralysis; unpublished data).

When a facial paralysis develops in a child who has chronic suppurative otitis media with or without cholesteatoma, immediate surgical intervention is indicated (see Chap. 13).

CHOLESTEROL GRANULOMA

Cholesterol granuloma is a sequela of chronic otitis media with effusion. It has been described as "idiopathic hemotympanum," since clinically the tympanic membrane appears to be dark blue, a so-called "blue eardrum." Unfortunately, this term is a misnomer, since there is no evidence that bleeding within the middle ear is related to the etiology of this disease, nor is the presence of fresh blood or microscopic amounts of old blood (Sade et al., 1980). The condition is rare in all age groups but does occur in children and is most likely due to long-standing changes associated with chronic otitis media with effusion (Paparella and Lim, 1967; Sheehy et al., 1969). The blue color of the tympanic membrane as visualized through the otoscope is probably due to the reflection of light from the thick liquid (granuloma) within the middle ear. The condition must be differentiated from an uncovered high jugular bulb and a glomus tumor, either tympanicus or jugulare (Valvassori and Buckingham, 1974) and, more commonly, chronic otitis media with effusion or barotitis.

The tissue has been described as being composed of chronic granulations, with foreign body giant cells and foam cells within the middle ear or mastoid, or both. Cholesterol crystals are usually present. The condition is similar to a chronic middle ear effusion except that a soft brownish material that contains shining golden-yellow specks is present. The pathologic process present with cholesterol granuloma should not be confused with that of a cholesteatoma (Schuknecht, 1974). Similar granulomas have been described in other parts of the body: atheromatous and dermoid cysts, periapical and follicular cysts of the jaw, old infarcts, and hematomas (Korthals Altes, 1966). When the granulomas are stained, prominent iron deposits or hemosiderin may be found (Bak-Pederson and Tos, 1972; Nager and Vanderveen, 1977), but not in sufficient quantities to account for the otoscopic appearance of the blue tympanic membrane.

The condition has been reproduced in experimental animals by injecting foreign material into the middle ears of guinea pigs (Friedmann, 1959) and rabbits (Dota et al., 1963), by obstructing the long bones of birds (Ojala, 1957; Beaumont, 1966, 1967), and after chronic obstruction of the eustachian tube in monkeys (Main et al., 1970). The pathogenesis described in the latter experimental model is similar to that known to occur in humans when the eustachian tube was obstructed by a muscle pedicle flap (Linthicum, 1971) or by a tumor (Sheehy et al., 1969). In addition to occurring as an isolated pathologic entity, cholesterol granuloma can be associated with chronic suppurative otitis media with or without cholesteatoma or any inflammation that may obstruct portions of the middle ear or mastoid, or both.

The condition will not respond to medical treatment, middle ear inflation, or myringotomy with tympanostomy tube insertion. However, when a child is observed to have a tympanic membrane that has a dark blue appearance and is unresponsive to nonsurgical management, a myringotomy under general anesthesia should be performed, since on occasion, chronic otitis media with effusion may also be associated with a blue tympanic membrane (again, probably as the result of the way light from the otoscope is reflected from the middle ear effusion). However, if a thick brown liquid is found during the procedure, successful aspiration of the material will not be possible, and if a tympanostomy tube is inserted, it will become occluded immediately. The treatment of choice for a cholesterol granuloma is middle ear and mastoid surgery. The granuloma in the mastoid can be removed by performing a complete simple mastoidectomy, and the middle ear portion can be removed by using a tympanomeatal approach. There is no reason to remove the canal wall unless a cholesteatoma is present. A tympanostomy tube should be inserted into the tympanic membrane at the time of the procedure and reinserted as often as needed, that is, until the middle ear remains normally aerated following spontaneous extubation.

It would appear from what is known of the pathogenesis and pathology of cholesterol granuloma that the best management is prevention, which should consist of active treatment and prevention of chronic otitis media with effusion.

INFECTIOUS ECZEMATOID DERMATITIS

Otitis media with perforation (also a patent tympanostomy tube) can be associated with an infection of the external auditory canal (external otitis) secondary to a discharge from the middle ear and mastoid. An infection in the mastoid may also erode the bone of the ear canal or the postauricular area, resulting in a dermatitis (see Fig. 17–1*A*). The ear canal skin is erythematous, edematous, and filled with purulent drainage, and yellow-crusted plaques may be present. The organisms involved are usually the same as those found in the middle ear–mastoid infection, but the flora of the external canal may contribute to the infectious process. *Pseudomonas* sp and *Proteus* sp are frequently present. Fungi may also be present in chronic cases; most commonly, *Aspergillus niger* or *alba* is found. A culture of the external auditory canal should be obtained, and the results should be compared with those of a needle aspiration of the middle ear discharge through the tympanic membrane perforation or the tympanostomy tube, which will aid in determining the offending organisms. Antimicrobial therapy can then be selected by the results of the culture and sensitivity testing. The infection may spread to the auricle, periauricular area, or other parts of the body, possibly as a result of direct implantation of the organisms or possibly as an autosensitivity phenomenon. Coagulase-positive *S. aureus* is the most frequently involved bacterium (Senturia et al., 1980b).

Severe inflammatory stenosis of the external auditory meatus is uncommon and, therefore, can be differentiated from the extreme tenderness and pain that are so commonly present in acute diffuse external otitis. Also included in the differential diagnosis would be impetigo contagiosa and a secondary infection associated with contact, or seborrheic, dermatitis. Management should be directed toward resolving the middle ear–mastoid infection, which may require medical treatment

Table 17–3 OTOTOPICAL AGENTS AVAILABLE TO TREAT OTITIS MEDIA WITH PERFORATION, DISCHARGE, AND SECONDARY ECZEMATOID EXTERNAL OTITIS

Generic Name	Product Name
Chloramphenicol	Chloromycetin Otic
Colistin sulfate; neomycin sulfate; thonzonium bromide	Coly-Mycin S Otic
Polymyxin B; neomycin sulfate; gramicidin; hydrocortisone	Cortisporin Cream and Cortisporin Ointment
Polymyxin B; neomycin sulfate; hydrocortisone	Cortisporin Otic Solution and Suspension
M-cresyl acetate	Cresylate
Gentamycin sulfate	Garamycin Ophthalmic Solution Sterile Cream, Ointment
Polymyxin B sulfate; bacitracin; gramicidin	Neosporin G Cream
Neomycin; polymyxin B; hydrocortisone; glycerin	Otobione Otic Suspension
Neomycin; glycerin	Otobiotic Otic Solution
Polymyxin B; hydrocortisone	Pyocidin-Otic

or surgery, or both. If the skin of the ear canal is the only area of involvement, then a combination of an antibiotic with or without hydrocortisone otic drops is usually sufficient to reduce the inflammation (Table 17–3). Polymyxin B, neomycin sulfate with hydrocortisone (Cortisporin Otic Suspension) or colistin sulfate, neomycin sulfate, and thonzonium bromide (Coly-Mycin S Otic) are the most commonly employed drugs; however, the ototopical agents may be ototoxic to the cochlea if they penetrate the middle ear and, therefore, should be used with caution. If a fungal infection is present, M-cresyl acetate eardrops (Cresylate) may need to be prescribed. Irrigation of the ear canal with 2 per cent acetic acid or frequent suctioning of the ear canal may also hasten the resolution of the external canal infection.

If the adjacent skin around the auricle or other parts of the body is involved, the skin should be cleansed with saline solution or aluminum acetate and treated with a local antibiotic-corticosteroid cream (see Table 17–3). The child should be cautioned about spread of the infection from the ear canal to other parts of the body and should refrain from putting his or her finger in the ear or scratching the infected skin. Cotton in the external ear canal can be helpful if profuse drainage is present but should be changed as frequently as necessary.

NECROTIZING ("MALIGNANT") EXTERNAL OTITIS

Necrotizing external otitis is a severe form of external otitis caused by *P. aeruginosa* that can extend to and invade the middle ear and other contiguous tissues. This complication has inappropriately been termed "malignant external otitis" in the literature, but no tumor is involved in the pathologic process (Chandler, 1968). This severe form of disease chiefly affects elderly diabetics but may rarely occur in children as a complication of otitis media and mastoiditis. The skin and cartilage may slough, leaving the bone exposed, and necrosis of the eardrum produces a perforation. The infection can cause osteomyelitis of the temporal bone and base of the skull, and intracranial extension of the disease may result in death. Profuse purulent drainage is present (Joachims, 1976). Management consists of intensive parenteral administration of antibiotics effective against *P. aeruginosa,* such as gentamycin and carbenicillin (see Table 16–32), and débridement. Surgery, usually a radical mastoidectomy and wide débridement, may be required when osteomyelitis is severe and unresponsive to the antimicrobial agents.

SELECTED REFERENCES

McCabe, B. F., Sade, J., and Abramson, M. (Eds.). 1977. Cholesteatoma: First International Conference. New York, Aesculapius Pub.
This is the state of knowledge of the epidemiology, pathogenesis, management, and complications of cholesteatoma.

Paparella, M. M., and Meyerhoff, W. L. 1980. Mastoidectomy and tympanoplasty. *In* Paparella, M. M., and Shumrick, D. A. (Eds.). *Otolaryngology,* Vol. 2. Philadelphia, W. B. Saunders Co., pp. 1510–1547.
This chapter has an excellent description of procedures employed for the intratemporal complications and sequelae of otitis media.

Saunders, W. H., Paparella, M. M., and Miglets, A. 1980. Atlas of Ear Surgery, 3rd ed. St. Louis, The C. V. Mosby Co.
The current techniques for surgery of the middle ear and mastoid are illustrated and described in detail.

Schuknecht, H. F. 1974. Pathology of the Ear. Cambridge, MA, Harvard University Press, pp. 215–244, 251–254.
This is the best description of the pathology of the intratemporal complications and sequelae of otitis media.

Shambaugh, G. E., and Glasscock, M. E. 1980. Surgery of the Ear, 3rd ed. Philadelphia, W. B. Saunders Co., pp. 251–287, 326–347, 408–453.
The indications for surgery and the techniques for the procedures are described in detail.

REFERENCES

Abramson, M. 1969. Collagenolytic activity in middle ear cholesteatoma. Ann. Otol. Rhinol. Laryngol., *78*:112–124.

Abramson, M., Lachenbruch, P. A., Press, B. H. J., et al. 1977. Results of conservative surgery for middle ear cholesteatoma. Laryngoscope, *87*:1281–1287.

Allam, A. F., and Schuknecht, H. F. 1968. Pathology of petrositis. Laryngoscope, *78*:1813–1832.

Andreasson, L., and Harris, S. 1979. Middle ear mechanics and eustachian tube function in tympanoplasty. Acta Otolaryngol., Suppl. *360*:141–147.

Armstrong, B. W. 1965. Tympanoplasty in children. Laryngoscope, *75*:1062–1069.

Austin, D. F. 1976. The retraction pocket in the treatment of cholesteatoma. Arch. Otolaryngol., *102*:741–743.

Avery, A. D., et al. 1976. Quality of Medical Care Assessment Using Outcome Measures: Eight Disease-Specific Applications. Prepared for the Health Resources Administration, Department of Health, Education and Welfare by the Rand Corp., Santa Monica, CA.

Bailey, T. H., Jr. 1976. Absolute and relative contraindications to tympanoplasty. Laryngoscope, *86*:67–69.

Bak-Pederson, K., and Tos, M. 1972. The pathogenesis of idiopathic haemotympanum. J. Laryngol. Otol., *86*:473–485.

Baron, S. H. 1969. Management of aural cholesteatoma in children. Otolaryngol. Clin. North Am., *2*:71–88.

Baxter, J. D., and Ling, D. 1974. Ear disease and hearing loss among the Eskimo population of the Baffin zone. Can. J. Otolaryngol., *3*:110–122.

Beaumont, G. D. 1966. The effects of exclusion of air from pneumatized bones. J. Laryngol. Otol., *80*:236–249.

Beaumont, G. D. 1967. Cholesterol granuloma. J. Laryngol. Soc. Aust., *2*:28–35.

Beery, Q. C., Doyle, W. J., Cantekin, E. I., et al. 1980. Eustachian tube function in an American Indian population. Ann. Otol. Rhinol. Laryngol., *89*(68):28–33.

Bezold, F. 1889. Cholesteatom, Perforation der Membrana Flaccida Shrapnelli und Tubenverschluss, eine Atiologische Studie. Ztschrf. Ohrenheilk., *20*:5–28.

Bluestone, C. D. 1971. Eustachian tube obstruction in the infant with cleft palate. Ann. Otol. Rhinol. Laryngol., *80*(2):1–30.

Bluestone, C. D., Beery, Q. C., Cantekin, E. I., et al. 1975. Eustachian tube ventilatory function in relation to cleft palate. Ann. Otol. Rhinol. Laryngol., *84*:333–338.

Bluestone, C. D., Beery, Q. C., and Paradise, J. L. 1973. Audiometry and tympanometry in relation to middle ear effusions in children. Laryngoscope, *83*:594–604.

Bluestone, C. D., Cantekin, E. I., Beery, Q. C., et al. 1977. Functional Eustachian tube obstruction in acquired cholesteatoma and related conditions. *In* McCabe. B. F., Sade, J., and Abramson, M. (Eds.). Cholesteatoma: First International Conference. New York, Aesculapius Pub., pp. 325–335.

Bluestone, C. D., Cantekin, E. I., Beery, Q. C., et al. 1978. Function of the Eustachian tube related to surgical management of acquired aural cholesteatoma in children. Laryngoscope, *88*:1155–1163.

Bluestone, C. D., Cantekin, E. I., and Douglas, G. S.

1979. Eustachian tube function related to the results of tympanoplasty in children. Laryngoscope, 89:450–458.

Bluestone, C. D., Casselbrant, M. L., and Cantekin, E. I. 1982. Functional obstruction of the Eustachian tube in the pathogenesis of aural cholesteatoma in children. In Sade, J. (Ed.). Cholesteatoma and Mastoid Surgery. Proceedings of the Second International Conference on Cholesteatoma and Mastoid Surgery. Amsterdam, Kugler Pub., pp. 211–224.

Bluestone, C. D., Wittel, R. A., and Paradise, J. L. 1972. Roentgenographic evaluation of the Eustachian tube function in infants with cleft and normal palates. Cleft Palate J., 9:93–100.

Brandow, E. C., Jr. 1977. Implant cholesteatoma in the mastoid. In McCabe, B. F., Sade, J., and Abramson, M. (Eds.). Cholesteatoma: First International Conference. New York, Aesculapius Pub., pp. 253–256.

Buchwach, K. A., and Birck, H. G. 1980. Serous otitis media and type I tympanoplasties in children. Ann. Otol. Rhinol. Laryngol., 89(68):324–325.

Cambon, K., Galbreath, J. D., and Kong, G. 1965. Middle ear disease in Indians on the Mount Currie Reservation, British Columia. Can. Med. Assoc. J., 93:1301–1305.

Cantekin, E. I., Saez, C. A., Bluestone, C. D., et al. 1979. Airflow through the Eustachian tube. Ann. Otol. Rhinol. Laryngol., 88:603–612.

Cawthorne, T., and Griffith, A. 1961. Primary cholesteatoma of the temporal bone. Arch. Otolaryngol., 73:252–261.

Chandler, J. R. 1968. Malignant external otitis. Laryngoscope, 78:1257–1294.

Cody, D. T. 1977. The definition of cholesteatoma. In McCabe, B. F., Sade, J., and Abramson, M. (Eds.). Cholesteatoma: First International Conference. New York, Aesculapius Pub., pp. 6–9.

Cohn, A. M., Schwaber, M. K., Anthony, L. S., et al. 1979. Eustachian tube function and tympanoplasty. Ann. Otol. Rhinol. Laryngol., 88:339–347.

DeBlanc, G. B. 1975. Otologic problems in Navajo Indians of the Southwestern United States. Hear. Instrum., 26:15–16, 40–41.

Derlacki, E. L. 1973. Congenital cholesteatoma of the middle ear and mastoid. A third report. Arch. Otolaryngol., 97:177–182.

Derlacki, E. L., and Clemis, J. D. 1965. Congenital cholesteatoma of the middle ear and mastoid. Ann. Otol. Rhinol. Laryngol., 74:706–727.

Diamant, M. 1952. Chronic Otitis. A Critical Analysis. New York, S. Karger.

Dota, T., Nakamura, K., Saheki, M., et al. 1963. Cholesterol granuloma: Experimental observations. Ann. Otol. Rhinol. Laryngol., 72:346–356.

Downs, M. P. 1975. Hearing loss: Definition, epidemiology and prevention. Pub. Health Rev., 4:255–280.

Doyle, W. J. 1977. A functiono-anatomic description of Eustachian tube vector relations in four ethnic populations: An osteologic study. Microfilm, Ann Arbor, MI, University of Michigan.

Doyle, W. J., Cantekin, E. I., and Bluestone, C. D. 1980. Eustachian tube function in cleft palate children. Ann. Otol. Rhinol. Laryngol., 89(68):34–40.

Ekvall, L. 1970. Eustachian tube function in tympanoplasty. Acta Otolaryngol. (Stockh.), Suppl. 263:33–42.

Fairbanks, D. N. 1981. Antimicrobial therapy for chronic suppurative otitis media. Ann. Otol. Rhinol. Laryngol., 90(84):58–62.

Fisher, B. 1966. The social and emotional adjustment of children with impaired hearing attending ordinary classes. Br. J. Educ. Psychol., 36:319–321.

Friedman, I. 1957. The pathology of otitis media (III) with particular reference to bone changes. J. Laryngol. Otol., 71:313–320.

Friedmann, I. 1959. Epidermoid cholesteatoma and cholesterol granuloma: Experimental and human. Ann. Otol. Rhinol. Laryngol., 68:57–79.

Fry, J., Dillane, J. B., McNab Jones, R. F., et al. 1969. The outcome of acute otitis media. (a report to the Medical Research Council). Br. J. Prev. Soc. Med., 23:205–209.

Glasscock, M. E. 1969. Middle fossa approach to the temporal bone: An otologic frontier. Arch. Otolaryngol., 90:15–27.

Glasscock, M. E. 1972. Chronic petrositis: Diagnosis and treatment. Ann. Otol. Rhinol. Laryngol., 81:677–685.

Glasscock, M. E. 1976. Symposium: Contraindications to tympanoplasty: II. An exercise in clinical judgment. Laryngoscope, 86:70–76.

Glasscock, M. E. 1977. Results in cholesteatoma surgery. In McCabe, B. F., Sade, J., and Abramson, M. (Eds.). Cholesteatoma: First International Conference. New York, Aesculapius Pub., pp. 401–403.

Goetzinger, C. P., Harrison, C., and Baer, C. J. 1964. Small perceptive hearing loss: Its effect in school age children. Volta Rev., 66:124–131.

Goodey, R. J., and Smyth, G. D. 1972. Combined approach tympanoplasty in children. Laryngoscope, 82:166–171.

Grundfast, K. M., and Bluestone, C. D. 1978. Sudden or fluctuating hearing loss and vertigo in children due to perilymph fistula. Ann. Otol. Rhinol. Laryngol., 87:761–771.

Habermann, J. 1888. Zur Entstehung des Cholesteatoms des Mittelohrs (Cysten in der Schleimhaut der Paukenhohle, Atrophie der Nerven in der Schnecke). Arch. f. Ohrenh. (Leipz.), 27:42–50.

Harker, L. A., and Koontz, F. P. 1977. The bacteriology of cholesteatoma. In McCabe, B. F., Sade, J., and Abramson, M. (Eds.). Cholesteatoma: First International Conference. New York, Aesculapius Pub., pp. 264–267.

Heermann, J., Jr., Heermann, H., and Kopstein, E. 1970. Fascia and cartilage palisade tympanoplasty. Arch. Otolaryngol., 91:228–241.

Hellman, K. 1925. Studien uber das Sekundare Cholesteatom des Felsenbeins. Z. Hals. Nas Ohrenheilk., 11:406.

Hinchcliffe, R. 1977. Cholesteatoma: Epidemiological and quantitative aspects. In McCabe, B. F., Sade, J., and Abramson, M. (Eds.). Cholesteatoma: First International Conference. New York, Aesculapius Pub., pp. 277–286.

Holm, V. A., and Kunze, L. H. 1969. Effects of chronic otitis media on language and speech development. Pediatrics, 43:833–839.

Holmquist, J. 1968. The role of the Eustachian tube in myringoplasty. Acta Otolaryngol. (Stockh.), 66:289–295.

Igarashi, M., Konishi, S., Alford, B. R., and Guilford, R. F. 1970. The pathology of tympanosclerosis. Laryngoscope, 80:233–243.

Ingelstedt, S., Flisberg, K., and Ortegren, U. 1963. On the function of middle ear and Eustachian tube. Acta Otolaryngol. (Stockh.), Suppl. 182.

Jaffe, B. F. 1969. The incidence of ear disease in the Navajo Indians. Laryngoscope, 79:2126–2134.

Jansen, C. 1963. Cartilage-tympanoplasty. Laryngoscope, 73:1288–1302.

Joachims, H. Z. 1976. Malignant external otitis in children. Arch. Otolaryngol., 102:236–237.

Juselius, H., and Kaltiokallio, K. 1972. Complications of acute and chronic otitis media in the antibiotic era. Acta Otolaryngol. (Stockh.), 74:445–450.

Kaplan, G. J., Fleshman, J. K., Bender, T. R., et al. 1973. Long-term effects of otitis media: A ten-year cohort study of Alaskan Eskimo children. Pediatrics, 52:577–585.

Karma, P., Jokipii, L., Ojala, K., et al. 1978. Bacteriology of the chronically discharging middle ear. Acta Otolaryngol. (Stockh.), 86:110–114.

Kessner, D., Snow, C. K., and Singer, J. 1974. Assessment of Medical Care for Children. Contrasts in Health Status, Vol. 3. Washington, DC, Institute of Medicine, National Academy of Sciences.

Khanna, S. M., and Tonndorf, J. 1972. Tympanic membrane vibrations in cats studied by time-averaged holography. J. Acoust. Soc. Am., 51:1904–1920.

Kinney, S. E. 1978. Postinflammatory ossicular fixation in tympanoplasty. Laryngoscope, 88:821–838.

Kodman, F. 1963. Educational status of hard of hearing children in the classroom. J. Speech Hear. Disord., 28:297–299.

Korthals Altes, A. J. 1966. Cholesterol granuloma in the tympanic cavity. J. Laryngol. Otol., 80:691–698.

Lange, W. 1932. Tief Eingezogene Membrana Flaccida und Cholesteatom. Z. Hals. Nas. Ohrenheilk., 30: 575–582.

Lee, K., and Schuknecht, H. F. 1971. Results of tympanoplasty and mastoidectomy at the Massachusetts Eye and Ear Infirmary. Laryngoscope, 81:529–543.

Lewis, N. 1976. Otitis media and linguistic incompetence. Arch. Otolaryngol., 102:387–390.

Linthicum, F. H., Jr. 1971. Cholesterol granuloma (iatrogenic), further evidence of etiology, a case report. Ann. Otol. Rhinol. Laryngol., 80:207–210.

Lowe, J. F., Bamforth, J. S., and Pracy, R. 1963. Acute otitis media: One year in a general practice. Lancet, 2:1129–1132.

Main, T. S., Shimada, T., and Lim, D. J. 1970. Experimental cholesterol granuloma. Arch. Otolaryngol., 91:356–359.

Mawson, S. R., and Ludman, H. 1979. Diseases of the Ear: A Textbook of Otology. Chicago, Year Book Medical Pub., pp. 378–380.

Maynard, J. E. 1969. Otitis media in Alaskan Eskimo children: An epidemiological review with observations on control. Alaska Med., 11:93–98.

McCafferty, G. J., Coman, W. B., Shaw, E., et al. 1977. Cholesteatoma in Australian aboriginal children. In McCabe, B., Sade, J., and Abramson, M. (Eds.). Cholesteatoma: First International Conference. New York, Aescapulius Pub., pp. 293–301.

McGuckin, F. 1961. Concerning the pathogenesis of destructive ear disease. J. Laryngol. Otol., 75:949–961.

McKenzie, D. 1931. The pathogeny of aural cholesteatoma. J. Laryngol. Otol., 46:163–190.

Miller, G. F., Jr., and Bilodeau, R. 1967. Preoperative evaluation of Eustachian tube function in tympanoplasty. South. Med. J., 60:868–871.

Muenker, G. 1980. Results after treatment of otitis media with effusion. Ann. Otol. Rhinol. Laryngol., 89(68):308–311.

Nager, F. 1925. The cholesteatoma of the middle ear. Ann. Otol. Rhinol. Laryngol., 34:1249–1258.

Nager, G. T., and Vanderveen, T. S. 1976. Cholesterol granuloma involving the temporal bone. Ann. Otol. Rhinol. Laryngol., 85:204–209.

Needleman, H. 1977. Effects of hearing loss from early recurrent otitis media on speech and language development. In Jaffe, B. F. (Ed.). Hearing Loss in Children. Baltimore, University Park Press, pp. 640–649.

Neil, J. F., Harrison, S. H., Morbry, R. D., et al. 1966. Deafness in acute otitis media. Br. Med. J., 1:75–77.

Ojala, L. 1957. Pneumatization of the bone and environmental factors: Experimental studies on chick humerus. Acta Otolaryngol. (Stockh.), Suppl. 133.

Ojala, L., and Saxen, A. 1952. Pathogenesis of middle ear cholesteatoma arising from Shrapnell's membrane (attic cholesteatoma). Acta Otolaryngol. (Stockh.), Suppl. 100:33–54.

Olmstead, R. W., Alvarez, M. C., Moroney, J. D., et al. 1964. The pattern of hearing following acute otitis media. J. Pediatr., 65:252–255.

Palva, A., Karma, P., and Karja, J. 1977. Cholesteatoma in children. Arch. Otolaryngol., 103:74–77.

Paparella, M. M. 1977. Otologic surgery in children. Otolaryngol. Clin. North Am., 10:145–151.

Paparella, M. M., and Lim, D. J. 1967. Pathogenesis and pathology of the "idiopathic" blue eardrum. Arch. Otolaryngol., 85:249–258.

Parapella, M. M., Goycoolea, M. V., and Meyerhoff, W. L. 1980. Inner ear pathology and otitis media: A review. Ann. Otol. Rhinol. Laryngol., 89(68):249–253.

Paparella, M. M., Goycoolea, M. V., Meyerhoff, W. L., et al. 1979. Endolymphatic hydrops and otitis media. Laryngoscope, 89:43–54.

Paparella, M. M., Oda, M., Hiraide, F., et al. 1972. Pathology of sensorineural hearing loss in otitis media. Ann. Otol. Rhinol. Laryngol., 81:632–647.

Paradise, J. L., Bluestone, C. D., and Felder, H. 1969. The universality of otitis media in fifty infants with cleft palate. Pediatrics, 44:35–42.

Peckham, C. S., Sheridan, M., and Butler, N. R. 1972. School attainment of seven-year-old children with hearing difficulties. Dev. Med. Child. Neurol., 14:592–602.

Ranier, A. 1938. Development and construction of the pyramidal cells. Arch. Ohren.-Nasen-U., Khelkopfh., 145:3.

Ratnesar, P. 1977. Aeration: A factor in the sequelae of chronic ear disease among the Labrador and Northern Newfoundland coast. In McCabe, B., Sade, J., and Abramson, M. (Eds.). Cholesteatoma: First International Conference. New York, Aesculapius Pub., pp. 302–307.

Reed, D., Struve, S., and Maynard, J. E. 1967. Otitis media and hearing deficiency among Eskimo children. A cohort study. Am. J. Public Health, 57:1657–1662.

Ritter, F. N. 1977. Complications of cholesteatoma. In McCabe, B. F., Sade, J., and Abramson, M. (Eds.). Cholesteatoma: First International Conference. New York, Aesculapius Pub., pp. 430–437.

Ruedi, L. 1958. Cholesteatosis of the attic. J. Laryngol. Otol., 72:593–609.

Sade, J. 1977. Pathogenesis of attic cholesteatoma: The metaplasia theory. In McCabe, B. F., Sade, J., and Abramson, M. (Eds.). Cholesteatoma: First International Conference. New York, Aesculapius Pub., pp. 212–232.

Sade, J., Halevy, A., Klajman, A., et al.: 1980. Cholesterol granuloma. Acta Otolaryngol. (Stockh.), *89*:233–239.

Schiff, M., Poliquin, J. F., Catanzaro, A., et al. 1980. Tympanosclerosis: A theory of pathogenesis. Ann. Otol. Rhinol. Laryngol., *89*(70):1–16.

Schuknecht, H. F. 1974. Pathology of the Ear. Cambridge, MA, Harvard University Press, pp. 227–233.

Senturia, B. H., Bluestone, C. D., Limb, D. J., et al. 1980a. Recent advances in otitis media with effusion. Ann. Otol. Rhinol. Laryngol., *89*, Suppl. 68.

Senturia, B. H., Marcus, M. D., and Lucente, F. E. 1980b. Diseases of the External Ear: An Otologic-Dermatologic Manual, 2nd ed. New York, Grune and Stratton.

Severeid, L. R. 1977. Development of cholesteatoma in children with cleft palate: A longitudinal study. *In* McCabe, B. F., Sade, J., and Abramson, M. (Eds.). Cholesteatoma: First International Conference. New York, Aesculapius Pub., pp. 287–292.

Shambaugh, G. E.. and Glasscock, M. E. 1980. Surgery of the Ear, 3rd ed. Philadelphia, W. B. Saunders Co., pp. 432–436.

Sheehy, J. C. 1978. Management of cholesteatoma in children. Adv. Otorhinolaryngol., *23*:58–64.

Sheehy, J. L., and Anderson, R. G. 1980. Myringoplasty: A review of 472 cases Ann. Otol. Rhinol. Laryngol., *89*:331–334.

Sheehy, J. L., Brachman, D. E., and Graham, M. D. 1977. Complications of cholesteatoma: A report on 1024 cases. *In* McCabe, B. F., Sade, J., and Abramson, M. (Eds.). Cholesteatoma: First International Conference. New York, Aesculapius Pub., pp. 420–429.

Sheehy, J. L., Linthicum, F. H., Jr., and Greenfield, E. C. 1969. Chronic serous mastoiditis, idiopathic hemotympanum and cholesterol granuloma of the mastoid. Laryngoscope, *79*:1189–1217.

Sheehy, J. L., and Patterson, M. E. 1967. Intact canal wall tympanoplasty with mastoidectomy: A review of 8 years' experience. Laryngoscope, *77*:1502–1542.

Siedentop, K. H. 1968. Eustachian tube dynamics, size of the mastoid air cell system, and results with tympanoplasty. Otolaryngol. Clin. North Am., *1*:33.

Smyth, G. D. 1972. Tympanic reconstruction. Otolaryngol. Clin. North Am., *5*:111–125.

Smyth, G. D. 1977. Postoperative cholesteatoma. *In* McCabe, B. F., Sade, J., and Abramson, M. (Eds.). Cholesteatoma: First International Conference. New York, Aesculapius Pub. pp. 355–362.

Sobol, S. M., Reichert, T. J., Faw, K. D., et al. 1980. Intramembranous and mesotympanic cholesteatomas associated with an intact tympanic membrane in children. Ann. Otol. Rhinol. Laryngol., *89*:312–317.

Solomon, N. E., and Harris, L. J. 1976. Otitis media in children: Assessing the quality of medical care using short-term outcome measures. Quality of medical care assessment using short-term outcome measurement: Eight disease-specific applications. Rand Report R-2021/2-HEW, Rand Corp., Santa Monica, CA, p. 589.

Sorensen, H. 1977. Antibiotics in suppurative otitis media. Otolaryngol. Clin. North Am., *10*:45–50.

Stool, S. E., and Randall, P. 1967. Unexpected ear disease in infants with cleft palate. Cleft Palate J., *4*:99–106.

Storrs, L. A. 1976. Contraindications to tympanoplasty. Laryngoscope, *86*:79.

Teed, R. W. 1936. Cholesteatoma verum tympani. Its relationship to first epibranchial placode. Arch. Otolaryngol., *24*:455–474.

Tschopp, C. F. 1977. Chronic otitis media and cholesteatoma in Alaskan native children. *In* McCabe, B., Sade, J., and Abramson, M. (Eds.). Cholesteatoma: First International Conference. New York, Aesculapius Pub., pp. 290–292.

Tumarkin, A. 1938. A contribution to the study of middle ear suppuration with special reference to the pathogeny and treatment of cholesteatoma. J. Laryngol. Otol., *53*:685–710.

Valvassori, G. E., and Buckingham, R. A. 1974. Middle ear masses mimicking glomus tumors: Radiographic and otoscopic recognition. Ann. Otol. Rhinol. Laryngol., *83*:606–612.

Virtanen, H., Palva, T., and Jauhiainen, T. 1980. The prognostic value of Eustachian tube function measurements in tympanoplastic surgery. Acta Otolaryngol. (Stockh.), *90*:317–323.

vonTroltsch, A. F. 1869. Handbuch der Ohrenheilkunde. Lepzig, W. Engelmann.

Wendt, H. 1873. Desquamative Entzundung des Mittelohrs (Cholesteatom des Felsenbeins). Arch. Ohren-heilk. (Leipzig), *14*:428.

Wiet, R. J. 1979. Patterns of ear disease in the Southwestern American Indian. Arch. Otolaryngol., *105*:381–385.

Wiet, R. J., DeBlanc, G. B., Stewart, J., et al. 1980. Natural history of otitis media in the American native. Ann. Otol. Rhinol. Laryngol., *89*(68):14–19.

Wishik, S. M., Kramm, E. R., and Koch, E. M. 1958. Audiometric testing of school children. Public Health Rep., *73*:265–278.

Wittmaack, K. 1933. Wie ensteht ein genuines Cholesteatom? Arch. f. Ohren-Nasen-u. Kehlkopfh., *137*:306–332.

Young, C., and McConnell, F. 1957. Retardation of vocabulary development in hard of hearing children. Except. Child Ann., 368–370.

Zinkus, P. W., Gottlieb, M. I., and Schapiro, M. 1978. Developmental and psychoeducational sequelae of chronic otitis media. Am. J. Dis. Child., *132*:1100–1104.

Zollner, F. 1956. Tympanosclerosis. J. Laryngol. Otol., *70*:77–85.

Zonis, R. D. 1970. Chronic otitis media in the Arizona Indian. Arizona Med., *27*:1–6.

Chapter 18

INTRACRANIAL SUPPURATIVE COMPLICATIONS OF OTITIS MEDIA AND MASTOIDITIS

Charles D. Bluestone, M.D.
Jerome O. Klein, M.D.

There has been an overall decline in the incidence of suppurative intracranial complications of otitis media since the advent of antimicrobial agents. Today, these complications occur more often in association with chronic suppurative otitis media and mastoiditis, with or without cholesteatoma, than in association with acute otitis media (Juselius and Kaltiokallio, 1972).

The middle ear and mastoid air cells are adjacent to important structures, including the dura of the posterior and middle cranial fossa, the sigmoid venous sinus of the brain, and the inner ear. Suppuration in the middle ear or mastoid, or both, may spread to these structures, producing the following suppurative intracranial complications: meningitis, extradural abscess, subdural empyema, focal encephalitis, brain abscess, lateral (sigmoid) sinus thrombosis, and otitic hydrocephalus (Fig. 18–1).

Multiple complications are frequently dependent on the route of infection. Thus, a patient may have meningitis, lateral sinus thrombosis, and a cerebellar abscess or other combinations of suppurative disease involving adjacent areas.

Any child who has acute or chronic otitis media who develops one or more of the following signs or symptoms, especially while receiving medical treatment, should be suspected of having a suppurative intracranial complication: persistent headache, lethargy, malaise, irritability, severe otalgia, onset of fever, nausea, and vomiting. The following would be definitive signs and symptoms demanding an intensive search for an intracranial complication: stiff neck, focal seizures, ataxia, blurred vision, papilledema, diplopia, hemiplegia, aphasia, dysdiadochokinesia, intention tremor, dysmetria, and hemianopsia. Conversely, children with intracranial infection, such as meningitis or a brain abscess, must have middle ear–mastoid disease ruled out as the origin of or concomitant with the central nervous system disease.

In children who have acute or chronic suppurative otitis media, the presence of headache, even though a nonspecific symptom, should indicate a potential complication. Irritability, lethargy, or other changes in personality may be secondary to intracranial spread of the infection. Even though fever is common when acute infection of the ear is present, persistent or recurrent fever may be a potentially dangerous sign. Fever is rarely present in children with chronic suppurative otitis media and, when present, may be a hallmark of an impending intracranial complication.

The diagnosis of intracranial complications has been greatly improved since the advent of the widespread availability and use of computerized tomography, but when not available,

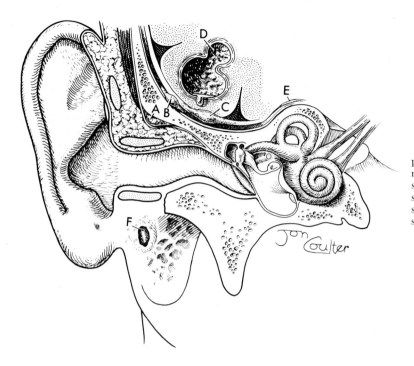

Figure 18–1 Suppurative complications of otitis media and mastoiditis. *A*, Subperiosteal abscess; *B*, extradural abscess; *C*, subdural empyema; *D*, brain abscess; *E*, meningitis; *F*, lateral sinus thrombosis.

then arteriography should be used. For lesions above the tentorium, electroencephalography and radionuclide brain scanning may be of value as diagnostic procedures. When the lesions are below the tentorium, these methods are not as helpful (du Boulay, 1979).

Intracranial extension of infection may take place because of (1) progressive thrombophlebitis permitting the inflammatory process to spread through the intact bone (osteothrombophlebitis), (2) erosion of the bony walls of the middle ear or mastoid (osteitis), and (3) extension along preformed pathways — the round window, dehiscent sutures, skull fracture, or congenital or surgically acquired bony dehiscences (mastoidectomy with dura exposure).

In this chapter, the incidence, pathogenesis, etiology, diagnosis, management, and outcome for each of these complications as they relate to children will be presented. Following the description of the specific complications, a section on timing and type of otologic surgery appropriate for children is provided, but a detailed description of the operative procedures has not been included, since the latest otologic and neurologic surgical techniques are adequately described and illustrated in currently available texts that are listed at the end of the chapter (see Selected References).

INCIDENCE

Prior to the introduction of antimicrobial agents, 2.3 per cent of all patients with acute and chronic suppurative otitis media developed intracranial complications, and two thirds of the cases were due to chronic middle ear disease (Turner and Reynolds, 1931). In the antibiotic era, intracranial complications are uncommon, but approximately two thirds are still caused by chronic ear disease (Jeanes, 1962). However, Dawes (1979) reported that most intracranial complications in children were secondary to acute otitis media. Ritter (1977) reviewed 152 cases of cholesteatoma, about half of which were present in patients younger than 20 years of age. The study, which represented cases seen between 1965 and 1970, included four cases with suppurative intracranial complications: two patients with sigmoid sinus thrombosis and one patient each with an extradural abscess and a brain abscess. In a review by Sheehy et al. (1977), of 1024 operations in 949 patients, 17.7 per cent of whom were 15 years of age or younger, performed during the years 1965 through 1974, only one patient had meningitis and in only two patients was an extradural abscess present; however, neither of these complications occurred in children. The relative incidence of suppurative intracranial complications of acute and chronic otitis

Table 18–1 SUPPURATIVE INTRACRANIAL COMPLICATIONS OF ACUTE OR CHRONIC OTITIS MEDIA IN 29 CHILDREN AND ADULTS TREATED AT THE VASA CENTER HOSPITAL (VASA, FINLAND)

	Acute Otitis Media	Chronic Otitis Media	Total
Meningitis	9	5	14
Extradural or perisinuous abscess	3	5	8
Lateral sinus thrombosis	2	3	5
Temoral lobe abscess	0	2	2
TOTAL	14	15	29

(Adapted from Juselius, H., and Kaltiokallio, K. 1972. Complications of acute and chronic otitis media in the antibiotic era. Acta Otolaryngol. (Stockh.), 74:445–450.)

media is indicated in a report of 29 consecutive cases treated at a medical center in Finland during the years 1956 through 1971 (Table 18–1). Meningitis was the most common of these complications. This has also been the case in other reports in the antibiotic era (Krajina, 1956; Proctor, 1966).

MENINGITIS

Meningitis may be associated with infections of the middle ear in three circumstances: (1) direct invasion, in which a suppurative focus in the middle ear or mastoid spreads through the dura and extends to the pia-arachnoid, causing generalized meningitis; (2) inflammation in an adjacent area, in which the meninges may become inflamed if there is suppuration in an adjacent area such as a subdural abscess, brain abscess, or lateral sinus thrombophlebitis; (3) concurrent infection, in which otitis media arises by contiguous spread from an infectious focus in the upper respiratory tract and meningitis results from invasion of the blood from the upper respiratory focus. The infections are simultaneous, but meningitis does not arise from the middle ear infection.

The most common route is the third, hematogenous spread. Less common is direct invasion through congenital preformed pathways or by thrombophlebitis, which usually extends to the middle cranial fossa through the petrosquamous suture or to the posterior cranial fossa through the subarcuate fossa, that is, the first route. In the preantibiotic era, Lindsay (1938) examined the histopathology of temporal bones of patients who had had acute otitis media and meningitis and found

that most of the specimens had evidence of direct spread of the infection through the petrous apex. However, since the advent of the widespread use of antimicrobial agents, extension of the infection has been thought to be along preformed pathways or by direct extension through the dura. Spread of infection from the middle ear and mastoid through the inner ear to the meninges is another pathway but is thought to be rare compared to the other pathogenic mechanisms.

The symptoms of meningitis caused by any of the three mechanisms include fever, headache, neck stiffness, and altered consciousness. Examination of cerebrospinal fluid reveals pleocytosis and elevation of protein concentration in all routes of infection, but depression of sugar levels is common in only the first and third routes. Polymorphonuclear leukocytes are the predominant cell type in the early phase of meningitis caused by the first and third mechanisms. When infection occurs by the second mechanism, it is likely to be more chronic; therefore, lymphocytes usually predominate. Organisms are usually isolated from the spinal fluid when meningitis is caused by the first and third mechanisms but not by the second one. Thus, meningitis from the second mechanism may be defined as an aseptic meningitis (clinical signs of meningitis associated with cells in the cerebrospinal fluid but without bacteria isolated by usual laboratory techniques).

The organisms associated with meningitis arising from acute otitis media are the common agents of meningitis, *Streptococcus pneumoniae* and *Haemophilus influenzae* type b. There has been an overall increase in the frequency of bacterial meningitis in children, which has been due mostly to an increase in cases in which *H. influenzae* type b is the causative organism. About 20 per cent of all cases of acute otitis media are due to *H. influenzae*, but less than 10 per cent of these are type b (Harding et al., 1973). Feigin (1981) reported that 14 per cent of children with *H. influenzae* type b otitis media also had meningitis.

Initial management of menigitis involves the administration of high doses of antimicrobial agents. If the causative agent is unknown, ampicillin and chloramphenicol are started (see Chap. 16, Table 16–32). The regimen may be modified after the results of cultures are known. If the cultures are negative and there is concern that a suppurative focus may be producing the aseptic process, diagnostic tests should be performed to identify the focus, to obtain material for culture, and to clear, usually by incision and drainage, the local infection. If acute or chronic otitis media with effusion is present, then tympanocentesis, for identification of the causative organism within the middle ear, and myringotomy, for drainage, should be performed immediately. If acute mastoiditis with osteitis is present, a complete simple mastoidectomy is indicated as soon as the child is able to tolerate a general anesthetic. If chronic suppurative otitis media with or without cholesteatoma is present, then a radical mastoidectomy is frequently required and should be performed when the patient is stable. Appropriate management of any of the suppurative intratemporal complications, such as petrositis or labyrinthitis, or intracranial complications, such as an extradural abscess, will also require surgical intervention.

Occasionally, following trauma to the temporal bone, acute otitis media develops that is complicated by meningitis. Tympanocentesis and myringotomy should be performed immediately for culture and drainage or culture of the otorrhea, if present. However, exploration of the middle ear and mastoid may be necessary later to search for and repair possible defects in the dura, especially if cerebrospinal fluid otorrhea is present.

Appropriate management of both the meningitis and the suppurative focus within the temporal bone should result in a favorable outcome, although many studies still report a considerable mortality associated with otitic meningitis. Kessler et al. (1970) reported a mortality rate of 33 per cent in their series of 51 cases of otitic meningitis.

EXTRADURAL ABSCESS

Extradural (epidural) abscess usually results from the destruction of bone adjacent to dura by cholesteatoma or infection, or both. This occurs when granulation tissue and purulent material collect between the lateral aspect of the dura and adjacent temporal bone. Dural granulation tissue within a bony defect is much more common than an actual accumulation of pus. When an abscess is present, a dural sinus thrombosis or, less commonly, a subdural or brain abscess may also be present. If extensive bone destruction has occurred when acute mastoid osteitis (acute "coalescent" mastoiditis) is present, an extradural abscess may develop in the area of the sigmoid dural sinus.

Symptoms can include severe earache, low-grade fever, and headache in the temporal region with deep local throbbing pain, but the more common extradural abscess encountered today may produce no signs or symptoms. Frequently, an asymptomatic extradural abscess is found in patients undergoing elective mastoidectomy for cholesteatoma.

When otorrhea accompanies an extradural abscess, it is characteristically profuse, creamy, and pulsatile. Compression of the ipsilateral jugular vein may increase the rate of discharge and the degree of pulsation. Usually there is not accompanying fever, but malaise and anorexia may be observed. Usually there are no neurologic signs, the intracranial pressure is normal, and it is difficult to detect any displacement of the brain. Cerebrospinal fluid cell count and pressure are normal unless meningitis is also present. Computerized tomography may demonstrate a sizable extradural abscess (Fig. 18–2).

Although identification of the infecting organism and appropriate antimicrobial therapy can help to prevent the development of an intradural complication from an extradural abscess, the treatment of extradural abscess itself consists of surgical drainage. A mastoidectomy is performed, enough bone is removed so that the dura of the middle and posterior fossae may be inspected directly, the extradural abscess is identified and drained, and the otologic procedure that will provide optimal exteriorization of the diseased area is completed by removing all the granulation tissue until normal dura is found.

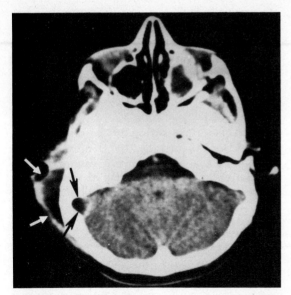

Figure 18–2 Computerized tomogram of a 9-year-old girl showing a right perisinuous extradural abscess (black arrows) as a complication of acute mastoiditis with osteitis and a subperiosteal abscess (white arrows). There had been a one-week history of hearing loss, otalgia, and a profuse, foul-smelling otorrhea, and a three-day history of high fever, postauricular swelling, disorientation, and irritability, which persisted in spite of parenterally administered antimicrobial agents. A complete simple mastoidectomy and drainage of the extradural abscess resulted in a favorable outcome.

SUBDURAL EMPYEMA

A subdural empyema is a collection of purulent material within the potential space between the dura externally and arachnoid membrane internally. Since the pus collects in a preformed space, it is correctly termed empyema rather than abscess. Subdural empyema may develop as a direct extension of infection or, more rarely, by thrombophlebitis through venous channels. It is one of the rarer complications of otitis media and mastoiditis.

Children with subdural empyema are extremely toxic and febrile. There are usually the signs and symptoms of a locally expanding intracranial mass. Severe headache in the temporoparietal area is usually present. Central nervous system findings may include seizures, hemiplegia, dysmetria, belligerent behavior, somnolence, stupor, deviation of the eyes, dysphagia, sensory deficits, stiff neck, and a positive Kernig sign. Hemiplegia and jacksonian epilepsy in a child with suppurative disease of the middle ear and mastoid usually are indicative of a subdural empyema. Computerized tomography is often diagnostic of the process. The peripheral white blood cell count is high and there is a predominance of polymorphonuclear leukocytes. The cerebrospinal fluid glucose concentration is normal, and no microorganisms are seen on smear or culture of the cerebrospinal fluid.

Treatment of subdural empyema includes intensive intravenous antimicrobial therapy and neurosurgical drainage of the empyema through burr holes or craniectomy. Mastoid surgery to locate and drain the source of infection is usually delayed until after neurosurgical intervention has yielded some improvement in neurologic status. The condition still has a high mortality rate, and more than half of those children who recover will have some neurologic deficit.

FOCAL OTITIC ENCEPHALITIS

Focal areas of the brain may become edematous and inflamed as a complication of acute or chronic otitis media or of one or more of the suppurative complications of these disorders, such as an extradural abscess or dural sinus thrombophlebitis. This localized inflammation is called focal otitic encephalitis, the signs and symptoms of which may be similar to those that are characteristic of a brain abscess, except that suppuration within the brain is absent. Ataxia, nystagmus, vomiting, and giddiness would indicate a possible focus within the cerebellum, whereas drowsiness, disorientation, restlessness, seizures, and coma may indicate a cerebral focus. In both sites, headache may be present. However, since these signs and symptoms are also commonly associated with a brain abscess or subdural empyema, needle aspiration may be necessary to rule out the presence of an abscess. Computerized tomography is helpful in making this distinction. If an abscess is not thought to be present, then the focal encephalitis should be treated by administering therapeutic doses of antimicrobial agents and by an appropriate otologic surgical procedure to remove the infection performed as soon as possible, since failure to control the source of the infection within the temporal bone, as well as the focal encephalitis, may result in the development of a brain abscess. Anticonvulsive medication is given when there is cerebral involvement.

BRAIN ABSCESS

Of all age groups, infants and children have the highest incidence of brain abscess (Brewer et al., 1975). However, the incidence of brain abscess has decreased significantly in the antibiotic era. During the period from 1930 to 1960, there were 89 cases of otogenic brain abscess at the Otolaryngological Hospital of the University of Helsinki, whereas between 1961 and 1969, there were only three cases (Tarkkanen and Kohonen, 1970). Infection of the middle ear and mastoid, however, remains the predominant source of infection when abscess in the brain does occur (Liske and Weikers, 1964; Morgan et al., 1973; Beller et al., 1973).

Otogenic abscess of the brain may follow directly from acute or chronic middle ear and mastoid infection or may follow the development of an adjacent infection, such as lateral sinus thrombophlebitis, petrositis, or meningitis. The dura overlying the infected mastoid is invaded either along vascular pathways or by adherence of the dura to underlying infected bone. Chronic otitis media or mastoiditis with or without cholesteatoma may lead to erosion of the tegmen tympani by pressure necrosis and perforation of the bone with resultant inflammation of the dura and invasion by pathogenic organisms. An extradural abscess occurs with subsequent infiltration of the dura and spreads to the subdural space. A localized subdural abscess or leptomeningitis ensues. Invasion of brain tissue follows, and the various stages of abscess formation take place: inflammatory reaction, suppuration, necrosis and liquefaction, and development of a fibrinous capsule. If delimitation of the abscess does not occur, infection may extend to the meninges or may rupture into the ventricles.

The site of the abscess is the area closest to the primary source of infection. Thus, temporal lobe abscesses occur following invasion through the tegmen tympani or petrous bone. Cerebellar abscesses occur when the infectious focus is the posterior surface of the petrous bone or thrombophlebitis of the lateral sinus. An abscess in the temporal lobe occurs more commonly than does one in the cerebellum, and multiple abscesses are not uncommon.

The natural history of brain abscesses includes resorption and healing through gliosis and calcification, spontaneous rupture through a fistulous tract, or spillage into the ventricles or subarachnoid space, producing encephalitis or meningitis.

The bacterial pathogens responsible for brain abscesses include the virulent invasive strains associated with acute disease or the more indolent strains associated with chronic disease (Brewer et al., 1975). These include the following: (1) gram-positive cocci — group A *Streptococcus, S. pneumoniae, S. viridans,* and *Staphylococcus aureus;* (2) gram-negative coccobacilli — *H. influenzae* and *H. aphrophilus;* (3) gram-negative enteric bacilli — *Escherichia coli, Proteus* species, *Enterobacter aerogenes, E. cloacae,* and *Pseudomonas aeruginosa;* (4) anaerobic bacteria — *Eubacterium* species, *Bacteroides* species, *Peptostreptococcus* species, and *Propionibacterium acnes* (Heineman and Braude, 1963).

Signs of invasion of the central nervous system usually occur about a month after an episode of acute otitis media or an acute exacerbation of chronic otitis media. Systemic signs, including fever and chills, are variable and may be absent. Signs of a generalized central nervous system infection include severe headache, vomiting, drowsiness, seizures, irritability, personality changes, altered levels of consciousness, anorexia and weight loss, and meningismus. In addition to these signs of an expanding intracranial lesion, there may be specific signs of involvement of the temporal or cerebellar lobes, including symptoms of involvement of cranial nerves, vertigo, focal seizures, visual field defects, and nystagmus. Temporal lobe abscesses may be silent. There may be persistent purulent ear drainage, suggesting the primary site of infection. Terminal signs include coma, papilledema, or cardiovascular changes.

Diagnosis is based on development of clinical signs, the results of electroencephalography, and roentgenographic evidence. Computerized tomography is an invaluable aid in diagnosis (Fig. 18–3). Radionuclide brain scans can be abnormal when focal encephalitis or a brain abscess is present. Of particular concern is the sudden appearance of signs of acute disease — fever and headache — in a patient with chronic middle ear disease.

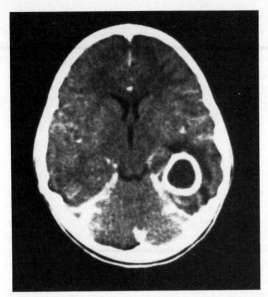

Figure 18–3 Computerized tomogram of a 14-year-old boy showing a brain abscess as a complication of chronic suppurative otitis media with an attic cholesteatoma. There had been an eight-week history of persistent aural discharge, lethargy, and progressive hearing loss, and a four-week history of vomiting and headache. Physical examination revealed papilledema and bilateral abducens palsy. Complete recovery followed neurosurgical removal of the abscess and a radical mastoidectomy.

Lumbar puncture is not universally recommended owing to the possibility of herniation of the brain and death; however, when it is performed, the cerebrospinal fluid may be normal if the abscess is deep in the tissue and does not produce inflammation of the meninges, or if it does, there may be an increased number of cells, initially a predominance of polymorphonuclear leukocytes, then lymphocytes. The concentration of protein may be high, but the sugar level is not usually reduced unless there is bacterial invasion of the meninges. Cultures of the spinal fluid are usually negative in the absence of suppurative meningitis.

Treatment includes use of antimicrobial agents, drainage or resection of the brain abscess, or both, as well as the surgical débridement of the primary focus, the mastoid, or adjacent infected tissues such as thrombophlebitis of the lateral sinus. The choice of the most appropriate antimicrobial regimen is difficult because of the varied bacteriology of otogenic brain abscess. Aspiration of the abscess to define the etiology is most helpful (Garfield, 1979). Initial therapy should include administration of a penicillin for gram-positive cocci, an aminogylcoside for gram-negative enteric pathogens, and chloramphenicol to combat gram-negative organisms and, more importantly, anaerobic bacteria (see Chap. 16, Table 16–32). Even with the administration of antimicrobial agents, the mortality of brain abscess has been approximately 30 per cent (McGreal, 1962; Morgan et al., 1973). The best results, a zero mortality, were reported in brain abscesses in children treated by catheter drainage (Selker, 1975).

LATERAL SINUS THROMBOSIS

Lateral and sigmoid sinus thrombosis or thrombophlebitis arises from inflammation in the adjacent mastoid. The superior and petrosal dural sinuses also are intimately associated with the temporal bone, but they are rarely affected. The mastoid infection in contact with the sinus walls produces inflammation of the adventitia followed by penetration of the venous wall. Formation of a thrombus occurs after the infection has spread to the intima. The mural thrombus may become infected and may propagate, occluding the lumen. Embolization of septic thrombi or extension of infection into the tributary vessels may produce further disease.

This complication is still common in children. Of the 13 patients who had otogenic lateral sinus disease at the Groote Schurr Hospital in South Africa during the period from 1967 to 1970, nine were younger than 20 years of age; six children had chronic ear infections, and three had acute ear infections (Seid and Sellars, 1973).

The clinical signs of lateral sinus thrombosis may be grouped as follows: (1) general — fever, headache, and malaise; with the formation of the infectious mural thrombus, the patient may have spiking fever and chills; (2) central nervous system — headache, papilledema, signs of increased intracranial pressure, altered states of consciousness, and seizures; (3) metastastic disease caused by infected thrombi and septic infarcts — pneumonia, septic infarcts, empyema, bone and joint infection, and, less commonly, thyroiditis, endocarditis, ophthalmitis, and abscess of the kidney (Rosenwasser, 1945); (4) spread to skin and soft tissues—cellulitis or abscess; and (5) signs of intracranial complications, including meningitis, cavernous sinus thrombosis, and brain abscess.

Bacteremia is frequent. In Rosenwasser's series of 100 patients published in 1945, the specific years of the cases are not mentioned, but only 19 patients received sulfonamides, so presumably most were evaluated prior to 1935. Bacteremia was frequent; 80 of 100 patients had presurgical cultures of the blood that were positive, and the cultures of 8 of 17 patients that were negative preoperatively were positive postoperatively. Bacteremia persisted after the operation in 36 cases for a median of 4 to 5 days and a range of 1 to 24 days. The predominant organism was beta-hemolytic streptococci (68 patients), with *S. pneumoniae* type 3 (3), Proteus sp. (2), *S. aureus* (1), and *P. aeruginosa* (1) also being found.

Computerized tomography is an invaluable aid in making the diagnosis and should precede a lumbar puncture. Variations in cerebrospinal fluid pressure occur and can be demonstrated by the Queckenstedt test, which measures changes in cerebrospinal fluid pressure with compression and release of the jugular vein. If the sinus is occluded, there is no rise in pressure when the jugular vein of the affected side is compressed, whereas compression of the contralateral jugular vein results in a brisk rise and fall in pressure. However, if the intracranial pressure is increased, the brain may herniate. In addition to this potential danger, the Queckenstedt test may be negative or inconclusive (Juselius and Kaltiokallio, 1972). There are usually no other abnormalities in the cerebrospinal fluid, although in some cases, leakage of red cells and subsequent xanthochromia may occur (Greer and Berk, 1963).

Management includes use of antimicrobial agents (as described in the section on mastoiditis in Chap. 17) and surgery. The administration of anticoagulant medication has also been advocated. The sinus should be uncovered, and any perisinuous abscesses should be drained. The lateral sinus should be opened and the thrombus removed. On rare occasions, the internal jugular vein may have to be ligated. For a complete description of the surgical technique, see Shambaugh and Glasscock (1980).

The mortality in the Rosenwasser series was 27 per cent, with an increased risk in patients over age 30. The mortality rate is still high and has been reported in a large series of cases to be between 10 and 40 per cent. Not much has changed with regard to mortality of this intracranial complication 40 years after the introduction of antimicrobial agents.

OTITIC HYDROCEPHALUS

The term "otitic hydrocephalus" was introduced by Symonds in 1931 to describe a syndrome of increased intracranial pressure but with no abnormalities of the cerebrospinal fluid complicating acute otitis media. The pathogenesis of the syndrome is unknown, but since the ventricles are not dilated, the term benign intracranial hypertension also seems appropriate. The disease is virtually always associated with lateral sinus thrombosis.

Symptoms include a headache that is often intractable, blurring of vision, nausea, vomiting, and diplopia. Signs include a draining ear, abducens paralysis of one or both lateral rectus muscles, and papilledema.

Computerized tomography must be performed prior to lumbar puncture to prevent brain herniation. When performed, the cerebrospinal fluid pressure is high, sometimes above 300 mm water, but protein, cells, and sugar concentrations are normal, and the ventricles are of normal or small size. Although thought of as benign, otitic hydrocephalus in some cases has proceeded to loss of vision secondary to optic atrophy.

Treatment includes use of antimicrobial agents and mastoidectomy. An aggressive surgical approach would appear to be warranted because of the possibility of optic atrophy.

TYPE AND TIMING OF OTOLOGIC SURGICAL INTERVENTION

In general, an aggressive approach to surgical management should be taken when a suppurative intracranial complication of otitis media and mastoiditis is present. If an acute or chronic middle ear effusion is present, an immediate tympanocentesis for culture of the middle ear effusion and myringotomy for drainage are mandatory. A tympanostomy tube should also be inserted to promote continued drainage of the middle ear and mastoid. The tympanostomy tube can be inserted even though a purulent middle ear effusion is present. If the tube is subsequently spontaneously extruded owing to profuse otorrhea, it can always be replaced if the perforation closes, but the insertion of a tympanostomy tube that remains in place will eliminate the need for subsequent myringotomies if the myringotomy incision heals during the course of the illness (when a tube is not inserted). There is no reason to withhold this procedure even in the critically ill child, since a tympanocentesis-myringotomy can be invaluable in the diagnosis and management of the infection, and if the child is toxic, the procedure can be performed without general anesthesia. The technique should include a culture of the ear canal followed by sterilization of the external ear canal prior to the tympanocentesis, since an unusual organism may be present (see Chap. 16, Tympanocentesis and Myringotomy, pp. 423 to 476).

When more extensive otologic surgery is required to eliminate the infection within the temporal bone, the timing of the surgical intervention will depend upon the status of the child. Ideally, the otologic surgery should be performed as soon as the diagnosis of intracranial complication is confirmed. However, this is frequently not possible, since the neurologic status of the patient or the presence of sepsis, or both, may make the child an anesthesia risk. For such cases, otologic surgical intervention may not be possible until the child's condition has stabilized. When neurosurgical intervention is required immediately, as when a brain abscess or subdural empyema is present, the otologic surgery can be performed at the same time if the child's condition is stable at the end of the neurosurgical procedure. However, if the patient's condition does not warrant prolonging the anesthesia, then the otologic surgery should be performed as soon as the child is able to tolerate a second surgical procedure. This usually is within a few days or a week but should not be delayed so long that the primary source of the infection is not controlled, as lack of control of the primary source of infection can interfere with the resolution of the intracranial infection or can even result in another intracranial complication.

The type of otologic surgical procedure chosen will depend on the type of pathologic process present. If acute mastoid osteitis is present, then a complete simple (cortical) mastoidectomy should be performed and a drain inserted into the mastoid cavity. The middle ear must also be drained, which may be accomplished by inserting a tympanostomy tube if a perforation is not present. If a subperiosteal abscess is present, a drain should also be used. If a child has an ear infection that has resulted in a suppurative intracranial complication, drainage of the mastoid may not be achieved by a myringotomy alone because of an aditus ad antrum obstruction, and, therefore, performance of a mastoidectomy should be considered in order to drain the infection; in these cases, the mastoidectomy is performed as an emergency procedure. Occasionally, when such an obstruction exists between the middle ear and the mastoid air cell system, the middle ear will be found to be free of effusion (as confirmed by a myringotomy), but the mastoid will be infected. In such cases, the mastoid infection must be drained as soon as possible.

When the suppurative intracranial infection is secondary to chronic suppurative otitis media, especially when a cholesteatoma is present, performance of a radical mastoidectomy is invariably indicated. A possible exception to this rule would be the incidental finding of extradural granulation tissue or an abscess during mastoid surgery to remove cholesteatoma. If an intratemporal complication is present, such as petrositis or labyrinthitis, definitive surgery must be performed. A search for a labyrinthine fistula, an extradural abscess, or extension of infection into the sigmoid sinus should always be part of the surgical procedure.

PREVENTION

The life-threatening complications of middle ear disease in children are relatively uncommon. Our goal should be to reduce the incidence of these complications still further by effective management of acute and chronic otitis media with effusion and prevention of chronic suppurative otitis media and cholesteatoma. Multiple factors may influence the extension of infection from the middle ear and mastoid to the intracranial cavity, such as the virulence of the bacteria, efficacy of antimicrobial therapy, defects in anatomy, altered host immunity, and surgical drainage. An impending complication may be prevented from developing into a life-threatening condition if tympanocentesis and myringotomy are performed to identify the causative organism and provide adequate drainage when children with acute otitis media have persistent or recurrent fever, otalgia, or other signs and symptoms of toxicity that are not responding to medical management. In such cases, the results of the culture from the middle ear effusion should guide the clinician in the selection of the appropriate antimicrobial agent. If persistent or recurrent discharge through a perforation is present, then a culture should be obtained by needle aspiration of the purulent material that is within the middle ear cavity. The antimicrobial agent chosen should be administered in a dose that is adequate by the route appropriate to prevent a suppurative complication.

In children who have had an episode of meningitis as a complication of acute otitis media, presence of a perilymphatic fistula (cerebrospinal fluid fistula) must be ruled out, especially if more than one episode of meningitis has occurred. The fistula may be in the area of the oval or round window, or both, and may be of congenital origin or may be due to an acquired defect (Grundfast and Bluestone, 1978). Suppurative labyrinthitis is usually present, and the fistula must be repaired to prevent recurrence of the intracranial complication. Acute mastoid osteitis and petrositis are other possible intratemporal complications of acute otitis media in which the infection may spread to the intracranial cavity. Early diagnosis and appropriate management of these conditions can prevent intracranial complications.

A suppurative complication should be suspected in children who have the signs and symptoms of acute infection or when preexisting chronic suppurative otitis media is present with or without a cholesteatoma. An acute exacerbation in a chronically infected ear may destroy bone and permit bacteria to enter the intracranial cavity. A persistent aural discharge may indicate the presence of this type of pathologic process.

In children who have chronic suppurative otitis media and in whom the discharge from the ear is persistent in spite of medical treatment, such as ototopical medication and orally administered antimicrobial agents, hospitalization may be required to provide more aggressive therapy. A parenterally administered antimicrobial agent may be necessary, depending upon the results of the culture of the discharge, and direct instillation through the tympanic membrane perforation of appropriate ototopical medication after thorough aspiration of the middle ear may be warranted. This procedure is best performed using the otomicroscope. If the suppurative process continues in spite of this type of medical management, then surgical intervention is indicated. Frequently, a cholesteatoma is found in the middle ear and possibly the mastoid, which could not be identified by inspection of the tympanic membrane even when visualized with the aid of the otomicroscope. Even if a cholesteatoma is not present, then middle ear and mastoid surgery is still indicated in such cases in order to drain the ear and decrease the possibility of further complications. Tympanoplasty surgery, which may be performed at the time of the initial procedure or as a second-stage operation, may be required to prevent subsequent episodes of discharge.

When a cholesteatoma is present, the diagnosis should be made as soon as possible, and surgery is indicated, since structural damage to the middle ear and mastoid is usually progressive and suppurative complications are an ever-present danger. The most important goals of surgery on such ears are complete eradication of the cholesteatoma (or its exteriorization), elimination of the infection, and prevention of potential intratemporal or intracranial complications. If these goals are met, the ear is "safe." Prolonged follow-up of children who have had cholesteatoma is mandatory, since recurrence is common. In patients who have had middle ear and mastoid surgery performed and in whom infection in the middle ear or mastoid cavity, or both, persists in spite of medical management, surgical intervention may again be necessary. In cases in which a radical mastoidectomy has been performed, the middle ear–mastoid discharge may be the result of reflux of nasopharyngeal secretions through a patent eustachian tube into the middle ear. Surgical closure of the middle ear end of the eustachian tube may be required to eliminate the reflux and chronic infection (see Chap. 17). Likewise, identification of an extradural abscess can prevent spread of the infection further into the intracranial cavity. During surgery, a thorough examination of the tegmen tympani should be performed, since such an abscess may be present as a result of cholesteatoma or infection, or both, being present in the area. If the cholesteatoma is in the area of the lateral semicircular canal, the possibility of a labyrinthine fistula must be ruled out. Juselius and Kaltiokallio (1972) reported that of 42 patients with labyrinthine fistulas, 5 had suppurative labyrinthitis and meningitis.

Antimicrobial agents have greatly reduced the incidence of intracranial complications of infections of the middle ear and mastoid, but the physician must remain alert to the possibility of an unusual event. In underdeveloped areas of the world, where availability of medical facilities is still limited, complications occur with significant morbidity and mortality (Raikundalia, 1975).

SELECTED REFERENCES

Alford, B. R., and Cohn, A. M. 1980. Complications of suppurative otitis media and mastoiditis. *In* Paparella, M. M., and Shumrick, D. A. (Eds.). Otolaryngology, Vol. 2. Philadelphia, W. B. Saunders Co., pp. 1490–1509.
The descriptions of the intracranial suppurative complications of otitis media are presented in a clear and concise manner.

Dawes, J. D. K. 1979. Complications of infections of the middle ear. *In* Ballantyne, J., and Groves, J. (Eds.). Diseases of the Ear, Nose, and Throat, 4th ed., Vol. 2. London, Butterworth and Co., pp. 305–384.
This section of an authoritative four-volume otolaryngology text contains a detailed description of the intracranial complications of otitis media by a clinician with extensive experience.

McCabe, B. F., Sade, J., and Abramson, M. (Eds.). 1977. Cholesteatoma: First International Conference. New York, Aesculapius Pub., pp. 420–437.
The papers presented at this meeting on the complications of cholesteatoma represent the current state of our knowledge.

Saunders, W. H., Paparella, M. M., and Miglets, A. W. 1980. Atlas of Ear Surgery, 3rd ed. St. Louis, The C. V. Mosby Co., pp. 164–219.
This atlas provides clear illustrations of otologic surgical procedures.

Schuknecht, H. F. 1974. Pathology of the Ear. Cambridge, MA, Harvard University Press, pp. 247–251.
This text has the best description of the pathology of intracranial suppurative complications of otitis media written for the otolaryngologist.

Shambaugh, G. E., and Glasscock, M. E. 1980. Surgery of the Ear, 3rd ed. Philadelphia, W. B. Saunders Co., pp. 289–326.
The description in this text of the otologic surgical techniques employed for patients with suppurative disease in the intracranial cavity is excellent.

Symon, L. (Ed.). 1979. Neurosurgery. *In* Rob, C., and Smith, R. (Eds.). Operative Surgery Series, 3rd ed. London, Butterworth and Co., Ltd., pp. 13–49, 330–340, 398–406.
This represents the current state of the art, as described in a textbook, of the neuroradiologic and neurologic surgical procedures employed for the suppurative intracranial complications of otitis media and related conditions.

REFERENCES

Beller, A. J., Sahar, A., and Praiss, I. 1973. Brain abscess: Review of 89 cases over a period of 30 years. J. Neurol. Neurosurg. Psychiatry, *36*:757–768.

Brewer, N. S., MacCarty, C. S., and Wellman, W. E. 1975. Brain abscess: A review of recent experience. Ann. Intern. Med., *82*:571–576.

Dawes, J. D. K. 1979. Complications of infections of the middle ear. *In* Ballantyne, J., and Groves, J. (Eds.). Scott-Brown's Diseases of the Ear, Nose, and Throat, 4th ed, Vol. 2. London, Butterworth and Co., Ltd., pp. 305–384.

du Boulay, G. H. 1979. Current practice in neurosurgical radiology. *In* Symon, L. (ed.). Neurosurgery. *In* Rob, C., and Smith, R. (Eds.). Operative Surgery Series, 3rd ed. London, Butterworth and Co., Ltd., pp. 13–45.

Feigin, R. D. 1981. Bacterial meningitis beyond the neonatal period. *In* Feigin, R. D., and Cherry, J. D. (Eds.). Textbook of Infectious Diseases, Vol. I. Philadelphia, W. B. Saunders Co., pp. 293–308.

Garfield, J. 1979. Intracranial abscess. *In* Symon, R. (Ed.). Neurosurgery. *In* Rob, C., and Smith, R. (Eds.). Operative Surgery Series, 3rd ed. London, Butterworth and Co., Ltd., p. 335.

Greer, M., and Berk, M. S. 1963. Lateral sinus obstruction and mastoiditis. Pediatrics, *31*:840–844.

Grundfast, K. M., and Bluestone, C. D. 1978. Sudden or fluctuating hearing loss and vertigo in children due to perilymph fistula. Ann. Otol. Rhinol. Laryngol., *87*:761–771.

Harding, A. L., Anderson, P., Howie, V. M., et al. 1973. *Hemophilus influenzae* isolated from children with otitis media. *In* Sell, S. H., and Karzon, D. T. (Eds.). *Hemophilus influenzae*. Nashville, TN, Vanderbilt University Press, pp. 21–28.

Heineman, H. S., and Braude, A. I. 1963. Anaerobic infection of the brain: Observations on eighteen consecutive cases of brain abscess. Am. J. Med., *35*:682–697.

Jeanes, A. 1962. Otogenic intracranial suppuration. J. Laryngol. Otol., *76*:388–402.

Juselius, H., and Kaltiokallio, K. 1972. Complications of acute and chronic otitis media in the antibiotic era. Acta Otolaryngol. (Stockh.), *74*:445–450.

Kessler, L., Dietzmann, K., and Krish, A. 1970. Beitrag zur otogenen meningitis. Z. Laryngol. Rhinol. Otol., *49*:93–100.

Krajina, Z. 1956. Observations on endocranial complications of the ear and sinuses in the era of antibiotics. Pract. Oto-rhino-laryngol, (Basel), *18*:1–22,

Lindsay, J. R. 1938. Suppuration in the petrous pyramid. Ann. Otol. Rhinol. Laryngol., *47*:3–36.

Liske, E., and Weikers, N. J. 1964. Changing aspects of brain abscesses: Review of cases in Wisconsin 1940 through 1962. Neurology, *14*:294–300.

McGreal, D. A. 1962. Brain abscess in children. Can. Med. Assoc. J., *86*:261–268.

Morgan, H., Wood, M. W., and Murphey, F. 1973. Experience with 88 consecutive cases of brain abscess. J. Neurosurg., *38*:698–704.

Proctor, C. A. 1966. Intracranial complications of otitic origin. Laryngoscope, *76*:288–308.

Raikundalia, K. B. 1975. Analysis of suppurative otitis media in children: Aetiology of non-suppurative otitis media. Med. J. Aust., *1*:749–750.

Ritter, F. N. 1977. Complications of cholesteatoma. *In* McCabe, B. F., Sade, J., and Abramson, M. (Eds).

Cholesteatoma: First International Conference. New York, Aesculapius Pub., pp. 430–437.

Rosenwasser, H. 1945. Thrombophlebitis of the lateral sinus. Arch. Otolaryngol., *41*:117–132.

Seid, A. B., and Sellars, S. L. 1973. The management of otogenic lateral sinus disease at Groote Schuur Hospital. Laryngoscope, *83*:397–403.

Selker, R. G. 1975. Intracranial abscess: Treatment by continuous catheter drainage. Child's Brain, *1*:368–375.

Shambaugh, G. E., and Glasscock, M. E. 1980. Surgery of the Ear, 3rd ed. Philadelphia, W. B. Saunders Co., pp. 302–312.

Sheehy, J. L., Brackmann, D. E., and Graham, M. D. 1977. Complications of cholesteatoma: A report on 1024 cases. *In* McCabe, B. F., Sade, J., and Abramson, M. (Eds.). Cholesteatoma: First International Conference. New York, Aesculapius Pub., pp. 420–429.

Symonds, C. P. 1931. Otitic hydrocephalus. Brain, *54*:55–71.

Tarkkanen, J., and Kohonen, A. 1970. Otogenic brain abscess. Arch. Otolaryngol., *91*:91–93.

Turner, A. L., and Reynolds, E. E. 1931. Intracranial Pyogenic Diseases. Edinburgh, Oliver and Boyd.

Chapter 19

DISEASES OF THE INNER EAR AND SENSORINEURAL DEAFNESS

Robert J. Ruben, M. D.

The diseases of the inner ear can become manifest at any time during childhood. There are, at the present time, no cures for these maladies; the physician can only prevent or care for them. This chapter will discuss the more common and serious of these diseases. The child's physician must know that the condition exists, and the best intervention is dependent on early detection and recognition of a hearing loss. All children affected can be significantly helped by the use of hearing aids and proper education, but unless the hearing loss is recognized, these interventions cannot be instituted. Lack of proper care for these children may condemn them to irreversible loss of language and other cognitive functions.

CLASSIFICATION OF SENSORINEURAL DEAFNESS

I. Congenital
   A. Genetic
   B. Acquired
      1. Infection
      2. Other teratogens, e.g., ototoxic drugs
   C. Unknown

II. Postnatal
   A. Genetic
   B. Acquired
      1. Infection
      2. Traumatic
      3. Ototoxic medication
      4. Other
   C. Unknown

Congenital sensorineural hearing loss is classified into those types that occur before birth and those that occur after birth. This is perhaps, in the area of genetic disease, an artificial nosology because the genetic diseases that phenotypically manifest themselves after birth really occur before birth. However, the differentiation between congenital and postnatal disease is important in terms of the management of the child. It is important to remember always that when etiology cannot be established, it also cannot be said that genetic disease has been ruled out. Many of the unknowns will, with further examination or in subsequent children in the same family, prove to be genetic.

CONGENITAL INNER EAR PROBLEMS

Pathoembryology

The histopathology of congenital sensorineural deafness can be divided into two groups: cases in which the bony labyrinth is normal and the neuroepithelium (organ of Corti) is abnormal (Fig. 19–1) and cases in which the bony labyrinth is abnormal and in which there may or may not be normal neuroepithelium (Fig. 19–2). These two types of histopathology have their bases in the development of the inner ear and also have

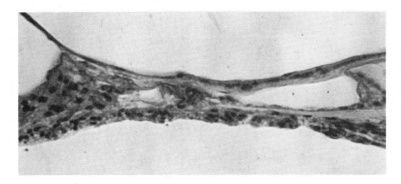

Figure 19–1 Degeneration of the organ of Corti in the temporal bone of a deaf patient. The organ of Corti, tectorial membrane, and nerve fibers are absent. The scala media is collapsed.

clinical consequences for the management of the patient.

The types of pathology in which there are major malformations of the bony labyrinth are rare and are most likely due to faulty induction of the inner ear. The primary inductor of the bony labyrinth is probably the developing central nervous system, as demonstrated by a number of experimental studies in amblystoma (Yntema, 1950) and mice (Deol, 1964). If there is an abnormality in the developing brain stem, it appears that this will result in an abnormal bony labyrinth. The operation of this principle has also been

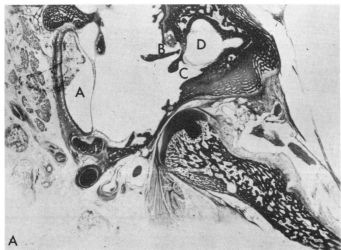

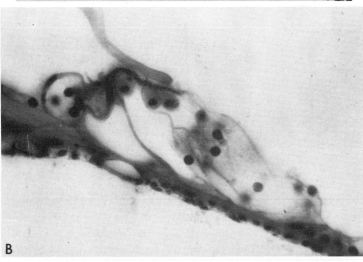

Figure 19–2 *A*, Cross-section through a malformed human temporal bone. The patient had an associated central nervous system malformation. On the left (A) are the external auditory canal and the tympanic membrane. On the right side of the picture is a large, sac-like cochlea (D) in which the round window (C) and the oval window can be seen. There is an abnormal columella-like stapes present (B). *B*, A higher power photomicrograph from the same specimen, part *A*, which shows the organ of Corti in this severely malformed cochlea. Note that three outer hair cells and an inner hair cell can be identified.

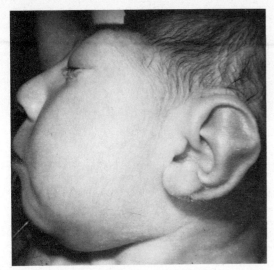

Figure 19–3 Anencephalic child. This patient had a bony labyrinthine abnormality diagnosed by radiography. The patient responded to sound.

observed in humans (Henke and Lubarsch, 1926). It would appear that human fetuses with anencephaly have abnormal bony labyrinths (Fig. 19–3), a condition that can be detected clinically by the use of various forms of radiography (Jensen, 1974). Faulty induction of the bony labyrinth by an abnormally developing central nervous system implies that if a child has an abnormally shaped bony labyrinth, he or she may also have an abnormal central nervous system. This clinical correlation appears to be most constant in children with severe labyrinthine malformations. Radiographic examination of the inner ear of a deaf neonate should lead the physician to suspect a malformation of the central nervous system and to perform appropriate studies. The prognosis for such a neonate may be guarded.

The second general type of inner ear histopathology is pathology of the sensory epithelium, most often evidenced by absence of the organ of Corti and pathologic changes in the membranous structures that surround the organ of Corti. The mechanism for this loss of hair cells has been considered to be either lack of development or degeneration. Four separate areas of observation indicate that lack of the organ of Corti is the result of premature cell death. The first, a study of the cell kinetics of the inner ear (Ruben, 1967b), showed that the organ of Corti is composed of end-state cells; i.e., after the cells are formed they are unable to reproduce them-

selves. Since the cells of the organ of Corti in humans are probably formed during the second month of intrauterine life, any loss of cells after this time would result in a hearing loss.

A second set of observations concerns the fact that malformations of the bony labyrinth still result in labyrinths with sensory epithelia (Fig. 19–2). Thus, even the most severely congenitally malformed ears will have sensory structures.

The third group of data comes from observations of the development of genetically determined sensorineural deafness in the cat (Bosher and Hallpike, 1966), mouse (Mikaelian and Ruben, 1965) and dog (Anderson et al., 1968). In all of these instances, hair cells are present during development, and they degenerate either before birth or sometime after birth (Fig. 19–4).

The last piece of evidence that indicates premature cell death as the probable cause of pathologic conditions of the organ of Corti is found in the few studies of human fetuses that had a high probability of being deaf, since they were infected with the rubella virus (Bordley et al., 1968). All of these fetuses were found to have sensory epithelia. The histopathology of rubella sensorineural deafness is well known and shows, among other findings, a lack of sensory cells (Schuknecht, 1974).

The evidence strongly indicates that an important mechanism for the lack of the organ of Corti in congenital sensorineural hearing loss is premature cell death. This is the most probable explanation of all sensory deafness that occurs after birth, including genetically determined deafness that comes about through acquired diseases of the inner ear.

Another aspect of developmental pathology of the inner ear with important clinical application is the effect of the loss of the organ of Corti and/or sound deprivation on the auditory pathways of the central nervous system. One of the earliest studies of this subject (Levi-Montalcini, 1949) showed that when the otocyst was removed from a chick embryo and the embryo was allowed to develop, there was a decrease in the number of the structures comprising the auditory pathways. These findings were restudied and expanded (Jackson and Rubel, 1976; Parks and Robinson, 1976). More recently (Webster and Webster, 1977) it has been shown that there

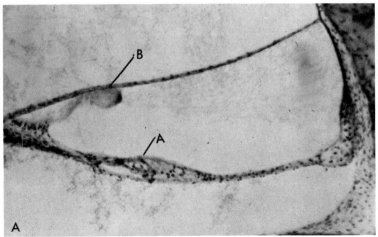

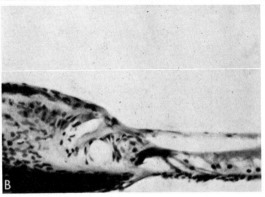

Figure 19–4 *A,* The organ of Corti of a Dalmatian puppy showing the beginning of the pathologic changes in the organ of Corti (A) and the scala media. The hair cells are present but appear abnormal. The tectorial membrane (B) is adherent to Reissner's membrane. *B,* Organ of Corti from a deaf, mature Dalmatian dog showing the end stage of degeneration of the organ of Corti and a collapsed scala media. The hair cells, nerve fibers, and tectorial membrane are absent.

will be structural changes in the central auditory pathways when destruction of the inner ear or sound deprivation occurs at later stages of development. Behavioral expressions of these probable anatomic changes in the central nervous system secondary to auditory deprivation have also been reported (Gottlieb, 1975; Riesen and Zilbert, 1975).

These observations have two clinical implications. The first is that very early loss of the organ of Corti, or of hearing, may induce anatomic changes in the central nervous system in humans. Thus, the normal development of the central nervous system may be impaired. Secondly, some of the central nervous system anatomic changes, with their subsequent behavioral deficits, may be ameliorated by the use of sound stimuli as early as possible. This supposition makes imperative the need for early detection and initiation of hearing aid therapy in deaf infants.

Etiology of Deafness

Determining the etiology of deafness in an individual has particular utility in the man-

agement of the patient and his or her family, as will be discussed later in this section. At the present time, it is felt that of all congenital deafness, about 50 per cent is due to acquired disease, 15 per cent is due to autosomal dominant inheritance, 34 per cent is due to autosomal recessive inheritance, and 1 per cent is due to X-linked inheritance. When these percentages are based on actual observations of patients, they may include a group of cases, amounting to 40 per cent of the total, in which the etiology is unknown (Ruben and Rozycki, 1971). It has been suggested (Fraser, 1976) that most of the unknown cases are probably due to autosomal recessive inheritance.

Genetic Deafness

There are more than 70 different genetic syndromes associated with congenital sensorineural deafness. These have been catalogued and described (Fraser, 1976; Konigsmark and Gorlin, 1976; McKusick, 1966), and most of them are very rare. The most common or important of the genetically de-

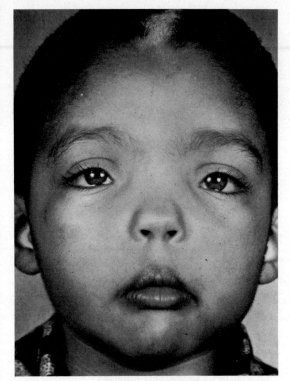

Figure 19–5 This patient is profoundly deaf in both ears, has a white forelock, an increased intercanthal distance, and an antimongoloid slant of both eyes. The patient's family members show other stigmata of the Waardenburg syndrome.

termined sensorineural deafnesses found in humans are Waardenburg syndrome (a dominant gene) and the Jervell and Lange-Nielsen, Pendred, and Usher syndromes (gene recessive). There are also dominant, recessive, and X-linked genetically transmitted diseases that have no other signs or symptoms than deafness.

Waardenburg syndrome (Fig. 19–5) was first described by Waardenburg (1951). This syndrome is transmitted as an autosomal dominant, and it is felt to be responsible for approximately 1 to 2 per cent of all cases of congenital deafness (Fraser, 1976). The description of the syndrome includes six features: (1) lateral development of the internal canthi with dystrophia of the lacrimal punctum and horizontal shortening of the palpebral fissures; (2) a prominent, broad, nasal root; (3) hypertrichosis of the eyebrows; (4) white forelock; (5) heterochromia of the irides; and (6) sensorineural deafness, either total or subtotal. Since the syndrome was identified, several other associated features have been defined, including a cleft lip, cleft palate, or both, and high-arched palate (Fisch,

1959); patchy depigmentation of the skin that can best be seen under ultraviolet light; changes in iris pigmentation in one eye during the first year of life (Settlemayer and Hogan, 1961); absent vestibular response (Stoller, 1962); pigmentary heterochromia of the fundus (Goldberg, 1966); and disappearance of the white forelock after the first year of life (Hansen et al., 1965). The syndrome has been found throughout the world and in all races, and the expression of this dominant gene is quite variable. A study of 523 affected individuals in 81 families (Parithe and Cohen, 1971) demonstrates some of the variability of expressivity (Table 19–1). These data were derived from patients who were suspected of having this syndrome and who had profound sensorineural hearing losses. It can be seen that, of the group of families, 44 per cent had profound sensorineural hearing losses and 9 per cent had partial hearing losses. These partial hearing losses included unilateral hearing losses.

The diagnosis of Waardenburg syndrome can be made by observing any of the stigmata of the syndrome in the propositi or the family. Dystrophic canthi and an abnormal intercanthal distance are two of the most common expressions of this syndrome. An excellent table of interpupillary distance in various racial groups and at various ages has been compiled by Pryor (1969) and helps to determine the normality of this factor. A difference in color of the irides should not be confused with heterochromia, which results from lesions of the cervical sympathetics (Calhoun, 1919).

Table 19–1 VARIABILITY OF EXPRESSIVITY OF WAARDENBURG SYNDROME[*]

Finding	Incidence
Dystrophic canthus	83
Hypertelorism	17
Laterally displaced lacrimal punctum	59
Dacrocystitis	19
Broad nasal root	68
Hyperplasia of eyebrows	57
Heterochromia of iris	51
White forelock (poliosis)	48
Vitiligo	16
Premature graying of hair	33
Congenital deafness, profound	44
Congenital deafness, partial	9
Cleft lip and palate	10
High, arched palate	27

[*]From Parithe, O. A., and Cohen, M. M. J., 1971.

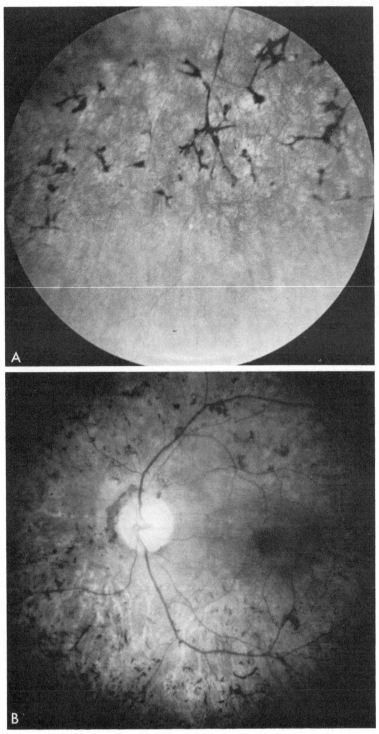

Figure 19–6 *A*, The retina of a patient with Usher disease (retinitis pigmentosa) at the onset of the visual deficits. *B*, The retina of a patient with Usher disease in its late stage. (Courtesy of Dr. Paul Henkind, Professor of Ophthalmology, Albert Einstein College of Medicine and the Montefiore Hospital and Medical Center of New York.)

It is felt (Fraser, 1976) that the degree of penetrance for profound congenital sensorineural deafness in Waardenburg syndrome is about 0.20 and that the mutation rate for this syndrome is about 0.5 per 100,000 gametes. There is a possible linkage of the Waardenburg gene to the ABO gene (Simpson et al., 1974).

The histopathology of one case of Waardenburg syndrome has been reported (Fisch, 1959) to show a normal bony labyrinth, lack of the organ of Corti and spiral ganglion cells, and atrophy of the stria vascularis. The vestibular labyrinth was normal.

Usher disease (retinitis pigmentosa) was first described in 1858 by Von Graefe. This disease is transmitted as an autosomal recessive and is felt to be responsible for approximately 4 per cent of congenital deafness cases (Fraser, 1976). The syndrome consists of congenital sensorineural deafness, progressive retinitis pigmentosa, night blindness and tunnel vision, cataracts, vestibular impairment, mental retardation, psychosis, spinocerebellar ataxia, and nystagmus (Hallgren, 1959; Nuutila, 1970). Additionally, a decrease in olfaction (Vernon, 1969) and an increased incidence of branchial cleft cysts (Kloepfer et al., 1966) have been noted in these patients. The retinal findings show granular accumulations of pigment that begin at the optic fundus and extend toward the periphery (Fig. 19–6). Although these symptoms are due to an autosomal recessive gene, there is a significant amount of variability in the expression of the gene (Table 19–2). It appears that most but not all of the individuals homozygotic for Usher disease have a severe to profound sensorineural hearing loss, although some may have only a mild to moderate hearing loss, and there is

one report in which the hearing loss was progressive (Sirles and Slasghts, 1943). The retinal signs and symptoms are progressive throughout life. Nuutila (1970) showed that night blindness is the first retinal sign in 92 per cent of cases and will be evident before the age of 10. At the end of the second decade of life, 2 in 63 people will be blind, 5 in 63 will have tunnel vision, and 34 in 63 will have decreased visual acuity.

The diagnosis of retinitis pigmentosa can be made early in life with an ophthalmoscope or by means of electroretinography (Vernon, 1969). An infant born with sensorineural hearing loss for which there is no definite etiology should be examined with the ophthalmoscope and, if available, by electroretinography. If electroretinography is not available and if there is no history of retinitis pigmentosa, routine fundoscopic examinations should be made throughout the first two decades of life. It is very important to determine whether or not the patient will lose his or her vision, because if the patient is deaf and will then lose his or her vision, special habilitative intervention must be initiated. It is also important for the parents to be aware that they are carrying the gene. The use of electroretinography and audiology has enabled the retrospective identification of some of the heterozygote carriers of the syndrome (Kloepfer et al., 1970). These techniques for identification of heterozygote carriers should be undertaken in all members of the family to determine the carriers of the disease.

The high prevalence of mental retardation and psychosis in this syndrome has, in part, been accounted for by abnormal electroencephalograms and pneumoencephalograms (Nuutila, 1970). Some of the psychoses may be the result of the extreme sensory depriva-

Table 19–2 INCIDENCE OF DEFECTS IN 177 INDIVIDUALS WITH RETINITIS PIGMENTOSA AND 304 NONAFFECTED SIBLINGS IN 102 FAMILIES*

Sign or Symptom	Number	Per Cent
Glaucoma	3/88	3
Nystagmus	11/158	7
Profound to severe deafness	155/177	88
Moderate to severe deafness	22/177	12
Vestibular impairment**	6/7	86
Mental deficiency	41/172	24
Psychosis	26/113	23

*From Hallgren, B., 1959.
**This testing was carried out in children with gait impairment by caloric testing.

tion occurring with both deafness and blindness.

The histopathology of retinitis pigmentosa was reported by Belal (1975). This report showed that degeneration of the organ of Corti and spiral ganglion cells, mainly in the basal turn, occurs in patients with this disease, although the remainder of the inner ear structures were not noticeably diseased. An earlier report (Nager, 1927) described marked degeneration of the organ of Corti and supporting structures, including the stria vascularis in the basal turn, with retinitis pigmentosa. The saccular and vestibular apparatuses were abnormal, and atrophy was noted in the primary auditory portion of the central nervous system in the ears studied.

The *Jervell and Lange-Nielsen syndrome* involves autosomal recessive sensorineural deafness (Jervell and Lange-Nielsen, 1957). This syndrome consists of hearing impairment associated with syncopal episodes and sudden death. It is one of the genetic syndromes that must be detected early, as there are efficacious interventions to preserve the life of the patient.

The frequency of this disease is variable, perhaps depending upon the thoroughness of the diagnostic workup of the population and the early death of affected individuals. It is felt that the variability of symptoms and frequency of early death may account for a number of crib deaths in families in which there are other affected members. It is estimated that the frequency may be as high as 1 in 1 million births or 1 per cent of the deaf population (Fraser et al., 1964b). Another survey in Canada (Fay et al., 1971) showed an incidence of about 1 in 1000 deaf children or 0.1 per cent of severely hearing impaired patients. The syndrome has been reported to have a wide geographic distribution in North America, Western Europe, and India (Fraser, 1976). It presents as severe congenital sensorineural hearing loss; the average hearing levels for nine cases were 125 Hz, 60 dB; 250 Hz, 65 dB; 500 Hz, 75 dB; 1000 Hz, 85 dB; 2000 Hz, 100 dB; 2000 Hz, no response; 4000 Hz, no response; and 8000 Hz, no response (Fraser et al., 1964a). The ECG anomalies (Fraser et al., 1964a) are large T waves, and the QT interval may not be too prolonged. The QT interval has also been found to vary among and within individuals. The most marked feature of the syndrome is the syncopal episodes, which

may begin in the second to third year of life or earlier. They may last from five to ten minutes and can vary in frequency from one per day to one per year or less often. Without therapy, approximately half of the patients die before the age of 15.

The cardiac abnormalities that appear to result in death can be treated, if diagnosed. There are at least two reports of the effectiveness of propranolol in treating this syndrome. Olley and Fowler (1970) stated that during a syncopal attack, the electrocardiogram shows asystole, followed by ventricular tachycardia, which can lead to ventricular fibrillation. The latter would respond to defibrillation. They recommended that patients with the Jervell and Lange-Nielsen syndrome be given 5 mg of propranolol each day and also discussed the use of phenobarbital in these patients. It is apparent that all patients with either idiopathic sensorineural hearing loss or autosomal recessive disease in which a specific syndrome has not been identified should have at least one electrocardiogram. One series (Fay et al., 1971) found that there were 28 abnormal electrocardiograms in a population of 1126 severely to profoundly deaf children. The 27 cases included one with the Jervell and Lange-Nielsen syndrome, four with a prolonged QT interval that was not as long as those found in the Jervell and Lange-Nielsen syndrome, five with wandering pacemakers and a predominant sinus rhythm, one with an A-V nodal rhythm, two with first-degree heart block, three with an occasional ectopic ventricular premature beat, one with Wolff-Parkinson-White type B pattern, and ten with isolated QRS frontal axis abnormalities.

The possibility of identifying heterozygote carriers by means of a prolonged QT interval has been suggested (Fraser et al., 1964b; Sanchez-Cascos et al., 1969). This technique may have its limitations, and there are some suggestions that the QT interval may normalize in the young adult (James, 1967), but this has not been proved, and the usefulness of identifying heterozygotic carriers is so great that it appears advisable for relatives of known patients with the Jervell and Lange-Nielsen syndrome to have an electrocardiogram.

The histopathology of both the inner ear and the heart in this syndrome has been described (Fraser et al., 1964a; Friedmann et al., 1966). The bony labyrinth is normal, the organ of Corti shows degeneration in all turns with a decrease in the number of spiral ganglion cells, and there are large periodic acid–Schiff (PAS) hyaline deposits in a partially atrophic stria vascularis. The macula of the utricle and the three cristae show degeneration and PAS-positive hyaline nodules. The cardiac findings reveal hypertrophy of the tunica intima of the artery of the sino-atrial node, infarction of the sinoatrial node with fibrosis, a marked decrease in the perinuclear clear zone of Purkinje's fibers, and abnormalities of the A-V node; the parasympathetic ganglia near the nodes were noted to be hemorrhagenic and appeared to be degenerating.

Pendred disease is an autosomal recessive form of sensorineural deafness associated with goiter, first described in 1896 by Pendred. The diagnosis of this disease was further advanced in 1958 by Morgans and Trotter by the use of the perchlorate test, which showed an abnormal organification of non-organic iodine. The disease is found throughout the world (Fraser, 1976) and may account for deafness in from 1 to 7 per cent of severely to profoundly deaf children (Thould and Scowen, 1964). This author's experience has not confirmed the high frequency, but this may be due to the difference in populations examined.

This disease is clearly inherited as an autosomal recessive, with some variability of expressivity of the effect of the gene in the homozygote. The hearing loss is sensorineural and is usually static, but there have been observations of possible progression (Fraser, 1976). The hearing loss is usually severe to profound, mainly affecting the high tones, but there may be some cases of unilateral hearing loss and others in which significant hearing may remain. Thould and Scowen (1964), after reviewing the audiograms of 23 patients with Pendred disease, stated that 1 of 23 had no response; 12 of 23 were very severely deaf; 8 of 23 were less severely deaf; and 2 of 23 had low levels of hearing. Vestibular responses are quite variable in these patients.

The goiters will usually be apparent before the age of eight and in some instances may be found at birth (Thould and Scowen, 1964). The patients are usually eurythyroid (Fraser, 1976; Thould and Scowen, 1964). It has been found that the goiter in this syndrome is not associated with cancer and is easily treated with exogenous thyroid hormone. Many patients have undergone multiple and partial thyroidectomies, and the goiter has returned (Smith, 1960). It is felt from a review of the literature that in almost all cases a total or partial thyroidectomy is contraindicated.

Fraser (1976) feels that the frequency of the allele in this disease is approximately 0.008 and that the mutation rate may be 56/1,000,000 loci per gamete (Fraser, 1965a). It has also been noted (Fraser, 1965a) that heterozygotes may show a decrease in protein-bound iodine. Statistically this decrease in the protein-bound iodine is significant at the 2 per cent level.

A set of temporal bones from a patient who may have had Pendred disease has been reported (Hvidberg-Hansen and Jorgensen, 1968). The patient had recurrent goiter and an abnormal perchlorate test. The family history is suggestive of Pendred disease but not pathognomonic, and study of sections of the abnormal thyroids showed findings consistent with but not pathognomonic for Pendred disease. Temporal bone histopathologic studies indicated that the cochlea contained only two turns and that the neuro-epithelium of the cochlea and the spiral ganglion cells was absent. The macula was normal, but periotic connective tissue was found with ossification of the endosteum of the labyrinthine wall.

Pathologic conditions of the thyroid consisted of colloid tissue, and there was fibrous scarring of the nodules in all 14 cases studied; epithelial proliferation was a dominant feature in 9 of the cases, while there were focal areas of proliferation in five cases and occasional focal calcifications (Smith, 1960).

There are a number of congenital sensorineural deafness syndromes that are inherited by autosomal recessive, autosomal dominant, or X-linked mechanisms and in which there are no other associated stigmata (Konigsmark and Gorlin, 1976). These cases may account for 16 per cent of the total population of those who suffer congenital sensorineural deafness. Of this 16 per cent, approximately 66 per cent inherited the disorder by a dominant gene, 33 per cent inherited the gene recessively, and in less than 1 per cent of these cases was the deafness sex-linked (Ruben and Rozycki, 1971).

There were two reports of dominantly inherited sensorineural hearing loss without stigmata as early as 1883 and 1898 (Bell,

1969; Fay, 1898). However, even before the acceptance of mendelian genetics, there was an appreciation of the inheritance of deafness that was clinically characterized by consanguinity or familial deafness (Wilde, 1853). The incidence of congenital sensorineural deafness without stigmata has been reported for different populations throughout the world, and there are several aspects of these inherited forms of sensorineural deafness that should be noted. The first is the variability of penetrance in those with a dominant form of transmission; it appears that unilateral sensorineural deafness represents incomplete penetrance of a dominant gene for sensorineural hearing loss (Smith, 1939). Everberg (1960) found that about 25 per cent of unilateral sensorineural deafness was genetic and that the family members of these individuals suffered varying degrees of sensorineural hearing loss.

X-linked sensorineural hearing loss has frequently been reported (Sataloff et al., 1955). Fraser (1965b) points out that X-linked inheritance with the appearance of the disease in the male may account for the greater percentage of males than females with severe to profound congenital sensorineural hearing loss. It is of interest to note that Wilde (1853) also found a higher percentage of deaf males than females in all of the populations he studied. X-linked inheritance contributes to the difficulty of making a correct genetic diagnosis, since families at the present time are usually small, and many times there may be no further pregnancies after a deaf child is born. In families with only one male child who is deaf, the possibility of X-linked inheritance must be considered when there is no other diagnosis. Fraser (1965b) estimates that this form of inheritance could account for 6.2 per cent of deafness in males and 3.2 per cent of the congenitally sensorineurally deaf population.

The diagnosis of genetically transmitted sensorineural deafness without associated stigmata can be made if there are (1) two or more siblings affected, (2) a consanguinous marriage, (3) a family history of sensorineural deafness, and (4) audiometric indications of sensorineural hearing loss that cannot be attributed to another cause in relatives of the deaf child (Johnsen, 1952).

The preceding are only some of the most common of the genetic diseases that result in congenital sensorineural hearing loss. Other defined syndromes, when aggregated, account for a larger number of the cases.

Acquired Congenital Diseases

There are two major perinatal types of acquired sensorineural hearing loss. The first is from the ingestion of various ototoxic and teratogenous substances, thalidomides being the best known of the latter group. Maternal ingestion of streptomycin during pregnancy has been found to cause sensorineural hearing loss in the fetus (Robinson and Cambon, 1964); quinine and chloroquine phosphate are also thought to cause congenital sensorineural hearing loss (Fraser, 1976).

The second major cause of acquired congenital sensorineural hearing loss is intrauterine infection. Syphilis, toxoplasmosis, and possibly cytomegalic inclusion disease are relatively infrequent causes of infection, whereas the most common cause of acquired congenital sensorineural hearing loss is maternal infection with rubella. Congenital rubella infection as a cause of congenital sensorineural hearing loss was first reported in 1943 (Swan et al.), although perhaps the earliest cases of probable rubella deafness were described by Wardrop in 1813. Fetuses that have been infected with the rubella virus will exhibit a constellation of abnormal findings, and the earlier the infection occurs in intrauterine life, the more severe the effects tend to be. Manifestation of the syndrome varies not only with each child but also in different populations, depending upon both the susceptibility of the population and the variability of the virus. Table 19–3 summarizes some of the findings in a group of 41 Australian patients aged 5 to 19 years whose mothers contracted rubella during pregnancy.

Congenital rubella may be diagnosed by means of physical examination and immunologic techniques. The most common and consistent finding is the clumped pigmentary retinitis that may or may not be associated with cataracts (Fig. 19–7). Other abnormal findings are microcephaly, intrauterine growth retardation, jaundice, and lesions of the long bones. Any mother with a history of a rash during pregnancy or who may have been exposed to rubella should be considered as possibly having had a rubella infection. It has been suggested that all pregnant women have rubella titers taken routinely at the

Table 19–3 FREQUENCY OF RUBELLA-INDUCED
ABNORMALITIES IN 41 CHILDREN°

Defects	Number	Per Cent
Ocular defects	37	90
Deafness	31	76
Congenital heart disease	15	37
Central nervous system involvement	13	32
Low birth weight	17	41
Neonatal difficulties	14	34
Skeletal defects	27	66
Small stature	22	54
Dental defects	16	39
Dermatoglyphic changes	18	44

°From Forrest, J. M., and Menser, M. A. 1970.

beginning of their pregnancies and that follow-up titers be taken as pregnancy progresses (Ruben, 1970). The results of testing an infant for an increase in rubella titers can be misleading, but the presence of rubella-specific IgM antibodies in the cord, the mother's, or the infant's serum during the first six months of life is diagnostic of congenital rubella (Forrest and Menser, 1975), although the test may not discover all cases of congenital rubella. The diagnosis of congenital rubella in older children may be difficult, as they may have been infected with a wild type of virus or vaccinated. If children over

two years of age with a low rubella antibody titer do not respond to vaccine, they may have had rubella congenitally (Cooper et al., 1971). A rubella antibody titer should be obtained from all patients and their mothers when etiology for the congenital sensorineural hearing loss cannot be established, unless the child has been immunized with the rubella vaccine.

The hearing loss found in congenital rubella is predominantly sensorineural in nature. Most of the patients will have severe to profound sensorineural hearing losses, although the loss might be different for each ear

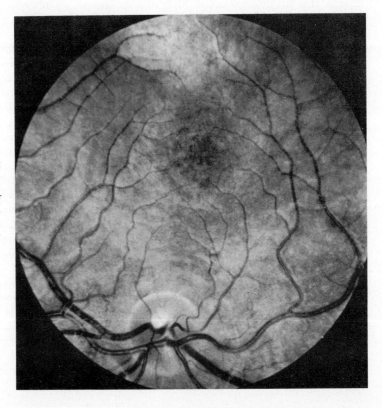

Figure 19–7 The retina of a patient with congenital rubella who has typical "salt and pepper" retinitis. (Courtesy of Dr. Paul Henkind, Professor of Ophthalmology, Albert Einstein College of Medicine and the Montefiore Hospital and Medical Center of New York.)

(Bordley et al., 1968). Other patients will have a lesser loss, and in some cases the hearing loss may be progressive (Alford, 1968; Bordley and Alford, 1970). The hearing loss may also be conductive, owing either to a fixed stapes (Richards, 1964) or to serous otitis media, which is consistent with the frequent finding of a high-arched palate in these patients. The presence of progressive and conductive middle ear disease emphasizes the need for constant audiometric and impedance monitoring of all patients with deafness due to congenital rubella.

Another aspect of the rubella syndrome is that a number of patients have been reported to have significant language retardation (Weinberger et al., 1970) without an associated hearing loss. The possibility exists that some cases of language impairment may be attributed to mild or moderate sensorineural hearing loss, a fluctuating conductive hearing loss, or both.

The variability of findings in cases of congenital rubella is thought to have a possible genetic basis. Both Fraser (1976) and Anderson et al. (1970) have reported data indicating that there is an increased incidence of sensorineural hearing loss, secondary to rubella, in families with a genetic predisposition to sensorineural hearing loss. The hypothesis is that the predisposition to deafness is increased by the presence of both etiologic factors.

Vaccination for rubella is widespread in the United States at present, but the program could be expanded, as it was estimated that in 1975, 19 per cent of children 5 to 9 years of age were not immune to rubella, accounting for not less than 16,000 new cases of rubella in 1975 (Salisbury and Ma, 1976). New cases of congenital sensorineural hearing loss resulting from intrauterine rubella infection may still present to the physician, who must consider this possible etiology in any differential diagnosis of congenital sensorineural hearing loss.

The ears of patients who suffered congenital rubella infection show a normal bony labyrinth, degeneration of the organ of Corti, granulation at the junction of the stria vascularis and Reissner's membrane and collapse of the saccule (Bordley and Alford, 1970; Friedmann, 1974; Michaels, 1964). All of these findings are not the same in each case and reflect the clinical variability of the hearing losses found in these patients.

Genetic Counseling

Auditory habilitation must be instituted as soon as possible for each patient with congenital sensorineural hearing loss. The physician must also be able to offer the family guidance concerning the risks of having other deaf children. The previous paragraphs have stressed the need for exact delineation of the etiology of the hearing loss, although when this is done in a clinical setting about 40 per cent of the cases will not be found to have a known cause. In all of these "idiopathic" cases, the relatives should be further examined, a review of the family history should be made, and a search for consanguinity, physical examination of the family members for the stigmata of known genetic syndromes, and audiometric examination of the family members should be performed. The audiometric examination appears to be the best, albeit a far from satisfactory, way to detect heterozygotes in recessive disease and partial penetrance in dominant disease (Deraemaeker, 1960; Anderson and Wedenberg, 1968). The age of the parents must also be taken into account, as children born to older parents may be affected through new, dominant mutations (Fraser, 1976).

The risk in proved cases of autosomal dominant deafness of having other children with the same problem is 50 per cent; for having other children with autosomal recessive deafness, the risk is 25 per cent. Those cases of deafness for which there is no known etiology must be presumed to be genetic, either dominant, recessive, or X-linked. The possibility of having another affected child in such a family is greater than 1 in 1000 and less than 1 in 2 or 1 in 4, depending upon the mode of transmission of the deafness (Fraser, 1976). Some probable recurrence rates, based on a number of different factors, have been calculated by Fraser (1976), who states that the overall risk of deafness for another child is approximately 10 per cent, a figure that varies according to the birth order. For the first child born after an affected sibling, the risk of recurrence is 12.5 per cent; the recurrence risk for the second child is 10 per cent; for the third child it is 7.5 per cent; and for the fourth child it is 5 per cent. These figures, although they are only estimations, are very useful in informing parents of the risks of having other affected children.

POSTNATAL DEAFNESS

There are no adequate data on the frequency of postnatal sensorineural hearing loss in children, although it is a common clinical finding. Many of the children have a moderate to severe hearing loss, not severe to profound. Thus, the diagnosis may be delayed, and the presenting problems, especially in a younger child, may not be recognized. The importance of early diagnosis of postnatal sensorineural hearing loss is twofold. First, a habilitation program should be instituted so that the child's auditory ability will be improved. This is even more important in the progressive types of sensorineural hearing loss. If the deficit is recognized early, habilitation may be instituted before the sensorineural hearing loss becomes profound, and the child will have the advantage of a period of auditory learning while there is still useful hearing. The second major reason why early diagnosis is important is that a number of sensorineural hearing losses are associated with life-threatening diseases for which effective medical and surgical interventions are available. The hearing loss may be the first clinical symptom of these disease states.

Genetic Causes of Deafness

There are over 30 different genetically determined syndromes in which sensorineural hearing loss is involved, either wholly or in part, most of which are characterized by progressive sensorineural hearing loss.

Alport disease, probably the most common of these, is an inherited condition that consists of progressive sensorineural hearing loss and progressive nephritis. It was first described in 1927 by Alport and is one of a series of genetically transmitted renal diseases associated with sensorineural hearing loss. The disease has been found throughout the world and in many different racial groups.

Some of the other syndromes in which genetic sensorineural hearing losses are associated with renal disease are hypertension, renal failure, abnormal steroidogenesis, hypogenitalism, and sensorineural deafness; Charcot-Marie-Tooth syndrome with nephritis and sensorineural deafness; macrothrombocytopathia, nephritis, and sensorineural deafness; infantile renal tubular acidosis and congenital sensorineural deafness; adolescent or young adult renal tubular acidosis and slowly progressive sensorineural deafness; renal disease, hyperprolinuria, ichthyosis, and sensorineural deafness; and nephritis, urticaria, amyloidosis, and sensorineural deafness.

Alport disease is more severe in males than in females, although the symptoms are variable in a given patient. Conditions characteristic of Alport disease include hematuria, pyuria, uremia, sensorineural hearing loss, and ocular pathology (consisting of myopia, cataracts, lenticonus, and spherophakia). The age of onset of sensorineural hearing loss is usually after the first decade of life, although the renal symptoms have been found, retrospectively, in infants and have been characterized by the appearance of a "red diaper" as a consequence of the hematuria. If the disease is untreated, affected males usually die by the third decade of life. Females usually have a longer or normal life span but will have toxemia during pregnancy. The advanced renal lesions can be noted by an intravenous pyelogram that shows atrophy, a lobulated kidney, or both. Occasionally there may be ureteral abnormalities.

The possibility of Alport disease should be considered in any child with a sensorineural hearing loss of recent onset, regardless of sex. Urinalysis and either a serum creatinine or blood urea nitrogen level should be obtained. More than three red blood cells or five white cells per high power field, or protein in the urine, is considered abnormal.

The hearing loss characteristic of Alport disease progresses with age, as demonstrated by the data of Cassidy et al. (1965) (Table 19–4). The sensorineural hearing loss is pre-

Table 19–4 FREQUENCY OF SENSORINEURAL HEARING LOSS IN ALPORT DISEASE*

Age (Years)	Per Cent With Significant Hearing Loss	
	Male	*Female*
0–19	25	10
20–39	74	33
40–59	64	55
>60	86	83

*From Cassidy, G., Brown, K., Cohen, M., and DeMaria, W. 1965.

dominant in the higher frequencies, showing characteristics of a cochlear lesion (positive short increment sensitivity index [SISI], recruitment, and a lack of tone decay). There appears to be some direct correlation between the severity of the hearing loss and the severity of the renal disease. Patients seldom have more than a severe hearing loss and can usually be helped significantly with a hearing aid. There are two reports that have shown an improvement in the hearing levels of patients with Alport disease after renal dialysis or renal transplantation (Johnson et al., 1976; Mitschke et al., 1975).

The ocular abnormalities occurring in Alport disease are important in that, as in Usher disease and congenital rubella, there is a possibility that the patient may have impairment of two sensory modalities, hearing and vision. Ocular defects, as reported by Faggioni et al. (1972), can occur in 23 per cent of the cases and are four times more frequent in males than in females. They involve the lens in 14 per cent of patients, and lenticonus is a feature in 6 per cent, cataracts in 7 per cent, and spherophakia in 1 per cent of patients.

The classic forms of mendelian inheritance do not explain the inheritance of Alport disease: There is a propensity for sons of affected mothers to be more affected than sons of affected fathers (Preus and Fraser, 1971). The most tenable hypothesis at this time to explain the transmission of Alport disease is that it is an autosomal dominant with decreased penetrance in sons of affected fathers. Table 19–5 presents the risks of renal failure developing in the offspring of affected parents: Renal failure will develop in about 50 per cent of sons and daughters of affected females, in about 50 per cent of daughters of affected males, and in 13 per cent of sons of affected males.

Table 19-5 RISKS OF DEVELOPMENT OF MICROSCOPIC SIGNS OF KIDNEY DISEASE FOR OFFSPRING OF PARENTS WITH SYMPTOMS OF ALPORT DISEASE°

Affected Parent	Sons	Daughters
Mother	42	45
Father	13	53

° From Preus, M., and Fraser, F. G. 1971.

The disease can also be transmitted by an apparently asymptomatic parent, although it is probable that with a more precise definition of the phenotype the asymptomatic parents can be shown to be affected. Inheritance of Alport disease by the offspring of asymptomatic parents follows the same pattern as inheritance from symptomatic parents.

The histopathology of the ears and kidneys in Alport disease has often been reported; there was no consistent temporal bone pathology, although in all cases the middle ears and bony labyrinths were normal. The pathology in four pairs of temporal bones ranged from minor changes in the macula (Fujita and Hayden, 1969) to degeneration of the organ of Corti, atrophy of the spiral ligament, and foam cells in the endolymphatic sac (Crawfurd and Toghill, 1968). Fujita and Hayden (1969) reported on a number of patients who suffered severe sensorineural hearing loss as evidenced on audiograms; even though in another instance the patient had had good cochlear microphonics and acoustic nerve action potentials, as recorded from the round window, he had a significant high-frequency hearing loss with a speech reception threshold of 40 dB (Ruben, 1967a).

The renal lesions occurring in Alport disease have been examined by light and electron microscopy (Kaufman et al., 1970; Spear and Gussen, 1972) and show thickening of the basement membrane of the glomerulus, flocculent precipitates in the basilar membrane, extrinsic thickening of the lamina densa, focal sclerosis, interstitial fibrosis (which was progressive in serially studied cases), interstitial infiltration, centrolobular proliferation, epithelial proliferation, glomerular hyalinization, tubular atrophy, and a variable appearance of foam cells, both within and between patients. There also appears to be a decrease in the dense deposits in the glomeruli that is correlated with a decrease in immunoglobulins.

Hicks disease: There are more than 15 different genetic diseases that have central and peripheral nervous system degeneration associated with progressive sensorineural hearing loss (Konigsmark and Gorlin, 1976). Hicks disease—sensory radicular neuropathy and sensorineural deafness—has been reported to be associated with sensorineural hearing loss developing in the second decade (Fitzpatrick et al., 1976) and now must be considered to be one of the progressive sensorineural disease syndromes of childhood.

Refsum disease, consisting of retinitis pigmentosa, hypertrophic peripheral neuropathy, motor and sensory deficits, ataxia, ichthyosis, and sensorineural hearing loss, is the only sensorineural hearing disease in which the biochemical abnormality is known. It was first described by Refsum in 1946. The disease is transmitted as an autosomal recessive and is rare; approximately 50 cases have been reported in the world's literature from Western Europe and North America.

The disease usually manifests itself during the first decade of life or at the beginning of the second decade. The patient will usually have night blindness that is progressive and results in severe visual difficulties due to decreased visual fields and posterior cataracts (Richterich et al., 1965). The patients develop weakness, especially in the limbs, and moderate to marked muscle wasting. There will be associated cerebral ataxia, and in about 80 per cent of the patients electrocardiographic changes are found, including an increased P–Q interval and nodal and auricular extrasystoles. Clinically these changes are evidenced by tachycardia, gallop rhythm, and cardiac insufficiency. In many patients there are bony changes, including spondylitis, kyphoscoliosis, hammer toes, and pes cavus. These bony changes are probably secondary to the peripheral neuropathy that is similar to that seen in Hicks disease. More than half of these patients will have mild ichthyosis.

The hearing loss accompanying Refsum disease usually begins in the second decade. Bergsmark and Djupesland (1968) noted a clinical hearing loss in 34 of their 44 patients with this disease. Audiometric data were obtained in 34 of the patients with a hearing loss, and, of these, 22 had a sensorineural hearing loss as shown by the presence of recruitment, a decreased middle ear reflex threshold, and a lack of tone decay. Vestibular testing, consisting of cold water caloric testing, was performed in only a few patients, and the results were normal.

The biochemical basis of Refsum disease was reported in 1963 (Klenk and Kahlke) to be an accumulation of phytic acid. Patients were placed on diets free of phytic acid, phytol, and phytanic acid (eliminating all chlorophyll, butterfat, and so forth), and the phytic acid levels fell, in seven to eight months, to within 25 or 30 per cent of the prediet levels (Eldjarn et al., 1966). None of the patients' conditions worsened, and the peripheral nerve conduction time of one patient improved. Another report on two patients showed a considerable improvement in ulnar nerve conduction time, increased strength of muscle groups, return of reflexes, lessened pain, and improvement in light touch, position sense, and coordination. There was no improvement in vision or hearing (Steinberg et al., 1970).

Hernoon and Steinberg (1969) defined the enzymatic defect in cultured fibroblasts of patients with Refsum disease: deficiency in the enzyme involved in the alpha hydroxylation of phytanate. The enzymes for subsequent steps in the degradation of phytic acid appear to be normal or near normal.

Temporal bone pathology has been reported in two cases of Refsum disease (Friedmann, 1974; Hallpike, 1967). Both reports describe a normal middle ear and bony labyrinth but note degeneration of the organ of Corti and of the saccule. In one case there was a marked decrease in spiral ganglion cells, and in the other they were normal. The cristae and maculae were normal in both specimens, but in one (Hallpike, 1967) the disease was associated with a sudden hearing loss.

The neuropathology of Refsum disease (Refsum, 1952) includes fibrous thickening of the leptomeninges and infiltration by lipid macrophages, moderate degeneration of the peripheral nerve, axonal changes in the anterior horn cells of the spinal cord, degeneration of the fiber tracts from the pontobulbar region to the cerebellar white matter, and Sudan-positive fat in moderate amounts in the nerve cells and ependyma. Electron microscopic studies of the nerves (Fardeau and Engle, 1969) showed frequent nonspecific lipid deposits in Schwann cell cytoplasm.

Sensorineural hearing loss without other stigmata. There is a large group of patients with genetically transmitted sensorineural hearing loss without any other stigmata. This group includes patients with bilateral acoustic neuromas that are inherited as an autosomal dominant. Such cases have been described by Feiling and Ward (1920) and by Gardner and Frazier (1930). This disease entity may be different from von Recklinghausen's neurofibromatosis in that it is less frequently associated with pigmentary changes and cutaneous neurofibromatosis (Alliez et al., 1975). This form of acoustic neuroma may account for 1 to 4 per cent of all patients with acoustic neuromas and has been found in Western Europe and North America.

Young et al. (1971) studied the relatives of the patients studied by Gardner and Frazier (1930) and obtained information on 1500 family members, of which 648 were alive at the time of the study. The onset of the symptoms of hearing loss or unsteadiness can be as early as two years of age, with a mean age of 21 years. The initial symptoms were decreased hearing in 11 of 21 patients, tinnitus in 6 of 21, unsteadiness in 3 of 21, and facial weakness in 1 of 21 patients. Café au lait spots were usually small and solitary. Autopsy findings in 4 of 14 cases showed that there were other asymptomatic central nervous system tumors. Those individuals who were not operated on lived an average of 18.5 years, and those who were operated upon lived for an average of 9.2 years after the operation.

The hearing loss associated with congenital acoustic neuromas can initially be unilateral and progress to a bilateral loss. There is some variability in the nature of the loss, and the audiometric characteristics appear to be similar to those of other cerebropontine angle tumors. Most tumors, when of sufficient size, will lead to tone decay, a high-frequency hearing loss, difficulty in speech discrimination, and absent middle ear reflexes.

Individuals with acoustic neuromas have abnormal or absent vestibular responses. It has been noted that the numbers of drownings and near drownings in the children of these patients were remarkably high (Young et al., 1971); three individuals nearly drowned as a result of losing their sense of direction while under water, and three teenagers did drown. They were all children of affected parents. It seems reasonable to assume that the pathology of congenital acoustic neuroma is similar to that of other acoustic neuromas and that growth of the tumor begins on the superior vestibular nerve. Thus, we might also assume that the patients who drowned had vestibular deficits. Since our own clinical experience has shown that children with vestibular impairment have a greater propensity for drowning than others, we feel that tests of vestibular function should be performed on all children with sensorineural hearing loss. If an impairment of the vestibular system is found, the parent and the child should be warned about the risk of swimming, especially underwater, and precautions, such as close supervision, use of life jackets, and avoidance of underwater swimming, should be instituted.

The diagnosis of acoustic neuroma in a child should be made by means of audiometric, vestibular, and radiographic examinations. The tumors can be detailed with special radiographic techniques (Fritz and Harwood-Nash, 1974).

The histopathology of acoustic neuromas is similar to that of other neuromas (Nager, 1964), with bundles of elongated cells forming palisades. Acoustic neuromas invade the internal auditory meatus, infiltrate the modiolus and scala tympani of the basal turn, and leave proteinaceous precipitate in the scalae tympani and vestibuli. A typical case of bilateral acoustic neuroma is illustrated in Figure 19–8. The patient first had symptoms at 10 years of age and died at age 15.

There are numerous other genetically transmitted sensorineural hearing losses that

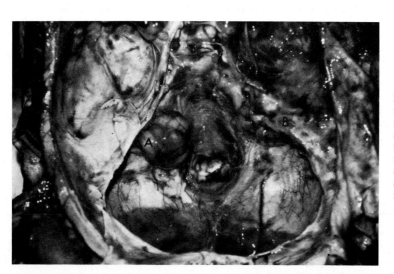

Figure 19–8 The base of the cranium of a 14 year old who died of multiple brain tumors. A large acoustic neuroma can be seen on the left (A). On the right in the region of the temporal bone there is a surgical deficit (B) where another acoustic neuroma was successfully removed three years before death.

Table 19–6 PREVALENCE OF OTHER ABNORMALITIES WITH SENSORINEURAL DEAFNESS DUE TO FIVE CAUSES*

Etiology	Cerebral Palsy or Hemiplegia, Per Cent	Mental Retardation (IQ below 70), Per Cent	Aphasic Disorders, Per Cent	Visual Defects, Per Cent	Orthopedic – Excluding Cerebral Palsy, Per Cent	Seizure, Per Cent
Prematurity	18	17	36	28	9	2
Heredity	0	0	2	21	2	0
Meningitis	10	14	16	6	5	3
Rubella	4	8	22	30	5	0
Rh incompatibility	51	5	23	24	2	7

*From Vernon, M. 1967.

have their onset after birth with no associated stigmata (Konigsmark and Gorlin, 1976). Most of these are progressive and seldom result in profound deafness. They are inherited as autosomal dominant, autosomal recessive, or X-linked characteristics. Children with progressive sensorineural hearing loss can present a diagnostic problem in that they may not have symptoms directly referable to their hearing. This is especially true of younger children, who may exhibit social and psychologic changes. Another indication of possible sensorineural hearing loss may be marked changes in school achievement. Many of these children are not deaf but have moderate losses and/or high-frequency losses that may be impairing their social relationships. The histopathology and expressivity of the gene for such sensorineural loss is variable (Rapoport and Ruben, 1974).

Acquired Sensorineural Hearing Loss

Acquired sensorineural hearing losses in children occur mainly during the perinatal period, the most common cause being prematurity. "Prematurity" is defined in many ways and is really nothing more than a statement about the size and gestational age of an infant. A number of different factors associated with prematurity could result in sensorineural hearing loss: anoxia; kernicterus, which probably acts through anoxia; ototoxic medication; labyrinthitis; meningitis; and temporal bone fractures. The last four will be discussed under separate headings because they contribute in large part to postnatal acquired sensorineural hearing loss in children.

The incidence of prematurity as a factor in sensorineural hearing loss has been reported in a clinical outpatient population to be approximately 10 per cent (Ruben and Rozycki, 1970) and as high as 23 per cent in a total population of deaf children (Johnsen, 1952). It has been established that about 2 per cent of children with birth weights under 1.36 kg (3 lb) may have significant sensorineural hearing loss (Fraser, 1976). The chance of a premature infant being deaf is 20 times greater than that of the child with a normal birth weight.

Premature sensorineural hearing-impaired children will usually have a severe sensorineural hearing loss, a high-frequency hearing loss, or both. These children have been found to have a high percentage of multiple handicaps: Vernon (1967) found in a deaf school population that 33 per cent of premature children had one other handicap, 27 per cent had two other handicaps, and 8 per cent had three other handicaps. Thus, 68 per cent of the children had multiple handicaps, which included aphasia, mental retardation, visual pathology, emotional disturbance, and orthopedic abnormalities. Table 19–6 presents comparable data concerning multiple handicaps compared with other etiologic factors. It may be noted from Table 19–6 that those children who were premature had the highest percentage of single handicaps in three of the six categories and were the only group that had the highest percentage in more than one category. These data indicate that a premature child who has sensorineural deafness may be expected to have other difficulties, and this information must be considered in planning any habilitative program for the child. This also means that, in general, the prognosis for normal development of a premature sensorineural hearing-impaired child must be more guarded than for other children.

There are a number of factors that may

bring about sensorineural hearing loss in the premature infant, of which anoxia is probably the most important. Hall (1964) examined the inner ears and cochlear nuclei of 39 children who had undergone prolonged periods of neonatal anoxia; 32 could be considered premature. The findings revealed that the inner ears were either normal or showed changes compatible with histologic or postmortem artifacts. The changes found in the inner ears were not similar to those found in experimental anoxia. The cochlear nuclei showed a decrease in cell number and a decrease in volume proportional to the length of time of the anoxia. The cochlear nuclei, both dorsal and ventral, showed a decrease in cell population of 20 per cent after 10 hours of anoxia, 40 per cent after 24 hours of anoxia, and 45 per cent after two days of anoxia. These findings agree with the histopathology of kernicterus; in prematurity associated with anoxia, they suggest that the pathologic lesion resulting in sensorineural hearing loss may not lie in the cochlea but in the cochlear nucleus complex and perhaps in other portions of the central nervous system. This information also agrees with the observation that premature infants with respiratory distress syndrome develop more neurologic anomalies than weight-controlled premature infants who do not have the respiratory distress syndrome (Fisch et al., 1968). The hypothesis that central nervous system pathology is the underlying mechanism for sensorineural hearing loss in the premature infant is also congruent with the high rate of multiple central nervous system handicaps found in these children (Vernon, 1967).

The problems encountered with kernicterus are similar to those seen with prematurity, and many children with kernicterus are also premature. The frequency of a history of kernicterus in a population of sensorineurally deaf children today is about 0.5 to 1.5 per cent (Ruben and Rozycki, 1970; Vernon, 1967). Owing to improved perinatal care, fewer cases of Rh incompatibility are seen, but ABO and other blood group incompatibilities are found to be associated with kernicterus and sensorineural hearing loss. The hearing loss in these cases is usually a high-frequency loss with little loss of speech discrimination. The acoustic characteristics are those of a cochlear loss (Matkin and Carhart, 1966), but in one study a number of the subjects heard the signals in the binaural median plane localization tests as separate signals and not as a fused signal. This was felt to be a possible indication of central auditory pathology (Matkin and Carhart, 1966).

A long-term follow-up study of children with kernicterus (Walker et al., 1974) found that 22 per cent of the children had severe sensorineural hearing loss consistent with the severity of the hemolytic disease. This report noted that children with the greatest sensorineural hearing losses had multiple handicaps as well.

Histopathologic examination of the ears and brains of patients with kernicterus shows the middle and inner ears to be normal, with the abnormalities occurring in the central nervous system (Dublin, 1976). Changes are noted throughout the central nervous system, and whereas the auditory system shows the greatest amount of nerve cell injury in the ventrocochlear nucleus, there appears to be a sparing of the dorsal cochlear nucleus. The dorsal olivary complex, inferior colliculus, medial geniculate body, and auditory cortex show variable degrees of pathology.

Meningitis is one of the common causes of postnatal sensorineural hearing loss and may account for 4 to 7 per cent of the cases seen in a clinical setting (Barr and Wedenberg, 1965; Ruben and Rozycki, 1970). Meningitis may also play a role in the sensorineural hearing loss associated with prematurity in infancy, since the incidence of meningitis appears to be higher in the premature than in the full-term infant. A serial autopsy study of 101 infants showed that of five infants with meningitis who died, three had bacterial labyrinthitis that probably would have resulted in a severe to profound sensorineural hearing loss (Johnson, 1961). Only one of the three patients had pathologic evidence of otitis media, although otitis media was found in 55 per cent of the total population studied. Meningitis occurs throughout the pediatric age range, and the incidence of bilateral sensorineural hearing loss may be as high as 3 per cent of cases (Dahnsjo et al., 1976). Unilateral sensorineural hearing loss may also result from meningitis, and, in the report mentioned, this was found in 8 per cent of the patients. The hearing loss following meningitis can either remain static or be progressive. The author has observed that the onset of severe to profound sensorineural hearing loss has also been noted to be delayed several weeks or

Table 19-7 MEAN PURE TONE LOSS, FROM 512 TO 2048 Hz, ASA, IN DEAFNESS DUE TO FIVE CAUSES, 1951*

Etiology	Mean Hearing Loss (dB)
Kernicterus	76
Rubella	82
Prematurity	83
Genetic	88
Meningitis	93

*From Vernon, M. 1967.

months after the meningitis has resolved. Improvement in hearing has been reported after meningococcal meningitis (Liebman and Ronis, 1963) and *Haemophilus influenzae* meningitis (Roeser et al., 1975).

Children with deafness secondary to meningitis show symptoms similar to those with deafness due to prematurity. Vernon (1967) states that 28 per cent of such children will have one other significant handicap, 4 per cent will have two handicaps, 4.3 per cent will have three handicaps, and 1 per cent will have four handicaps. Overall, 38 per cent of the group will have one or more additional handicaps, including cerebral palsy, aphasia, mental retardation, visual pathology, emotional disturbance, and orthopedic pathology. The severity of the deafness is, on the average, greater in these children than in those who are deaf from other causes (Table 19–7). Patients with meningitic sensorineural hearing loss almost invariably have an absence of vestibular function. Thus, the same precautions apply concerning swimming that were cited for patients with acoustic neuromas.

The histopathology of hearing loss following meningitis has been well described (Friedmann, 1974; Schuknecht, 1974). The bacteria can invade the inner ear through various pathways, including the nerves, vessels, cochlear aqueduct, and the endolymphatic duct and sac. This results in a labyrinthitis that destroys the neuroepithelium. The inner ear is then replaced by granulation tissue, fibrous scars, and new bone (Fig. 19–9). Occasionally the diagnosis of postmeningitis deafness can be made radiographically, because part of the membranous labyrinth will be replaced by bone; this abnormal bone can be detected by suitable radiographic techniques.

Labyrinthitis without meningitis today is commonly of viral origin and is only infrequently due to bacterial or fungal infection. The incidence of labyrinthitis without meningitis, in a clinical population of patients with deafness, has been reported as about 2 per cent (Ruben and Rozycki, 1970). Various viruses, including mumps (Vuori et al., 1962), herpes zoster (Blackley et al., 1967), perhaps the coxsackievirus, and others have been implicated in sensorineural hearing loss (Rowson, 1975). The incidence of significant hearing loss in the childhood population is probably less than 1 per cent, secondary to viral labyrinthitis. The hearing losses are usually unilateral but, as previously mentioned (Everberg, 1960), many unilateral hearing losses are genetic in origin. A study of an epidemic of mumps in 298 Finnish servicemen revealed that 13 men, or 4 per cent, developed sensorineural hearing loss (Vuori et al., 1962). The hearing returned to normal or near normal in 13 of the 14 affected pa-

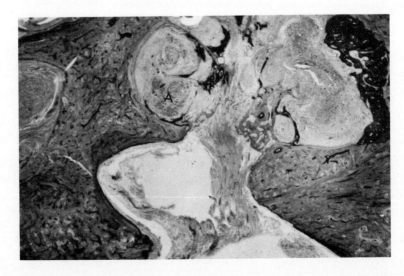

Figure 19–9 A cross-section through the temporal bone demonstrating the end stage of labyrinthitis. The entire cochlea has been replaced by granulation tissue and new bone formation (A).

tients, and only one, or less than 1 per cent of the total population, had a persistent, unilateral, significant sensorineural hearing loss.

The histopathology of viral infection has often been reported, but documentation of the virus as a definitive cause of the hearing loss is less than certain. One of the more accurately documented cases is that reported by Blackley et al. (1967) in which the patient had a history of herpes zoster infection associated with the Ramsay Hunt syndrome (facial paralysis, herpetic eruption on the face, and sensorineural hearing loss). The histopathology in this case showed perivascular, perineural, and intraneural round cell aggregations in the facial nerve, cochlea, and mastoid process. The organ of Corti was absent, and the scala media was collapsed.

Patients with sickle cell anemia have been found to have sensorineural hearing loss (Todd et al., 1973; Urban, 1973). Todd et al. (1973) showed that 15 per cent of patients with this disorder between the ages of 10 and 19 years had sensorineural hearing losses of more than 25 dB at one or more frequencies from 500 to 8000 Hz ISO. However, some of these hearing losses may be spontaneously reversible (Urban, 1973). The ears of one 10 year old boy with sickle cell disease and sensorineural hearing loss, with a pure tone audiogram of 35 dB and a positive SISI at 1000 and 4000 Hz, showed degenerative changes in the organ of Corti and stria vascularis but normal spiral ganglion cells (Morgenstein and Manace, 1969). The changes were felt to be due to repeated hypoxic episodes during sickle cell crises.

There are numerous other causes of sensorineural hearing loss in children, perhaps the most prevalent of which are head trauma, ototoxic drugs, and noise trauma. Patients who suffer head injury may have fractures of the temporal bone, which may result in conductive, mixed, or sensorineural hearing loss with or without associated facial paralysis. If the fracture goes through the bony labyrinth, there will usually be a profound sensorineural hearing loss. Fractures of the bony labyrinth heal by a nonbony fibrous union. If the fracture extends into the middle ear, for the rest of their lives these patients will be at risk for developing meningitis from otitis media, as the infection can spread from the middle ear cleft via the fibrous fracture line to the meninges. It has been suggested (Ma-

kishima and Snow, 1975) that some of the sensorineural hearing loss following head trauma may be the result of hemorrhage into the statoacoustic nerve. These cases would not show radiographic signs of temporal bone fracture, and they may have no otologic signs of fracture, such as hemotympanum or ruptured tympanic membrane.

Sound trauma is another cause of sensorineural hearing loss and is usually associated with workers exposed to sudden, loud noises, such as explosions. Occasionally a child will be seen who has had a firecracker explode next to his or her ear. Such a child may have a tympanic membrane perforation and may also exhibit a temporary threshold shift. Another possible cause of sound trauma is the high sound levels in incubators (American Academy of Pediatrics, 1974). These sound levels have not been proved to be harmful but may be a contributing factor to deafness in a premature infant who is also receiving ototoxic medication. It has been noted that young guinea pigs are more susceptible to noise trauma than are adult guinea pigs (Douek et al., 1976).

Another cause of sensorineural hearing loss is ototoxic medications, the most common of which are the aminoglycosides, including neomycin, kanamycin, streptomycin, dihydrostreptomycin, vancomycin, and gentamicin, and ethacrynic acid and furosemide (Worthington, 1973). Most of these drugs are excreted by the kidneys, to which they may also be toxic. A patient who is administered any of these drugs must have his or her renal function carefully monitored. The most common situations in which sensorineural deafness is observed with the use of these drugs are when an overdose is inadvertently given, when there is unrecognized renal impairment, and when the drug is used to preserve life, even with the knowledge of the possibility of sensorineural hearing loss. If possible, all patients taking these medications should have serial audiometric and vestibular studies performed. If these patients have symptoms of auditory or vestibular impairment or if the objective testing shows a deficit in either the auditory or vestibular system, then the treatment plan should be reconsidered. Some of the medications, for instance, neomycin, will continue to cause irreversible hearing loss after the first signs of deficiency are noted and the drug is discontinued. Others, such as ethacrynic acid, will usually cause a hearing loss that is resolved when the medication is stopped. Some experimental evidence would suggest a synergistic effect with ethacrynic acid and some of the aminoglycosides.

There are numerous causes of sensorineural hearing loss in children, each of which accounts for only a small portion of the total number of those affected with this condition. The physician must be able to establish the cause of the sensorineural hearing loss, because a knowledge of the etiology will, in many instances, mandate a specific form of intervention. Whether the intervention is genetic counseling, renal dialysis, or intensive, nonvisual aural habilitation is dependent upon knowledge of the etiology of deafness or impairment.

DIAGNOSIS AND MANAGEMENT OF SENSORINEURAL DEAFNESS

Diagnosis

The prompt diagnosis of sensorineural deafness in the infant or child is one of the most important interventions a physician can make. If the diagnosis is delayed, the result may be irreversible abnormal patterns of speech, language cognition, and socialization. Figures 19–10 and 19–11 give some strategies for diagnosis and management of sensorineural deafness in children.

There are three ways in which a child can be identified as being at risk for sensorineural hearing loss: by referral from an infant or school screening program, by identification of the child through a high risk registry, or, perhaps the most common, by parental identification of a possible hearing problem. All too often this last method of possible identification is ignored by the physician (Ruben, 1978); the physician should assume in all cases that the parent is probably correct and should investigate the child thoroughly for a sensorineural hearing loss.

It is now possible, through the use of electrocochleography, brain stem–evoked potentials, cortex-evoked potentials, acoustic reflexes, and various behavioral techniques, to make a diagnosis of significant hearing loss in any child at any age. The differential diagnosis of sensorineural hearing loss in an infant or child who does not respond to sound or in one with delayed or abnormal language development must include peripheral hearing loss, central auditory processing abnormality, mental retardation, and, in some instances, maturational delay in responsiveness to sound. In many cases the final diagnosis may include both peripheral hearing loss and mental retardation. After a diagnosis of the site of the deficit is made, the etiology of the hearing loss should be determined, and the child should be further evaluated to determine what other organ systems may be affected. It is important to establish the etiology of the deafness in order to offer genetic counseling to the parents and the child, to assess other organ systems that may be involved, to determine the possible medical treatment, and to provide for optimal habilitation of the patient.

The diagnosis of the etiology of a sensorineural hearing loss in infants and children begins with the medical history. This must include a family history, and special inquiries should be made to elicit the possibility of consanguinity, even if it is not readily apparent. This will, in the usual American family, involve tracing the origins of both sides of the family for three or four generations. Careful attention should be given to any history of hearing impairment in other family members and to evidence of any other stigmata of genetic disease. If the family history is negative and no acquired etiology is evident, then audiometric assessment of the parents, siblings, and grandparents should be undertaken to determine if there are any carriers of a deafness gene that may lead to a diagnosis of genetic hearing loss.

The prenatal history is examined to determine whether there is any history of possible infection (viral or bacterial), administration of ototoxic medication, or attempted abortion. The perinatal history is obtained to determine if the child was premature or had kernicterus or if there was significant birth trauma or anoxia. The past history of the child is obtained to determine whether the child had meningitis, ototoxic medication, labyrinthitis, or head trauma.

In about half of the cases, a probable etiology may be established from the history and physical examination; in the remainder the etiology will remain a mystery. Almost all infants with a diagnosis of sensorineural hearing loss will undergo further laboratory investigation to determine the etiology and to ascertain the integrity of other organ systems. Each patient should have mastoid radio-

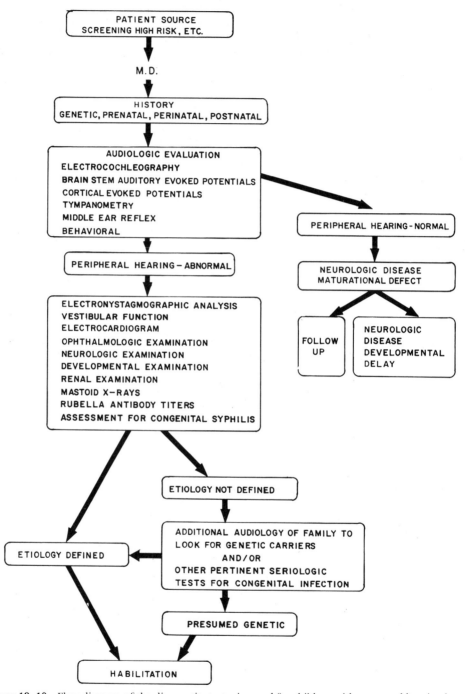

Figure 19–10   Flow diagram of the diagnostic strategies used for children with suspected hearing losses.

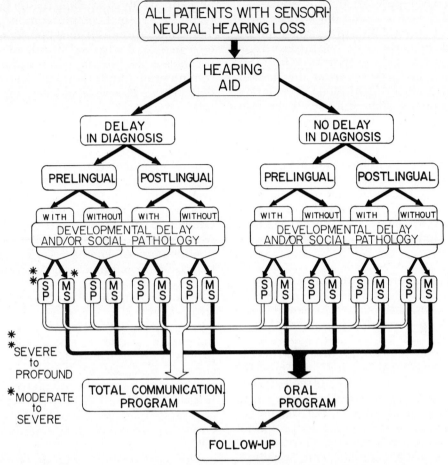

Figure 19–11 Flow diagram for the management of children with hearing loss.

graphs to determine if the bony labyrinth is normal. If it is abnormal, other neurologic deficits may be expected. Vestibular testing is performed in all cases to assess the integrity of the vestibular system. As previously mentioned, an absent vestibular response can be dangerous if the child goes swimming. Also of importance is the observation that patients with decreased vestibular responses will have delayed motor development, which can be confused with early signs of developmental delay (Rapin, 1974).

The high incidence of neurologic, ophthalmologic, cardiac, and renal diseases in children with sensorineural deafness makes it imperative that each patient also undergo appropriate evaluation of these other organ systems. In our clinic, this consists of a pediatric neurologic and developmental examination, a complete ophthalmologic examination, an electrocardiogram, and urinalysis

accompanied by measurement of serum creatinine levels. These examinations have been useful in making a diagnosis and in defining other systemic abnormalities.

Congenital infection by rubella is still a primary cause of sensorineural deafness, even though many times the infection in the mother may be subclinical. Because of the importance of being able to diagnose the cause of deafness, all mothers and children should have rubella antibody titers obtained if there is no history of previous immunization. Other intrauterine infections, such as toxoplasmosis and cytomegalic inclusion disease, are assessed by serum studies and physical examination if the history indicates that this may be a cause. Congenital syphilis resulting in sensorineural hearing loss in infants has been, in our experience, an uncommon occurrence. However, owing to the increase in the incidence of venereal disease in the general population, this source of congenital deafness should not be disregarded. Most often, syphilis can be ruled out by examining the obstetric and birth records, in which there is usually a report of at least one test for syphilis performed on the mother and/or the umbilical cord blood. The infant with congenital syphilis will usually, but not invariably, be stigmatized, and the diagnosis can then be confirmed.

The older child is investigated in a similar manner, but more emphasis should be placed on the renal, ophthalmologic, and neurologic examinations. The older child must have, in addition to the investigations already described, an evaluation of speech, language cognition, and socialization.

Intervention and Health Maintenance

After the diagnosis of a sensorineural hearing loss has been made, the otorhinolaryngologist has only begun his or her task of caring for the patient. The diagnosis of the degree and type of hearing loss must be considered in its relationship to the patient's general health and psychologic and social status. Those patients who are diagnosed prelingually as having severe to profound hearing loss need at least three interventions. The first is proper amplification, usually a binaural hearing aid, at the earliest possible time. The second necessary intervention is an infant auditory training program. There is wide debate concerning two types of auditory habilitation. There are those who feel that habilitation should be based solely on oral training, perhaps reinforced with speech reading (lipreading). The other group advises a total communication program that includes both sign language and oral training with the aid of speech reading. The experiences gathered over a number of years and with many hundreds of patients have caused our own group at Albert Einstein College of Medicine, in most instances, to recommend total communication habilitative therapy if it is available. This advice is given to the parent, for it is strongly felt, but not proved, that it is most important for the infant to learn language. Our experience with infant auditory programs, both oral training and total communication, has shown that those infants with total communication develop better language skills as they mature. There is a second and

perhaps equally compelling reason for recommending the total communication program: The child's social relations appear to be better when he is involved in this program. It becomes easier for the parents and child to communicate, and they can more clearly demonstrate their love and affection for each other.

The recommendation for a total communication program is made even more strongly when the patient has or is suspected of having a developmental delay. It is felt that these patients need all the communicative input available to learn the maximum amount of language. Additionally, those children from families in which there is significant social stress will also need the additional help in the development of language and socialization that a total communication program can afford.

A total communication program is also advocated for all patients for whom there has been a significant delay in diagnosis. Many times the diagnosis may not be made until the patient is two to five years of age, and these children have lost what may be the most critical and important years for language formation and will have great difficulty in acquiring language. Every means should be employed to optimize their acquisition of language.

The recommendation for an oral program is usually reserved only for those children with moderate to severe hearing losses who have no developmental delays and no significant social problems. The oral program is also recommended for children who are postlingually deaf and who have no developmental delay or significant social pathology.

There are many communities in which there is no choice between a total communication program and an oral program. In these communities, attempts should be made to provide a comprehensive program for infant auditory training that allows all patients to be exposed to an optimal educational program.

The third intervention is to inform the parents about the child's disability; i.e., why the child has the problem and how the child is to be cared for. This is usually done in an informing interview. The parents, with or without the child, depending on the child's age, meet with the professionals who have performed the diagnostic assessment of the child. This group should, before the meeting with the parents, review the material and decide among themselves the best plan for the child. One to two hours should be allowed for the interview, for the professionals must explain to the parents in understandable terms what has been ascertained and the rationale for habilitation of the child. One member of this group should then become the responsible professional for the continued long-term care of the child. The parents will contact this person to ask questions and seek advice concerning the development of the child for many years after the diagnosis and plan for management have been made. This person should also reassess the child continually as he or she develops. This is done by means of a hearing test, given at least once a year, and by reassessment of cognitive, language, and social development. The long-term care of the child must also include a careful assessment for serous otitis media; if this develops in addition to the sensorineural hearing loss, there will be even greater impairment (Ruben and Math, 1978). The patient must also be followed for possible progression of the sensorineural hearing loss. All patients wearing hearing aids need to have their aids checked frequently, and molds for the hearing aids will need to be remade often for infants, as the size and shape of the external auditory canal will change rapidly. Occasionally an external otitis will occur, which must be treated properly so the child can wear the aid and not be deprived of hearing.

There is one special category of patients, those in whom no etiologic diagnosis is made and in whom the possible etiology may be a recessive genetic gene. Some of these patients will have Usher disease (retinitis pigmentosa), and the possibility of this diagnosis must always be considered so that a proper habilitative program can be instituted for a child who is deaf and will become blind. The development of blindness in a child who has been taught to depend on visual cues will cause the child to lose much of what he or she has learned. All children with deafness of unknown etiology should be routinely examined ophthalmologically in order to detect impending blindness as soon as possible.

Periodic assessment of the child should be undertaken, for there is always a possibility that the original diagnosis was incorrect. One can be sure of the diagnosis if, over time, the clinical and laboratory findings are consistent. Although there have been substantive advances in the diagnosis of communication disorders in infants and young children over the past decade, there is still the possibility of error. If an error has been made, the habilitative therapy should be corrected as soon as possible.

SELECTED REFERENCES

Fraser, G. R. 1976. The Causes of Profound Deafness in Childhood. Baltimore, Johns Hopkins University Press.

This is an excellent book that reviews the genetic components of deafness and evaluates them in terms of the other etiologies of this impairment. This is probably the best book in the field of deafness etiology.

Friedmann, I. 1974. Pathology of the Ear. London, Blackwell Scientific Publications.

This is an excellent book on pathology of the ear, containing many valuable references and many case histories.

Konigsmark, B. W., and Gorlin, R. J. 1976. Genetic and Metabolic Deafness. Philadelphia, W. B. Saunders Co.

This book is a catalog of different types of genetic deafness. It contains many illustrations that will help to identify various syndromes.

Schuknecht, H. 1974. Pathology of the Ear. Boston, Harvard University Press.

This is an excellent text of pathology of the ear that lists many of the types of congenital hearing losses. There is also an excellent treatment of the pathophysiology underlying the various sensorineural hearing losses. The illustrations in this work are of the highest caliber.

REFERENCES

Alford, B. R. 1968. La bete noire de la medecine. Laryngoscope, 78:1623.

Alliez, J., Masse, J. L., and Alliez, B. 1975. Tumeurs bilaterales de l'acoustique et maladie de Recklinghausen observees dans plusieurs generations. Rev. Neurol. (Paris), 131:545.

Alport, A. C. 1927. Hereditary familial, congenital, hemorrhagic nephritis. Brit. J. Med., 1:504.

American Academy of Pediatrics Committee on Environmental Hazards. 1974. Noise pollution: neonatal aspects. Pediatrics, 54:476.

Anderson, H., Barr, B., and Wedenberg, E. 1970. Genetic disposition as a prerequisite for maternal rubella deafness. Arch. Otolaryngol., 91:141.

Anderson, H., Henricson, B., Lundquist, P. G., et al. 1968. Genetic hearing impairment in the Dalmatian dog. Acta Otolaryngol., Supplement 232.

Anderson, H., and Wedenberg, E. 1968. Audiometric identification of normal hearing carriers of genes for deafness. Acta Otolaryngol., 65:535.

Barr, B., and Wedenberg, E. 1965. Prognosis of perceptive hearing loss in children with respect to genesis and use of hearing aid. Acta Otolaryngol., 59:462.

Belal, A. 1975. Usher's syndrome (Retinitis pigmentosa and deafness). J. Laryngol. Otol., *89*:175.

Bell, A. G. 1969. Memoirs upon the Formation of a Deaf Variety of the Human Race. Report to the National Academy of Science, 1883. Washington, D. C., A. G. Bell Association for the Deaf.

Bergsmark, J., and Djupesland, G. 1968. Heredopathia atactica polyneuritiformis (Refsum's disease). Eur. Neurol., *1*:122.

Blackley, B., Friedmann, I., and Wright, I. 1967. Herpes zoster auris associated with facial nerve palsy and auditory nerve symptoms. Acta Otolaryngol., *63*:531.

Bordley, J. E., and Alford, B. R. 1970. The pathology of rubella deafness. Int. Audiol., *9*:58.

Bordley, J. E., Brookhouser, P. E., Hardy, J., et al. 1968. Prenatal rubella. Acta Otolaryngol., *66*:1.

Bosher, S. K., and Hallpike, C. S. 1966. Observations of the histogenesis of the inner ear degeneration of the deaf white cat and its possible relationship to the aetiology of certain unexplained varieties of human congenital deafness. J. Laryngol. Otol., *80*:222.

Calhoun, F. P. 1919. Causes of heterochromic irides with special reference to paralysis of the cervical sympathetics. Am. J. Ophthalmol., *2*:255.

Cassidy, G., Brown, K., Cohen, M., et al. 1965. Hereditary renal dysfunction and deafness. Pediatrics, *35*:967.

Cooper, L. Z., Florman, A. L., Ziring, P. R., et al. 1971. Loss of rubella hemagglutination inhibition antibody in congenital rubella. Am. J. Dis. Child., *122*:397.

Crawfurd, M. D., and Toghill, P. J. 1968. Alport's syndrome of hereditary nephritis and deafness. Q. J. Med., *37*:563.

Dahnsjo, H., Andersson, H., Hallander, H. O., and Rudberg, R. D. 1976. Tone audiometry control of children treated for meningitis with large intravenous doses of ampicillin. Acta Paediatr. Scand., *65*:733.

Deol, M. S. 1964. Abnormalities of inner ear in Kreisler mice. J. Embryol. Exp. Morphol., *12*:475.

Deraemaeker, R. 1960. Recessive congenital deafness in a North Belgian province. Acta Genet. (Basel), *10*:295.

Douek, E., Bannister, L. H., Dodson, H. C., et al. 1976. Effects of incubator noise on the cochlea of the newborn. Lancet, *2*:1110.

Dublin, W. B. 1976. Fundamentals of Sensorineural Auditory Pathology. Springfield, Ill., Charles C Thomas.

Eldjarn, L., Try, K., Stokke, O., et al. 1966. Dietary effects on serum–phytanic acid levels and on clinical manifestations in heredopathia atactica polyneuritiformis. Lancet, *1*:691.

Everberg, A. 1960. Unilateral anacusis: clinical, radiological and genetic investigations. Acta Otolaryngol., Suppl., *158*:366.

Faggioni, R., Scouras, J., and Streiff, E. B. 1972. Alport's syndrome: clinicopathological considerations. Ophthalmologica (Basel), *165*:1.

Fardeau, M., and Engel, W. K. 1969. Ultrastructural study of a peripheral nerve biopsy in Refsum's disease. J. Neuropathol. Exp. Neurol., *28*:278.

Fay, E. A. 1898. Marriages of the Deaf in America. Washington, D.C., Volta Bureau.

Fay, J. E., Olley, P. M., Partington, M. W., et al. 1971. Surdo-cardiac syndrome: Incidence among children

in schools for the deaf. Can. Med. Assoc. J., *105*:718.

Feiling, A., and Ward, E. A. 1920. A familial form of acoustic tumor. Br. Med. J., *1*:496.

Fisch, L. 1959. Deafness as part of an hereditary syndrome. J. Laryngol. Otol., *73*:355.

Fisch, R. O., Gravem, H. J., and Engel, R. R. 1968. Neurological status of survivors of neonatal respiratory distress syndrome. J. Pediatr., *73*:395.

Fitzpatrick, D. B., Hooper, R. E., and Seife, B. 1976. Hereditary deafness and sensory radicular neuropathy. Arch. Otolaryngol., *102*:552.

Forrest, J. M., and Menser, M. A. 1970. Congenital rubella in school children and adolescents. Arch. Dis. Child., *45*:66.

Forrest, J. M., and Menser, M. A. 1975. Recent implications of intrauterine and postnatal rubella. Aust. Paediat. J., *11*:65.

Fraser, G. R. 1976. The Causes of Profound Deafness in Childhood. Baltimore, Johns Hopkins University Press.

Fraser, G. R. 1965a. Association of congenital deafness with goitre (Syndrome of Pendred) — study of 207 families. Ann. Hum. Genet., *28*:201.

Fraser, G. R. 1965b. Sex-linked recessive congenital deafness and the excess of males in profound childhood deafness. Ann. Hum. Genet., *29*:171.

Fraser, G. R., Froggatt, P., and James, T. N. 1964a. Congenital deafness associated with electrocardiographic abnormalities, fainting attacks and sudden death — a recessive syndrome. Q. J. Med., *33*:361.

Fraser, G. R., Froggatt, P., and Murphy, T. 1964b. Genetic aspects of the cardioauditory syndrome of Jervell and Lange-Nielsen. Ann. Hum. Genet., *28*:133.

Friedmann, I. 1974. Pathology of the Ear. London, Blackwell Scientific Publications.

Friedmann, I., Fraser, G. R., and Froggatt, P. 1966. Pathology of the ear in the cardio-auditory syndrome of Jervell and Lange-Nielsen (recessive deafness with electrocardiographic abnormalities). J. Laryngol., *80*:451.

Fritz, C. R., and Harwood-Nash, D. C. 1974. Radiology of the ear in children. Radiol. Clin. North Am., *2*:433.

Fujita, S., and Hayden, R. C. 1969. Alport's syndrome. Arch. Otolaryngol., *90*:453.

Gardner, W. J., and Frazier, C. H. 1930. Bilateral acoustic neurofibromas: a clinical study and field survey of a family of five generations with bilateral deafness in 38 members. Arch. Neurol. Psychiatr., *23*:266.

Goldberg, M. F. 1966. Waardenburg's syndrome with fundus and other anomalies. Arch. Ophthalmol., *76*:797.

Gottlieb, G. 1975. Development of species identification in ducklings. (1) Nature of perceptual deficit caused by embryonic auditory deprivation. J. Comp. Physiol. Psychol., *89*:387.

Hall, J. G. 1964. The cochlea and the cochlear nuclei in neonatal asphyxia. Acta Otolaryngol., Suppl., 194.

Hallgren, B. 1959. Retinitis pigmentosa combined with congenital deafness; with vestibulo-cerebellar ataxia and mental abnormality in a proportion of cases. Acta Psychiat. Scand., *34*, Suppl. 138.

Hallpike, C. S. 1967. Observations on the structural basis of two rare varieties of hereditary deafness. *In* de Reuck, A. V., and Knight, J. (Eds.) Myotatic, Kinesthetic and Vestibular Mechanisms. Ciba Foundation Symposium. Boston, Little, Brown & Co., 1967.

Hansen, A. C., Ackaouy, G., and Crump, E. P. 1965. Waardenburg's syndrome: Report of a pedigree. J. Nat. Med. Assoc., *57*:8.

Henke, F., and Lubarsch, O., 1926. Handbuch der Speziellen Pathologischen Anatomie und Histologie. Berlin, Springer-Verlag.

Hernoon, J. H., and Steinberg, D. 1969. Refsum disease — characterization of enzyme defect in cell culture. J. Clin. Immunol., *58*:1017.

Hvidberg-Hansen, J., and Jorgensen, M. B. 1968. The inner ear in Pendred's syndrome. Acta Otolaryngol., *66*:129.

Jackson, J. R., and Rubel, E. W. 1976. Rapid transneuronal degeneration following cochlear removal in the chick. Anat. Rec., *184*:434.

James, T. N. 1967. Congenital deafness and cardiac arrhythmias. Am. J. Cardiol., *19*:627.

Jensen, J. 1974. Congenital anomalies of the inner ear. Radiol. Clin. North Am., *12*:473.

Jervell, A., and Lange-Nielsen, F. 1957. Congenital deafmutism, functional heart disease with prolongation of Q–T interval and sudden death. Am. Heart J., *54*:59.

Johnsen, S. 1952a. Natal causes of perceptive deafness. Acta Otolaryngol., *42*:51.

Johnsen, S. 1952b. The heredity of perceptive deafness. Acta Otolaryngol., *42*:439.

Johnson, D. W., Wathen, R. L., and Mathog, R. H. 1976. Effects of hemodialysis on hearing threshold. ORL, *38*:129.

Johnson, W. W. 1961. A survey of middle ears: 101 autopsies of infants. Ann. Otol. Rhinol. Laryngol., *70*:377.

Kaufman, D. B., McIntosh, R. M., and Smith, F. G. 1970. Diffuse familial nephropathy: a clinical pathological study. J. Pediatr., *97*:37.

Klenk, E., and Kahlke, W. 1963. Uber das Vorkommen der 3, 7, 11, 15-Tetramethylhexadecansaure in den Cholesterinestern und anderen Lipoidfraktionen der Organe bei einem Krankheitsfall unbekannter Genese. Hoppe-Seyler's Z. Phys. Chem., *333*:133.

Kloepfer, H. W., Hallpike, C. S., De Hass, E. B., et al. 1970. Usher's syndrome with special reference to heterozygote manifestations. Docum. Ophthalmol., *28*:166.

Kloepfer, H. W., Laguaite, J. K., and McLaurin, J. W. 1966. The hereditary syndrome of deafness in retinitis pigmentosa. Laryngoscope, *76*:850.

Konigsmark, B. W., and Gorlin, R. J. 1976. Genetic and Metabolic Deafness. Philadelphia, W. B. Saunders Co.

Levi-Montalcini, R. 1949. Development of the acousticovestibular centers in chick embryo in the absence of the afferent root fibers and descending fiber tracts. J. Comp. Neurol., *91*:209.

Liebman, E., and Ronis, M. L. 1963. Hearing improvement following meningitis deafness. Arch. Otolaryngol., *90*:470.

McKusick, V. A. 1966. Mendelian Inheritance in Man (Catalogs of Autosomal Dominant, Autosomal Recessive and X-linked Phenotypes). Baltimore, Johns Hopkins University Press.

Makishima, K., and Snow, J. B. 1975. Pathogenesis of hearing loss in head injury. Arch. Otolaryngol., *102*:426.

Matkin, N. D., and Carhart, R. 1966. Auditory profiles associated with Rh incompatibility. Arch. Otolaryngol., *84*:502.

Mikaelian, D., and Ruben, R. J. 1965. Development of hearing in the normal CBA-J mouse. Acta Otolaryngol., *59*:451.

Mitschke, H., Schmidt, P., Kopsa, H., and Zazgornik, J. 1975. Reversible uremic deafness after successful renal transplantation. N. Engl. J. Med., *292*:1062.

Morgans, M. E., and Trotter, W. R. 1958. Association of congenital deafness with goitre. Lancet, *1*:607.

Morgenstein, K. M., and Manace, E. D. 1969. Temporal bone histopathology in sickle cell disease. Laryngoscope, *79*:2172.

Nager, F. R. 1927. Zur Histologie der Taubstummheit bei Retinitis pigmentosa. Beitr. Path. Anat., *77*:288.

Nager, G. T. 1964. Association of bilateral VIIIth nerve tumors with meningiomas in von Recklinghausen's disease. Laryngoscope, *74*:1220.

Nuutila, A. 1970. Dystrophia retinae pigmentosadysacusis syndrome (DRD). A study of the Usher or Hallgren syndrome. J. Genet. Hum., *18*:57.

Olley, P. M., and Fowler, R. S. 1970. The surdo-cardiac syndrome and therapeutic observations. Brit. Heart J., *32*:467.

Parithe, O. A., and Cohen, M. M. J. 1971. The Waardenburg syndrome. Birth Defects, original article series, *7*:147.

Parks, T. N., and Robinson, J. 1976. The effects of otocyst removal on the development of chick brain stem auditory nuclei. Anat. Rec., *184*:497.

Pendred, V. 1896. Deaf mutism and goitre. Lancet, *2*:532.

Preus, M., and Fraser, F. G. 1971. Genetics of hereditary nephropathy with deafness (Alport's disease). Clin. Genet., *2*:331.

Pryor, H. B. 1969. Objective measurement of interpupillary distance. Pediatrics, *44*:973.

Rapin, I. 1974. Hypoactive labyrinth and motor development. Clin. Pediatr., *13*:922.

Rapoport, Y., and Ruben, R. J. 1974. Dominant neurosensory hearing loss: Genetic, audiologic and histopathologic correlates. Trans. Am. Acad. Ophthalmol. Otol., *78*:423.

Refsum, S. 1946. Heredopathia atactica polyneuritiformis. Acta Psychiatr. Neurol. Scand., Suppl, *38*.

Refsum, S. 1952. Heredopathia atactica polyneuritiformis. J. Nerv. Mental Dis., *116*:1046.

Richards, C. S. 1964. Middle ear changes in rubella deafness. Arch. Otolaryngol., *80*:48.

Richterich, R., Moser, H., and Rossi, E. 1965. Refsum's disease (heredopathia atactica polyneuritiformis). Humangenetik, *1*:322.

Riesen, A. H., and Zilbert, D. E. 1975. Developmental Neuropsychology of Sensory Deprivation. New York, Academic Press.

Robinson, G. C., and Cambon, K. G. 1964. Hearing loss in infants of tuberculous mothers treated with streptomycin during pregnancy. N. Engl. J. Med., *271*:949.

Roeser, R. J., Campbell, J. D., and Daly, D. D. 1975. Recovery of auditory function following meningitic deafness. J. Speech Hearing Dis., *40*:405.

Rowson, K. E. K., Hinchcliffe, R., and Gamble, D. R. 1975. A virological and epidemiological study of patients with acute hearing loss. Lancet, *1*:471.

Ruben, R. J. 1967a. Cochlear potentials as a diagnostic test in deafness. Symposium on Sensory Neural

Hearing Processes and Disorder. Boston, Little, Brown & Co., pp. 313–338.

Ruben, R. J. 1967b. Development of the inner ear of the mouse: A radioautographic study of terminal mitosis. Acta Otolaryngol., Suppl., *220.*

Ruben, R. J. 1970. Screening for rubella during pregnancy. N. Engl. J. Med. *283*:1292.

Ruben, R. J. 1978. Delay in diagnosis (editorial). Volta Review #4, *80*:201–202.

Ruben, R. J., and Rozycki, D. 1970. Diagnostic screening for the deaf child. Arch. Otolaryngol., *91*:429.

Ruben, R. J., and Rozycki, D. 1971. Clinical aspects of genetic deafness. Ann. Otol. Rhinol. Laryngol., *80*:255.

Ruben, R. J., and Math, S, 1978. Serous otitis media associated with sensorineural hearing loss in children. Laryngoscope, 7:1139.

Salisbury, A. J., and Ma, P. 1976. Reported rubella in the United States, 1975. National Foundation — March of Dimes.

Sanchez-Cascos, A., Sanchez-Harguindey, L., and de Rabago, P. 1969. Cardio-auditory syndromes. Brit. Heart J., *31*:26.

Sataloff, J., Pastore, P. N., and Bloom, E. 1955. Sex-linked hereditary deafness. Am. J. Hum. Genet., 7:201.

Schuknecht, H. 1974. Pathology of the Ear. Boston, Harvard University Press.

Settlemayer, J. R., and Hogan, M. 1961. Waardenburg syndrome — Report of a case in a non-Dutch family. N. Engl. J. Med., *261*:500.

Simpson, J. L., Falk, C. T., Morillo-Cucci, et al. 1974. Analysis for possible linkage between loci for the Waardenburg syndrome and various blood groups and serological traits. Am. J. Hum. Genet., *13*:45.

Sirles, W. A., and Slasghts, H. 1943. Pigmentary deafness of retina and neural type deafness. Am. J. Ophthalmol., *26*:961.

Smith, A. B. 1939. Unilateral hereditary deafness. Lancet, *2*:1172.

Smith, J. F. 1960. The pathology of the thyroid in the syndrome of sporadic goitre and congenital deafness. Quart. J. Med., *29*:297.

Spear, G. S., and Gussen, R. 1972. Alport's syndrome, emphasizing electron microscopic studies of the glomeruli. Am. J. Pathol., *69*:213.

Steinberg, D., Mize, C. E., Hernoon, J. H., et al. 1970. Phytic acid in patients with Refsum's syndrome and response to dietary treatment. Arch. Intern. Med., *125*:75.

Swan, C., Tostevin, A. L., Moore, B., et al. 1943. Congenital defects in infants following infectious diseases during pregnancy. With special reference to the relationship between German measles and cataract, deaf-mutism, heart disease and microcephaly, and to the period of pregnancy in which the occurrence of rubella is followed by congenital abnormalities. Med. J. Aust., 2:201.

Thould, A. K., and Scowen, E. F. 1964. The syndrome of congenital deafness and simple goiter. J. Endocrinol., *30*:69.

Todd, G. B., Serjeant, F. R., and Larson, M. R. 1973. Sensorineural hearing loss in Jamaicans with sickle cell disease. Acta Otolaryngol., *76*:268.

Urban, G. E. 1973. Reversible sensorineural hearing loss associated with sickle cell crisis. Laryngoscope, *83*:633.

Vernon, M. 1967. Prematurity and deafness: The magnitude and nature of the problem among deaf children. Except. Child., *33*:289.

Vernon, M. 1969. Usher's syndrome — deafness and progressive blindness. Clinical cases, prevention, theory and literature survey. J. Chron. Dis., *22*:133.

von Graefe, A. 1858. Vereinzelte Beobachtungen und Bemerkungen. Exceptionelles Verhalten des Gesichtsfeldes bei Pigmentenartung der Netzhaut. Albrecht von Graefe's Arch. Klin. Ophthalmol., *4*:250.

Vuori, M., Lahikainen, E. A., and Peltonen, T. 1962. Perceptive deafness in connection with mumps. Acta Otolaryngol., *55*:232.

Waardenburg, P. J. 1951. A new syndrome combining developmental anomalies of the eyelids, eyebrows and nose root with pigmentary defects of the iris and head hair and with congenital deafness. Am. J. Hum. Genet., *3*:195.

Walker, W., Ellis, M. I., Ellis, E., et al. 1974. A follow-up study of survivors of Rh hemolytic disease. Dev. Med. Child Neurol., *16*:592.

Wardrop, J. 1813. History of James Mitchell, a Boy Born Blind and Deaf with an Account of the Operation Performed for Recovery of His Sight. London, Murray.

Webster, D. G., and Webster, M. 1977. Neonatal sound deprivation affects brain stem auditory nuclei. Arch. Otolaryngol., *103*:392.

Weinberger, M. M., Masland, M. W., Asbed, R. A., et al. 1970. Congenital rubella presenting as retarded language development. Am. J. Dis. Child., *120*:125.

Wilde, W. R. 1853. Practical Observations on Aural Surgery and the Nature and Diagnosis of Diseases of the Ear. Philadelphia, Blanchard and Lea.

Worthington, E. L. 1973. Index-Handbook of Ototoxic Agents, 1966–1971. Baltimore, Johns Hopkins University Press.

Yntema, C. L. 1950. Analysis of induction of the ear from foreign ectoderm in the salamander embryo. J. Exp. Zool., *113*:211.

Young, D. F., Eldridge, R., Nager, G. T., et al. 1971. Hereditary bilateral acoustic neuroma — central neurofibromatosis. Birth Defects, original article series, *7*:73.

Chapter 20

DISEASES OF THE LABYRINTHINE CAPSULE

LaVonne Bergstrom, M.D.

The labyrinthine or otic capsule consists of persistent or primary bone overlaid both internally and externally with perichondrial or lamellar bone. The ossicles, although of branchial origin, have a similar composition. Most diseases of the otic capsule also affect the skeleton generally; only one, otosclerosis, seems to occur only in the otic capsule. Many of these disorders are seen in the preadult years; some are present at birth. When they occur in the temporal bone they may be silent or latent, but when symptomatic they profoundly affect a child's school and social life.

OSTOSCLEROSIS (OTOSPONGIOSIS)

Clinical otosclerosis is rare under the age of five years and is extremely rare in people of Oriental or black heritage (McKenzie, 1948; Larsson, 1960; Friedmann, 1974; Schuknecht, 1974). Symptoms begin between the ages of 11 and 30 in 70 per cent of individuals but in only 2 to 3 per cent prior to age 15. The youngest recorded case was one year of age (Nager, 1969). Otosclerosis is genetic, probably of autosomal dominant inheritance with reduced penetrance, although this may be more apparent than real, since histologic otosclerosis may occur in "silent" areas of the labyrinthine capsule. Polygenic inheritance, possibly involving genes affecting collagen, calcium, parathormone, and bony structure, has also been postulated (Mendlowitz et al., 1976). Low fluoride content in drinking water has been hypothesized to contribute to the development of otosclerosis (Daniel,

1969), but its relationship to genetic factors has yet to be clarified. Otosclerotic foci occurred in only 0.6 per cent of temporal bones in patients under age five and 4 per cent over age five, rising to an incidence of 10 per cent in males and 18 per cent in females between the ages of 30 and 50. However, stapes ankylosis occurred in only 15 per cent of bones with histologic findings of otosclerosis (Guild, 1944).

Clinically, the otosclerosis patient experiences insidious, usually bilaterally symmetric, progressive hearing loss. Tinnitus and vertigo are unusual in young individuals. Upon examination, the tympanic membranes of these patients are intact and mobile, and the nose and throat examination is normal. The patient's articulation and voice quality are good unless the hearing loss occurred very early and was rapidly progressive. Bone conduction may be louder than air conduction as measured by tuning fork tests, but in early cases only audiometry may demonstrate an air-bone gap. The acoustic impedance instrument will show normal middle ear pressure, but the acoustic reflex will either show a peculiar on-off negative deflection in early cases or will be absent, and impedance may be high (Terkildsen et al., 1973; Van Wagoner and Campbell, 1976). Concurrent sensorineural hearing loss may also occur. The accelerating effects of pregnancy and possibly of birth control pills on the symptomatic onset of otosclerosis in about 25 per cent of cases must be noted, since more teenage girls are using contraceptives or becoming pregnant.

Otosclerosis often begins in the endochondral bone anterior to the oval window. An active or immature focus, often thought to represent an earlier phase in the evolution of the lesion (Nager, 1969), is sometimes visible through an intact tympanic membrane as an area of reddish glow on the promontory, referred to as "Schwartze's sign." When examined during surgery such a focus is soft and bleeds readily; histologically it stains blue with hematoxylin and eosin and is quite vascular and spongiotic. Nager reported an extensive, active lesion in the temporal bone of an 8½ year old girl with normal hearing (Nager, 1969). In young patients with otosclerosis, otologic surgeons may encounter active vascular lesions that tend to refix the stapes after mobilization or to obliterate the oval window. Mature, inactive, or "healed" foci are grossly white, avascular, stain red or pink with hematoxylin-eosin, and more closely resemble normal compact bone than otosclerotic bone. Active and inactive foci may be seen at different locations in the same individual. Circumferential confluent or multiple lesions have been described in these types of bones (Black et al., 1969).

Ankylosis of the stapes may involve only the fibrous annulus; if the ankylosis is bony, it may involve only the anterior footplate, or if it is obliterative it may bury the crura and footplate in a mound of otosclerosis. An otosclerotic focus may invade labyrinthine spaces and may be associated with spiral ligament and strial atrophy, organ of Corti hair cell loss, neural atrophy, and vestibular pathology (Sando et al., 1968; Sando et al., 1974). Rüedi and Spoendlin believe that blood shunts from the middle ear circulation to the spiral ligament, causing congestion of its vessels and resultant cochlear neuroepithelial damage (Rüedi and Spoendlin, 1966). Other theories are that an otosclerotic focus releases toxic substances into the inner ear or that its effect is purely mechanical, distorting basilar membrane movement or propagation of the traveling wave (Altmann et al., 1966; Sando et al., 1968).

The differential diagnosis of otosclerosis is congenital ossicular fixation, which may present identical clinical findings and a positive family history. Petrous pyramid polytomography may demonstrate gross congenital ossicular lesions or large, active otosclerotic lesions. Ossicular discontinuity, which may be congenital or postinflammatory, may cause increased compliance on the tympanogram and may be demonstrable by tomography. Most sequelae of otitis media are evident on otologic examination, and other disorders of the otic capsule have systemic or regional manifestations.

The treatment of significant hearing loss due to otosclerosis in early life deserves special consideration, although very little authoritative information on this subject is available. Some clinicians believe that surgery should be postponed until active foci become inactive in order to decrease the risk of inner ear damage or recurrent stapes fixation. Amplification of hearing could tide over the individual until the disease stabilizes and surgery is indicated. Some espouse treatment with fluoride, calcium, and vitamin D for adults who develop progressive sensorineural hearing loss and who show roentgenographic evidence of labyrinthine invasion by otosclerosis (Shambaugh and Causse, 1974; Parkins, 1974). Such a regimen should probably be undertaken only after consultation with an endocrinologist because no longitudinal data on children or adolescents treated in this manner are available. Stapes surgery may give good long-term results in those patients whose otosclerosis seems mature and inactive, but long-term hearing improvement is maintained at a 10 dB or smaller air-bone gap in less than 70 per cent of patients of all ages (Schuknecht, 1974). It would seem wise to avoid operating on the only ear through which the patient can hear or on unilaterally involved ears and to reserve operating on the second ear until adult life, since operative techniques may improve. A child or teenager who may not be capable of fully informed consent deserves consultation with the most experienced and skillful otologic surgeon available before a decision for or against surgery is made. Complications of stapes surgery include sensorineural hearing loss, oval window fistula (Hemenway et al., 1968), granuloma (Gacek, 1970), and suppurative labyrinthitis (Schuknecht, 1974). The child operated upon for otosclerosis might be particularly at risk for this last complication, since the incidence of upper respiratory infections and otitis media is highest in the early school years.

OSTEOGENESIS IMPERFECTA

Osteogenesis imperfecta occurs in two forms. The more severe congenital type is distinguished by craniotabes, multiple wormian bones of the skull, and congenital and many postnatal fractures that cause stunting and deformities of the torso and limbs (Fig. 20–1). Affected neonates may not survive. In the less severe form, osteogenesis imperfecta tarda, congenital fractures may occur, but deformity is less pronounced. Hearing loss, which may be sensorineural, conductive, or mixed, typically begins in the second or third decade of life. Three types of middle ear pathology have been described. The ossicles, especially the stapes, are very fragile, with such thinning of the structures that ossicular discontinuity or fracture occurs. A second finding has been that of a bulky, soft, crumbly stapes footplate that may be lightly ankylosed. Occasionally, thin crura and a bulky footplate occur together. Since there is abundant histologic, biochemical, and other evidence to show that osteogenesis imperfecta and otosclerosis are distinct dysplasias of the temporal bone, it is of considerable interest that they may occur together. Lesions compatible with congenital conductive hearing loss have been reported. Lopping, outward slanting, posterior rotation, or notching of the posterosuperior helical margin of the pinnae and salmon-pink flush of the promontory are other otologic features of interest. Other head and neck findings may include blue sclerae, dentinogenesis imperfecta, and epistaxis. These children, who may undergo many surgical procedures, are at risk for hemorrhage, malignant hyperthermia, hypertrophic scar formation, incompetent or floppy heart valves, and cor pulmonale (Bergstrom, 1977).

Older children and teenagers may develop enough hearing loss to require treatment. Measures such as preferential seating in school and speech reading training may suffice, but amplification or middle ear surgery might be desirable.

When examined histologically, osteogenesis imperfecta bone appears to be very porous and has poor matrix surrounding a few cancellous trabeculae containing numerous osteocytes. There is an increased amount of osteoid and woven bone; microfractures may be seen, and the collagen of this type of bone is defective in some way. In the temporal bone there is widespread deficiency of ossification of the ossicles and the area around membranous labyrinthine end-organs and nerves. As a result of deficient laying down of bone the internal auditory canal may appear to be widened and the mastoid air cells to be

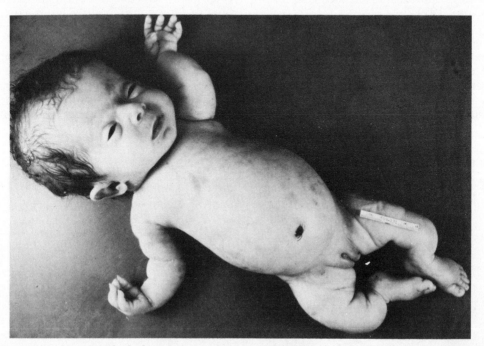

Figure 20–1 Neonate who had severe osteogenesis imperfecta congenita and died of respiratory complications. Note short, bent extremities. (Used by permission of F. O. Black et al. and Colorado University Associated Press.)

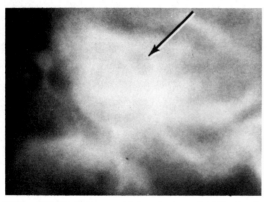

Figure 20–2 Petrous polytomogram of patient who has van der Hoeve syndrome of osteogenesis imperfecta tarda and hearing loss. Note widened appearance of the cochlea owing to deficient laying down of bone, giving a "cochlea within a cochlea" appearance (arrow). (Used by permission of W. Hanafee, M.D.)

unusually well pneumatized. Fractures may occur. Inner ear pathology includes calcific deposits in, and acute degeneration of, the cochlear vascular stria; swelling and distortion of the tectorial membrane; and degeneration of the organ of Corti and vestibular neuroepithelium. Petrous pyramid polytomography duplicates some of the above findings. In addition, a widened cochlea or "cochlea within a cochlea" may be seen (Fig. 20–2) (Bergstrom, 1977).

There appear to be fewer fractures of facial bones than of the skeleton generally, but there is some evidence to suggest that facial fractures may occur more frequently in osteogenesis imperfecta than has heretofore been suspected (Bergstrom, 1977).

The inheritance of osteogenesis imperfecta

tarda may be dominant or recessive. Subclinically affected parents may have affected children. Osteogenesis imperfecta congenita offspring have been born to normal parents, to carriers of the trait, and to those affected by the tarda form.

OSTEOPETROSIS
(ALBERS-SCHÖNBERG DISEASE)

Osteopetrosis, also called marble bone or chalk bone disease, is a sporadic or recessively inherited general bone dyscrasia characterized by hard, brittle bones. There is no race, sex, or geographic predisposition to the disease, and two clinical forms exist. The malignant form is characterized by progressive cranial compression causing blindness, deafness, facial palsy, anosmia, mental retardation, and medullary compression (Fig. 20–3). These and severe anemia, hepatosplenomegaly, long bone fractures, and hypocalcemic tetany cause death in the early months or years of life. The benign variant of this disease is compatible with a normal life span and normal intelligence but is expressed clinically in excessive height, a leonine appearance, conductive or mixed hearing loss, and facial palsy that may begin in the teenage years (Fig. 20–4). Headaches, optic atrophy, clubbing of long bones, genu valgum, coxa vara, proptosis, and osteomyelitis may become manifest later in life (Klintworth, 1963; Hamersma, 1970, 1973).

The pathophysiology of this disease is based on the observation that primitive fetal bone does not resorb, and the resulting increase in bone density that characterizes os-

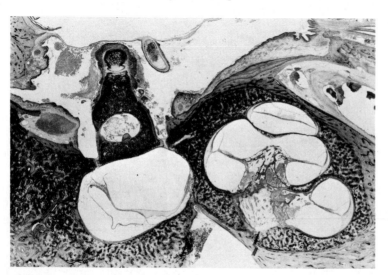

Figure 20–3 Horizontal temporal bone section from a young child who, prior to death, had been blind and deaf owing to the malignant form of osteopetrosis. Note the stapes, the bulk of which is due to lack of resorption of cartilage, thus preventing remodeling into the adult form. (×12) (Courtesy of S. E. Stool, M.D.)

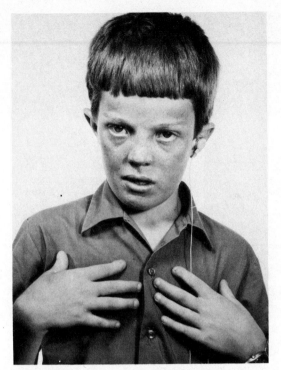

Figure 20–4 Twelve year old boy with the benign form of osteopetrosis. He had several episodes of facial palsy with nerve degeneration prior to undergoing facial nerve decompression at age six. Note his relatively expressionless, somewhat asymmetric face. He also underwent surgical widening of narrowed external auditory canals and exploratory tympanotomy for fixation of malleus and incus in the epitympanum. Subsequently the stapes has fixed. He also has syndactyly, absent fingernails and an enlarging skull. (Courtesy of H. Hamersma, M.D.)

teopetrosis may be seen on late prenatal roentgenograms. Calcium salts are deposited in the bone in large quantities, but the resultant hard bone lacks the adult structure designed to withstand stress and hence breaks readily at right angles to the long axis (Myers and Stool, 1969). The bone has small haversian canals and a relatively poor blood supply; hematopoietic marrow encroachment, neutropenia, and poor vascular supply predispose to osteomyelitis (Sofferman et al., 1971). Cranial foramina, including the foramen magnum, fail to enlarge during growth.

Roentgenograms are essential to the diagnosis of osteopetrosis. They show homogeneous bone density, loss of the diploë, and thickening of the base and dome of the skull. Mastoid and petrous pyramid films show obliteration of the air cell system and may show narrowed external and internal auditory canals, oval and round windows, middle ear space, and dense bone engulfing the malleus and incus in the epitympanum. Cholesteatoma may form behind bony external auditory canal masses.

Examination of postmortem temporal bone specimens of patients with osteopetrosis has shown shallow middle ear spaces, dehiscent fallopian canals, a bulky stapes of fetal form, and cochlear and saccular endolymphatic hydrops (Myers and Stool, 1969). Other postmortem temporal bone findings include exostoses of the middle ear cavity and downgrowth of a greatly thickened epitympanic plate, narrowed internal autitory canal, and incomplete temporal bone fractures (Hamersma, 1970, 1973; Suga and Lindsay, 1976).

CRANIOMETAPHYSEAL DYSPLASIA (PYLE DISEASE)

This autosomal, dominantly inherited disorder affects the temporal bone in childhood. Its overall features include widening of the metaphyseal part of the long bones and overgrowth of the craniofacial bones (leontiasis ossea) (Fig. 20–5). Progressive conductive and/or sensorineural hearing loss, eustachian tube obstruction, nasal deformity, obliteration of nasal passages and paranasal sinuses, nasolacrimal duct obstruction, mandibular overgrowth, defective dentition and occlusion, hypertelorism, facial paralysis, other cranial nerve palsies, cerebellar tonsil compression with resultant nystagmus, and brain stem compression due to narrowing of the foramen magnum complete the clinical picture. Physical findings include narrow external auditory canals and hypoactive vestibular responses. Roentgenograms may show narrowing of the middle ear, internal carotid canal, jugular foramen, and internal auditory canal; encroachment on the cochlea, and oval and round windows; fusion of ossicles; and obliteration of mastoid air cells. These more detailed findings are best delineated by petrous pyramid polytomography (Kietzer and Paparella, 1969; Kim, 1974).

Microscopically, these temporal bones show increased amounts of subperiosteal and subendosteal bone that produce a very compact laminar bone, the dilated haversian canals which contain osteoblasts and osteocytes but no osteoclasts. There is an increased amount of intercellular ground substance in these bones (Kietzer and Paparella, 1969).

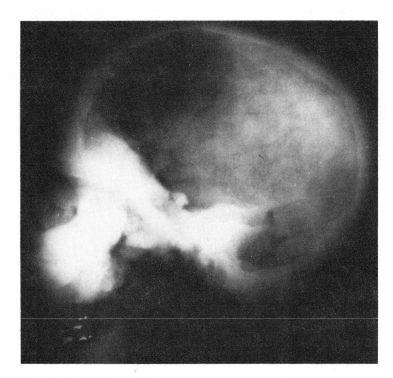

Figure 20–5 Skull film of patient with far-advanced craniometaphyseal dysplasia. The overgrowth of facial and cranial bones, especially around the cranial base, is extreme. Note obliteration of labyrinthine spaces. (Used by permission of Dr. Lorraine Smith.)

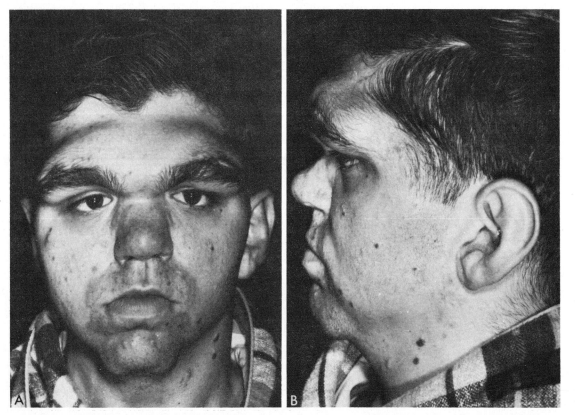

Figure 20–6 Patient who has frontometaphyseal dysplasia demonstrates overgrowth of the supraorbital ridges, especially laterally. (From Gorlin et al., 1976. Used by permission of the authors and the publisher, The American Medical Association.)

FRONTOMETAPHYSEAL DYSPLASIA (GORLIN-HOLT SYNDROME)

This entity is thought to be due to failure to absorb secondary spongy bone, and a number of features distinguish it from craniometaphyseal dysplasia. Cases may be sporadic or may result from a rare autosomal recessive gene. Patients with this dysplasia exhibit severe overgrowth of the supraorbital ridges, especially laterally, agenesis of the frontal sinuses, hypodevelopment of the mandible, defective dentition, a high arched palate, decreased vision, and a conductive or mixed hearing loss (Fig. 20–6). Also seen are hirsutism, winged scapulae, flaring of the iliac bones, a limited range of motion of the joints (especially in elbow extension) and poorly developed muscles. However, these individuals seem to be of normal intellect (Gorlin et al., 1976).

Roentgenograms show metaphyseal splaying of tubular bone, internal hyperostosis, perisutural sclerosis, thoracic scoliosis, irregular rib and vertebral contours, disproportionately long limbs and digits, and absence or atrophy of temporal muscles. Frequently in these patients the frontal ridge is hyperostotic, the frontal sinuses are absent, the foramen magnum is enlarged, and the cervical vertebrae may be abnormal (Arenberg et al., 1974; Gorlin et al., 1976). Petrous pyramid polytomography may show fused and/or fixed malleus and incus, a malformed stapes, and irregular thickness of the cochlear capsule (Arenberg et al., 1974). No temporal bone histopathology has been reported in these cases.

FIBROUS DYSPLASIA (OSSIFYING FIBROMA)

Fibrous dysplasia occurs in three forms, any one of which may involve the temporal bone: (1) monostotic, in which, as the name implies, bony involvement is confined to one bone, usually in the craniofacial region; (2) polyostotic, in which multiple bones are involved; however, the disorder is nonsyndromal and affects only bony tissue; and (3) polyostotic, or the McCune-Albright syndrome (Talbot et al., 1974; Rimoin et al., 1973). Common associated abnormalities include precocious sexual development and café au lait spots. The proportion of females suffering from this disease exceeds that of males for all forms of the disease.

The clinical symptoms of temporal bone involvement are external hard swelling in the temporal and periauricular area, sometimes with associated pain and fever; external auditory stenosis; hearing loss that is usually conductive, although total sensorineural hearing loss has been reported; and facial nerve paresis or paralysis. Characteristically, bone swelling begins in childhood or adolescence, may progress to grotesque proportions, and tends to become quiescent after general skeletal growth stops, although it does not regress spontaneously. Cases of adult onset have been reported. Hearing loss may be present for some time before bone swelling, and it is not clear from published reports whether in all such instances the hearing loss was due to fibrous dysplasia or an unrelated cause. Otorrhea may occur and may herald the development of cholesteatoma behind an occluding mass of fibrous dysplastic bone in the external auditory canal, the middle ear, or the mastoid. Postauricular fistula has been reported, and although vestibular symptoms have not been emphasized in published reports, in one patient the lateral semicircular canal was eroded (Cohen and Rosenwasser, 1969; Sharp, 1970; Tembe, 1970; Chatterji, 1974).

General roentgenographic findings in these cases may be categorized as follows: (1) cystic changes (21 per cent); if teeth are involved the lamina dura may be absent and tooth roots separated; (2) sclerotic (23 per cent); and (3) pagetoid (56 per cent), characterized by a "cotton-wool" appearance. This last symptom tends to be found in older patients. The mastoid air cell system, middle ear space, and internal auditory canal may be obliterated (Talbot et al., 1974) (Fig. 20–7).

When these patients are examined during surgery, dense sclerotic bone or gritty vascular tissue is found to be eroding the otic capsule or invading and filling available spaces, including the external ear canal, the mastoid, and the labyrinthine cavities (Cohen and Rosenwasser, 1969). Cholesteatoma may be found in nearly 50 per cent of cases (Sharp, 1970).

The pathologic picture of this disease varies. In its active form, very cellular connective tissue composed of stellate or fusiform cells and numerous mitoses is seen. The margin between the connective tissue matrix and the bony islands is marked by a scroll edge to the bone, and the bone has been likened to the pieces of a jigsaw puzzle. The quiescent

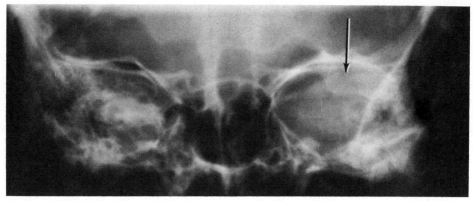

Figure 20–7   Fibrous dysplasia of the left petrous bone (arrow). Note the obliteration of the mastoid air cell system and the external auditory canal as well as the heavy osseous density in general. (Used by permission of W. Hanafee, M.D.)

stage shows more mature fibrous tissue with few mitoses and more bone, but osteoblasts, osteoclasts, and osteoid are not present. The inactive stage shows degeneration of the connective tissue matrix and no bone islands (Batsakis, 1974). The underlying etiology of these histologic changes is unknown.

OTHER DYSPLASIAS

Hearing loss of varying degrees and types has been reported in other disorders, including craniofacial dysostosis (Crouzon) (Baldwin, 1968), diastrophic dwarfism (Bergstrom, 1971), and an unclassified bone dysplasia associated with retinal detachment and deafness (Roaf et al., 1967).

EVALUATION AND THERAPY

Many of the dysplasias can be differentiated by characteristic radiographic findings. The extent and type of involvement of the middle ear, mastoid, fallopian canal, or labyrinthine capsule can be demonstrated best by plain mastoid films and petrous pyramid polytomography, the latter taken in axial, lateral, and basal projections. Occasionally, as in fibrous dysplasia, biopsy of the affected bone may be necessary for confirmation of the diagnosis. Functional disturbances can be detected and quantified by the use of tuning forks, audiometry, tympanometry, vestibular testing, and facial nerve conduction studies. Occasionally, retrocochlear testing may be indicated.

Conductive hearing loss in these cases may

be caused by surgically correctable external ear canal or middle ear lesions. Where cholesteatoma is known or suspected, surgery to exteriorize or remove it along with obstructing bony masses is essential, regardless of the state of the hearing. Where bony compression of the fallopian or internal auditory canal exists and has caused facial weakness or seems likely to be a cause of sensorineural hearing loss, surgical decompression may be feasible but should be preceded by thorough neurosurgical and roentgenographic evaluation.

When surgery is not possible or has been unsuccessful, hearing amplification and other measures to improve communication should be instituted. In young children in whom surgery can be deferred, amplification should be used if hearing loss interfering with normal language development exists. Hearing conservation measures should be urged for sensorineural losses, and genetic counseling should be offered to individuals and families affected by inherited bony disorders. Every attempt to detect hearing loss early should be made in those children at risk for the disorder or already known to have it.

At present there is no acceptable chemotherapy for any of the known bony dysplasias affecting the labyrinthine capsule in childhood or adolescence.

SELECTED REFERENCES

Gorlin, R. J., Pindborg, J. J., and Cohen, M. M. 1976. Syndromes of the Head and Neck. New York, McGraw-Hill Book Co.
  This new edition of a by now classic reference work is notable for its systematic presentation of syndromes, a few of

which are included in this chapter. The illustrations of pertinent craniofacial features are excellent.

Schuknecht, H. F. 1974. Pathology of the Ear. Cambridge, Mass. Harvard University Press, pp. 351–364, 378–383.

A large format, superb illustrations from the author's large collection of temporal bone specimens, and a writing style that clearly communicates years of careful study and observation of an extensive otologic patient population make this reference unique and indispensable for an understanding of the pathology of some of the entities described in this chapter.

REFERENCES

Altmann, F., Kornfeld, M., and Shea, J. 1966. Inner ear changes in otosclerosis. Ann. Otol. Rhinol. Laryngol., 75:5–32.

Arenberg, I. K., Shambaugh, G. E., Jr., and Valvassori, G. E. 1974. Otolaryngologic manifestations of frontometaphyseal dysplasia. The Gorlin-Holt syndrome. Arch. Otolaryngol., 99:52–58.

Baldwin, J. L. 1968. Dysostosis craniofacialis of Crouzon. Laryngoscope, 78:1660–1676.

Batsakis, J. G. 1974. Tumors of the Head and Neck. Baltimore, The Williams and Wilkins Company, pp. 306–308.

Bergstrom, L. 1971. A high risk register to find congenital deafness. Otolaryngol. Clin. North Am., 4:369–399.

Bergstrom, L. 1977. Osteogenesis imperfecta: otologic and maxillofacial aspects. Laryngoscope, 87:Suppl. No. 6.

Black, F. O., Sando, I., Hildyard, V. H. et al. 1969. Bilateral multiple otosclerotic foci and endolymphatic hydrops. Ann. Otol. Rhinol. Laryngol., 78:1062–1073.

Chatterji, P. 1974. Massive fibrous dysplasia of the temporal bone. J. Laryngol. Otol., 88:179–183.

Cohen, A., and Rosenwasser, H. 1969. Fibrous dysplasia of the temporal bone. Arch. Otolaryngol., 89:447–459.

Daniel, H. J. III. 1969. Stapedial otosclerosis and fluorine in drinking water. Arch. Otolaryngol., 90:585–589.

Friedmann, I. 1974. Pathology of the Ear. London, Blackwell Scientific Publications, pp. 245–278.

Gacek, R. R. 1970. The diagnosis and treatment of poststapedectomy granuloma. Ann. Otol. Rhinol. Laryngol., 79:970–975.

Gorlin, R. J., Pindborg, J. J., and Cohen, M. M. 1976. Syndromes of the Head and Neck. New York, McGraw-Hill Book Co., pp. 315–318.

Guild, S. R. 1944. Histologic otosclerosis. Ann. Otol. Rhinol. Laryngol. 53:246–266.

Hamersma, H. 1970. Osteopetrosis (marble bone disease) of the temporal bone. Laryngoscope, 80:1518–1539.

Hamersma, H. 1973. Total decompression of the facial nerve in osteopetrosis. ORL, 36:21–32.

Hemenway, W. G., Hildyard, V. H., and Black, F. O. 1968. Post-stapedectomy perilymph fistulas in the Rocky Mountain area. Laryngoscope, 78:1687–1715.

Kietzer, G., and Paparella, M. M. 1969. Otolaryngological disorders in craniometaphyseal dysplasia. Laryngoscope, 79:921–941.

Kim, B. H. 1974. Roentgenography of the ear and eye in Pyle disease. Arch. Otolaryngol., 99:458–461.

Klintworth, G. K. 1963. The neurologic manifestations of osteopetrosis (Albers-Schönberg's disease). Neurology, 13:512–519.

Larsson, A. 1960. Otosclerosis, a genetic and clinical study. Acta Otolaryngol., Suppl. 154.

McKenzie, W. 1948. Otosclerosis in childhood. J. Laryngol. Otol., 62:661–670.

Mendlowitz, J. C., and Hirschhorn, K. 1976. Polygenic inheritance of otosclerosis. Ann. Otol. Rhinol. Laryngol., 85:281–285.

Myers, E. N., and Stool, S. E. 1969. The temporal bone in osteopetrosis. Arch. Otolaryngol., 89:460–469.

Nager, G. T. 1969. Histopathology of otosclerosis. Arch. Otolaryngol., 89:341–363.

Parkins, F. M. 1974. Fluoride therapy for osteoporotic lesions. Ann. Otol. Rhinol. Laryngol., 83:626–634.

Rimoin, D. L., and Hollister, D. W. 1973. Polyostotic fibrous dysplasia. In Birth Defects. Atlas and Compendium. Baltimore, Williams and Wilkins Co., pp. 739–740.

Roaf, R., Longmore, J. B., and Forrester, R. M. 1967. A childhood syndrome of bone dysplasia, retinal detachment and deafness. Dev. Med. Child. Neurol., 9:464–473.

Rüedi, L., and Spoendlin, H. 1966. Pathogenesis of sensorineural deafness in otosclerosis. Ann. Otol. Rhinol. Laryngol., 75:525–552.

Sando, I., Hemenway, W. G., Hildyard, V. H., et al. 1968. Cochlear otosclerosis: a human temporal bone report. Ann. Otol. Rhinol. Laryngol., 77:23–36.

Sando, I., Hemenway, W. G., Miller, D. R., et al. 1974. Vestibular pathology in otosclerosis, temporal bone histopathological report. Laryngoscope, 84:593–605.

Schuknecht, H. F. 1974. Pathology of the Ear. Cambridge, MA, Harvard University Press, pp. 351–364.

Shambaugh, G. E., and Causse, J. 1974. Ten years' experience with fluoride in otosclerotic (otospongiotic) patients. Ann. Otol. Rhinol. Laryngol., 83:635–642.

Sharp, M. 1970. Monostotic fibrous dysplasia of the temporal bone. J. Laryngol. Otol., 84:697–708.

Sofferman, R. A., Smith, R. O., and English, G. M. 1971. Albers-Schönberg's disease (osteopetrosis), a case with osteomyelitis of the maxilla. Laryngoscope, 81:36–46.

Suga, F., and Lindsay, J. R. 1976. Temporal bone histopathology of osteopetrosis. Ann. Otol. Rhinol. Laryngol., 85:15–24.

Talbot, I. C., Keith, D. A., and Lord, I. J. 1974. Fibrous dysplasia of the craniofacial bones. J. Laryngol. Otol., 88:429–443.

Tembe, D. 1970. Fibro-osseous dysplasia of temporal bone. J. Laryngol. Otol., 84:107–114.

Terkildsen, K., Osterhammel, P., and Bretlau, P. 1973. Acoustic middle ear muscle reflexes in patients with otosclerosis. Arch. Otolaryngol., 98:152–155.

Van Wagoner, R. S., and Campbell, J. D. 1976. The use of electro-acoustic impedance measurements in detecting early clinical otosclerosis. J. Otolaryngol., 5:33–36.

Chapter 21

INJURIES OF THE EAR AND TEMPORAL BONE

Simon C. Parisier, M.D.

INTRODUCTION

Accidental injuries have become a major problem in modern mechanized society. Vehicular or pedestrian accidents account for more than 50 per cent of the deaths of persons in the first two decades of life (Vital Statistics, 1974). Falls continue to be a leading cause of injuries to children under 5 years of age (Hendrick et al., 1965). Moreover, the head injuries which commonly occur in such accidents are often accompanied by damage to the ear (Podoshin and Fradis, 1975; Hough and Stuart, 1968). The popularity of scuba diving, water skiing, and other sports has exposed an additional number of young people to possible ear injuries. When we add the above hazards to such existing problems as the fetish of cleaning wax from the ear canals of infants, or the apparent sensual satisfaction which young children experience when playing with their ears, we begin to understand the extent of the problem. This chapter reviews the variety of injuries that involve the ear and temporal bone. Trauma to the auricle is covered in Chapter 15, Diseases of the External Ear.

The Physician and the Injured Child

Traumatic injuries to the ear and temporal bone occur more commonly to children and adolescents than to adults (Hough and Stuart, 1968; Tos, 1973). In dealing with children, the physician must establish himself as a gentle, concerned person. Any examina-

tion, no matter how routine, should be explained or demonstrated beforehand so that it can be understood, thus eliminating fear of the unknown. For example, the otoscope or ear speculum can be introduced to the child by examining his hand with it before placing it in his ear. You can familiarize the patient with the wax curette by first tickling his hand with it, then touching the auditory meatus, before using the metal instrument to clean the canal. The child can be prepared for the loud noise of the suction aspirator by a demonstration of its function with a cup of water. When a procedure is expected to be painful, a general anesthetic is recommended, even in small infants who can be restrained effectively. The child who is confident that the physician will not cause unnecessary pain is usually a cooperative patient.

Trauma to the ear, even a minor scratch that causes bleeding from the·external canal, will generally seem catastrophic to the injured patient and his parents. The physician treating the child must enroll the family's full cooperation by explaining the problem in terms the family understands. It must be remembered that the attitude of the parent towards the physician is transmitted to the injured child.

INJURIES AND FOREIGN BODIES OF THE EXTERNAL AUDITORY CANAL

The cleaning of wax from the ears seems to be a cultural phenomenon. In order to gain access to the ear canal, a variety of objects, ranging from bobby pins to match sticks, is used. It is not uncommon for a new mother in this country to be given free samples of products for her newborn. Included in the gift package may be cotton-tipped applicators, which are often used to clean the baby's ear canals. Thus, from infancy, the individual is taught that the ever-present cerumen is a form of dirt and must be removed regularly.

During the ear-cleansing ritual, the mother's manipulations may be painful, causing the child to jerk his head, and the ear may be injured. Ordinarily, only a minor laceration of the ear canal will result. While the bleeding may be profuse at the onset, it usually stops spontaneously, forming a clot that may obstruct the external canal. In order to determine if the tympanic membrane has been damaged, the debris should be removed gently. It may not be possible to clean the canal if a child is unable to cooperate adequately or if the blood has formed a tenacious crust that is firmly attached to the skin of the canal wall or to the drum. In such instances, rather than risk inflicting further damage by traumatic manipulations, the physician should observe the child's progress. In order to prevent infection, the ear must be kept dry. When bathing the child, the parents are instructed to prevent water from getting into the auditory canal by occluding the meatus with a nonabsorbent cotton (lamb's wool) impregnated with petroleum jelly.

During play, young children between one and three years of age will frequently place small beads, paper, peanuts, or other foreign bodies into their external ear canals. Even an older child may innocently stick something into a friend's ear canal. If the child does not complain of the intromitted material, its presence may be detected only later, during a routine examination or because the ear has become secondarily infected.

Removal of these foreign bodies can be both technically difficult for the physician and painful to the child, especially when the foreign body is wedged in the ear canal. The problem may be compounded if an unskilled person has unsuccessfully attempted to remove the material, thereby producing local trauma and swelling within the ear canal. Should a secondary infection be present, the problem would be complicated by inflammatory changes characterized by swelling of the canal wall skin, otorrhea, and, if the inflammation is severe, granulation tissue. These findings, which can mimic a chronic mastoid infection, generally will not respond to local or systemic antibiotics and will completely resolve only after the offending object is removed.

As a rule, the removal of a foreign body requires that the patient be extremely cooperative, since an inappropriate movement can result in further injury with damage to the eardrum and the ossicular chain. Therefore, the use of a general anesthetic for removal of the foreign body should be considered if the physician anticipates that the process may be technically difficult and painful, or if the child is not able to hold still without being restrained.

TRAUMATIC MIDDLE EAR INJURIES

Trauma to the delicate tympanic membrane resulting in a tympanic membrane perforation occurs quite often and may be caused by a variety of injuries (Silverstein et al., 1973; Wright et al., 1969). An explosive blast, such as a firecracker going off near an ear, will produce a violent shock wave capable of rupturing the drum (Sudderth, 1974; Singh and Ahluwalia, 1968). A damaging shock wave can be produced if a child is slapped with an open hand across the ear, e.g., by an angry parent or when fighting with another child. If the blow occludes the external auditory meatus, the resulting inward displacement of the air column contained in the external canal will cause a rupture of the membrane. A similar type of injury occurs during dives or falls into swimming pools, during water skiing, while surfboarding, or while tumbling in a rough surf. A perforation may occur if the ear hits the water in such a way that the column of air contained within the external canal is forcibly displaced, or if the water strikes the ear with considerable impact.

Tympanic membrane lacerations frequently occur when a cotton-tipped applicator or other object being used to relieve an itch or clean out wax is accidentally pushed through the drum. Iatrogenic tears of the drum have occurred in the process of removing foreign bodies from the ear of a struggling child. Additionally, the tympanic membrane can be perforated during ear syringing to remove wax. Occasionally, the pressure of the water being instilled into the external canal is enough to drive a hard waxy pellet through the drum.

Following an uncomplicated tympanic membrane perforation, a mild conductive hearing loss will be observed on audiometric testing (10 to 35 dB). While small children rarely complain of loss of acuity, occasionally a tympanic membrane laceration will occur in a child who has an unrecognized pre-existing hearing loss in the opposite ear, thus causing a bilateral loss. In such cases, behavioral changes may reveal the change in hearing.

When a traumatic tympanic membrane perforation occurs, there is generally considerable pain, accompanied by bleeding from the ear that stops spontaneously. If water gets into the ear, a secondary infection may occur that should be treated with systemic antibiotics (e.g., ampicillin) and local nonirritating eardrops, (e.g,, Cortisporin Otic Suspension).

Injuries severe enough to rupture the tympanic membrane may also damage the ossicular chain (Silverstein et al., 1973; Wright et al., 1969). A dislocation of the incus is the most commonly observed injury. Usually, the incudostapedial joint will be separated or the stapes arch fractured (Sadé, 1964) or both. This trauma may cause a transient subluxation of the stapes into the inner ear vestibule, resulting in a tear of the annular ligament and a perilymphatic fluid leak into the middle ear space (Silverstein et al., 1973; Fee, 1968).

Generally, this fluid leak produces a significant sensory hearing loss and/or severe vertigo (Fig. 21–1).

Traumatic perilymph fistulas can also occur without ossicular involvement. The force of an injury sufficient to cause a tympanic membrane perforation may result in an accompanying rupture of the round window membrane. Such a defect will allow the leakage of perilymph into the middle ear, producing the characteristic symptoms of sensory hearing loss and vertigo (Fig. 21–2).

Ear injuries that result in the production of excessive stapedial vibrations can also produce intracochlear damage (Igarashi et al., 1964). Such trauma may be caused by a sudden explosive noise, an excessive excursion of the intact tympanic membrane, or a direct force applied to the stapes. These injuries cause a damaging piston-like movement of the stapes that produces a forceful perilymphatic fluid wave. This movement results in traumatic excursions of the basilar membrane that can lead to a loss of hair cells and even avulsion of the organ of Corti (Fig. 21–3).

Treatment of Middle Ear Injuries

Most traumatic tympanic membrane perforations will heal spontaneously. Small perforations may repair themselves within a few weeks. Occasionally, however, a very large perforation will persist. In such cases, the lacerated epithelial margins of the defect do not grow across the drum defect to bridge the

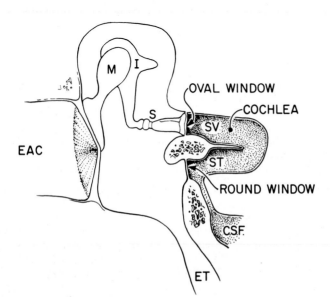

Figure 21–1 Diagrammatic representation of the ear. Movement of the stapes (**S**) in the oval window produces a perilymphatic fluid wave that travels from the scala vestibuli (**SV**) through the scala tympani (**ST**) and causes a displacement of the round window membrane. The perilymph communicates with the cerebrospinal fluid (**CSF**) through the cochlear aqueduct. **EAC** — external auditory canal. **M** — malleus. **I** — incus. **ET** — eustachian tube.

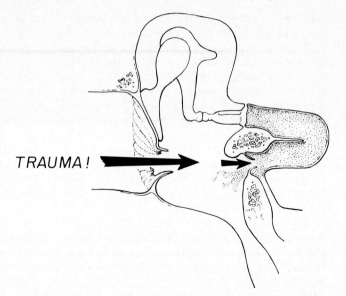

Figure 21–2 Trauma sufficient to rupture the tympanic membrane may also cause a round window membrane rupture with a resulting leak of perilymph (stippling) into the middle ear.

TRAUMA!

existing gap. Instead, the edges curl under the remaining drum remnant, forming a healed epithelial rim; thus, the perforation becomes a permanent one.

If the child is seen shortly after suffering a tympanic membrane perforation, an attempt can be made to realign the torn edges. The procedure can be performed either using general anesthesia or, in a cooperative child, under local anesthesia. The edges of the perforation, which frequently become inverted below the residual drum remnant, should be approximated and the fragments supported by gelfoam placed in the middle ear.

A persistent tympanic membrane perforation can often be encouraged to heal. The epithelialized edge of the drum remnant can be debrided chemically by cauterization, using minute quantities of 50 per cent trichloroacetic acid. A mildly irritating topical medication is prescribed to stimulate spontaneous reparative processes (Juers, 1963; Derlacki, 1973). Generally, the treatment has to be repeated several times; it is somewhat painful and therefore may not be well tolerated by young children.

Although most traumatic tympanic membrane perforations will heal spontaneously, in certain specific instances immediate surgery is necessary (Silverstein et al., 1973). If, following a middle ear injury, the patient suffers a neurosensory hearing loss and vertigo, the

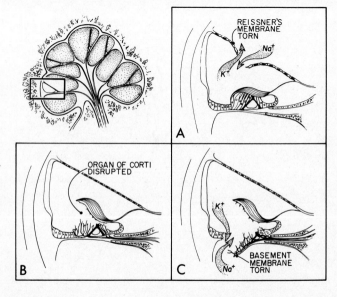

Figure 21–3 Excessive vibrations of the stapes can produce a forceful perilymphatic fluid wave that may result in intracochlear damage. A, Reissner's membrane, which normally separates the endolymph (high potassium–low sodium) from the perilymph (low potassium–high sodium), may be torn. The resulting changes in the K–Na concentration damage the affected hair cells, producing a sensory hearing loss. B, Excessive vibrations of the basilar membrane may produce a disruption of the organ of Corti. C, Tears of the basilar membrane will be associated with severe injuries to the organ of Corti and a profound hearing loss.

middle ear should be explored for a possible perilymphatic leak (Fig. 21–4). If a stapedial subluxation is present, it should be corrected by returning the stapes to its original position. Additionally, the oval window area should be sealed with a tissue graft. The possibility of round window membrane rupture should be explored; the presence of this condition is confirmed by the observation of clear fluid welling up from the round window niche or by the visualization of an actual tear in the round window membrane. In such cases, the area should be packed with a tissue graft. Another indication for immediate surgery would be a complete facial paralysis the onset of which was noted immediately following the middle ear trauma. This problem is discussed in the section on temporal bone fractures (p. 621).

Should ossicular chain involvement be suspected following injury to the middle ear, elective surgery to correct the hearing mechanism may be advantageous (Armstrong, 1970). Generally, patients who have a tympanic membrane perforation will present with a 30 to 40 dB conductive hearing loss. In these situations, a patch test may be useful in determining whether the hearing loss is due to the existing tympanic membrane perforation. This test is performed by first documenting the existing hearing loss with a preliminary audiogram. Next, a patch made of cigarette paper is placed over the entire drum defect. If the perforation is very large, it may not be possible to cover it entirely; moreover, in some cases, the anterior edge of the defect may be obscured by a prominent overhang of the canal wall. After the patch is applied, a repeat audiogram is obtained. A significant improvement in hearing indicates that the ossicular chain is intact and that the hearing loss is due to the perforation. However, when the hearing acuity is unchanged or is worse, the presence of a coexisting ossicular discontinuity should be suspected.

The radiologic examination of the ossicular chain using polytomography has been found to be very useful in evaluating patients who have suffered trauma to the middle ear (Wright et al., 1969). This technique will reveal a dislocated incus or malleus 90 per cent of the time. However, it should be noted that the delicately structured stapes cannot be adequately visualized (Fig. 21–5).

When the ossicular chain is disrupted, elective surgical correction may be considered. The immediate repair of traumatic injuries to the ossicular chain allows the surgeon to reduce an existing dislocation and to restore an essentially normal condition before fibrotic adhesions form. Additionally, at the time of the ossicular repair, the tympanic membrane perforation may be grafted to restore hearing to a normal level.

Prior to undertaking elective repair of a traumatic middle ear defect, one must carefully evaluate the child's ability to cooperate with the surgeon who will care for the ear postoperatively. In younger children particularly, the past medical background must be reviewed for problems suggestive of an underlying eustachian tube dysfunction that would jeopardize the chances for successful otologic surgery. A history of recurrent serous or purulent otitis media, an allergic background, symptoms suggestive of chronic

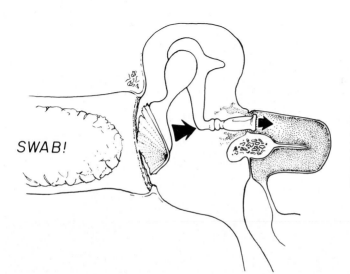

Figure 21–4 An injury to the middle ear, caused by a cotton-tipped swab accidentally pushed through the drum, displaced the stapes *(arrow)* into the vestibule and produced an oval window perilymphatic *(stippled area)* leak.

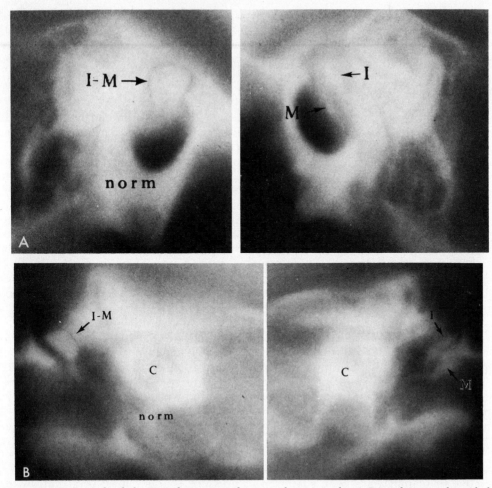

Figure 21–5 Ossicular dislocation demonstrated using polytomography. *A*, Lateral section through the middle ear. On the normal side (**norm**), the incus-malleus complex (**I-M**) has a molar tooth appearance. A dislocation of the ossicles produces a separation of the incus (**I**) from the malleus (**M**). *B*, Frontal section. On the normal side (**norm**), the incus and malleus produce a single density (**I-M**). On the opposite side, a traumatic ossicular discontinuity is present. The malleus (**M**) and incus (**I**) are seen as individual structures. The malleus is rotated laterally, with its head in the external canal and its long process pointing to the promontory. C = cochlea.

nasal congestion, and a history of frequent upper respiratory infections with otalgia would indicate that the child is not a suitable candidate for elective middle ear reconstructive surgery (see Chapter 17). In such children, especially if they are very young, the most suitable therapeutic alternative may be to temporize and accept the presence of a chronic tympanic membrane perforation. One must not overlook the clinical reality that the treatment for many children with eustachian tube dysfunction and serous otitis media is a myringotomy, i.e., creation of a perforation that is kept open by insertion of a middle ear ventilating tube.

When a child has a tympanic membrane

perforation, it is essential that water be prevented from entering the ear. Water irritates the exposed middle ear mucosa, producing a profuse seromucinous otorrhea. When infection supervenes, an acute bacterial otitis media will occur. Fungi, whose growth is stimulated by the moist environment of these draining ears, are a common cause of superficial infections. These problems can be avoided by occluding the external ear canal with lamb's wool and petroleum jelly when there is any chance of water getting into the ear. When swimming, the child should wear a bathing cap to assure that the lamb's wool is not displaced. Definitive surgery to close the tympanic membrane perforation may be performed when the child has "outgrown" the frequent ear problems associated with respiratory infections.

Surgical Repair of Middle Ear Injuries

Fracture of the ossicles can be corrected by tympanoplastic surgery in which the conductive mechanism is reconstructed, often dramatically improving the hearing level. Thus, when the long process of the incus has been fractured, the continuity of the ossicular chain can be restored by appropriately reshaping the incus and interposing it between the malleus handle and the stapes capitulum (Pennington, 1973). An alternative technique would be to use a stainless steel wire to connect these two structures (Bellucci, 1966). When both the stapes superstructure and the long process of the incus are fractured, the body of the incus can be sculpted so as to extend from the malleus handle to the stapes footplate. Malleolar fractures are usually associated with fracture or dislocation of the incus. In such cases, the sound-conducting mechanism can be reconstituted by placing a strut of conchal cartilage onto the stapes capitulum or the footplate, thereby enabling it to make contact with the tympanic membrane.

In comminuted temporal bone fractures, the patient's incus may have been shattered and therefore may not be available for ossicular reconstruction. In such cases, homograft incudi (Wehrs, 1974) and conchal cartilage have been utilized. In children the use of cortical bone for ossicular replacement is discouraged since there is a tendency for a bony ankylosis to form, with fixation to adjacent bony structures that results in recurrence of the conductive hearing loss.

Tympanic membrane defects can be repaired by grafting. The most common type of tissue used is the fascia that covers the temporalis muscle. The perichondrium obtained from the tragal cartilage is also a useful material for closing small defects or for reconstructing the ossicular mechanism when cartilage is required.

OTITIC BAROTRAUMA

As has been previously noted, snorkeling and scuba diving have become popular in recent years, with many adolescents participating in underwater diving as a recreational activity. Even more common is travel by plane. These activities, however, require that the individual be able to adapt to rapid changes in pressures (Graves and Edwards 1944; Elner et al., 1971).

During ascent in an airplane, the pressure in the middle ear increases until it reaches a point at which the eustachian tube is forced open. On descent, as the plane prepares to land, a negative middle ear pressure builds. Since the eustachian tube is normally closed while at rest, this pressure difference will persist until the person swallows. With the muscular activity of swallowing, the tensor veli palatini muscle contracts, the tubal lumen is opened, and the tympanic pressure is equalized. When diving underwater, the reverse sequence occurs: positive pressure is experienced on descent and negative pressure occurs on ascent.

If the eustachian tube fails to open, the resulting negative middle ear pressure causes a retraction of the tympanic membrane. In order to equilibrate the induced negative pressure, a transudation of serous fluid from the mucosal surface fills the middle ear (Flisberg et al., 1963). If the pressure changes are sudden, bleeding into the middle ear space may result or the tympanic membrane may rupture (Schuknecht, 1974). In adults, these pressure changes have been known to produce traumatic perilymphatic leaks due to round and/or oval window ruptures (Pullen, 1972; Goodhill et al., 1973) (Fig. 21–6).

Eustachian tube function is generally compromised when a person has an upper respiratory disorder. Thus, diving or flying — both of which require good eustachian tube function to equilibrate the middle ear pressure — may cause certain individuals to experience the difficulties described in the preceding paragraph. Many young children have borderline eustachian tube function and should not fly when they have a cold. Even on commercial airlines, as descent takes place, a negative middle ear pressure will result that may produce severe pain and a hearing loss. These problems can be minimized by using both oral and topical nasal decongestants to shrink the nasal and the eustachian tube mucosal linings before the plane begins to descend. Encouraging the child to swallow repeatedly or giving him chewing gum or giving an infant a bottle will keep the normal

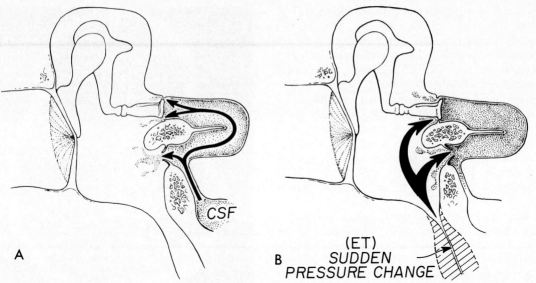

Figure 21–6 Perilymphatic leaks due to round or oval window ruptures. *A,* Sudden increases in cerebrospinal fluid (CSF) pressures occur during vigorous physical activity, sneezing, etc. The cerebrospinal and perilymph fluid spaces communicate through the cochlear aqueduct. Abrupt increases in cerebrospinal fluid pressure may be transmitted to the labyrinth, producing ruptures and leakage of perilymph into the middle ear (Explosive Route, Goodhill, 1971). *B,* Sudden air pressure changes transmitted through the eustachian tube (ET) into the middle ear space can produce ruptures of the round window membrane or of the annular ligament in the oval window and leakage of perilymph into the middle ear (Implosive Route, Goodhill, 1971).

forces that are necessary to open the eustachian tube operating. Additionally, the child should be kept in an erect position with his head elevated to decrease the passive venous mucosal congestion that tends to further compromise eustachian tube patency (Rundcrantz, 1970).

TEMPORAL BONE FRACTURES

Care of the Accident Victim

Head trauma is frequently associated with a simultaneous injury to the ear. In a motor vehicle or pedestrian accident, the victim may suffer multiple injuries that are life threatening and require urgent medical attention. When treating these patients, primary consideration must be given to assuring an adequate airway, preventing shock due to blood loss, controlling bleeding, and maintaining a stable neurological state.

In treating the unconscious patient, the first priority must be to establish an unobstructed airway. Oral and tracheal secretions must be cleared; tracheal toilet must be carried out if there is a suggestion of aspiration.

Assisted ventilation must be provided when respirations are inadequate. If there is evidence of a chest injury, such as a pneumothorax, a flail chest, or a cardiac tamponade, the condition must be immediately corrected.

Once adequate ventilation is assured, the patient should be evaluated for bleeding. It must be emphasized that hypotensive shock is rarely caused by a head injury alone. The common signs and symptoms of acute blood loss are a rising pulse rate and falling blood pressure. Generally, the opposite findings are seen with increased intracranial pressure — the pulse rate slows and the blood pressure rises. The treatment for hypovolemic shock is immediate replacement of the intravascular volume. Initially, an appropriate intravenous solution should be given until compatible whole blood transfusions are obtained. The source of bleeding, whether it is a ruptured spleen or kidney, a lacerated liver, or a pelvic fracture, must be identified and the hemorrhage controlled.

After stabilizing the patient's respiratory and circulatory systems, the neurological status should be evaluated. It is important that the patient's level of consciousness be explicitly documented. The fundi should be evaluated for papilledema as an indication of increased intracranial pressure. Pupil size, equality, and reactivity, and corneal reflexes should be recorded. Spontaneous or induced extraocular movements and the presence of nystagmus should be noted. Facial movements, either spontaneous or provoked by painful stimuli, should be documented. Moreover, symmetry of limb movements, muscle tone, and reflexes must be evaluated. Additionally, the possibility of a vertebral fracture should be considered, and if it is suspected, special care must be taken to prevent possible spinal cord injury.

The initial neurological evaluation establishes a baseline. The patient's clinical status will be determined by any changes in these primary observations. Thus, an improving level of consciousness and the absence of asymmetric lateralizing findings are hopeful signs. Increasing coma, dilatation of a pupil, and hemiparesis suggest a deteriorating condition that may be caused by cerebral edema or an expanding intracranial hematoma that may require neurosurgical intervention.

The care of accident victims suffering from head and other bodily injuries requires the

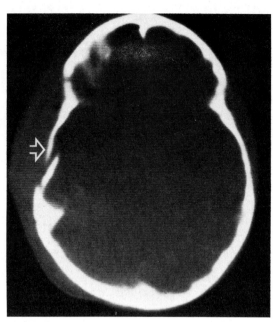

Figure 21-8 Computerized axial tomography. Arrow shows fracture of temporal squama.

specialized attention of physicians from various disciplines who must work as a team in a cooperative endeavor. Generally, the otolaryngologist has the dual responsibilities of establishing and maintaining proper ventilation, as well as evaluating the otoneurological status.

The radiological examination of a patient with head injury should be performed only after the patient's acute problems have been stabilized. The computerized axial tomographic study of the head is useful for demonstrating the presence of intracranial damage, such as an intracerebral or subdural hematoma and pneumocephalus (Fig. 21-7). Additionally, it may clearly demonstrate a fracture of the skull and/or temporal bone (Fig. 21-8). Skull radiographs should be obtained to observe for sutural splitting, a linear or depressed skull fracture, and the existence of pneumocephalus.

Classification of Temporal Bone Fractures

Temporal bone fractures were thoroughly studied and categorized during the end of the 19th and beginning of the 20th centuries (Grove, 1928). The fractures, which occasionally may be bilateral, are classified according to their course relative to the axis of the temporal bone (Grove, 1939; Proctor et al.,

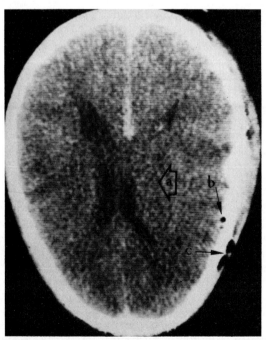

Figure 21-7 Computerized axial tomography performed because of a head injury. (a) Intracerebral edema with compression of the lateral ventricle, (b) pneumocephalus, (c) subcutaneous emphysema.

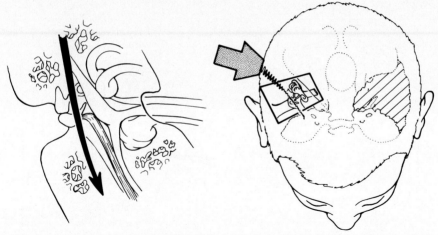

Figure 21–9 Longitudinal fractures of the temporal bone usually occur as a result of a circumscribed blow delivered to the temporoparietal area. The fracture line follows a course parallel to the long axis of the petrous apex.

1956; Hardwood-Nash, 1970; Ward, 1969). The longitudinal fracture that follows a course parallel to the long axis of the petrous apex is the most common; it accounts for 80 per cent of the temporal bone fractures seen (Fig. 21–9). Clinically, this type of fracture occurs following a circumscribed blow delivered to the temporoparietal region. The individual may not be knocked unconscious. However, the injury causes a bending inward of the skull and results in a fracture that follows a characteristic pathway. The separation extends from the squama to involve the posterior superior bony canal wall, lacerating the attached skin and causing bleeding from the ear. Evidence of the defect can sometimes be seen otoscopically, appearing as a steplike deformity with notching of the tympanic ring. The fracture continues anteriorly through the area of the tegmen. The bony rent that involves the roof of the middle ear causes mucosal bleeding that produces a hemotympanum. When the force of the impact is sufficient to cause a separation of the bony segments, significant middle ear injuries can result. In such a case, the tympanic membrane may be torn and the ossicles may be dislocated, fractured, or both. The facial nerve is involved in 25 to 30 per cent of patients suffering longitudinal temporal bone fractures. Injury to the facial nerve generally occurs in its horizontal portion between the geniculate ganglion and the second genu (McHugh, 1963). The fracture line continues anteriorly and parallel to the eustachian tube towards the foramen lacerum.

Transverse fractures, which run perpendicular to the long axis of the temporal bone, are much less common (Fig. 21–10). They occur as a result of forceful blows that usually produce serious head injury and loss of consciousness. Such blows may be fatal. Generally, the impact is exerted over the occipital or frontal area, which causes a compression of the calvarium in an anteroposterior direction. This results in a fracture where the skull is structurally weakest, i.e., in the area of the foramen magnum and at the base of the petrous bone, where it is perforated by many canals and foramina. The resulting bony rent characteristically crosses the pyramid at a right angle, extending into the area of the internal auditory canal, the cochlea, and the vestibule. This injury to the auditory and vestibular system immediately produces profound neurosensory hearing loss and vertigo. In 50 per cent of these cases, a severe facial nerve injury occurs that results in an immediate facial paralysis. The fracture may or may not extend into the middle ear. If the promontory surface is involved, rupture of the round and oval windows may occur, accompanied by dislodgement of the stapes.

Since the tympanic membrane generally remains intact, a hemotympanum may also be observed. Moreover, the fracture can extend to involve the jugular bulb area and other structures of the base of the skull.

The classification of temporal bone fractures into longitudinal and transverse is useful in that it emphasizes the various important anatomical structures likely to be injured

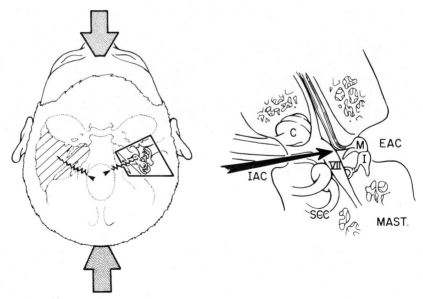

Figure 21–10 Transverse fractures of the temporal bone usually occur as a result of a forceful blow, the impact of which is exerted over the frontal or occipital area. This causes a compression of the calvarium in an anteroposterior direction with a fracture where the skull is weakest, i.e., the foramen magnum and the foramen within the petrous bone, The fracture line crosses the long axis of the petrous apex at right angles and may be bilateral. C = cochlea; M = Malleus; I = incus; IAC = internal auditory canal; EAC = external auditory canal; MAST = Mastoid; SCC = superior semicircular canal.

(Table 21–1). However, radiographically the fracture may not fall into either classification. The small child's skull is elastic, and following significant head trauma, inward compression of the convex surface can result in extensive lines of fracture. This may produce a comminuted type of fracture having both a longitudinal temporoparietal component and a transverse, base of the skull component (Hardwood-Nash, 1970; Potter, 1971) (Fig. 21–11). Additionally, in spite of the presence of cerebrospinal otorrhea, a temporal bone fracture may not be seen radiographically (Hardwood-Nash, 1970; Potter, 1972). Occasionally, even with polytomography, when the fragments are not greatly displaced or separated, it may not be possible to demonstrate a fracture (Mitchell and Stone, 1973).

Table 21–1 CLASSIFICATION OF TEMPORAL BONE FRACTURES

	Longitudinal Fractures	Transverse Fractures
Per cent of temporal bone fractures	80%	20%
Point of impact	Temporoparietal area	Frontal or occipital area
Force of impact	Moderate to severe	Severe
Loss of consciousness	Not always present	Present
Associated Otologic Findings		
Ear canal bleeding	Frequent	Infrequent
Tympanic membrane perforation	Frequent	Infrequent
Hemotympanum	Common	Less common
Hearing loss	Variable: conductive, mixed, and neurosensory	Profound neurosensory loss
Vertigo	Variable frequency and severity	Frequent; severe
Facial nerve:		
Injury	Variable severity	Severe
Incidence	25%	50%
Paralysis	May be incomplete; onset may be delayed	Immediate onset; complete paralysis

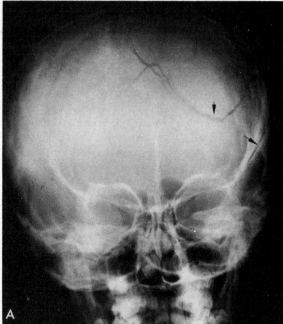

Figure 21-11 Frontal *(A)* and lateral *(B)* views of nine-year-old boy involved in a bicycle-automobile accident; he suffered a head injury with a period of unconsciousness. An extensive comminuted skull fracture that involves the temporal bone is present (arrows).

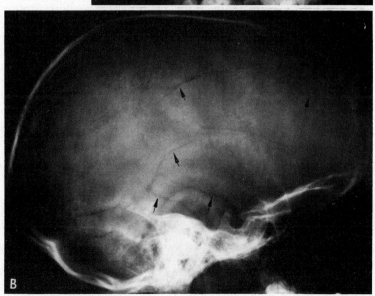

Therefore, it should be emphasized that serious damage can occur to the tympanic membrane, ossicular chain, and cochleovestibular systems without radiographic evidence of either a skull or a temporal bone fracture. Furthermore, it may be difficult to keep a small child properly positioned for the length of time necessary for adequate radiographic examination of the temporal bone without using sedation or a general anesthetic (see Chapter 8C for a complete discussion of temporal bone radiography). In spite of these inherent difficulties, radiographs of the tem-

poral bones will be useful to the clinician since they may show an ossicular dislocation. Furthermore, in the presence of a facial paralysis, visualization of the responsible fracture may help determine the operative approach and also may indicate the complexity of the existing problem. Thus, if a transverse fracture is observed, the surgeon will be alerted preoperatively that the facial nerve may have been torn and will be prepared for the possibility of nerve grafting. Nevertheless, it must be stressed that, although the radiographic studies can be useful, the demonstration of a temporal fracture in itself does not mean treatment is required.

Treatment of Temporal Bone Fractures

The comprehensive care of the accident victim has been discussed. However, depending on the severity of any coexisting trauma, it may be necessary to postpone such diagnostic procedures as audiometric evaluation, caloric tests, radiographs, and facial nerve testing. Even minor operative procedures may have to be deferred until the patient's condition is stable, especially with small children who require general anesthesia. Occasionally, when a serious concomitant condition requires operative intervention with general anesthesia, it may be possible to evaluate and treat existing otologic problems at the same time. For example, while the child is under general anesthesia, the external ear canal can be cleaned of blood clots and ceruminous debris and the tympanic membrane can be examined. If there has been a perforation, the edges can be reapproximated and the drum defect repaired. At the same time, minor ossicular defects can be corrected.

Evaluation and Management of Signs and Symptoms Associated with Temporal Bone Injuries

When considering the management of temporal bone fractures, the saying, "It's what's inside that counts" is appropriate. Therapy is aimed at restoring the function of the injured structures. Therefore, treatment must be guided by the individual victim's signs and symptoms.

Bleeding

Bleeding from the ear commonly occurs following acute trauma to the temporal area (Grove, 1939; Proctor et al., 1956; Mitchell and Stone, 1973; Røhrt, 1973). In order to determine its significance, the exact source of the hemorrhage must be identified. Glancing blows that displace the pinna from its soft tissue attachments to the scalp can produce a shearing effect that may lacerate the skin of the bony external canal and produce bleeding even with an intact tympanic membrane. Injuries of sufficient violence to produce a

temporal bone fracture will frequently be associated with a tear of the external canal that extends to and perforates the adjacent drum. Finally, severe trauma to the chin can cause the mandibular condyle to fracture through the anterior wall of the external auditory canal, causing bleeding from the ear and severe otalgia when the mouth is opened. Generally, the bleeding noted is self-limiting and requires no active therapy. Instilling a few drops of a sterile vasoconstrictor (1:100,000 adrenaline, 1 per cent Neo-Synephrine) can usually control the bleeding. Only rarely will significant hemorrhaging result, with bleeding coming from the ear as well as going through the eustachian tube into the nose and pharynx. In such cases, packing for hemostasis is required.

Following an ear injury, the external ear canal should be cleansed of ceruminous debris and blood clots. As soon as the more pressing injuries have been treated and the child is stable, the extent of injury to the ossicles and drum should be assessed. Admittedly, this task may be extremely difficult when dealing with a frightened child who is unable to cooperate. As discussed above, if an associated injury has required general anesthesia, the ear can be evaluated and treated efficiently while the child is asleep.

Four or five days after a base of the skull fracture, it is not unusual for an ecchymotic area to appear in the area of the mastoid process (Battle's sign). This is caused by the extravasation of blood pigments into the area and is evidence of an existing fracture but, in itself, is not an indication for any therapy.

Cerebrospinal Fluid Otorrhea·

A cerebrospinal fluid (CSF) otorrhea noted after head trauma is a definite sign that the skull has been fractured and a meningeal tear has occurred. This traumatic communication can be the pathway for bacterial contamination and the cause of meningitis. Cerebrospinal fluid otorrhea has been reported as occurring much more frequently in children than in adults following a temporal bone fracture (Hardwood-Nash, 1970; Mitchell and Stone, 1973). The higher incidence of this clinical sign in youngsters is probably related to the elastic properties of the child's skull. Following significant trauma, the displacement of the highly malleable bony structures results in a stretching, with tearing of the underlying attached meningeal structures.

A cerebrospinal fluid leak may be obscured by active bleeding coming from the injured ear. When a cerebrospinal fluid leak is suspected, the bloody material from the ear should be collected and a sample placed on a filter paper. If cerebrospinal fluid is present, it will separate from the blood, forming a clear ring around the central hemorrhagic spot. As the coexisting bleeding ceases, the character of the otorrhea changes. Moreover, as the fluid becomes more watery and clearer, the presence of a cerebrospinal fluid leak becomes more obvious. In cases where the tympanic membrane has remained intact, the presence of cerebrospinal fluid behind the drum will mimic the otoscopic findings observed in serous otitis media, i.e., a dull, immobile drum. In such cases, if the patient is instructed to bend over or is held upside down, clear fluid may pass down the eustachian tube and drip out the nose. An alternative way of obtaining a sample of the fluid is to perform a myringotomy and to collect the fluid directly from the middle ear. The material obtained should be analyzed for sugar. A sugar concentration of greater than 40 gm per 100 ml suggests that the material is cerebrospinal fluid.

In most cases, traumatic cerebrospinal fluid otorrhea will stop spontaneously within two weeks and rarely requires surgical intervention. The use of prophylactic antibiotics to prevent meningitis is controversial (Mac Gee et al., 1970; Klastersky et al., 1976). Bedrest, avoidance of activity, and elevation of the head to decrease the intracranial cerebrospinal fluid pressure is recommended.

A persistent or recurrent cerebrospinal fluid leak is a common cause for recurrent meningitis. When this possibility is suspected, the presence of the leak should be documented and its exact location identified. The area from which the contrast material extravasates into the temporal bone may be pinpointed by performing a posterior fossa contrast study (Schultz and Stool, 1970; Kaufman et al., 1969). The presence of a cerebrospinal fluid leak may also be detected by using radioisotopes (Parisier and Birken, 1976): [111]Indium DTPA* is injected into the cerebrospinal fluid spaces, and if a tympanic membrane perforation is present, a cottonball is placed

adjacent to the drum opening. Additional cottonballs are inserted intranasally to absorb any cerebrospinal fluid leaking down the eustachian tube. Serial scans of the patient's head area are performed to observe suspected extravasation into the temporal bone. If the cerebrospinal fluid leak persists for more than four weeks, or if it recurs, surgery should be considered. Using an appropriate temporal bone operative technique, the area from which the cerebrospinal fluid is leaking must be identified and securely packed off using temporalis fascia and a free muscle plug. Occasionally, in refractory cases, a neurosurgical approach to seal the leak from within the cranial cavity may be required.

Hearing Loss

Following a significant head injury, the focus of medical attention is directed towards controlling life-threatening problems and closely monitoring the patient's neurological status. When there is no bleeding from the ear and the tympanic membrane is intact, it may be erroneously concluded that no significant ear damage has occurred. Indeed, infants and young children generally will not complain of having suffered a hearing loss. As a result, traumatic hearing losses may not be detected at the time of the injury, especially when they are unilateral and the child suffers no functional impairment. Thus, it is common for the effect of the trauma not to be recognized until much later. For example, it may first be detected when the child's hearing acuity is screened in school, or even later during a military preinduction or a pre-employment physical examination when the individual is noted to have an unusual hearing loss of undetermined origin. Therefore, following significant head injury, an attempt should be made to establish accurate auditory thresholds. In infants, this may require repeated evaluations performed over many months, until reliable thresholds can be obtained (see the discussion of audiologic assessment in Chapter 8B).

The hearing losses that occur as a result of head trauma vary considerably (Table 21–2). The most common type of hearing impairment following head and temporal bone trauma is a neurosensory hearing loss (Table 21–3), which has been reported in from 13 to 83 per cent of patients with these injuries (Podoshin and Fradis, 1975; Hough and

---

*[111]Indium diethylenetriamine pentaacetic acid

Table 21–2   INCIDENCE OF TRAUMATIC CONDUCTIVE HEARING LOSS
DUE TO OSSICULAR DISRUPTION

	Fracture of Temporal Bone (per cent)	Head Injury (per cent)
Podoshin and Fradis, 1975		1.4
Cremin, 1969		1
Røhrt, 1973	1	
Mitchell and Stone, 1973°	6	
Proctor et al., 1956	32	
Hough and Stuart, 1968	37	

°Pediatric series.

Stuart, 1968; Tos, 1973; Grove, 1947; Mitchell and Stone, 1973; Røhrt, 1973; Barber, 1969). Audiometric analysis of the hearing loss by complete site-of-lesion tests has demonstrated that some patients develop a cochlear loss, while others exhibit a retrocochlear loss. Additionally, even when a conductive hearing disorder is present, a coexisting neurosensory type of loss will frequently be observed.

Pathogenesis of Cochlear Loss. When significant trauma occurs to the head, with or without fracture, the force of the impact will momentarily compress the child's relatively elastic skull, which rapidly regains its original configuration. The pressure wave involves the encased cochlear structures and is thought to cause an excessive displacement of the basilar membrane (Igarashi et al., 1964; Schuknecht, 1969; 1950). This displacement produces a hearing loss similar to that caused by intense acoustic stimulation, that is, a discrete drop in acuity in the 4000 to 8000 Hz range. Generally, the discrimination scores will be good, recruitment may be present, and there will not be any abnormal tone decay. Similar hearing losses were produced experimentally in animals (Schuknecht et al., 1951). A powerful blow to a cat's head held in

a fixed position, produced a loss of acuity confined to the 3000 to 8000 Hz range. The pathologic findings observed in these temporal bones resembled those of patients with a history of head trauma. Histologically, there were varying degrees of damage to the organ of Corti. This damage was most marked in the midbasal cochlear turn.

A traumatic cochlear-type of hearing loss may occur as a result of leakage of perilymph from the inner ear vestibule (Fig. 21–12) (Fee, 1968). A blow to the skull may produce a shock wave that will distort the area of the round window niche and disrupt the attachment of the round window membrane, thereby causing it to tear. Following a significant head injury, the stapes, which is suspended within the air-containing middle ear cleft, will be exposed to a different compressional force than will the surrounding temporal bone. Moreover, the trauma may stimulate the simultaneous contraction of the stapedius muscle, which acts to rotate the stapes posteriorly and laterally out of the oval window. As a result of these forces, a subluxation of the stapes occurs that produces a tear of the annular ligament. Following either of these injuries involving the round or oval window, there is a resulting perilymphatic fluid leak

Table 21–3   INCIDENCE OF TRAUMATIC NEUROSENSORY HEARING LOSS

	Fracture of Temporal Bone (per cent)	Head Injury (per cent)
Hough and Stuart, 1968	62	
Barber, 1969	63	46
Proctor et al., 1956	56	83
Tos, 1973	27	
Røhrt, 1973	14	
Mitchell and Stone, 1973°	13	
Grove, 1939	63	24 to 45
Podoshin and Fradis, 1975		19

°Pediatric series.

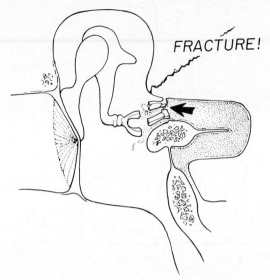

Figure 21–12 Temporal bone fracture with disruption of the stapes and a perilymph leak producing a sensory hearing loss.

which is associated with a hearing loss of varying severity. Furthermore, the traumatic distortion of the cochlear configuration following a blow to the head can produce a rupture of the relatively delicate basilar or Reissner's membrane. This results in a disruption of the partition between the cochlear duct and the scala tympani or vestibuli. As a consequence, the potassium-rich endolymph mixes with the sodium-rich perilymph, producing biochemical changes that cause a significant labyrinthine disorder (see Fig. 21–3).

Symptomatically, vertigo usually occurs following cochlear membrane tears and/or perilymphatic leaks. The spinning and accompanying nausea with vomiting may be so unpleasant that the patient will not immediately be aware of the associated hearing loss. The treatment of traumatic perilymphatic leaks was discussed in the part of this chapter dealing with treatment of middle ear injuries.

Pathogenesis of a traumatic retrocochlear hearing loss. Following a head injury, the patient may suffer a hearing loss characterized audiometrically by a discrimination score that is surprisingly low and the presence of pathologic tone decay. These findings indicate the existence of a retrocochlear process. Recent animal experiments have demonstrated that, following trauma to the freely mobile head, a retrocochlear or central auditory

hearing loss occurs (Makishima and Snow, 1975a; 1975b; 1976). At the moment of impact, the brain, which is suspended in cerebrospinal fluid, moves independently within the rigid skull, causing a substantial amount of swirling. This rotational displacement of the brain around the brain stem frequently results in a contrecoup cerebral injury. Moreover, this movement can severely stretch the cranial nerves where they leave the brain to enter their respective foramina (Strich, 1961). The abducens and the auditory-vestibular nerves seem to be particularly susceptible to this type of shearing force. As a result of this type of injury, multiple unilateral or bilateral cranial nerve deficits may occur even without skull fractures.

Pathologic examination of temporal bones obtained from persons who died as a result of head trauma have shown hemorrhages of the eighth cranial nerve at the fundi of the internal auditory canal (Grove, 1928; Makishima and Snow, 1975a). Recently, animal experiments were performed that were designed to simulate the kind of injury that occurs to man (Makishima and Snow, 1975a; 1976). Guinea pigs with freely mobile heads were shaken within a padded cell. None of the experimental animals suffered a skull fracture. Nevertheless, the experiments did produce retrocochlear and/or central types of hearing losses. The pathological findings were similar to those observed in human temporal bones. Areas of hemorrhage were present in the cerebrum, cerebellum, brain stem, eighth nerve, and seventh nerve.

The extent of the neurosensory hearing loss that occurs following head trauma is not always consistent with the severity of the blow or with the extent of the resulting neurological trauma. Occasionally, a patient who has suffered a mild head injury will have a surprisingly severe neurosensory hearing loss, whereas the victim with a serious concussion may not experience a significant loss of acuity. In addition, the neurosensory hearing loss observed following trauma is not always permanent. Frequently, there is some return of hearing acuity. Low-frequency losses, for instance, have a greater tendency to resolve than do higher frequency losses. Indeed, depending on the mechanism of the injury, spontaneous improvement of hearing may occur. The hemorrhage and edema within a nerve that is caused by stretching may also resolve, leaving little permanent damage. Finally, the healing of intracochlear membrane tears and the sealing off of traumatic oval or round window leaks may be accompanied by the recovery of hearing.

Conductive Hearing Loss. A longitudinal fracture of the temporal bone is often associated with middle ear injuries since bleeding into the middle ear space frequently occurs as a result of the trauma. When the drum remains intact, a hemotympanum results (Podoshin and Fradis, 1975; Hendrick et al., 1965). This has been estimated to occur in 3 to 5 per cent of patients with skull fractures and in 20 per cent of patients with temporal bone fractures (Mitchell and Stone, 1973). The condition is usually temporary, improving spontaneously when the blood is either resorbed from the tympanic cavity or evacuated from the area through the eustachian tube into the nasopharynx. Occasionally, the fluid collection persists for many weeks. In these cases, when a myringotomy is performed, the fluid aspirated will resemble serum. In such cases, a tube should be inserted in order to ventilate the middle ear cleft.

When the force of an injury fractures the temporal bone, a gap results between the fragments as they momentarily separate. Characteristically this rent will extend through the posterior superior canal wall and will produce a rupture of the tympanic membrane, with bleeding from the ear canal. Tympanic membrane perforations occur in

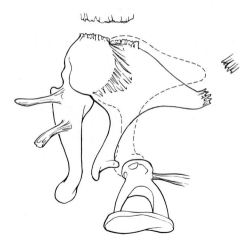

Figure 21–14 Dislocation of the incus with a separation of the incudostapedial joint is the most common type of ossicular injury.

about 50 per cent of patients with temporal bone fractures (Grove, 1939; Mitchell and Stone, 1973). Often, the traumatic drum defect will heal spontaneously. In some cases, the traumatic fragmentation of the temporal bone can damage the contained ossicles (Fig. 21–13) (Hough, 1959; Hough and Stuart, 1968; Wright et al., 1969; Spector et al., 1973; Elbrond and Aastrup, 1973; Cremin, 1969). Usually, this type of injury occurs with head trauma of sufficient intensity to cause unconsciousness (see Table 21–3). The most common type of ossicular injury associated with temporal bone fractures is a separation of the incudostapedial joint (Fig. 21–14). Dislocation of the incus occurs almost as often. In fact, it is not unusual for these two types of injuries to

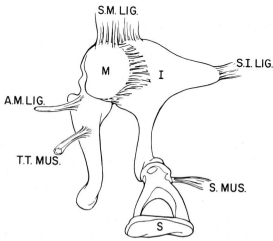

Figure 21–13 Ossicular chain — Malleus (**M**), Incus (**I**), Stapes (**S**). Middle ear muscles — Tensor tympani muscle (**T.T. MUS.**), Stapedius muscle (**S. MUS.**). Ossicular ligaments — Anterior malleolar ligament (**A.M. LIG.**), Superior malleolar ligament (**S.M. LIG.**), Short incudal ligament (**S.I. LIG.**).

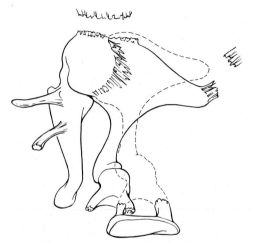

Figure 21–15 Dislocation of the incus; fracture of the stapes crura.

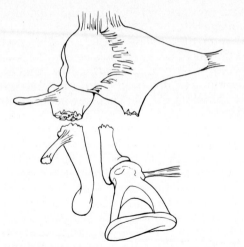

Figure 21–16 A fracture of the malleus is generally accompanied by other ossicular injuries.

occur simultaneously. Stapedial crural fractures are less common (Fig. 21–15), with the malleus being the ossicle least likely to be injured (Fig. 21–16).

There are several anatomical reasons that may explain these observations (Hough, 1959; Hough and Stuart, 1968). The malleus and stapes have firmer points of attachment than the incus. Moreover, the malleolar handle is supported by the tympanic membrane and has attachments to the anterior malleolar ligament and to the tensor tympani muscle, which give this ossicle ample support. The stapes is also anchored in the oval window niche by the annular ligament, and it gains further support from the attachment of the stapes muscle. Therefore, of the three ossicles, the incus is the most vulnerable to traumatic injuries since it is suspended between the malleus and stapes with only one firm point of attachment — the posterior incudal ligament.

The vulnerability of the incus is compounded by the contraction of the middle ear muscles. A traumatic blow causes an abrupt reflex muscular contraction. The stapedius muscle rotates the stapes posteriorly and laterally out of the oval window. The tensor tympani muscle contraction simultaneously pulls the malleus handle and the attached incus medially toward the promontory. Following a severe blow to the head, the uncontrolled reflex muscular contraction may produce an unstable ossicular situation, making the incudostapedial joint the most vulnerable link in the ossicular chain (Fig. 21–17).

In many case reports describing the surgical correction of traumatic ossicular disruptions in adults, the damage actually occurred in childhood (Hough, 1959; Hough and Stuart, 1968; Spector et al., 1973; Wright et al., 1969). Such an ear injury may not be detected, since most small children will not complain of the resulting loss of hearing. Therefore, following any otologic trauma, an audiometric evaluation should be obtained routinely.

Vertigo

The trauma that produces a neurosensory hearing loss may simultaneously cause vertigo (Podoshin and Fradis, 1975; Silverstein et al., 1973; Grove, 1939; Proctor et al., 1956; Barber, 1969; Schuknecht, 1969). The pathogenesis of traumatic vestibular and auditory injuries involves common sensory organ and neural innervation. Thus, for example, when the eighth nerve is damaged by a shearing force or when a perilymph leak occurs, vestibular symptoms as well as hearing loss may occur.

A labyrinthine concussion may result following a head injury especially when the otic capsule is fractured. The victim, if conscious,

Figure 21–17 A traumatic blow to the head causes an abrupt contraction of the middle ear muscles. *A,* The stapedius rotates the stapes laterally and posteriorly out of the oval window. The tensor tympani pulls the malleus handle medially toward the promontory. T.T. = tensor tympani muscle; S. MUS. = stapedius muscle. *B,* The simultaneous reflex contraction of these two muscles creates a tension that pulls the malleus in an opposite direction from the stapes and that may be a factor in producing a dislocation of the incus.

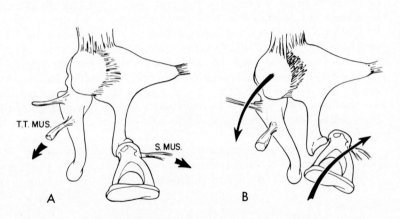

will immediately experience a violent spinning sensation which will be accompanied by a neurosensory hearing loss, nausea, and vomiting. Characteristically, following a peripheral labyrinthine injury, the patient will be more comfortable when positioned with the head turned so that the injured ear is up. The rapid phase of nystagmus will beat toward the uninvolved ear. However, in many instances, in spite of the patient's subjective complaint of vertigo, the observer will fail to see the expected nystagmus. In such cases, the absence of nystagmus is due to its suppression by visual fixation: when the patient is examined with eyes open, nystagmus due to a peripheral labyrinthine disorder may be markedly suppressed or abolished by visual fixation. This effect of the visual system may be abolished by examining the patient with eyes closed using electronystagmography (refer to Chapter 11). Another way of overcoming visual fixation is by using Frenzel glasses, which contain +20 diopter lenses embedded in a goggle-like frame (Cohen, 1966). Within the frame are small light bulbs. The purpose of these glasses is to blur the vision and effectively prevent visual fixation. Additionally, they magnify and illuminate the patient's eyes, making it easier for the examiner to detect even a fine nystagmus. The Frenzel glasses can easily be carried in a medical bag, and are extremely useful when the physician is required to perform a bedside evaluation of the vertiginous patient who either cannot be transported to a vestibular laboratory for electronystagmography because of associated injuries, or is unwilling to move since the slightest change in position produces violent spinning and vomiting.

Following a traumatic labyrinthine injury, the patient generally will be unwilling to move. The central nervous system gradually compensates for the injury and a characteristic recovery phase occurs. For the first two to four days, the vertigo will be constantly present. After a few days the patient will be dizzy with any movement. Slowly, the vertigo diminishes so that it only occurs transiently during head movement. After a few weeks, it will be present only when the head is turned so that the affected ear is facing downward. In children, complete symptomatic recovery usually occurs within three to six weeks.

An otoneurologic evaluation should be performed routinely to differentiate between imbalance and vertigo caused by injury to the brain stem or cerebellum, and that due to damage of the peripheral end organ (see Chapter 8D). Following an ear injury, when vestibular damage is suspected, the caloric test is useful in evaluating the functional status of a traumatized labyrinth. Caloric testing should not be performed when a perilymphatic or a cerebrospinal fluid leak is suspected. When a tympanic membrane perforation is present, unless air is used for the caloric test, special precautions must be taken before water is instilled into the ear. In cooperative children and adolescents with external canals of adequate size, finger cots are inserted into both the ear canals. This will prevent water from getting into the middle ear space through a drum defect. An equal volume of ice water is instilled into each finger cot; the nystagmus produced by the caloric stimulation can then be evaluated. Sterile saline can be used to perform a caloric examination in smaller children with a perforated ear drum in whom a finger cot cannot be inserted. A 30 cc sterile saline vial is chilled in a beaker of iced water, the ear canal is carefully cleaned of any wax or debris, and then the minimum amount of iced sterile saline that will produce a definite nystagmus is instilled into the normal ear (0.2 to 0.6 cc). The volume of the same solution necessary to induce nystagmus in the affected ear is determined for comparison. The functional status of both labyrinths is qualitatively evaluated by comparing the volume of iced saline required in each ear to produce nystagmus.

Post-traumatic positional vertigo has been reported to occur in children (Eviatar and Eviatar, 1974). In this condition, the vertigo is induced when the head is placed in a supine or hyperextended position. When the patient is placed in this position, the nystagmus appears after a latency period of a few seconds, builds to a crescendo, and then disappears. Clinically, the Frenzel glasses are extremely helpful in observing these characteristic eye movements. If the patient's head is moved and then returned to the original position, the nystagmus will not occur since it is fatigable. In adults, this condition is common. It has been attributed to the jarring loose of the utricular otoliths, which gravitate to the most dependent portion of the vestibular system and come to rest on the ampullated end of the posterior semicircular canal (Schuknecht, 1969). Clinically, however, this condition seldom seems to occur in children.

Facial Paralysis

Overall, a facial paralysis occurs in 21 to 33 per cent of children suffering from temporal bone fractures (Hardwood-Nash, 1970; Mitchell and Stone, 1973; Alberti and Biagioni, 1972). A facial paralysis occurs in half of the patients who have a transverse type of fracture (Grove, 1939; Proctor et al., 1956). However, since 75 to 80 per cent of temporal bone fractures are of the longitudinal type, the majority of facial nerve injuries occur as a result of this latter injury. Anatomically, the facial nerve is most commonly injured where it is most vulnerable (McHugh, 1963). Regardless of the type of temporal bone fracture, damage to the facial nerve usually occurs in its horizontal portion between the geniculate ganglion and the second genu where it turns to assume a vertical course. In this area, the thin, relatively fragile bone that covers the facial nerve affords little protection. In longitudinal fractures, the damage to the facial nerve is frequently mild, and most patients recover spontaneously. The more serious transverse fractures of the temporal bone that are caused by violent head trauma occur infrequently; 50 per cent of persons with these fractures suffer a severely traumatized or torn facial nerve.

When examining a patient following significant head trauma, the physician must evaluate facial movement. Specific detailed observations describing the movements of the upper and lower face, including eye closure, should be recorded when the patient is initially seen. Admittedly, this may be extremely difficult when severe facial lacerations, ecchymotic changes, and swelling are present. If the patient is unconscious, an attempt to produce facial grimacing should be made by using a painful stimulus. The symmetry of facial muscle tone should be assessed. When a facial paralysis is present, it must be determined whether the paralysis is complete or partial. Even in the unconscious patient, an assessment of tear production should be attempted by performing the Schirmer test. When the patient is conscious, complete topographic testing should be performed to try, anatomically, to localize the site of injury to the facial nerve (see Chapter 13, Facial Paralysis). Thus, when a patient with a facial paralysis does not tear on the affected side, this indicates that the facial nerve has been injured at, or proximal to, the geniculate ganglion.

The facial paralysis following severe head injury may be caused by an injury to the central nervous system rather than to the peripheral nerve. In one study of 115 cases of traumatic facial paralysis occurring in children, 55 per cent were attributable to upper motor neuron injury (Hendrick et al., 1965). Frequently, but not invariably, the central type of facial paralysis will be more marked in the lower two thirds of the face. Additionally, in spite of the paralysis, movement on the affected side may occur in association with involuntary emotional expressions.

If a patient is noted to have a complete facial paralysis immediately following a temporal bone injury, it is necessary to perform only topographic testing in order to determine the site of injury. Additionally, a complete polytomographic radiologic examination may help to pinpoint the site and extent of involvement. In these patients, electrical testing is unnecessary since the results observed will be misleading for at least 48 to 72 hours after the acute injury. As soon as the patient is able to tolerate surgery, the facial nerve should be explored to determine the cause of injury. Bony fragments impinging on the nerve should be removed. Since damage to the nerve is frequently caused by edema, the neurolemmal sheath should be incised. If the nerve is lacerated, immediate nerve grafting should be performed. When topographic tests demonstrate that tearing is absent on the affected side, a complete exploration with decompression of the facial nerve into the internal auditory canal is indicated.

When the facial paralysis is of delayed onset or is incomplete, the prognosis for spontaneous recovery is better. The status of the facial nerve should be monitored carefully using the tests of facial function described in Chapter 13. If, on serial testing, nerve degeneration is observed, exploration of the facial nerve with decompression should be performed.

FACIAL PARALYSIS IN NEONATES

Infrequently, a newborn infant is noted to have a peripheral facial paralysis, which may be due to several causes (Alberti and Biagioni, 1972; Miehlke, 1973; Hepner, 1951; Kornblut, 1974). During the last months of pregnancy, the increased intrauterine pressure may continuously press the side of the embryo's face against its own shoulder, resulting in a facial paralysis. During delivery, damage to the facial nerve can occur either when the neonate's head is squeezed against the mother's sacral prominence or when obstetrical forceps are applied traumatically. In such cases, the nerve may be injured by direct pressure either in the facial-parotid area or within the temporal bone. In the latter instance, the trauma may occur as a result of either a forceful indentation of the elastic skull or an actual fracture. Frequently, the intrapartum traumatic facial paralysis will improve spontaneously (Alberti and Biagioni, 1972). However, facial nerve decompression has been required in selected cases (McHugh, 1963; Kornblut, 1977).

ACOUSTIC TRAUMA

One of the most common causes of loss of hearing is acoustic trauma. An explosive blast near a child's ear, such as the detonation of a firecracker, cap gun, or weapon, can produce an immediate loss of hearing that occasionally is severe. Repeated, frequent exposure to the loud noises produced by snowmobiles, motorcycle engines, power tools, or model gasoline engines can also damage the inner ear. The popularity of loudly amplified music has made headphone amplifiers and loud electronic rock music a part of our youth culture. However, it has been suggested that this fad can damage hearing.

A loud, explosive blast produces a sound wave causing a large excursion of the tympanic membrane, which is translated through the ossicular chain into a forceful inner ear perilymphatic traveling fluid wave. As a result, an excessive displacement of the basilar membrane occurs that causes a shearing force that damages the hair cells.

Prolonged exposure to loud noises produces enzymatic and biochemical activity within the organ of Corti. Moderate auditory stimuli produce increased metabolism of the hair cells, which after a period of time leads to exhaustion of energy sources and results in a loss of auditory acuity. Although these changes are initially reversible, a permanent hearing loss will occur when a person is repeatedly exposed to loud noises (Schuknecht, 1974).

The severity of the hearing loss following chronic noise exposure is related to the intensity of the sound and daily duration of exposure; for example, exposure to a constant noise of 100 dB for two hours is equivalent to exposure to a noise of 115 dB for 15 minutes. Thus, it has been estimated that 41.5 per cent of individuals 50 years of age who have been habitually exposed to a 100 dB noise will suffer a noise-induced hearing handicap (Guide for Conservation of Hearing in Noise, 1969).

Noise-induced hearing losses can be prevented by use of ear protectors that reduce the exposure of the inner ear to traumatic acoustic stimuli. Earplugs designed to occlude the ear canal are an inexpensive way of obtaining personal protection. Contrary to popular opinion, filling the ear canal with dry cotton is not effective, since it does little to attenuate sound levels. Another approach is to control noise exposure environmentally — preventing children from playing with cap guns or exploding fire crackers and controlling the intensity of amplified music.

SELECTED REFERENCES

Hardwood-Nash, D. C. 1970. Fractures of the petrous and tympanic parts of the temporal bone in children: A tomographic study of 35 cases. Am. J. Roentgenol. Radium Ther. Nucl. Med. *110*:598–607.

Hough, J. V. D., and Stuart, W. D. 1968. Middle ear injuries in skull trauma. Laryngoscope, *78*:899–937.

A comprehensive, well-organized clinical review which describes the authors' experiences with 31 cases of temporal bone fractures with accompanying middle ear damage.

Mitchell, D. P., and Stone, P. 1973. Temporal bone fractures in children. Can. J. Otolaryngol., *2*:156–162.

Both these excellent articles review the clinical experience with temporal bone fractures at the Hospital for Sick Children, Toronto, Canada. Unlike most reports, which are based on patients of all ages, these authors' observations are derived exclusively from a pediatric population.

REFERENCES

Alberti, P. W., and Biagioni, E. 1972. Facial paralysis in children. A review of 150 cases. Laryngoscope, *82*:1013–1020.

Armstrong, B. W. 1970. Traumatic perforations of the tympanic membrane: Observe or repair? Laryngoscope, *82*:1822–1830.

Barber, H. O. 1969. Head injury. Audiological and vestibular findings. Ann. Otol. Rhinol. Laryngol., *78*:239–252.

Bellucci, R. J. 1966. Tympanoplasty, the malleus stapes wire and total defect skin graft. Laryngoscope, *76*:1439–1458.

Cohen, B. C. 1966. The examination of vestibulo-oculomotor function. Mt. Sinai J. Med. N.Y., *33*: 243–251.

Cremin, M. D. 1969. Injuries of the ossicular chain. J. Laryngol. Otol., *83*:845–862.

Derlacki, E. L. 1973. Office closure of central tympanic membrane perforations: A quarter century of experience. Trans. Am. Acad. Ophthalmol. Otolaryngol., 77:(ORL) 53–65.

Elbrond, E., and Aastrup, J. E. 1973. Isolated fractures of the stapedial arch. Acta Otolaryngol., *75*:357–358.

Elner, A., Ingelstedt, S., Ivarsson, A. 1971. Normal function of the eustachian tube. Acta Otolaryngol., *72*:320–328.

Eviatar, L., and Eviatar, A. 1974. Vertigo in childhood. Clin. Pediatr., *13*:940–941.

Fee, G. A. 1968. Traumatic perilymphatic fistulas. Arch. Otolaryngol., *88*:477–480.

Flisberg, K., Ingelstedt, S., and Ortegren, V. 1963. On middle ear pressure. Acta Otolaryngol., (Suppl) *182*:43–56.

Goodhill, V., Harris, I., Brockman, S. J., and Hantz, O. 1973. Sudden deafness and labyrinthine window ruptures. Ann. Otol. Rhinol. Laryngol., *82*:2–12.

Goodhill, V. 1974. Sudden deafness and round window rupture. Laryngoscope, *81*:1462–1474.

Graves, G. O., and Edwards, E. F. 1944. The eustachian tube. Arch. Otolaryngol., *39*:359–397.

Grove, W. E. 1928. Otological observations in trauma of the head. A clinical study based on 42 cases. Arch. Otolaryngol., *8*:249–299.

Grove, W. E. 1939. Skull fractures involving the ear. A clinical study of 211 cases. Laryngoscope, *49*:678–707, 833–870.

Grove, W. E. 1947. Hearing impairment due to craniocerebral trauma. Ann. Otol. Rhinol. Laryngol., *56*:264–269.

Guide for Conservation of Hearing in Noise. 1969. American Academy of Ophthalmology and Otolaryngology. Rochester, Minn.

Hardwood-Nash, D. C., 1970. Fractures of the petrous and tympanic parts of the temporal bone in children: A tomographic study of 35 cases. Am. J. Roentgenol. Radium Ther. Nucl. Med., *110*:598–607.

Hendrick, E. B., Hardwood-Nash, D. C., and Hudson, A. R. 1965. Head injuries in children: Survey of 4,465 consecutive cases at Hospital for Sick Children, Toronto, Canada. Clin. Neurosurg., *11*:46–65.

Hepner, W. R., Jr. 1951. Some observations of facial paresis in the newborn infant: Etiology and incidence. Pediatrics, *8*:494–497.

Hough, J. V. D. 1959. Incudostapedial joint separation: Etiology, treatment and significance. Laryngoscope, *69*:644–664.

Hough, J. V. D., and Stuart, W. D. 1968. Middle ear injuries in skull trauma. Laryngoscope, *78*:899–937.

Igarashi, M., Schuknecht, H., and Myers, E. 1964. Cochlear pathology in humans with stimulation deafness. J. Laryngol., *78*:115–123.

Juers, A. L. 1963. Perforation closure by marginal eversion. Arch. Otolaryngol., 77:76–80.

Kaufman, B., Jordan, V. M., and Pratt, L. L. 1969. Positive contrast demonstration of a cerebrospinal fluid fistula through the fundus on the internal auditory meatus. Acta Radiol., *9*:83–90.

Klastersky, J., Sadeghi, M., and Brihaye, J. 1976. Antimicrobial prophylaxis in patients with rhinorrhea or otorrhea: A double blind study. Surg. Neurol., *6*: 111–114.

Kornblut, A. D. 1974. Facial nerve injuries in children. J. Laryngol. Otol,, *88*:717–730.

Kornblut, A. D. 1977. Facial nerve injuries in children. Ear Nose Throat J., *56*:369–376.

Mac Gee, E. E., Cauthen, J. C., and Brackett, C. E. 1970. Meningitis following acute traumatic cerebrospinal fluid fistula. J. Neurosurg., *33*:312–316.

Makishima, K., and Snow, J. B., Jr. 1975a. Pathogenesis of hearing loss in head injury. Arch. Otolaryngol., *101*:426–432.

Makishima, K., and Snow, J. B., Jr. 1975b. Electrophysiological responses from the cochlea and inferior colliculus in guinea pigs after head injury. Laryngoscope, *85*:1947–1956.

Makishima, K., and Snow, J. B., Jr. 1976. Effect of head blow on the development of hearing loss. Laryngoscope, *86*:971–978.

McHugh, H. F. 1963. Facial paralysis in birth injury and skull fractures. Arch. Otolaryngol., *78*:443–455.

Miehlke, A. 1973. Surgery of the facial nerve, 2nd ed. Philadelphia, W. B. Saunders Co., pp. 86–87.

Mitchell, D. P., and Stone, P. 1973. Temporal bone fractures in children. Can. J. Otolaryngol., *2*:156–162.

Parisier, S. C., and Birken, E. A. 1976. Recurrent meningitis secondary to idiopathic oval window CSF leak. Laryngoscope, *86*:1503–1515.

Pennington, C. L. 1973. Incus interposition techniques. Ann. Otol. Rhinol. Laryngol., *82*:518–531.

Podoshin, L., and Fradis, M. 1975. Hearing loss after head injury. Arch. Otolaryngol., *101*:15–18.

Potter, G. D. 1971. Fractures of the temporal bone. *In* Jensen, J., and Roysing, H.: Fundamentals of Ear Tomography. Springfield, Ill., Charles C Thomas, pp. 106–118.

Potter, G. D. 1972. Temporal bone fractures. Problems in radiologic diagnosis. Laryngoscope, *82*:408–413.

Proctor, B., Gurdjian, E. S., and Webster, J. E. 1956. The ear in head trauma. Laryngoscope, *66*:16–59.

Pullen, F. W. II. 1972. Round window membrane rupture: A cause of sudden deafness. Trans. Am. Acad. Ophthalmol. Otolaryngol., *76*:1444–1450.

Røhrt, T. 1973. Fracture of temporal bone, early or retrospective diagnosis and surgical hearing reconstruction. Acta Otolaryngol., *75*:355–356.

Rundcrantz, H. 1970. The effects of position change on eustachian tube function. Otolaryngol. Clin. North Am., *3*:103–110.

Sadé, J. 1964. Traumatic fractures of the stapes. Arch. Otolaryngol., *80*:258–262.

Schuknecht, H. F. 1950. A clinical study of auditory damage following blows to the head. Ann. Otol. Rhinol. Laryngol., *59*:330–358.

Schuknecht, H. F. 1969. Mechanism of inner ear injury from blows to the head. Ann. Otol. Rhinol. Laryngol., *78*:253–262.

Schuknecht, H. F. 1974. Pathology of the Ear. Cambridge, Mass., Harvard University Press, pp. 309–310.

Schuknecht, H. F., Neff, W. D., and Perlman, H. B. 1951. An experimental study of auditory damage following blows to the head. Ann. Otol. Rhinol. Laryngol., *60*:275–289.

Schultz, P., and Stool, S. E. 1970. Recurrent meningitis due to a congenital fistula through the stapes footplate. Am. J. Dis. Child., *120*:553–554.

Silverstein, H., Fabian, R. L., Stool, S. E., and Hong, S. W. 1973. Penetrating wounds of the tympanic membrane and ossicular chain. Trans. Am. Acad. Ophthalmol. Otolaryngol. (ORL), 77:125–135.

Singh, D., and Ahluwalia, K. S. 1968. Blast injuries of the ear. J. Laryngol. Otol. 82:1017–1028.

Spector, G. J., Pratt, L. L., and Randall, G. 1973. A clinical study of delayed reconstruction in ossicular fractures. Laryngoscope, 83:837–851.

Strich, S. J. 1961. Shearing of nerve fibers as a cause of brain damage due to head injury. A pathological study of 20 cases. Lancet, 2:442–448.

Sudderth, M. F. 1974. Tympanoplasty in blast induced perforation. Arch. Otolaryngol., 99:157–159.

Tos, M. 1974. Course of sequelae of 248 petrosal fractures. Acta Otolaryngol., 75:353–354.

Vital Statistics of the United States 1974. Volume II. Mortality Part B. National Center for Health Statistics, Rockville, Md., 1976.

Ward, P. H. 1969. Histopathology of auditory and vestibular disorders in head trauma. Ann. Otol. Rhinol. Laryngol., 78:227–238.

Wehrs, R. E. 1974. The homograft notched incus in tympanoplasty. Arch. Otolaryngol., 100:251–255.

Wright, J. W., Jr., Taylor, C. E., and Bizal, J. A. 1969. Tomography of the vulnerable incus. Ann. Otol. Rhinol. Laryngol., 78:263–279.

Chapter 22

TUMORS OF THE EAR AND TEMPORAL BONE

John R. Stram, M.D.

Tumors of the external ear and temporal bone constitute a relatively small percentage of the tumors of the head and neck seen in the pediatric patient: Of 25,000 cases of pediatric neoplasms on file at the Armed Forces Institute of Pathology (AFIP), there are approximately 100 examples of primary involvement of the temporal bone. Textbooks of pediatric otolaryngology by Ferguson and Kendig (1972) and by Jaffe (1977) have only briefly discussed the more common neoplasms that occur in this region, apparently because there was insufficient material available from which to develop a more extensive presentation. In a review in 1954 of 54 neoplasms of the temporal bone and middle ear, Bradley and Maxwell identified only four tumor examples in pediatric patients. Of the 38 cases of malignant tumors of the middle ear and mastoid process reported by Figi and Hempstead in 1943, only one tumor in the temporal bone occurred in a child.

Unfortunately, temporal bone neoplasms in children are often diagnosed late in the course of disease and usually only after treatment for another suspected illness has failed. Early, accurate diagnosis, confirmed by histologic evaluation of a biopsy specimen, is essential to the planning of effective treatment for such tumors. Once the correct diagnosis has been made, improved surgical and anesthesia techniques, radiotherapy control, and an expanding inventory of chemotherapeutic agents make control of these neoplasms possible.

As Sections 1 and 2 of this text indicate, the temporal bone contains structures that are fully developed at birth, whereas other parts are vestigial at birth and assume their adult configurations through later growth and development. Tremble's (1977) observations suggest that little growth occurs in the membranous labyrinth following birth. In his publications on meningioma and temporal bone epidermoids, Nager (1964, 1975) demonstrated that neither the tympanic membrane nor the fibrous annulus undergoes significant postnatal growth. It is not surprising, therefore, that mesenchymal tumors of these structures are not reported. Nager has demonstrated that the centers of most active growth in the temporal bone include the suture lines of the temporal bone, the tympanic bone, and the tympanic annulus, as well as the soft parts of the auricle, the ear canal, and the vascular and nerve supplies to these areas. Most tumors in pediatric patients develop in these anatomic areas of greatest growth activity. Rhabdomyosarcoma, plexiform neurofibroma, mesenchymoma, osteosarcoma, chondrosarcoma, and fibrosarcoma are tumor types commonly associated with growing tissue and are also the types of tumors most frequently reported to occur in the temporal bones of children (Bradley and Maxwell, 1954; Figi and Hempstead, 1943).

The temporal bone develops as an enlarging tissue mass that either invests or displaces adjacent organs and tissues. This mode of development helps to explain the occurrence of choristomas and meningiomas in the temporal bone. A popular theory of tumor development is that tissue anlagen of organs adjacent to the temporal bone become separated from their normal tissue masses and are included in the developing temporal bone. With growth this tisssue becomes a recognizable tumor mass of histologically normal tissue in an alien location. Frequent literature reports of the presence of arachnoid villi, central nervous system tissue, primitive neurectoderm, and salivary gland tissue in the temporal bone support this theory of temporal bone tumor formation (Guzowski and Paparella, 1976; Nager, 1964). This heterotopic tissue is benign, and its anatomic location in the temporal bone, as well as the size of the mass, will govern the presenting signs and symptoms and dictate the therapeutic approach. Occasionally, heterotopic arachnoid tissue may give rise to primary meningiomas of the temporal bone as described by Nager (1964) and Guzowski and Paparella (1976).

An understanding of the embryology of tissues contained within the temporal bone is essential to an understanding of the histologic variations possible in a biopsy specimen of a tumor of this region. The accurate diagnosis of neoplasms of the temporal bone requires that histologic material be examined by experienced pathologists who are familiar with the histology of developing tissues of this region. Frequently, sophisticated diagnostic techniques, such as electron microscopy, and tissue culture techniques, such as those described by Wigger and Mitsudo in their 1976 report of a congenital malignant fibrous histiocytoma, may be necessary to arrive at an accurate diagnosis.

EXOSTOSES

Benign bony occlusion of the external auditory canal (exostosis) has been associated by Van Gilse (1938) and by Fowler and Osmun (1942) with cold water entering the external auditory canal. Exostoses are hard, bony masses that have either a sessile or pedunculated configuration and that commonly occur in the suture lines of the external auditory canal. They are seldom seen before the age of 10 years. According to Mawson (1963), they are often bilateral and are three times more common in males than in females. They are probably the commonest bony proliferation found in the external ear canal. Ash (1960) distinguishes between this lesion and a true osteoma, the latter being considered rare, usually presenting in the inferior aspect of the ear canal at the junction of bone and cartilage of the external auditory canal. There are reports in the literature of giant

cell tumors occurring in the temporal bones of newborn infants (Japanese) and of chondrosarcomas occurring in the first decade of life (Leédham, 1972), but these represent single case reports and are quite uncommon.

FIBROUS DYSPLASIA

In a 1970 review of monostotic fibrous dysplasia, Sharp states that this entity has been known to occur in the temporal bones of pediatric patients since 1946. Five of the eleven cases reviewed and reported in the world literature occurred in children, in whom the tumor developed at the beginning of the second decade of life. Histologically the tumor tissue was sclerotic, with expansion in size of the involved bone in all cases reported. Occlusion of the external auditory meatus was a· common finding, and in half the cases in which the dysplastic bone occluded the external auditory canal, cholesteatomas were also present. The differential diagnosis of this entity includes osteoblastoma, osteoma, osteomyelitis, and local reaction to a meningioma. Conservative local therapy provided control in the cases reported. In only one of these eleven cases of monostotic fibrous dysplasia was trauma associated with the recognition of this tumor. A hearing loss was a common primary complaint in these cases. Confusion exists in the literature as to whether or not valid clinical and histologic distinctions can be made between monostotic fibrous dysplasia and a benign fibro-osseous lesion, ossifying fibroma (juvenile ossifying fibroma), which can involve the temporal bones in children. Respected authorities feel there are grounds for separation of the two entities, particularly on clinical, radiologic, therapeutic, and prognostic grounds (Hyams, 1976; Lichtenstein and Jaffe, 1942; Lichtenstein, 1972).

TUMORS OF BONE AND CARTILAGE

There are no pediatric case reports of cartilaginous neoplasms of the external ear or external auditory canal; and there is but one reference, by Piepgras (1972), to a chondroblastoma occurring in the temporal bone of a patient who was close to the second decade of life. In 1974 Ronis reported on the incidence of osteoblastoma of the temporal bone in the pediatric age group. This histologically bizarre but benign osteoid-producing tumor, although rare, has been reported specifically in the temporal bone by Lichtenstein and Sawyer (1964), Dahlin and Johnson (1954), and Byers (1968). Although they occur more commonly in the vertebrae and the long bones, 15 to 20 per cent of these lesions involve the calvarium, and two thirds of the cases reported by Lichtenstein and Sawyer (1964) were in children between 6 and 12 years of age and showed no racial or sexual predilections. Osteoblastomas presented clinically as radiologically osteolytic lesions associated with primary complaints of vascular tinnitus or a conductive hearing loss. Surgical removal of the tumor provided relief of these symptoms in the cases reported.

METASTATIC TUMORS

Metastatic tumors and secondary malignant tumors of the temporal bone were reported by Schuknecht and colleagues in 1968, but none of the tumors reported occurred in children. These tumors may, however, occur in the pediatric age group. The primary tumors include renal cell carcinomas; adenoid cystic carcinomas of the parotid; carcinomas of the larynx, thyroid, and nasopharynx; meningeal sarcomas; gliomas of the pons; lymphosarcomas; and melanosarcomas. The metastatic forms of these tumors in the temporal bone were characterized by bone destruction and scattered involvement throughout the temporal bone.

SOFT TISSUE TUMORS — RHABDOMYOSARCOMAS

By far the most common tumor of mesenchymal origin in the temporal bone is rhabdomyosarcoma. A review of the world literature prior to 1973 by Deutsch and Felder (1974) revealed 73 cases that presented in the ear or mastoid region. In 1958, in what is essentially a histologic classification, Horn and Enterline divided rhabdomyosarcomas of the head and neck, including the temporal bone, into embryonal rhabdomyosarcoma, alveolar rhabdomyosarcoma, and sarcoma botryoides. In a 1976 review of AFIP

otolaryngologic pathology material, Hyams reported that the majority of the cases with involvement of the temporal bone by rhabdomyosarcoma occurred in the pediatric age group. From a review of a published series of case reports, there appears to be no difference in the clinical presentations of the different histologic types of this entity. The mean age for establishment of the diagnosis is 6.1 years; the age range is 16 months to 16 years. Approximately half the individuals reported in the literature sought medical care and examination after sustaining trauma to the region of the ear and mastoid. The average interval between initial symptoms and establishment of the diagnosis and institution of therapy was 3.5 months. The most common presenting sign was a tumor or swelling; the most common presenting symptom was pain. Physical findings usually revealed the tumors to be in the ear canal or postauricular region. On gross examination there was a characteristic, superficial blood vessel dilatation over the tumor mass. Unfortunately, these entities have frequently been initially diagnosed as hematomas, otitis media, or aural polyps. Subsequently, at the time of definitive diagnosis, the tumor had already spread to the nasopharynx, pharynx, cranial cavity, dura, cervical lymph nodes, and orbit, lessening the chances of cure. The majority of the patients reported in the literature and in the AFIP otolaryngologic pathology registry died as a result of uncontrolled primary tumor. A 1973 report by Jaffe and coworkers and a 1976 report by Liebner support the effectiveness of the current philosophy of treating the primary tumor and its most common sites of spread initially with intensive radiotherapy or combining radiotherapy with surgical debulking and chemotherapy.

TUMORS OF HEMATOPOIETIC ORIGIN — HISTIOCYTOSIS

Histiocytosis X is the term used to identify a composite common to eosinophilic granuloma, Hand-Schuller-Christian disease, and Letterer-Siwe disease. The common single or multiple bone lesion appears to be lytic on radiography and is histologically benign, with a proliferation of lipid-laden histiocytes, giant cells, and eosinophils. Eosinophilic granuloma is the most likely of these entities to present as a solitary lesion and is therefore reported as a tumor that occurs in the temporal bone. In a review of 16 cases of eosinophilic granuloma of the temporal bone by Toohill in 1973, 14 occurred in the pediatric age group. The age range was 1 to 12 years with a male predominance. In four cases the temporal bone lesions were bilateral. The commonest presenting symptoms were otorrhea, pain, and postauricular swelling; one patient presented with facial paralysis. The commonest physical findings were granulation tissue polyps of the external ear canal with evidence of bone erosion primarily involving the posterosuperior external canal wall. The majority of patients responded to either surgical or radiation therapy. A review of the AFIP Temporal Bone Inventory by Hyams in 1976 identified 10 cases of histiocytosis X in children aged 1 to 10 years, with an equal distribution of males and females.

The etiology of histiocytosis is unknown. Clinicians can draw few clues to aid in management of the disease from the philosophic arguments for differentiation of acute disseminated and localized multifocal histiocytosis or from the arguments that morphologically the acute and chronic forms are the same. However, he or she should be encouraged that this condition responds well to supportive treatment, whether it be radiotherapy or surgical extirpation.

LYMPHORETICULAR NEOPLASMS (LYMPHOMA AND LEUKEMIA)

Lymphomatous involvement of the temporal bone has been comprehensively reported on by Shambron and Finch in 1958, Zechner and Altman in 1969, and Paparella in 1973. These authors suggest an incidence of temporal bone involvement by this malignant neoplastic entity of from 16 to 35 per cent. Histologically, acute leukemic infiltration of the temporal bone is manifested as perivascular infiltration of the submucosal stroma of the mucous membrane of the middle ear and of the pneumatized cells of the mastoid. Temporal bone studies have demonstrated similar infiltration of the external auditory canal, the tympanic membrane, the middle ear mucosa, the facial nerve, the eustachian tube, and the mastoid air cell system. Occasionally, the membranous labyrinth may be involved by the leukemic infiltrate or at

least by hemorrhage precipitated by the disease. Paparella (1973) points out that approximately 28 per cent of the clinical problems in leukemic patients were directly attributable to leukemic infiltrates of the ear and temporal bone. Interestingly, 48 per cent of the leukemic patients studied had otologic signs and symptoms in the course of their disease that were not directly attributable to postmortem temporal bone involvement by the leukemic process. Paparella (1973) recommends routine otologic, audiologic, and vestibular evaluation of all patients with leukemia. The common presenting signs and symptoms of leukemic involvement of the temporal bone include ear canal and middle ear ulceration and hemorrhage, thickened tympanic membrane and middle ear mucosa, and lesions of the major nerve trunks in the temporal bone, producing hearing loss, facial paralysis, and vertigo. Acute lymphocytic leukemia, acute myelogenous leukemia, and erythroleukemia are the diagnoses associated with temporal bone involvement.

Although no clinical reports of a lymphoma involving the temporal bone of a child by metastatic spread or by contiguous spread could be found in the literature, it should be understood that lymphosarcoma and Hodgkin disease are forms of lymphoma commonly found in children. These entities rarely occur primarily in the temporal bone but may encroach upon the temporal bone from without, particularly from the region of the parotid gland and parotid lymph nodes.

TUMORS OF NERVE TISSUE ORIGIN

Tumors of nerve tissue origin are rare in the pediatric age group, although peripheral nerve schwannomas (neurilemomas) and neurofibromas (plexiform neuromas) have been recognized in the external ear canal and middle ear. Tumors of the eighth nerve, either in association with neurofibromatosis (von Recklinghausen disease) or as primary neurilemomas of the eighth nerve, are rare in children but must be considered in the differential diagnosis of retrocochlear hearing loss. Previous mention has been made of the presence of heterotopic brain tissue in the middle ear, the so-called glioma. Extensive review by Nager (1964), Guzowski and Paparella (1976), and Buehrle (1972) have identified arachnoid tissue in the petrous apex, along the course of the greater superficial petrosal nerve, in the semicanal of the tensor tympani muscle, in the anterior middle ear, the genu of the facial nerve, the internal auditory meatus, and in the jugular foramen. The potential for aberrant meningeal tissue in these locations to develop into meningiomas is supported in the extensive review of this tumor by Nager (1964). Histologically, this tumor can be mistaken for a glomus jugulare tumor (jugulotemporal extraadrenal paraganglioma), but the problem of differential diagnosis has not presented itself in the pediatric age group because glomus jugulare tumors rarely occur before the end of the second decade of life.

TUMORS OF THE SKIN AND SKIN APPENDAGES

The tissue components of the external ear and temporal bone are those of the body in general. Squamous cell carcinomas, squamous papillomas, sweat gland tumors, melanomas, basal cell carcinomas, and hair follicle tumors have all been reported to occur in the skin of the external ear and ear canal by Ash and Raum (1956) and Batsakis (1974), but essentially only single case reports occur in the pediatric population. In general, the observations of Bradley and Maxwell (1954) are supported: Tumors of the temporal bone in children are more often sarcomas. However, a 1976 report by Conley and Schuller indicates that 6.5 per cent of all ear canal malignancies occur in children under the age of 20 years; cerumen gland adenocarcinomas predominate in this series. MacComb and Fletcher (1968) reported that melanomas rarely occur before the age of 16 years but that 20 to 30 per cent of pediatric melanomas involve the head and neck. Xeroderma pigmentosa most often involves the skin of the head and neck in the pediatric patient and is a precursor of squamous cell and basal cell carcinoma. This entity tends to be more common in Negroes.

EPIDERMOID TUMORS (CONGENITAL CHOLESTEATOMA)

Congenital cholesteatomas or epidermoids of the temporal bone are considered aberrant epithelial tissue or teratomatous malformations found in the temporal bone from birth to the eighth decade (Nager, 1975). The peak age for symptom development is 15 years. These lesions are pearly or shiny epithelial masses, usually developing behind an intact tympanic membrane in the petrotympanic suture line. They tend to expand with general body growth toward the cerebellopontine angle. There is a characteristic absence of a history of chronic middle ear disease in these patients. The recommended management is surgical with protracted follow-up care.

MISCELLANEOUS ENTITIES

Tumors of blood vessels and superficial lymphatics are apparently of relatively minor occurrence and are not reported in the literature. The observed regression of these entities with total body growth should govern the decision for timing of surgical therapy, if any.

Nodular fasciitis and fibromatosis are histologic entities that present as postauricular swellings and are difficult to classify accurately. When found in a neonate or a very young child, they may have benign courses, but fibromatosis may be persistently aggressive and destructive despite its benign histology. Electron microscopy and tissue culture techniques, as well as careful histologic study, may be necessary to establish the cell of origin of this entity. A review of the subject by Vogel and Karmody (1979) emphasizes the difficulty in predicting the clinical course and response to therapy of this lesion.

Table 22–1 is a compilation of the neoplasms seen in the temporal bone area in the pediatric age group in the AFIP material from 1955 to 1975 (Hyams, 1976). Because of the relatively small number of cases in the entire study, statistical analysis by sex or age is not possible.

CLINICAL CORRELATIONS

A review of the literature shows that temporal bone neoplasms have been recorded as presenting with the following signs and symptoms: (1) external auditory canal obstruction, (2) discharge, (3) recognizable tumor in the ear canal, (4) ulceration, (5) a fixed mass over the mastoid process or canal

Table 22–1 NEOPLASMS OF THE TEMPORAL BONE AREA IN THE PEDIATRIC AGE GROUP (AFIP 1955–1975)

Neoplasms	External Ear	Occurring In The: Middle Ear	Temporal Bone
Squamous papilloma	1 (10 yrs)M°	—	—
Squamous cell carcinoma	1 (6 yrs)M	1 (10 yrs) F	—
Pilomatrixoma	4 (4–14 yrs) 2F, 2M	—	—
Basal cell carcinoma	1 (12 yrs) M	—	—
Ceruminoma	—	1 (10 yrs)	—
Juvenile xanthogranuloma	3 (1–6 yrs) 1F, 2M	—	—
Nodular fasciitis	2 (4, 5 yrs) 2M	—	—
Dermatofibroma	2 (8, 10 yrs) 1F, 1M	—	—
Fibromatosis	2 (6, 8 yrs) 2M	—	—
Fibromyxoma (sarcoma)	—	—	1 (? yrs) M
Lymphangioma	1 (6 yrs) M	—	—
Embryonal rhabdomyosarcoma	10 (2–11 yrs) 3F, 7M	6 (2–11 yrs) 3F, 3M	10 (2–12 yrs) 5F, 5M
Lymphoma	—	1 (8 yrs) F	—
Neurilemoma	—	1 (13 yrs) M	—
Neurofibroma	2 (1, 7 yrs) 2M	—	—
Glioma	—	1 (11 yrs) M	—
Meningioma	—	1 (8 yrs) M	—
Giant cell tumor	—	—	1 (4 yrs) M
Histiocytosis X	—	—	10 (1–10 yrs) 5F, 5M
Ossifying fibroma	—	—	8 (5–12 yrs) 3F, 5M
Chondrosarcoma	—	—	1 (4 yrs) M
Hamartoma	—	1 (11 yrs) F	—

° The first number is the number of cases reported, the age in parentheses is the age or ages of the patients reported, and M and F denote the sex of the patients.

wall, (6) facial paralysis, (7) mastoid tenderness, and (8) chronic and unremitting pain.

With the exception of facial paralysis, any clinician recognizes these as the primary complaints of a multiplicity of inflammatory disorders involving the ear and mastoid. Even the most sophisticated outpatient department would soon tire of comprehensively evaluating each case with this symptom complex to detect possible temporal bone neoplasms at the initial clinical evaluation. Table 22–2 attempts to identify the tumor types found in

Table 22–2 SYMPTOMS OF VARIOUS TUMORS OF THE TEMPORAL BONE

	Chronic, unremitting pain	Mastoid tenderness	Facial paralysis	Mastoid or canal swelling	Ulceration	Ear canal tumor	Ear discharge	Ear canal obstruction	Hearing loss	Tinnitus	Vertigo
Tumors of bone and cartilage	X		X	X	X	X	X	X	X	X	
Tumors of blood and lymph vessels				X	X			X			
Tumors of nerve tissue			X	X					X	X	X
Tumors of skin and appendages	X	X		X	X	X	X				
Leukemia and lymphoma	X	X	X	X	X		X	X	X	X	X
Tumors of mesenchymal tissue	X	X	X	X	X	X	X	X	X	X	
Metastatic tumors	X	X	X	X					X	X	X

the temporal bone by signs and symptoms associated with neoplasms in this anatomic region. It is hoped that this presentation will help the clinician to identify these tumors by their clinical presentations.

BIOPSY DIAGNOSIS

The 1962 study by Dito and Batsakis, as well as a more recent work by Liebner (1976), suggests that an inverse relationship exists between duration of symptoms and survival after therapy. There is a lack of reassurance in their observation that the initial tissue biopsy report was possibly neither accurate nor tumor-specific in a large number of the cases that presented as ear canal masses and later were proved to be primary temporal bone neoplasms. The cases reported in the literature are also characterized by a significant delay in obtaining surgical biopsy specimens. A thorough knowledge of the expected courses of inflammatory disease and familiarity with the expected responses to therapy of each of these inflammatory entities will serve to alert the clinician to a disease process that is quite different from an inflammatory disease. The fact that these tumors were not identified in the initial specimens may be explained by inaccuracies or deficiencies in the biopsy procedure or by artifacts in the specimen submitted to the pathologist for sectioning; inflammation and granulation tissue play a role in the pathologic appearance of any tumor that presents to an external surface with ulceration or superficial necrosis. Biopsy specimens that are too small or that fail to sample tissue deep to the surface ulceration and inflammation may not include tissue characteristic of these tumor types. The use of cupbiting forceps or mechanical compression of a biopsy fragment after it is obtained may introduce crushing artifacts that mask the true morphology of the tissue. The last, and perhaps most common, artifact in small tissue biopsies is dessication artifacts produced by drying of very small tissue specimens between the time they are obtained and the time they are placed in formalin. Three guidelines for maximizing the amount of information that can be obtained from specimens follow.

1. Obtain a biopsy specimen from deeply enough in the tumor that it is representative of the tumor.
2. Avoid crushing the biopsy specimen in cupbiting forceps or compressing it mechanically.
3. Avoid dessicating the specimen by placing the biopsy specimen in formalin solution as rapidly as possibly after it is obtained.

Pathologists should be alerted to the clinical differential diagnosis of the tissue mass biopsied. Special histologic stains and additional pathology consultations should be obtained for any case in which the morphology of the lesion is less than characteristic of an entity that explains the patient's clinical course. With the advent of polytomography, radiographic evaluation of the temporal bone can be carried out with great precision. Mastoid survey radiographs are indicated in every case of facial paralysis and in cases presenting as periauricular tumor masses. Complete audiometric studies with tympanometry will alert the clinician to the presence of middle ear tissue masses associated with a conductive hearing loss. The recognition of a middle ear mass should be followed by a comprehensive radiologic evaluation of the temporal bone in order to plan definitive surgical biopsy procedures.

MANAGEMENT

The treatment modalities available to the clinician treating neoplasms of the temporal bone are surgery, radiotherapy, and chemotherapy. Solitary lesions that lend themselves to surgical extirpation include monostotic fibrous dysplasias, eosinophilic granulomas, epidermoids, meningiomas, choristomas, neurilemomas, and gliomas. Radiation therapy alone, or combined radiation therapy and surgical debulking procedures, are the recommended approaches to rhabdomyosarcoma, cerumen gland carcinoma, and extensive eosinophilic granuloma. It should be emphasized that in treating sarcomatous lesions, radiation therapy should include the sites to which the tumors commonly spread as a part of the initial therapy. The addition to the treatment possibilities of acute and chronic chemotherapy with an ever-expanding inventory of drugs has led to a major increase in the survival of these tumor patients. Drug regimens change too rapidly to be included in a textbook, but their significance in treating tumors of the temporal bone cannot be overlooked. Thus, the management of a child with a malignancy or mass should always be handled by a team that includes a chemotherapist.

Tumors of the temporal bone in children are rare. They are seen more commonly in the muscle, blood vessels, and growing bone than in the skin and nerve tissue of the temporal bone. These entities should be suspected whenever more common disease entities fail to respond to conventional therapy.

Accurate, early diagnosis is facilitated by anatomically appropriate biopsy material properly fixed and processed by a pathologist alerted to the clinical suspicion of these entities.

SELECTED REFERENCES

Batsakis, J. G. 1974. Tumors of the Head and Neck. Baltimore, Williams and Wilkins Co.
     This anatomically specific work provides concise, current information as well as a comprehensive bibliography for further reading.

Nager, G. T. 1975. Epidermoids of the temporal bone. Laryngoscope, *85*, Suppl. 2.
     This is an excellent source of information on temporal bone development and growth as well as an excellent reference source on this subject.

Sharp, M. 1970. Monostotic fibrous dysplasia of the temporal bone. J. Laryngol. Otol. *84*:697–708.
     This is a comprehensive clinical review of this subject.

REFERENCES

Ash, J. E. 1960. Pathology of the Ear. *In* Schenk, H. P. (Ed.) Otolaryngology, Hagerstown, Vol. I, Chap. 4.

Ash, J. E., and Raum, M. 1956. An Atlas of Otolaryngolic Pathology. Washington, American Registry of Pathology.

Batsakis, J. G. 1974. Tumors of the Head and Neck. Baltimore, Williams and Wilkins Co.

Bradley, W., and Maxwell, N. J. 1954. Neoplasms of the middle ear and mastoid. Laryngoscope, *64*:533–566.

Buehrle, R. 1972. Meningioma in the temporal bone. Can. J. Otol., *1*:16–20.

Byers, P. D. 1968. Benign osteoblastic lesions of bone. Cancer, *22*:43–57.

Conley, J., and Schuller, D. 1976. Malignancies of the ear. Laryngoscope, *86*:1147–1163.

Dahlin, D. C., and Johnson, E. W., Jr. 1954. Giant osteoid osteoma. J. Bone and Joint Surg., *36A*:559–572.

Deutsch, M., and Felder, H. 1974. Rhabdomyosarcoma of the ear and mastoid. Laryngoscope, *84*:586–592.

Dito, W. R., and Batsakis, J. G. 1962. Rhabdomyosarcoma of the head and neck: An appraisal of the biologic behavior in 170 cases. Arch. Surg., *84*:582.

Ferguson, C. F., and Kendig, E. L. 1972. Pediatric Otolaryngology. Philadelphia, W.B. Saunders Co.

Figi, F. A., and Hempstead, B. E. 1943. Malignant tumors of middle ear and mastoid. Arch. Otolaryngol., *37*:149–168.

Fowler, E. P., Jr., and Osmun, P. M. 1942. New bone growth due to cold water in ears. Arch. Otolaryngol., *36*:455–466.

Guzowski, J., and Paparella, M. 1976. Meningiomas of the temporal bone. Laryngoscope, *86*:1141–1146.

Horn, R. C., Jr., and Enterline, H. T. 1958. Rhabdomyosarcoma, a clinical pathological study and classification of 39 cases. Cancer, *11*:181–199.

Hyams, V. J. 1976. AFIP symposium: Pediatric neoplasms of the temporal bone in the pediatric age group. Otolaryngologic Pathology, December 6–8.

Jaffe, B. F. 1977. Hearing Loss in Children. Baltimore, University Park Press.

Jaffe, N., Filler, R. M., Farber, S., et al. 1973. Rhabdomyosarcoma in children: Improved outlook with a multidisciplinary approach. Am. J. Surg., *125*:482–487.

Leedham, P. W. 1972. Chondrosarcoma with subarachnoid dissemination. J. Pathol., *107*:59–61.

Lichtenstein, L. 1972. Bone Tumors, 4th ed. St. Louis, C. V. Mosby Co.

Lichtenstein, L., and Jaffe, H. L. 1942. Fibrous dysplasia of bone. Arch. Pathol., *33*:777–816.

Lichtenstein, L., and Sawyer, W. R. 1964. Benign osteoblastoma, further observations and report of 20 additional cases, J. Bone and Joint Surg., *46A*:755–765.

Liebner, E. J. 1976. Embryonal rhabdomyosarcoma of head and neck in children: Correlation of stage, radiation dose, local control, and survival. Cancer, *37*:2777–2786.

MacComb, W. S., and Fletcher, G. H. 1968. Cancer of the Head and Neck. Baltimore, Williams and Wilkins Co.

Mawson, S. R. 1963. Diseases of the Ear. Baltimore, Williams and Wilkins Co.

Nager, G. T. 1964. Meningiomas involving the temporal bone. Springfield. IL, Charles C Thomas.

Nager, G. T. 1975. Epidermoids of the temporal bone. Laryngoscope, *85*:Suppl. 2.

Paparella, M. 1973. Otologic manifestations of leukemia. Laryngoscope, *83*:1510–1526.

Piepgras, U. 1972. Chondroblastoma of the temporal bone, an unusual cause of increasing intracranial pressure. Neuroradiology, *4*:25–29.

Ronis, M. L. 1974. Benign osteoblastoma of the temporal bone. Laryngoscope, *84*:857–863.

Schuknecht, H. F., Allam, A. F., and Murakami, Y. 1968. Pathology of secondary malignant tumors of the temporal bone. Ann. Otol. Rhinol. Laryngol., *77*:5–22.

Shambron, E., and Finch, S. C. 1958. The auditory manifestations of leukemia. Yale J. Biol. Med., *31*:144.

Sharp, M. 1970. Monostotic fibrous dysplasia of the temporal bone. J. Laryngol. Otol. *84*:697–708.

Toohill, R. 1973. Eosinophilic granuloma of the temporal bone. Laryngoscope, *83*:877–889.

Tremble, G. E. 1977. Observations made in the labyrinths of adults. J. Otolaryngol., *6*(4):327–333.

Van Gilse, P. H. G. 1938. Des observations ultereures sur le genese des exostoses due conduit externe par l'irritation d'eau froide. Acta Otolaryngol., *26*:343.

Vogel, D. H., and Karmody, C. S. 1979. Congenital fibrous lesion of the temporal bone. Arch. Otolaryngol., *105*:215–219.

Wigger, H. J., and Mitsudo, S. M. 1976. Fibrous histiocytoma simulating congenital fibromatosis. Virchows Arch. (Pathol. Anat.), *370*(3):255–266.

Zechner, G., and Altman, F. 1969. Histological studies of the temporal bone in leukemia. Ann. Otol. Rhinol. Laryngol., *78*:375–387.

THE NOSE, PARANASAL SINUSES, FACE, AND ORBIT

Chapter 23

EMBRYOLOGY AND ANATOMY

David N. F. Fairbanks, M.D.

CHRONOLOGY

The period of development of the nose and paranasal sinuses is a continuum spanning from the third week of gestation, when the primordia of these structures first appear, through early adulthood when sinus pneumatization and nasal bony growth ceases. The events and the timing of development of these structures may be outlined in the following manner.

Fetus at three weeks: Olfactory placodes appear in frontonasal process.

Fetus at four weeks: Olfactory placodes become nasal pits. Maxillary processes appear.

Fetus at five weeks: Nasal pits deepen into clefts separated by primitive septum (frontonasal process). Vomeronasal organ appears.

Fetus at six weeks: Oronasal membranes rupture, forming primitive choanae. Primitive palate forms by fusion of maxillary process with medial and lateral nasal processes. Upper lip forms by fusion of medial nasal and lateral nasal maxillary processes. Naso-optic furrow (to become lacrimal apparatus) disappears. Maxillary and ethmoidal folds appear (to become turbinates).

Fetus at seven weeks: Definitive septum begins growth. Second ethmoidal fold appears.

Fetus at eight weeks: Olfactory nerve bundles appear. Palatine processes fuse in midline anteriorly. Uncinate process and ethmoidal infundibulum appear.

Fetus at three months: Palate fusion completed. Maxillary sinus outpouching appears. Cartilaginous nasal capsule forms from mesenchymal condensation. Nasal glands appear.

Fetus at four months: Ethmoidal sinus outpouching appears. Sphenoidal sinus outpouching appears. Bulla ethmoidalis becomes well defined.

Fetus at five months: Vomeronasal organ begins degeneration.

Fetus at six months: Cartilaginous nasal capsule divides into alar, lateral, and septal cartilages. Maxillary ossification begins.

Fetus at seven months: Maximal development of ethmoidal turbinates (up to five) occurs; turbinates begin coalescence.

BIRTH: Frontal sinus furrows appear.

Only two to three ethmoidal turbinates remain.

Craniofacial ratio is 8:1.

six months: Nares double their birth dimensions.

one year: Maxillary sinus reaches infraorbital nerve.

two years: Frontal sinuses reach frontal bone.

Ethmoidal sinuses approximate each other and lamina papyracea.

three years: Nasal growth spurt occurs.

Ossified union occurs between perpendicular plate of ethmoid, lamina papyracea, cribriform plate, and vomer.

four years: Sphenoidal sinus begins invasion of sphenoid bone.

five years: Craniofacial ratio is 4:1.

six years: Frontal sinuses are visible on radiographs in frontal bone.

Sphenoidal sinus is pneumatized to vidian canal.

Nasal growth spurt occurs.

seven years: Nose doubles its birth length.

Maxillary sinus begins inferiorly directed growth.

Ethmoidal sinuses extend beyond boundaries of ethmoids.

eight years: Maxillary sinus approximates inferior nasal meatus.

Frontal sinus reaches level of orbital roof in 50 per cent of children.

nine years: Maxillary sinus pneumatizes zygomatic process.

12 years: Floor of maxillary sinus is level with floor of nose.

Puberty: Accelerated nasal and maxillary growth occurs.

Nose triples its birth length.

End of puberty: Sphenoidal sinus growth ceases.

Frontal sinus growth ceases.

Ethmoidal sinus growth ceases.

Maxillary sinus growth ceases except at area of third molar, which will become pneumatized when the molar erupts.

Adulthood: Closure of spheno-occipital synchondrosis occurs.

Craniofacial ratio is 2:1.

50 years: Fusion of perpendicular plate of ethmoid with vomer is completed.

THE NOSE AND FACE

Early Development

The nose originates in the cranial ectoderm near the embryonic anterior neuropore. The cellular thickening of sensory epithelium that becomes the paired olfactory placodes is recognizable as early as the third fetal week. As the surrounding mesoderm increases in thickness, the nasal placodes become passively depressed, forming the nasal pits in a broad mass of tissue, the frontonasal process (Fig. 23–1).

Further deepening of the pits separates the frontonasal process into paired medial and lateral boundaries of the nasal walls. The medial processes fuse in the formation of the central portion of the upper lip, the premaxillary process, and the primitive nasal septum. By the fifth week, the nasal pits are cleft-like, blindly ending epithelial pouches with smooth lateral nasal walls and a thick "septum" of frontonasal process showing the early vomeronasal organ of Jacobson.

The inferior boundary of the nasal cavity is deficient until the paired maxillary processes of the first (mandibular) arches grow anteriorly and medially to abut against, and later fuse with, the medial nasal processes. Fusion also takes place laterally between the maxillary and lateral nasal processes to obliterate the naso-optic furrow.

Posterior extension of the nasal cavities thins out the membrane separating them from the oral cavity. By the 38th day this bucconasal membrane is so thin that it has only two layers, the nasal and oral epithelia. It becomes so attenuated that rupture ensues, forming the choanae. Failure of rupture results in choanal atresia. These early choanae do not correspond in position to the definitive choanae, which will ultimately be more posterior and are not established until the third month when the definitive palate is completed. This accounts for the observation that the anterior extent of choanal atresia is unexpectedly far anterior in the nasal cavity.

Between the 40th and 60th fetal days, the nares are temporarily obstructed by proliferating epithelial cells. These cells must later degenerate and shed, and if they fail to do so, atresia of the nares with bony and membranous closure occurs.

Details of the formation of the lips and palate are covered in Section I in this text. It is sufficient to say that the primitive choanae become elongated by posterior extension and then by progressive posteriorly directed fusion of the palatal processes. In formation of the definitive palate, the final position of the choanae is established. During this process, a portion of the buccal cavity becomes incorporated into the nose on the nasal side of the hard palate and in the inferior nasal meatus. The palatal processes fuse not only with each other but also with the definitive nasal septum, which is concurrently growing posteriorly from the primitive septum toward the buccal pituitary outpouching.

During the third fetal month, condensation of mesenchyme results in formation of the primitive nasal capsule (Fig. 23–2), a cartilaginous structure from which, or upon which, will develop all the bony and cartilaginous nasal and paranasal structures. Just as Meckel's cartilage is the primary skeleton of the lower face, so is the nasal capsule the primary skeleton of the upper face. Its continuity is short-lived. In the sixth fetal month ingrowth of connective tissue divides it into individual alar (lower lateral) cartilages, septal, and (upper) lateral cartilages. The greater part of the posterior capsule becomes ossified as the ethmoid bone, encompassing the ethmoidal turbinates, sinus walls, and perpendicular plate. Portions of the sphenoid bone ossify from this capsule. Upon its lateral surfaces form the nasal bones and maxillae. Ossification and absorption of this capsule is a process that begins early in fetal life, progresses well into adulthood, and is never completed (inasmuch as the cartilage of the anterior nose and septum persists as remnants of the capsule).

The Internal Nose, Lateral Wall

Simultaneous with palatal formation, the nasal walls begin to develop into the complex configuration that ultimately characterizes them. There is an inherent tendency for the nasal cavity to increase its surface area. The 40 day old embryo shows shallow grooves, which will become inferior and middle meatuses. The intervening tissue proliferates, bulges into the nasal cavity, and becomes the inferior or maxillary turbinate. The ethmoidal turbinates (e.g., middle, superior, and supreme) initially arise on the nasal septum, but the direction of growth in the nasal cavity shifts them to the lateral wall. Initially, there is a single ethmoidal fold in each nasal cavity. By 48 days, there is a second; by 100 days, a third. By the seventh to ninth fetal months, there may be as many as five ethmoidal turbinates with intervening meatuses, but after birth the uppermost and less developed ones coalesce and disappear (Schaeffer, 1920).

The typical number of ethmoidal turbinates is three: middle, superior, and supreme. The supreme turbinate has been identified in 88 per cent of fetuses, 73 per cent of nine year old children, and 26 per cent of adults (Zimmerman, 1938). Rarely, an even higher turbinate persists.

Posterior and superior to the highest ethmoidal turbinate lies the sphenoethmoidal recess, which is limited by the angle formed by the cribriform plate superiorly and the anterior surface of the sphenoid posteriorly. In the recess is found the ostium of the sphenoid sinus.

The agger nasi is a slight elevation above the inferior turbinate and anterior to the middle turbinate that develops more or less parallel to the bridge of the nose. The olfactory sulcus is a channel-like space anterior and superior to the agger nasi, limited by the arched confluences of the medial and lateral nasal walls. It leads from the nasal vestibule to the olfactory area in the roof of the nose and then posteriorly into the sphenoethmoidal recess.

Under cover of the middle turbinate, the middle meatus of the nose begins its complex development. As early as the 60th day of fetal life, a crescent-shaped fold (the uncinate process) appears with a furrow (the ethmoid infundibulum) immediately above it. Shortly thereafter, another bulge (the ethmoid bulla)

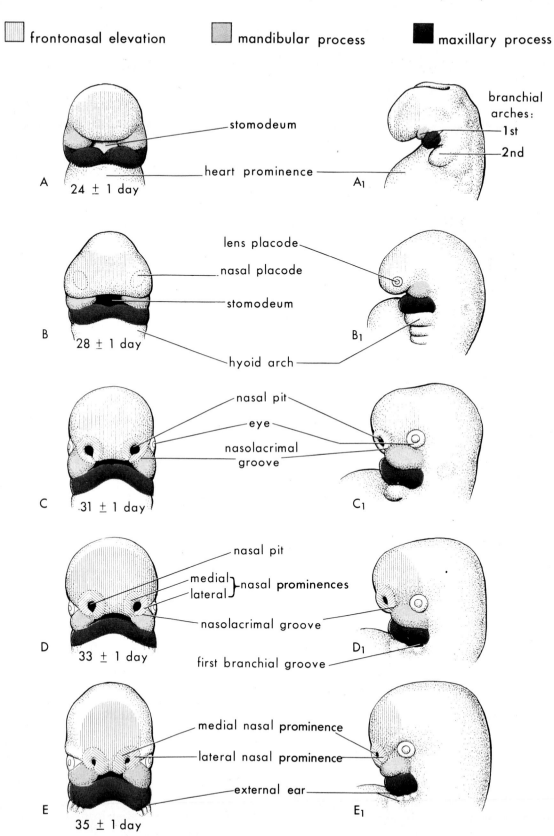

Figure 23–1   Diagrams illustrating progressive stages in the development of the human face during the embryonic and fetal periods. (From Moore, K. L., 1973. The Developing Human. Philadelphia, W. B. Saunders Co.)

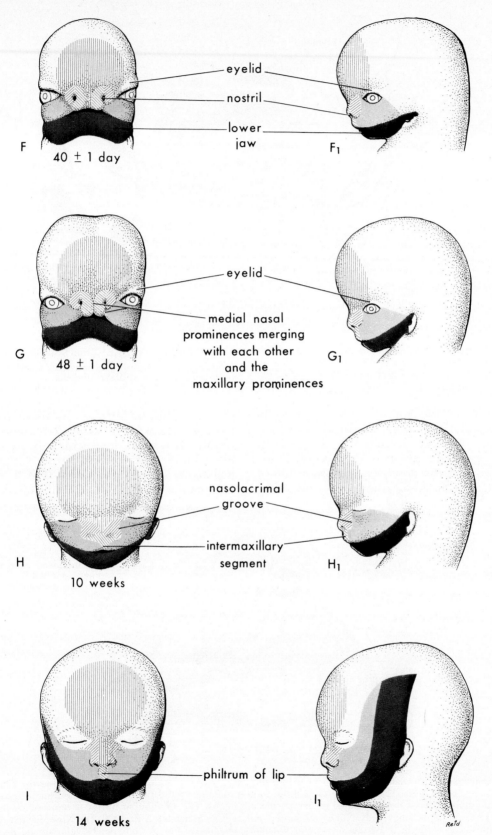

F   eyelid   F₁

nostril

lower jaw

40 ± 1 day

G   eyelid   G₁

medial nasal prominences merging with each other and the maxillary prominences

48 ± 1 day

H   nasolacrimal groove   H₁

intermaxillary segment

10 weeks

I   philtrum of lip   I₁

14 weeks

Figure 23–1 *Continued*

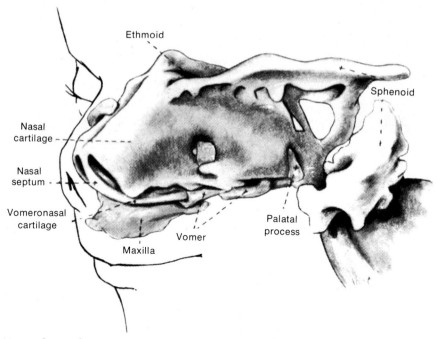

Figure 23–2   The cartilaginous nasal capsule from a human fetus aged 4 months. (From Schaeffer, J. P., 1920. The Nose, Paranasal Sinuses, Nasolacrimal Passageways, and Olfactory Organ in Man. A Genetic, Developmental and Anatomico-Physiological Consideration. Philadelphia, Blakiston Co.)

arises above the furrow. Above the bulla appears the suprabullar furrow, from which anterior ethmoid air cells will develop. In ensuing weeks, a variety of folds and furrows develop as if the nose would develop into a complex turbinate–meatus system as in other mammals, but by birth or shortly thereafter, most of them have coalesced and disappeared. However, the uncinate process, ethmoid bulla, and ethmoid infundibulum remain constant and prominent (Fig. 23–3).

From the infundibulum the maxillary sinus

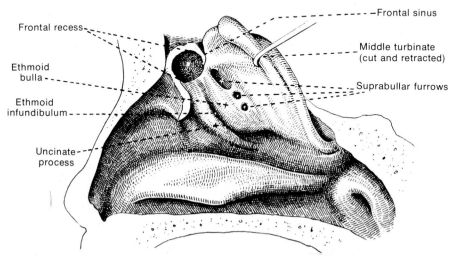

Figure 23–3   The lateral wall of a 14 month old child with the middle turbinate turned aside. The whole frontal recess is expanding toward the frontal region in the establishment of the frontal sinus. The infundibulum and the frontal recess are discontinuous. The suprabullar furrow is represented by a series of depressions, rudimentary ethmoidal cells. (From Schaeffer, J. P., 1920. The Nose, Paranasal Sinuses, Nasolacrimal Passageways, and Olfactory Organ in Man. A Genetic, Developmental and Anatomico-Physiological Consideration. Philadelphia, Blakiston Co.)

will develop, as will some ethmoid air cells, including those that pneumatize the ethmoid bulla. The frontal sinus forms from the superior extent of the infundibulum or, more commonly, from separate furrows superior to the infundibulum.

Continued development of the ethmoid bulla and the uncinate process so narrows the communication of the infundibulum with the nose that it becomes a slit-like opening, the hiatus semilunaris.

The superior nasal meatus contains ostia of the posterior ethmoid cells and is much less complicated than the middle meatus. Occasionally, however, various recesses and folds are present. When a supreme meatus is found, it usually contains an ostium of a posterior ethmoid air cell.

The Nasal Septum

The nasal septum is first apparent as the thick, fused, medial processes of the frontonasal process between the nasal pits. By the third month of fetal life, mesenchymal condensation occurs, and cartilage grows in from the body of the sphenoid to form two adjacent plates. These plates subsequently fuse

with one another (except in the case of the bifid nose) and fuse ventrally with the lateral nasal walls to complete the primitive nasal capsule.

The cartilaginous septum is formed by the septal (quadrilateral) cartilage, the vomeronasal cartilages, and the medial crura of the alar (lower lateral) cartilages (Fig. 23–4). The septal cartilage is roughly quadrangular in shape with a tail-like posterior extension, the sphenoidal process. In infancy, the sphenoidal process is in continuity with the sphenoid bone, completely separating the vomer and perpendicular plate of the ethmoid (Fig. 23–5). Fusion between the latter two bones begins posteriorly and extends forward by progressive absorption of the sphenoidal process or sometimes by displacement of it to one side.

Superiorly, the septal cartilage is continuous with the (upper) lateral cartilages, which extend like wings from it. As it projects anteriorly, it separates from them and extends between the alar cartilages to within 1 cm of the tip of the nose.

The vomeronasal cartilages are two narrow, longitudinal strips, 7 to 15 mm long, lying along the inferior margin of the septal cartilage, attached to the vomer posteriorly

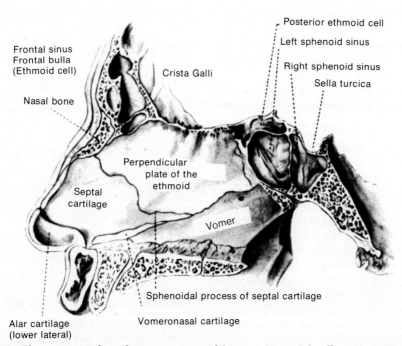

Figure 23–4 The osseous and cartilaginous septum of the nose. (From Schaeffer, J. P., 1920. The Nose, Paranasal Sinuses, Nasolacrimal Passageways, and Olfactory Organ in Man. A Genetic, Developmental and Anatomico-Physiological Consideration. Philadelphia, Blakiston Co.)

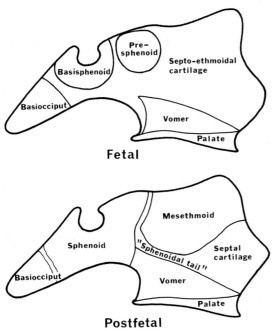

Figure 23–5 The nasal septum and basicranium during fetal and early postnatal life. Not to scale. (From Moore, W. J., and Lavelle, C. L., 1974. Growth of the Facial Skeleton in the Hominoidea. London, Academic Press, Inc.)

and to the maxillary crest anteriorly. They are not always differentiated from the septal cartilage and may appear only as lateral processes or spurs from its inferior border.

The membranous septum (mobile septum) is the portion anterior to the end of the septal cartilage. It is formed by skin and subcutaneous tissue of the nasal columella.

The bony septum is composed of two major elements: the vomer and the perpendicular plate of the ethmoid, and their articulating points with the nasal spine of the frontal bone, the rostrum of the sphenoid, and the crests of the nasal, maxillary, and palate bones, as shown in Figure 23–4.

The perpendicular plate of the ethmoid (mesoethmoid) is the ossified upper to midline portion of the primitive nasal capsule. Ossification begins in the fifth fetal month and is not completed until the 17th year. Ossification means replacement of thick, infantile cartilaginous septum with thin bone. The perpendicular plate is thin except at points of articulation with adjacent bone and septal cartilage, where it remains thick and may even contain marrow spaces.

At the nasal roof it articulates with the cribriform plate and even extends above it

into the cranial cavity as the crista galli (Fig. 23–4). The cribriform plate is a fibrous structure until it becomes ossified in the third year, providing a firm union between the lateral and medial ethmoidal elements. The anterior extent of ossification of the perpendicular plate is quite variable. It may extend no further forward than the anterior extent of the nasal spine of the frontal bone, or as far forward as the distal border of the nasal bones, or any distance in between. Obviously, its size is reciprocally related to the size of the septal cartilage.

The vomer, by contrast, develops not by ossification of cartilage but rather from connective tissue membrane on each side of the septal cartilage. For the opposing lamellae of the vomer to fuse, the intervening cartilage must be absorbed, a process that begins about the third fetal month and may not be completed until mid-adulthood. The lamellae grow upwards toward the perpendicular plate of the ethmoid, imprisoning the sphenoid process (tail) of the septal cartilage. Ideally, absorption and fusion proceed in an orderly fashion, and the remaining cartilage lies in a V-shaped groove on top of the two plates of the vomer. However, any inequality of growth between the plates will allow the cartilage to escape its imprisoned position and to buckle laterally, creating the posterior septal spur, a common irregularity of the septal surface.

Even on the normal, fully matured septum, elevations and ridge-like protuberances interrupt the smooth surface. The most constant is the tuberculum septi, an area of thickened mucosa appearing opposite the anterior end of the middle nasal turbinate. Occasionally, oblique mucosal ridges are notable on the posteroinferior septum. These are septal plicae, remnants of mucosal folds prominent up to eight months of fetal age, which generally regress and disappear in infancy. They may persist and may even hypertrophy into tumor-like obstructing masses.

Anomalies and Variations, The Internal Nose

Asymmetry of the Nasal Septum

Approximately 80 per cent of humans have some deformity of the nasal septum. The asymmetry may affect any or all parts of the septum except for the posterior free border at the choanae where it is always midline. A common area of deflection is along the articulation between the vomer and perpendicular plate of the ethmoid, especially when these two bones are separated for a considerable distance by the sphenoidal process of the septal cartilage. Ridge-like deflections and spurs may occur there even if the rest of the septum is straight. Sometimes the septum bows entirely into one nasal cavity; at other times a double buckling occurs with an S-shaped deformity affecting both cavities. The septal cartilage is often dislocated out of the midline groove of the maxillary crest (Fig. 23–6).

No one hypothesis is adequate to explain all cases of septal deformity. Twin studies do not suggest that septal deformity is genetically determined. However, it is a trait that is characteristic of the family of humans and some other primates, species that exhibit a prominent forward extension of the cranial cavity above the face. Even prehistoric *Australopithecus boiseii*, who lived 1,750,000 years ago, appears to have had the deformity. Gray (1978) studied more than 3000 skulls of various mammals and found only one case (in a Pekinese dog) of septal deformity in 642 nonprimates. He found septal deformities in 7 per cent of lower apes (baboons and mandrils), 37 per cent of higher apes (chimpanzees and gorillas), and 73 to 87 per cent of

humans of various races. Two theories are postulated to explain these observations:
1. The erect posture of the gravid female results in a lengthy period during which the fetus' head is engaged in the pelvis, which creates external pressures against the nose and face.
2. Vertical growth of the septum is impeded by its fixed position between an unyielding hard palate below and an overhanging cranial cavity above, which causes the growing septum to buckle.

Even passage of the head through the birth canal causes significant nasal injury. Gray (1978) found nasal and septal deformities in 4 per cent of infants born of normal vaginal deliveries and in 13 per cent of difficult deliveries (e.g., occipitoposterior presentations), but only rarely in infants delivered by cesarean section. Although most newborn nasal deformities can be corrected easily by gentle, close reduction, occasionally the deformed pyramid is immobile and resistant to corrective manipulations. Kirchner (1955) and Cottle (1951) observed that such solid deformities are self-correcting and that the nose will return to the midline position within the first year, sometimes even within the first few months. This solid deformity is likely due to a long-standing intrauterine position where some unusual pressure is placed against one side of the face (such as an arm or

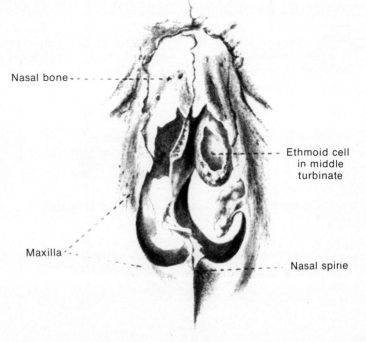

Figure 23–6 Septal deformity with compensatory turbinate hypertrophy. Note the ethmoid air cell in the middle turbinate. (From Schaeffer, J. P., 1920. The Nose, Paranasal Sinuses, Nasolacrimal Passageways, and Olfactory Organ in Man. A Genetic, Developmental and Anatomico-Physiological Consideration. Philadelphia, Blakiston Co.)

Nasal bone

Ethmoid cell in middle turbinate

Maxilla

Nasal spine

a shoulder) during development. Gray regards this type of pressure against the maxilla as responsible not only for nasal and septal deformities but also for deformities of the palate and teeth. He notes that when the deformity of the septum results in shortening of its height, the palate will fail to grow downwards, and a high-arched palate with abnormalities in dental occlusion will occur.

Nasal injury accounts for most cases of nasal and septal deformity, but the injury may be remote in time and often not remembered. Indeed, the prominent, unprotected position of the nose on the face makes injury almost impossible to avoid throughout life. Frequently, a deformity resulting from a childhood injury may appear to be insignificant, but it becomes prominent during adolescence when asymmetries become exaggerated under the pressure of accelerated septal growth.

Turbinate Deformity

Extra space available in one nasal cavity, due to long-standing displacement of the septum into the other, is likely to become occupied by overdeveloped inferior or middle turbinates (Fig. 23–6). Both bone and mucosal elements participate in this compensatory hypertrophy. Additionally, an ethmoid air cell may invade the middle turbinate, giving it a rounded, bullous look, often creating airway obstruction. Whether the turbinate enlargement forces the septum to become deformed or the turbinate simply enlarges to fill the space created by the septal deformity is a developmental puzzle. Although such turbinate invasion by ethmoid air cells is

common in adults (12 per cent or more), it is only occasionally seen in children (see Ethmoid Sinuses).

The Vomeronasal Organ

The vomeronasal organ (organ of Jacobson) is an accessory olfactory organ in some mammalian species, but it is rudimentary in man. It reaches its maximal development in the 20th fetal week and usually degenerates in late fetal life. It is sometimes detectable even in adulthood as a blind mucosal pocket 2 to 6 mm deep on each side of the septum just above the orifice of the nasopalatine canal.

Other anomalies of the internal nose, such as nasopalatine cysts and choanal atresia, are described in other chapters of this text. The nasal encephalocele is described in Surgical Hazards.

The External Nose

Nasal landmarks are illustrated in Figure 23–7. It should be noted that the superoanterior surface of the nose is termed the nasal dorsum even though it occupies a ventral position with respect to the rest of the body. The glabella is the point between the eyebrows, or more specifically, the smooth body triangular portion of frontal bone between the supraorbital ridges. The nasion is the point where the internasal suture meets the frontal bone.

Three paired bones form the external nasal skeleton: the nasal bones, the frontal processes of the maxillae, and the nasal portions of the frontal bones (Fig. 23–8). The last

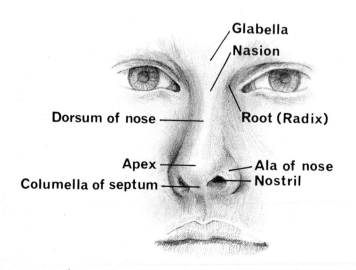

Figure 23–7 Nasal topography.

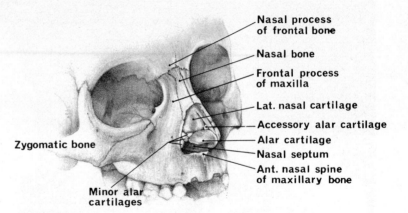

Figure 23–8 Cartilaginous and bony nasal skeleton.

Labels: Nasal process of frontal bone · Nasal bone · Frontal process of maxilla · Lat. nasal cartilage · Accessory alar cartilage · Alar cartilage · Nasal septum · Ant. nasal spine of maxillary bone · Zygomatic bone · Minor alar cartilages

named articulate with and project beneath the nasal bones (Fig. 23–4) and frontal processes of the maxilla so that both frontal and maxillary bones lend support to the nasal bridge. The point of articulation is named the nasal root or radix. When the nasal bones grow unequally or are absent, the frontal processes of the maxillae grow anteriorly to fill in the defect. The nasal bones are paired, arched structures that articulate with each other at their apex, where they also articulate with the frontal spine of the frontal bone and the perpendicular plate of the ethmoid. They are thickest at this point and are narrowed laterally where they articulate with the frontal processes of the maxillae. Their free anterior margins articulate with and overlie the fused (upper) lateral and septal cartilages. That they must overlie the lateral cartilages is a developmental imperative. They develop in membrane on the surface of the cartilaginous nasal capsule. The cartilage of the capsule can be demonstrated as late as the first postfetal month before it is absorbed. The lacrimal bone forms in a similar manner.

Maxillary ossification begins at about the sixth fetal week from a center above the canine tooth germ and spreads in all directions. At about the fourth fetal month, the maxilla invades the cartilaginous nasal capsule and participates in formation of the lateral nasal wall and ethmoidal boundaries. The cartilaginous capsule is absorbed beneath the maxilla so that the latter receives the evaginating maxillary sinus pouch. Cartilaginous masses that are occasionally seen in the alveolar processes of the developing maxilla may represent cartilaginous capsule remnants.

Four major cartilages and a variable number of minor or accessory cartilages participate in the formation of the external nose (Fig. 23–8). The septum also participates, as described in previous paragraphs. The lateral nasal cartilage (also termed upper lateral or triangular cartilage) is a flattened triangular plate in the middle of the nose. It is fused in the midline with the septum and with its fellow of the opposite side. The paired alar cartilages (also termed greater alar, lobular, or lower lateral cartilages) partially encircle the nares and assist in keeping them open and in giving shape to the base of the nose. Each consists of two crura, which are continuous at the apex, giving the nasal tip an arched contour. The medial crura approximate each other, bounding a deep median groove, extend posteroinferiorly in the nasal columella, and end in a free out-turned border.

Each lateral crus extends posterolaterally in the ala towards the maxilla but does not reach it, the interval being filled with a strong sheet of fibrous tissue in which are embedded the minor nasal cartilages. In some cases, the lateral crus is so prolonged that it replaces the minor (lesser, accessory) cartilages.

The lateral crura are bound by fibrous tissue to the septum anteriorly and to the lateral cartilages superiorly. At the connection between lateral and alar cartilages, the latter overlies the former in most instances (77 per cent), and they are often interlocked by their scroll-like curling margins. Occasionally (in 17 per cent of cases), they do not overlap at all, or the lateral may overlie the alar cartilage at the articulation (11 per cent) (Dion et al., 1978).

Postnatal Growth and Development

At birth, the face is small relative to the cranium, as illustrated in Figure 23–9. The craniofacial ratio is 8:1 compared to 4:1 at 5

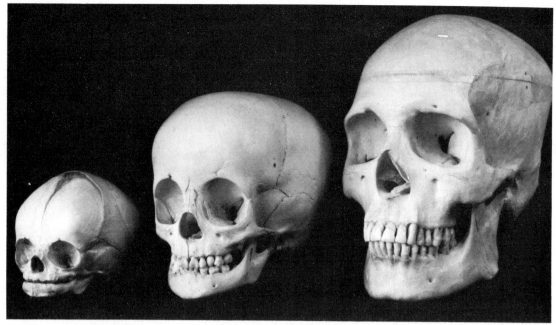

Figure 23–9 Skulls of newborn, 5 year old child, and adult demonstrate decreasing craniofacial ratios.

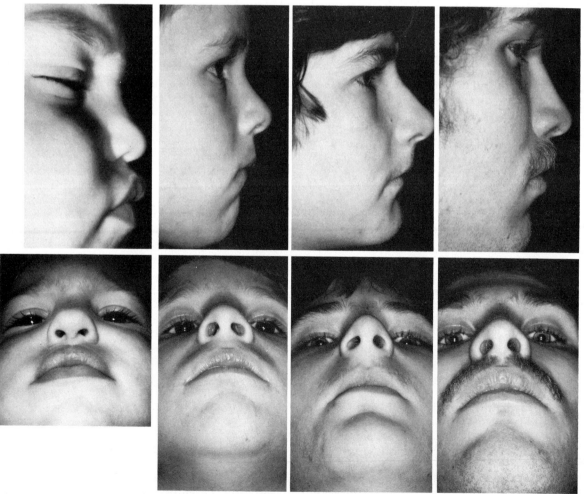

Figure 23–10 Changing shape of nose from infancy through adolescence. From left to right: Infant, 7 years, 13 years, 17 years.

years and 2:1 in adulthood. At birth, the nasal fossae are as wide as they are high, and their lower border is just below the plane of the orbit. The ethmoidal part of the nasal fossa is twice as high as the maxillary portion, but since the latter grows faster after birth, the two portions are equal by the time dentition is completed in the late teens.

The nares are small at birth, measuring 5 to 7 mm vertically and 7 to 8 mm horizontally. By 6 months of age they have doubled their dimensions, but they retain their roughly circular shape until puberty when the vertical diameter becomes greater and the nares become oval or oblong in shape (Fig. 23–10). The nose grows in several spurts, with maxima at ages three, six, and seven years, and then from puberty to age 20 (Reichert, 1963). The nose reaches twice its birth length by seven years, and at 14 years it is triple its birth length.

The maxilla grows forward and downward at a rate of 1 mm per year in childhood, slowing to 0.25 mm in the 11th year, then accelerating to 1.5 mm per year in adolescence, eventually ceasing at about age 17. Its direction of growth is 51 degrees forward and downward from an imaginary line between the nasion and the sella (Moore and Lavelle, 1974).

As early as 1857 it was recognized that a major force in the projection and growth of the upper face is the thrust of the growing nasal septum (Scott, 1953). Facial growth occurs as a complex interaction of four processes: (1) cartilaginous expansion, specifically the septal cartilage, which grows as a sheet, creates forward projection of the nose, and forces the maxilla and palate forward and downward (Fig. 23–11); (2) conversion of cartilage into bone at bony–cartilaginous junctions, a process most active in the fetal period and first three years; (3) intersutural periosteal bone deposition, which is stimulated by external forces (e.g., the force of the expanding septum) that create intersutural separation; (4) surface periosteal bone deposition, which is a constant remodeling process in which, for the most part, internal surfaces are resorbed and new bone is deposited on outer surfaces. The outer deposition accounts for facial growth and the internal resorption allows the sinuses to invade the facial bones (Enlow, 1978).

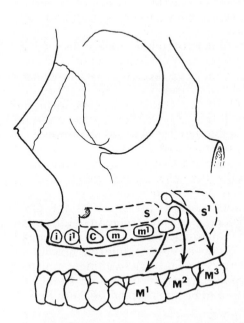
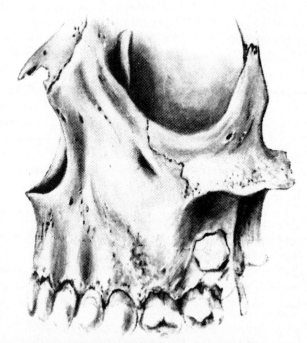

Figure 23–11 *Left,* Postnatal growth of the maxilla is downward and forward. The broken line outlines the maxilla at birth; the adult bone is shown in solid lines. *c,* deciduous canine; *i* and *i*¹, deciduous incisors; *m* and *m*¹, deciduous molars; *M*¹, *M*², and *M*³, permanent molars; *s,* maxillary sinus at birth; *s*¹, maxillary sinus at maturity. *Right,* Arrested development in rotation may result in an impacted third molar, high and posterior in the maxilla. (From Schaeffer, J. P., 1920. The Nose, Paranasal Sinuses, Nasolacrimal Passageways, and Olfactory Organ in Man. A Genetic, Developmental and Anatomico-Physiological Consideration. Philadelphia, Blakiston Co.)

Anomalies and Variations, the External Nose

The external nose characteristically exhibits individual, familial, and racial variability. These differences are not pronounced in the early childhood years. Even in persons destined to have prominent noses with "hump" deformities, the dorsum is usually straight or concave during childhood. Not until the period of rapid nasal (especially septal) growth in puberty does the nose assume its individual characteristics, which are the result of a combination of genetic and traumatic influences.

A common developmental defect is the nasal dermoid cyst, a hair-bearing epidermal inclusion cyst appearing in the midline over the nasal dorsum (Pratt, 1965). Its surface opening is usually a pinpoint depression, but it may be deep and long, even as a midline cleft or fissure. It represents a failure of fusion of the medial processes. Other manifestations of that failure include the bifid nasal tip and the median nasal cleft.

Developmental failures can lead to unilateral or bilateral nasal absences, deficient cartilage and bone formation, and other abnormalities. Nasal deformity always accompanies a cleft lip since development of the upper lip and nares is a process of fusion of portions of the frontonasal process with the maxillary process, all occurring simultaneously.

These and other deformities are detailed in other chapters of this volume.

Surgical Hazards

The primary hazard of nasal surgery in children is interruption of nasal growth. In early puberty nasal growth outdistances that of the face and produces exaggerated nasal features that tempt both patient and surgeon to correct them. Since the final result of growth is difficult to predict, premature surgery may produce a nose disproportionately small with respect to the fully grown face.

Bony growth occurs on subperiosteal surfaces as well as at all points of union between the various osseous and cartilaginous elements of the nose. Disruption of these suture lines and periosteal coverings can hardly be avoided during rhinoplastic procedures. For the same reason, nasal fractures in children should be reduced by the closed method.

Cartilaginous growth occurs throughout the entire plate of the quadrilateral cartilage. Therefore, removal of any portion of that plate reduces the total growth capacity of the septum, which is the determining factor for projection not only of the nasal profile but also of the facial profile. Gilbert and Segal (1958) suggest that the degree of saddle formation is proportional to the amount of resected cartilage and that when surgery is required for nasal obstruction in a child, only small buttons of cartilage should be removed, only at the point of maximal obstruction. Furthermore, the mucoperichondrial incision and elevation should be made close to the resection site so that there is minimal interference with the blood supply that the mucoperichondrium provides to surrounding cartilage. They also warn against disrupting the attachments of the upper and lower lateral cartilages to the septum or maxillae.

Elective surgery on the external nose is generally avoided until full facial growth is achieved, usually by age 16 for females and 18 for males. Certain exceptions to this rule are notable. Severe congenital deformities, such as those associated with cleft lip, should be corrected early, lest growth exaggerate the deformity (Farrior and Connolly, 1970). The same applies to severe traumatic deformities.

Intracranial complications are also a hazard in nasal surgery. The perpendicular plate of the ethmoid at the nasal roof articulates with the cribriform plate, then extends into the floor of the cranial cavity to form the crista galli (Fig. 23–4). This structure should not be subjected to vigorous manipulations such as twisting and pulling during a septal resection for fear that hazardous communications into the intracranial cavity will be opened. Another potential pathway to the intracranial space is presented by the nasal encephalocele, a rare congenital intranasal mass that masquerades as a polyp. True nasal polyps occur rarely in children (except in those with cystic fibrosis), so a single unilateral polyp-like structure in a child should be considered to be an encephalocele until proven otherwise.

Septal perforations usually occur in the cartilaginous septum. The cartilage is entirely dependent on overlying mucosa for its blood supply, and it will disintegrate if mucosa is damaged on both sides of the septum in corresponding areas. Simultaneous bilateral nasal cautery for epistaxis is inadvisable for this reason. Septal surgery is the most common cause of perforations (Fairbanks and Chen, 1970).

THE MAXILLARY SINUSES

Growth and Development

The maxillary sinus is first evident about the 70th fetal day as an evagination in the lateral wall of the ethmoidal infundibulum. Although usually a single pouch, it may be two pouches that develop into two sinus cavities that later fuse but leave two ostia.

The fetal maxillary sinus is a slit-like space in the middle meatus between the lateral wall of the nose and the inferior turbinate. Even before birth enough resorption of the cartilaginous capsule takes place so that the sinus comes into contact with the maxilla and pneumatization commences. At birth the sinus is 7 to 8 mm deep (anterior to posterior), half as wide, and slightly more than half that dimension in height. It is a tubular sac, the lower margin of which lies slightly below the level of the upper border of the interior meatus. Anteriorly it extends to the lacrimal duct. It is not always demonstrable on radiographs, although it is of considerable size. Facial growth and maxillary sinus growth proceed together.

Not until the end of the first year has the sinus extended laterally below the orbit to the position of the infraorbital nerve. Growth in width lags behind growth in other dimensions, for until the teeth erupt there is little room in the maxilla into which the sinus can grow (Fig. 23–12). During the third and fourth years conspicuous growth in width occurs. At five years the sinus reaches consid-

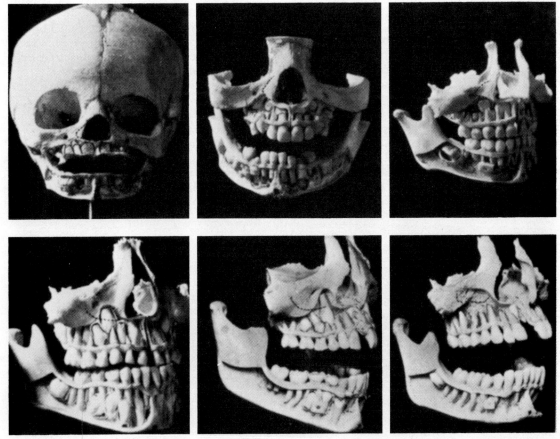

Figure 23–12 Dissections showing the relationship of the teeth to the developing maxillary sinus indicated by a dotted line. (From Schaeffer, J. P., 1920. The Nose, Paranasal Sinuses, Nasolacrimal Passageways, and Olfactory Organ in Man. A Genetic, Developmental and Anatomico-Physiological Consideration. Philadelphia, Blakiston Co.)

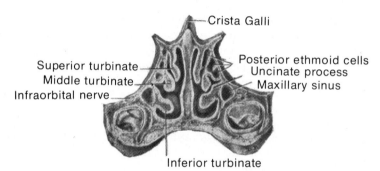

—Crista Galli

Superior turbinate
Middle turbinate
Infraorbital nerve

Posterior ethmoid cells
Uncinate process
Maxillary sinus

Inferior turbinate

Figure 23–13 Coronal section from a 38 day old child showing extent of superoinferior and lateral development of the maxillary sinus and proximity of the developing teeth to the orbital floor. (From Davis, W. B., 1918. Anatomy of the nasal accessory sinuses in infancy and childhood. Ann. Otol. Rhinol. Laryngol., 27:940–967.)

erably beyond the infraorbital canal, and by nine years it has pneumatized the zygomatic process of the maxilla (Figs. 23–13, 23–14, 23–15, and 23–16).

Inferiorly directed expansion accelerates between the seventh and ninth years with the eruption of the permanent teeth, particularly the canines and molars, which leaves vacant spaces that the sinus pneumatizes. This growth brings the sinus in proximity to the inferior nasal meatus by age eight. It reaches the level of the nasal floor variably between ages eight and 12 years.

By the 15th year the sinus reaches its adult size except for some expansion that will occur in height. The lowest extension of the cavity occurs when the third molar erupts and the space is pneumatized by the sinus.

As the sinus expands posteriorly, the posterior part of the maxilla, which contains the rudiments of the permanent molar teeth, undergoes a rotation inferiorly, as illustrated in Figure 23–11. What was located posteriorly ultimately comes to occupy a position on the alveolar border of the maxilla. An impacted

third molar, placed high posteriorly on the posterior maxilla, is due to arrested development in rotation.

Anomalies and Variations

The walls of the maxillary sinus are often smooth and even. Yet almost 50 per cent of adult maxillary sinuses have ridges, crescentic projections, and septa incompletely dividing the cavity into various-sized compartments. They are probably due to uneven bone resorption during pneumatization or possibly may have been duplicated cavities that failed to fuse completely.

True duplication of the maxillary sinus (with two separate ostia, both of which enter the nasal infundibulum) is developmentally explainable, as mentioned in previous paragraphs. More often, however, the ostium of the superior or posterior compartment enters the superior meatus, and the cell is actually a posterior ethmoid sinus that invaded the maxilla. Considering true duplications and

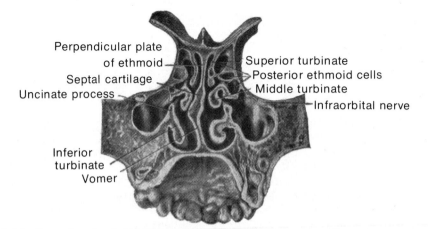

Perpendicular plate
of ethmoid
Septal cartilage
Uncinate process

Superior turbinate
Posterior ethmoid cells
Middle turbinate
Infraorbital nerve

Inferior
turbinate
Vomer

Figure 23–14 Coronal section from a 3½ year old child showing the extent of lateral and superoinferior development of the maxillary sinus and the posterior ethmoid cells. Note the deflection of the septum and its influence on the turbinates. (From Davis, W. B., 1918. Anatomy of the nasal accessory sinuses in infancy and childhood. Ann. Otol. Rhinol. Laryngol., 27:940–967.)

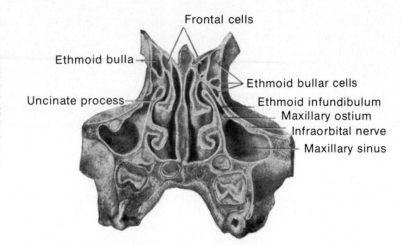

Figure 23–15 Coronal section from a 4½ year old child showing the extent of lateral and superoinferior development of the maxillary sinus and its relation to developing teeth. Note the ridge beneath the left infraorbital nerve. (From Davis, W. B., 1918. Anatomy of the nasal accessory sinuses in infancy and childhood. Ann. Otol. Rhinol. Laryngol., 27:940–967.)

maxillary ethmoid cells together, Schaeffer (1920) described the incidence of this phenomenon as occurring in 2.5 per cent of specimens.

The clinical significance of these separated compartments is that during irrigations and surgical explorations, the surgeon may enter one cavity and neglect disease in an adjacent one.

The maxillary sinus ostium lies in the ethmoid infundibulum, which is reached by traversing the hiatus semilunaris deep in the middle meatus of the nose (Figs. 23–14, 23–15, and 23–16). Bounding the hiatus is the ethmoid bulla above and the uncinate process below. These structures are often pneumatized by ethmoid air cells. When enlarged, they narrow the hiatus to slit-like dimensions and not only impede maxillary sinus drainage but also direct frontal and anterior ethmoid sinus drainage into the maxillary sinus ostium.

When the uncinate ridge is high (25 per cent of cases), or the ethmoid bulla is low and overhanging (11 per cent), or the middle turbinate is low and bulky (17 per cent), cannulation of the natural ostium is difficult or impossible (Van Alyea, 1951). Indeed, Schaeffer (1920) concluded, after dissecting a large number of specimens, that cannulation of the natural ostium in the live patient would have been anatomically impossible in the vast majority of cases. But Van Alyea (1951) claimed that the ostium was easily accessible in 40 per cent of cases, and both authors conceded that the cannula may succeed in entering the sinus, not through the natural ostium but rather by penetrating the lateral nasal wall posterior to the hiatus in an area of thin or absent bone termed the "undefended area."

This area is in the medial wall of the maxillary sinus where the perpendicular plate of the palate bone, the uncinate process

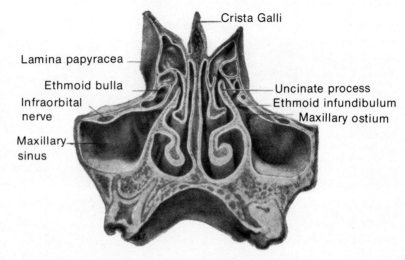

Figure 23–16 Coronal section from a 10 year old child showing the size and relations of the maxillary sinus, the maxillary ostium, and its relationship with the ethmoid infundibulum, the bulla, the uncinate process and the anterior ethmoid cells. (From Davis, W. B., 1918. Anatomy of the nasal accessory sinuses in infancy and childhood. Ann. Otol. Rhinol. Laryngol., 27:940–967.)

of the ethmoid bone, the maxillary process of the inferior turbinate, and a portion of the lacrimal bone are all loosely and incompletely articulated. There are numerous dehiscences and defects there; the area is held intact only by membrane on the sinus and nasal side. In dried skulls, the area is usually found devoid of bone, as a large dehiscence.

The accessory maxillary ostium (or ostia) that is so common in adults occurs in this "undefended area." It drains directly into the middle meatus of the nose and not into the ethmoid infundibulum, which distinguishes it from the natural or the duplicated maxillary sinus ostium. It develops by the gradual thinning of bone in the advanced stages of maxillary sinus pneumatization until the bone is finally absorbed and the thinned membranes rupture spontaneously (a situation analogous to the rupture of the bucconasal membrane in the formation of the choana). This accounts for the frequency of accessory ostia in adulthood (variously reported at 25 to 50 per cent) and the rarity before the age of 15 years (15 per cent in children) (Van Alyea, 1951) (Fig. 23–17).

The size of the maxillary sinus varies considerably among patients of the same age and even from side to side in the same patient. Small sinuses occur when there is deficient absorption of cancellous bone in the sinus floor, a deep canine fossa with encroachment of the anterior sinus wall, excessive bulging of the nasal wall, or imperfect dentition. Minor differences in size and shape between the right and left maxillary sinuses are commonplace. Dixon (1959) claims that true absence of the

sinus never occurs, but in his series of 200 dissections he found one sinus with a capacity of only 1 cc, and Maresh (1940) reports the incidence of hypoplasia to be 6.3 per cent.

Sinuses can be unusually large when pneumatization extends into the alveolar, frontal, or zygomatic processes of the maxilla, the orbital process of the palatine bone, or underneath the nasal floor into the palatal recess.

Thickness of sinus walls varies from 5 to 8 mm down to a papery thin delicacy or absence, especially on the nasal wall and in the canine fossa. There are many exceptions to the idea that large sinuses have the thinnest walls and vice versa.

Ectopic teeth in the maxillary sinuses are regularly reported, especially in the dental literature. Developmental errors may be causative but so also could injuries to the maxilla, such as facial trauma or difficult dental manipulations. Any absent tooth in the maxilla with unusually long delayed eruption should suggest eruption into the nose or sinus. Ectopic incisors and canines may appear in the nasal floor. Ectopic molars are found in the floor of the maxillary sinus; the third molar is most frequently involved, as explained in a previous paragraph.

Anatomic Relationships and Surgical Hazards

The floor of the maxillary sinus is the alveolar process of the maxilla. Spongy bone separates the sinus cavity from the roots of the teeth and their sockets. Even though this

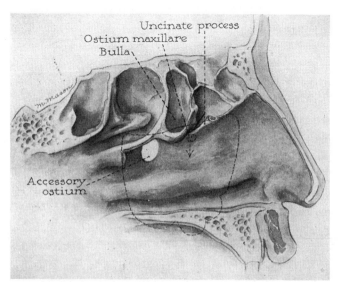

Figure 23–17 Low overhanging ethmoid bulla makes the maxillary ostium inaccessible. However, a large accessory ostium is available for cannulation. (From Van Alyea, O. E., 1951. Nasal Sinuses, An Anatomic and Clinical Consideration, 2nd ed. Baltimore, Williams & Wilkins Co.)

is the thickest of the sinus walls, it is frequently thin enough to show irregular elevations in the sinus floor overlying the tooth roots. Thinning to the point of direct communication of tooth roots with the maxillary sinus sometimes occurs in young adulthood, but usually not until advanced age.

Dr. Nathaniel Highmore, after whom this antrum has been called, gave a detailed description of the cavity as early as 1651. He had a patient whose abscess in the sinus was drained by extraction of the canine tooth. That particular sinus must have been exceptionally large because the canine tooth does not usually come into close relationship with the sinus; neither do the incisors. Even the first and second premolars are often not in close proximity to the floor of the cavity. The three molar teeth are most constantly and intimately related to the sinus, but in small sinuses even the first molar may be omitted.

In children, surgical procedures through the canine fossa should be done with great consideration for developing teeth. Injury to them leads to either death of the teeth or ultimate eruption of deformed teeth. Radiographs should locate their position, and the approach should be high and lateral enough to avoid them. Endonasal approaches to the sinus in children are best carried out through the middle meatus, since the floor of the sinus may not reach the level of the nasal floor until the 12th year. Furthermore, the inferior meatus is exceedingly narrow because of the relatively large inferior turbinate and its heavy mucosa.

The anterior wall of the sinus contains the infraorbital foramen at the upper aspect of the canine fossa. It is approximately the same distance from the midline as the palpable supraorbital notch, and it is 0.5 cm or less below the infraorbital rim. The nerve and vessel that exit through this foramen should be protected during periosteal elevation in the Caldwell-Luc approach. Damage to the nerve results in sensory loss to the cheek and upper lip and occasionally neuroma formation that can be painful.

The roof of the maxillary sinus is the thin plate of bone forming the orbital floor. Not infrequently it is modeled into a ridge by the infraorbital canal (Fig. 23–15). In some instances the ridge is replaced by a groove covered only by thin membrane.

The infraorbital nerve and artery are in jeopardy when curettage is performed on the roof of the sinus cavity. The orbital periosteum is a sufficiently thick and recognizable barrier between the orbital contents and the sinus. However, in orbital floor fractures the periosteum is often lacerated and orbital fat protrudes into the roof of the sinus, mimicking a mucosal polyp. It should not be removed lest enophthalmus be exaggerated by a further loss of orbital contents.

Innervation of the maxillary teeth may also be jeopardized by sinus surgery. The posterosuperior dental nerves, branches of the maxillary nerve, enter the maxilla posteriorly through tiny foramina and run through spongy bone covering the tooth roots of the molars and premolars. They may be immediately submucosal so that curettage of the sinus floor leaves the teeth numb.

Canine and incisor teeth are innervated by the anterosuperior dental nerve, which branches off the infraorbital nerve midway in its canal. In some instances, it runs obliquely (anteromedially) across the roof of the maxillary sinus in a raised, thin bony canal, but often it is covered only by mucous membrane. Otherwise, it remains in the infraorbital canal until it reaches the anterior sinus wall where it turns medially. In the medial wall of the sinus, at the level of the anterior end of the inferior turbinate, the nerve turns downward toward the nasal spine and gives off its branches to the teeth. When surgery requires removal of the anterior wall of the sinus high and medially or removal of the antral roof, injury to this nerve may occur.

The posterior boundary of the sinus is the anterior wall of the pterygopalatine fossa, which contains the ramifying maxillary nerve and artery. One branch of that artery, the greater palatine, courses toward the palate through a canal in the posteroinferior medial wall of the maxillary sinus. It may be encountered by the surgeon as he or she takes down the posteroinferior bony ridge during nasoantral fenestration. Bleeding can be troublesome.

Sometimes the posterior or superior wall is divided into two plates separated by an invading ethmoid air cell. Indeed, the ethmoid sinus field is the most medial superior boundary of the maxillary sinus cavity. It requires only gentle pressure to crack through the thin, shell-like bone to perform the transantral ethmoidectomy, an operation that affords good, safe visualization of the posterior ethmoid complex.

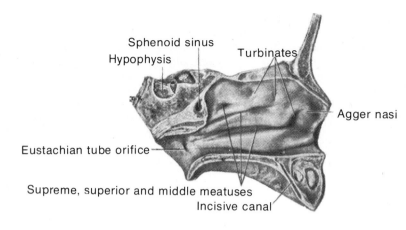

Sphenoid sinus
Hypophysis
Turbinates
Agger nasi
Eustachian tube orifice
Supreme, superior and middle meatuses
Incisive canal

Figure 23–18 Sagittal section from an 8 day old child shows the left lateral nasal wall and the extent of development of the sphenoid sinus. Note the anteroinferior wall of the sphenoid sinus, termed the sphenoid concha or ossiculum Bertini. (From Davis, W. B., 1918. Anatomy of the nasal accessory sinuses in infancy and childhood. Ann. Otol. Rhinol. Laryngol., 27:940–967.)

Figure 23–19 Sagittal section from a child nearly 2 years old. The sphenoid sinus appears small, but in a more lateral plane it was developed more extensively in the posterolateral direction, its inferolateral wall being only 1 mm from the pterygopalatine fossa. (From Davis, W. B., 1918. Anatomy of the nasal accessory sinuses in infancy and childhood. Ann. Otol. Rhinol. Laryngol., 27:940–967.)

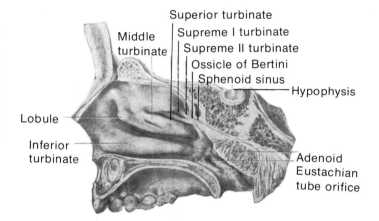

Superior turbinate
Supreme I turbinate
Supreme II turbinate
Middle turbinate
Ossicle of Bertini
Sphenoid sinus
Hypophysis
Lobule
Inferior turbinate
Adenoid
Eustachian tube orifice

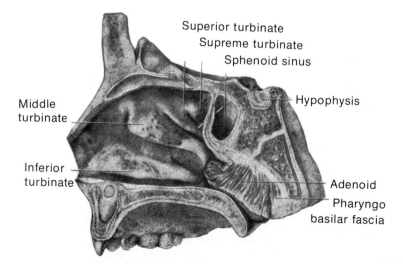

Superior turbinate
Supreme turbinate
Sphenoid sinus
Hypophysis
Middle turbinate
Inferior turbinate
Adenoid
Pharyngo basilar fascia

Figure 23–20 Sagittal section from a 6 year old child showing presellar sphenoidal pneumatization. (From Davis, W. B., 1918. Anatomy of the nasal accessory sinuses in infancy and childhood. Ann. Otol. Rhinol. Laryngol., 27:940–967.)

Table 23-1 THE OCCURRENCE OF DIFFERENT TYPES OF SPHENOID SINUSES AMONG VARIOUS AGE GROUPS

Type of Sinus	0–3 yrs	4–12 yrs	13–20 yrs	21–30 yrs
Presellar	100%	57%	13%	6%
Sellar	0	43%	65%	72%
Sellar–extensive	0	0	22%	22%

(Modified from Vidic, B. 1968. The postnatal development of the sphenoidal sinus and its spread into the dorsum sellae and posterior clinoid processes. Am. J. Roentgenol., *104*:177–183.)

THE SPHENOID SINUSES

Growth and Development

The sphenoid sinus arises in the posterior cupola or dome of the cartilaginous nasal capsule; its origin is suggested as early as the fourth fetal month. It develops as a constricted portion of the nasal fossa, its ostium always to remain cephalic to the highest nasal concha.

Although this sinus remains in its nasal position until the fourth postnatal year, it may be large enough to retain infectious material in its cavity. During the fourth year, the nasal capsule resorbs and the sinus comes in contact with the sphenoid bone, allowing ingrowth and sphenoid pneumatization. Its early growth is posterolateral rather than ventral, leading to early thinning of the lateral walls and an early intimate relationship with the ophthalmic and maxillary nerves. By the age of 6 or 7 years, it establishes a close relationship with the pterygoid (vidian) canal and its vessels and nerve. The growth rate averages 0.25 mm per year in the posterior direction, but it progresses in irregular spurts (Hinck and Hopkins, 1965).

Sphenoid sinuses have been classified into three categories that reflect the degree of pneumatization into the sphenoid bone.

1. *Conchal type.* Pneumatization does not extend into the body of the sphenoid bone but is arrested in its infantile position (Figs. 23–18 and 23–19). The small right and left sinuses are widely separated by a thick bony septum. Persistence of this type of sinus into late childhood is rare and is observed in only 2.5 per cent of adults (Hammer and Radberg, 1961).

2. *Presellar type.* Pneumatization extends only as far posteriorly as the sella turcica, or more specifically not beyond the vertical plane of the tuberculum sella (Fig. 23–20). This is the usual condition of childhood (Table 23–1), but pneumatization proceeds with age so that by adulthood the frequency of this type drops below 10 per cent.

3. *Sellar type.* Pneumatization advances beyond the tuberculum sella in 90 per cent of cases by the end of adolescence,

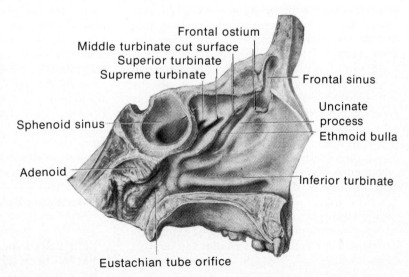

Figure 23–21 Sagittal section from a 10 year old child showing sellar-type pneumatization, which has extended beneath the anterior portion of the sella turcica. The anterior portion of the middle turbinate and a portion of the medial wall of the frontal sinus have been removed to demonstrate continuity from the sinus into the ethmoid infundibulum. (From Davis, W. B., 1918. Anatomy of the nasal accessory sinuses in infancy and childhood. Ann. Otol. Rhinol. Laryngol., 27:940–967.)

Frontal ostium
Middle turbinate cut surface
Superior turbinate
Supreme turbinate
Frontal sinus
Uncinate process
Ethmoid bulla
Sphenoid sinus
Adenoid
Inferior turbinate
Eustachian tube orifice

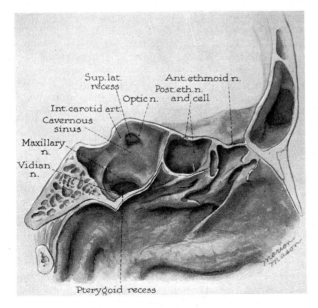

underneath the sella in over 20 per cent of cases (Fig. 23–21), and even posterior to the sella in up to 10 per cent of cases (Fig. 23–22).

The sphenoid is the first of all the paranasal sinuses to achieve full development. Growth ceases in early adulthood; 50 per cent are mature at age 15.

Anomalies and Variations

The sinus cavity is generally limited to the anterosuperior part of the sphenoid bone, although extensive sinuses have been described with pneumatization of the entire sphenoid bone, lesser and greater wings, basilar process of the occipital bone, supermedial aspect of the orbit, and orbital process of the palatal bone, and otherwise crowding spaces ordinarily occupied by posterior ethmoid cells.

In a small sinus the interior walls are usually even and regular. However, of all the paranasal sinuses, the sphenoid is most likely to have the most irregular internal topography. Partial septa and recesses vary from slight elevations to bridge-like osseous barriers incompletely dividing the sinus into subcompartments. Diverticula may extend into outlying portions of the sphenoid, even into the epidural spaces of the hypophysis, cavernous sinus, and optic nerves. Mounds and raised areas give evidence and warning of externally bordering neural and vascular structures (Fig. 23–22).

The intersinus septum is variable in both thickness and location. It is midline only at its anterior origin where it is in line with the nasal septum. Elsewhere it deviates to one side or the other or may even be situated in an oblique semihorizontal plane, so that the sinus of one side may seem to rest on top of the other. The sphenoid sinuses do not communicate with each other. If there appears to be no septum at all, it is likely due to agenesis of one sinus with compensatory pneumatization of the other with only one ostium.

The size and location of the sphenoid ostia are quite variable, even from one side to the other in the same specimen. However, they are always located in the sphenoethmoidal recess, cephalic to the uppermost turbinate that is present. Usually they are slightly superior to the midplane of the anterior sinus wall and 35 to 40 mm above the floor of the nasal cavity at maturity. The usual ostium is 2 by 3 mm in diameter, is placed 2 mm lateral to the nasal septum, and is hidden from anterior view by the superior turbinate. Large ostia, up to 6 mm in diameter, are occasionally seen opening immediately lateral to the septum. The ostium may be as far as 7 mm distant from the septum and may be as small as 1 by 1.5 mm in diameter (Fig. 23–23).

Anatomic Relationships and Surgical Hazards

The paired sphenoid sinuses are located in what has been termed the danger position in

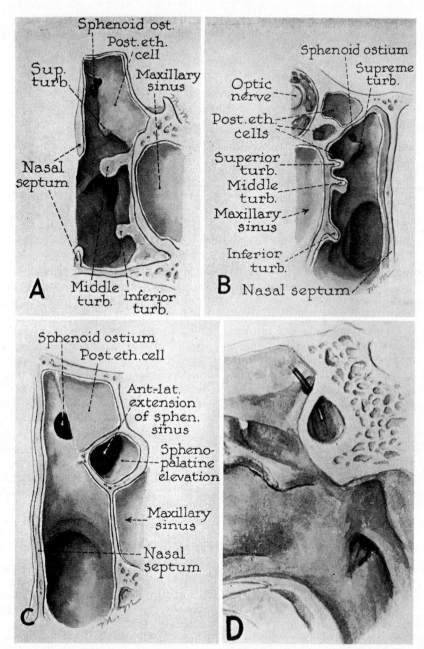

Figure 23–23 Types of sphenoid ostium. *A*, Average type. The orifice shown measures 3.5 by 2.5 mm. It is located in a shallow sphenoethmoid recess less than 2 mm from the nasal septum. *B*, Small ostium deep in the recess. *C*, Large opening in typical location. *D*, Ostium in roof of sinus. (From Van Alyea, O. E., 1951. Nasal Sinuses, An Anatomic and Clinical Consideration, 2nd ed. Baltimore, Williams & Wilkins Co.)

Table 23-2   ELEVATIONS IN THE SPHENOID SINUS WALL

Structure	Incidence	Anatomic Position
Hypophysis	87%	Midline, posterior (presellar sinus) Midline, superior (sellar sinus)
Internal carotid artery°	53%	Lateral wall, as a raised serpentine mound
Optic nerve and artery	40%	Superolateral (chiasm is anterior to hypophysis in roof)
Maxillary nerve°	40%	Lateral wall
Vidian nerve and artery	36%	Floor
Nerves of superior orbital fissure	35%	Lateral wall
Sphenopalatine artery and ganglion	30%	Anterior floor
Mandibular nerve°	4%	Lateral wall

°Several of the above structures actually course through or lateral to the cavernous sinus, which lies between them and the sinus lumen on the lateral wall of the sphenoid sinus.

(Modified from Van Alyea, O. E. 1941. Sphenoid sinus, anatomic study, with consideration of the clinical significance of the structural characteristics of sphenoid sinus. Arch. Otolaryngol., *34*:225–253, and Van Alyea, O. E. 1951. Nasal Sinuses, An Anatomic and Clinical Consideration, 2nd ed. Baltimore, Williams & Wilkins Co.)

the skull, owing to their proximity to important vascular and neurologic structures, as listed in Table 23–2 (Fig. 23–22).

Van Alyea's studies (1941, 1951) were from observations on mature sinuses, which exhibit more advanced pneumatization than do those of children. The interior of the sinus lumen often exhibited elevated ridges or mounds, which indicated important underlying neurovascular structures, separated from the sinus by as little as 0.2 mm of bone. Occasionally, bone was even dehiscent (absent) in the adult specimens. More often in children, however, the bone is thicker, and there may be no landmarks on the interior sinus walls to suggest the position of such structures.

THE ETHMOID SINUSES

Growth and Development

The ethmoid air cells are evaginations of nasal mucosa from the middle, superior, and first supreme nasal meatuses. As dimple-like depressions, they are in evidence as early as the fourth fetal month. By the seventh fetal month, they are hollowed-out blind sacs with ostia into their respective meatuses.

Ethmoid cells grow relatively rapidly in the early years. At birth they are all present as widely separated, rounded epithelial recesses. During the second year they approach each other and alter their shape by mutual compression and become flattened laterally by the lamina papyracea. Growth is then directed upward toward the cribriform plate. There is little uniformity of development in what has been termed a "struggle for space." Even though one cell may have its origin inferior to another, it may outgrow its neighbor and force it to progress in a direction other than that in which it was primarily growing. But each cell will always communicate with the meatus from which it originated; cells from unlike meatuses never communicate with each other.

By the seventh year, the enlarged ethmoid cells begin to pneumatize all available space, extending into the turbinates and the frontal and sphenoid bones. Between the 12th and 14th years, they attain their final forms.

There is an early division of the ethmoid labyrinth into anterior and posterior groups. Anterior cells arise inferior to the attachment of the middle turbinate and posterior cells arise superior to it. The anterior ethmoid cells develop from three areas in the middle meatus (Fig. 23–3).

1. *Frontal recess.* The most ventral and cephalic of the anterior group develop from furrows on the lateral wall of the frontal recess. They vary in number; one or more may become frontal cells, or the group may be absent altogether. The agger nasi is commonly pneumatized by the most ventral of these cells.

2. *Infundibulum.* From the ventral end of the

ethmoid infundibulum grow the infundibular cells, which may number as many as seven but usually are not more than three. They variably pneumatize the agger nasi and the uncinate process and may grow sufficiently into the frontal bone to become frontal sinuses or frontal bullae. It should be recalled that the maxillary sinus ostium also drains into the infundibulum. This explains why suppurative disease may coexist in the frontal, maxillary, and infundibular ethmoid sinuses yet not involve the bullar and posterior ethmoid cells, which have separate ostia.

3. *Bullar furrows.* The ethmoid bulla, also termed the accessory concha, is hollowed out by cells originating in the furrows above and below it. Such bullar cells frequently also pneumatize the supraorbital plate of the frontal bone and the infraorbital plate of the maxilla. Their size greatly influences the width of the hiatus semilunaris and, therefore, the natural drainage channel of the maxillary sinus.

The posterior ethmoid cells gradually pneumatize and make the superior and supreme turbinates appear as shell-like structures. They may extend into the supraorbital plate of the frontal bone, the infraorbital plate of the maxilla, the middle nasal turbinate, and the orbital process of the palate.

Pneumatization of the ethmoid bulla is the most constant feature of ethmoid sinus development; it can be demonstrated in all anatomic dissections. Posterior ethmoid cells were found in 96 per cent of Van Alyea's (1951) specimens and pneumatization of the agger nasi in 89 per cent (Figs. 23–24 and 23–25).

Anomalies and Variations

By adulthood the ethmoid labyrinth is seldom entirely confined within the ethmoid bone. Even before puberty, significant encroachments into neighboring areas can be demonstrated. Particularly common are supraorbital extensions into the frontal bone (15 per cent of cases studied) and infraorbital extensions into the maxilla (11 per cent). An extension into the maxilla could be termed a supernumerary maxillary sinus, but, in fact, it is a posterior ethmoid cell with its natural ostium draining into the superior meatus.

Posterior ethmoid cells may encroach on the sphenoid sinus lumen (9 per cent) and may erode into the palate bone (the inappropriately named palatal sinus).

Anterior cells may crowd the lacrimal bone, encroach upon the frontal sinus lumen as frontal bullae (see Frontal Sinuses), and invade the middle turbinate (concha), hollowing it out and making it shell-like (Fig. 23–6). These conchal cells develop from either anterior or posterior ethmoid cells. They are

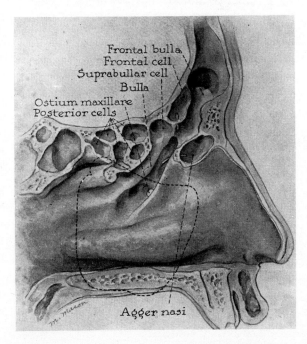

Figure 23–24 Ethmoid cells invading the frontal bone, encroaching upon the frontal sinus (frontal bulla). Note also the large cell in the agger nasi. (From Van Alyea, O. E., 1951. Nasal Sinuses, An Anatomic and Clinical Consideration, 2nd ed. Baltimore, Williams & Wilkins Co.)

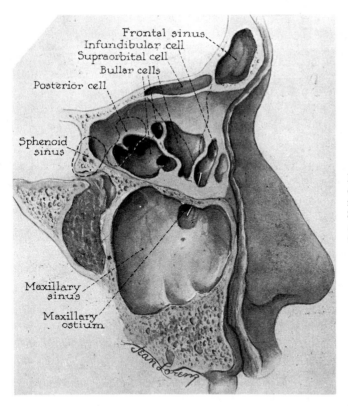

Frontal sinus
Infundibular cell
Supraorbital cell
Bullar cells
Posterior cell
Sphenoid sinus
Maxillary sinus
Maxillary ostium

Figure 23–25 Large bullar cells crowd other ethmoid cells. Note also the supraorbital ethmoid cell. (From Van Alyea, O. E., 1951. Nasal Sinuses, An Anatomic and Clinical Consideration, 2nd ed. Baltimore, Williams & Wilkins Co.)

quite common in adults (12 per cent of skulls dissected by Schaeffer, 1920). Although such extensions have been demonstrated in fetal and childhood specimens, their development is not pronounced until puberty or later. Other than their location, they do not differ from other ethmoid cells. However, their dependent position with respect to their ostia makes them disadvantageously placed for natural drainage; hence, they are frequently involved in suppurative disease. Their ostia may be located in either the superior or middle meatus (in approximately equal proportions) according to their origins.

Dehiscences (deficient osseous boundaries) occur frequently, particularly in the lamina papyracea (orbital plate) and occasionally in the floor of the anterior cranial fossa. Thus, ethmoid membrane may be contiguous with periorbitum and dura mater, respectively. Likewise, ethmoid membranes may be in actual contact with the lacrimal sac.

Anatomic Relationships and Surgical Hazards

The anatomic position of the ethmoidal field accounts for not only surgical hazards but also the hazard of extension of uncontrolled infection. The ethmoid sinus complex is a roughly pyramidal shaped mass, wide posteriorly, narrowed anteriorly, inconstantly contained within the following boundaries.

Superiorly: The fovea ethmoidalis is a plate of bone separating the floor of the anterior cranial fossa from the ethmoid complex. This plate descends in a posterior to inferior direction at an angle of 15 degrees from horizontal. Therefore, anterior ethmoid cells extend higher than posterior cells even when they do not encroach upon the frontal sinuses. The superior boundary of the most anterior cells is the floor of the frontal sinus.

Anteriorly: The lacrimal bone houses the lacrimal sac on its anterolateral surface and the agger nasi medially.

Inferiorly: The most medial aspect of the roof of the maxillary sinus is adjacent to the ethmoid sinus complex. The relationship is narrow anteriorly, but it widens posteriorly.

Laterally: The lamina papyracea (orbital plate or *os planum*) separates the orbit from the ethmoid complex. It articulates with the lacrimal bone anteriorly, the maxilla inferiorly, the frontal bone superiorly, and the lesser wing of the sphenoid posteriorly.

Medially: The nasal turbinates and meatuses form the lateral wall of the nose and medial boundaries of the sinuses.

Posteriorly: The posterior ethmoid cells share a common wall with the sphenoid sinuses anterolaterally.

It is common for ethmoid cells in their pneumatization to push their boundaries beyond the usual anatomic positions.

Separating the ethmoid field from the orbit is the lamina papyracea, which is, as its name implies, of paper-thin delicacy and which may even be dehiscent in places. The optic nerve at the optic foramen is separated from the most posterior and superior ethmoid cells by bone of only 2 to 5 mm thickness, and it may be seen prominently in 4 per cent of specimens (Dixon, 1959) (Fig. 23–26). Sometimes aggressive posterior ethmoid cells pneumatize the body and lesser wing of the sphenoid bone at the expense of the sphenoid sinus (ethmosphenoidal cell). Then the proximity of these cells to the optic nerve exists for much of its distance from the orbital foramen to the optic chiasm. The intervening bone may be of tissue paper thickness or it may be absent.

Such an ethmosphenoidal cell will replace the sphenoid as the superior and posterior boundary of the pterygomaxillary fossa with its neurovascular contents. A "supernumerary maxillary sinus," which is, in fact, an extended posterior ethmoid sinus, will replace the maxillary sinus as the anterior boundary of the same fossa.

Two small neurovascular bundles penetrate the lamina papyracea to supply the ethmoid complex: the anterior and posterior ethmoidal arteries and branches of the trigeminal nerve (Fig. 23–27). They will be encountered during an external surgical approach to the ethmoid. The anterior is the larger of the two arteries and may require ligation or application of a surgical clip to achieve hemostasis. The ligature should be placed on the orbital side of any anticipated division since arterial flow is from lateral to medial. The posterior branch should be the posterior limit of dissection, for it lies only a few millimeters in front of the optic nerve (3 to 8 mm in an adult). A line connecting these two foramina is on a parallel with and is just inferior to the floor of the anterior cranial fossa and the cribriform plate. The anterior and posterior ethmoidal arteries arise from

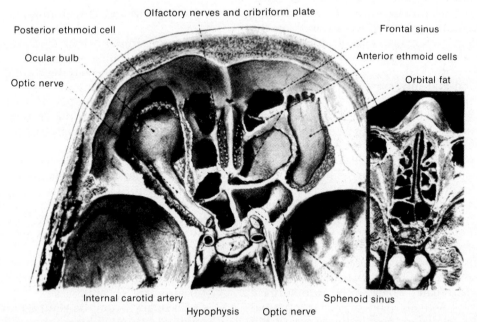

Figure 23–26   Exposure of the ethmoid and sphenoid sinuses, optic nerves and eyeballs by removal of the floor of the anterior cranial fossa. Note the right optic nerve in the sphenoid sinus, which extends above and below it. The left optic nerve bears a more common relationship to the posterior ethmoid and sphenoid sinuses. The insert is a transection of the ethmoid and sphenoid sinuses showing a larger number of ethmoid cells and the relationship of the optic nerve to the posterior ethmoid cells and sphenoid sinuses. (From Schaeffer, J. P., 1920. The Nose, Paranasal Sinuses, Nasolacrimal Passageways, and Olfactory Organ in Man. A Genetic, Developmental and Anatomico-Physiological Consideration. Philadelphia, Blakiston Co.)

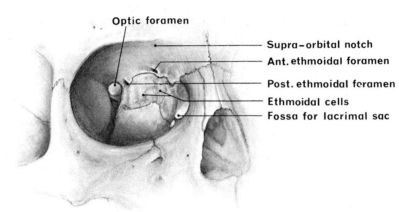

Optic foramen

Supra-orbital notch

Ant. ethmoidal foramen

Post. ethmoidal foramen

Ethmoidal cells

Fossa for lacrimal sac

Figure 23–27 Medial view of the orbit demonstrates foramina of the anterior and posterior ethmoid neurovascular bundles, which serve as surgical landmarks, indicating the proximity of the optic nerve and cribriform plate.

the ophthalmic artery as it courses along the medial wall of the orbit. Although the posterior branch passes directly into the ethmoid sinuses and nasal fossa, the anterior branch takes a more circuitous route. It courses through its foramen to enter the anterior cranial fossa. It then passes forward on top of the cribriform plate to a slit-like foramen at the side of the crista galli where it enters the nasal fossa. It descends on the interior lateral nasal wall and finally exits between the nasal bone and the lateral cartilage to reach the tip of the nose. Coursing with the arteries are corresponding ethmoidal veins that communicate freely with the dural veins, including the superior saggital sinus, as well as the ophthalmic vein, which empties into the cavernous sinus. These pathways afford easy extension of nasal and sinus infection into periorbital and intracranial areas (Fairbanks et al., 1975).

During ethmoid surgery the cribriform plate is at a risk. Damage to it not only jeopardizes the olfactory sense but also can cause cerebrospinal fluid leakage and intracranial spread of infection. The cribriform plate actually lies lower than the roof of the ethmoid labyrinth. In fact, in 70 per cent of specimens it lies 4 to 7 mm below the level of the orbital roof.

To avoid injury to the cribriform plate, surgeons are usually admonished to dissect no further medially than the origin of the middle turbinate, which is the safe surgical landmark. Actually, the posterior ethmoid cells arise medial to the middle turbinate, but they are lateral to the origin of the superior turbinate, which becomes the landmark in the deeper recesses of the nasal cavity.

The external ethmoidectomy carries an added risk of disrupting the attachment of the medial canthal ligament of the orbit,

which leads to unilateral widening of the intercanthal distance. However, since surgical exposure is limited in children and since the surgical hazard to the optic nerve is so great with poor exposure, the external approach is most widely recommended in children. Furthermore, the usual indication for ethmoidectomy in children is orbital cellulitis or abscess, which requires an external approach in any instance.

THE FRONTAL SINUSES

Growth and Development

The frontal sinuses originate as outgrowths of the ventral cephalic ends of the middle meatuses in an area termed the frontal recess. This area, operculated by the middle turbinate, is identifiable in the late third to early fourth fetal month. Both the frontal sinuses and the anterior ethmoid cells develop in this area.

By the time of birth, the area has developed only to the stage of pits or furrows in that recess (Fig. 23–28). It is from one or more of these furrows that the sinuses will develop. They develop variously:

1. By direct extension of the whole frontal recess (Fig. 23–3).
2. From one or more of the anterior ethmoid cells, which originate in the frontal furrows (Fig. 23–29).
3. Occasionally, from the ventral end of the ethmoid infundibulum.

In the first instance there will be no true nasal duct but instead a wide communication with the nose anterior and superior to the hiatus semilunaris. This is the most common finding. In the latter two instances a frontal duct will develop, the tortuosity of which will de-

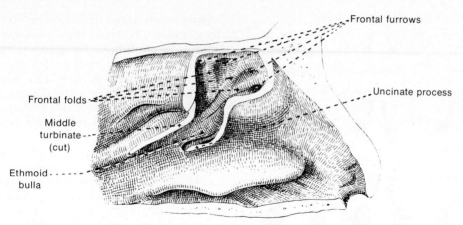

Figure 23-28 Lateral nasal wall of a term fetus. The middle turbinate has been removed, which exposes the accessory folds and furrows of the frontal recess. (From Schaeffer, J. P., 1920. The Nose, Paranasal Sinuses, Nasolacrimal Passageways, and Olfactory Organ in Man. A Genetic, Developmental and Anatomico-Physiological Consideration. Philadelphia, Blakiston Co.)

pend on the cell from which the sinus originated and the degree of development and disposition of neighboring ethmoid cells. Furthermore, the relationship of that duct to the ethmoid infundibulum may be so intimate that drainage from the duct could find its way into the infundibulum and from there through the maxillary ostium into the maxillary sinus (Fig. 23–24). This may explain the old clinical dictum that the maxillary sinus is a cesspool for frontal sinus drainage. Anatomically, however, that should be the case in less than 50 per cent of cases.

At birth, the frontal sinuses still may not be demonstrable. Although the rudiments are advanced, they are not topically frontal. The appearance of the frontal sinus is not certain until the sixth to 12th postfetal month. By the 20th month the frontal sinus has eroded into and begun to ascend the vertical portion of the frontal bone. By the middle of the third year the cupola of the sinus is visible above the level of the nasion, and by the eighth year at least one frontal sinus reaches the level of the orbital roof in 50 per cent of subjects (Maresh, 1940). The sinus grows vertically at an average rate of 1.5 mm per year (Davis, 1918), more slowly in early years and more rapidly after the seventh or eighth year (Fig. 23–30). It reaches its mature size during puberty and thereafter grows a small amount into old age.

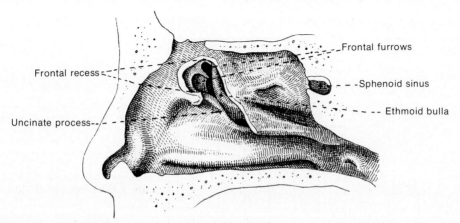

Figure 23-29 The frontal recess of a 5 month old child. Note the pouching of the frontal furrows and the frontal recess in the formation of the anterior ethmoidal cells and the frontal sinus. The sphenoid sinus is also well established. (From Schaeffer, J. P., 1920. The Nose, Paranasal Sinuses, Nasolacrimal Passageways, and Olfactory Organ in Man. A Genetic, Developmental and Anatomico-Physiological Consideration. Philadelphia, Blakiston Co.)

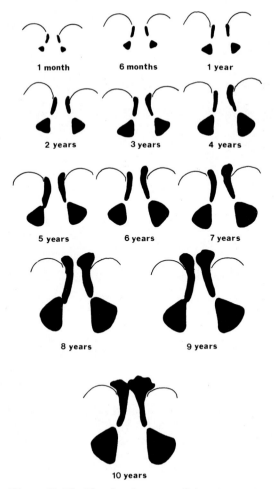

Figure 23–30 The development of the sinuses in a series of radiographs of one child over a 10 year period. (From Maresh, M. M., 1940. Paranasal sinuses from birth to late adolescence. Am. J. Dis. Child., 60:58–75.)

Anatomists agree that there is no constant or so-called "normal" type anatomy of the sinuses. According to Schaeffer (1920), "adherence to a single fixed and arbitrary normal is fraught with danger since with variations come altered size, altered shape, altered anatomic relations." Maresh's longitudinal radiographic study of 100 children demonstrates this variability in Figures 23–31 and 23–32; he noted that growth proceeds at an irregular pace. In many instances, a cell would begin to bud upward and after reaching a point above the nasion would fail to increase for several years. Later it would increase in size again very rapidly and either equal the size of the other frontal sinus or even become larger in a comparatively short time.

Early vertical invasion is nearer the inner plate of the frontal bone than the outer. This leads to a thin inner plate of almost entirely compact bone as opposed to the thick outer (anterior) wall of both compact and cancellous bone. Invasion is, from the outset, variable and asymmetrical. The intersinus septum is midline only at its base. Although it becomes paper-thin, it is not normally perforated.

Anomalies and Variations

In many instances the frontal sinus never invades far into the vertical portion but grows extensively into the horizontal portion of the frontal bone, forming large air spaces over the orbits. This leads to the erroneous belief that there is frequently an agenesis of the

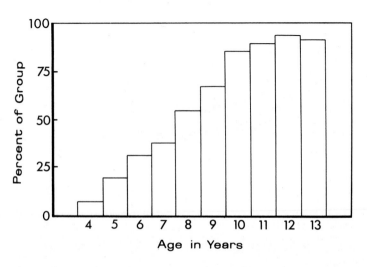

Figure 23–31 Percentage of children who had one or both frontal sinuses at the level of or above the orbital roof in the radiographs made at the indicated ages. (From Maresh, M. M., 1940. Paranasal sinuses from birth to late adolescence. Am. J. Dis. Child., 60:58–75.)

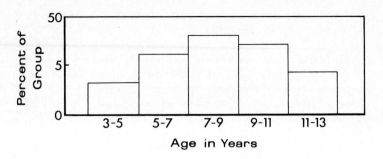

Figure 23–32 Time of appearance of frontal sinuses above the orbital roofs as shown by radiographs taken at the age intervals indicated, when one or both frontal sinuses first reached the level of the orbital roof. (From Maresh, M. M., 1940. Paranasal sinuses from birth to late adolescence. Am. J. Dis. Child., 60:58–75.)

frontal sinus. True bilateral agenesis occurs in no more than 4 per cent of skulls, but unilateral absence is seen in 11 per cent (Dixon, 1959). In as many as 30 per cent of skulls, the frontal sinuses are considered to be underdeveloped or hypoplastic (Maresh, 1940).

Supernumerary frontal sinuses are common in both the horizontal and the vertical portions of the frontal bone. They can be placed side by side or one posterior to the other, a confusing situation for the surgeon. Schaeffer (1920) has described as many as six frontal sinuses in one skull, two on one side and four on the other. Each sinus is normally independent of another (developed from a different furrow) and has its own ostium of communication with the anterior middle meatus.

Not infrequently an anterior ethmoid cell encroaches upon the frontal sinus floor, pushing it upwards, balloon-like, into the sinus lumen. This is called a frontal bulla (Figs. 23–24 and 23–33). At times, several such cells will arrange themselves, tier-like, in the floor of the frontal sinus. Bullae may be so prominent and so located that the usual trephine operation could enter a bulla instead of the frontal sinus.

Asymmetry between right and left frontal sinuses is the rule rather than the exception, and asymmetry of the intersinus septum may be so exaggerated that one frontal sinus overlies the other, the latter appearing as a bulla. Extensive pneumatization of the sinus is described as far laterally as the temporal bones and into the nasal bones, but this condition occurs in adulthood.

Figure 23–33 Invasion of the horizontal portion of the frontal bone by both frontal and ethmoid air cells. Note supraorbital extension of frontal sinus and bulge in its floor by ethmoid cell. (From Van Alyea, O. E., 1951. Nasal Sinuses, An Anatomic and Clinical Consideration, 2nd ed. Baltimore, Williams, & Wilkins Co.)

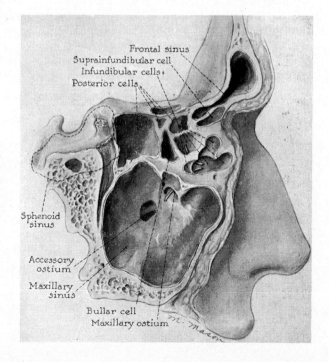

Anatomic Relationships and Surgical Hazards

Only the thin layer of compact bone of the inner (posterior) table of the frontal sinus separates it from the dura mater and frontal lobe of the brain. The floor of the sinus overlies the orbit and some of the anterior ethmoid cells (Fig. 23–33). If the horizontal portion of the frontal bone has been extensively pneumatized, the sinus can overlie posterior ethmoid cells as well. Posteromedially a mound may be seen that overlies the olfactory area. Infection spreads readily from the frontal sinuses to the orbit and intracranial space, either by osteitis of their common walls or through the thrombophlebitic intercommunications. The proximity of these structures to the frontal sinus should be considered during surgery to avoid entering and spreading disease into uninvolved areas.

In the diseased state, especially when a mucocele is present, any of the bony walls may be eroded (Fairbanks et al., 1975). However, dura and periorbita are usually recognizable if the surgical exposure is wide enough. When the sinuses are extremely small, finding the lumen may represent the greatest challenge of the surgical procedure. Preoperative tomography is helpful.

The supraorbital and supratrochlear nerves and vessels, branches of the ophthalmic nerve and artery, exit the orbit superficial to the periosteum of the supraorbital ridge. If a brow incision requires penetration of the periosteum and is carried as far laterally as the supraorbital notch, numbness and paresthesia of the forehead will result.

REFERENCES

Cottle, M. H. 1951. Nasal surgery in children. E.E.N.T. Monthly, 30:32–38.

Davis, W. B. 1918. Anatomy of the nasal accessory sinuses in infancy and childhood. Ann. Otol., Rhinol. Laryngol., 27:940–967.

Dion, M. C., Jafek, B. W., and Tobin, C. E. 1978. The anatomy of the nose, external support. Arch. Otolaryngol., 104:145–150.

Dixon, F. W. 1959. Clinical significance of anatomical arrangement of paranasal sinuses. Ann. Otol. Rhinol. Laryngol., 67:736–741.

Enlow, D. H. 1978. Handbook of Facial Growth. Philadelphia, W. B. Saunders Co.

Fairbanks, D. N. F., and Chen, S. C. A. 1970. Closure of large nasal septum perforations. Arch. Otolaryngol., 91:403–406.

Fairbanks, D. N. F., Vanderveen, T. S., and Bordley, J. E. 1975. Intracranial complications of sinusitis. In Maloney, W. H. (Ed.) Otolaryngology, Vol. III. Hagerstown, Md., Harper & Row, Chap. 19.

Farrior, R. T., and Connolly, M. E. 1970. Septorhinoplasty in Children. Otolaryngol. Clin. North Am., 3:345–364.

Gilbert, J. G., and Segal, S. 1958. Growth of the nose and the septorhinoplastic problems in youth. Arch. Otolaryngol., 68:673–682.

Gray, L. P. 1978. Deviated nasal septum, incidence and etiology. Ann. Otol. Rhinol. Laryngol., 87, Suppl. 50.

Hammer, G., and Radberg, C. 1961. Sphenoidal sinus: Anatomical and roentgenologic study with reference to transsphenoid hypophysectomy. Acta Radiol., 56:401–422.

Hinck, V. C., and Hopkins, C. E. 1965. Concerning growth of the sphenoid sinus. Arch. Otolaryngol., 82:62–66.

Kirchner, J. A. 1955. Traumatic nasal deformity in the newborn. Arch. Otolaryngol., 62:139–142.

Maresh, M. M. 1940. Paranasal sinuses from birth to late adolescence. Am. J. Dis. Child., 60:58–75.

Moore, K. L. 1973. The Developing Human. Philadelphia, W. B. Saunders Co., pp. 150–151.

Moore, W. J., and Lavelle, C. L. 1974. Growth of the Facial Skeleton in the Hominoidea. London, Academic Press, Inc.

Pratt, L. W. 1965. Midline cysts of the nasal dorsum: Embryologic origin and treatment. Laryngoscope, 75:968–980.

Reichert, H. 1963. Plastic Surgery of the nose in children. Plast. Reconstr. Surg., 31:51–54.

Ritter, F. N. 1973. The Paranasal Sinuses: Anatomy and Surgical Technique. St. Louis, The C.V. Mosby Co.

Schaeffer, J. P. 1920. The Nose, Paranasal Sinuses, Nasolacrimal Passageways, and Olfactory Organ in Man. A Genetic, Developmental and Anatomico-Physiological Consideration. Philadelphia, Blakiston Co.

Scott, J. H. 1953. The cartilage of the nasal septum. Brit. Dent. J., 95:37–43.

Van Alyea, O. E. 1941. Sphenoid sinus, anatomic study, with consideration of the clinical significance of the structural characteristics of sphenoid sinus. Arch. Otolaryngol., 34:225–253.

Van Alyea, O. E. 1951. Nasal Sinuses, An Anatomic and Clinical Consideration, 2nd ed. Baltimore, Williams & Wilkins Co.

Vidic, B. 1968. The postnatal development of the sphenoidal sinus and its spread into the dorsum sellae and posterior clinoid processes. Am. J. Roentgenol., 104:177–183.

Zimmerman, A. A. 1938. Development of the paranasal sinuses. Arch. Otolaryngol., 27:793–795.

Chapter 24

PHYSIOLOGY

Kenneth Grundfast, M.D.

The nose is a mucosa-lined space through which inspired and expired air passes, and it is the sense organ for olfaction.

It is important to realize that the nose is not merely a hollow conduit through which air passes. While passing through the nose, air from the ambient environment is altered and made suitable for entrance into the bronchi and lungs. The shape of the nasal turbinates causes the formation of airstreams within the nose. The richly vascular nasal mucous membrane is capable of rapidly cleansing, warming, and humidifying inspired air. Also, the nasal mucous membrane is capable of initiating a localized immune response to inhaled antigens or pathogens. The nose interacts with the lungs via neural reflexes and provides a certain resistance to airflow that is necessary for normal lung function.

An understanding of nasal and paranasal sinus function is based upon knowledge of functional anatomy and a familiarity with relevant physiologic mechanisms.

FUNCTIONAL ANATOMY

Structures and Spatial Relationships

The *anterior nares* are the skin-lined portions of the nose between the nostrils and the ciliated mucosa at the anterior ends of the nasal septum and turbinates. The cross-sectional diameter at the anterior nares is the smallest in the respiratory tract. The *intranasal cavity,* divided in the midline by the septum, extends posteriorly from the nares to the choanae. The lateral walls of the nose are formed by the turbinates and corresponding meatuses. The inferior turbinate, or concha, is a separate bone, whereas the middle and superior turbinates (conchae) are portions

of the ethmoid bone. Posterior to the middle turbinate is the sphenopalatine foramen, through which vessels and nerves pass into the pterygopalatine fossa.

Ostia from the maxillary, frontal, anterior, and middle ethmoid sinuses are located in the middle meatus. Secretions from the posterior ethmoid sinus cells empty into the superior meatus, and secretions from the sphenoid sinus empty into the portion of the nose known as the *sphenoethmoidal recess.*

The turbinates and septum occupy significant space so that the room for air to pass through the nose is relatively small in comparison to the transverse width of the nose. The nasal airway undergoes significant change in shape in early infancy (Livingstone, 1932), but by the age of approximately one year, the shape of a child's nose is similar to the shape seen in adults (Negus, 1958).

Histology and Microanatomy

The *mucous membrane* is composed of tall columnar ciliated cells and basal cells lying on a basement membrane. The basement membrane varies in thickness. Capillary loops extend through the basement membrane in certain areas. The stroma contains mucous and serous glands with ducts extending to the surface. Interstitial cells that are present include eosinophils, mast cells, polymorphonuclear leukocytes, plasma cells, and lymphocytes. Aggregations of lymphocytes can be dense enough to form lymphoid nodules.

Cilia are long, thin, hair-like mobile organelles that project from the luminal surface of some columnar epithelial cells. The cilia (Fig. 24–1) in the human nose are approximately 0.7 mm long and 0.3 mm thick, and they are composed of sheaves of microtubules (My-

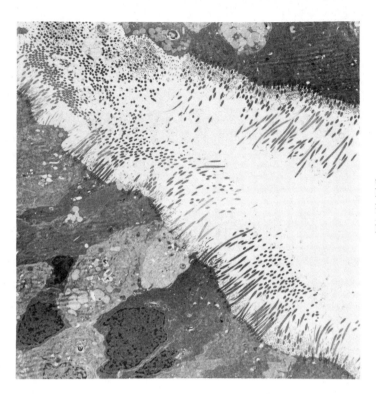

Figure 24–1 Ciliated columnar epithelial cells are seen in this biopsy of human nasal mucosa (× 2800). (Electron micrograph courtesy of the Pathology Department, Children's Hospital of Pittsburgh.)

gind, 1978). The number of cilia on the surface of the columnar cells in the nose varies. Biopsies from the anterior part of the nose reveal only single islands of cilia covering about 10 per cent of each cell's surface, whereas the surface of the cells located more posteriorly in the nose is virtually covered by cilia (Mygind and Bretlau, 1974). The cilia bend and move as the coaxial microtubules slide past one another. The energy that

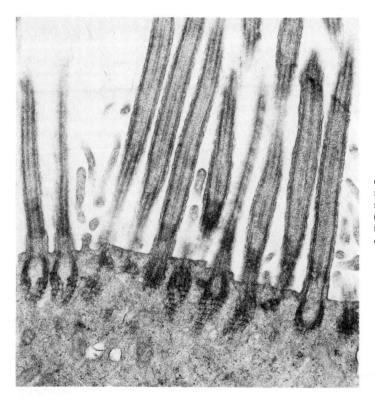

Figure 24–2 Longitudinal profiles of cilia showing central and peripheral microtubules and basal bodies with striated roots. Human nasal mucosa (× 28,000). (Electron micrograph courtesy of the Pathology Department, Children's Hospital of Pittsburgh.)

Figure 24–3 *A*, Cross-sectional profile of cilium with the normal axonemal configuration: 9 + 2 microtubular arrangement, dynein arms (responsible for ciliary motion — arrowheads), and radial spokes (arrow). Human nasal mucosa (× 215,000). *B*, Cross-sectional profiles of cilia from patient with Kartagener syndrome. Dynein arms are lacking on the outer microtubular doublets. Absence of dynein arms is found in patients with immotile cilia syndrome, which includes Kartagener syndrome. A few doublets have short spurs in the position of the dynein arms (arrows). Human nasal mucosa (× 215,000). (Electron micrographs courtesy of the Pathology Department, Children's Hospital of Pittsburgh.)

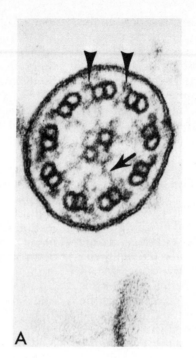
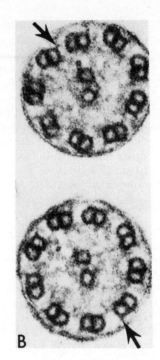

A

B

powers the movement of the cilia comes from adenosine triphosphate (ATP) produced in mitochondria at the base of the cilium. In most areas of the nose, cilia move surface secretions backward toward the nasopharynx, but the cilia in a small area at the anterior end of the inferior turbinates carry material forward to the anterior nose, where it can be removed from the body by nose blowing or wiping. The cilia beat in a wave-like motion that has two components, a quick, straight-armed, "effective" motion that propels surface mucus, and a "curling" recovery stroke that is a slower motion opposite to the direction of mucous flow. The cilia stroke about 600 to 1500 times per minute (Huizing, 1967). Ciliary motion can be affected by changes in moisture content, pH, temperature, and the presence of topically applied drugs.

The *tubuloalveolar gland system* produces mucoprotein and mucopolysaccharide that flow onto the epithelial surface via large ducts. Even some of the cells lining the large ducts have secretory activity so that the composition of secretions emanating from the gland system can be modified as the secretion flows toward the mucosal surface.

Goblet cells present in the epithelium are another source of mucus. Mucus produced by the goblet cells has a sulfate radical attached as a side chain of the mucopolysaccharide molecule, whereas the mucus produced by the tubuloalveolar system is nonsulfated. As a result, the mucous sheet on the surface of the epithelium is composed of both sulfated and nonsulfated mucopolysaccharides and mucoprotein, the density of which may be altered by changes in the rate of secretion of the component cell systems or by dilution with transudate directly from the capillary bed (Taylor, 1980).

Microvilli are finger-like expansions of cytoplasm that significantly increase the surface area of the epithelial cells. All columnar epithelial cells, ciliated and nonciliated, are covered by 300 to 400 microvilli (Mygind, 1978). The presence of the microvilli enhances the ability of each cell to transport substances and water between the intracellular space and the nasal fluid, thus providing a mechanism for maintaining proper moisture on the epithelial surface. As a lawn holds dew more than a paved road, so microvilli-covered cells maintain surface moisture better than plain squamous epithelial cells (Mygind, 1978).

The *basement membrane* is permeable not only to fluids but also to particulate matter trapped within the surface mucus (Munzel, 1972). There is a difference between the basement membrane in the nose and basement membranes located elsewhere in the body. By definition, basement membranes are periodic acid-Schiff (PAS)–positive, except in the nose, where the basement membrane has a negative PAS reaction at birth and during early infancy. Possibly, the sulfated mucopolysaccharides migrating through the basement membrane are responsible for the PAS-positive reaction. As sulfated mucopolysaccharide molecules remain within the mesh of reticulin composing the basement membrane, the basement becomes more PAS-positive. There is some evidence that sulfation and migration of mucopolysaccharides across the basement membrane are associated with estrogen activity and carbohydrate metabolism. Therefore, the production of nasal secretions may, at least partially, be controlled by normonal and metabolic factors.

The nasal epithelium in children with chronic mucopurulent nasal discharge contains large amounts of the enzyme succinic dehydrogenase, whereas infected epithelia elsewhere in the body show no increase in succinic dehydrogenase. The presence of this enzyme indicates a *localized increase* in the level of the metabolic activity. The increased metabolic activity is associated with increased numbers of goblet cells in the epithelium. These goblet cells synthesize their sulfated mucus from components that migrate through the basement membrane. The fact that these components are PAS-positive accounts for the marked PAS-positive reaction seen in the nasal basement in children with chronic nasal discharge. Thus, it seems that the nasal mucous membrane is capable of manifesting a localized cellular response to environmental stimuli mediated by metabolic pathways.

Blood Supply and Nerve Supply

Blood vessels supplying the mucous membrane are most numerous in the anterior region of the nose. The arterioles of the nasal respiratory mucosa lack an internal elastic membrane, and the vascular endothelial basement membrane is continuous with the basement membrane of smooth muscle cells in the wall of the arteriole (Mygind, 1978). As a result, the subendothelial musculature of these vessels may be influenced more readily than other vessels by pharmacologic agents such as histamine or systemically administered vasoconstrictors.

Small, regular capillaries are located in the lamina propria. The capillaries below the surface epithelium are larger and have *fenestrations*. The fenestrae are small areas in the endothelial lining where the endothelial cell consists of only a thin single membrane. This membrane and the porous basement membrane, reinforced by pericytes, constitute the only barrier between blood plasma and tissue fluid, thus providing for rapid passage of fluid throughout the vascular wall.

Veins within the nose form a cavernous plexus underneath the mucous membrane. The plexus is especially well developed over the middle and inferior turbinates and the lower portion of the septum. Venous drainage is principally through the ophthalmic, anterior facial, and sphenopalatine veins. The venous systems of the nose, paranasal sinuses, and orbit communicate freely through valveless veins. Therefore, venous stasis related to nasal congestion can cause dark circles or discoloration beneath the eyes known as "allergic shiners."

In some areas of the nose, cavernous sinusoids are interposed between the capillaries and venules. These cavernous sinusoids can be regarded as specialized capillaries that enable the nasal mucosa to adapt its thickness and temperature to varying environmental factors.

Nerve supply to the nose is complex. The olfactory mucosa, located high in the nose, is characterized by the presence of "special sense" receptor nerve cells with central processes that unite to form the small nerve fiber bundles that pass through the cribriform plate to enter the brain. These nerves constitute the neuronal pathway for olfactory sensation. The anterior and posterior ethmoid nerves, branches of the ophthalmic division of the trigeminal nerve, supply pain, temperature, and touch sensations to the mucous membrane on the lateral wall of the nose anterior to the turbinates and meatus and the corresponding area of the septum. Nasal branches of the sphenopalatine ganglion containing fibers of the maxillary division of the trigeminal nerve supply pain, temperature, and touch sensation to most of the rest of the nasal mucosa. Parasympathetic supply originates in the facial nerve, where preganglionic fibers course to the sphenopalatine ganglion. The postsynaptic parasympathetic fibers enter all branches of the sphenopalatine ganglion and are distributed to the glandular epithelium within the nose. It is stimulation of the fibers that results in secretion from the glands in the nasal mucosa. Sympathetic fibers course through the sphenopalatine ganglion without synapsing. Stimulation of the sympathetic fibers causes vasoconstriction of blood vessels supplying the nasal mucosa.

The subepithelial cavernous sinusoids are kept partially constricted by continuous sympathetic stimulation. As the sinusoids account for a large part of nasal blood volume in the turbinates, autonomic regulation can rapidly cause considerable change in the thickness of the nasal mucosa, and, in turn, autonomic regulation can affect the degree of nasal patency (Mygind, 1978).

Both the secretory and contractile myoepithelial elements of the human nasal glands are under parasympathetic control, in contrast to the dual autonomic control of salivary gland secretion. However, since the secretion of glands depends upon their blood supply, secretion of the nasal glands is indirectly affected by sympathetic stimulation mediated through the innervation of blood vessels within the nose. The sympathetic innervation maintains a tonic vasoconstrictor action. Stimulation of the sympathetic supply results in additional vasoconstriction.

Autonomic innervation plays an important role in the function of nasal mucous membranes. As the autonomic regulation of blood flow in the arterioles and cavernous spaces varies, the temperature and thickness of the mucosa change.

PHYSIOLOGIC MECHANISMS

Although the nose is usually not considered to be a complex organ, it plays an important role in respiratory function, and several rather complicated processes take place in the nose. Inspired air is filtered, changed in temperature, and humidified. The nose contains the special sensory receptors for olfaction. Immunologic protective reactions and hypersensitivity (allergic) reactions occur within the nose. An understanding of nasal function depends upon familiarity with several important physiologic mechanisms.

Aerodynamic Factors

Nasal valve. As air passes through the nose both with inspiration and expiration, a stream of air is formed. Approximately 1.5 to 2.5 cm posterior to the nostril, the airstream converges to pass through an area with a relatively narrow cross-sectional diameter known as the "nasal valve" or the "liminal valve" (Proctor, 1977). With deep inspiration, the upper lateral cartilages are sucked toward

the septum, and the aperture through which air enters the nose is narrowed. If the upper and lower lateral cartilages are excessively weak for any reason, then the cartilaginous "valve" will collapse when a relatively small amount of negative intranasal pressure develops. If the weak area is limited to the upper lateral cartilages, the central portion of the nose assumes a pinched appearance, while weakness in both the upper and lower lateral cartilages may lead to intermittent collapse of the soft tissue walls of the nose, and the nostrils may assume a narrowed, slit-like shape. Thus, there is a definite relationship between the position of the alar cartilages relative to the nasal septum and inspiratory effort. The greater the negative pressure required to produce collapse in the "valve" region of the nose, the greater is the airflow. More simply, the wider the aperture and the stiffer the cartilages in the valve area, the greater is the amount of air that can flow through the nose per unit of time. Although they are not anatomically distinct, there are two other areas of the nose termed "valve" areas — one in the area between the nasal septum and the anterior part of the inferior turbinate and the other in the region where erectile tissue comprises the mucosa covering the septum.

The liminal valve is the most important segment for the regulation of air inflow (Bridger and Proctor, 1970). It affects the direction, volume, and velocity of the current of inspired air. As the liminal valve retards the inflow of air, adequate time is provided for the nose to condition the air that passes posterior to the valve region. Deformities of the nasal septum, the alae, or both can cause severe obstruction when deformity involves any of the nasal valve areas.

Airstream. After passing the valve area, the airstream bends at an angle of 60 to 130 degrees from its initial direction to pass mostly along the middle meatus and somewhat along the floor of the nose (Proctor, 1977). As the air passes through constricted areas in the nose, velocity of the airstream changes. There is an increase in linear velocity as the inspired airstream passes through the valve region and a decrease in velocity when the airstream enters the larger area of the nose posterior to the valve, then another decrease in velocity when the air enters the nasopharynx. As air is inspired, only a small portion of the airstream enters the deeper recesses of the meatuses or the area cephalad to the middle turbinate. At very low flow rates, air moves in streamlines through the nose, but at peak flow in quiet breathing, some turbulence develops (Olariu and Teodorescu, 1973). After air enters the nasopharynx, it moves in a straight line into the pharynx, larynx, and trachea unless there is obstruction from enlarged adenoids or tonsils.

Airflow Resistance

As air passes through the nose, certain factors impede the flow of air. Collectively, the impeding factors are referred to as "resistance." The resistance provided by anatomic structures in the nose, pharynx, and larynx keeps sufficient air in the alveoli to enable absorption of oxygen from the air during respiration. Nasal airflow resistance during inspiration helps to maintain the negative intrathoracic pressure that is necessary for proper cardiopulmonary function.

The nose accounts for approximately one half of the total respiratory resistance to airflow (Proctor, 1977). When nasal mucosa is markedly congested, resistance to airflow increases. The degree of nasal vascular congestion varies with changes in ambient temperature and body position. When the ambient temperature is lower than 7 degrees C, significant nasal congestion with an increase in airflow resistance can occur (Drettner, 1961). Changes in body position alter resistance through hydrostatic effects on the vasculature. Change from a standing to a sitting position and change from a sitting to a recumbent position increase nasal airflow resistance (Rao and Potdar, 1970). When lying in a lateral position, the downside nasal passage is more congested. In infants, the pulmonary resistance varies inversely with nasal resistance (Lacourt and Polgar, 1971). Yet, maintaining adequate pulmonary resistance is important, especially in infants. Apparently, the efficiency of pulmonary function is reduced when there is a significant decrease in nasal airway resistance (O'Neil, 1959).

Nasal cycle. Most people are aware of the fact that patency of one side of the nose varies in relation to patency of the other side. There is some evidence that this fluctuation occurs in regular cycles (Stocksted, 1952). Each phase of this cycle may last from 50 minutes to four hours; however, studies have shown that a normal adult male will breathe mainly through one nostril for three hours while the mucous membrane of the other is slightly

engorged, and then the relative engorgement occurs on the opposite side of the nose (Taylor, 1980). This cycle is controlled by the autonomic nervous system. Sympathetic stimulation causes vasoconstriction with shrinkage of the turbinates, while the parasympathetic system mediates swelling of the turbinates.

Interrelationship with pulmonary function. Increased resistance to airflow through the nose may be associated with decreased pulmonary alveolar ventilation and resultant hypoxia (Ogura and Harvey, 1971). Experimental studies reveal that dogs forced to breathe through the mouth develop a decrease in the Po_2 of arterial blood (Ohnishi et al., 1972). This experimental finding may explain the observation that some children who are mouthbreathers have a disturbance of acid-base balance in which their blood alkali reserve is reduced, with a corresponding increase in pH (Taylor, 1980). If there is significant prolonged obstruction of the upper airway, cor pulmonale can develop. In some children with obstructive hypertrophy of the tonsils and adenoids, hypoxia, hypercarbia, and respiratory acidosis may lead to pulmonary vascular constriction, causing increased pulmonary vascular resistance and pulmonary artery hypertension (Levy et al., 1967; Luke et al., 1966). This hypertension increases the work of the right ventricle and leads to hypertrophy of the cardiac muscle and eventual heart failure.

Nasal airflow in the newborn. It is generally recognized that the newborn infant breathes exclusively through the nose. Although the exact reason for obligate nose-breathing in the newborn is not known, the high cephalad position of the larynx and trachea with close apposition of the soft palate to the tongue and epiglottis may make mouthbreathing more difficult than nose-breathing. Experiments on sleeping infants encased in a whole body plethysmograph revealed a marked decrease in tidal volume when an infant's pharynx was obstructed (Taylor, 1980). Despite the decreased tidal volume, some infants were not aroused from sleep.

Nasal airway resistance is much higher in infancy and early childhood than in adult life. Infants also tend to maintain a constant pulmonary resistance that is related via reflexes to nasal airflow. This may have special significance for the newborn, who breathes only through the nose. Should severe nasal obstruction occur, respiratory distress can develop, and even death may follow. Although nasal obstruction *per se* has not been shown to be the cause of sudden infant death syndrome, one study demonstrated distinct obstruction of the nose by mucosal swelling, secretions, or both in every infant examined after death that had been attributed to sudden infant death syndrome (Lacourt and Polgar, 1971).

NEUROENDOCRINE CONTROL

Vasomotor reaction. The term "vasomotor reaction" refers to the complex response of the nasal mucous membrane to various nonallergic stimuli. It is characterized by swelling of the nasal mucous membrane, which results in increased nasal obstruction, increased secretions, and sometimes sneezing. The nervous system receives information regarding changes in the internal and external environment via sense organs; then adjustments of these changes are brought about through effector mechanisms that include not only direct neuronal stimulation but also changes in the rate at which hormones are secreted (Taylor, 1980). The response of the nasal mucosa to various stimuli is an integrative action involving neuroendocrine control.

Any vasodilator drug can induce a vasomotor reaction. With intranasal bacterial infections, vasodilators are released, and the intermediate metabolites of many viral infections have much the same effect. In allergic individuals, the intranasal antigen-antibody reaction results in the localized release of such powerful vasodilators as histamine, serotonin, and various slow-reacting substances. The most important vasodilator substance, however, under both normal and pathologic conditions, is acetylcholine, which is produced at the parasympathetic nerve endings (Taylor, 1980). Acetylcholine and the substance that rapidly destroys it at nerve endings, acetylcholinesterase, are controlled by the hypothalamus. Thus, emotional factors and hormonal factors may influence the vasomotor reaction.

Mucociliary Flow

Mucous blanket. The term "mucous blanket" is used to describe the all-important thin layer of mucus that constantly covers the nasal mucous membrane. The composition of the mucus is approximately 96 per cent water, 1 per cent inorganic salts, and 2.5 to 3 per cent mucin (Taylor, 1980). Small changes in the content of the mucin produce significant changes in the viscosity of the mucus. The so-called "mucous blanket" consists of an outer layer of viscous mucus resting on a thin layer of serous fluid. Since the cilia of the columnar epithelial cells lining the nose extend into the thin layer of serous fluid, motion of the cilia effectively moves the layer of more viscid fluid, the mucus, that rests on the layer of serous fluid. Thus, there is a layer of mucus covering the lining of the nose like a "blanket," and the ciliated epithelial cells are constantly propelling the mucus in a posterior direction toward the nasopharynx, where the mucus leaves the nose and is swallowed.

Rate of mucociliary flow. In terms of the rate of flow of mucus along the epithelial surface of the nose, normal individuals fall into the following three main groups: (1) smooth mucociliary flow at an average rate of 0.84 cm per min; (2) jerky, interrupted flow at an average rate of 0.3 cm per min; (3) slower than 0.3 cm per min (Bang et al., 1967; Proctor et al., 1973). Thus, the normal nose has a rapidly moving stream of mucus capable of entrapping foreign particles and removing them from the airstream before air reaches the lungs. If the flow of mucus is not sufficiently rapid, then *mucostasis* occurs, and bacteria or pollen may remain on the surface of a cell long enough to penetrate the cell body rather than being transported toward the pharynx. When parasympathetic activity is increased, as in the vasomotor reaction, the rate of mucous flow increases.

IMMUNOLOGIC REACTIONS

Particulate matter filtered from inspired air may be organic or inorganic allergenic particles. In addition, bacteria, viruses, dust, fumes, or other foreign bodies may be removed from air and deposited in the mucous blanket. Some of these substances remain within the mucous layer and are quickly removed from the nose, whereas others penetrate the mucosal layer and react with submucosal structures. The type of reaction that occurs once a substance reaches the submucosal structures is variable. There may be no reaction, minimal inflammation, or a full allergic type of response. Of course, the antigen-antibody reaction that takes place in the nasal submucosa is an important bodily defense mechanism, yet release of histamine and other substances can cause troublesome symptoms.

Immunoglobulins. The circulating antibodies that are so important in nasal physiology are found in the gamma globulin fraction of plasma protein. The immunoglobulins are manufactured principally in the plasma cells of the reticuloendothelial system in response to an antigenic stimulus such as the presence in the nose of bacteria, viruses, or pollens.

IgA is the major immunoglobulin of external secretions from the mucous and serous glands of the nasal mucosa. It is produced locally within the nasal submucosa, and it is capable of neutralizing viruses as well as promoting phagocytosis and intracellular destruction of organisms by macrophages.

The development of IgA plasma cell collections in lymphoid tissue and around the serous and mucous glands of the nose is dependent on the presence of bacteria within the gland lumen. Animals reared in germ-free environments have a greatly reduced amount of IgA cell production and IgA in the serum (Taylor, 1980). In fact, since the newborn has a sterile nasal mucous membrane, the development of IgA immunity is dependent upon colonization of the nose by bacteria. Consequently, the nasal defense mechanisms for the newborn human consist mostly of filtration and mucociliary clearance of particulate matter. Immunity is derived from circulating maternal antibodies until the local production of IgA begins in response to bacterial colonization of the nose. Usually, bacterial colonization occurs within a few hours after birth, and lymphoid tissue forms in the mucosa and nasopharynx within days.

IgE binds to tissue mast cells and blood basophils, leading to the release of histamine and other mediator substances. Similar to the IgA-producing cells, the cells that produce IgE are found in the lymphoid tissue of the nose, mostly around the mucous and serous glands. In the genetically predisposed individual, IgE is produced when various allergenic substances permeate the mucosal surface. The mucociliary blanket prevents penetration of all insoluble particles, including potential allergens of more than 3 millimicrons (μ) in diameter. Allergen particles smaller than 3 μ in diameter form a soluble fraction in the liquid phase and in this form easily penetrate to the subepithelial layer, where they are neutralized by an immune reaction. The presence of free antibody in the sol-gel layer further inhibits the passage of allergens. When there is a vasomotor response, the transudate from capillary loops carries in it free antibody. Although the presence of excessive amounts of transudate fluid in the nose may cause symptoms of rhinorrhea, attempts to suppress fluid transudation may lessen the amount of free antibody present in the sol-gel layer, in turn impairing a local defense mechanism.

Eosinophils present in the nasal mucosa, in the nasal secretions, and in the peripheral blood are recognized features of an IgE-mediated reaction occurring in the nose. Eosinophils migrate toward certain chemical stimuli known as eosinotactic factors. Release of the eosinotactic factor of anaphylaxis (ECF/A) from allergan-challenged mast cells accounts for local eosinophilia in hay fever (Mygind, 1978). Although eosinophilia is characteristic of allergic disease, it is not pathognomonic.

In nasal allergy, eosinophils are transported from the bone marrow to the mucous membrane via the blood stream. Counting eosinophil cells in peripheral blood mostly gives information about the size of the shock organ affected rather than the severity of an allergic reaction in a specific location. That is, a child with chronic asthma would be expected to manifest greater eosinophilia in the peripheral blood than a child with acute allergic rhinitis. In fact, if the nose is the only organ affected by an allergic reaction, then the blood eosinophil count will usually be within normal limits.

Eosinophils can be detected on nasal smears. However, the significance of eosinophils detected on nasal smears may be difficult to interpret. Although most adults without symptoms of nasal allergy have no eosinophils present in a nasal smear, 25 to 30 per cent of infants do have eosinophils present in a smear from the nasal mucosa (Matheson et al., 1957; Crawford, 1960). Also, asymptomatic young children are found to have eosinophils on nasal smears more often (17 per cent) than are adults (Murray and Anderson, 1969). This is particularly true for children who have had breast-feeding supplemented in the first month of life (Murray, 1971). Nasal eosinophilia in children with atopic dermatitis is indicative of the subsequent development of allergic airway symptoms (Crawford, 1960).

Mast cells contain granules that are active in

the nasal allergic response. Morphologically and functionally, there are many similarities between mast cells found in nasal mucosa and basophil leukocytes, which act as "circulating mast cells" (Mygind, 1978). The mast cell can "degranulate," releasing the histamine contained in granules, in response to specific immunologic factors (allergens), nonselective immunologic factors (anti-IgE) and nonspecific, nonimmunologic factors (drugs, anaphylatoxin, venoms, lysosomal enzymes, or mechanical trauma).

"Specific immunologic degranulation" occurs in response to the reaction between allergen and IgE on the cell membrane. Although the IgE in normal individuals has no known allergen specificity, IgE molecules on a mast cell of an allergic individual vary in allergen specificity to form a heterogeneous population (Mygind, 1978). Some molecules may have specificity for animal disorder, others for grass pollen, and others for unknown factors. Juxtaposition of two IgE molecules with identical allergen specificity seems to be a prerequisite for mast cell degranulation with release of histamine because the degranulation is initiated when the allergen molecule forms a bridge between adjacent IgE molecules (Stanworth, 1971, 1973). The degranulation occurs only in the areas of the cell membrane where allergen and antibody interact.

"Nonselective immunologic degranulation" occurs in response to the presence of animal antibody against human IgE. The intranasal application of anti-IgE antibody causes nasal symptoms with nasal eosinophilia in patients with allergic rhinitis but not in normal subjects (Okuda, 1975). Since it is generally accepted that anti-IgG antibody (rheumatoid factor) plays a role in the pathogenesis of rheumatoid arthritis, it is possible that anti-IgE antibodies may be significant in causing perennial rhinitis (Assem, 1975).

"Nonimmunologic factors" can cause mast cell degranulation with release of histamine. Agents known to cause degranulation include polymixin B, chlorpromazine, atropine, acetylsalicylic acid, morphine, curare, plasma substitutes, and anesthetics (Mongar, 1956; Lorenz, 1975).

The primary mediators of an allergic reaction that are released when mast cells degranulate are histamine, slow-reacting substance of anaphylaxis (SRS-A), eosinophil chemotactic factor of anaphylaxis (ECF-A), and platelet activating factor (PAT). Secondary mediators of the immediate type of allergic reaction released from mast cells are prostaglandins, serotonin, and kinins. The nucleotides that are intracellular regulators of a mast cell's tendency to react to an allergen are cyclic adenosine monophosphate (cyclic AMP) and cyclic guanosine monophosphate (cyclic GMP). A high ratio of cyclic AMP to cyclic GMP reduces the mast cells' tendency to degranulate. Patients with perennial rhinitis have abnormal mucosal reactions when challenged with chemical mediators. Also, there is suggestive evidence that an abnormality of intracellular regulators contributes to the development of nasal symptoms in allergic patients (Mygind, 1978).

REFERENCES

Assem, E. S. K. 1975. Circulating IgE levels in patients with cancer. Lancet, 2:34–35.

Bang, B. G. Mukherjee, A. L., and Bang, F. B. 1967. Human nasal mucus flow rates. Johns Hopkins Med. J., 121:38–48.

Bridger, G. P., and Proctor, D. F. 1970. Maximum nasal inspiratory flow and nasal resistance. Ann. Otol. Rhinol. Laryngol., 79:481–488.

Crawford, L. V. 1960. A study of the nasal cytology in infants with eczematoid dermatitis. Ann. Allergy, 18:59–64.

Drettner, B. 1961. Vascular reactions of the human nasal mucosa on exposure to cold. Acta Otolaryngol. (Stockh.), Suppl. 166:1.

Huizing, E. H. 1967. Pathophysiology of the ciliary epithelium. Int. Rhinol., 5:73–78.

Lacourt, G., and Polgar, G. 1971. Interaction between nasal and pulmonary resistance in newborn infants. J. Appl. Physiol., 30:870–873.

Levy, A. M., Tabakin, B. S., Hanson, J. S., and Narkewicz, R. M. 1967. Hypertrophied adenoids causing pulmonary hypertension and severe congestive heart failure. N. Engl. J. Med., 277:506–511.

Livingstone, G. 1932. The nasal airway in the newborn child: Demonstration of model. Proc. R. Soc. Med., 25:1761–1763.

Lorenz, W. 1975. Histamine release in man. Agents Actions, 5:402–416.

Luke, M. J., Mehrizi, A., Folger, G. M., Jr., and Rowe, R. D. 1966. Chronic nasopharyngeal obstruction as a cause of cardiomegaly, cor pulmonale, and pulmonary edema. Pediatrics, 37:762–768.

Matheson, A., Rosenblum, A., Glazer, R., and Dacanay, E. 1957. Local tissue and blood eosinophils in newborn infants. J. Pediatr., 51:502–509.

Mongar, J. L. 1956. Measurement of histamine-releasing activity. In Ciba Foundation Symposium. Histamine. Boston, Little, Brown and Company, pp. 74–91.

Munzel, M, 1972. The permeability of intercellular spaces of the nasal mucosa. Z. Laryngol. Rhinol. Otol., 51:794–798.

Murray, A. B. 1971. Infant feeding and respiratory allergy. Lancet, 1:497.

Murray, A. B., and Anderson, D. O. 1969. The epidemiologic relationship of clinical nasal allergy to eosinophils and to goblet cells in the nasal smear. J. Allergy, 43:1–8.

Mygind, N. 1978. Nasal Allergy. Oxford, England, Blackwell Scientific Publications.

Mygind, N., and Bretlau, P. 1974. Scanning electron microscopic studies of the human nasal mucosa in normal persons and in persons with perennial rhinitis. II. Secretion. Acta Allergy (Kbh.), 29:261–280.

Negus, V. E. 1958. The Comparative Anatomy and Physiology of the Nose and Paranasal Sinuses. Edinburgh, E. & S. Livingstone, Ltd.

Ogura, J. H., and Harvey, J. E. 1971. Nasopulmonary mechanics: Experimental evidence of the influence of the upper airway upon the lower. Acta Otolaryngol., 71:123–132.

Ohnishi, T., Ogura, J. H., and Nelson, J. R. 1972. Effects of nasal obstruction upon the mechanics of the lung in the dog. Laryngoscope, 82:712–736.

Okuda, M. 1975. Response of the human nasal mucous membrane to anti-human IgE serum. Arch. Otorhinolaryngol. 211:25–33.

Olarin, B., and Teodorescu, M. L'écoulement biphas au niveau des fosses nasales. Acta Otorhinolaryngol. Belg., 27:60–68.

O'Neil, J. J. 1959. Pulmonary function tests as an adjunct in bronchology. Ann. Otol. Rhinol. Laryngol., 68:897–905.

Proctor, D. F. 1977. The Upper Airways: I. Nasal physiology and defense of the lungs. Am. Rev. Resp. Dis., 115:97–129.

Proctor, D. F., Anderson, I., Lundgvist, G., and Swift, D. L. 1973. Nasal mucociliary function and the indoor climate. J. Occup. Med., 15:169–174.

Rao, S., and Potdar, A. 1970. Nasal airflow with body in various positions. J. Appl. Physiol., 28:162–165.

Stanworth, D. R. 1971. Immunoglobulin E (reagin) and allergy. Nature (London), 233:310–316.

Stanworth, D. R. 1973. Immediate Hypersensitivity: The Molecular Basis of Allergic Response. New York, American Elsevier Publishing Company.

Stocksted, P. 1952. The physiologic cycle of the nose under normal and pathologic conditions. Acta Otolaryngol. (Stockh.), 42:175–179.

Taylor, M. 1980. Physiology of the nose, paranasal sinuses, and nasopharynx. In English, G. M. Otolaryngology, Vol. 2. Hagerstown, MD, Harper and Row, Chap. 3N.

Chapter 25

METHODS OF EXAMINATION

Gerald B. Healy, M.D.

INTRODUCTION

Examination of the pediatric patient requires a careful, gentle approach. One must remember that the child is usually apprehensive and afraid when approaching any physician. This is probably due to strange surroundings filled with multiple gadgets. This fear can frequently be alleviated by placing familiar objects, such as puppets, toys, and cartoon characters, in the examining area.

One of the essential parts of the examination is the time spent talking to the patient. Obviously, with the infant this may not be rewarding, but with the older child it will help to alleviate some of his or her fears. Time should be taken to show the patient the various objects to be used in the examination, such as the head mirror or nasal speculum. In fact, it is wise to allow the child to handle the instruments and perhaps even to let him or her examine a toy animal. If a head mirror will be used, the child should be allowed to see his or her reflection in the mirror to alleviate the fear of this large, awesome object sitting on the physician's head. It is a matter of tell, show, and do!

It is essential that the physician be truthful with the patient regarding what is going to be done. If the examination will be uncomfortable, the physician should tell the patient. The child should never be confronted by sudden, unexpected maneuvers. Each part of the examination should be explained to the child. This will play a large role in gaining the patient's trust.

Parental participation is most important. The physician must take time to obtain a good history and display genuine concern and interest when speaking with the parents. A complete history, including questions about other organ systems, as well as a family history, is frequently invaluable in arriving at a precise diagnosis.

General anesthesia may be required to do an adequate examination of the nose and paranasal sinus region. This often occurs in cases in which foreign bodies are present or with uncontrollable epistaxis, when absolute cooperation is required. The physician should not hesitate to use this mode of examination if the individual problem warrants it.

Palpation plays a very important role in examining the nose, sinuses, and face, and at times the examination can be done without the use of any instruments whatsoever.

EQUIPMENT

The head mirror, a 150 watt light bulb for illumination, the hand-held otoscope, and the hands of the examiner are the primary pieces of examining equipment. Other sources of illumination, such as the electric head lamp or flashlight, may be used when circumstances warrant it. A nasal speculum may occasionally be required in the examination. The nasopharyngeal mirror and tongue depressor are also essential.

Topical vasoconstrictors with various means of application, including aerosol delivery systems, cotton-tipped applicators, and cotton pledgets, should be available.

Sinus transillumination is of limited value in the pediatric patient, but the completely equipped examining area should have this means of evaluation available.

The operating microscope may be required for more precise examination and when

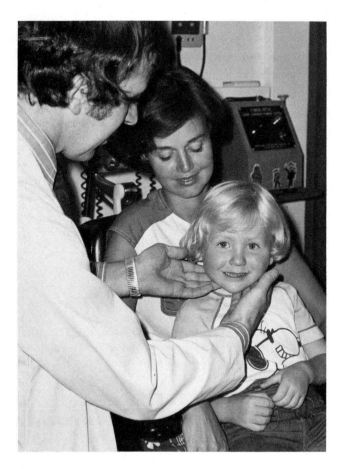

Figure 25–1 Positioning of child in mother's lap is most appropriate for examining pediatric patients.

available is helpful. An ordinary ear speculum used with the microscope may well allow examination of the entire length of the nasal passage, especially in the very small child.

Positioning of the patient is most important. The patient must feel as comfortable and secure as possible. Often this requires the parent to hold the child in his or her lap and provide reassurance frequently during the examination (Fig. 25–1). It is usually not advisable to hold the child down on the table and restrain him or her, as most children can be examined in the upright position. Infants, however, may need to be placed in the supine position for evaluation. It is advisable that the infant be adequately restrained so that there will be no unexpected movement.

CLINICAL EXAMINATION

The Face

Examination of the face must be preceded by an adequate history. Mass lesions in the region of the face and orbit should prompt questions regarding their duration, changes in size, the presence or absence of pain, or any evidence of infection. A history of trauma is most important in the evaluation of facial swelling. History of exposure to infectious disease, such as tuberculosis, is quite important. When the orbital region is involved, questions regarding vision must be asked, and the presence or absence of diplopia must be ascertained, especially in cases related to trauma.

Facial asymmetry should lead to questions regarding facial function or evidence of muscular weakness. Asymmetry of the face secondary to seventh cranial nerve dysfunction should obviously prompt a search into the patient's neurologic and otologic history. Any swelling of the parotid or submaxillary regions requires questioning regarding a possible relationship of eating to fluctuation in size of the swelling. The dental history must also be considered when determining the cause of swellings around the face and upper neck.

Clinical examination of this region begins by careful observation. Any asymmetry or masses should be noted. Attention should be given to the location of the masses, which frequently will be helpful in the differential diagnosis. The examiner should also be aware of any draining sinuses, as this can be indicative of congenital defects. Such a sinus, occurring on the dorsum of the nose, may be indicative of a dermoid cyst.

Sinuses occurring on the lateral portion of the face or neck may indicate first or second branchial groove anomalies. These anomalies in the neck may also lead to cystic defects of the branchial cleft system.

The punctum of the lacrimal sac should be inspected to rule out the presence or absence of debris or purulence in this region.

Any patient with periorbital swelling or pain should have a complete ophthalmologic examination, as well as radiographic evaluation of the sinuses.

Examination of the face should also include the region of the salivary glands. This requires gentle palpation to determine the relationship of the gland in question to underlying structures. A finger cot is placed over the index finger, and then the finger is placed into the oral cavity over the gland in question. The first and second fingers of the opposite hand are placed on the outside, and bimanual palpation is undertaken. This allows for estimation of the presence or absence of a mass, as well as tenderness and mobility. External massage of the glands should always be undertaken to determine flow from the salivary ducts. The appearance and consistency of the secretions should be noted carefully (Chap. 51).

Evaluation of facial swelling should include examination of the teeth, oral cavity, pharynx, and nasopharynx. Note should be made of any distortion of the parapharyngeal structures, as this may indicate extension of disease from the deep facial structures. The examiner must inspect the tonsils and observe for any medial displacement secondary to such underlying pathologic conditions. The presence or absence of trismus should be noted, as this may indicate pathologic conditions involving the pterygoid muscles.

The presence of facial masses often requires a search for systemic disease. Any nodular mass, especially if associated with drainage, should prompt a suspicion of tuberculosis or atypical microbacteria. No biopsy specimen should be obtained from a mass until a thorough search for systemic disease has been carried out. Skin testing, as well as

hematologic evaluation, may be necessary. Rapidly changing massses deserve immediate attention because of the ever-present possibility of neoplasm.

Trauma can present a puzzling and challenging problem to the examiner. Distortion and asymmetry due to swelling can confuse the issue and prevent absolute definition of underlying pathologic states. Observation, palpation, and the help of roentgenograms may be necessary to delineate completely the extent of the problem.

Bimanual palpation of the bony structures of the face should be undertaken in an attempt to ascertain defects. This should be done simultaneously on both sides of the face. Trauma to the maxillary or mandibular region should prompt an evaluation of occlusion. Any question of maxillary fracture requires digital palpation of the palate to assess the presence or absence of mobility (Fig. 25–2). A finger cot is placed on the examiner's index finger and thumb and the upper alveolus is firmly grasped and rocked with a to-and-fro motion to establish the presence or absence of freely floating components.

Injuries to the cervical spine often accompany severe facial trauma. The patient should not be manipulated needlessly until this possibility has been ruled out.

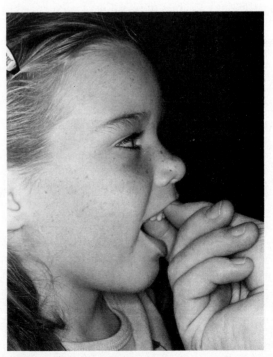

Figure 25–2 Digital palpation of the maxilla to establish the presence of fracture.

The Nose

Evaluation of the nose must be done in a systematic and organized fashion. One method of examination should be adopted, and a mental checklist should be employed so that no area is left out.

History should be sought from the parents, and, if the age of the child warrants, it is frequently possible to get useful information by merely asking the patient. Questions related to trauma, prior nasal disease, pain, nasal obstruction, nasal discharge, allergy, and distortion of olfaction should be asked. It is most important to ascertain sleeping habits and breathing patterns during sleep. Snoring and mouth breathing may signal nasal obstruction. This may warrant further examination of the nasopharynx.

Syndromes related to the cardiovascular system have had their origins traced directly to nasal obstruction. Therefore, the patient with a history suggesting severe obstruction may require more investigation, including cardiopulmonary evaluation, in addition to examination of the nasopharynx.

External Examination. Inspection plays an important role in examining the external nose. This will give an indication of the relative size and contour of the nose, which may be important in assessing breathing capabilities. Visible deformities, such as skin lesions, fistulae, swellings, or deviations should be noted. The presence or absence of a supratip crease should be noted. This may indicate the "nasal salute" of allergy (Chap. 37).

The bony and cartilaginous framework must be carefully examined not only for their relationships to each other but also for their relationships to the rest of the face. Such observations may explain the cause of nasal obstruction. The nasal bones should be palpated carefully, and the junction of the nasal bones with the upper lateral cartilages, as well as the junction of the cartilages with each other, should be noted.

The vestibular region should be inspected for gross lesions and for patency of the air passage. This is particularly important in the newborn infant, in whom evaluation of airflow is very critical inasmuch as these children are obligate nose breathers. A small wisp of cotton may be placed under the naris on each side to test for airflow. It is also possible to place a small nasopharyngeal mirror under each naris to watch for "fogging," which will indicate the presence or absence of airflow.

Internal Examination. The internal examination of the nose begins with careful inspection of the vestibular region. This is frequently overlooked by the passage of a nasal speculum, which obscures the first 1.0 to 1.5 cm of the nose.

Examination of the internal nose may be accomplished in a number of ways. Gentle upward rotation of the tip of the nose by the thumb of the examiner gives access to the vestibular region as well as to the anterior portion of the septum and the anterior segment of the inferior turbinates (Fig. 25–3). Illumination must be adequate and can be provided by a head mirror, head light, an otoscope with a nasal speculum attached, or even a flashlight.

Location of the septum is a critical element in evaluating the nose for nasal obstruction. The caudal septum must be evaluated carefully for discoloration, as it may play a major role in impeding free breathing. This portion is frequently bypassed by the insertion of a nasal speculum or the nasal head of the otoscope.

Inspection of the distal portion of the septum is important in evaluating the patient with epistaxis. The anterior portion has a rich vascular supply and is frequently the site of bleeding. This is also the site of septal perfo-

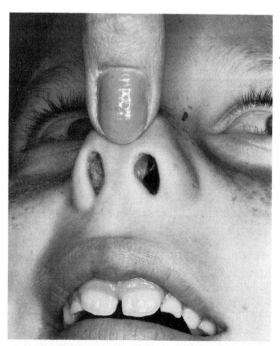

Figure 25–3 Elevation of the nasal tip by the examiner for inspection of the vestibule and septum. This maneuver avoids need for nasal speculum.

ration, which occasionally can be hidden by small crusts. If crusts are present in this area, they must be removed gently with a bayonet forceps or similar instrument to gain complete visualization of the internal nose.

Palpation of the septum is often necessary, especially after trauma. A small cotton swab may be used to compress the mucosa delicately in order to decide whether or not hematoma or abscess is present. These usually present as soft, doughy swellings either with or without tenderness.

Adequate examination of the nasal passage must be undertaken in any neonate with respiratory distress. These children are obligate nose breathers, and conditions such as choanal atresia or subluxation of the septum must be ruled out (Chap. 31).

This examination begins by an estimation of the amount of airflow through the nasal passage. A small, No. 8 catheter is gently passed along the floor of the nose into the pharynx. Frequently, it is necessary to apply a vasoconstrictor to the nasal mucous membrane in the form of 0.125 per cent phenylephrine hydrochloride solution. This is especially true in the newborn, in whom mucous membrane swelling is quite common. After appropriate shrinkage, it is possible to examine the internal nose by the use of an appropriate small ear speculum on the head of the hand-held otoscope.

Neonatal evaluation requires adequate illumination so that the entire internal framework of the nose can be inspected. An adequate evaluation of the septum must be undertaken to determine the presence or absence of dislocation.

Evaluation of the mucous membrane is an important part of the internal examination. Healthy mucosa is usually pink and moist, while pale, cyanotic, excessively moist mucosa may signal allergy or some other pathologic condition. Usually the neonate has slightly more edematous and moist mucosa than the older child.

In the presence of severely swollen mucosa, an adequate assessment of the internal nose cannot be undertaken without the use of vasoconstrictors. The use of a rapid aerosol spray is probably the most advisable way to obtain vasoconstriction. A 0.125 or 0.25 per cent solution of phenylephrine hydrochloride is usually adequate to obtain this. Occasionally, 1 or 2 per cent cocaine can be used where topical anesthesia is required. It is not advisable to pack the nose of a very young child with cotton pledgets, as this may frighten and alienate the patient.

Full lateral examination of the internal nose is frequently overlooked. This involves a visualization of the turbinates, noting their size, color and shape. Often, patients with a severe nasal septal deviation will present with compensatory hypertrophy of the turbinate facing the concavity of the deviation.

The middle turbinate region should be observed for the presence of a discharge and, if one is present, its appearance and location should be recorded. The anterior nasal sinuses (maxillary and anterior ethmoid) open into the middle meatus, and discharges from infections in these regions will present themselves in this area (Fig. 25–4). Posterior sinuses (the sphenoid and posterior ethmoid) drain into the superior meatus. The swollen, edematous mucosa associated with sinusitis must be shrunken in order to get an adequate estimation of the type and location of discharge. This material should be cultured, although the value of these cultures is somewhat controversial.

Clear, watery discharge may signify a vasomotor condition, or, on occasion, can represent cerebrospinal fluid. This is especially true after trauma or in patients with recurrent meningitis. If one suspects the presence of cerebrospinal fluid, analysis of the fluid is necessary. Radioisotope studies can be helpful in ruling out the presence or absence of a cerebrospinal fluid leak in the region of the cribriform plate.

Mucosa should be observed for other changes. A polypoid appearance or frank polyps may signal an allergic condition. Cystic fibrosis often presents with nasal polyps or polypoid changes in the nose, and thus, any child presenting with nasal polyps should have a sweat test to rule out the possibility of this disease (Chap. 36).

Mass lesions, such as gliomas and encephaloceles, can be mistaken for nasal polyps in the young child, and their presence must be considered in any patient with a nasal mass. A biopsy specimen of mass lesions in the nose should not be taken without consideration of this diagnosis. If one entertains the diagnosis, radiographic and radioisotopic studies should be undertaken to confirm its presence or absence.

Unilateral nasal discharge may signal the presence of a foreign body or unilateral choanal atresia. If one suspects a foreign body, it may be unwise to attempt its removal

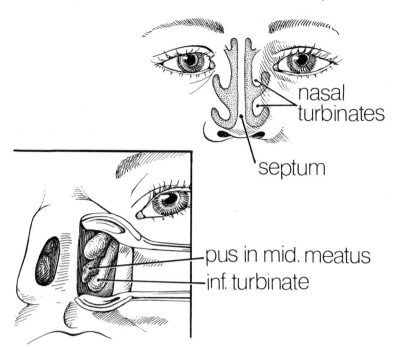

nasal
turbinates

septum

pus in mid. meatus
inf. turbinate

Figure 25–4 Internal nasal anatomy showing location of discharge in infections of the anterior sinuses (middle meatus).

without the use of general anesthesia. In this instance especially, this adjunct to examination becomes important and should not be overlooked.

If possible, an estimation of the adequacy

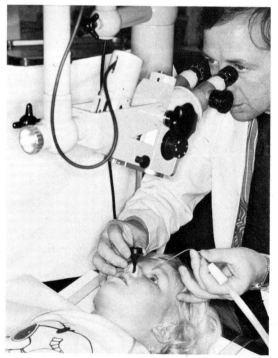

Figure 25–5 Use of the surgical microscope for detailed examination of the nose.

of olfactory function should be made. An easy and accurate method has yet to be developed, but gross testing should be attempted whenever possible. Any condition causing mucosal changes in the nose may well distort the sense of smell.

If precise examination of the nose is required, the surgical microscope and an ear speculum may be used (Fig. 25–5). This will give an excellent view after appropriate vasoconstriction and is especially useful in the cooperative patient.

The Sinuses

The development of the sinuses is variable in the pediatric patient. The ethmoids represent the most often clinically involved sinus in the patient under 10 years of age. The ethmoids and extremely small maxillary sinuses are present at birth. The frontal sinus does not begin to develop until approximately the age of eight years. It never develops in approximately 5 per cent of the population, and has only unilateral development in about 15 per cent. The sphenoid sinus begins to pneumatize at approximately three years of age, but full pneumatization is not complete until adolescence.

History of disease of the paranasal sinuses should be taken in conjunction with the history of the nasal status. Prior history of allergy is not uncommon. Perhaps the most common symptoms of acute sinus pathology are pain and nasal obstruction. The patient may often complain of nasal discharge as well. Occasionally, the only presenting manifestation of the disease in children will be a history of progressive swelling in the periorbital region; this can occur early with ethmoid sinusitis, especially in the young patient.

Examination. Palpation plays a large role in examination of the sinuses of any young child. The supraorbital region must be palpated carefully, and gentle tapping with the index finger should be undertaken to determine the presence or absence of tenderness. The ascending process of the maxilla and the canine fossa must be inspected. After gloving, the index finger is placed in the gingivobuccal sulcus, and gentle pressure is applied over the anterior and lateral walls of the maxillary sinus. These maneuvers may be unrewarding in the very young infant, however, and reliance on other clinical signs may be necessary.

Transillumination of the sinuses plays no significant role in examination of the pediatric patient, although it may be helpful in the adolescent.

Diagnostic surgical procedures involving the sinuses are rarely indicated in the pediatric patient. Occasionally, a diagnostic tap and irrigation of the maxillary sinus may be necessary to obtain material for culture and perhaps for cytologic evaluation. Radiographic studies of the maxillary sinuses to ascertain their size and relationship to erupted and unerupted teeth are necessary as a first step.

Antral puncture always requires general anesthesia in children. An appropriate vasoconstrictor is applied, and the sinus is entered with a trocar and cannula. Puncture is made through the inferior meatus, approximately 1.5 cm posterior to the anterior tip of the inferior turbinate (Fig. 25–6). The needle is gently advanced until the posterior wall is reached, then gently withdrawn approximately 0.5 cm. A syringe is attached and saline solution is gently instilled into the sinus. Fluid should be observed entering the nasal cavity through the natural ostium of the sinus. If this is not observed, the procedure should be immediately stopped, as the needle may not be in the proper position. In the young child with unerupted teeth, entrance may need to be made through the middle meatus rather than through the inferior meatus.

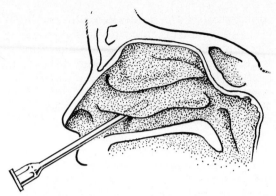

Figure 25–6 Position of trocar in inferior meatus for antral puncture.

Other methods of sinus irrigation have been advocated in the past. The technique described by Proetz (1939) uses the principle of displacement whereby air is drawn from the sinuses by suction and the fluid to be introduced into the sinus lies over the ostium when pressure is returned to normal. This will allow the fluid to flow into the sinus from which the air has been withdrawn. This technique is rarely used now because of the fear that infection may be transferred to previously healthy sinuses. It should be used only after cultures of the sinus have been obtained and appropriate antimicrobial therapy has been instituted. On occasion, it can be of great value in treating subacute or chronic ethmoiditis.

The Proetz method requires vasoconstriction. The patient's head is held back so that the chin and the external auditory canal are in the same vertical plane. The nose is then filled with a solution of ephedrine and saline. Negative pressure is applied to one nostril while the other is closed by a finger, and the patient is asked to occlude his pharynx by repeating the letter "k-k-k-k-k" or "kitty-kitty-kitty."

Exploratory sinus surgery may on rare occasion be required, especially if the presence of a neoplasm is suspected. Any bony destruction noted on roentgenograms of the sinuses requires further investigation in the form of surgical exploration. This may well represent either chronic infection or the presence of malignancy.

Nasopharynx

Roentgenography and rhinoscopy are the two primary means of evaluating the nasopharynx (see Diagnostic Procedures). Digital examination is not advocated because bleeding may be precipitated, which can be frightening to the patient and difficult to control. Palpation of the soft palate is advised, however, to ascertain the presence or absence of a submucous cleft. The presence of such a defect would obviously alert the physician against removing any of the lymphoid tissue in the nasopharynx.

The nasopharynx should be observed for the presence or absence of any mass lesion, which in children commonly represents adenoid tissue. The possible presence of lesions such as angiofibromas and neoplasms of other types must be kept in mind during the examination. The size, configuration, and surface appearance of all masses must be noted. Posterior rhinoscopy by the direct or indirect method should be attempted on all patients in whom a lesion might be present. If the patient is unable to tolerate this procedure, then direct examination under general anesthesia is required. This is accomplished by placing small catheters through the nose into the pharynx. The palate is then gently retracted laterally, and a large mirror is used to give a full panoramic view of the nasopharyngeal vault and the eustachian tube orifices.

Radiographic evaluation may also determine the presence or absence of a mass lesion when posterior rhinoscopy is not possible.

DIAGNOSTIC PROCEDURES

Posterior Rhinoscopy.   Posterior rhinoscopy is often overlooked in young children because many believe it cannot be accomplished. Contrary to this opinion, young children will frequently cooperate for this examination if they are reassured and if time is spent to gain their confidence. The use of a 00 or 000 mirror with gentle tongue depression will accomplish this. The child may be distracted by asking him or her to "breathe like a doggy" while the physician proceeds with the examination (Fig. 25–7).

Fiberoptic flexible or rigid endoscopic equipment may be used but frequently requires the use of topical or general anesthesia. Obtaining the cooperation of the child may be difficult, especially if he or she is very young. The advent of the small, flexible rhinolaryngoscope is making this evaluation somewhat more feasible. This instrument is gently passed over the floor of the nose while the examiner carefully observes the nasopharynx (Fig. 25–8).

Roentgenography.   A radiographic evaluation is part of any comprehensive examination of the sinuses. Radiographic evaluation of the nose is somewhat less informative, except in cases in which the presence of a foreign body is suspected. All children with periorbital cellulitis or swelling, nasal discharge, or edema of the nasal mucosa that do

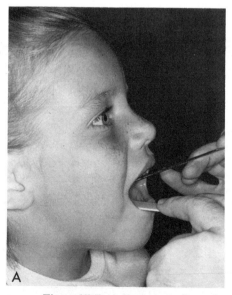
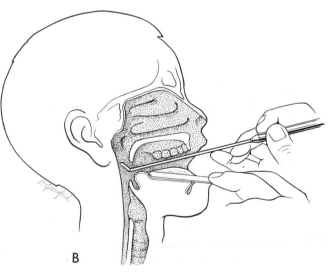

A   B

Figure 25–7   A, Posterior indirect rhinoscopy in the young child. B, Schematic drawing of the proper location of a mirror for view of the nasopharyngeal vault.

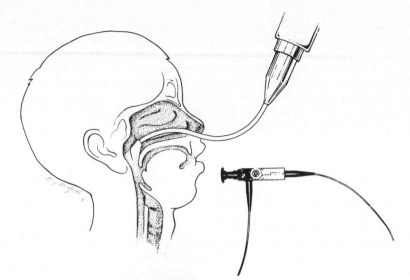

Figure 25–8 Location of the flexible fiberoptic nasopharyngoscope along the floor of the nose for view of the nasopharynx and pharynx. (Insert shows a full view of the instrument.)

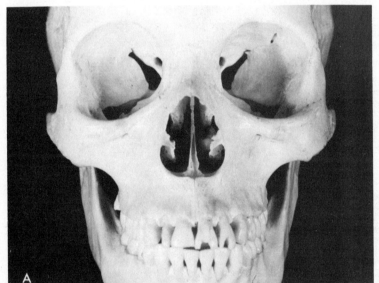

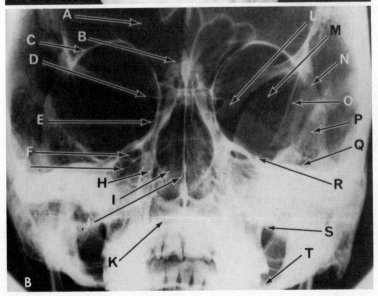

Figure 25–9 A, Photograph of the dried skull in the Caldwell projection. B, Caldwell view: A, frontal sinus; B, crista galli; C, superior orbital margin; D, optic foramen; E, ethmoid sinus; F, foramen rotundum; G, maxillary sinus; H, pyriform aperture; I, nasal cavity; J, nasal septum; K, floor of the nose; L, lesser wing of the sphenoid bone; M, greater wing of the sphenoid bone; N, zygomatic-frontal suture; O, temporal line; P, zygomatic bone; Q, petrous ridge of temporal bone; R, infraorbital foramen; S, lateral wall of maxillary sinus; T, floor of posterior cranial fossa. (Courtesy of Arch. Otolaryngol., 87:184–195, 1968 and the American Academy of Ophthalmology and Otolaryngology.)

not respond to conventional therapy should have radiographic evaluation of their sinuses.

A dental view of the nasal bones may be helpful in estimating the degree of trauma to the nasal framework. The gross appearance of the external nose, as well as estimation of the internal framework, are far more valuable than questionable roentgenograms of the nasal bones.

Roentgenographic evaluation of the paranasal sinuses is somewhat more valuable, however. The four traditional views — Caldwell, Waters, lateral, and submentovertical — are the most helpful in the estimation of diseases of the sinuses and facial bones.

The Caldwell or occipitofrontal view best delineates the ethmoid and frontal sinuses. The temporal bones and base of the skull are projected onto the maxillary antrum, thereby concealing it and making this an undesirable view for evaluating the maxillary sinuses (Fig. 25–9).

The Waters or occipitomental view best delineates the maxillary sinus and the orbital floor. It is an important view in the estimation of facial trauma as it gives a fairly panoramic view of the facial bones (Fig. 25–10).

The lateral view gives good visualization of the anterior and posterior ethmoid cells, as well as of the frontal and sphenoid sinuses. It also shows the thickness of the antral walls

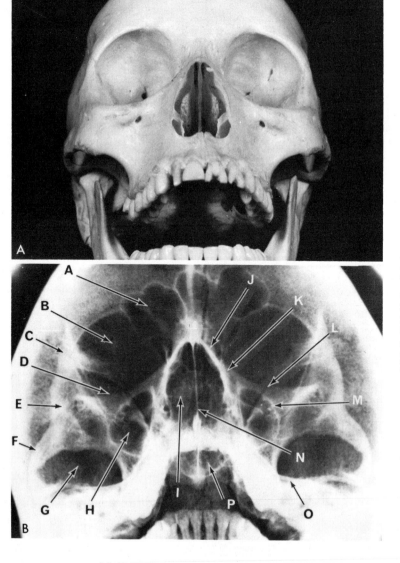

Figure 25–10 *A*, Dried skull in Water's projection. *B*, Water's view: A, frontal sinus; B, orbit; C, zygomatic-frontal suture; D, inferior orbital rim; E, zygoma; F, zygomatic arch; G, infratemporal fossa; H, maxillary sinus; I, nasal cavity; J, nasal bone; K, frontal process of maxilla; L, superior orbital fissure; M, infraorbital foramen; N, nasal septum; O, petrous ridge of temporal bone; P, sphenoid sinus. (Courtesy of Arch. Otolaryngol., 87:196–209, 1968 and the American Academy of Ophthalmology and Otolaryngology.)

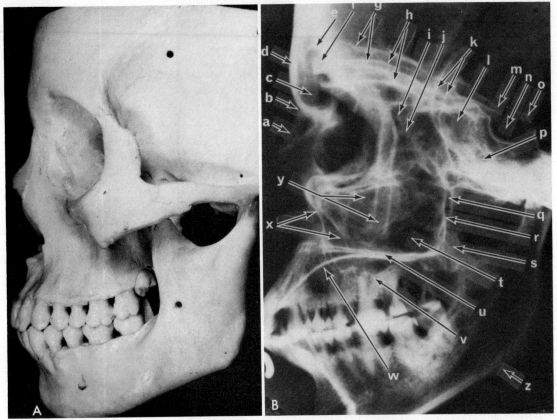

Figure 25–11 *A*, Dried skull on lateral projection. *B*, Lateral view showing: a, nasal bone; b, nasofrontal suture; c, frontal sinus; d, anterior wall of frontal sinus; e, posterior wall of frontal sinus; f, supraorbital margin; g, cerebral surface orbital plate; h, orbital surface of orbital plate; i, cribriform plate; j, anterior ethmoid air cells; k, anterior wall of middle cranial fossa (greater wing of sphenoid bone); l, posterior ethmoid cells; m, anterior clinoid process; n, sella turcica; o, posterior clinoid process; p, sphenoid sinus; q, turgomaxillary fissure; r, posterior wall of maxillary sinus; s, pterygoid plates; t, maxillary sinus; u, floor of the nose; v, floor of the maxillary sinus; w, roof of the mouth; x, anterior wall of the maxillary sinus; y, zygomatic process of the maxilla; z, mandible. (Courtesy of Arch. Otolaryngol. 87:299–310, 1968 and the American Academy of Ophthalmology and Otolaryngology.)

and the relationship of the antral floor to the teeth (Fig. 25–11). This is especially important in the young patient. This view can be used conveniently to estimate the presence or absence of a nasopharyngeal mass lesion.

A submentovertical view estimates the extent of the posterior ethmoid and sphenoid sinuses and gives an excellent panoramic view of the base of the skull (Fig. 25–12).

Polytomography. Polytomography of the paranasal sinus region can on occasion give useful information, especially if there is a possibility of fracture or bony destruction (Fig. 25–13). Defects in the region of the cribriform plate can occasionally be demonstrated with this technique as well.

Radiopaque Media. Special studies utilizing radiopaque material can aid in the diagnosis of lesions of the nose or facial region. Conditions such as choanal atresia can be demonstrated by the use of the "choanogram." In this technique, the opaque material is placed in the nasal cavity in order to demonstrate the presence or absence of material in the pharynx (Fig. 25–14).

Sialography. Sialography may be used to study both the parotid and submaxillary glands. With this technique, radiopaque material is gently injected into the duct of the salivary gland to be studied, and films are taken of the gland in question (Fig. 25–15). Occasionally, the use of fluoroscopy is helpful

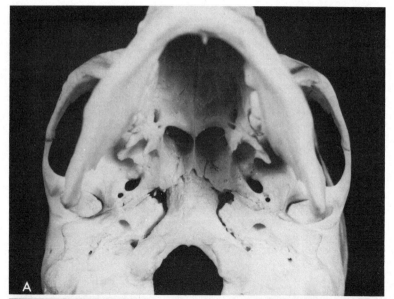

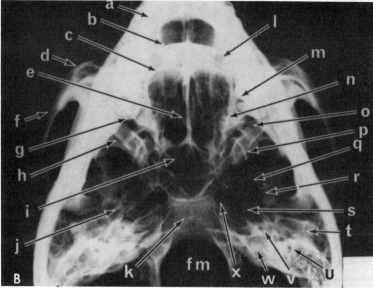

Figure 25–12 *A*, Dried skull in submentovertical projection. *B*, Submentovertical view: a, mandible; b, anterior wall of frontal bone; c, posterior wall of frontal bone; d, zygoma; e, nasal septum; f, zygomatic arch; g, lateral wall of antrum; h, lateral wall of orbit; i, sphenoid sinus; j, eustachian tube; k, clivus; l, lacrimal canal; m, maxillary sinus; n, greater palatine foramen; o, inferior orbital fissure; p, pterygoid plates; q, foramen ovale; r, foramen spinosum; s, carotid canal; t, external auditory canal; u, stylomastoid foramen; v, cochlea; w, internal auditory canal; x, foramen lacerum; fm, foramen magnum. (Courtesy of Arch. Otolaryngol., 87:311–322, 1968 and the American Academy of Ophthalmology and Otolaryngology.)

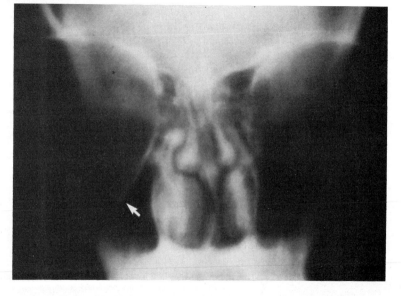

Figure 25–13 Polytomograph of maxillary sinuses showing orbital floor fracture (*arrow.*)

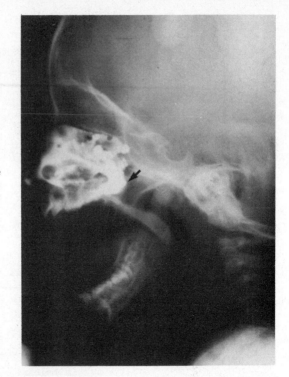

Figure 25–14 Choanogram showing nonfilling of the nasopharynx secondary to choanal atresia. (*Arrow* indicates point of atresia plate.) The child is placed in the supine position for study.

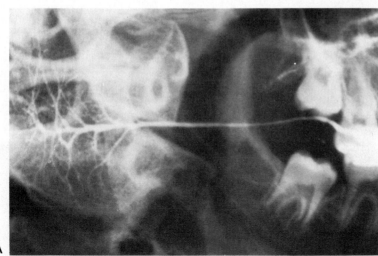

A

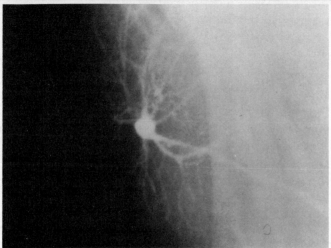

B

Figure 25–15 *A*, Normal parotid sialogram (lateral view); *B*, Normal parotid sialogram (AP view).

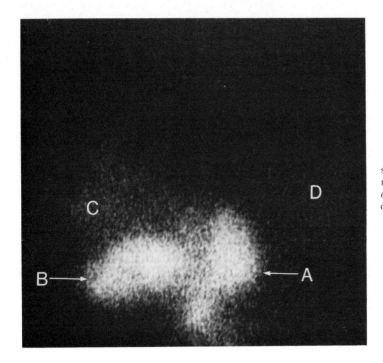

Figure 25–16 Normal lateral radiosialogram following administration of 2 microcuries of technetium ^{99m} showing a, parotid gland; b, submaxillary gland; c, nose; d, posterior occiput.

as an adjunct to this study. Preliminary films include stereoposteroanterior and lateral films of the mandibular region. After these are reviewed and the contrast material is injected, the same views are repeated.

The analysis of the sialogram includes a detailed examination of the main secretory ducts (Wharton's or Stensen's), the smaller ducts branching within the gland, and the parenchyma of the gland itself. Deep sedation or even general anesthesia may be required in the very young child in order to undertake this study (Gates, 1977).

Radioisotopic Examination. The use of radioisotopic evaluation in the region of the face has its greatest application in examination of the salivary glands. The ductal cells of these structures have the ability to extract iodide from the peritubular capillaries and to secrete it into the ductal lumen. Iodine^{125} or technetium^{99m} can be recorded from salivary gland tissue, thus providing the basis for salivary gland scanning (Gates, 1977).

The material is injected intravenously, and then the structures to be examined are scanned at varying intervals thereafter. Normal outlines of the glandular structures can be seen easily and the presence of mass lesions can be detected (Figs. 25–16 and 25–17).

Computerized Axial Tomography. Computerized axial tomography (CT or CAT) was

introduced in 1972. This method of evaluation makes it possible to identify different soft tissue structures that vary by 1 to 2 per cent in their absorption of x-rays. This new equipment is much more sensitive than radiographic film in the differentiation of

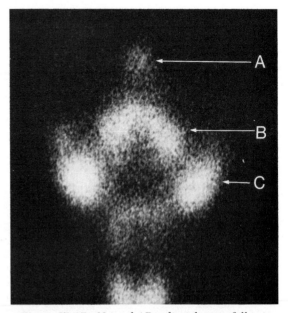

Figure 25–17 Normal AP radiosialogram following administration of 2 microcuries of technetium^{99m} showing: a, nose; b, submaxillary gland; c, parotid gland.

various anatomic structures. The images are made in a transverse plane rather than in the traditional coronal or sagittal planes.

The computed tomographic scanner is a roentgenographic machine capable of producing a cross-sectional image on a television monitor. Mathematical formulas are used to calculate very slight differences in absorption coefficients of different tissue to an x-ray beam that passes through the body from a number of directions around a parallel to the transverse axis. The computer is then utilized to sort out the large number of equations presented by this technique (Carter et al., 1977).

The use of computerized axial tomography in examination of the region of the nose and paranasal sinuses is rapidly becoming widespread. Various anatomic structures can be delineated in the nose and paranasal sinus region by this computer examination technique (Figs. 25–18 and 25–19).

Contrast material (enhancement technique) has been used frequently in conjunction with CAT scans of the head. Its major value is in delineating lesions of the brain, and it has limited usefulness in the discovery of pathologic conditions of the nose and paranasal sinuses.

Ultrasonography. Ultrasonography is a technique for examining the acoustic proper-

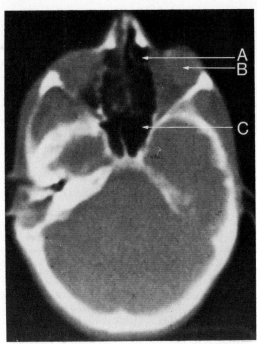

Figure 25–19 Normal transverse computerized tomograph showing: *a*, ethmoid sinuses; *b*, orbit; *c*, sphenoid sinus. (Courtesy of Barbara Carter, M.D.)

ties of tissues. Sound waves are generated by a piezoelectric crystal placed in close contact with the skin, and a short pulse of ultrasound (usually 1 to 5 MHz) is transmitted. A returning echo is then received by the crystal. Inasmuch as the velocity of sound through most tissues is fairly uniform (1500 m per sec), it is possible to compute the distance of the echo from the transducer. This is done by means of a cathode ray tube, which displays both the starting point of the signal and the location of the echo on an oscilloscope screen.

A linear recording showing the amplitude and time relationship of the echo to the original pulse is called an *A Scan.* If the echo is stored, it can be assimilated to produce a composite picture called a *B Scan* (Noyek et al., 1977).

This technique has been shown to be quite useful in delineating orbital lesions (Chap. 29). Its usefulness in the remainder of the face and sinus region has been somewhat limited up to this point, although it has been used to differentiate solid from cystic lesions in the parotid gland and thyroid.

The usefulness of this technique in diagnosing pathologic sinus conditions is now being investigated.

Miscellaneous Procedures. Other help-

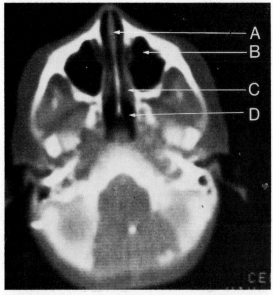

Figure 25–18 Normal transverse computerized tomograph showing: *a*, nasal septum; *b*, maxillary sinus; *c*, turbinates; *d*, nasopharynx. (Courtesy of Barbara Carter, M.D.)

ful diagnostic procedures in the region of the nose and paranasal sinuses may occasionally be required. The use of nasal smears for cytologic evaluation is often helpful in ascertaining the presence or absence of an allergic state. A specimen of nasal mucus is obtained by swabbing with a cotton-tipped applicator just below the inferior turbinate and along the floor of the nose. The material is then gently rolled onto a glass slide and immediately sprayed with fixative solution. Wright's stain is then applied for approximately 15 seconds, followed by a buffered solution for 15 seconds. The slide is then rinsed with distilled water and allowed to dry. It is then ready for examination under the oil immersion microscope. The relative numbers and types of cells seen on the slide are tabulated in a *cytogram* (Bryan and Bryan, 1974).

Large numbers of eosinophils may be indicative of an allergic state. However, patients with vasomotor rhinitis may occasionally have eosinophilia as well. Eosinophilia is also seen on the nasal smears of infants under three months of age.

A negative cytogram does not necessarily rule out allergy. Serial cytograms may be necessary. This test is just one in the armamentarium of the examiner, and it should be coupled with the assessment of the history and appearance of the nose and sinuses before an allergy is diagnosed or ruled out.

Cultures of the nasopharynx can occasionally be helpful in treating patients with persistent rhinitis or chronic sinusitis. These may be obtained by gently passing a small wire nasopharyngeal swab along the floor of the nose into the nasopharynx after the mucous membrane has been treated with appropriate vasoconstrictors.

REFERENCES

Bryan, M. P., and Bryan, W. T. K. 1974. Cytologic diagnosis in allergic disorders. Otolaryngol. Clin. North Am., 7(3):637–666.

Carter, G., et al. 1977. Cross-Sectional Anatomy —Computed Tomography and Ultrasound Correlation. New York, Appleton-Century-Crofts.

Gates, G. A. 1977. Sialography and scanning of salivary glands. Otolaryngol. Clin. North Am., 10 (2):379–390.

Noyek, A. M., Holgate, R. C., et al. 1977. Sophisticated radiology in otolaryngology. J. Otolaryngol., Supp. 3, 6:95–117

Proetz, A. W. 1939. The Displacement Method. St. Louis, Annals Pub. Co.

Chapter 26

NASAL OBSTRUCTION AND RHINORRHEA

Walter M. Belenky, M.D.

INTRODUCTION

The importance of nasal obstruction and rhinorrhea in nasal function and disease was well known by and was the concern of many physicians in ancient times. Among the earliest writings on this subject, the Hindu Arthava-Veda Sanhita (1500–800 B.C.) (Wise, 1898) listed causes of nasal discharge. Although Hippocrates described nasal discharge in his humoral theory in 415 B.C. and this problem was again mentioned by Celsus (c. 30 A.D.), Galen was the first to postulate on the etiology of rhinorrhea around 160 A.D. (Brock, 1916). He suggested that nasal discharge contained waste products from the brain that had been filtered by the pituitary and entered the nose by the cribriform and ethmoid plates. This theory was accepted for 1500 years until Schneider in 1600 A.D. pronounced that nasal discharge is a product of the membrane lining of the nose (cited by Schaefer in 1932).

This concern of the ancient physicians with nasal discharge was well taken, as the obstructed or draining nose is the most common complaint the otolaryngologist is faced with in evaluating nasal problems in all patients, including the pediatric patient. The nose acts as the "guardian of the lower respiratory tract" and "the initiator of the immune response to inhaled antigens and pathogens" (Taylor, 1979). Nasal obstruction and rhinorrhea may appear as both symptoms and signs, reflecting the anatomic and physiologic importance of the nose in both health and disease. Frequently occurring together, they may vary sufficiently in their characteristics to aid the observant clinician in his diagnosis.

The presence of one without the other may be equally significant.

Nasal obstruction and rhinorrhea present in a variety of ways. The onset of symptoms may be acute as in the common cold or chronic as in the older child's suffering from the stuffy, runny nose of perennial allergic rhinitis. These complaints may be the symptoms of a life-threatening disease, such as bilateral choanal atresia, or they may be due simply to the bothersome but normal physiologic changes that occur in the nose during puberty. The symptoms of nasal obstruction and rhinorrhea that may prompt parents to bring a child to the physician for treatment are often accompanied by the non-nasal symptoms of dry, coated tongue, bad breath, snoring, mouth-breathing, and postnasal drip.

The clinician must recognize the symptoms of nasal obstruction and rhinorrhea and, through the taking of a thorough history and the performance of a physical examination, must assess the entire patient, particularly the internal and external nose and related structures, in order to determine whether the pathology is of local or systemic origin. In evaluating nasal obstruction, the clinician must first determine if it is unilateral or bilateral, complete or partial, intermittent or constant, congenital or acquired, and of sudden or gradual onset. Examination of the nose may determine the anatomic site of obstruction. Cottle (1968) described five areas of the nose where abnormalities may occur: (1) the vestibular area; (2) the "liminal valve" area, or the relationship of the caudal end of the upper lateral cartilage to the nasal septum, the os internum, the narrowest portion of the nasal passage; (3) the attic, or area of the septum under the bony vault; (4) the anterior turbinates; and (5) the posterior turbinates and posterior choanae. For completeness a sixth area, the nasopharynx, might be added. Physiologically, certain areas appear to be more important during nasal inspiration and have been described by Bridger (1970) and others (Bridger and Proctor, 1970) as nasal valves. These include the "liminal valve" considered by many to be the most important part during inspiration in the Caucasian nose (Bridger, 1970; von Dishoeck, 1942, 1965); the erectile tissue of the nasal turbinates (turbinate valve); and the nasal septum (septal valve).

To aid the clinician in measuring the degree of obstruction objectively and in quantifying nasal functions, rhinomanometry procedures have developed to measure the amount of air pressure and rate of airflow in the nasal channel during respiration. These procedures have been helpful in substantiating clinical findings of nasal obstruction; for example, significant airway obstruction may occur with minimal anatomic abnormality in areas 1 and 2, while larger deformities in areas 3, 4, and 5 may cause minimal obstructive symptoms (Bridger, 1970; Bridger and Proctor, 1970). Further, such data have highlighted the importance of the streamlined airflow in the nose with reduction of eddy currents and resistance. However, rhinomanometry is still of limited clinical value, as the data obtained do not appear to reflect overall respiratory function, nor do they establish respiratory dysfunction as being caused by the nose (Kern, 1973).

In some cases the clinical impression of nasal obstruction can be confirmed by lateral radiographs of the nose and nasopharynx. Such radiographs may show obstruction of the airway by hypertrophic adenoids if they are taken with the mouth closed. Contrast nasograms can demonstrate choanal atresia.

As with nasal obstruction, rhinorrhea must first be evaluated by the clinician as to its extent, frequency, duration, time and nature of onset, and quantity. By classical definition, rhinorrhea is the "free discharge of a thin nasal mucus" (Dorland, 1974).

The vasomotor reaction is the primary response of the nasal mucosa to a variety of stimuli. The ratio of acetylcholine production to acetylcholine enzymatic destruction is important in determining the intensity and duration of the vasomotor reaction. Numerous factors influence this ratio, but primary control is exerted by the hypothalamus by direct stimulation via the autonomic nervous system to release acetylcholine, and indirect control is established via the hypothalamic pituitary axis and estrogen release, which inhibits acetylcholinesterase function. As is well documented (Stoksted, 1952; Chladek et al., 1972; Taylor, 1961a, 1973, 1979), the control of nasal respiration regulates the oxygen intake of the lungs and thus influences cellular respiration throughout the body. This control is neuroendocrine in nature, originating in the hypothalamus in response to afferent stimuli from body receptors monitoring the internal and external environments of the body. Control is effected via chemical mediators working directly at cell surface nerve endings or indirectly via hormonal activity.

The primary target site effecting control of nasal respiration is the nasal mucosa, which is in a dynamic state, changing constantly under normal and abnormal conditions in response to internal and external stimuli. This complex, integrated neuroendocrine pathway utilizes the autonomic nervous system efferents and hormonal mediators of the pituitary axis to effect a primary functional response of the nasal mucosa known as the vasomotor reaction.

The vasomotor reaction is the end result of these multiple interactions and is characterized by increased nasal mucosal surface area, increased nasal obstruction, and increased nasal secretions (Taylor, 1973, 1979). The vasomotor reaction is chemically initiated at the end organ by vasodilating agents; the most important and powerful dilating agent in normal and disease states is acetylcholine, which is produced at parasympathetic nerve endings. Its action in turn is regulated by acetylcholinesterase activity at the nerve ending.

Nasal obstruction is produced by vasomotor reaction and in many diseases is controlled by the autonomic nervous system, which acts on the erectile tissue of the nasal lining.

The increased nasal secretions of the vasomotor reaction are largely composed of mucus from the nasal mucosa. Nasal mucus is the basic ingredient of nasal discharge and consists of 2.5 to 3 per cent nonsulfated and sulfated mucoproteins and mucopolysaccharides, 1 to 2 per cent inorganic salts, and 96 per cent water (Taylor, 1979). It is produced by nasal mucosa from goblet cells, stromal mucosa, serous glands, and duct cells. Transudation can quickly occur via the semipermeable basement membrane and from the capillary loops that pierce the membrane, thus bringing fluid and debris directly onto the surface epithelium and contributing to mucus formation (Taylor, 1974). This fluid may be seen as the sudden, diffuse, watery discharge occurring in several diseases.

Excessive mucus formation or increased viscosity of mucus in response to internal and external stimuli may lead to stasis and poor drainage from the nose. Such stasis frequently leads to secondary infections, chronic changes in the nasal mucosa, or both. The normal nasal secretion rate is 0.1 to 0.3 ml per kg per day.

The significance of the mucus and increased nasal secretions that are a part of the vasomotor reaction and that accompany nasal disease lies in the relationship of the specific physiochemical qualities of mucus to nasal function. Along with the erectile nature of the nasal mucosa, nasal mucus provides temperature regulation of the internal environment and inspired air, humidification of inspired air, and vasorespiration control. The peculiar adhesiveness and surface electrical activity of nasal mucus, the result of sulfated mucins, combines with the vibrissae to keep particulate matter from the lower airway. Mucus acts as a primary defense mechanism in inflammatory disease by retaining immunoglobulins and bacteriolytic enzymes (lysozymes) as well as agents or allergens to which this response is initiated. Taylor has written excellent reviews of nasal physiology if the reader wishes to obtain further information on the subject (1971, 1973, 1974, 1979).

NORMAL PHYSIOLOGIC STATE

The clinician is at times confronted with infants and children complaining of nasal obstruction and rhinorrhea but without any evidence of local or systemic disease. In these cases, nasal obstruction and rhinorrhea may represent a normal physiologic nasal function or may be symptoms of a pathologic condition. The frequency of such complaints increases as the child approaches adolescence, and this fact must be taken into consideration when making a differential diagnosis. Table 26–1 lists a number of normal physiologic states in which increased rhinorrhea and nasal obstruction may occur.

Table 26–1   NORMAL PHYSIOLOGIC CAUSES OF INCREASED NASAL OBSTRUCTION AND RHINORRHEA

Nasal cycle
Paradoxic nasal obstruction
Nasopulmonary reflex
Puberty
Menses
Psychosomatic factors
External environmental stimuli

The Nasal Cycle

The nasal cycle is a rhythmic alternating side-to-side congestion and decongestion of the cavernous tissue of the nasal turbinates. Although it occurs in 80 per cent of the population, it is usually unnoticed because the total nasal resistance remains constant. Occasionally the cycle will increase in intensity and produce signs of obstruction without any significant increase in nasal secretions (Taylor, 1979).

Paradoxic Nasal Obstruction

The older child and adolescent with longstanding, severe unilateral obstruction (such as that due to a septal deformity) will often complain of intermittent obstruction of the patent nasal airway. The patent side has functioned as the entire nasal airway, and complaints are elicited only when factors such as the nasal cycle intermittently obstruct the patent side (Arbour, 1975).

The Nasopulmonary Reflex

Often children with a common cold will complain of breathlessness out of proportion to the degree of nasal obstruction observed by the examiner. This is probably the result of reduced vital capacity secondary to stimulation of a nasopulmonary reflex by increased nasal obstruction (Taylor, 1973). Similarly, hypothalamus-mediated nasopulmonary reflexes account for a common complaint of dependent nasal obstruction in the recumbent position; compression of the dependent lung elicits an ipsilateral nasal obstruction (Sercer, 1930). Ogura and others have studied the nasopulmonary reflexes and have documented a relationship between nasal resistance and pulmonary resistance. They found that increased nasal resistance produces increased pulmonary resistance and decreased pulmonary compliance with probable decreased alveolar ventilation (Ogura et al., 1964, 1966, 1968, 1973; Ogura and Nelson, 1968; Ogura and Harvey, 1971). This may result in aberration of blood gases, acid-base imbalance, and tissue hypoxemia, which may account for the generalized symptoms of fatigue, restlessness, and irritability seen in children with severe upper airway obstruction (Ohnishi and Ogura, 1969; Ohnishi et al., 1972).

Puberty and Menses

Adolescent females, and even males, will occasionally complain of intermittent nasal obstruction and rhinorrhea during the pubescent period as a result of increases in the level of estrogen and, in part, testosterone, which increase the normal vasomotor reaction by decreasing the activity of acetylcholinesterase. Similarly, periodic complaints will occur in the postpubescent female with relationship to menstruation (Taylor, 1973, 1979; Mortimer et al., 1936; Parkes and Zuckerman, 1931).

Psychosomatic Causes

Teenagers especially may present with symptoms of intense vasomotor reactions related to emotional states such as anxiety, stress, fatigue, and anger. These are mediated through reflexes centered in the hypothalamus. These symptoms may be accompanied by unilateral migraine headaches, which are mediated by similar reflexes (Taylor, 1973, 1979; Holmes et al., 1950).

External Environmental Stimuli

Numerous complaints of obstruction and rhinorrhea are nothing more than an expression of the nasal vasomotor reaction to external stimuli and reflect the nasal mucosa's normal function as an interface between the body's internal and external environments. Thus, such symptoms may be dependent upon the composition of gases and particulate matter (such as dust, fur, and smog) or upon the temperature and water content of the inspired air. The watery discharge one

experiences on going outside during the winter is a good example of this type of vasomotor reaction (Taylor, 1973).

NASAL OBSTRUCTION AND RHINORRHEA IN DISEASE

The significance of nasal obstruction and rhinorrhea in nasal diseases that may occur in the pediatric patient cannot be stressed too greatly. As discussed, both may be a manifestation of the basic vasomotor reaction to abnormal internal or external stimuli. However, obstruction may occur with little contribution from the vasomotor reaction but from a single mass blockage of the nasal airway as seen in choanal atresia. Similarly, rhinorrhea may lack the usual mucus component and instead may be distinctly pathologic in nature, as when it is composed of cerebrospinal fluid.

Nasal obstruction and rhinorrhea vary in nature according to their etiology. Table 26–2 classifies these according to their pathogenesis.

Congenital

In view of the varied and complicated plications and involutions that tissues involved in the formation of the face and nose undergo, it is remarkable how infrequently congenital abnormalities of the nose occur. Such abnormalities are most likely due to a combination of exogenous teratogenic factors and inherited gene patterns. In some cases in which nasal development is limited, the cause of the symptoms of obstruction is obvious: Total nasal agenesis, although rare, has been reported (Wilson, 1962). Proboscis lateralis similarly is an extreme congenital anomaly (Wilson, 1962; Biber, 1949). Congenital occlusion of the anterior nares seldom occurs, but when it does it may be unilateral or bilateral, complete or partial, and nasal obstruction may vary accordingly (Wilson, 1962). Rhinorrhea plays a limited role in the complaints that result from these rare anomalies (Chap. 31).

The total dependency of neonates and infants upon nasal respiration is highlighted by the acuteness and severity of the symptoms of nasal obstruction in these children. Adaptation of the infant to oral breathing may take

Table 26-2 NASAL OBSTRUCTION AND RHINORRHEA IN DISEASE

Congenital
Total nasal agenesis
Proboscis lateralis
Congenital occlusion of anterior nares
Posterior choanal atresia
Mandibulofacial dysostoses
  Treacher-Collins syndrome
  Crouzon disease
Coronal craniosynostosis
Cleft palate
Congenital cysts of nasal cavity
  Dermoid
  Nasoalveolar
  Dentigerous
  Mucous cysts of floor of nose
  Jacobson organ cysts
Meningoencephalocele
Encephalocele
Pharyngeal bursa (Tornwaldt)
Hamartomas
Craniopharyngiomas
Chordomas
Teratoid tumors
Epignathus
Possible third branchial cleft cyst (Frazer, 1940)
  (presenting in Rosenmueller fossa.)

Inflammatory
Infectious
  Bacterial
    Secondary invaders
    Primary agent
      Diphtheria
      Pertussis
      Tuberculosis
      Rhinoscleroma
      Leprosy
  Viral
    Primary agent
      Acute viral rhinonasopharyngitis
      Rhinovirus
      Adenovirus
      Coxsackieviruses A and B
      Myxoviruses
        Influenza
        Parainfluenza
        Respiratory syncytial virus
    Prodromal stage of virus disease
      Mumps
      Poliomyelitis
      Measles (rubella, rubeola)
      Roseola infantum
      Erythema infectiosus
      Infectious mononucleosis
      Hepatitis
  Spirochetal
    Congenital "snuffles"
    Acquired "snuffles"

Protozoan
  Leishmaniasis
Fungal
  Moniliasis
  Mucormycosis
  Aspergillosis
Parasitic
Allergic
  Acute—type I (anaphylactic, reagin-dependent)
  Chronic-Nasal polyposis
Toxic
  External stimuli
    Inhalants (urban pollutants, etc.)
    Ingested (hormones, iodides, bromide, aspirin)
    Topically applied (nose drops, cocaine) (rhinitis
      medicamentosa)
Nasopharyngeal
  Adenoid hyperplasia

Traumatic
External deformity
  Neonatal
  Acquired in childhood
Internal deformity
  Neonatal
  Septal hematoma acquired in childhood
  Septal abscess acquired in childhood
Foreign bodies
  Rhinolith
Cerebrospinal fluid rhinorrhea
  Traumatic
  Spontaneous

Neoplastic
Ectodermal origin
Mesodermal origin
Neurogenic origin
  Olfactory neuroblastoma
Odontogenic origin
Idiopathic origin
  Juvenile angiofibroma

Metabolic
Cystic fibrosis
Calcium abnormalities
Magnesium abnormalities
Thyroid disease
  Hypothyroidism
  Hyperthyroidism
Diabetes mellitus
Immune deficiency disease

Idiopathic
Atrophic rhinitis
Chronic catarrhal rhinitis

weeks to several months. Although not completely understood, the obligatory nasal breathing of the neonate may be due to "a high cephalic position of cervical viscera with closed opposition of the soft palate to the tongue and epiglottis" (Taylor, 1979; Swift and Emery, 1973). Also, it has been postulated that this early dependence on nasal breathing may be nature's way of insuring maximal exposure of nasal and nasopharyngeal lymphoid tissue to inspired pathogens and allergens, thus promoting the early development of the immune response (Taylor, 1979). In general, nasal airway resistance is higher in children than in adults, and their resistance remains more constant (Lacourt and Polgar, 1971). The sleeping child will show patterns of rapid eye movement (REM) sleep with increased episodes of periodic breathing with decreased amplitude accompanied by apnea (Taylor, 1979). Unilateral nasal obstruction in the sleeping child will also reflexly produce periodic major body movements, seemingly attempting to decrease the airway obstruction (Masing and Horsbach, 1969). Nasal obstruction in obligatory nasal breathers, such as infants, along with delays in body movement may lead to sufficient hypoxia to produce apnea during REM sleep (Taylor, 1979).

Choanal atresia is the most common congenital nasal anomaly, and it may be unilateral or bilateral, complete or incomplete, bony or membranous. Unilateral presentation is most common, and in 90 per cent of the cases atresia is bony rather than membranous (Skolnik et al., 1973). Newborns with bilateral, complete choanal atresia present in acute respiratory distress, as might be expected with complete nasal obstruction in an obligatory nose breather. The nasal mucosa of such children may secrete thick, glary mucus. Unilateral atresia, although producing a persistent unilateral discharge, may remain asymptomatic from an obstructive standpoint until later in life, although occlusion of the normal side by acquired disease may produce marked symptomatology, especially in infancy.

Congenital nasal deformity and obstruction may occur as part of the various mandibulofacial dysostoses (e.g., Treacher-Collins syndrome and Crouzon disease) secondary to intrauterine disturbance in the first and second branchial arch development. There may be associated hypoplasia of the external nose or nasal obstruction secondary to malar, maxillary, and palatal hypoplasia. Coronal craniosynostosis, accompanied by a brachycephalic skull with shortened anteroposterior dimensions, may result in midface contracture and subsequent nasal and nasopharyngeal airway obstruction. Cleft palate deformities also alter the structure of the nasal cavity, as they are accompanied by nasoseptal deformities (Longacre, 1968).

Congenital cysts may occur in the nasal cavity, and, depending upon their size and location, may present with degrees of nasal obstruction. Such cysts may be dermoid, nasoalveolar (incisive canal cysts), or dentigerous and mucous cysts of the floor of the nose and Jacobson's organ. Nasal discharge may be present from a draining sinus tract and may consist of epithelial debris and ectodermal gland secretions (Furstenberg, 1936; Proctor and Proctor, 1979). Nasal obstruction in the neonatal period may occur secondary to congenital cerebral herniation into the nose in the form of a meningocele (meninges alone), meningoencephalocele (meninges and a portion of the brain), or encephalocele (glial tissue with no persistent brain connection). Rhinorrhea may be present as a vasomotor response to altered airflow with a purulent component from secondary bacterial infection; however, in herniations with central connections, clear, watery cerebrospinal fluid rhinorrhea may occur spontaneously (Furstenberg, 1936; Proctor and Proctor, 1979).

Nasopharyngeal lesions may present at birth with obstruction, minimal rhinorrhea, mucopurulent crusting, and postnasal discharge secondary to mucostasis. The pharyngeal bursa (Tornwaldt's bursa) in the midline of the nasopharynx may be patulous at birth, although this is rarely noted, but later may become cystic, inflamed, and symptomatic (Proctor and Proctor, 1979; Dorrance, 1931). Other uncommon lesions of the nasopharynx include hamartomas, craniopharyngiomas, chordomas, and teratoid tumors (embryomas and epignathus). Frazer and others have even postulated that a third branchial cleft cyst could present in the fossa of Rosenmuller (Dorrance, 1931).

Inflammatory Nasal Disease

By far, the most common nasal disease in children is that due to inflammatory responses of the nasal mucosa to infectious, allergic, or toxic agents. Obstruction and rhinorrhea occur in response to the nasal vasomotor reaction, which is initiated as a specific defense mechanism to dilute the offending agents and bring specific antibodies into action. Since the majority of offending agents are airborne, the nasal vasomotor reaction is the first line of body defense. Typically the reaction works to increase the nasal surface area and increase nasal secretions, which result in increased obstruction; the total effect represents the prodromal symptomatology of many common illnesses in children (Chaps. 32 & 37).

The obstruction produced enhances the retention of the offending agents in the nose and allows for appropriate sensitization and antibody response from cells in the nasal mucosa.

In acute inflammation, vascular dilatation, along with arteriolar constriction, occurs, accompanied by exudation of protein-rich fluid and the emigration of polymorphonuclear leukocytes and monocytes into the inflamed tissue (Taylor, 1979). Immunoglobulin A(IgA), the major immunoglobulin in nasal secretions, is synthesized by plasma cells in the mucosa and nasal lymphoid tissues (Ogra and Karzon, 1970). It is produced locally to a variety of bacterial and viral antigens. It is virus-neutralizing and may be active in promoting phagocytosis and intracellular destruction of organisms by macrophages.

Following the acute inflammation, there is usually resolution or repair and regeneration if tissue necrosis has occurred. Chronic inflammation may occur with prolongation of the symptoms of rhinorrhea and obstruction.

Bacterial infection in the nose is most commonly a secondary infection, often a result of the prolongation of the vasomotor reaction with mucus stasis. Acute and chronic sinusitis may subsequently occur for the same reasons as a result of the continuity of nasal and sinus mucosa. Rhinorrhea becomes more purulent and reflects the increased inflammatory exudate. Obstruction results from the swollen turbinates and mucosa. Offending organisms include *Diplococcus, Streptococcus, Staphylococcus,* and *Haemophilus influenzae.* Pre-existing nasal problems that result in nasal obstruction commonly progress to bacterial rhinosinusitis (Taylor, 1979; Wilson, 1962).

Special mention must be made of diphtheritic rhinitis. Although uncommon today, it is a grave disease that if untreated may be fatal. Caused by *Corynebacterium diphtheriae,* acute nasal diphtheria may present with a foul, possibly bilateral nasal discharge that often excoriates the upper lip and nostrils. Chronic nasal diphtheria also occurs and is often called membranous rhinitis. A thin, glary discharge is frequently seen. Nasal obstruction is found in both diseases. The classical pale yellow or whitish membranous exudate of diphtheria may be seen covering the mucous membranes of the nose, and the nasal discharge may contain shreds of membranes along with blood (Wilson, 1962).

Other specific bacterial infections producing nasal symptoms in children include pertussis, tuberculosis, rhinoscleroma, and leprosy. The first stage of pertussis is called the catarrhal phase, with symptoms similar to those of the common cold (Wilson, 1962; Lederer, 1952).

In tuberculosis of the skin (lupus vulgaris), involvement of the nasal vestibule and subcutaneous structures of the nose, including cartilage, may be present. This is usually endogenic, with bacilli of *Mycobacterium tubercula* produced via the blood, although the organisms may be introduced externally. Obstruction and mucopurulent secretions may characterize the presence of the disease in the nose (Lederer, 1952).

Primary tuberculosis of the nose is rare, but it may occur as a result of direct contamination by bacilli in the air or from fingers and instruments or via blood and lymphatic routes. The primary granulomas formed by reaction to the bacilli may ulcerate and obstruct the nose. The symptoms of primary tuberculosis of the nose are related to the degree of nasal ulceration present. When ulceration occurs, the resultant rhinorrhea is usually mucopurulent and blood-tinged (Lederer, 1952).

Other causes of chronic granulomatous disease of the nose include rhinoscleroma and leprosy. However, the obstruction that occurs as a result of these illnesses is usually the first sign of the disease, with mucopurulent and semisanguineous discharge developing later secondary to tissue necrosis (Lederer, 1952).

Viruses may be present but remain inactive in the nasal cavities of children. Under the proper circumstances, such as cooling of the limbs, a decrease in mucosal temperature may occur, which may activate the virus and produce symptoms of infection. Viruses present extracellularly, stimulating a vasomotor reaction, and may take part in antigen-antibody reactions (Taylor, 1979).

Acute viral rhinitis or rhinonasal pharyngitis, the "common cold," is the most frequently seen cause of nasal obstruction and rhinorrhea in children. This self-limiting disease is caused by a number of different viruses, including rhinovirus (the most common), adenovirus, Coxsackie A, and Coxsackie B (Nelson, 1975). The myxoviruses, including influenza, parainfluenza, and respiratory syncytial virus (RSV), may also cause colds. Respiratory syncytial virus is especially prevalent in infants under two months of age (Taylor, 1979; Kim et al., 1969), although newborns may have a high concentration of antibodies to RSV from their mothers. The nasal obstruction resulting from infection by the respiratory syncytial virus may cause problems in these obligatory nose breathers, but such infection may help them develop active immunity to the virus.

Nasal obstruction and rhinorrhea may appear in the prodromal periods of a variety of other childhood viral illnesses, including mumps, poliomyelitis, measles (both rubella and rubeola), roseola infantum, erythema infectiosus, infectious mononucleosis, and hepatitis (Nelson, 1975).

Spirochetal disease may also occur in the nasal cavities of children. Nasal syphilis may appear in two stages. Symptoms of the early stage develop between the second and third weeks of life and resemble those of acute viral rhinitis. There is a thin, watery nasal discharge that becomes mucopurulent. Marked nasal obstruction develops with characteristic noisy breathing termed "snuffles." The later stage of congenital syphilis occurs in children three years or older and is marked by a gummatous involvement of the nose with resultant obstruction and purulent, sanguineous discharge. In acquired syphilis, the secondary stage may present with symptoms of acute rhinitis, while tertiary stage symptoms are secondary to tissue destruction (Wilson, 1962; Lederer, 1952).

In tropical environments, leishmaniasis from the protozoa Leishmania tropica may produce symptoms similar to those of syphilis (Lederer, 1952).

Fungal disease may also produce symptoms of obstruction and rhinitis but often occurs secondary to injury of the nasal mucosa (Lederer, 1952).

Parasitic diseases in children cause nasal reactions similar to those seen when an organic foreign body is present in the nose. Parasites that may infect the nose include leeches and maggots.

Allergic rhinitis is another common cause of nasal obstruction and rhinorrhea in the pediatric patient. Although there are four basic types of allergic reactions, the Type I (anaphylactic-reagin-dependent) hypersensitivity is predominant in most inhalant allergies and allergic rhinitis (Gell and Coombs, 1968). A vasomotor reaction occurs in response to an antigen (allergen)–antibody (IgE) reaction in the nasal mucosa. In genetically predisposed individuals, continuous exposure to an inhalant allergen results in the production of antibodies of the reagin type (IgE) from plasma cells in the nasal tissue. IgE becomes attached to mast cells. When additional antigen is inhaled, it is trapped by the nasal mucosa and is passed to the tissue level where the reaction occurs. Subsequently there is a release of chemical mediators (called vasoactive amines) from the mast cells. These mediators include histamine, serotonin, slow-reacting substances of anaphylaxis (SRS-A), and eosinophilic chemostatic factor (ECF-A). These in turn produce vasodilatation, increased capillary permeability, and an intense vasomotor reaction (Taylor, 1979; Stahl, 1974).

Clinically, the result of such an intense vasomotor reaction is nasal obstruction and a profuse watery rhinorrhea, often associated with sneezing and nasal pruritus. Mucostasis can occur with resultant secondary bacterial infection. The symptoms usually occur chronically with a specific periodicity.

With chronic inflammation of the mucous membrane of the nose and paranasal sinuses, manifested by hypersecretion and hyperplasia, nasal polyps can form. They represent a focal exaggeration of hyperplastic rhinosinusitis in which stromal binding of the intracellular fluid results in the formation of tissue polyps. The obstruction increases, and both watery and mucoid secretions become more abundant (Stahl, 1974).

Nasopharyngeal adenoid hyperplasia is another common cause of nasal obstruction in the pediatric patient. As part of Waldeyer's ring, the adenoids occupy a key position in the development of the immune process. Adenoids are minimal in size at birth, increase in size at one to three years of age when active immunity is being established, and may recede at puberty (Taylor, 1979; Hollender, 1959). In the nasopharynx, they are in constant contact with inspired air and are continually bathed by nasal mucus cleared from the posterior choanae by the nasal ciliary mechanism. Thus, they are continually exposed to antigens (bacterial, viral, or allergens) inhaled by the individual. They react by forming their own complement of antibodies to these antigens, and it has been postulated that "they modify the microorganisms encountered and release them or their toxins into the reticuloendothelial system of the body as an antigen stimulus for exciting active immunization" (Taylor, 1979). This activity may account for the increase in size of adenoidal tissue with increasing antigen stimulation and may explain the occurrence of adenoid hypertrophy. Nasal obstruction and chronic purulent rhinorrhea may result from such hypertrophy.

The severest form of nasal obstruction may occur in the presence of marked hypertrophy of adenoidal tissue with or without tonsil enlargement. Increased nasal airway resistance may lead to increased pulmonary resistance and alveolar hypoventilation, which is mediated by nasopulmonary reflexes. The result may be hypoxia causing secondary pulmonary vasoconstriction with increased pulmonary vascular resistance. Eventually, prolongation of these symptoms may lead to cor pulmonale (Levy et al., 1967; Luke et al., 1966).

A toxic nasal inflammatory response may occur in children in response to stimulation by a variety of external substances, both inhaled and ingested. Inhaled substances may act as chemical irritants and react with the nasal mucosa to cause defensive vasomotor responses. Such responses may be difficult to distinguish from those occurring as part of type I–mediated allergic reactions (Taylor, 1979).

Children may inhale from 10,000 to 15,000 liters of air per day, much of this polluted in our present environment. The urban pollutants may include oxides of nitrogen, carbon monoxide, ozone, aldehydes, ketones, chlorine, sulfur dioxide, ammonia, and hydrocarbons. These plus cigarette smoke may lead to increased nasal discharge as a result of the vasomotor reaction (Taylor, 1979; Taylor, 1973).

Locally applied prescribed and over-the-counter preparations containing sympatho-

mimetic agents may produce a quick nasal toxic reaction due to the rebound phenomenon of rhinitis medicamentosa. Although such a phenomenon is less commonly seen in children than in adults, it may account for persistent obstruction and rhinorrhea following a cold. Currently, adolescents are being seen with nasal problems resulting from cocaine usage. The local vasoconstriction with subsequent reactive hyperemia that occurs when cocaine is snuffed may produce mucoid rhinorrhea. Prolonged use of the drug will result in tissue necrosis, and the mucoid drainage may become more purulent (Blue, 1969; May and West, 1973).

Ingested substances that may produce rhinorrhea and symptoms of nasal obstruction include hormones, iodides, and bromides. Aspirin sensitivity may be the cause of intermittent profuse watery rhinorrhea and nasal obstruction in adolescents. Such sensitivity may be the result of the inability of some individuals to counteract the effects of prostaglandin release or inhibition (Stahl, 1974).

Traumatic Disease

The necessity to diagnose traumatic nasal disease in children early has been emphasized in recent years owing to the recognition of the importance of nasal respiration and the nasopulmonary reflex on lung physiology and the realization of the influence of abnormal nasal functions on subsequent facial, dental arch, and palatal growth. Conservative management of abnormal nasal function or deformities of the nose is still advocated, but treatment should not be delayed if "marked disturbance in function or distortion exists that also interferes with growth and facial development" (Farrior and Connolly, 1970).

Nasal obstruction is the primary symptom of external and internal nasal trauma. The severity of the effects of such obstruction are dependent upon the extent and location of the injury and the age of the child. Obstruction may be evident and total or more subtle and intermittent depending upon such factors as "paradoxical nasal obstruction" and the nasal cycle (Chap. 35).

Alteration of the normal "streamlined" flow of air through the nose may lead to turbulence and eddies in airflow and a resultant vasomotor reaction. Mucosal injury and mucostasis may lead to bacterial invasion, which could result in mucopurulent nasal discharge. This may be further aggravated by mucociliary damage. Atrophic mucosa may be the end result with further accentuation of rhinorrhea and obstructive symptoms.

With increased turbulence and stasis of air in the nose, particulate matter and allergens accumulate in the mucosa, causing more intense vasomotor, allergic, and inflammatory reactions.

This pathogenesis has led to the treatment maxim of restoring the normal streamlining of nasal respirations in order to improve alveolar ventilation and to avoid interference with nasal mucosal function, especially in children.

Nasal obstruction from traumatic deformities may occur at any age but may not be symptomatic in the young infant or neonate unless it is severe enough to cause respiratory distress in the obligatory nosebreather. Such obstruction may be obvious in cases of severe external trauma but more occult in the younger patient with only septal trauma. Marked septal deformities may occur in up to 70 per cent of newborns secondary to intrauterine or birth trauma (Kirchner, 1955; Hinderer, 1976). Such defects may be asymptomatic until adolescence when the deformity is accentuated by nasal growth. The symptomatology at that time will depend upon the age of the child and the degree and location of the deformity.

In the acute traumatic period, intermittent bleeding and the development of nasal obstruction sometime after the trauma suggests development of a septal hematoma. Subsequent throbbing pain and elevated temperature may indicate the presence of a septal abscess. Untreated, this abscess may lead to septal perforation with resultant airway turbulence and subsequent increased obstruction and rhinorrhea.

Internal trauma may be the result of the introduction of foreign materials into the nasal cavity, which would cause an intense vasomotor reaction, rhinorrhea, and obstruction. Such trauma characteristically is seen in children up to the age of three years, who frequently stuff foreign objects into their nostrils. Less frequently, foreign material enters the nose through the posterior choanae secondary to regurgitation (Lederer, 1952) (Chap. 34).

The symptoms of a foreign body in the nose are dependent upon the nature of the foreign material, its size, the number of objects, and the location of the foreign body. However, a child presenting with unilateral, purulent, fetid nasal discharge is highly suggestive of a foreign body. Symptoms of a foreign body reaction may be delayed but are earlier in onset when the foreign body is organic. Long-standing symptoms of obstruction may indicate that calcareous deposits have formed about the foreign body and that a rhinolith has developed (Lederer, 1952).

In traumatic nasal disease, special attention must be paid to determining the presence or absence of rhinorrhea of cerebrospinal fluid. Cerebrospinal fluid rhinorrhea is most commonly seen after skull trauma, although it may occur spontaneously either with or without increased intracranial pressure. It may also be a manifestation of cerebrospinal fluid otorrhea presenting in the nasal cavity via the eustachian tube. Spontaneous cerebrospinal fluid rhinorrhea has been seen with a variety of intracranial lesions, especially intrasellar tumors, but it may also be present in young infants secondary to congenital bone dehiscences (Montgomery, 1973; Briant and Snell, 1967; Kaufman, 1909; Duckert and Mathog, 1977).

The presence of cerebrospinal fluid rhinorrhea is first suggested by history and the gross nature of the nasal discharge. A clear, salty, often unilateral drainage from the nose, especially after a head injury, is highly suggestive of cerebrospinal fluid rhinorrhea. When such fluid flows profusely from the nose and when the drainage increases in quantity with changes in position of the head, during a Valsalva maneuver, and with jugular compression, the possibility that the rhinorrhea is cerebrospinal fluid is significant. A rapid method of analyzing such nasal drainage is to test it with glucose oxidase-impregnated test sticks. However, since these sticks will react to as little as 10 mg per 100 ml of glucose, they may give false positive reactions due to the presence of lacrimal secretions or the products of an allergic reaction or infectious rhinosinusitis in the nasal secretions. A negative test is highly significant in ruling out the presence of cerebrospinal fluid rhinorrhea, while a strongly positive reaction to nasal secretions shows the presence of 50 mg per 100 ml or more of glucose, indicating that the presence of cerebrospinal fluid in the nasal discharge is quite likely (Kaufman,

1909). If sufficient fluid can be collected, biochemical analysis for the presence of protein, glucose, and electrolytes will confirm the diagnosis of cerebrospinal fluid rhinorrhea. Demonstration of the area of the fistula is best achieved by evaluating the results of radiography, tomography, placement of an intrathecal tracer with intranasal pledgets, and cisternography (Duckert and Mathog, 1977).

Neoplastic Disease

Primary neoplasms of the nasal cavity are rare; they account for less than 0.3 per cent of tumors of the body (Axtell et al., 1972). When they do occur, they may be of ectodermal, mesodermal, neurogenic, or odontogenic origin (Bortnick, 1973). Any tumor that occurs in adults may also occur in children, but a few are more commonly seen in and, indeed, tend to be specific to the pediatric patient (Chap. 36).

Nasal obstruction and rhinorrhea are the two most common symptoms of nasal tumors. These symptoms are related to the increasing size of the neoplastic mass and the effect of the tumor on the nasal mucosa. In neoplasms primary to the nasal cavity, symptomatology arises early, but symptoms are delayed in tumors of the nasopharynx and sinuses until nasal cavity invasion occurs (Bortnick, 1973).

Rhinorrhea may occur as a typical vasomotor reaction to nasal airway invasion. Such nasal discharge may become purulent with stasis and secondary infection, sanguineous with tissue necrosis, and eventually may contain cerebrospinal fluid as a result of extension of the pathologic lesion into the cranial cavity. The triad of symptoms, including nasal obstruction, rhinorrhea, and epistaxis, is common in neoplasms. Nasal polyposis may also arise as a secondary sign of nasal neoplasm.

Juvenile nasopharyngeal angiofibromas are specific to the adolescent male with symptoms usually arising between seven and 17 years of age, at an average age of 14. The symptoms are progressive, partial unilateral obstruction followed by progressive obstruction of the involved side and then partial obstruction on the opposite side. Epistaxis attacks occur with increasing frequency along with pathologic symptoms in adjacent structures (Patterson, 1965; Patterson, 1973).

Olfactory neuroblastoma is another uncommon neoplasm but one that frequently presents in the pediatric patient. Originating primarily in the area of the olfactory mucosa, it may not produce signs of obstruction until it has grown to considerable size. Epistaxis due to tissue destruction is the usual presenting symptom (Cantrell et al., 1977; Schenck and Ogura, 1972; Ogura and Schenck, 1973). In children, neoplasms of the hematopoietic system rarely present in the nasal cavity, but when they do they are usually secondary to metastatic invasion from leukemic disease (Sanford and Becker, 1967).

Metabolic Disease in the Nasal Cavity

Nasal symptoms of obstruction and rhinorrhea may be important in the early diagnosis of cystic fibrosis or mucoviscidosis. In mucoviscidosis, an inherited systemic disease in which the alimentary and respiratory tracts are involved, abnormally viscid mucus is produced. Histologically the nasal submucosal glands are hypoplastic and appear to be dilated with eosinophilic staining material. Nasal mucous secretions exhibit marked adhesiveness and a changed water-binding capacity and permeability related to an increased calcium concentration (Gharib et al., 1964). The viscid, tenacious mucus and nasal obstruction characteristic of mucoviscidosis leads to stasis and secondary infection by *Staphylococcus aureus, Pseudomonas, Streptococcus viridans, Haemophilus influenzae,* or *Neisseria catarrhalis.* Nasal polyps frequently occur in association with the problems just mentioned (Baker and Smith, 1970).

The nasal obstruction of mucoviscidosis is produced by (1) the thick, tenacious mucus; (2) the chronic, thickened nasal mucosa; and (3) nasal polyps. Chronic sinusitis may aggravate the situation, as upward of 90 per cent of children with cystic fibrosis have evidence of severe opacification of the sinuses on radiographic examination (Baker and Smith, 1970; Gharib et al., 1964). The result is that a child presenting with thick, foul-smelling, purulent, bilateral nasal secretions, chronic nasal obstruction, nasal polyps, and a broad nasal bridge must be considered to have mucoviscidosis until proved otherwise.

In other metabolic diseases, obstruction and rhinorrhea are produced as a result of modification of the normal vasomotor reaction. The effects of endogenous hormones on nasal mucosa have been discussed earlier. Exogenous hormones may have a similar effect on the vasomotor reaction (Schreiber, 1973).

Calcium and magnesium potentiate the action of acetylcholinesterase in nasal mucosa, and the former will modify the permeability of the basement membrane. Deficiencies of these elements may intensify the vasomotor reaction, while exogenous calcium has been used in the past to alleviate symptoms of vasomotor rhinitis (Taylor, 1973, 1979).

In hypothyroid states, low ionic calcium levels will be seen and can modify the vasomotor reaction. In hyperthyroidism, thyroxin, through its influence on lung dynamics, may hypothalamically influence the nasal mucosa and produce symptoms of vasomotor rhinitis (Taylor, 1979; May and West, 1973).

Disorders in carbohydrate metabolism often lead to chronic nasal infection in children. This may be the result of impairment in the system by which carbohydrate metabolism releases antibodies from cells in the nasal mucosa (Taylor, 1979; May and West, 1973).

In immune deficiency diseases, there is a general increased incidence of infections. However, with isolated IgA deficiency, these infections are mostly confined to the upper respiratory tract. In response to pathogens, a more intense and prolonged vasomotor reaction will be seen as the lack of IgA allows the invasion of the nasal mucosa by the pathogens (Taylor, 1979).

Idiopathic Nasal Disease

Among nasal diseases of unknown etiology, there are two that may present in the pediatric patient with characteristic symptoms of obstruction and rhinorrhea.

Atrophic rhinitis (ozena, rhinitis fetida, rhinitis crustosa) is a chronic nasal disease with onset in childhood that features progressive atrophy of nasal mucosa and underlying bone. The presenting symptoms are obstruction of the nasal airway due to enlargement of the nasal cavity and disturbance of normal streamline airflow. Characteristically, the nasal mucosa is foul-smelling, green, and crusted, although there is minimal purulent discharge. The secretions are characteristically composed of exfoliated nasal mucosal

cells. Vitamin, iron, endocrine, and nutritional deficiencies have been implicated. The principal organisms that are responsible for the purulence of the secretions are *Klebsiella ozaenae*, a form of *Corynebacterium diphtheriae*, and the Perez-Hofer bacillus (Wilson, 1962; Goodman and DeSouza, 1973).

Chronic catarrhal rhinitis is a chronic nasal disease of children occurring most commonly in the lower socioeconomic groups. This disease is characterized by chronic mucopurulent discharge. It tends to resolve spontaneously at puberty and has been felt to be a basement membrane disease, metabolic in origin with an endocrine defect as its underlying etiology (Taylor, 1961a, 1979; Wilson, 1962).

REFERENCES

Arbour, P. L., and Kern, E. B. 1975. Paradoxical nasal obstruction. Can. J. Otolaryngol., *4*:333.

Axtell, L. M., Cutter, S. J., and Meyers, M. H. 1972. End results in cancer. Report no. 4. Washington, D.C., U.S. Dept. of Health, Education and Welfare, Public Health Service, N.I.H., 85–88.

Baker, D. C., and Smith, J. T. 1970. Nasal symptoms of mucoviscidosis. Otolaryngol. Clin. North Am., *3*:257–264.

Biber, J. J. 1949. Proboscis lateralis: Rare malformation of nose; its genesis and treatment. J. Laryngol. Otol., *63*:734–741.

Bickmore, J. T., and Marshall, M. L. 1976. Cytology in nasal secretions: Further diagnostic help. Laryngoscope, *86*:516.

Blue, J. A. 1969. Over-medication of nasal mucosa. Mod. Med., *37*:90.

Bortnick, E. 1973. Neoplasms of the nasal cavity. Otolaryngol. Clin. North Am., *6*:801.

Briant, T. D. R., and Snell, D. 1967. Diagnosis of cerebrospinal rhinorrhea and the rhinologic approach to its repair. Laryngoscope, *77*:1390–1409.

Bridger, G. P. 1970. Physiology of the nasal valve. Arch. Otolaryngol., *92*:543–553.

Bridger, G. P., and Proctor, D. F. 1970. Maximum nasal inspiratory flow and nasal resistance. Ann. Otol. Rhinol. Laryngol. *79*:481–489.

Bryan, M. P., and Bryan, W. T. K. 1969. Cytologic and cytochemical aspects of ciliated epithelium in differentiation of nasal inflammatory diseases. Acta Cytol., *13*:515.

Bryan, W. T. K., and Bryan, M. P. 1959. Cytologic diagnosis in otolaryngology. Trans. Am. Acad. Ophthalmol. Otolaryngol., *63*:597–612.

Cantrell, R. W., Ghorayeb, B. Y., and Fitz-Hugh, G. S. 1977. Esthesioneuroblastoma: Diagnosis and treatment. Ann. Otol. Rhinol. Laryngol., *86*:760–765.

Celsus, A. C. *De Medicina,* trans. Spencer, W. G.

Chladek, V., Pihrt, J., and Engler, V. 1972. Vasomotor reactions in nasal mucosa in adolescents. C.S. Hyg., *17*:241.

Cottle, M. H. 1968. Rhino-manometry: An aid in physical diagnosis. Int. Rhinol., *6*:7–26.

Dorland's Illustrated Medical Dictionary, 25th ed. Philadelphia, W. B. Saunders Co., 1974.

Dorrance, G. M. 1931. The so-called bursa pharyngea in man. Arch. Otolaryngol., 13:187–224.

Duckert, L. G., and Mathog, R. H. 1977. Diagnosis in persistent cerebrospinal fluid fistulas. Laryngoscope, 87:18–25.

Farrior, R. T., and Connolly, M. E. 1970. Septorhinoplasty in children. Otolaryngol. Clin. North Am., 3:345.

Frazer, J. E. 1940. A Manual of Embryology, 2nd ed. London, Bailliere, Tindall and Cox.

Furstenberg, A. C. 1936. A Clinical and Pathological Study of Tumors and Cysts of the Nose, Pharynx, Mouth and Neck of Teratological Origin. Ann Arbor, Edward Brothers.

Galen, C. 1916. On the Natural Faculties, trans. Brock, A. J. London, W. Heinemann Ltd.

Gell, P. G. H., and Coombs, R. R. A. 1968. Clinical Aspects of Immunology, 2nd ed. Philadelphia, F. A. Davis Co.

Gharib, R., Allen, R. P., Joos, H. A., et al. 1964. Paranasal sinuses in cystic fibrosis. Am. J. Dis. Child., 108:499.

Goodman, W. S., DeSouza, F. M. 1973. Atrophic rhinitis. Otolaryngol. Clin. North Am., 6:773–782.

Hinderer, K. H. 1976. Nasal problems in children. Pediatr. Ann., 52:499.

Hippocrates The Aphorisms, trans. Jones, W. H. S., and Withington, E. T. 1922. London, W. Heinemann Ltd.

Hollender, A. R. 1959. The lympoid tissue of the nasopharynx. Laryngoscope, 69:529.

Holmes, T. H., Goodell, H., Wolf, S., et al. 1950. The Nose: An experimental study of the reactions within the nose in human subjects during varying life experiences. Springfield, IL, Charles C Thomas.

Kaufman, H. H. 1909. Non-traumatic cerebrospinal fluid rhinorrhea. Arch. Neurol., 21:59.

Kern, E. B. 1973. Rhinomanometry. Otolaryngol. Clin. North Am., 6(3):863–873.

Kim, H. W., Bellanti, J. A., Arrobio, J. O., et al. 1969. Respiratory syncytial virus neutralizing activity in nasal secretions following natural infection. Proc. Soc. Exp. Biol. Med., 131:658.

Kirchner, J. A. 1955. Traumatic nasal deformity in the newborn. Arch. Otolaryngol., 62:139.

Lacourt, G., and Polgar, G. 1971. Interaction between nasal and pulmonary resistance in newborn infants. J. Appl. Physiol., 30:870–3.

Lederer, F. L. 1952. Diseases of the Ear, Nose and Throat, 6th ed. Philadelphia, F. A. Davis Co.

Levy, A. M., Tabakin, B. S., and Hanson, J. S. 1967. Hypertrophied adenoids causing pulmonary hypertension and severe congestive heart failure. N. Engl. J. Med., 277:506.

Longacre, J. J. 1968. Craniofacial Anomalies: Pathogenesis and Repair. Philadelphia, J. B. Lippincott Co.

Lorin, M. I., Pureza, F. G., Irwin, D. M., et al. 1976. Composition of nasal secretions with cystic fibrosis. J. Lab. Clin. Med., 88:114–17.

Luke, M. J., Mehrizi, A., Folger, G. M., Jr., et al. 1966. Chronic nasal obstruction as a cause of cardiomegaly, cor pulmonale and pulmonary edema. Pediatrics, 37:762.

Masing, H., Horbasch, G. 1969. The influence of the nose on the sleeping habits of infants. Int. Rhinol., 7:41.

May, M., and West, J. W. 1973. The stuffy nose. Otolaryngol. Clin. North Am., 6:655.

Montgomery, W. W. 1973. Cerebrospinal fluid rhinorrhea. Otolaryngol. Clin. North Am., 6:757.

Mortimer, H., Wright, R. P., Bachman, C., et al. 1936. Effect of estogenic hormones on nasal mucosa of monkeys. Proc. Soc. Exp. Biol. Med., 34:535.

Nelson, W. E. 1975. Textbook of Pediatrics, 10th ed. Philadelphia. W. B. Saunders Co.

Ogra, P. L., and Karzon, D. T. 1970. The role of immunoglobulins in the mechanism of mucosal immunity to virus infection. Pediatr. Clin. North Am., 17(2): 385.

Ogura, J. H., and Harvey, J. E. 1971. Nasopulmonary mechanics — experimental evidence of the influence of the upper airway upon the lower. Acta Otolaryngol., 71:123.

Ogura, J. H., and Nelson, J. R. 1968. Nasal surgery: Physiologic considerations of nasal obstruction. Arch. Otolaryngol., 88:288.

Ogura, J. H., Dammkuehler, R., and Nelson, J. R. 1966. Nasal obstruction and the mechanics of breathing. Arch. Otolaryngol., 83:135.

Ogura, J. H., Nelson, J. R., Dammkuehler, R., et al. 1964. Experimental observations of the relationships between upper airway obstruction and pulmonary function. Ann. Otol. Rhinol. Laryngol., 73:381.

Ogura, J. H., Nelson, J. R., Suemitsu, M., et al. 1973. Relationship between pulmonary resistance and changes in arterial blood gas tension in dogs with nasal obstruction and partial laryngeal obstruction. Ann. Otol. Rhinol. Laryngol., 82:668.

Ogura, J. H., and Schenck, N. L. 1973. Unusual nasal tumors. Otolaryngol. Clin. North Am., 6:813–837.

Ogura, J. H., Unno, T., and Nelson, J. R. 1968. Baseline values in pulmonary mechanics for physiologic surgery of the nose: Preliminary report. Ann. Otol. Rhinol. Laryngol., 77:367.

Ohnishi, T., and Ogura, J. H. 1969. Partitioning of pulmonary resistance in the dog. Laryngoscope, 79:1847.

Ohnishi, T., Ogura, H. H., and Nelson, J. R. 1972. Effects of nasal obstruction upon the mechanics of the lung in the dog. Laryngoscope, 82:712.

Parkes, A. S., and Zuckerman, S. 1931. Menstrual cycle of primates: II. Some effects of oestin on baboons and macaques. J. Anthropol., 65:272.

Patterson, C. N. 1965. Juvenile nasopharyngeal angiofibroma. Arch. Otolaryngol., 81:270–277.

Patterson, C. N. 1973. Juvenile nasopharyngeal angiofibroma. Otolaryngol. Clin. North Am., 6:839.

Proctor, B., and Proctor, C. 1979. Congenital lesions of the head and neck. Otolaryngol. Clin. North Am., 3(2):221–248.

Sanford, D. M., and Becker, G. D. 1967. Acute leukemia presenting as nasal obstruction. Arch. Otolaryngol., 85:102–104.

Schenk, N. L., and Ogura, J. H. 1972. Esthesioneuroblastoma: An enigma in diagnosis, a dilemma in treatment. Arch. Otolaryngol., 96:322–324.

De Catarrhis Libri, Vol. I (cited by Schaeffer, 1932).

Schreiber, U. 1973. Vasomotor rhinitis with hormonal contraception. H. N. O. 21:180.

Sercer, A. 1930. Researches on the reflex influencing of each lung from its corresponding nasal cavity. Acta Otolaryngol., 14:99.

Skolnik, E. M., Kotler, R., and Hanna, W. A. 1973.

Choanal atresia. Otolaryngol. Clin. North Am., 6(3):83.

Stahl, R. H. 1974. Allergic disorders of the nose and paranasal sinuses. Otolaryngol. Clin. North Am., 7:703.

Stoksted, P. 1952. The physiologic cycle of the nose under normal and pathologic conditions. Acta Otolaryngol., 42:175.

Swift, P. G., and Emery, J. L. 1973. Clinical observations on response to nasal occlusion in infancy. Arch. Dis. Child., 48:947–951.

Taylor, M. 1961a. Catarrhal rhinitis in children. Proc. R. Soc. Med., 54:1961.

Taylor, M. 1961b. An experimental study of the influence of the endocrine system on nasal respiratory mucosa. J. Laryngol. Otol., 75:972.

Taylor, M. 1973. The nasal vasomotor reaction. Otolaryngol. Clin. North Am., 6:645.

Taylor, M. 1974. The origin and function of nasal mucus. Laryngoscope, 84:612–636.

Taylor, M. 1979. Physiology of the nose, paranasal sinuses and nasopharynx. In English, G. M. (Ed.) Otolaryngology, Vol. 2, Ch. 3N. Hagerstown, Md., Harper & Row.

von Dishoeck, H. A. E. 1942. Inspiratory nasal resistance. Acta Otolaryngol., 30:31–39.

von Dishoeck, H. A. E. 1965. The part of the valve and the turbinate in total nasal resistance. Int. Rhinol., 3:19–26.

Wilson, T. G. 1962. Diseases of the Ear, Nose and Throat in Children, 2nd ed., ch. 10. London, W. Heinemann Ltd.

Wise, T. A. 1898. Arthava Veda Samhita. In Commentary on the Hindu System of Medicine. Calcutta. (cited by Mackenzie).

Chapter 27

EPISTAXIS

M. C. Culbertson, Jr., M.D.

The respiratory system is widely discussed in the writings of ancient philosophers and medical practitioners; only the poorly understood vascular system receives more attention from these early writers. Prehippocratic references to rhinologic subjects include such topics as removal of foreign bodies from the respiratory passages, pain of inflammatory diseases, and the inconvenience of catarrhs. The "Corpus Hippocraticum" frequently mentions epistaxis specifically.

Although epistaxis may occur at any age, at any time, and in any season, nosebleed is a common complaint in the pediatric population and occurs more frequently in the winter months. In a major study of 1734 patients, 175 cases of epistaxis were recorded in the worst winter month and 110 cases occurred in July (Juselius, 1974). A nosebleed may result from nasal trauma at birth or in infancy, but children aged 2 to 10 years are more commonly affected than are infants.

Epistaxis in children often produces parental concern out of proportion to the actual danger to the child, although the bleeding may herald a serious illness, such as a nasopharyngeal angiofibroma or leukemia. Usually epistaxis is associated with no more than a mild irritation or excoriation of the mucosa. The alert physician, when procuring a history and conducting an examination of the nose while firmly quieting the patient and relatives, can assess the seriousness of the episode of bleeding.

ANATOMY

In children the bleeding site is almost always the anterior portion of the nose, usually on the septum in Little's area or adjacent to this site. The nose receives terminal branches from both the internal and external carotid artery systems (Figs. 27–1 and 27–2). The internal carotid artery supplies blood to the nose through the anterior and posterior ethmoidal arteries, which arise in the posterior orbit from the ophthalmic artery. The anterior ethmoidal artery, the larger of the two, supplies the lateral wall of the nose, the nasal septum, and the nasal tip; and the posterior ethmoidal artery supplies the posterior lateral wall of the nose, including the superior turbinate and the superior portion of the septum. The sphenopalatine artery, which is a branch of the internal maxillary artery, is the major terminal artery of the external carotid artery system supplying the nose. The major branch enters the nose through the sphenopalatine foramen, and another exits the greater palatine foramen to the palate and into the nose through the incisive canal. The sphenopalatine artery supplies the posterior septum and the inferior and middle turbinate area of the lateral nasal wall. The anterior portion of the upper lip is supplied by a branch of the labial artery. These all coalesce in an area of the septum known as Kiesselbach's plexus. The nasal epithelium especially that of the cartilaginous septum, has little cushioning submucosal tissue so that vessels are offered very little protection, and contraction of an injured vessel to close its lumen may be quite limited owing to the lack of an elastic submucosal layer.

Protruding as it does, the nose is a common target for traumatic injury, and by its very function the nasal mucosa is traumatized. In a distance of about 7 cm the nose conditions inspired air. The air entering the nose may be

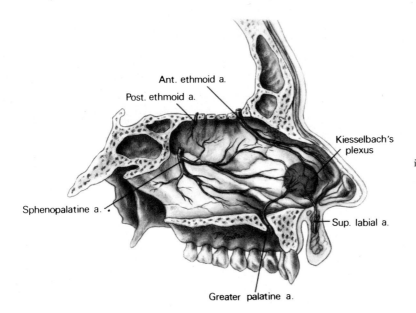

Figure 27–1 Arteries supplying the nasal septum.

−20° C with a relative humidity of 20 per cent, and when the air reaches the posterior pharynx it is almost free of particulate matter, its temperature is about 37° C, and its relative humidity is approximately 100 per cent (Chaps. 23 & 24).

ETIOLOGY

Inflammation

As noted in Table 27–1, inflammation or infection of the upper respiratory tract is probably the most common cause of epistaxis. Increased vascularity of the nasal mucosa and crusting in the anterior nares occur during an upper respiratory infection, so it is not surprising that childhood exanthems are associated with epistaxis. In fact, epistaxis is a common accompaniment to rubella and varicella (Chap. 32).

Children with nasal allergies experience nasal congestion, discharge, and at times superimposed infections of the nose. In addition, occasionally epistaxis will accompany allergic rhinitis (Chap. 37).

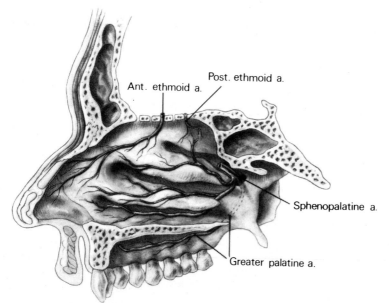

Figure 27–2 Arterial supply of the lateral wall of the nasal cavity.

Table 27–1 ETIOLOGY OF EPISTAXIS
IN CHILDREN

I. Common causes
  A. Inflammation
    1. Upper respiratory infections
      a. Viral
      b. Bacterial
    2. Childhood exanthems
    3. Rheumatic fever
  B. Trauma
    1. Dry air
    2. Injury, external, with or without fracture
    3. Patient-induced (nose picking)
    4. Foreign body
  C. Allergic rhinitis with or without accompanying inflammation
II. Uncommon causes
  A. Alterations of intravascular factors of hemostasis
    1. Platelet abnormalities
      a. Idiopathic thrombocytopenic purpura (quantitative change in platelets)
      b. Thrombocytopathic purpuras (qualitative change in the platelets, such as occurs with von Willebrand disease or Glanzmann thrombasthenia)
    2. Coagulation defects
      a. Hemophilia A and B (Christmas disease)
      b. Bleeding caused by anticoagulant drugs such as coumarin
  B. Hypertension (not in the author's experience)
  C. Idiopathic
  D. Inflammatory
    1. Lethal midline granuloma
    2. Bacterial granuloma
  E. Neoplasms
    1. Benign
      a. Juvenile nasopharyngeal angiofibroma
      b. Polyps
      c. Meningocele and meningomyelocele
    2. Malignant leukemias
  F. Parasite in nasal or nasopharyngeal space
  G. Structural
    1. Deviation of the septum
    2. Adhesions between septum and lateral nasal wall
  H. Trauma
    1. Postsurgical bleeding
    2. Chemical and caustic agents

Trauma

Trauma to the nose is a principal cause of epistaxis in children and adults. Dry air, as well as physical injury, are sources of nasal trauma. In fact, forced-air central heating systems reduce the humidity in our homes to levels below those of our driest deserts, and excessive cooling of air can produce the same lowering of relative humidity. Our modern lifestyle could be more a source of nasal trauma than actual physical injury.

Foreign bodies in the nose are discussed fully in Chapter 34. Epistaxis is a common presenting symptom in cases of foreign body obstruction of the nose, and attempts to remove the foreign body without proper patient preparation and restraint, illumination, and adequate instrumentation can result in more severe nasal bleeding (Chap. 35).

Although nasal surgery in children is not common, bleeding can occur after surgery. Surgical procedures in contiguous areas, including adenoidectomy and dacryocystorhinostomy, can result in epistaxis postoperatively (Brenner, 1974).

Trauma to the face and nose with or without nasal bone fracture is a common cause of epistaxis. However, it is important to beware of repeated epistaxis following head trauma without visual evidence of damage to the nose or an obvious bleeding site (Pathak, 1972), as this may indicate more extensive damage of non-nasal structures, requiring more aggressive management.

Barotrauma of the paranasal sinuses, septal perforations, and exposure of the nose to chemicals and caustics, although uncommon, can all cause nasal bleeding. Parasites of the nasal cavity are very rarely seen in this country, but in Southeast Asia their presence in the nose is a common cause of epistaxis. Granulomas of the nose are seldom encountered in pediatric patients (Roback, et al., 1969), but when they are present the presenting symptom is usually epistaxis. Rare inflammatory conditions that cause nosebleeds are leprosy, atrophic rhinitis, tuberculosis, glanders, and certain fungus infections such as rhinosporidiosis.

Tumors

Tumors of the nose occur more commonly in adults than in children, but nasal growths in all age groups cause epistaxis and nasal obstruction. Meningoceles, malignant tumors, papillomata, and nasal polyps can cause nosebleeds (Chap. 36).

Juvenile nasopharyngeal angiofibroma is an uncommon neoplasm of the nasopharynx found almost exclusively in adolescent males. The most frequent symptom (occurring in 86 per cent of cases) is epistaxis. This is generally recurrent and brisk, but only rarely life-threatening. Nasal obstruction is the second most common symptom (occurring in 80 per cent of patients) (Jafek, 1978). Fewer than 25 per cent of patients with juvenile nasopharyngeal angiofibroma have associated rhinorrhea, conductive hearing loss, or neurologic deficits (as vision changes). Upon examination the tumor in the nasopharynx and nasal cavity is obvious. It is felt that this neoplasm may originate in the vascular stroma of the connective tissue elements at the base of the sphenoid and the pterygoid prominences, and that it might begin to regress around age 20. However, no reference in the recent literature has suggested waiting for the tumor to regress. Because of its locally destructive nature, its nearness to intracranial structures, and its known tendency to extend laterally and intracranially, this tumor should be treated aggressively and without delay. In fact, 20 per cent of these tumors are reported to have extended intracranially, and 80 per cent have extended into the sphenoid sinus by the time of discovery (Jafek et al., 1973).

Most authors do not recommend obtaining a biopsy from this tumor; in fact, there are several reports of "massive hemorrhage" resulting from surgery to obtain a biopsy specimen or even from palpation of the tumor. Plane radiographic films of the skull will show the soft tissue mass in the nasopharynx. On the skull views, evidence of erosion of the posterior wall of the antrum, the hard palate, the sphenoid body, and the superior orbital fissure and enlargement of the pterygomaxillary space may indicate extension of the tumor. Extension of the tumor into the sphenoid sinus is also easily seen by plane radiographs. Angiography with the subtraction technique of both the internal and external carotid systems is essential in outlining the extent of the tumor and is even helpful in its diagnosis. Occasionally vertebral arteriography and intracranial venography (to assess the status of the cavernous sinus) may be indicated. Preoperative occlusion of the arterial blood supply and hormonal therapy (for males only) with diethylstilbesterol may also be considered.

Surgical excision is the treatment of choice of the great majority of physicians who treat this neoplasm, although one author (Briant et al., 1970) reported radiation as his only form of treatment. Owens' transpalatal approach, described by Jafek (1978) is used to approach the tumor. If an extension laterally cannot be extirpated with the nasopharyngeal tumor mass, a lateral extension of the palate incision or an additional gingivobuccal incision is made. Occasionally a lateral extension may require an external incision to remove it, but even then the tumor should be removed as one piece whenever possible.

Management of a neoplasm with intracranial extension requires a surgical team approach by the otolaryngologist and the neurosurgeon. The extracranial tumor should be removed first and then, through a separate surgical approach, the intracranial neoplasm should be explored and resected. Three months postoperatively, angiography should be repeated to identify any residual neoplasm, which is then treated with radiation therapy. In such cases, 3000 to 4000 rads with carefully defined ports is used. These patients must be followed through maturity to detect and treat early any further recurrences of the tumor.

Other (Rare) Causes

Changes in the blood vessels that occur with hereditary hemorrhagic telangiectasia result in epistaxis. In a series of 80 patients studied from 1962 through 1976, the median age of onset of this familial disease was 17 years, and the earliest incidence of associated epistaxis occurred at two years of age (Letson and Birck, 1973).

Hypertension is a possible cause of epistaxis, and in older adult patients the severity of the epistaxis may be related to the degree of hypertension.

Epistaxis may be a manifestation of a bleeding disorder. However, one author concluded that, "If on careful history and physical examination and family history, epistaxis proves to be the only manifestation of bleeding, it is most likely that the child does not have an underlying hemorrhagic disorder" (Schulman, 1959).

One must remember to include the ingestion of drugs, especially aspirin, as a possible cause of epistaxis.

Other very rare causes of epistaxis in childhood include spontaneous intracavernous (infraclinoid) aneurysm of the internal carotid artery, aneurysm of the vein of Galen communicating with dilated arterioles derived from the posterior cerebral arteries, and primary idiopathic thrombocytopenic purpura. Aplastic anemia associated with drugs and other toxic agents and leukemias are other rare causes of epistaxis.

MANAGEMENT

Proper management of the child who presents with nosebleed begins with the attitude toward the child and his relatives. A quick assessment of the patient's general condition (the degree of blood loss) and history from the parents or the child (the circumstances surrounding the onset, cause, past history of epistaxis, and family history) will help to reassure all parties (Stool and Kemper, 1969).

At the time of the initial visit and treatment of the epistaxis or later during follow-up treatment, hematologic evaluation should be considered. This may involve simple laboratory procedures such as complete blood count (cbc), prothrombin time, and partial thromboplastin time. Consultation with the child's primary physician or even consideration of referral to a pediatric hematologist for further studies is possible. These further steps depend on the cause and the course of the nosebleed in the past and as the child is treated.

Many times the bleeding has stopped by the time the physician sees the child, but these patients should still be examined carefully. If the area from which the bleeding occurred is obvious and it appears that active bleeding could recur, cauterization and packing might be indicated.

Active bleeding from the anterior nose can often be stopped by the application of pressure of the thumb and index finger over the soft parts of the nose for about five minutes. If bleeding persists, the nose should carefully be cleaned of blood clots, using suction with adequate illumination (the magnification of the Zeiss otologic microscope is often helpful) (Fig. 27–3) and irrigated with a weak vasoconstrictor such as .125 per cent neosynephrine isotonic. After such cleansing, examination

usually reveals bleeding in or around Kiesselbach's plexus area on one side. A cotton pledget dampened with 4 per cent xylocaine, with or without a vasoconstrictor such as epinephrine 1:10,000, may be placed against the bleeding point and left in place with pressure applied for five minutes. Immobilization of the patient and good illumination of the bleeding area during these procedures are essential.

If it appears that the bleeding will recur after these measures have been taken, the offending vessel may be cauterized. In children electrocautery is usually not recommended. A silver nitrate stick may be used, but for very small nares a small-diameter metal applicator sparingly tipped with cotton dipped in trichloroacetic acid is usually safer. Care must be used to place the damp cotton wisp only on the specific area. Petrolatum can be used to cover adjacent mucosa and skin to localize the cauterized area. Repeated cauterizations may be complicated by septal perforations.

In some patients, the bleeding point cannot be found, and simple pressure or cauterization will not control the bleeding. In these children, packing of one or both sides of the nose should be the next step.

For most children, sedation or, on occasion, general anesthesia is necessary for complete examination, reduction of a fracture, or for packing procedures. Chloral hydrate (Noctec) has been found to be superior to barbiturates, tranquilizers, or narcotics, used singly or in combination, for this purpose. The initial oral dose given is 40 mg per kg of body weight, and 15 to 20 mg per kg may be

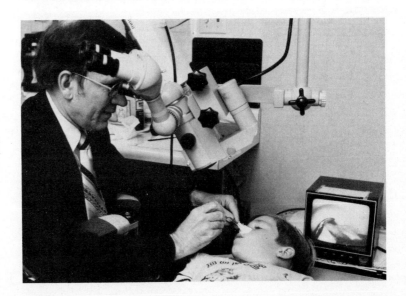

Figure 27–3 Use of the Zeiss otomicroscope for illumination and magnification of the bleeding site.

added in 30 to 40 minutes if the child is not tranquil.

The rare cases in which nasal packing is necessary to control epistaxis occur as the result of trauma, with or without a fracture, or in children with blood dyscrasias. When nasal packing must be done, long-fiber or rayon cotton soaked in a mild vasoconstrictor can be fashioned into any length or width pack and placed in the nasal cavity (Fig. 27–4). If the cotton is to be left for any period of time, it should be impregnated with an antibiotic ointment. Gauze can be placed more tightly in the nasal space than can cotton as it is packed in layers from the anterior opening of the nose posteriorly to the posterior border of the middle turbinate, and from the floor of the nose to the superior extent of the nasal vault. Oxidized regenerated cellulose gauze or cotton (Oxycel) may be put in the area of active bleeding and then supported. If this absorbable material is used alone it need not be removed later. Packing of other material is usually removed within three days and, even when the nose has not been infected, the patient is given an antibiotic prophylactically.

If packing of both anterior nasal chambers does not suffice to stop the bleeding, then a posterior pack may be used. This may consist of a carefully inflated Foley catheter, which should be inflated with a measured amount of liquid outside the nose to judge its size before insertion. Or one of the specially prepared postnasal balloons (such as the Gotts-

chalk Nasostat) may be used for the posterior portion of the combined anterior and posterior packing. These newly designed, prefabricated, latex rubber balloons may be obtained in small sizes. The use of a tonsil–adenoid hemostatic sponge passed through the mouth to the nasopharynx with ties through one nostril to the anterior nares is illustrated in Figure 27–5. The posterior pack provides a stable mass against which the carefully placed anterior packing may provide pressure to stop the bleeding (Fig. 27–6). The nasal packing should be impregnated with an antibiotic ointment (without steroids), and antibiotics should be administered parenterally or orally while the packs are in place and for a few days after removal of the packs.

Careful examination of the nasal cavity under general anesthesia using the Zeiss otomicroscope (lowest power) and suction can help to isolate a bleeding point otherwise inaccessible to view (Fig. 27–3). Bleeding from an ostium of the maxillary antrum, a vessel hidden by the inferior turbinate, or one high in the vault can better be identified and treated in this manner. Nasal bleeding that persists despite the treatment described may come from a sinus cavity. In these cases further studies to exclude the possibility of bleeding from the sinuses must include radiographic evaluation.

The measures just discussed will almost always be adequate to control bleeding in the majority of children with epistaxis. Bleeding from extensive fractures, tumors, telangiecta-

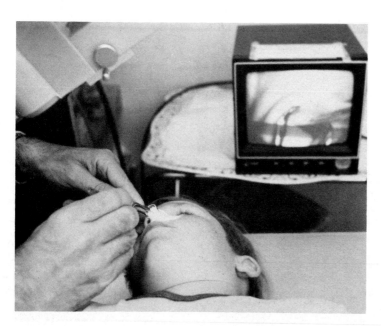

Figure 27–4 Placing of long-fiber cotton pack in nasal cavity.

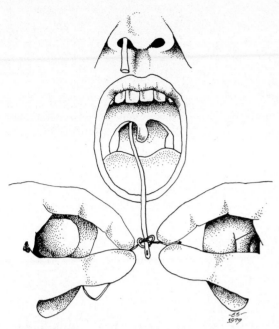

Figure 27–5 Insertion into the nasopharynx of the adenoid hemostatic sponge. A rubber catheter is threaded through the nasal cavity into the pharynx and out of the mouth. The double string on the sponge is tied to the catheter and drawn retrograde through the nose and tied securely but with little pressure over a flexible tube.

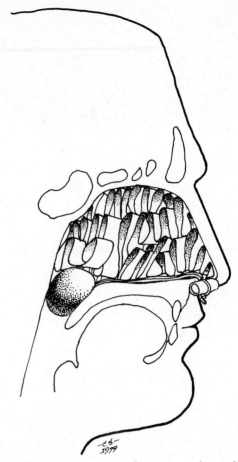

Figure 27–6 Posterior and anterior packs in place. The string holding the posterior pack is illustrated.

sia, surgical procedures, and bleeding disorders can be exceptions.

Nasal septal surgery may be necessary to stop bleeding in rare instances. Recently we have recognized that septoplasty with replacement of cartilage is an acceptable procedure even in preadolescent patients. Repair of a septum that blocks the airway and also is the cause of recurrent nasal bleeding is an effective and reasonable treatment.

Arterial ligation for epistaxis in children is very rarely indicated (Chandler and Serrins, 1965). For anterior and superior bleeding, occlusion of the anterior and posterior ethmoidal arteries is employed. For bleeding arising from the posterior portion of the nose, occlusion of the appropriate branches of the internal maxillary artery is the preferred procedure (Figs. 27–7 and 27–8).

Arterial ligation is carried out if other measures discussed previously have not proved successful in stopping the epistaxis. Septal dermoplasty (Sanders, 1970) is a surgical procedure that may be indicated in children with recurrent epistaxis in hereditary telangiectasia and von Willebrand's disease (Letson and Birck, 1973). Cryosurgery has

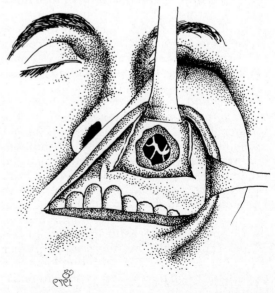

Figure 27–7 View of the internal carotid artery through a fenestra of the posterior wall of the antrum through a Caldwell-Luc approach.

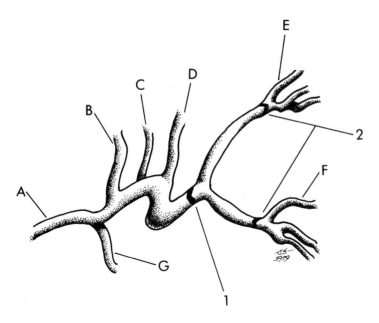

Figure 27–8 Diagram of the third part of the course of the left internal maxillary artery (pterygopalatine portion). *A,* Internal maxillary artery. *B,* Artery of the pterygoid canal (Vidian). *C,* Infraorbital artery. *D,* Pharyngeal artery. *E,* Sphenopalatine artery. *F,* Descending palatine artery. *G,* Dental artery. The areas labeled 1 and 2 are locations of clip application.

been used to treat epistaxis on occasion (Bluestone and Smith, 1967).

PREVENTION

The treatment of a bleeding episode should be extended to measures designed to prevent recurrence of the bleeding. These measures consist of educational and common-sense advice given to the patient and his family by the treating physician.

One of the simplest and most effective of these measures is humidification of the child's home environment. In our homes in past years, humidity levels were controlled by evaporation of water from vessels placed on radiators and space heaters. Also, house plants played a real part in providing humidity in our living quarters (Fig. 27–9).

Year-round control of temperature in large numbers of our homes began in the warmer climates in the 1950s. Recent changes in methods of home temperature conditioning, particularly heating, have led to the need for humidity control also. In dwellings with forced-air central heat furnaces, the relative humidity level in dry cold weather can drop to 5 per cent; the relative humidity level in the heating season *should* be between 40 and 50 per cent. In the heating season, proper insulation and mechanical humidifiers are important to maintain a proper humidity level (Fig. 27–10).

Humidifiers come in a variety of types, but almost all central heating units can be provid-

ed with one of two basic types of humidifiers: the most efficient and trouble-free are evaporative humidifiers; the spray type is less desirable for homes. These humidifiers are usually controlled by a humidistat. Portable humidifiers, which are filled with water automatically or manually, vary in capacity from many liters to as little as two liters. Since humidified air travels about a space rapidly

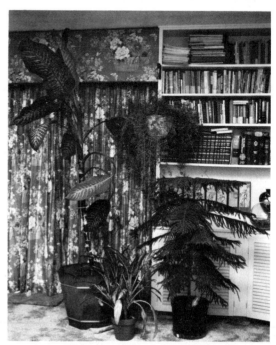

Figure 27–9 Houseplants — humidification by natural means.

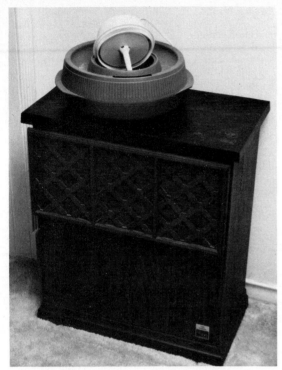

Figure 27-10 Two types of portable humidifiers — "cool mist" and forced air evaporative.

without air circulation, one or several of these portable units can serve a home quite well.

Some humidifiers operate by air forced through water-soaked material, supplying the humidity. Another type produces cool mist by breaking the water into very small particles. Portable boiling water humidifiers (steam) are not recommended because of the danger of injury from the hot water and their greater use of fuel. Too great a difference between inside and outside temperature in summer cooling can drop the humidity below the healthful level. A temperature spread of no more than 12° C is probably optimal.

When dry crusts occlude the nasal airway, petroleum jelly or a similar substance may be put in the anterior nares at bedtime. If an infection is present, an antibiotic or antibiotic–steroid ophthalmic ointment (not water miscible) may be used. Steroid-containing ointments should be used no longer than two weeks without follow-up care by the physician.

Prevention of epistaxis also includes the control of nasal and paranasal sinus infections, treatment of allergies affecting the nose, and prevention of nose picking. All of these measures require the cooperation of parents and patients but are worthwhile to prevent an annoying and sometimes frightening episode of bleeding from the nose.

SELECTED REFERENCES

Hansen, J. 1974. Disorders of nasal septum and related structures. *In* Otolaryngology, Vol. 3, Chap. 9, New York, Harper and Row.

Hansen gives a good review of coagulation and platelet disorders, as well as an extensive table listing causes of epistaxis.

Stool, S. E., and Kemper, B. 1969. Brenneman's practice of pediatrics, Vol. 4, chap. 54. New York, Harper and Row.

This chapter is written for the pediatrician and gives an overview of epistaxis in children.

For further information on this subject, see the following references.

REFERENCES

Adams, D. M. 1973. Transantral internal maxillary artery ligation in prolonged or severe posterior epistaxis. J. La. State Med. Soc., *125*:389.

Alavi, K. 1969. Epistaxis and hemoptysis due to hirudo medicinalis (Medical leech). Arch. Otolaryngol., *90*:178.

Bell, M., Hawke, M., and Jahn, A. 1974. New device for the management of postnasal epistaxis. Balloon Tamponade. Arch. Otolaryngol., *99*:373.

Bluestone, C. D., and Smith, H. C. 1967. Intranasal freezing for severe epistaxis. Arch. Otolaryngol., *85*:445.

Blumfeld, R., and Skolnik, E. M. 1965. Intranasal encephaloceles. Arch. Otolaryngol., *82*:527.

Brenner, R. L. 1974. Dacryocystorhinostomy in children. Tex. Med., *70*:71.

Briant, T. D. R., Fitzpatrick, P. J., and Book, H. 1970. The radiological treatment of juvenile nasopharyngeal angiofibromas. Ann. Otol. Rhinol. Laryngol., *79*:1108.

Chandler, J. R., and Serrins, A. 1965. Transantral ligation of the internal maxillary artery for epistaxis. Laryngoscope, *75*:1151.

Coleman, C. C., Jr. 1973. Diagnosis and treatment of congenital arteriovenous fistulas of the head and neck. Am. J. Surg., *126*:557.

El bitar, H. 1971. The etiology and management of epistaxis. A review of 300 cases. Practitioner, *207*:800.

English, G. M., Hemenway, W. G., and Cundy, R. L. 1972. Surgical treatment of invasive angiofibroma. Arch. Otolaryngol., *96*:312.

Falter, M. S., and Kaufman, M. F. 1971. Congenital factor VII deficiency. J. Pediatr., *79*:298.

Goldstein, A. 1970. Postvaricella bleeding presenting as epistaxis. Arch. Otolaryngol., *92*:173.

Goode, R. L., and Spooner, T. R. 1972. Management of nasal fractures in children. A review of current practices. Clin. Pediatr., *119*:526.

Hansen, J. 1974. Disorders of nasal septum and related structures. *In* Otolaryngology, Vol. 3, chap. 9.

Huggins, S. 1969. Control of hemorrhage in otorhinolaryngologic surgery with oxidized regenerated cellulose, EENT Mo., *48*:420.

Iwamura, S., Sugiura, S., and Nomura, Y. 1972. Schwannoma of the nasal cavity. Arch. Otolaryngol., *96*:176.

Jafek, B. 1978. Personal communication with author.

Jafek, B., Nahum, A., Butler, R., et al. 1973. Surgical treatment of juvenile nasopharyngeal angiofibroma. Laryngoscope, *83*:707.

Juselius, H. 1974. Epistaxis. A clinical study of 1,734 patients. J. Laryngol. Otol., *88*:317.

Kadish, S. P. 1971. Epistaxis in a teen-age boy. J.A.M.A., *216*:508.

Kahn, A. A., Khaleque, K. A., and Huda, M. N. 1969. Rhinosporidiosis of the nose. J. Laryngol. Otol., *83*:461.

Leslie, J., and Ingram, G. I. 1971. The diagnosis of long-standing bleeding disorders. Semin. Hematol., *8*:140.

Letson, J. A., Jr., and Birck, H. G. 1973. Septal dermoplasty for von Willebrand's disease in children. Laryngoscope, *83*:1078.

Malcomson, K. G. 1963. The surgical management of massive epistaxis. J. Laryngol. Otol., *77*:299.

Mettler, C. C. 1947. History of Medicine, Philadelphia, Blakiston Co.

Montgomery, W. W., Lofgren, R. H., and Chasin, W. D. 1970. Analysis of pterygopalatine space surgery. Laryngoscope, *80*:1179.

Pathak, P. N. 1972. Epistaxis—due to ruptured aneurysm of the internal carotid artery. J. Laryngol. Otol., *86*:395.

Pearson, B. W., MacKenzie, R. G., and Goodman, W. S. 1969. The anatomical basis of transantral ligation of the maxillary artery in severe epistaxis. Laryngoscope, *79*:969.

Pinsker, O. T., and Holdcraft, J. 1971. Surgical management of anterior epistaxis. Trans. Am. Acad. Ophthalmol. Otol., *75*:492.

Quick, A. J. 1967. Telangiectasia: its relationship to the Minotvon Willebrand syndrome. Am. J. Med. Sci., *254*:585.

Roback, S. A., Herdman, R. C., Hoyer, J., et al. 1969. Wegner's treatment. Am. J. Dis. Child., *118*:608.

Rowe, N. L. 1968. Fractures of the facial skeleton in children. J. Oral Surg., *26*:505.

Sanders, W. H. 1970. Septal dermoplasty—its several uses. Laryngoscope, *80*:1342.

Schulman, I. 1959. The significance of epistaxis in children. Pediatrics, *24*:489.

Stool, S. E., and Kemper, B. 1969. Brenneman's Practice of Pediatrics, Vol. 4, Chap. 54. New York, Harper and Row.

Chapter 28

FACIAL PAIN AND HEADACHE

Frank E. Lucente, M.D.

Complaints of facial pain and headache in the child are often difficult to assess if one cannot obtain an accurate history or establish the precise location of the pain. Many of these complaints will disappear quickly and do not require evaluation by a physician. However, patients with persistent or recurrent symptoms should have complete head and neck examinations. Such evaluation may require a multidisciplinary approach by the otolaryngologist, pediatrician, neurologist, ophthalmologist, dentist, psychiatrist, and social worker. It is the responsibility of the otolaryngologist to explore the potential etiologic role of otolaryngologic structures in facial pain and headache.

Pain in the head may result from stimulation, traction, or pressure on any of the pain-sensitive structures of the head, which include the trigeminal, glossopharyngeal, vagal, and upper cervical nerves; the large arteries at the base of the brain and their major branches; the dura mater at the base of the skull; the cranial sinuses and afferent veins; the arteries of the dura mater; and some extracranial structures such as the scalp, arteries, and muscles (Lagos, 1971).

Headache may be a recognizable symptom in children three years of age and older. The infant or younger child may present with irritability or unusual behavior rather than with complaints of headache when experiencing the pathologic processes we will describe.

Although most pains in the head and neck region result from a pathologic process at or close to the area indicated by the patient, the physician might consider the phenomenon of referred pain when no abnormalities are found in this area. A common example of referred pain is the otalgia produced by inflammatory, infectious, and neoplastic lesions of the pharynx. The external ear and middle ear receive sensory innervation from the fifth, seventh, ninth, and tenth cranial nerves and from the second and third cervical nerves. An irritative process anywhere along the distribution of any of these nerves can present as a referred otalgia.

A thorough history will often provide the diagnosis for the pain. It should include questions about severity, duration, location, character, circumstances of onset, exacerbating or remitting factors, repetition, frequency, and associated symptoms in the head and neck region and elsewhere. In taking the history the physician should also attempt to become more familiar with the child as a social being by inquiring about his family, social, and educational settings. It is often helpful to talk with the child in the absence of the parents, particularly when psychologic factors appear to cause, exacerbate, or modify the headache symptoms. The patient should have a complete head and neck examination, including skull, facial bones, eyes, ears, temporomandibular joint, nose, nasopharynx, oral cavity, teeth, oropharynx, larynx, cervical muscles, and associated soft tissues. In palpating the head and neck region, one should begin in asymptomatic areas and move slowly toward symptomatic or tender areas, in order to avoid frightening or hurting the child any more than necessary. Percussion of the teeth, sinuses, and mastoids should also be included. A thorough neurologic examination should also be performed with particular attention to the cranial nerves.

The performance of ancillary laboratory

tests and radiographs is guided by the clinical impression obtained from the history and physical examination. There are few, if any, mandatory screening tests, and indiscriminate ordering of tests should be avoided.

In this chapter we shall present a differential diagnosis for headache and facial pain (Tables 28–1, 28–2, and 28–3), consider a few of the more common causes or conditions associated with these complaints, and suggest that more extensive discussion is found in related chapters.

MUSCULAR CONTRACTION HEADACHE (TENSION HEADACHE)

This is probably the most common headache in childhood. It is usually bilateral, steady, nonpulsatile, and less intense than a migraine. The pain tends to present in the occipital region or as a band around the head. Since it probably results from prolonged contraction of muscles of the head and neck, it generally occurs later in the day and after

Table 28–2 ANATOMIC–ETIOLOGIC CLASSIFICATION OF FACIAL PAIN

Forehead	**Midfacial (cheek)**
Frontal sinus	Maxillary sinus
Ocular	Maxillary teeth
	Periodontal structures
Periorbital	Intranasal
Ocular	Parotid gland
Ethmoid sinus	
	Nasal
Preauricular	Nasal bones
Temporomandibular joint	Ethmoid sinus
External ear canal	Intranasal
Parotid gland	
	Jaw
Periauricular	Mandibular teeth
Middle ear	Periodontal structures
External ear (auricle)	Submandibular gland

periods of physical or emotional stress or intense intellectual activity. Although less common in children than in adults, it is sometimes seen in hard-working students. The failure of the pain to be intensified by coughing, straining at stool or placing the head in a dependent position distinguishes this type of headache from those due to intracranial causes (Dyken, 1975).

On examination, one may find restriction and pain with movement of the neck and tenderness over the occipital nerves. Tenderness in the upper border of the trapezius and intrinsic cervical muscles is also found.

Management varies with the underlying cause. Oral analgesics and local treatment with heat may help, but elimination of the underlying physical or psychologic strain is most important. As with other headaches in children, complete and repeated explanation and reassurance are most important.

Table 28–1 ETIOLOGIC CLASSIFICATION OF HEADACHE

Environmental	**Toxic – Metabolic**
Heat	"Pseudotumor"
Humidity	Steroids
Noxious fumes	Tetracycline
Noise	Vitamin A
Infectious	Other drugs
Extracranial	Sulfa
Teeth	Indomethacin
Sinus	Heavy metals
Pharynx	Lead
Ear	Arsenic
Septicemia	Mercury
Viral exanthems	Hypoglycemia
Musculoskeletal	Hyperammonemia
Intracranial	Metabolic acidosis
Meningitis	Hypoxia
Encephalitis	Anemia
Brain abscess	CO poisoning
Vascular	Hypercarbia
Migraine	Porphyria
Hypertension	**Congenital**
Aneurysm	Arnold-Chiari syndrome
Vascular malformation	**Cervical**
Horton syndrome	**Neuralgic**
(Histamine cephalgia)	Herpetic
Traumatic	Postherpetic
Neoplastic	Idiopathic
Extracranial	**Psychologic**
Intracranial	
Epileptic	
Psychomotor	
Postictal	
Ocular	
Allergic	

Modified from Meloff, K. L.: Headache in pediatric practice. Headache 13: 125–129, 1973.

MIGRAINE HEADACHE

Migraine headaches commonly begin during adolescence, but this syndrome may occasionally be seen in younger children. Migraine is very uncommon before the age of four years.

Although the adolescent may experience classic migraine headaches similar to those found in adults — with prodromal anorexia and scotomata, severe unilateral pulsatile headache lasting 4 to 8 hours and followed by diffuse head pain, photophobia, abdominal discomfort, nausea, vomiting, and postictal lethargy — younger children more frequent-

Table 28–3 CLINICAL SUMMARY OF FACIAL PAIN AND HEADACHE

Disease or Disorder	Location	Character	Usual Frequency	Accompanying Symptoms	Usual Time of Day	General Therapy	Duration
Sinusitis	Frontal Midfacial Periorbital	Dull	Inconsistent	Nasal congestion Nasal drainage	Morning Evening	Decongestant Antibiotic	More than one day
Migraine Classic Common	Unilateral Frontotemporal Periorbital	Severe Throbbing	Weekly or monthly	Nausea Vomiting Scotomata	Any time	Ergotamine Tranquilizer Anticonvulsant	Classic: Less than 8 hours Common: Hours to days
Psychogenic (Tension)	Frontal Occipital Band-like	Inconsistent	Daily	Nervousness Anxiety Withdrawn behavior	During or after stress	Analgesic Tranquilizer	Variable
Brain tumor	Frontal Parietal Occipital	Dull	Daily	Ataxia Behavior change Visual disturbance	Morning Evening	Relief of intra-cranial pressure	More than one day
Ocular disorders	Ocular Frontal	Dull	Daily	Squint Refractive errors	Afternoon Evening	Visual correction	Several hours
Convulsive equivalent	Frontal Temporal	Dull	Daily or weekly	Vomiting Staring episodes Hyperactivity	Any time	Anticonvulsant	Minutes to hours
Meningitis Encephalitis	Frontal Occipital	Dull	Constant	Fever Nuchal rigidity Convulsions	Any time	Antibiotics	Constant

Modified from Jabbour, J. T., et al. 1976. Pediatric Neurology Handbook. Flushing, N.Y., Medical Examination Publishing Co.

ly have common (atypical) migraines which lack the prodromal signs and which may last from hours to days. For this reason, the diagnosis may be elusive until symptoms have been present for several months. A family history of migraine or convulsive disorders is often obtained (McNaughton, 1975).

Occasionally the child will present only with paroxysmal vomiting, hemiparesis, diplopia, or ataxia. Headache may appear later in the clinical course. The attacks usually last two to three hours but may last up to 48 hours. They are often followed by a period of sleep and tend to recur at irregular intervals.

The disease appears more frequently in boys than in girls, and the patients are often compulsive, intense, hard-working perfectionists. While emotional stress may precipitate a migraine episode, it should not be considered a psychiatric disorder. The pathogenesis is thought to involve initial cerebral vasoconstriction followed by rapid vasodilation.

Mild attacks may be relieved with salicylates or codeine taken at the very onset. Ergot preparations used in treating adult migraines may produce more intense and prolonged effects, possibly resulting in cerebral ischemia. Minor tranquilizers may interrupt the headache if given over a period of several months. The child should also be reassured that there is no neoplastic or psychologic cause for the headaches.

Ophthalmoplegic migraine is a rare variant of this clinical picture, in which partial or complete third-nerve palsy appears 6 to 24 hours after the onset of the headache. Although the ophthalmoplegia generally subsides within a few days, repeated episodes may leave the patient with some residual paralysis.

CONVULSIVE EQUIVALENT

Headaches may be associated with a paroxysmal cerebral dysrhythmia or psychomotor seizure. They usually have an acute onset during the day or night and last several minutes to several hours. They are characteristically dull and are located in the frontotemporal region. Pallor, abdominal discomfort, nausea, and vomiting follow onset of the headache. The pain may disappear after a brief period of sleep, and the child then usually feels quite well. Anticonvulsant medications, such as diphenylhydantoin (Dilantin) or barbiturates, usually produce a dramatic response.

TRACTION HEADACHE (BRAIN MASS HEADACHE)

Traction on intracranial pain-sensitive structures caused by brain tumor, hematoma, aneurysm, or abscess will result in a traction headache. Brain tumors usually produce a steady, aching headache that may be more severe in the morning and in the erect position. It rarely has the pulsatile pattern of the vascular headache. Brain tumor headache tends to be more severe when the child is lying down and may awaken the child from sleep (Dyken, 1975).

VASCULAR MALFORMATION HEADACHE

Vascular malformation is a very uncommon cause of a headache, which usually lasts several days and which may be accompanied by seizures or periods of decreased levels of consciousness. Scotomata may also be present, but they are concomitant rather than antecedent as with migraine. The headache reaches its maximum intensity more quickly than the migraine headache, usually within seconds. In determining the etiology of the headache, it is important to look for coincident neurologic abnormalities that may persist long after the headache has disappeared. This type of headache is also associated with seizures and with cerebral hemorrhage.

HYPERTENSION HEADACHE

Hypertension is rarely seen in childhood and is consequently a rare cause of headaches among children. The headaches tend to resemble the hypertension headaches experienced by adults and the brain mass headache. They occur more commonly in the morning and fluctuate rapidly in intensity during the day, sometimes in relationship to the amount or intensity of physical activity. Among the disorders that may be associated with hypertensive headaches are acute and chronic renal disease, neuroblastoma, pheochromocytoma, and adrenal adenomas. Diagnosis is usually simple if the blood pressure is monitored.

Therapy involves analgesics and correction of the hypertension.

NEURALGIAS

The severe pain of trigeminal or glossopharyngeal neuralgia that is seen in adults is extremely rare in children.

NASAL AND PARANASAL SINUS DISEASE

The common viral upper respiratory infection is a frequent cause of headache, which may be diffuse or limited to the midfacial region. The pain is usually a dull ache that is exacerbated by placing the head in a dependent position. Associated symptoms and signs, including sneezing, nasal congestion, serous drainage, sore throat, malaise, cough, mild fever, and boggy nasal mucous membranes, will usually confirm the diagnosis. Recovery is usually spontaneous within 4 to 5 days if there are no bacterial complications (Chap. 32).

If the nasal drainage becomes cloudy and the nasal mucous membranes become markedly inflamed, purulent rhinitis should be suspected. It is usually caused by hemolytic *Staphylococcus aureus, Haemophilus influenzae,* or *Diplococcus pneumoniae.* When nasal drainage is persistently unilateral, the presence of a foreign body must be excluded (Chap. 34).

Inflammation, infection, or tumors in the paranasal sinuses produce localized or diffuse facial pain more commonly than headache. Pain from the maxillary sinus is experienced in the midface, cheek, or maxillary teeth. Ethmoid pain is felt between the eyes, and frontal pain is felt in the supraorbital region. Pain from the sphenoid sinus is poorly localized, occasionally being described as coming from deep within the head or at the cranial vertex. The frontal and sphenoid sinuses develop slowly and are usually not of clinical significance until adolescence (Strome, 1976).

Inflammation of the paranasal sinus probably causes far fewer headaches and facial pains than is commonly thought by patients. The sinus ostia, turbinates, and septum are more pain sensitive than the sinus mucosa itself, and before ascribing midfacial pain to the sinuses, the physician should find corroborative clinical evidence, such as purulent or watery nasal drainage, marked erythema of the nasal mucosa, or tenderness to percussion over the sinuses. Radiographic examination of the sinuses will be helpful in evaluating puzzling patients or in determining therapy.

Sinus disease in the child can be considerably more serious than in the adult owing to the incomplete development in children of the bony walls of the sinuses. The thinness of the lamina papyracea allows rapid extension of ethmoid infection into the orbit with production of orbital cellulitis or orbital abscess. Localized osteomyelitis may appear with spread of infection from any sinus into contiguous bone. Extension of infection through the posterior wall of the frontal sinus, roof of the ethmoid sinus, or any wall of the sphenoid sinus may lead to intracranial complications, such as extradural abscess, meningitis, or brain abscess. Persistent or severe headache in the child with clinical evidence of sinusitis mandates a thorough examination of areas adjacent to the sinuses.

OCULAR HEADACHE

When examining the patient complaining of headache or facial pain, it is important to consider ocular causes, to examine the eyes, and to obtain an ophthalmologic consultation when indicated. Extensive discussion of ocular causes of pain in this region will not be given here. However, several important disorders should be mentioned.

Refractive errors, especially hyperopia, may cause pain in the region of the eyes or anywhere in the head. A cycloplegic refraction, using drugs to paralyze the ciliary muscle, is required to confirm the diagnosis. In addition to mild eye pain or headache, symptoms in children may include blinking, rubbing the eyes, head tilting, photophobia, frowning, or closing one eye. Certain types of strabismus, especially exophorias, may also be associated with similar symptoms.

Acute glaucoma, which is rare in children, is characterized by sudden, severe pain in the eye and the supraorbital region. The pain is accompanied by blurring of vision, increased intraocular pressure, dilated pupil, and a cloudy cornea. More often the glaucoma occurring in childhood has an insidious onset and may be associated with tearing, photophobia, blurred vision, and less severe pain.

Acute iritis (anterior uveitis) may cause

photophobia, blurring, and extreme pain radiating from the eye to the forehead and temporal region. The eye is red (circumcorneal flush) and the pupil is small. Iritis in the child may have an insidious onset; it is essentially painless (Chap. 29).

Acute retrobulbar neuritis is usually associated with unilateral pain deep in the orbit. The pain occurs before blurring and is increased by rotation of the eye. The patient may complain of sudden loss of central vision. This disorder may be seen in teenagers but is uncommon in the young child.

Another rare childhood disorder is *Herpes zoster ophthalmicus,* which begins with severe pain in the region of distribution of the ophthalmic division of the trigeminal nerve. Several days later vesicles appear on the forehead and eyelids. Pain may persist after the acute infectious stage has passed.

Among the other ocular disorders to be considered with pain around the eyes are foreign bodies and inflammation of the lid or cornea (chronic blepharitis, conjunctivitis, or allergic reactions).

OTOLOGIC PAIN

Inflammatory, infectious, and neoplastic diseases in the external, middle, and inner ears may produce pain that the child may interpret or describe as headache or, rarely, facial pain. The numerous otologic causes for headache and facial pain are considered in chapters 9, 15, 16, 17, 18, 21, and 22. However, it is appropriate to reemphasize here the need for complete otologic and audiometric evaluation of any child with headache, even without associated otologic symptoms (Chap. 9).

DERMATOLOGIC INFECTIONS

Infections of the skin of the head and neck may produce pain. The areas involved can be overlooked in a cursory examination since they are often hidden. Among the bacterial infections that occur in children are facial cellulitis, nasal vestibulitis, and furunculosis of the external ear canal.

DENTAL DISEASE

Inflammation or infection of the teeth or their supporting structures may cause the child to complain of localized, diffuse pain. Inspection, palpation, and percussion of the teeth should be performed carefully and supplemented with radiographic examination when indicated. The condition of the gingivae should also be noted. Among the dental diseases that may present with headache or facial pain are caries, periapical abscess, periodontal disease, eruption of deciduous or permanent teeth, loss of deciduous teeth, dental impaction, infected dental cyst, and aphthous or herpetic stomatitis.

Children sometimes present with submandibular cellulitis and pain of no apparent cause except for radiographic evidence of beginning eruption of permanent dentition. These infections are usually responsive to broad-spectrum antibiotic therapy, although no actual etiologic factor ever becomes evident.

TEMPOROMANDIBULAR JOINT DISEASE

Pain from masticatory dysfunctions involving the temporomandibular joint is usually a dull ache experienced in the preauricular region. It is sometimes more diffuse and may be described by the patient as an earache. The pain is usually steady and is exacerbated by chewing or vigorous jaw motion. It may be seen in conjunction with any generalized or localized disease of synovial joints, such as rheumatoid arthritis.

HEAD TRAUMA

The elicitation of a history of cranial or maxillofacial trauma from the child or parent may be difficult. However, the presence of contusions, ecchymoses, abrasions, or bony tenderness may support the clinical suspicions. Thorough head and neck examination may disclose signs of trauma in regions less visible than the face and skull. Inconsistencies between the histories given by the child and parents may be noted. Radiographic evaluation should be performed if any trauma is suspected.

SYSTEMIC DISEASES

Headaches occur in association with fever, hypoxemia, hypercarbia, poisoning, systemic viral or bacterial infections, and postictal states. Distention of cerebral and pial vessels is the postulated mechanism for the pain. Headaches associated with systemic infections are often accompanied by fever, nausea, and vomiting.

PSYCHOGENIC HEADACHES

It is impossible to detail the psychologic significance with which the head, face, and neck are invested. However, the role of psychologic factors in the production, modification, and communication of painful sensations in this region cannot be overemphasized. Children learn very early that "headache" is a common somatic complaint used by adults to describe a discomfort that may have no relation to physical problems in or around the head. They may use the same phrases, "I have a headache," or "My head hurts," to describe their own experience of that same discomfort experienced by adults, or to provide an excuse for their unwillingness to perform a certain act (for instance, going to school, visiting a neighbor, doing household chores).

They may seek the secondary gain of increased attention that is usually given the sick child, or they may use this somatic complaint as a tool to manipulate parents, teachers, or other associates. Hopefully, careful questioning about both the circumstances of the pain and coincident factors will help to identify those patients in whom psychologic factors must be explored.

When the history is obtained from a parent, the physician should also be aware of the possibility that the parent is projecting his or her own concerns onto the patient, misstating the history or interpreting it prematurely, or seeking attention for his or her own problems. Inconsistencies in the history or the failure to find physical evidence for an abnormality (evidence of a physical abnormality) may suggest this situation.

However, just as one should not make psychogenic headache a diagnosis by exclusion, so also should one be careful not to eliminate physical causes before a thorough evaluation has been made. In ascribing pain in the head or face to a psychologic cause, one should be certain of both the absence of demonstrable organic disease and the presence of detectable emotional disturbance.

SELECTED REFERENCES

Alling, C. C., and Mahan, P. E. (Eds.) 1977. Facial Pain. Philadelphia, Lea & Febiger.
   This excellent text discusses the etiology and management of many types of facial pain. Among the subjects covered are functional anatomy, pharmacodynamics, vascular pain, paranasal sinuses, masticatory pain, occlusal disorders, psychosomatics, pain syndromes, and general patient examination.

Wolff, H. G. 1972. Headache and Other Head Pain. New York, Oxford University Press. (Revised by Dalessio, D. J.)
   This classic text provides a tremendous amount of clinical and experimental material relevant to the many causes of headache. Although headaches in infants and children are not discussed apart from adult disorders, the coverage of each condition includes pertinent aspects of the pediatric problems.

REFERENCES

Alling, C. C., and Mahan, P. E. (Eds.) 1977. Facial Pain. Philadelphia, Lea & Febiger.

Dyken, P. R. 1975. Headaches in children. Arch. Fam. Pract. *11*:106–111.

Jabbour, J. T., Duenas, D. A., Gilmartin, R. C., Jr., et al. 1976. Pediatric Neurology Handbook. Flushing, N.Y., Medical Examination Pub. Co.

Lagos, J. C. 1971. Differential Diagnosis in Pediatric Neurology. Boston, Little, Brown and Co.

McNaughton, F. L. 1975. Headache and other head pain. *In* Maloney, W. H. (Ed.) Otolaryngology, Vol. V. Hagerstown, MD. Harper & Row, Chap. 11N.

Meloff, K. L. 1973. Headache in pediatric practice. Headache, *13*:125–129.

Strome, M. 1976. Rhino-sinusitis and midfacial pain in adolescents. Practitioner, *217*:914–918.

Wolff, H. G. 1972. Headache and Other Head Pain. New York, Oxford University Press. (Revised by Dalessio, D. J.).

The author gratefully acknowledges the assistance in reviewing the text critically of the following members of the faculty of the Mount Sinai School of Medicine: Jonathan Z. Charney, M.D. (Department of Neurology); Roger G. Gerry, D.D.S. (Department of Dentistry); Alex Steigman, M.D. (Department of Pediatrics); and Alan Sugar, M.D. (Department of Ophthalmology).

Chapter 29

ORBITAL SWELLINGS

Thomas C. Calcaterra, M.D.

The child with an orbital swelling often represents a diagnostic challenge that may require the expertise of several medical specialists. The otolaryngologist is frequently consulted because many cases of orbital swelling are secondary to extracranial disease processes occurring adjacent to the orbit. It is important for the otolaryngologist to be familiar with the spectrum of diseases that may cause orbital swelling, the basic methods of orbital examination, and recently developed diagnostic studies applicable to the orbit.

The orbit is a pyramidal-shaped space, open anteriorly, but otherwise surrounded by thin bone. Any expansive disease, either within the orbit or from an adjacent site, may cause protrusion of the globe, a condition termed exophthalmos or proptosis. Accordingly, diseases that can cause exophthalmos may be classified into two major groups: intraorbital, consisting of lesions arising within the orbital space; and extraorbital, lesions involving the orbit by direct extension from adjacent structures or by metastasis from distant sites. The latter group can be subdivided into categories of intracranial and extracranial lesions. This latter group of extraorbital lesions, the extracranial lesions, are of major interest to the otolaryngologist because they frequently arise within the nose, paranasal sinuses, nasopharynx, or temporal fossa (see Table 29–1).

HISTORY

A comprehensive history is important to an evaluation of unilateral exophthalmos. The mode of onset and progression of the exophthalmos, the status of vision, and the presence of pain should be established. The patient should be questioned about previous sinus infections, allergies, nasal discharge, and facial numbness. Slow progression of proptosis suggests a benign tumor or cyst, whereas rapidly developing proptosis implies the presence of a primary or metastatic malignant tumor. Early loss of vision points to a lesion within the muscle cone involving the optic nerve, such as a glioma. Severe pain is generally symptomatic of an acute infection or hemorrhage.

Table 29–1 DISEASES CAUSING ORBITAL SWELLINGS: ANATOMIC CLASSIFICATION

Intraorbital Lesions
hyperthyroidism
histiocytosis
dermoid and teratoma
optic nerve glioma
rhabdomyosarcoma
melanoma
retinoblastoma
lacrimal gland tumors
hemangioma
metastatic tumors

Extraorbital — Extracranial Lesions
acute inflammation of any paranasal sinus
mucocele of any paranasal sinus
fibrous dysplasia
osteoma
angiofibroma of nasopharynx
nasopharyngeal cancer

Extraorbital – Intracranial Lesions
meningocele and encephalocele
cavernous sinus thrombosis
cavernous sinus fistula
anterior cranial fossa tumors
middle cranial fossa tumors

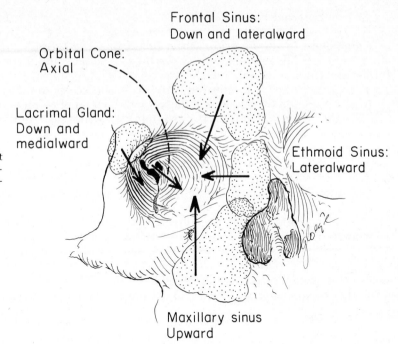

Orbital Cone:
Axial

Frontal Sinus:
Down and lateralward

Lacrimal Gland:
Down and
medialward

Ethmoid Sinus:
Lateralward

Figure 29–1 The arrows depict the direction of displacement typically encountered by a disease process within each paranasal sinus.

Maxillary sinus
Upward

PHYSICAL EXAMINATION

Direction of Displacement

The direction of displacment often indicates the site of the lesion (Fig. 29–1). Tumors within the muscle cone, such as an optic nerve glioma, may cause pure axial displacement. Acute inflammation or chronic mucopyocele arising from the frontal or ethmoid sinuses displaces the eye downward, laterally, or in both directions (Fig. 29–2). Displacement of the eye in a medial direction often denotes tumors of the lacrimal gland or the temporal fossa. Lesions arising in the maxillary sinus may push the globe upward.

Vertical displacement can be assessed by holding a ruler across both lateral canthi and determining the relationship of the pupils to this straight line. Horizontal displacement is determined by comparing the distance from a mark on the center of the bridge of the nose to each limbus (Chap. 15, The Eye in Childhood, 1967).

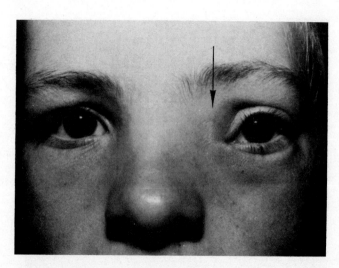

Figure 29–2 The arrow indicates fullness in the canthal region caused by an ethmoid mucocele, which displaces the left eye in a lateral direction.

External Examination

Examination of the anterior aspect of the globe and eyelids should be performed. While the child is quiet and the radial or carotid pulse is being monitored, any synchronous pulsation of the globe indicates loss of the bony partition between the frontal or temporal lobe and the orbital contents, allowing intracranial pulsations to be transmitted to the eye. Synchronous pulsations may also be observed with a carotid–cavernous sinus fistula. Auscultation over the closed eyelid or temporal region may reveal a bruit suggestive of an arteriovenous vascular malformation. Increased proptosis that becomes apparent while the child is crying suggests an orbital varix, particularly if there is concomitant dilation of the conjunctival veins. A palpable impulse that occurs when the child coughs suggests an encephalocele.

Chemosis, cellulitis, and fluctuation of the eyelids are signals of an inflammatory process, usually transmitted from the paranasal sinuses. Transillumination of the eyelid may disclose an underlying cyst. Although not as common in children as in adults, lid retraction, lid lag on upward gaze, lid restriction on elevation of the globe, and injection of the blood vessels over the lateral rectus muscle all imply the presence of endocrine exophthalmos.

Severe proptosis may prevent the lids from closing and thereby allow the cornea to dry (Calcaterra et al., 1974). The earliest sign of corneal exposure is the loss of normal corneal brightness. Moreover, persistent exposure can lead to ulceration, infection, and permanent scarring.

Palpation

Palpation of the orbital contents may yield important information, particularly regarding anteriorly located lesions such as mucoceles and lacrimal gland tumors. Ballottement of each globe should be performed in order to compare orbital resilience in each eye. Inflammatory lesions and tumors tend to feel resistant, whereas less resistance is noted with hemangiomas and endocrine exophthalmos (Fig. 29–3). Fullness in the infratemporal fossa suggests lateral extension of the disease process and irregularities of the orbital rim may represent bony destruction.

Ophthalmologic Examination

A complete ophthalmologic evaluation is mandatory. Decreased visual acuity is not characteristic of most intraorbital expansive processes unless the degree of proptosis is great or there is direct pressure on the optic nerve. A tumor directly behind the globe may indent the posterior wall of the retina in such a way as to induce a refractive error. A visual field defect suggests involvement of the optic chiasm. Fundoscopic examination may show the presence of retinal stria or scleral flattening, which usually indicates a discrete intraorbital tumor. Papilledema and optic atrophy generally imply direct involvement of the optic nerve by tumor pressure or infiltration (Kroll and Casten, 1966).

Limitation of ocular movement may reflect either direct mechanical infringement of the muscles or globe or involvement of the third, fourth, or sixth cranial nerves as they pass

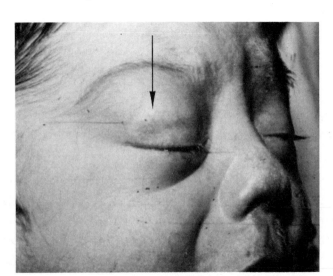

Figure 29–3 Infant with orbital and upper lid hemangioma. On palpation the hemangioma produced minimal resistance.

through the cavernous sinus or superior orbital fissure. The nature of this limitation of motion may be resolved by the forced duction test: after topical or general anesthesia, the limbus is grasped with conjunctival forceps. If the eye can be moved fully in the direction of limited motion, paralysis is the likeliest cause of the abnormal ocular movement, whereas if movement is restricted, mechanical infringement by tumor or inflammation probably is present.

Exophthalmometry

Exophthalmos may be established either by an absolute measurement that relates the distance of the corneal apex to a reference point on the skull, or by a relative measurement that compares the position of one cornea with the other (Calcaterra et al, 1974). Proptosis can be discerned easily by visualizing the eyes from above, over the forehead, or from below, over the malar eminences. Absolute measurements can be obtained with various instruments, the most common of which is the Hertle exophthalmometer, which uses the lateral orbital rim as a bony reference and projects a lateral view of the cornea on a millimeter scale. Testing variability may range between 1 and 2 mm, depending upon the consistent location of the instrument on the edge of the orbital rim, facial asymmetry, and thickness of the subcutaneous tissue over the bone. This instrument is especially useful in detecting smaller degrees of proptosis and for making objective measurements in serial examinations.

Proptosis is considered to be present when one globe is displaced 2 mm further forward than the other. This difference is usually accompanied by a widened palpebral fissure. However, a misleading appearance of proptosis may be present in patients with unilateral enophthalmos, lid retraction, or unilateral myopia.

Otolaryngologic Examination

Specific attention must be directed toward the nose, paranasal sinuses, nasopharynx, and neck. Inflammatory mucosal changes, purulent exudate, and polyps in the nose or nasopharynx all indicate possible sinusitis and a mucopyocele. Palpation and pressure over the sinuses may indicate inflammation or an underlying neoplasm.

The ears should be checked for a serous effusion inasmuch as it is well known that neoplasia and inflammation of the ethmoid sinuses and nasopharynx can impair function of the eustachian tube. The neck should be palpated carefully for the presence of enlarged lymph nodes that may harbor metastatic cells from a primary tumor in the region of the eye. An enlarged thyroid gland suggests hyperthyroidism and thus an endocrine basis for the exophthalmos.

An evaluation of cranial nerve function should be completed, particularly of the first and fifth cranial nerves. Lesions near the cribriform plate or sphenoid ridge may compromise olfaction. The first and second divisions of the fifth cranial nerve course behind, above, and below the orbital cavity, and adjacent lesions may cause deficient sensation over the forehead, cornea, or cheek.

DIAGNOSTIC STUDIES

Basic laboratory studies should include a complete blood count to ascertain possible evidence of inflammation or blood dyscrasia, as well as a chest radiograph to rule out granulomatous or metastatic disease. Other studies may include thyroid hormone assays to determine thyroid function, serum alkaline phosphatase to determine possible bone disease, and bone marrow aspiration if blood dyscrasia seems to be a possibility.

Radiologic Plain Films and Tomography

In order to provide a preliminary survey of more specific radiologic studies, routine films of the orbits and paranasal sinuses consisting of posteroanterior, Waters, lateral, basal, and optic foramina views should be taken. Occasionally such films can be diagnostic.

Tomography enables a three-dimensional perspective of the orbits to be studied, and it gives more precise information regarding their size, extent, and relationship to adjoining structures (Potter, 1972). Anteroposterior tomographic examination usually sections the orbital area every 5 mm, but narrower sections of 1 to 2 mm may be made if necessary. Basal-view tomography is particularly useful in evaluating the lateral walls of the orbit and optic canal.

Increased vertical distances greater than 2 mm between the infraorbital and supraorbital rims signify a space-occupying lesion. This concentric enlargement without bone erosion is typical of benign tumors (e.g., hemangiomas). Likewise, localized bone displacement without destruction of bone margin suggests a slow-growing benign tumor. Widening of the superior orbital fissure is mainly seen with tumors of neural origin (e.g., neurofibroma or glioma). Increased density of bone, particularly along the sphenoid wing, strongly suggests meningioma, whereas diffuse osteolysis or bone destruction is seen when there are malignant tumors such as metastatic lesions or primary orbital malignancies. Calcifications within the orbit are frequently encountered with retinoblastomas but are uncommon with hemangiomas or other venous malformations.

Tomography is especially helpful in distinguishing a sinus mucocele from sinusitis with orbital cellulitis. Displacement of the orbital contents by a mucocele necessarily produces a dehiscence of the lamina papyracea or the roof of the orbit, whereas cellulitis does not usually disturb the bone. Tomography also outlines structures such as the foramen rotundum, pterygopalatine fossa, inferior and superior orbital fissures, and the lacrimal fossa.

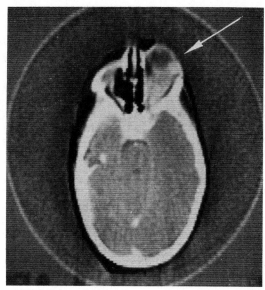

Figure 29–4 A computerized tomogram showing an intraorbital neurofibroma in a 1 year old infant. The arrow indicates proptosis and soft tissue density behind the globe.

mation regarding osseous anatomy, and angiography is a better means of defining vascular detail.

Computerized Tomography (CT)

The advent of computerized tomography has considerably improved the diagnosis of orbital lesions (Wright et al., 1975). In this procedure, the attainment of orbital detail is aided by the relatively large value differences in the absorption rates of fat, bone, and orbital soft tissue structures. When undergoing computerized tomography, children usually require general anesthesia.

The chief value of this type of scan is its reliability in localizing intraorbital lesions (Fig. 29–4). Both the optic nerves and extraocular muscles can be visualized readily, and any associated lesions can be outlined. Another advantage is the concomitant assessment of other anatomic sites, such as the ethmoid and sphenoid sinuses, nasopharynx, cranial cavity, and skull walls, thereby providing information about the origin and extent of the disease.

Computerized tomography undoubtedly surpasses other radiographic tests in the diagnosis of orbital lesions; however, present conventional tomography provides more infor-

Arteriography and Venography

The study of the arterial blood supply can be advantageous in evaluating certain orbital lesions (Vignaud et al., 1972). Selective contrast injection of the internal carotid artery delineates the ophthalmic arterial complex, and visualization is further enhanced by the subtraction technique, which eliminates surrounding osseous shadows (Fig. 29–5). Helpful information is also supplied by the capillary or late arterial phase of the arteriogram, which may outline pathologic vascularity of the lesion itself. Malignant lesions often demonstrate vascular lakes, tangles of tiny vessels, and arteriovenous shunts. However, hemangiomas and venous malformation are typically not visualized (Vignaud et al., 1972).

Venography is particularly valuable in cases of venous malformations and cavernous sinus inflammation or thrombosis (Fig. 29–6) (Hanafee, 1972). It may also help to determine the position of a mass above the muscle cone, an area not well visualized by the computerized tomography scan. Access to the orbital venous system is usually gained via

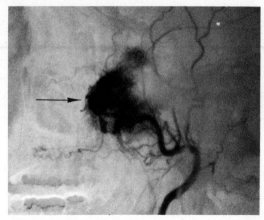

Figure 29–5 An arteriogram in an adolescent male with a nasopharyngeal angiofibroma extending to the orbit. The arrow points to the typical tangle of vessels feeding the tumor.

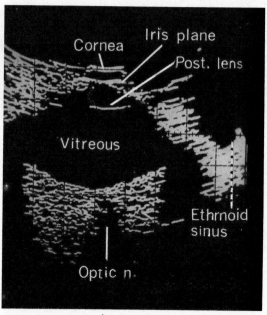

Figure 29–7 B-scan obtained through the midportion of the orbit. The most echo-dense anatomy appears opaque.

one of the forehead veins, although catheterization of the internal jugular vein and retrograde injection into the inferior petrosal sinus may be used. The lesion-localizing capability of this study is predicated on the relatively constant anatomy of the superior ophthalmic vein as it passes near the trochlea, under the medial rectus, and above the optic nerve to enter the cavernous sinus through the superior orbital fissure.

Ultrasonography

The orbital contents may also be scanned by the reflection of ultrasonic echoes (Gitter et al., 1968). These tracings can be recorded

on an oscilloscope as a linear display recording the amplitude and time relationship of the echo to the original pulse (A scan) or the storage of the echo pattern to produce a composite picture (B scan) (Fig. 29–7). The latter method provides two-dimensional acoustic sections of the orbit, which may be photographed. Information is obtained regarding the location, size, and margins of the lesion. Infiltrative lesions can often be distinguished from well-circumscribed lesions by this technique.

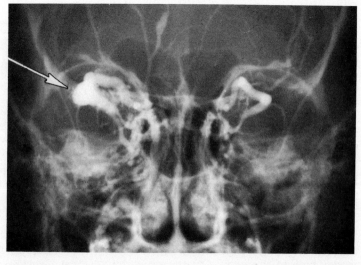

Figure 29–6 An orbital venogram demonstrating a varix of the superior ophthalmic vein as indicated by the arrow.

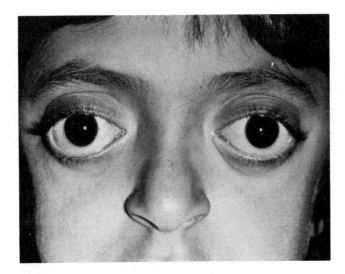

Figure 29-8 A child with Crouzon syndrome exhibiting bilateral proptosis secondary to hypoplasia of the maxillae.

CLINICAL FEATURES OF ORBITAL SWELLINGS

Arbitrarily the origin of proptosis in children can be categorized as being developmental, inflammatory, vascular, neoplastic, or metabolic. It is not the intent of this chapter to give details about each disease but rather to provide an overview of the types of diseases that may affect the orbit in the pediatric patient. Many of these diseases will be covered in the other chapters inasmuch as the orbit can be involved with disease in contiguous structures.

Developmental

Various developmental anomalies of the bony orbit produce proptosis simply by insufficient volume of the orbit, which causes the soft tissue of the eye to protrude. These include several types of craniostenosis (oxycephaly, turricephaly) owing to premature closure of one or more cranial sutures. Hereditary craniofacial dysostosis (Crouzon syndrome) also may produce proptosis due to foreshortening of the orbital floors and hypoplasia of the maxillae (Fig. 29-8).

Developmental defects in the orbital roof may allow a herniation of intracranial contents into the orbit. These are termed a meningocele, encephalocele, or hydroencephalocele, depending on what tissues are encompassed in the herniated sac (Kroll and Casten, 1966).

Dermoid cysts and teratomas may occur in the orbit. Dermoids consist entirely of ectodermal tissue and generally appear in the upper half of the orbit. On the other hand, teratomas, consisting of all three germ layers, are quite rare, although they may be large and are occasionally subject to malignant changes.

Inflammatory

Acute inflammatory disease of the orbit in children is likely to be secondary to infection in the paranasal sinuses. In children under the age of 10 years, the most common source is acute ethmoiditis (Fig. 29-9). In adolescents the frontal sinus may be the original site of the infection because at that stage it has reached nearly full development. Maxillary sinusitis less commonly produces orbital cellulitis. A more insidious inflammatory swelling may develop with mucocele erosion from any of the adjacent sinuses (Chap. 32).

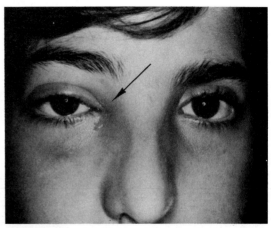

Figure 29-9 The arrow points to obital cellulitis and proptosis secondary to acute ethmoiditis.

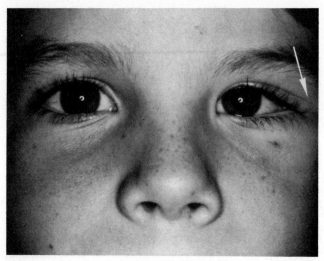

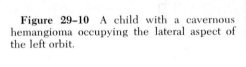

Figure 29-10 A child with a cavernous hemangioma occupying the lateral aspect of the left orbit.

On occasion, orbital inflammation arises from infections of the face or nose that extend to the orbit by retrograde thrombophlebitis. The dreaded complication in these instances is cavernous sinus thrombosis, which produces severe orbital pain, proptosis, and ophthalmoplegia.

Lacrimal sac infections can occur in children if the nasolacrimal duct is obstructed, causing an inflammatory swelling in the medial quadrant of the orbit. The lacrimal gland involvement may accompany mumps in children, and the inflammatory swelling is usually confined to the upper temporal portion of the orbit.

Several specific organisms may be responsible for chronic infection of the orbit. For example, tuberculosis may involve the orbital bone in the form of periostitis; mycotic infection such as mucormycosis and aspergillosis may affect the orbit in the juvenile diabetic patient as well as in those undergoing intensive chemotherapy for blood dyscrasias.

Vascular Abnormalities

Cavernous hemangioma is the most commonly seen vascular lesion of the orbit (Fig. 29–10). Although frequently congenital, this tumor may not grow noticeably until well after birth. Associated hemangiomas of the face, neck, and larynx may occur. Other related disorders are the lymphangiomas that are also seen in infancy and the orbital varices observed more frequently in older children. However, aneurysms of the ophthalmic artery and carotid cavernous sinus fistulas that produce pulsatile proptosis are rare in children.

Neoplasms

Orbital neoplasms may be primary within the orbit, secondary to direct extension from neighboring structures, or metastatic from a distant primary malignancy. The most common primary orbital neoplasms in children are optic nerve glioma and rhabdomyosarcoma. A large proportion of children with glioma will prove to have von Recklinghausen disease, which is characterized by slow growth and early loss of vision (Fig. 29–11). Rhabdomyosarcoma usually grows quite rapidly and appears during the first decade of life (Fig. 29–12). Other primary tumors are melanoma, retinoblastoma, and lacrimal gland tumors.

Secondary invasion of tumors from the paranasal sinuses and nasopharynx is much

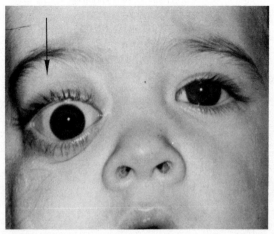

Figure 29–11 An infant with a large neurofibroma of the right posterior-superior aspect of the orbit with obvious proptosis and downward displacement of the eye.

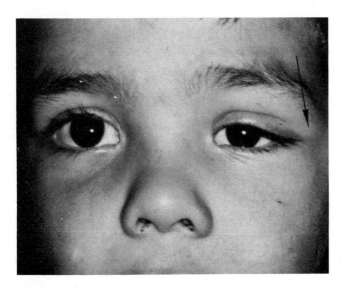

Figure 29–12   A child with a rhabdomyosarcoma involving the left lateral orbital space and temporal fossa.

less frequent in children than in adults. Extension of nasopharyngeal angiofibroma to the orbit is well known in male children. Sarcomas of the sinuses and adjacent structures involving the orbit are more common than squamous cell carcinomas in the pediatric age group. Fibrous dysplasia may involve the orbital bone and may decrease orbital volume, thus producing proptosis (Chap. 36).

The most common metastatic tumor found in the eye is a neuroblastoma from the adrenal gland, which usually occurs in children under five years of age (Kroll and Casten, 1966). Hematopoietic malignancies that may involve the orbit are lymphoma, Hodgkin disease, and chloroma (solid infiltration of cells in leukemia).

Metabolic Disease

Hyperthyroidism occurs much more commonly in adults, although several pediatric patients with Graves disease have been reported. The orbital involvement is usually bilateral and characterized by early lid retraction and eye fullness; eventually chemosis and diplopia may develop.

Other histiocytic diseases that may involve the orbit include eosinophilic granuloma, Hand-Schüller-Christian disease, and Letterer-Siew disease.

SELECTED REFERENCES

Calcaterra, T. C., Hepler, R. S., and Hanafee, W. N. 1974. The diagnostic evaluation of unilateral exophthalmos. Laryngoscope, *84*:231–242.

This article emphasizes those diseases that are otolaryngologic in origin but may present initially as unilateral exophthalmos. The steps in the diagnostic work-up are summarized.

Ophthalmologic Staff of the Hospital for Sick Children. 1967. Diseases of the Orbit, Chap. 15. The Eye in Childhood. Chicago Yearbook Medical Pub.
  This chapter provides a comprehensive review of diseases that may cause proptosis in children. The hospital's experiences with 257 cases serve as the source for the review.

Kroll, A. J., and Casten, V. G. 1966. Diseases of the orbit. *In* Liebman, G., and Gillis, P. (Eds.). The Pediatrician's Ophthalmology. St. Louis, The C. V. Mosby Co.
  This chapter discusses orbital disease in children from the standpoint of general disease categories, i.e., developmental, trauma, inflammation, and neoplasm. There is an excellent discussion of differential diagnosis.

REFERENCES

Calcaterra, T. C., Hepler, R. S., and Hanafee, W. N. 1974. The diagnostic evaluation of unilateral exophthalmos. Laryngoscope, *84*:231–242.

Gitter, R., Meyer, D., and Goldberg, R. 1968. Ultrasonography in unilateral proptosis. Arch. Ophthalmol., *79*:370–375.

Hanafee, W. N. 1972. Orbital venography. Radiol. Clin. North Am., *10*:63–82.

Kroll, A. J., and Casten, V. G. 1966. Diseases of the orbit. *In* Liebman, G., and Gillis, P. (Eds.). The Pediatrician's Ophthalmology. St. Louis, The C. V. Mosby Co.

Ophthalmologic Staff of the Hospital for Sick Children. 1967. Diseases of the Orbit, Chap. 15. The Eye in Childhood. Chicago Yearbook Medical Pub.

Potter, G. D. 1972. Tomography of the orbit. Radiol. Clin. North Am., *10*:21–38.

Vignaud, J., Clay, C., and Aubin, M. D. 1972. Orbital arteriography. Radiol. Clin. North Am., *10*:39–62.

Wright, J. E., Lloyd, G. A., and Ambrose, J. 1975. Computerized axial tomography in the detection of orbital space-occupying lesions. Am. J. Ophthalmol., *80*:78–84.

Chapter 30A

COSMETIC PROBLEMS INVOLVING THE FACE

Richard C. Webster, M. D.

INTRODUCTION

Authors of other chapters will touch on aspects of this chapter and, in many instances, will deal with subjects not covered here because of limitations of space. Thus, skeletal structures aside from those involving the ear will not be discussed, nor will abnormalities involving the deeper soft tissues be addressed, although what occurs in tissues beneath the surface may have profound effects on the face. Spacial limitations dictate selectivity; I have picked four examples from the many possible to illustrate aesthetic concepts and surgical principles as they apply to aspects of appearance. They should be considered as examples, not as an inclusive listing and an exhaustive discussion of the entities (Rees and Wood-Smith, 1973; Lewis, 1973) that can produce abnormality, disharmony, or ugliness in the faces of children.

Throughout this chapter, positional and directional terms are given with respect to the patient facing forward and with the head positioned so that the Frankfort plane is horizontal.

PSYCHOLOGIC, SOCIAL, AND ECONOMIC ASPECTS OF AESTHETIC SURGERY IN CHILDREN

Psychologic Aspects

Whatever the uncharted physicochemical arrangements in the brain are, the observable fact is that humans are social creatures. Most of us like to be different from others only in certain socially approved ways. Even overwhelming parental love and strong sibling support cannot totally overcome a normally intelligent child's observation that physical appearance is important in gaining or losing the approval of others. When what we try to achieve in interaction with others is hindered by what we come to know is something wrong with our appearance, we begin to resent it. When we want to be humorous, we appreciate the laughter of others. The social goal has been achieved. However, none of us likes to be laughed at. The boy with protruding ears quickly tires of hearing laughter and jibes of "Dumbo," "Monkey Ears," "Loving Cup," and "Jug Head." Patterns of inferiority, shyness, and resentment form early and are added to day by day. My observation, in over 30 years of practice, is that these reactions are normal in the otherwise normal individual; only an idiot or a nonperceiver of the world around him or her can escape these feelings. We all are products of our genetic and environmental backgrounds. When something about us separates us from others in a less than desirable way, its recognition affects us psychologically to varying degrees; these variations depend upon the rest of our genetic and environmental backgrounds.

If the reader will close his or her eyes for a moment and add to his or her own face unduly thick lips, to a spouse's face an ectropion from a burn scar, or to a child's face a humped nose, if he or she will then in the mind's eye watch each of these individuals in daily contacts with playmates and adults through the formative years and the sensitive teenage times into adulthood, the reader can imagine what the deformity might do to his or her own emotional life or those of loved ones. Physicians, as a group, dealing daily with "necessary" surgery for lessening of pain and discomfort and for preservation of life and function, tend to have little sympathy for those afflicted with problems of appearance, and perhaps rightly so, as they put things in order of importance. However, almost every surgeon dealing with problems of appearance has noted increased sympathy on the parts of physicians for those with aesthetic defects when disfigurement occurs in the families of the doctors themselves.

Obviously, elimination or improvement of the disfigurement as early as is possible or safe is the treatment of choice in preventing or minimizing psychologic sequelae. However, because complete elimination often is not feasible or safe early in life, parents and child alike should be given the support of a planned program for improvement as early as the surgeon can devise it. Even young children need hope, if it realistically can be provided: the unbearable can be borne, if there is a chance for surcease. The empathy developing between a sympathetic and sensitive physician and the child and family frequently brings all through truly trying times. Many of the most gratifying parts of an entire practice may involve children with long-term problems and the relationships established between them and their parents and the aesthetic surgeon.

Social Aspects

The psychologic aspects just mentioned cannot be divorced from the child's interaction with the society in which he or she must function. Although human behavior is too complex to classify simplistically, we observe three main reactions to aesthetic defects: the child becomes shy and retiring, sometimes to the point of seeming backward; the child becomes aggressive or destructive verbally, physically or both, or he or she becomes the class clown (it is better to be laughed *with* than *at*). In none of these roles is the child satisfied or happy. The earlier in life that he or she slips into one or more of these patterns of interaction, the more profound the effect seems to be later in life, and the more difficult it becomes to reverse. We all know of individuals in whom adversity has led to strengths and the assumption of roles of leadership. However, probably very few ugly leaders or "successes," if given that option, would choose to relive their earlier lives as ugly children.

Essentially every normal person would prefer to interact with others hardly having to think about appearance. In other words, most of us would like to be rated or accepted for what we are by character, intellect, energy, and talent. It is when appearance intrudes into this rating system, so that we are judged or judge ourselves to be undesirable on the basis of our appearances, that our social relationships become less positive or constructive. The frequently improved social life of individuals after aesthetic surgery is a measure of proof that their appearance before treatment affected their social life adversely.

Economic Aspects

Aesthetic deformities carried into the earning years diminish the individual's economic potential. There is no doubt that appearance plays a role in job applications and opportunities. Furthermore, advancement up the organizational ladder often is influenced by an individual's appearance and, in particular, by his or her reaction to aesthetic defects. Certain career opportunities are denied to some individuals largely or completely on the basis of appearance (such as modeling and certain acting and sales opportunities).

Most children are not wage earners, but those who wish or have to enter the employment market must compete with thousands of other young people with normal appearances. When an employer or a personnel department interviewer has a choice, he or she generally will pick the normal or undeformed individual; and in food handling (waiter and waitress), receptionist, and sales jobs, a healthy, wholesome appearance without gross blemishes is an asset, if not a requisite.

However, the main economic effect of aesthetic deformities in childhood comes from their role in preventing children from acquiring those skills and abilities necessary to realize full economic potentials in later life. Anything that gets in the way of the child's learning experience or that hinders social interactions with peers or older children is more likely than not to impede the person later in both choice of career and selection by others for employment or advancement.

The other economic aspect of disfigurement in childhood deals with actual direct and indirect costs of treatment. Costs of surgery, anesthesia, and hospitalization for treatment of many disfigurements of congenital, traumatic, or neoplastic origin are usually partially or completely covered by insurance or third parties. Frequently not covered are office visits and the cost attributable to others necessary in complete treatment of certain deformities. These include, for example, speech therapists, pedodontists, prosthodontists, and orthodontists, who often should be involved in the care of complex problems such as cleft lip and cleft palate. Developmental disproportions of growth, such as many nasal deformities and certain other aesthetic problems, are specifically excluded from coverage in many areas. These include acne scarring and protruding ears. Those portions of care not covered by insurance or other third parties can impose quite a burden on young parents just beginning their earning years and on those with many children and low incomes, particularly when, as is often the case, more than one operation is required for complete treatment. Fortunately, from an economic point of view, many of the procedures required in staged surgery must be spaced far enough apart so that budgeting over a period of time is possible. Many cosmetic surgeons take into account the financial limitations of the parents in burdensome circumstances and lower their fees from the standard ones charged for similar procedures in adults.

MEDICOLEGAL ASPECTS

In certain respects, medicolegal aspects of cosmetic surgery in children do not differ from those applying to aesthetic surgery in adults. However, more individuals are involved than in the typical adult patient–surgeon relationship. Problems of who is responsible for granting consent and undertaking financial obligations must be clarified before surgery, except in emergencies. Intricacies of guardianship, age of consent, and capacity to enter into contracts and assume financial responsibilities must be understood. Differences in statutes of limitations in children and adults exist because care in the child is provided to a growing and changing individual, one whose legal status will alter in the future. Thus, in a state in which the statute runs for two years in the adult, it may run for 21 plus two years in an infant. In another it may run for three years in the adult and seven years in the child. The surgeon must understand the increased medicolegal risk resulting from these realities. It may be wise medically to retain records of treatment permanently, but it is medicolegally mandatory that the surgeon keep them at least until the statute has run its course, and perhaps longer.

COSMETIC SURGICAL CONSULTATIONS, EXAMINATIONS, AND DIAGNOSIS

Cosmetic surgical consultations may be discussed in terms of emergency, newborn or inpatient status, and routine office circumstances. In all cases an accurate diagnosis—physical, psychologic, and aesthetic—must be made. A part of the diagnosis involves an assessment of the parents or guardian. Because appearance is involved, an aesthetic diagnosis must be made and related to what the surgeon believes will be the subsequent effects of the abnormality and its treatment on the child and the parents. Only then can the surgeon discuss prognosis, therapy, and other factors with the parents and with the child, if he or she is old enough.

Most emergency consultations are the result of trauma. When it is possible to speak with the parents before treatment must begin, the surgeon should indicate what has been found and what he or she thinks should be done. Limitations on the surgeon's ability to continue follow-up care should be mentioned if they exist. If the child's condition allows it, the parents should be granted their right to reject all or part of the suggested treatment and to select another surgeon or, at least, request and obtain consultation with other therapists. The cosmetic surgeon must keep in mind that often there is an enormous burden of guilt felt by the parents because of feelings of responsibility for maiming the child. It is natural to want to paint a "rosy" picture under these circumstances. However, no matter how one's heart goes out to the child and the parents, one must remember that lies or gross distortions ("there won't be a scar") ("you won't even notice it in a couple of months") will not be appreciated later on and are likely to lead to lack of confidence in later care or even to medicolegal problems. There is an art to putting parental grief in its place, to pointing out that no parent can watch a child 24 hours a day and that, if the parent could, he or she would produce a totally abnormal individual, and in observing that in no way can the accident be considered deliberate. It is unnecessary and unwise to describe every detail of the injury, but the diagnosis should be stated and then followed with a positive plan for immediate treatment. As soon after treatment as possible, the parents should be told what was found and done and given a tentative prognosis. Almost always, it is wise to point out at this time that further treatment will or may be required to get the best possible result. Still later, at the office, more details about future therapy should be given. In other words, this consultation should be considered a gradual one, not completed until one gets into real planning for the future. At each major step along the way the parents should be consulted and informed.

If one is to undertake cosmetic surgical care of a newborn or of a patient already admitted to the hospital but not now considered an emergency, one must go through many of the same processes just described. In these instances the surgeon usually can spend time outlining the future program and go into more detail. The physician should remember that, again, particularly in the newborn, there may be strong elements of parental guilt ("the sins of the fathers"). The parents of these children also should be given a chance to elect to have the care provided elsewhere and by someone else. If other consultants are needed, the parents should be so informed, particularly if the child has a defect that will require therapy for many years and if state or other agencies provide this care. When the child is old enough to understand, he or she should be told what will be done in the immediate future. When a long-term program will be necessary, it should be mentioned that at appropriate times further treatments will be needed. As the surgeon gets to know the child better, he or she should explain the goals and outline, in general terms, the amounts of time and discomfort involved, as well as the wearing of splints or bandages after surgery. The fewer

unpleasant surprises the better, if a good long-term relationship is to be established.

Consultation at the office involves many of the factors already discussed, although there are some differences relative to consultations dealing with functional or life-preserving surgery. Because so much aesthetic surgery is elective compared to noncosmetic surgery, much more detail must be gone into in providing the information necessary to obtain a truly informed consent. The anticipated effects of growth must be considered and discussed in relation to the proposed therapeutic program and prognosis. Greater attention must be paid to listing alternatives, including that of no treatment. Risks, tissue costs, estimated length of hospitalization, and times of total disability, partial disability, and bandaging or splinting must be provided. A full and honest discussion of financial aspects must take place. A patient who will die or lose an important function without treatment may have little choice as to therapy or, if the situation is somewhat of an emergency, as to surgeon. In cosmetic surgery, the patient and parents almost always have the time to exercise their rights to choose the surgeon and to participate in choices of time and alternative methods of treatment. Therefore, they must be given the information that most intelligent people would need to make these choices. This is what informed consent is all about. Obviously, it does not call for a listing of every possible problem that might arise; it does require a discussion of probabilities and of common or important severe risks or complications (Goldwyn, 1972). The relationship of estimated future growth and development and of changing aesthetics of the face to treatment and prognosis must be included in information provided to obtain informed consent.

In general, most surgery, other than cosmetic, produces results that can be measured easily or objectively. Either death or continued life is the result of life-preserving surgery; most surgery to improve or maintain function gives results that can be observed by others and quantified: it is possible to state that 20 per cent of the function of the hand has been restored. However, when appearance is involved, quantitative measurements are difficult or impossible to make. What is a 20 per cent disfigurement of the face? What would be a 100 per cent disfigurement? In fact, it is difficult even to define ranges of normal. Because of this, it is easy for contentious parents to claim that they are unhappy with the cosmetic result, that they would never have agreed to the surgery had they been informed of what the result would be, and that they are not about to pay the surgeon's bill. Certainly, it is human to have less than friendly feelings for those to whom money is owed until the indebtedness ceases. Much cosmetic surgery is paid for only partly, or not at all, by insurance and third parties. Because payment must be made by the patient or parents and because results are so difficult to quantify, this field, more than any other, lends itself to abuse by litigious, irresponsible, or dishonest parties. Long ago, the dental field became familiar with the statement "the happy denture is the one that is paid for." More and more cosmetic surgeons are insisting upon payment before surgery for those aspects of care dealing with appearance to avoid unhappy patients and litigation. It is almost routinely observed by physicians who have used both systems, payment before and payment after surgery, that parents are happier during the course of treatment and with the results when they owe the doctor nothing than they are when they are left to evaluate the treatment provided in the light of the unpaid bill. It also is felt by surgeons who have tried both systems that they have appreciably lessened their exposure to malpractice hazards in this field by requiring payment before treatment.

A word must be added in regard to aesthetic diagnosis. Proportions must be considered and those elements making for harmony or disharmony must be related to the original problem and to the estimated effects of treatment on future growth and development. A sense of ranges of normal must be developed by those doing this work and should take into account factors such as sex, age, height, body build, ethnic background, changing aesthetic fashions, career goals, social aspirations, other features, and so forth. The diagnosis of what is wrong leads to thinking through all applicable therapeutic modalities known to the surgeon in order to compose the particular operation for that individual with particular problems.

In all three consultation situations, photographic documentation (Wright, 1975; Webster and Smith, 1977) is mandatory. The only exception should be that of the emergency in which treatment must be started before photographs can be taken. Words cannot depict appearance; good photography remains our most accurate medium for recording what was wrong and, later, what the results of treatment have been.

SELECTED COSMETIC PROBLEMS

Elective Incisions and Excisions

All surgeons should choose carefully where to place incisions (Borges, 1973) made to expose underlying structures and to excise abnormalities of the surface. Whether scar lines result from incising or excising, they should be placed, when one has a choice, with consideration of the following factors.

1. Incisions in hair-bearing skin, beveled to transect as few hair follicles as possible, produce less visible scars than those in nearby non-hair-bearing skin.
2. Scar lines made exactly in facial furrows or creases or at the junction of one aesthetic landmark with another (nose with cheek, nose with upper lip, or lip with chin) are less easily observed than those made in the landmark itself.
3. Scars inside a lined structure will be less visible than those made outside.
4. Long, straight lines running across concavities produce elevated webs, and those made across convexities lead to depressions in the convex surfaces.
5. Long, straight lines ending at or near the free border of the ear, the eyelids, the nasal alae, or the lips, or at or near a normal facial line like the philtral crest, often produce distortions or notching as the scars contract.
6. Scars on the front of the face confront the observer; those placed farther back are at an angle to him or her and thus are often less apparent.
7. Scars placed on earlobes, postauricular surfaces, and the lower part of the face are more likely to form keloids or hypertrophic scars than are those positioned further superiorly and anteriorly.
8. When long scars must be positioned to run at angles to the most favorable directions, they are likely to be less visible when curved or broken into shorter segments, parts of which run in the favorable direction, than if they are made in long, straight lines.
9. In general, younger patients are more

likely to form overgrown scars and are less likely to cooperate in using antitension taping or splinting.

Many elective incisions are shown in Figures 30A–1 and 30A–2. Dotted lines show incisions made to excise abnormalities of the skin and vermilion border. Dashed lines show the approximate position of the scar line resulting from closure of the defects. One arrow is used to remind the surgeon of placement of incisions in hair-bearing tissue when possible; the other arrow is there to remind the surgeon that incisions made inside lined structures may be the ones of choice if they provide safe and adequate exposure. Thirty-degree to 45-degree angles are depicted at the ends of the excisions. In most facial areas, one must incise far enough away from a lesion to produce 30-degree angles to avoid protrusions or "dog ears." In the nasal alae and tip even less than a 30-degree angle must be provided; in loose eyelid skin even more than a 45-degree angle often can be made. Deep creases and expression lines usually are not present in children, but having the child move the face or grimace to the extreme may show where lines will develop at a later age.

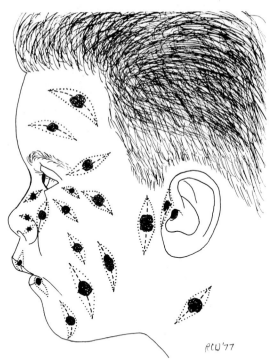

Figure 30A–2 Elective facial incisions and excisions in a child (side view).

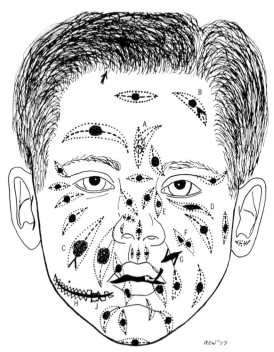

Figure 30A–1 Elective facial incisions and excisions in a child (front view). See text for details. Arrows should remind the surgeon that incisions that can be safely placed in hair-bearing skin or inside lined structures may be ones of choice.

Placing four fingers equidistant from the lesion and compressing the skin equally toward the lesion may produce creases or fine wrinkles indicating what the most favorable direction for a scar line may be. In general, Figures 30A–1 and 30A–2 show many of these favorable directions; but the illustrations should not be used as a substitute for checking in the individual patient each time for his variations from the averages shown in the drawings. There are numerous plastic surgical techniques available for avoidance of the long, uninterrupted lines produced by many of the excisions shown, including rotation, advancement, and transposition flaps (Grabb and Myers, 1975), but space does not allow discussion of these maneuvers here.

In Figure 30A–1, *A* depicts an area where the surgeon may have a choice between a vertical midline excision and one curving off to the side. Compressing the tissue with four fingers so that it moves as if the patient were frowning or elevating his brows will help in making the choice. *B* and *C* show, with heavy lines, how producing two 30-degree angles using an M-plasty (Webster et al., 1976) will allow the surgeon to shorten incision lines. In *C*, the dot below indicates how far the excision would have to go if this lower end were to consist of one 30-degree angle. Closure of the defect at *D* might produce an ectropion if sutures are placed in the usual fashion straight across the wound. If they are placed more horizontally to advance the skin above the wound medially and below laterally, the tendency toward ectropion will be minimized. Even so, this excision must be used with great care, and generally other flaps are safer at this point. *E* shows an excision that will produce a scar line at the junction of the nose with the lower lid and cheek, even though there are no creases or folds at this junction. Ordinarily, the scar line resulting from this type of excision is favorable. *F* illustrates separate excision of two lesions close to each other allowing closure with less tension than would be provided by a longer fusiform excision including both lesions. The offset, though it runs in an unfavorable direction, ordinarily would be inconspicuous as long as it is less than about 6 mm in length. Small excisions at the vermilion border may be handled as shown in the left upper lip, and larger ones may be handled as shown in the right upper lip. Even better may be provision of an offset as shown in the right lower lip. An offset is also shown in the junction of the lower lip with the chin and in Figure 30A–2 at the vermilion border of the upper lip.

Treatment of Nonelective Incisions and Surface Losses

At the time of a child's injury, it is almost impossible to obtain a truly informed consent for surgery from distraught parents. In general under these conditions, closure should be carried out as simply as possible, although wounds must be investigated and deeper structures must be treated before closure is effected. The minimum of sutures should be used to approximate important deeper structures, eliminate dead space that bandaging will not obliterate, and close the surface. If resurfacing requires flaps or grafts, these should be kept as simple as possible too. Far too large or too many stitches are used in many cases where appropriate taping and bandaging would avoid stitch necrosis and marking of surrounding normal tissues that may be needed greatly in later, more definitive repairs. As a rule, it is better to leave some parts of the wound open than to kill uninvolved surrounding tissue with brutal

tension. For skin closure, I prefer the use of sterile antitension paper taping combined with Davis and Geck 6–0 mild chromic catgut (when sutures are required at all); but, in some cases, continuous intradermal pull-out sutures of monofilament polypropylene or similar material may be used. Important landmarks such as free borders, vermilion borders, and philtral crests must be reapproximated accurately. Surface wound care postoperatively should be designed to keep the scar line as narrow as possible. Generally, this may be done with antitension paper tapes applied by the parents or patient to draw the wound edges together for up to six months.

Revisional work on contracting scars that produce distortions, depressions in convex areas, or web elevations in concave ones may involve insertion of grafts or transpositional flaps (Z-plasty is an example) across the scar. If the contraction is not too severe, use of zigzag plasties such as the running W-plasty or geometric broken line closure may prevent future linear contraction. Figure 30A–1 shows, at *G*, the use of the Z-plasty to correct a web scar crossing the cheek–lip groove. When designed as shown, the crossbar at the junction of the transposed flaps will restore the groove. *H* shows how normal tissue is removed on either side of a scar defect to produce triangular flaps that will fit into triangular defects on the opposite side. This technique is now called the running W-plasty. Note the narrow flaps on one side of the defect and the wide ones on the other where the defect curves. *J* depicts a geometric broken-line closure (Webster, Davidson, and Smith, 1977) in which the use of square, rectangular, and triangular flaps of varying widths produces a random pattern more difficult for the observer's eye to perceive and follow than the more regular and predictable running W-plasty. Note the treatment at each end of the scar to get approximately 30-degree angles.

It is permissible to add a small Z-plasty maneuver to an emergency closure if the patient's condition allows it and if the wound is so located and so long that it almost certainly will produce deformity as it contracts. Rarely would it be wise in an emergency to use geometric broken line closures or running W-plasties, particularly in children. One must always bear in mind that many children form hypertrophied scars. The parent who saw his child go into the emergency room with a straight wound will not look with favor

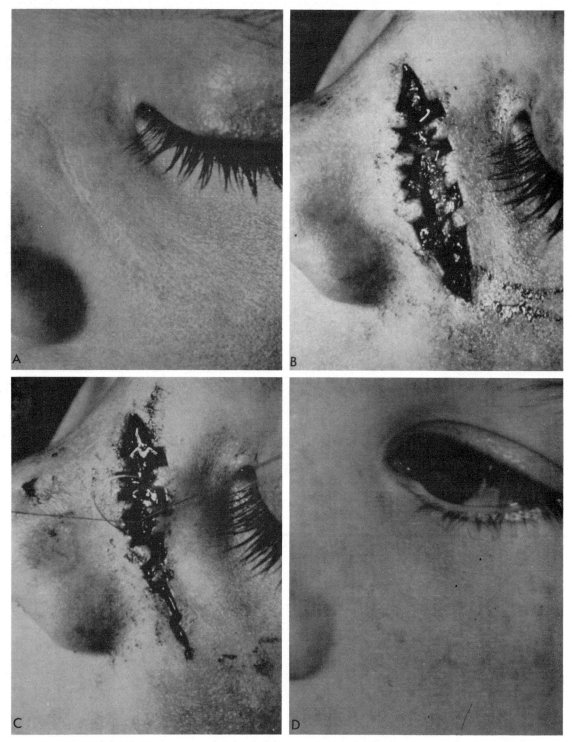

Figure 30A–3 *A*, Scar of nose and cheek running in unfavorable direction. Good plastic closure
was performed in the past in this 8 year old child. *B*, Tailoring for geometric broken line closure by
excision of scar and planned shapes of normal skin on each side of scar. *C*, White intradermal sutures
closing deeper skin edges. *D*, Random pattern makes it difficult to follow the scar.

on the surgeon who produced a long, light-ning-bolt hypertrophied scar in the initial closure. Almost all transposition or advancement flaps dictate more tension in closures of primary wounds, and increased tension is one of the factors producing hypertrophied scars. However, in revisional work, there are times when these procedures are of great value. In almost all cases, they should not be performed before revisional work on deeper structures is done. In cases in which the problem is one involving the surface only and despite meticulous plastic closure the patient has developed a grossly visible scar line, when the line is longer than 20 mm and does not run in a favorable direction and when the patient is well into adolescence, then Z-plasties, running W-plasties, or geometric broken-line closures, alone or in combination, may be most worthwhile. If good plastic closure in a straight line has produced a scar showing no hypertrophy but deformity more visible than it need be because of length, contraction, and direction, then it may be possible to carry out these revisional procedures much earlier in childhood (Fig. 30A–3).

Incisions and surface losses inevitably produce scarring, and there is no method known to get rid of scarring completely. Therefore, the best that can be done is to reduce a wide scar to a narrow one, with as many portions as possible flush with the surrounding normal surface and running in the most favorable directions and positions possible. Flaps from adjacent tissues usually allow revisional improvement of wide scars or of the often cosmetically unacceptable skin graft repairs used for coverage of defects too large to close primarily with adjacent tissues. Serial or multiple excision (Webster, 1969) is a valuable approach under these circumstances. Incisions are made just within the lesion, graft, or scar; the surrounding normal surfaces are undermined; the flaps thus produced are stretched over the abnormality as far as they will go; the overlapped portions of the abnormality are excised; and stitches are then placed to attach the flaps to the edges of the remaining abnormal surface. The stitches are not put into normal skin; they are placed into the lesion edges left attached to the normal surfaces of the flaps. Three to six or more months later, the same process may be repeated. Ordinarily, it will be found that the surrounding normal tissues now can be stretched to cover more of the abnormality. In the growing face, the surface tensions involved can affect the growth of underlying skeletal structures. Also, important aesthetic landmarks may be distorted or pulled toward the defect. Therefore, one must be circumspect in the use of serial excision. However, it still remains one of the most valuable tools in the armamentarium of the surgeon (Fig. 30A–4).

Hemangiomata and Lymphangiomata

Most hemangiomata observed early in childhood will regress spontaneously. Port-wine stains, those involving deeper structures including mucous membranes, and those at the junctions of skin with mucous membrane are less likely to disappear without treatment. Moreover, the last type of lesion mentioned is likely to consist of more mature vessels and to be more resistant to treatment with radiation therapy. Treatment with steroids, compression, ligation of feeding vessels, use of intense cold, embolization, and clotting agents has been carried out in conjunction with surgery. It is reported that all these modalities have been of some use, but all methods have dangers, some greater than others.

Some hemangiomata that ultimately will disappear rage out of control and menace important structures. The eyeball may be pushed out of the orbit or vision may be impeded so completely by a mass in front of the eye that visual function is damaged even though the lesion will regress later. Ulcerations may destroy major landmarks such as the lips or the nose. Treatment of these hemangiomata at this stage of medical science usually is best accomplished with small doses of radiation until a prompt response is obtained.

When infants with hemangiomata involving deeper structures such as the parotid or ones with cavernous elements involving the junctions of mucous membrane with skin are presented, we begin judicious injections with sclerosing agents. Thirty per cent invert sugar worked well; but, because it is not available at present, solutions of Morrhuate Sodium available for injections of varicose veins may be used. The dosage is small (less than 1 cc) at first but is increased with experience with the particular child. Usually a response is noted after the third to fourth

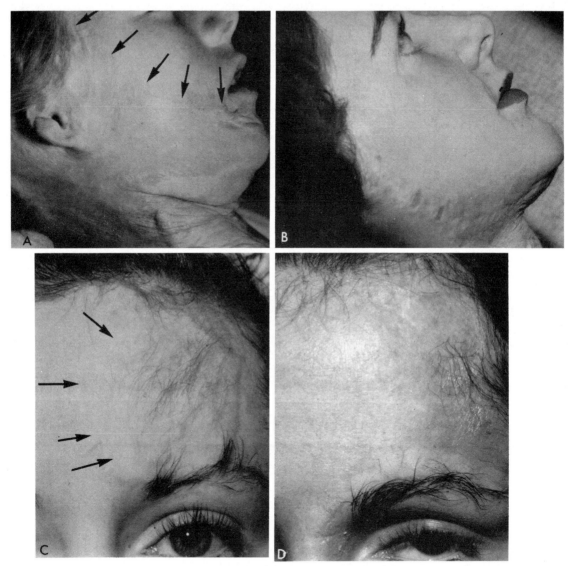

Figure 30A–4 *A*, Arrows point to junction of burn scar with unscarred parts of cheek and temple. *B*, Result of serial excision after several steps over a period of 10 years. *C*, Arrows point to medial edge of skin graft. Lateral edge shows. Forehead and temple skin to be stretched to cover grafted area by serial excisional approach. *D*, Results after 5 steps.

injection, in which case therapy will be continued, if necessary, even beyond six treatments. If there has been no response after six treatments, or if earlier than this it is apparent that the hemangioma is getting out of control and menacing life or important structures or functions, then this treatment is abandoned.

Whereas surgery has been used for embolization and the ligation of feeding vessels, most frequently it is employed for ultimate partial or total removal of lesions that have not regressed or for the treatment of parts of the face that have been scarred, distorted, or destroyed by the lesion in its earlier expanding or ulcerating phase. Lymphhemangiomata and lymphangiomata rarely subside on their own. Often they are extensive and continue to grow all through childhood, although the rate of growth usually slows as the child grows into adulthood. Partial excision of hemangiomata involves having an adequate team to control bleeding with pressure and the use of tourniquet sutures. Large lesions require prompt replacement of blood. Obviously, many plastic surgical techniques are needed, including the use of flaps, serial excisional approaches, and scar revisional modalities (Fig. 30A–5).

Otoplasty For Prominent Ears

In the treatment of prominent ears, the diagnosis dictates the techniques used. Stiffness of cartilage, age, shape of the head and face, the nature of scarring elsewhere, an assessment of the size of the ear, and just what structure protrudes in relation to another structure are among the factors that must be taken into account. Attempts must be made to provide a curved anthelix and a gently curved anthelical superior crus when these are missing. Correction of a protruding antitragus, lobe, or concha must be performed when indicated. Over 75 per cent of the ears that we have treated needed essentially no work to sharpen or increase the anthelical curvature: conchal set-back or pull-in procedures (Webster et al., 1974), combined with detachment or removal of the cauda helices for correction of prominent lobules when required, sufficed in these cases. Removal of discs of cartilage from the eminentia triangularis and conchae allows the ear to sit closer to the head. Soft tissue between the concha and the mastoid may be

excised to allow the auricle to sit even closer. Stitches running from conchal cartilage to the mastoid process may be added to increase the effect; however, care must be taken not to rotate the conchal cup so far forward with undermining, suturing, and skin closure that impingement on the external auditory canal occurs. Skin excision from the sulcus out to a line on the postauricular surface should be sufficient to allow closure under enough tension to add just slightly to the effects of the other maneuvers mentioned. If the lobe still protrudes, a flail may be made of the cauda by incising through it at its attachment to the rest of the auricular cartilage. Usually, then, the lower part of the helix and the lobule itself will be drawn in easily by closure of the skin defect posteriorly.

When the anthelical fold must be sharpened, when a superior crus must be provided, or when both procedures are necessary, this can be done in some instances by mere excision of more skin posteriorly, combined with less undermining of the auricle superiorly. In others, the cartilage must be weakened and/or provided with factors producing the desired curvatures. Among these are abrading the anterolateral surface of the cartilage, scoring it lightly, morselizing it gently, or using permanent mattress sutures, of 4–0 to 5–0 white Tevdek. It is vital that enough sutures be used to prevent the webbing that may otherwise be noticed in the posterior view, and that they be applied in such a fashion that a broadly, rather than sharply, curved superior crus is made. Attempts to correct conchal protrusion with suture techniques alone produce a wide and unaesthetic scapha. Most techniques that involve incising completely through cartilage in the anthelix area lead to sharp, abnormal anthelices. Much experience indicates that operations that correct prominent ears as early as four years of age do not affect growth of the ear adversely (Fig. 30A–6*A*, B).

CONCLUSIONS

This chapter has emphasized the psychologic, social, economic, and medicolegal aspects of aesthetic surgery in children, pointing out how these influence cosmetic surgical consultations, examinations, and diagnosis. It has shown selected examples to illustrate certain aesthetic surgical principles.

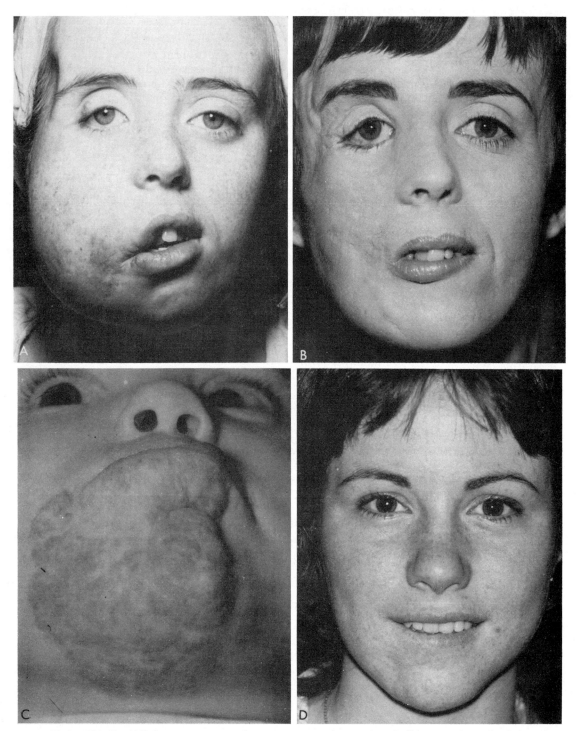

Figure 30A–5 *A*, Enlarging cavernous hemangioma involving orbit, skull, jaws, palate, cheek, lips, and pharynx. *B*, Fourteen years later after external carotid and other arterial ligations, resection of much of the mass, use of buried constricting sutures, and repair with rib bone and cartilage grafts and local flaps. *C*, Hemangioma involving cheek, lip, chin, and neck. *D*, Serial excisional and local flap techniques used (17 years later).

Illustration continued on the opposite page

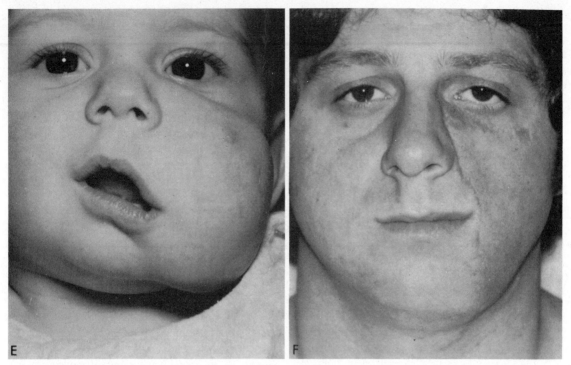

Figure 30A–5 *Continued* *E*, Lymphangioma of left cheek. *F*, Twenty-years later after partial excisions and local flap repairs.

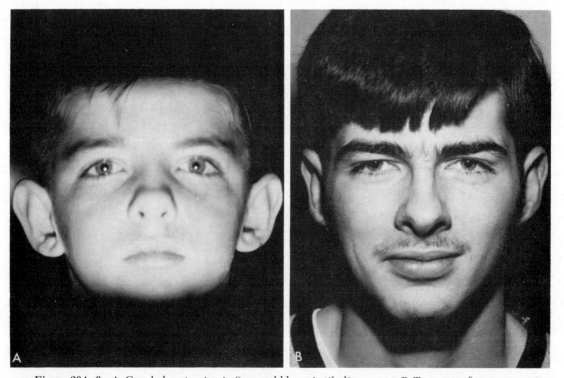

Figure 30A–6 *A*, Conchal protrusion in 9 year old boy. Antihelix present. *B*, Ten years after surgery.

Although there are differences between care involving the individual's appearance and that not devoted to changing appearance, fundamentally cosmetic surgery calls for the same meticulous attention to surgical detail and thoughtful and sympathetic general care that is required of good doctors in any other surgical specialty.

SELECTED REFERENCES

Goldwyn, R. M. 1972. The Unfavorable Result in Plastic Surgery. Boston, Little, Brown and Co.
This book describes many of the risks and complications in cosmetic surgery. Much of the information in it should be imparted to patients and parents before treatment to aid in obtaining informed consents.

Lewis, J. R., Jr. 1973. Atlas of Aesthetic Plastic Surgery. Boston, Little, Brown and Co.
This is a smaller book covering the field and emphasizing the viewpoints of another author experienced in aesthetic surgery.

Rees, T. D., and Wood-Smith, D. 1973. Cosmetic Facial Surgery. Philadelphia, W. B. Saunders Co.
This is the best book available covering most of the field of cosmetic surgery. In general, the illustrations are superbly done and the advice given is wise.

REFERENCES

Borges, A. F. 1973. Elective Incisions and Scar Revision. Boston, Little, Brown and Co.

Goldwyn, R. M. 1972. The Unfavorable Result in Plastic Surgery. Boston, Little, Brown and Co.

Grabb, W. C., and Myers, M. B. 1975. Skin Flaps. Boston, Little, Brown and Co.

Lewis, J. R., Jr. 1973. Atlas of Aesthetic Plastic Surgery. Boston, Little, Brown and Co.

Rees, T. D., and Wood-Smith, D. 1973. Cosmetic Facial Surgery. Philadelphia, W. B. Saunders Co.

Webster, R. C. 1969. Cosmetic concepts in scar camouflaging—serial excisional and broken line techniques. Trans. Am. Acad. Ophthalmol. Otol., *73*:256.

Webster, R. C., Davidson, T. M., and Smith, R. C. 1977. Broken line scar revision. Clin. Plast. Surg., *4*(2):263–274.

Webster, R. C., Davidson, T. M., Smith, R. C., et al. 1976. M-plasty techniques. J. Dermatol. Surg., *2*:393.

Webster, R. C., Smith, R. C., White, M. F., et al. 1974. Otoplasty: pull-in or pull-back techniques—25 year experience. Aesth. Reconstr. Facial Plast. Surg., *1*:1, (microfiche monograph).

Webster, R. C., and Smith, R. C. 1977. Devising evaluating systems for aesthetic procedures. Aesth. Reconstr. Facial Plast. Surg., *4*:1 (microfiche monograph).

Wright, W. K. 1975. Photographic documentation of cosmetic surgery. Aesth. Reconstr. Facial Plast. Surg., *2*:3 (microfiche monograph).

Chapter 30B

COSMETIC PROBLEMS INVOLVING THE NOSE

Richard C. Webster, M.D.

Remarks about psychosocial and medicolegal aspects of cosmetic care made in Chapter 30A apply to the nose as well. After all, it is the most prominent part of the face; disfigurements of it cannot be hidden easily by the victim or missed by the observer. I shall go into more detail in discussing the nose in order to make evident the relationships between the diagnosis of aesthetic problems and the establishment of cosmetic goals, and the processes then followed by the aesthetic plastic surgeon as he or she seeks to alter the anatomy to achieve those goals. Actually, similar processes are used in other cosmetic surgical procedures. No attempt will be made here to go into such technical detail that the novice could use this chapter as a "cookbook" to do a rhinoplasty by "recipe." Rather, I shall show that there is an order to rhinoplasty, that the surgeon sets the goals and then begins a *selecting* process, choosing certain technical modalities and rejecting others as he or she composes the operation for a particular patient with a particular combination of problems.

Throughout this chapter, positional and directional terms refer to a patient facing forward and with the head positioned so that the Frankfort plane is horizontal.

RHINOPLASTY IN EARLY CHILDHOOD

Obviously, in the space allowed here, one can only touch upon this enormous subject.

Congenital anomalies and severe effects of trauma or tumor growth may have to have treatment started early in childhood; but, in general, definitive treatment cannot occur until adolescence or adulthood. I usually prefer to wait to perform primary cosmetic rhinoplasty until the child has stopped growing in height; this guide is one that parents can measure easily. The nose does change some after height has reached its maximum but, in most cases, very little until middle age.

Early repair of trauma, congenital anomalies, or of distortions due to tumor growth, after removal or treatment of the tumor or cyst, should probably be confined to replacement of skeletal structures in as normal positions as possible and with as little undermining (producing sheets of scar) as possible. Contracting or distorting scars that interfere with growth will require treatment, but developmental abnormalities of the skeletal structures that would lead to a recommendation for aesthetic rhinoplasty probably should not be treated definitively until the child stops growing.

Trauma in childhood produces many deformities, which will be discussed later. The nose bent to the side, which may be observed at birth, usually will move to the midline in a few days. However, if examination shows that the septal cartilage is dislocated out of the vomerine groove and columella, then it should be replaced promptly. At any time during childhood, obvious fractures with displacement of bones should be reduced with open or closed techniques as indicated. The

759

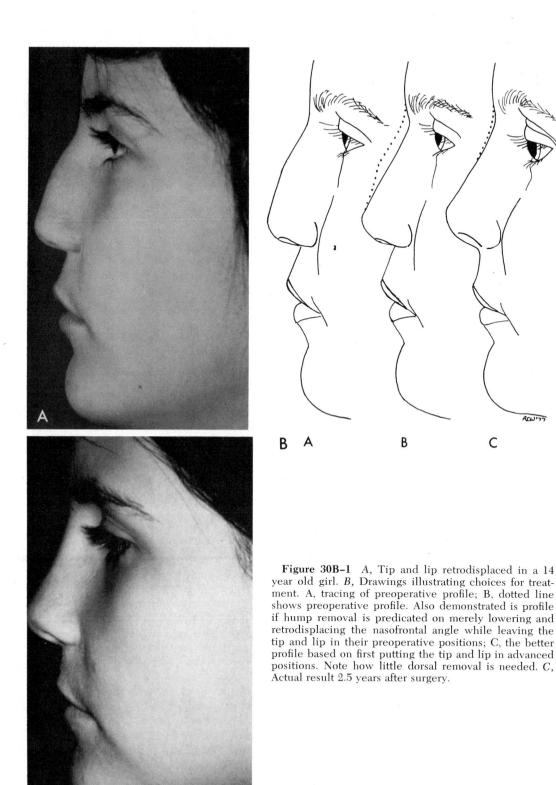

Figure 30B–1 *A*, Tip and lip retrodisplaced in a 14 year old girl. *B*, Drawings illustrating choices for treatment. A, tracing of preoperative profile; B, dotted line shows preoperative profile. Also demonstrated is profile if hump removal is predicated on merely lowering and retrodisplacing the nasofrontal angle while leaving the tip and lip in their preoperative positions; C, the better profile based on first putting the tip and lip in advanced positions. Note how little dorsal removal is needed. *C*, Actual result 2.5 years after surgery.

surgeon must always remember the possibility of septal hematoma or abscess being present in traumatic cases and must take steps to prevent these or treat them as they develop. Radiographs may be needed to help in diagnosis; but, even though it is perhaps medicolegally risky, I prefer not to expose the child to radiographs when my fingers, speculum, and eyes allow for full diagnosis and proper treatment. In cases of fracture that are detected late, a direct intranasal approach rather than undermining allows for separation of misaligned fragments and replacement in their proper positions; this may be followed by appropriate wiring, packing, or splinting.

I suspect that the most common injury leading to later deformity is tearing or peeling the upper lateral cartilages away from the nasal bones and pushing the septal cartilage back so that it fractures, dislocates from its attachments to bone, or both (Fig. 30B–1). Often the child is not seen at the time of injury; but even when he or she is, I find this entity a difficult problem to manage. All too often, splinting and packing are not effective in preventing the later development of a relative bony hump located just above a somewhat retrodisplaced cartilaginous dorsum. If obvious septal dislocation is noted at the time of injury, at least this much of the total injury should be corrected.

I do not believe that every slight difference in airflow through the nasal passages or in breathing capacity requires aggressive therapy in childhood. If a child with a septal deflection has recurring infections of the sinuses or middle ears, then I will do the most limited septoplasty or septorhinoplasty required to better the airway. Again, I undermine or resect as little bone and/or cartilage as possible.

RHINOPLASTIC TECHNIQUES

Septorhinoplasty for aesthetic improvement (Goldwyn, 1972; Lewis, 1973; Rees and Wood-Smith, 1973; Anderson, 1975; Beekhuis, 1974; Smith, 1974; Webster, 1975; Wright, 1974) is the most challenging of all cosmetic procedures and probably does more long-lasting good for more people than any other aesthetic operation. However, many inadequate or bad results still occur. Some are due to improper or incomplete aesthetic diagnosis, and some result from incompetent, inadequate, or overly aggressive surgery. I can only outline some of the concepts involved here; the subject, in reality, is complex and vast. However, I have worked out a point of view in over 30 years of doing thousands of rhinoplasties (Webster, 1975; Webster, Davidson, Rubin, et al., 1977 and 1978; Webster, Davidson, and Smith, 1977a and 1977b; Webster et al., 1975a, 1975b, and 1976; Webster, White, and Courtiss, 1972 and 1973), and I hope that the following brief remarks will be of value to younger or less experienced surgeons dealing with this procedure.

The nose must be related, in aesthetic planning, first to the brow, upper lip, and cheeks (Fig. 30B–1), and then to the rest of the facial features and the chin in particular (Fig. 30B–2*A* and *B*). Beginners should avoid excision of lining tissue except in septal shortening and hump removal. Insufficient draping or excessive contraction of the covering tissues may restrict the degree of perfection possible; but, within limits, excisions from skeletal structures will diminish certain dimensions and decrease the total external nasal size. Skeletal excisions produce voids; scar tissue forming in them pulls the more mobile skeletal components toward those less mobile. Incising completely through the tip cartilages or separating them from their attachments to the more fixed skeleton changes their mechanical characteristics. Overoperating frequently results from inability to control tip projection because of attempts to hide tip retrodisplacement by excessive excision of the dorsum. The widened alar base resulting from tip retrodisplacement leads to alar and nostril sill resections that might not be required were the surgeon able to keep the tip where he or she wanted it to be. A radix too prominent gives a masculine and often undesirable appearance, and a too-concave or retrodisplaced dorsal profile will lead to a feminine, weak, or "washed out" appearance. Inadequate projection of dorsum and tip leads to a blunted, uncouth appearance, and a tip too inferiorly positioned leads to an aged, tough, or avaricious look. There are exceptions, but a colummella–labial angle of 95 to 105 degrees is likely to be satisfactory in the male, and 105 to 115 degrees is likely to be pleasing in the female. Nostrils showing too much from the front (resulting from excessive superior rotation of the tip) produce a "pig snout" deformity, one most difficult to correct.

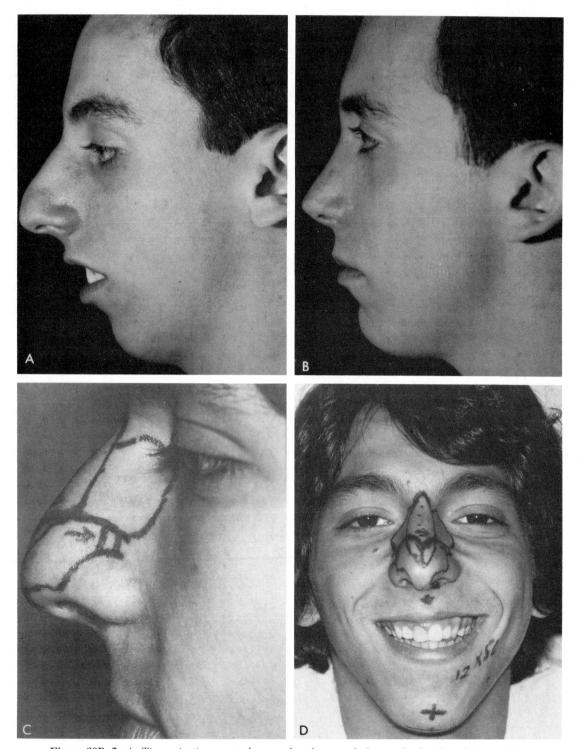

Figure 30B–2 *A,* Tip projecting, central upper lip short, and chin underdeveloped in an 18 year old boy. *B,* Tip retrodisplacement allowed central upper lip to slide downward. This and chin augmentation provide easly closure of lips to cover formerly grossly exposed teeth. *C,* Marking — rectangular excision of lateral crural cartilage will allow anterior part of lateral crus to retrodisplace and tip to rotate superiorly. *D,* Two 12 × 13 × 50 mm carved silicone rubber implants are to augment chin region. Observe fusiform excisions of cephalic lateral crura to allow narrowing.

In general, I perform at least three "operations" in rhinoplasty. The first is at the time of consultation; the second is that marked on the outside of the nose just before surgery (Fig. 30B–2C and D). These lend themselves to much easier correction than does the actual or third procedure. Almost the entire skeletal anatomy can be portrayed on the outside of the nose. Then, the proposed changes to achieve the desired effects can be added to the drawing. This marking is valuable in forcing the surgeon to think the procedure through from beginning to end; and, assuming that the marking was accurate and the procedure goes as planned, the photographs taken of the marked nose make the most accurate operative record possible.

Rhinoplastic techniques have been described in many texts and articles; this is not the place to discuss them in detail. Some, however, are more dangerous than others. Those relying heavily on septal shortening to pull the tip superiorly may lead to columellar retraction if the components in the lateral walls are not adequately treated. When they are adequately treated, often no excisions of septal cartilage and lining are needed to obtain the desired superior rotation of the tip. Many septorhinoplasties can be performed with no septal transfixion incision or with one made far enough anteriorly so that the posterior attachments of the medial crura to the septal cartilage are not destroyed. When the septum must be shortened in the vertical dimension by excision of septal cartilage and lining, the safest way to do it is to use a high septal transfixion incision. The scar that forms will have septal cartilage below and above it to limit its linear contraction and tip-retrodisplacing effect. Almost all septal work needed for airway improvement can be performed through a high septal transfixion or through the rhinoplastic incisions that expose the cartilaginous dorsum. The transfixion incision sweeping from the tip through the entire length of the membranous septum either to or beyond the anterior nasal spine introduces tip retrodisplacing factors and is unnecessary in most cases.

Narrowing

Essentially all rhinoplasties involve *narrowing* of one or more components. Hump removal almost always dictates narrowing of the remaining bony vault. Lateral osteotomies, which begin far posteriorly and well inferior to the level of the inferior turbinates, may lead to impingement on the important lower part of the airway. Curved lateral osteotomies (Fig. 30B–3H), which begin more anterosuperiorly so that intact bone holds the lateral walls out just above the alar lobules, tend to protect the patency of the airway here. Narrowing of the upper portion of the tip involves excision of widely flaring or recurving portions of the cephalic parts of the lateral crura (Fig. 30B–3G) and the caudal portions of the upper lateral cartilages, often combined with excisions of thick soft tissue at this level and of sesamoid cartilages when they are present between the upper and lower lateral cartilages. If medial crura at the foremost part of the tip are too far apart, those portions defining this part of the tip in both profile and frontal views must be allowed to move toward each other. This is done by excisions of soft tissue between them and by modifying the upper portions of the anterior medial crura by excisions, incisions, or morselization so that their laterally flaring tendencies are diminished or eliminated. Rarely is it necessary in narrowing maneuvers, and at times it can be dangerous, to transect the tip cartilages at the nostril margins. Most widening of the alar base can be improved or corrected fully with nostril sill resections, avoiding the dangers of cosmetic abnormalities and more visible scarring from more lateral excisions of alar tissues near the cheeks.

Profile Lines

The *establishment of profile lines* involves many factors (Fig. 30B–3). I find it helpful to plan the position of the nasofrontal angle and the columella–labial junction first; then the position of the tip is selected. Knowing these three positions, one then can decide how to go about achieving them surgically. Almost exact *positioning of the nasofrontal angle* can be achieved by appropriate excisions of bone and/or soft tissue, including procerus muscle, or by grafting either nasal or septal bone and cartilage. *Columella–labial junction and angle changes* can be made with plumping grafts or struts of cartilage behind and between medial crura, with tip advancing or retrodisplacing maneuvers, with excisions of caudal septal cartilage, or with a combination of these. Rarely is it wise to resect the anterior nasal

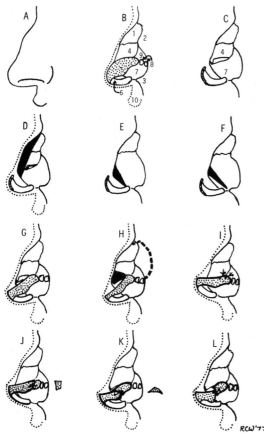

Figure 30B-3 Diagrams illustrating factors involved in superior rotation of tip. *A*, Brow, nose, and lip profile. *B*, Skeletal structures: 1, nasal bone; 2, frontal process of maxilla; 3, anterior nasal spine; 4, upper lateral cartilage; 5, lateral crus (stippled); 6, medial crus; 7, septal cartilage; 8, alar accessory cartilages; 9, fibrous tissue between cartilages and pyriform aperture; 10, central upper lip. *C*, Lateral crus removed to show more fixed skeletal structures. *D*, Removal of dorsal structures depicted in black will allow some superior rotation and tip retrodisplacement. *E*, Closure of septal void will pull upward on anterior columella and tip. *F*, The same applies to closure of the septal void above the high septal transfixion shown here. *G*, Narrowing resection of anterocephalic lateral crus produces complete strip. Recurving or flaring lower part of upper lateral cartilage is revealed. *H*, Narrowing resection here has set the tip-defining point closer to the junction of the lower margins of the medial and lateral crura. Dashes show curved lateral osteotomy. Large excision of upper lateral cartilage depicted introduces superiorly rotating forces but destroys valve and usually is unwise. *I*, Incising behind lateral crus and retrodisplacing complete strip with sutures as well as advancing medial crura (both techniques shown here) will superiorly rotate tip. Note changes in lip and columella-labial angle. *J*, Excising the segment of lateral crus shown shortens lateral crus horizontally and superiorly rotates tip. Excised cartilage shown at right. *K*, Excising somewhat triangular piece of cartilage from the rim strip or lateral crural flap allows superior rotation. *L*, This lateral crural flap variation allows superior tip rotation while thrusting the lower margin of the rim strip downward to improve high alar margin or acute angulation of alar margin.

spine. The tip can be pushed and rotated to the position desired with the surgeon's fingers after deciding the positions of the nasofrontal and columella–labial angles. This finger exercise will tell the operator whether tip-advancing, retrodisplacing, or rotating procedures will be wise and will give him or her an idea what the effect will be on the central upper lip. If the lower part of the tip and the anterior columella suddenly widen as the tip is pushed to the desired position, this flaring is caused by overriding of the caudal septal cartilage by the medial crura. To prevent this, superior portions of the medial crura or caudal septal cartilage must be excised (Fig. 30B–3*E*), or the septum must be shortened by excision of cartilage and lining, allowing the caudal edge of the septal cartilage to rotate or move superiorly (when high septal transfixion incisions are used) (Fig. 30B–3*F*).

Short of external incisions and major maxillofacial maneuvers (procedures rarely permissible in cosmetic rhinoplasty), it is only possible *to project the tip* or *lengthen the tip to radix distance* within limits (or to simulate these effects) by one or more of the following procedures: (1) setting the nasofrontal angle higher or the columella–labial angle more posteriorly; (2) grafting or implanting "pushers" or "fillers" beneath skin and overlying the nasal skeleton; (3) moving the medial crura forward (Fig. 30B–3*I*) by grafts or implants behind them, suturing them forward on the septal cartilage, or detaching the caudal septal cartilage to which they are attached and moving it forward on the fixed septal cartilage above; (4) detaching and advancing the lateral crura on the upper lateral cartilages and septum at the septal angle; (5) making boxy or widely flaring or obtuse junctions between medial and lateral crura more acute (thus more projecting); (6) increasing medial crural length by borrowing "turn-over" or "leaf-of-book" flaps from lateral crura or vice versa; and (7) setting tip-defining points lower (Fig. 30B–3*G* and *H*). Depending on how grafts or implants above and behind the columella–labial junction are placed and shaped and which of the techniques just mentioned are employed, the columella–labial junction may be moved in almost any selected direction, but the central upper lip can only be moved superiorly, inferiorly, or forward (Fig. 30B–1). If the cheek profiles are too flat or retrodisplaced or if the nostrils are made to look too long by any of the maneuvers just listed, grafts or implants may be placed behind the soft tissues where the ala–labial junction meets the cheek. In general, grafts are better than implants the closer to the surface they must be placed. In my experience, the patient's own septal cartilage, then nasal cartilage, then septal and nasal bone, are the best grafts for most rhinoplastic purposes. It is dangerous to discard any tissue removed until the entire operation is finished to the surgeon's satisfaction.

The *relationship of tip rotation to projection* forward from the facial plane depends on the attachments of skin and cartilage above, below, and behind the tip. It will rotate inferiorly and superiorly, and at some point along its somewhat peculiar arc of rotation it will project farthest forward from the facial plane. Often this point may be lower than it should be to be most aesthetic. Therefore, rotation to this ideal level will introduce a slight retrodisplacement as related to the facial plane. This is usually of little cosmetic consequence. On the other hand, a depressed tip positioned more inferiorly than it should be will become more projecting as it is rotated toward a more pleasing position unless other steps are taken to diminish the resulting increased projection.

Tip Retrodisplacement

Tip retrodisplacement beyond the control of the surgeon occurs all too easily. One can assume that the net effect of undermining in separating the tip cartilage from skin for exposure and draping, and of separating the tip cartilage from fixed skeleton in narrowing maneuvers, will be one of tip retrodisplacement. Short medial crura, long incisions separating medial crura from caudal septal cartilage and separating lateral crura from upper lateral cartilages and fibrous attachments at and near the pyriform aperture (carried well beyond the posterior extent needed merely for narrowing excisions), are tip retrodisplacing factors. Also, resection of the lower cartilaginous dorsum in setting its profile posteriorly (Fig. 30B–3D), transecting the tip cartilage completely from top to bottom, and larger excisions of cartilage than are needed for wise and precise narrowing and rotating of the tip (Fig. 30B–3H) are retrodisplacing factors. The more of these factors that are involved in the operation, the more need there is for the surgeon to use one or several of the maneuvers mentioned in the paragraph on achieving tip projection just to preserve the original projection or to minimize unwanted retrodisplacement. Desired tip retrodisplacement may be obtained by the calculated use of one or more of the retrodisplacing techniques just listed or by planned excisions of medial or lateral crural cartilage or both (Fig. 30B–3J), with or without lining or the use of permanent sutures, or both techniques, which retrodisplace the medial crura on the septal cartilage and/or lateral crura on the upper lateral cartilages and fibrous tissue near the pyriform aperture (Fig. 30B–3I).

Tip Rotation

Inferior rotation of the tip rarely is desired; it often happens inadvertently. When desired, it can be produced by using those factors listed earlier that produce retrodisplacement or shortening of the medial crura or advancement of the lateral crura.

A simulation of *superior tip rotation* can be given by deepening or lowering the nasofrontal angle or by advancing or inferiorly displacing the columella–labial junction. Shortening the skin between the radix and the tip or lengthening the columellar skin rotates the tip superiorly, and vice versa. In cosmetic rhinoplasty, most rotation results from changes in cartilaginous tissue. Turnover flaps, grafts, or excisions of tip cartilage so that remaining cartilage presses the skin forward and defines the tip farther up from the junction of the margin of the columella with the alar margin than it was defined preoperatively also will give the impression of superior tip rotation. These techniques are valuable when actual superior tip rotation would also elevate the anterior nostril edges so that too much nostril would show from the front.

Dynamically, most tip techniques fall into two main categories, those that transect the tip cartilage from above through the margin near the nostril edge and those that leave the margin intact. In general, the latter are safer. Tip-positioning procedures that cut completely through the tip cartilage near the nostril margin or that separate one or more of its components from support to fixed skeletal elements introduce more uncertainties in healing than do those that leave an intact strip of cartilage adjacent to columellar and alar borders or those that leave attachments to the fixed skeleton undisturbed. Procedures that produce large cartilaginous voids (Fig. 30B–3*H*) subject the patient to greater risks of asymmetric healing, dimpling, notching, and collapse than do those that leave more cartilage present to resist scar pulls and changes in atmospheric pressure during breathing. Rarely should cartilaginous excisional narrowing alone (Fig. 30B–3*G*) leave any appreciable voids when the remaining components are positioned where the surgeon wants them to remain. Almost never is it wise to excise any but the lowest and most anterior parts of the upper lateral cartilages to establish the profile of the dorsum and prevent overriding of the remaining upper lateral cartilages by the remaining lateral crural cartilage (Fig. 30B–3*D* and *H*).

Let us say that those excisions just to produce narrowing have been performed (Fig. 30B–3*G*). At this moment, still present is an intact strip of cartilage running from the attachments of the posterior medial crus to the septal cartilage, forward to the tip, and from it back and up to the intact attachments of the posterior lateral crus to the upper lateral cartilage and to the fibrous tissues near the pyriform aperture. This I call a *complete strip* (Fig. 30B–3*G*). It resists retrodisplacement, nostril notching, nostril rim collapse, and tip rotation. If its anterior portions are widely flaring, morselization and/or suturing of its medial crus to the other medial crus may allow further narrowing and slight projection of the tip. This complete strip can be superiorly rotated along with the tip by pushing or pulling the medial crus forward (Fig. 30B–3*I*) or by retrodisplacing the lateral crus (Fig. 30B–3*I*). At times, it is possible to vary the distance from the junction of the alar and columellar margins to the new tip-defining point produced by the most anterior part of the transecting incision (Fig. 30B–3*G* and *H*).

Transection at or near the dome breaks the spring and allows slight projection and narrowing if flaring portions are handled appropriately or if one crus is lengthened at the expense of the other. Also, superiorly rotating factors, such as vertical septal shortening, work against less resistance than with a complete strip. Transection of the lateral crus farther posteriorly than is required for flaps to lengthen the functioning medial crura or to narrow the tip breaks the spring and converts the lateral crus into two pieces of cartilage, one anterior to the transecting incision at the margin of the cartilage closest to

the nostril edge, and one posterior to it. The anterior segment continues close to the nostril rim into the tip and then posteriorly in the columella to the posterior end of the medial crus. This portion is called the *rim strip*. It rotates and retrodisplaces easily. When all or so much of the posterior portion of lateral crural cartilage is excised that a large void is left between the rim strip and the upper lateral cartilage and pyriform aperture, I call this the rim strip technique. Its large voids allow scar contraction to produce asymmetries, dimpling, and nostril collapse or retraction. I reserve this technique for certain revisions and for primary rhinoplasties in rare patients with exceedingly thick and porky skin.

Much safer, when rotation, retrodisplacement, or both are wanted, is the lateral crural flap technique. Here, the lateral crural cartilage posterior to and perhaps superior to the rim strip is left attached to fixed skeleton above and behind. This segment interposed between fixed skeleton and the rim strip is called the *lateral crural flap* (Fig. 30B–3*J* through *L*). Far too many factors are involved in the proper selection of the placement and shape of the transecting incisions that produce the rim strip and the lateral crural flap to go into here; but, with appropriate planning, it is possible to improve acute angulations or high arching of the alar margin. Pushing the tip to the position of superior rotation and/or retrodisplacement desired, the surgeon will find overlapping of parts of the rim strip and lateral crural flap. Excision of overlapped parts of one or both pieces of cartilage allows relatively precise tailoring in reshaping the new lateral crus. Permanent or catgut sutures or, in some cases, mere taping and splinting, may be used for reconstitution of the lateral crus.

In summary, then, *superior rotation of the tip* by modifying the lateral crus involves: (1) detaching it from the more fixed skeleton and suturing it with permanent sutures in a retrodisplaced position; (2) detaching a complete strip and permanently suturing it to more fixed skeleton in a retrodisplaced position (Fig. 30B–3*I*); or (3) transecting the lateral crus, placing the tip in the desired position, often excising overlapped or overlapping cartilage, so that the horizontal length of the lateral crus is shortened (Fig. 30B–3*J*) and/or the lateral crus is reshaped with at least its anterior portion rotated upward (Fig. 30B–3*K* and *L*), and joining the remaining portions of cartilage by sutures or taping and splinting. Although occasionally indicated, procedures transecting near or at the domes, or ones transecting farther back with excisions of most or all of the lateral crus behind and perhaps above the rim strip, are more dangerous than the others just mentioned and should not be used unless specific and overriding indications for their use are present.

Profile Adjustment

Sculpturing of flaring, thickened, drooping, or flabby alar lobules is hazardous for the beginner and can lead to asymmetries and scarring that are difficult to correct. The same is true of fine trimming and reshaping of the caudal margins of the medial crura for correction of slight hanging or drooping of the columella.

When the tip position has been established, hump removal and dorsal trimming allow controlled adjustment of the profile. Provision of adequate projection of lip and cheek profiles and projecting and rotating the tip to its desired position often make it clear that much less hump and dorsum need to be removed than was at first evident (Fig. 30B–1). The safest technique for the removal of the bony hump involves the use of sharp rasps, followed by shaving or trimming of the septal and upper lateral cartilages. When large humps must be removed or when the bone and cartilage must be saved and used, then I use an osteotome, followed by rasping and trimming. It should be emphasized that osteotomies or fracturing techniques required to correct gross curvatures or asymmetries of the bony components should be accomplished before the curved lateral osteotomies are performed. Final dorsal adjustments are made after performance of the curved lateral osteotomies (Fig. 30B–3H) and infracturing allow for moving the lateral walls against the septum. Deviations, curvatures, overriding of fractured portions, and unduly thickened parts of the bony and cartilaginous septal bridge against which the lateral walls are to be moved must be corrected and the lateral walls moved medially before final adjustment of the dorsum. Thinning, morselizing, incising, and resecting techniques all are employed in one case or another, as indicated, to obtain a straight septum. It will be found that many asymmetries may be corrected by the maneuvers described. After a final check of the dorsum and the tip, suturing, taping, and splinting finish the operation.

SUMMARY

Versatile and experienced rhinoplastic surgeons can perform most procedures under local or general anesthesia, with or without headlights. Most can vary the order of the steps in the surgery. I have tried to outline principles involved and have suggested the safest of the many choices and routines available. Along the same lines, I would recommend that the beginner start with general anesthesia and a headlight to supplement the lights available in the operating room. Bleeding will be greater under general anesthesia, but more precise judgments can be made when tissues are not swollen from injected medications. All packs used in surgery must be removed by count.

Every effort should be made to follow these patients for at least three years. It takes at least this long in many noses for approximate end results to be achieved. Defects of surgery and variations in healing can be appreciated only by following the patients until essentially all changes have occurred. Seek every opportunity to learn about facial aesthetics and the ranges of normal and to broaden one's knowledge as to how to change the anatomy to achieve desirable physiologic and aesthetic effects. Thoroughly analyze and inform patients and parents before surgery. The goal is more than a nose that looks good to the surgeon; it is a happy patient and a family satisfied in every way. Select the patients carefully. Leave demanding, difficult, or revisional cases to experienced operators; even they will have problems with these patients. One of the most valuable instruments in all of surgery is the telephone; use it early if help is needed.

Paying attention to the procedures recommended and avoiding the pitfalls mentioned should help the beginner or relatively inexperienced practitioner to develop an orientation and a practical philosophy that are likely to get him or her through those difficult early years until the surgeon has worked out individual approaches to rhinoplasty, the most difficult, challenging, and interesting of all cosmetic procedures. Using rhinoplasty as the example for all of cosmetic surgery, I have tried to show that the salient requisites are astute diagnosis of physical and aesthetic problems, full discussion before surgery, selection from among the best techniques in composing each operation, development of technical skills, and then rigorous and long follow-up. A fulfilling practice and many happier lives will be the result.

SELECTED REFERENCES

Goldwyn, R. M. 1972. The Unfavorable Result in Plastic Surgery. Boston, Little, Brown and Co.
> This book describes many of the risks and complications in cosmetic surgery. Much information in it should be imparted before treatment to patients and parents in obtaining informed consent.

Lewis, J. R., Jr. 1973. Atlas of Aesthetic Plastic Surgery. Boston, Little, Brown and Co.
> This is a smaller book covering the field and emphasizing the viewpoint of another author experienced in aesthetic surgery.

Rees, T. D., and Wood-Smith, D. 1973. Cosmetic Facial Surgery. Philadelphia, W. B. Saunders Co.
> This is the best book available covering most of the field of cosmetic surgery. In general, the illustrations are superbly done and the advice given is wise.

REFERENCES

Anderson, J. R. 1975. Cartilage-splitting tip techniques. Aesth. Reconstr. Facial Plast. Surg., 2 (microfiche monograph).

Beekhuis, G. J. 1974. Rhinoplasty: septo-rhinoplasty for the twisted nose. Aesth. Reconstr. Facial Plast. Surg., 1, (microfiche monograph).

Goldwyn, R. M. 1972. The Unfavorable Result in Plastic Surgery. Boston, Little, Brown and Co.

Lewis, J. R., Jr. 1973. Atlas of Aesthetic Plastic Surgery. Boston, Little, Brown and Co.

Rees, T. D., and Wood-Smith, D. 1973. Cosmetic Facial Surgery. Philadelphia, W. B. Saunders Co.

Smith, T. W. 1974. Nasal tip surgery. Aesth. Reconstr. Facial Plast. Surg., 1, (microfiche monograph).

Webster, R. C. 1975. Advances in surgery of the tip — intact rim cartilage techniques and the tip-columella-lip esthetic complex. Otolaryngol. Clin. North Am., 8:615–644.

Webster, R. C., et al. 1975a. Rhinoplastic techniques demonstrated in black cadaver — part I. Aesth. Reconstr. Facial Plast. Surg., 2, (microfiche monograph).

Webster, R. C., et al. 1975b. Rhinoplastic techniques demonstrated in black cadaver — part II. Aesth. Reconstr. Facial Plast. Surg., 2, (microfiche monograph).

Webster, R. C., et al. 1976. Atlas of tip rhinoplasty techniques on teaching model. Aesth. Reconstr. Facial Plast. Surg., 3, (microfiche monograph).

Webster, R. C., Davidson, T. M., Rubin, F. F., et al. 1977. Recording projection of nasal landmarks in rhinoplasty. Laryngoscope, 87:1207.

Webster, R. C., Davidson, T. M., Rubin, F. F., et al. 1978. Nasal tip projection changes related to cheeks and lip. Arch. Otolaryngol., 104:16.

Webster, R. C., Davidson, T. M., and Smith, R. C. 1977a. Curved lateral osteotomy for airway protection in rhinoplasty. Arch. Otolaryngol., 103:454.

Webster, R. C., Davidson, T. M., and Smith, R. C. 1977b. External marking in rhinoplastic planning. Laryngoscope, 87:126.

Webster, R. C., White, M. F., and Courtiss, E. H. 1972. Intact alar rim combined with septal transfixion in rhinoplasty — 20 year experience. Intern. Micro. J. Aesth. Plast. Surg. Corr. Rhinopl., E:1–60.

Webster, R. C., White, M. F., and Courtiss, E. H. 1973. Nasal tip correction in rhinoplasty. Plast. Reconstr. Surg., 51:384.

Wright, W. K. 1974. Hump removal, osteotomy, and recontouring of the bony cartilaginous pyramid. Aesth. Reconstr. Facial Plast. Surg., 1, (microfiche monograph).

Chapter 31

CONGENITAL MALFORMATIONS OF THE NOSE AND PARANASAL SINUSES

P. M. Sprinkle, M.D.

F. T. Sporck, M.D.

INTRODUCTION

Surgical procedures to correct major craniofacial congenital malformations are gradually being improved with increased experience and advances in surgical techniques. Such procedures usually involve a team approach since it is necessary to correct cosmetic, ophthalmic, respiratory, neurologic, and dental abnormalities and deformities in order to provide for optimal functioning of the multiple systems of the head and face.

Preoperative assessment of a child who is a candidate for such surgery must include an evaluation of the mental state of the patient and of the parents as well as an evaluation of the home environment in which the congenitally deformed child must live. The multiple problems of children with such deformities mandates an interdisciplinary approach to their management. One cannot make changes in a complex anatomic system such as the nose without seriously affecting adjoining anatomic structures.

MENINGOENCEPHALOCELES

A classification of meningoencephaloceles is shown in Table 31–1. It is difficult to diagnose meningoencephaloceles clinically because such diagnosis depends upon the results of microscopic examination of the excised tissue. Morphologic examination of a meningoencephalocele shows that it is composed of glial tissue and has a cerebrospinal fluid connection to the subarachnoid space.

Herniations of glial tissue are routinely classified according to the site at which and extent to which they bulge from the cranial cavity (Table 31–1). The meningoencephaloceles that are of the greatest interest to the otolaryngologist are of the sincipital and basal types. The sincipital meningoencephaloceles

Table 31–1 CLASSIFICATION OF MENINGOENCEPHALOCELES

I. Occipital meningoencephalocele
II. Meningoencephalocele of the cranial vault
   a. Interfrontal
   b. Anterior fontanelle
   c. Interparietal
   d. Posterior fontanelle
   e. Temporal
III. Frontoethmoid or sincipital meningoencephalocele
   a. Nasofrontal
   b. Nasoethmoidal
   c. Naso-orbital
IV. Basal meningoencephalocele
   a. Transethmoidal
   b. Sphenoethmoidal
   c. Transsphenoidal
   d. Frontosphenoidal or spheno-orbital
V. Cranioschisis
   a. Cranial upper facial cleft
   b. Basal lower facial cleft
   c. Occipitocervical cleft
   d. Acrania and anencephaly

include the following types: (1) nasofrontal — those passing between the frontal and nasal bones that present as round masses, usually covered with skin, in the midline of the root of the nose; (2) nasoethmoidal — those that exit the skull from between the frontal, nasal, and ethmoidal bones and that present on the side of the nose at the junction of the cartilaginous and bony portions; these may be bilateral; (3) spheno-orbital or frontosphenoidal — those that pass into the orbital cavity through the supraorbital tissue, causing exophthalmos; and (4) sphenomaxillary — those that pass through the superorbital fissure into the pterygopalatine side of the ramus of the mandible to produce a bulge of the cheek below the zygoma.

Embryology

It is probable that nasal gliomas and encephaloceles are related in origin. The fact that meningoencephaloceles are similar anatomically to nasal gliomas suggests that both are the result of defects in the closure of the foramen cecum about the third week of development, when the anterior neuropore usually closes. After the closure of the foramen cecum, the skin normally becomes separated from the cranium by an ingrowth of mesoderm from each side. Any residual connection between skin and cranium will prevent migration of the mesoderm, and a defect in the cranial cavity can result. Herniated glial tissue that maintains a connection with the cerebrospinal fluid of the brain would thus be defined as a meningoencephalocele.

Whereas nasofrontal meningoencephaloceles may be formed in this manner, basal and occipital meningoencephaloceles are the result of different developmental disturbances. Such meningoencephaloceles could be the result of anomalies in neural crest migration, although the contributions of factors such as infection, trauma, oxygen deprivation, and intrauterine and environmental influences have yet to be explored.

Diagnosis

Although ultimately making the diagnosis of meningoencephalocele will depend upon the results of the morphologic examination, the clinical diagnosis is usually straightforward. A pulsatile mass that transilluminates is the most frequent presentation, although the degree of transillumination and the pulsatility of the mass may be decreased if there are large amounts of glial tissue in the herniation. Routine skull radiographs and tomography of the involved area of the skull must be made in order to evaluate the symptoms properly.

Nasofrontal meningoencephaloceles must be differentiated from gliomas, congenital dermoid cysts of the nose, obstruction of the lacrimal sac apparatus, epidermal inclusion cysts, and other benign neoplasias of the nasofrontal areas.

Congenital dermoid cysts are differentiated by the accompanying pit, which usually contains hair. The pit may be located anywhere between the glabella and the columella of the nose.

Epidermal inclusion cysts are not usually seen until after puberty, whereas meningoencephaloceles are congenital defects. In addition to the conditions just mentioned from which nasofrontal meningoencephaloceles must be differentiated, nasoethmoid meningoencephaloceles must be distinguished from nasal polyposis.

Treatment

The treatment of meningoencephaloceles is primarily surgical and necessitates the early involvement of neurosurgeons in the management of such conditions. This is particularly true when the meningoencephalocele has arisen from an occipital cleft. The otolaryngologist is involved more commonly in the management of defects presenting in the area of the glabella and in the ethmoid regions.

The surgical approach most frequently utilized in these cases is a cranial incision followed by bifrontal craniotomy. Herniated brain tissue is removed, the bony defect is covered with bone or tantalum mesh, and the dural defect is then repaired with fascia. When a mass has herniated into the nose from a cranial defect, the intranasal mass may be removed transnasally after the cranial defect has been repaired.

Reconstruction of cosmetic defects resulting from treatment of meningoencephaloceles is obviously individualized and may be delayed until the child is much older rather

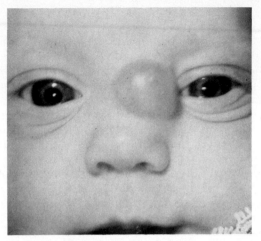

Figure 31–1 Nasal glioma.

than risk further interference with facial growth.

According to Matson (1969), patients with frontal meningoencephaloceles have good prognosis, since the herniated brain tissue usually arises from relatively "silent" areas of the frontal lobes. Thus, surgical excision of this tissue is unlikely to lead to serious neurologic deficit. However, Matson does advocate early treatment of these lesions.

NASAL GLIOMAS

Nasal gliomas are rare but interesting lesions of neurogenic origin. They initially form in utero in a manner similar to that in which an encephalocele forms, as herniations of ectodermal neural tissue of the brain into the nose or nasopharynx. These benign rests of neuroectodermal tissue then develop into nasal gliomas. Children with such masses may more appropriately be said to have congenital nasal neuroglial heterotopia. Figure 31–1 shows a child with a nasal glioma.

Etiology

Although nasal gliomas were first described by Reid in 1852, the term "glioma" was first used by Schmidt in 1900. Schmidt postulated that during fetal development, embryonic neuroectodermal tissue evaginated through the nasofrontal fontanel, under the developing nasal and frontal bones, in a manner similar to that in which an encephalocele develops (Fig. 31–2). During normal development, the evaginated tissue is retracted intracranially by the dura, and the area of the foramen cecum closes to separate the intracranial contents. However, closure of the cranial frontal sutures prior to the intracranial dural retraction would amputate a mass of neuroectodermal tissue while incomplete closure of the cranial sutures would be likely to result in a stalk of glial and fibrous tissue left attached to the neuroectodermal mass through the foramen cecum.

Other theories postulate that nasal gliomas result from (1) the amputation of portions of the olfactory bulb during closure of frontal bone sutures (Sussenguth, 1909); (2) the glial cells along the olfactory nerves during embryonic development (Dawson and Muir, 1955); (3) neuroectodermal rests becoming isolated in the nasal cavity early in embryonic development, leading to glial ectopia (Bratton and Robinson, 1946); and (4) teratomatous formation (Agarwal and Shrivastav, 1958).

Because encephaloceles and nasal gliomas are closely associated phenomena, and because stalks connected to the brain are frequently seen, we feel that nasal gliomas are

Figure 31–2. Etiology of nasal glioma.

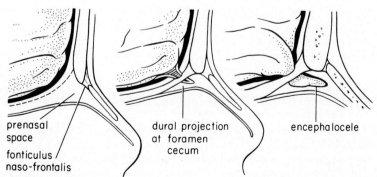

prenasal space

fonticulus naso-frontalis

dural projection at foramen cecum

encephalocele

TABLE 31–2 VARIATIONS OF BASAL AND SINCIPITAL ENCEPHALOCELES

Sincipital

1. Nasofrontal: protrusion between nasal and frontal bones
2. Nasoethmoidal: protrusion through foramen cecum; separated from nasal interior by ethmoid process
3. Naso-orbital: protrusion through medial wall of the orbit, involving frontal, ethmoid, and lacrimal bones

Basal

1. Transethmoidal: protrusion through defect in cribriform plate into the superior meatus
2. Sphenoethmoidal: protrusion into epipharynx through a defect between the posterior ethmoid cells and the sphenoid
3. Transsphenoidal: protrusion through a patent craniopharyngeal canal into the epipharynx
4. Sphenomaxillary: protrusion through the supraorbital fissure, through the infraorbital tissue, and then into the sphenomaxillary fossi; appears as a mass on the medial side of the mandibular ramus

probably formed in a manner similar to the way encephaloceles originate. Batsakis (1974) classifies nasal glial heterotopias as a variant of encephaloceles (Table 31–2). Of all such heterotopias, 75 per cent are occipital; 15 per cent are sincipital, located above the dorsum of the nose, the orbits, and the forehead; and 10 per cent are basal, presenting as masses protruding into the superior meatus of the nasal cavity, epipharynx, or sphenomaxillary fossa.

Differential Diagnosis

Congenital masses of the midface can be classified according to the type of cell of origin (neurogenic, ectodermic, or mesodermic) and must be differentiated from teratomas of multicellular origin. The neurogenic masses include true encephaloceles, nasal gliomas, meningoceles, and neurofibromas; the ectodermic masses include dermoid cysts, epidermoid inclusion cysts, sebaceous cysts, nasal polyps, lacrimal duct cysts, ethmoidal cysts, abscesses, and papillomas; the mesodermic masses include hemangiomas, lymphangiomas, lipomas, and angiofibromas. In addition to congenital masses, malignant tumors, including neuroblastomas, rhabdomyosarcomas, lymphomas, and nasopharyngeal carcinomas, should occasionally be considered in the differential diagnosis.

Therapeutic Approach

Clinical evaluation and treatment of nasal gliomas usually necessitates a team approach by the otolaryngologist and neurosurgeon. Because anomalies associated with encephaloceles have been reported in as many as 30 per cent of cases (Orkin and Fisher, 1966), evaluation of the patient should include assessment of the complete cardiovascular, pulmonary, gastrointestinal, urinary, and central nervous systems. Roentgenographic studies of the nasal region and base of the skull, including tomograms, should be performed on all patients. A history of cerebrospinal fluid rhinorrhea or meningitis should be sought, and all findings should be shared with the neurosurgical consultant. Evaluation and management of such patients requires the cooperation of the whole medical team.

Gliomas must be removed surgically, as they are not radiosensitive. Although they are not malignant neoplasms and do not retard growth and development, extranasal gliomas are cosmetically deforming and therefore should be treated promptly. If rhinorrhea is one of the presenting symptoms, neurosurgical exploration should be performed immediately, as there is an imminent risk of meningitis; occasionally patients have presented with meningitis. Preoperative evaluation should be completed and elective surgical treatment should be planned, keeping in mind that deformity of the facial bones may result from the mass effects of the tumor. Parents should be carefully educated as to the possible cosmetic deformity that could result from the condition and its treatment and to the possibility that facial plastic surgery may be required in the future.

Occasionally, intranasal gliomas may be resected surgically by an intranasal approach, but more frequently combined intranasal excision and craniotomy should be performed. A lateral rhinotomy enables the surgeon to visualize the cribriform plate area in order to remove the intranasal glioma and to determine if any glial stalk is present. In addition, any suspected intracranial connection or cerebrospinal fluid leak must be explored neurosurgically. The otomicroscope can be a very valuable aid in the dissection of all types of nasal gliomas. An extranasal glioma that shows no evidence of having any intranasal component or intracranial connection may simply be excised. However, if any intracranial connection is suspected, immediate neurosurgical exploration is necessary, although it should be noted that at the time of surgery only 20 per cent of all gliomas display recognizable intracranial connections (Karma et al., 1977).

CONGENITAL DERMOID CYSTS OF THE NOSE

Unlike teratomas, which contain all three embryonal germ layers, congenital dermoid cysts contain only ectodermal and mesodermal embryonic elements. The mesodermal elements in the wall of the cyst differentiate dermoid cysts from simple epidermoid cysts, the latter a clinically much more common entity (Fig. 31–3).

Nasal dermoids constitute slightly less than one per cent of all dermoid cysts. Nasal dermoids similarly account for about 10 per cent of the total number of dermoid cysts that occur in the head and neck.

Malignant change in a dermoid cyst of the nose has never been described in the English literature, but an increased incidence of other congenital abnormalities has been shown to be associated with congenital dermoid cysts of the nose. Nasal dermoids have been shown to have a familial tendency.

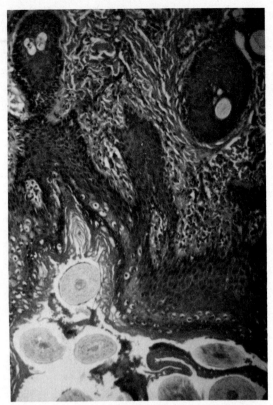

Figure 31–4 Photomicrograph of nasal dermoid cyst showing squamous epithelium, hairs, infectious material, and keratotic debris.

Morphology

Histologic sections of nasal dermoids, an example of which is shown in Figure 31–4, reveal typical stratified squamous epithelium and keratin. The presence of hair follicles and hair is an important differential finding, as such adnexal components are not a part of the usual simple epidermoid cyst. Adnexal sweat glands and sebaceous glands are also usually present in nasal dermoids, although smooth muscle in the walls of the cyst or adnexal hair follicles may be the only evidence of mesenchymal cell involvement in such anomalies. Varying degrees of inflammation are usually associated with these dermoids.

Etiology

It is appropriate at this point to review the embryogenesis of nasal gliomas. Although dural and neural elements that remain outside the embryonic midline foramen cecum

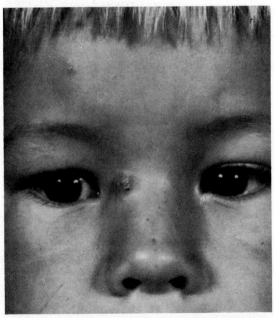

Figure 31–3 Nasal dermoid cyst with single pit on dorsum of nose and infected fistula at root of nose.

of the anterior cranial cavity have been implicated as leading to the formation of nasal gliomas, such elements may also be related to the occurrence of nasal dermoids. A potential prenasal space, normally obliterated by connective tissue, may also play a part in the etiology of nasal dermoids as well as nasal gliomas. Normally, neural elements protruding from the cranial cavity in the nasal region appear to be retracted through the embryonic foramen cecum. However, if the embryonic dura did not separate from the embryonic skin as retraction occurred, ectodermal elements could be pulled back or drawn into this prenasal space. Incomplete fusion of the rim of the foramen cecum would then lead to the formation of congenital dermoid cysts of the nose. For those more interested in the details of the etiology of such structures, Littlewood's (1961) excellent review is recommended.

Sites of Involvement

McCaffrey and colleagues (1979) reported on 21 patients with nasal dermoids, in some of whom more than one site was involved. However, nasal dermoids usually present only on the nasal dorsum; the single pit with extruding hair is the most common clinical appearance (Fig. 31–5).

Infection of a nasal dermoid with cystic extension may lead to the formation of single or multiple fistulae (Fig. 31–6); cystic remnants, either with or without associated infected fistulae, may present in the forehead, glabella, nasal tip, columella, and along the nasal system to the sphenoid sinus area, with varying degrees of involvement of these structures.

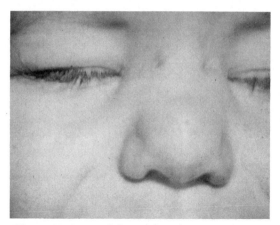

Figure 31–6   Nasal dermoid on dorsum with single fistula on each side of the root of the nose.

The astute physician should be aware that nasal dermoids may involve multiple sites and that at times neurosurgical consultation will be advisable in order to treat the patient optimally. Involvement of the cribriform plate with some separation of the frontal lobes can occur so that an innocent and benign-appearing pit on the dorsum of the nose could require extensive surgery to remove. Parents should be made aware of the reasons for performing such extensive surgery to avoid their feeling that the deformity resulting from such treatment occurred unnecessarily. The facial plastic reconstruction required to correct such defects may be delayed for years and will probably be time-consuming and expensive.

Diagnosis and Treatment

The diagnosis and treatment of nasal dermoids require a thorough understanding of their etiology. The extensions of this congenital deformity must be defined preoperatively in order to plan extirpative surgery properly. Likewise, the degree of cystic extension must be known in order that complete removal of the nasal dermoid can be accomplished with a single operation.

Diagnostic procedures in any individual case may include any or all of the following: preoperative or postoperative photography, routine sinus radiographs, laminography, CAT scan, injection of radiopaque media into cystic extensions, brain scan, neurosurgical evaluation, and full evaluation of any other coexisting congenital abnormality, such as a

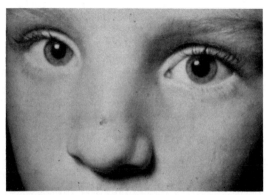

Figure 31–5   Single pit on dorsum of the nose.

congenital heart defect or renal, spinal, or extremity abnormalities.

Recurrences of such cysts have uniformly been due to incomplete removal of all elements at the time of initial surgery. Bone grafts inserted at the time of the initial surgery in an effort to repair immediately the cosmetic defect, which have become infected, have been confused with infected cystic remnants that might have been left behind. The physician's surgical skill, experience, ingenuity, and understanding may obviously be taxed in the management of any individual case.

Nasal dermoid cysts must be differentiated from sebaceous cysts, which are also attached to the skin but which are usually not seen prior to puberty. Nasal dermoid cysts may be differentiated from meningoceles by the fact that the latter characteristically transilluminate, whereas dermoids and gliomas do not. Gliomas, in addition, are solid masses. Laminography is usually quite helpful in differentiating between these midline structures and also will help the examiner to determine the extent to which the dermoid cyst underlies the nasal bones. This procedure is an essential part of complete diagnostic and preoperative evaluation. Injecting radiopaque media into these cysts will also demonstrate their extension beneath the nasal bone.

Other conditions from which nasal dermoid cysts must be differentiated include obstruction of the nasolacrimal system, hemangiomas, and simple lipomas. These last do not transilluminate and are freely movable in the subcutaneous tissue.

Complete removal of nasal dermoid cysts is necessary, as progressive expansion, infection, and fistula formation have occurred when such conditions have been ignored. Complete surgical removal must include the excision of cystic structures extending through and beneath the nasal bones or along the superior nasal septum posteriorly toward the pituitary. The surgeon must plan for plastic reconstruction of the area of excision before surgery is begun.

Usually, surgery for the removal of nasal dermoid cysts is not performed until the patient is two to five years old. Such surgery normally requires administration of a general anesthetic, as it is not always possible to determine preoperatively the full extent to which the cyst has invaded the subcribriform plate. Although cerebrospinal fluid may be encountered in the course of the dissection, this is not the rule.

In summary, congenital dermoid cysts and fistulas of the nose may occur at any point from the glabella to the base of the columella, but the most common site of presentation is at the inferior border of the nasal bone. These cysts may be superficial and may not involve the nasal bone, although many cysts may appear to be superficial but in fact extend through the nasal bone and superior nasal septum toward the region of the pituitary. The cysts probably represent the persistence of ectodermal elements in the line of fusion of the embryonic nose. Treatment of these cysts is complete surgical removal, with the extent of surgery varying according to the individual case.

HEMANGIOMAS

Hemangiomas are commonly occurring benign tumors that present during infancy or childhood. They may occur anywhere in the head and neck, including the nose. They are the single most frequently observed tumor in the region of the head and neck in childhood.

Historically, hemangiomas have been classified histologically as follows: (1) capillary, (2) cavernous, (3) mixed, and (4) hypertrophic or juvenile.

Batsakis (1974) feels that this classification is somewhat artificial and academic, as there is considerable overlap in category in any individual lesion. In addition, the histologic appearance of the tumor appears to have little bearing on the long-term behavior of these lesions. Batsakis (1974) also believes that the most important determinants of the prognosis in cases involving these lesions are (1) the anatomic site of the lesion; (2) the size, extent, and depth of the lesion; and (3) selection of the primary treatment.

While it is well documented that many, if not most, of these hemangiomas will resolve spontaneously, there has in the past been no good way of predicting which lesions will not regress and will thus need surgical intervention. A promising technique is to follow these children through serial Doppler examinations of the lesions at regular intervals. If the number of arteriovenous fistulas increases, the prognosis for spontaneous regression is poor.

Although hemangiomas commonly occur in the head and neck, they only infrequently involve the nose. Generally, conservative management with watchful waiting is the treatment of choice for these lesions. In a series of 19 patients with hemangiomas of the nasal tip whom Thomson and Lanigan (1979) reviewed, eight had been treated conservatively, and in all eight patients the hemangioma had spontaneously regressed to an aesthetically acceptable degree. In only three of the 11 patients treated surgically were the results attained aesthetically acceptable. Thus, it would appear that when dealing with lesions of the nose (unless the lesion is rapidly invasive or is causing a respiratory situation incompatible with life), the best course is watchful waiting.

COMPLETE AGENESIS OF THE NOSE

The complete absence of the nose and anterior nasopharynx is an exceptionally rare anomaly. Fewer than a dozen cases of such an anomaly have been reported in the literature. The most recent report was by Gifford and MacCollum (1972) and consisted of two cases. These patients had absence of the nasal bones and premaxilla. The soft tissue of the face was intact with no clefting, and there were no nostrils or evidence of any nasal development. In that report, a nasal airway was established at about age five or six years. Prosthetic noses were used until the nasal reconstruction could be carried out.

NASAL CLEFTING — NASAL DYSPLASIA

Actual clefting of the nose is a very rare deformity that is usually associated with some degree of hypertelorism and probably should fall under the broad term "frontonasal dysplasia" or "median cleft-face syndrome." The hallmarks of this disorder are (1) ocular hypertelorism; (2) broad nasal root; (3) lack of formation of the nasal tip; (4) widow's peak scalp bone anomaly; (5) anterior cranium bifidum occultum; (6) median clefting of the nose, lip, and palate; and (7) unilateral orbital clefting or notching of the nasal ala (Gifford and MacCollum, 1972).

The degree of involvement of the nose with this type of deformity is extremely variable, ranging between notching of the ala or notching between the alar cartilage and a wide separation of the two sides of the nose.

DeMyer and colleagues (1963) believe that there are strong associations between the degree of hypertelorism, cephalic anomalies, and the probability of mental deficiency in a given patient. According to their findings, the greater the degree of hypertelorism and the more extracephalic anomalies were present, the more likely the child was to be mentally deficient. If, on the other hand, the degree of hypertelorism was mild and there were no extracephalic anomalies, the chance that normal or near-normal CNS formation had occurred was good.

The surgical reconstruction of the more severe defects will probably require several procedures and a multidisciplinary approach, thus making it preferable that they be managed in a center where there is a craniofacial team.

MEDIAN FACIAL ANOMALIES

The group of defects lumped into the category of median facial anomalies was classified by DeMyer and colleagues (1963) into five categories of facies (Table 31–3). They found that individuals with these types of facies usually had associated holoprosencephaly.

The hallmarks of this group of facies are as follows: (1) ocular — may range from a single eye to orbital hypotelorism; (2) nasal — may range from arrhinia with proboscis to a flat nose; (3) cleft — there may be no cleft, there may be a median cleft of the lip with no premaxilla prolabium, or a bilateral lateral cleft of the lip with a rudimentary premaxilla prolabium may be present. Diagnostic evaluation of children with such ·characteristics should include skull radiographs, CAT scan, a transillumination, and genetic characterizations.

These defects are thought to originate embryologically as deficiencies of the prechordal mesoderm that lead to the deficiency in the central facial skeleton. Lack of induction of the rostral neuroectoderm results in the defect in the brain.

Children with median facial anomalies may have physiologic abnormalities, including poikilothermy, spasticity, hyperreflexia, ap-

Table 31-3   SEVERE DEGREES OF HOLOPROSENCEPHALY (ARRHINENCEPHALY)

Type of Facies	Facial Features	Cranium and Brain
I. Cyclopia	Single eye or partially divided eye in single orbit; arrhinia with proboscis	Microcephaly Alobar holoprosencephaly
II. Ethmocephaly	Extreme orbital hypotelorism but separate orbits; arrhinia with proboscis	Microcephaly Alobar holoprosencephaly
III. Cebocephaly	Orbital hypotelorism, proboscis-like nose but no median cleft of lip	Microcephaly; usually has alobar holoprosencephaly
IV. With median cleft lip	Orbital hypotelorism, flat nose	Microcephaly and sometimes trigonocephaly; usually has alobar holoprosencephaly
V. With median philtrum-premaxilla anlage	Orbital hypotelorism, bilateral lateral cleft of lip with median process representing philtrum-premaxillary anlage	Microcephaly and sometimes trigonocephaly. Semilobar or lobar holoprosencephaly

This table presents five facies diagnostic of holoprosencephaly. Although transitional cases do occur, the facies of each category are remarkably similar from patient to patient.

neic spells, seizures, poor growth, and psychomotor retardation. Because those with the more severe defects generally have a life expectancy of less than one year (Fig. 31–7), surgical treatment of these infants is generally not indicated. Rarely it may be necessary for the well-being of the family to perform a limited reconstruction. There have been sporadic reports of children with similar facies and normal CNS development (Pashayan and Lewis, 1980).

If the CNS development is normal, of course, a well thought out plan of reconstruction should be followed. The surgical reconstruction of these types of defects presents a two-fold problem of lack of both soft tissue and the underlying skeletal support. Post-

operatively, maintaining a nasal airway in these patients is a major problem. For this reason, artificial nasal airways should be left in place for the first 12 to 24 hours postoperatively.

PROBOSCIS LATERALIS

Proboscis lateralis is an unusual deformity. The proboscis is a tubular structure composed of skin and soft tissue that is attached at the inner canthus. There may be coexistent maldevelopment of the nasal cavity, varying from a normal nose to complete agenesis of the nasal cavity and the paranasal sinuses on that side (Figs. 31–8 and 31–9).

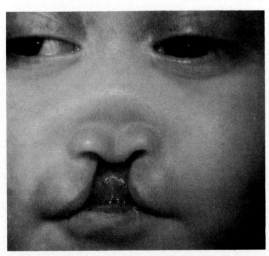

Figure 31-7   Central facial hypoplasia.

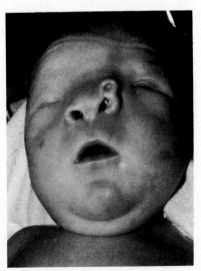

Figure 31-8   Proboscis lateralis.

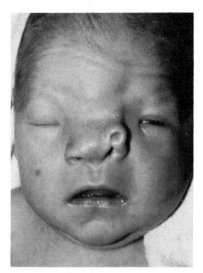

Figure 31–9 Proboscis lateralis.

The embryology of this lesion is uncertain. The most commonly accepted theory is that imperfect mesodermal proliferation occurs in the frontonasal and maxillary processes after formation of the olfactory pits. Epidermal breakdown then takes place, leaving the lateral nasal process sequestered as a tube arising in the frontonasal region. Also, as a result of the epidermal breakdown, no nasolacrimal duct is produced.

When these defects are reconstructed, as much of the soft tissue as is needed may be taken from the tube, the remainder being sacrificed. The skeletal deficiency may be corrected by use of bone or radiated costal cartilage.

CLEFT LIP NASAL DEFORMITY

Children with cleft lip and palate usually have a coexistent nasal deformity. With unilateral clefts, the nasal ala on the side of the cleft is laterally based, giving the appearance of a flat, flaring nostril. The columella is usually short on the cleft side. The maxilla on the cleft side is frequently hypoplastic, resulting in a relative retropositioning of the ala on that side. The nasal tip may also have a bifid appearance.

The most severe defects are those associated with a bilateral complete cleft. Individuals with such deformity frequently have very short columellas, 1 to 2 mm in length. They also may have bilateral maxillary hypoplasia with relative prognathism.

Children with clefts also may have severe nasal septal deformities, which may cause airway problems. If possible, it is best to wait until they have become teenagers before doing septal surgery, if at all. In some instances, this may not be possible, and a very conservative septal approach should be used. The surgeon should be cautioned that the resultant improvement in the nasal airway may have a deleterious effect on the individual's speech, leaving him with a velopharyngeal incompetence that had not been evident prior to surgery.

Many ways to handle cleft nasal deformities have been put forth. We prefer to perform an open tip rhinoplasty in combination with a velopharyngeal lengthening of the columellas as described by Bardach (personal communication). This technique is advantageous in that it allows excellent exposure of the lower lateral cartilages so that they may be aligned and trimmed and adjusted to the proper height, and it also permits lengthening of the columella. This procedure may be carried out any time after the child has reached the age of 8 or 10 years without the fear of impairment of normal growth of the face.

In those children in whom the degree of unilateral maxillary hypoplasia is so severe that there is obvious depression of the ala on that side, an implant under the ala of Supramid mesh or irradiated costal cartilage has been used to correct this defect. This implant is placed by a peroral route through the buccal sulcus.

CHOANAL ATRESIA

Choanal atresia is generally reported to occur about once in 8000 births. Recently this incidence has been questioned because many cases of bilateral choanal atresia may have gone undiagnosed and have resulted in death of the newborn. Mouth breathing is a learned phenomenon, and neonates do not generally learn to do this for several weeks.

The atresia may be unilateral or bilateral. Many cases of unilateral atresia may go undiagnosed until later in life when they may be evidenced by the presence of an intractable anterior nasal discharge. Bilateral atresia usually presents immediately in the neonate as respiratory distress.

The atresia in most cases is approximately 2 to 3 cm anterior to the posterior aspect of the hard palate. In about 90 per cent of cases the atresia is wholly or partly bony. The membranous atresias usually occur somewhat more posteriorly.

As the nasal placodes invaginate to form the nasal cavities, they form a membrane between the nasal and buccal cavities called the nasobuccal membrane. Should mesodermal tissue persist between the nasal and buccal ectoderm, this may result in bony atresia. This membrane normally ruptures during the sixth week of development. The buccopharyngeal membrane occurs more posteriorly, and failure of this structure to form may result in more posterior membranous stenosis.

The diagnosis of unilateral atresia is usually made later in life from a history of unilateral nasal discharge. The definitive diagnosis is made by inability to pass a catheter on the affected side. The atresia may be documented by instilling a small amount of radiopaque dye into the affected side with the patient in a supine position and then making a lateral radiograph of the skull.

Bilateral atresia usually presents with profound difficulty in breathing. If an infant survives the first few moments of life and the atresia still goes unnoticed, the infant will have difficulty feeding.

The immediate treatment of bilateral choanal atresia in the neonate involves establishing an artificial airway. This can be done with an oral airway, and tracheotomy should not be necessary unless there is some other coexisting condition that might compromise the airway. The method described by McGovern (1961) seems to be the best accepted. He described the use of a large, flanged rubber nipple with one or two large holes cut in it and strapped into the mouth with umbilical tape around the ears. This provides an airway while serving as well as a route for feeding.

Numerous surgical procedures have been described for correcting choanal atresia. The approaches used in these procedures are nasal, transseptal, and transpalatal.

The transnasal techniques range from blind puncture of the atretic membrane or plate to careful elevation of the anterior mucoperiosteum and removal of the bony plate with a microdrill under microscopic visualization. The posterior mucoperiosteum is preserved and is brought forward as flaps to cover the raw surfaces. A stent of appropriately sized plastic tubing is then put in place and left for approximately one month.

The blind puncture is to be condemned since there is a danger of perforating the spinal canal through the atlanto-occipital joint.

The approach that offers the best exposure and the best chance of success is the transpalatal approach. We favor an incision in the palate similar to that used for a velopharyngeal push-back. This allows for elevation of the palatal mucoperichondrium with wide exposure of the bony margin of the hard palate. In recent years several techniques have been described for removing the atretic plate through a transnasal route. These techniques involve the use of the otomicroscope and a drill or CO_2 laser.

REFERENCES

Agarwal, S., and Shrivastav, J. B. 1958. Neurogenic tumors of the nose. A report of two cases. Ann. Otol. Rhinol. Laryngol., 67:207–211.

Bardach, J., Professor, Department of Otolaryngology and Maxillofacial Surgery, University of Iowa Hospitals and Clinic, personal communication.

Batsakis, J. 1974. Tumors of the Head and Neck. Baltimore, Williams & Wilkins Co., p. 250.

Bratton, A. B., and Robinson, S. M. G. 1946. Gliomata of the nose and oral cavity: A report of two cases. J. Pathol. Bact., 58:643–648.

Dawson, R. L. G., and Muir, I. F. K. 1955. The frontonasal glioma. Br. J. Plast. Surg., 8:136–143.

DeMyer, W., Zeman, W., and Palmer, C. G. 1963. Familiar alobar holoprosencephaly (arrhinencephaly) with median cleft lip and palate. Neurology, 13:913–918.

Gifford, G. H., Jr., and MacCollum, D. W. 1972. Congenital malformations. In Ferguson, C. F., and Kendig, E. L., Jr. (Eds.) Pediatric Otolaryngology. Philadelphia, W. B. Saunders, p. 932.

Karma, P., Rasanen, O., and Karja, J. 1977. Nasal gliomas: A review and report of two cases. Laryngoscope, 87:1169–1179.

Littlewood, A. H. M. 1961. Congenital nasal dermoid cysts and fistulas. Plast. Reconst. Surg., 27:471–488.

Matson, D. 1969. Neurosurgery of Infancy and Childhood. Springfield, Ill., Charles C Thomas, Publ., pp. 61–76.

McCaffrey, T., McDonald, T. J., and Gorenstein, A. 1979. Dermoid cysts of the nose: Review of 21 cases. Otolaryngol. Head Neck Surg., 87:52–59.

McGovern, F. H. 1961. Bilateral choanal atresia in newborns: A new method of medical management. Laryngoscope, 71:480.

Orkin, M., and Fisher, I. 1966. Heterotopic brain tissue. Arch. Derm., 94:699–708.

Pashayan, H., and Lewis, M. B. 1980. Hypotelorism, nasomaxillary hypoplasia, and cleft lip and palate with normoaphely and normal intelligence. Cleft Palate J., *17*:62–64.

Reid. 1852. Uber angehoren Hirnbruche in den Stein und Nosengegend. Illus. M. Ztg., *1*:133.

Schmidt, M. B. 1900. Uber Seltene Spaltbildungen in Bereiche des Mittleren Strinfortsatzes. Virchows Arch. (Pathol. Anat.), *162*:340–370.

Sussenguth, L. 1909. Uber Nasengliome. Virchow Arch. (Pathol. Anat.), *195*:537–544.

Thomson, H. G., and Lanigan, M. 1979. The Cyrano nose: A clinical review of hemangiomas of the nasal tip. Plast. Reconstr. Surg., *63*:155–160.

Chapter 32

INFLAMMATORY DISEASES OF THE NOSE AND PARANASAL SINUSES

Paul A. Shurin, M. D.

NASAL DISORDERS

Introduction

Rhinitis, manifested by nasal congestion or discharge, is a major cause of morbidity in infants and children. At present we do not have enough information about the pathophysiology of rhinitis to make specific diagnoses or to prescribe therapy for the majority of patients suffering from this disorder. The most well-defined causes of rhinitis are the respiratory viruses. A viral cause of rhinitis is suggested by the acute onset of an illness with typical symptoms, often in conjunction with familial and community outbreaks of similar illness. Allergy is probably second only to infection as a cause of rhinitis. When allergy is the etiology, depending upon the nature of the child's exposure to the responsible allergen, the nasal disorder may be chronic or episodic; environmental, dietary, and pharmacologic agents have all been known to cause rhinitis. Allergic rhinitis has also been reported to occur as early as the first weeks of life. Drug-induced rhinitis may result from excessive use of local decongestants and the resulting vasomotor rebound; more rarely, drug-induced rhinitis may be seen as a neonatal problem following maternal drug use (narcotics, reserpine). So-called vasomotor rhinitis is manifested by chronic or episodic nasal obstruction, often in apparent response to changes in environmental temperature or humidity. Systemic diseases that may have nasal manifestations suggesting rhinitis in-

clude cystic fibrosis and hypothyroidism. Anatomic causes of obstruction or discharge include foreign bodies, polyps, and traumatic lesions (see Table 26–2).

The Common Cold Syndrome or Acute Nasopharyngitis

The importance of the common cold lies in its great frequency as a cause of acute morbidity in the general population. Surveys of acute symptomatic illnesses have shown more than 80 per cent of spontaneously occurring infections to consist of episodes of this syndrome. Colds occur more frequently in children than in adults: children average five colds a year in the first five years of life, whereas older children and their adult family members average two to three colds a year. Most colds are due to a rhinovirus infection.

Etiology. The common cold may be caused by a wide variety of viral agents (Table 32–1) (Loda et al., 1972; Gwaltney, 1975; Kaye et al., 1971; Monto and Ullman, 1974); however, even with use of the most sophisticated cultural and serologic procedures, the etiologic agent of many colds cannot at present be assigned. Rhinoviruses cause approximately 90 per cent of the colds for which an etiology can be determined. The role of respiratory viruses, particularly of the rhinovirus group, in producing colds has been elucidated through (1) controlled epidemiologic surveys with viral isolation and identification of specific antibody responses in infected

Table 32–1 ETIOLOGIC AGENTS OF THE COMMON COLD SYNDROME IN CHILDREN

Rhinoviruses (approximately 100 known types)
Respiratory syncytial virus
Parainfluenza virus (types 1–3)
Influenza A and B
Adenovirus (types 1–5)
Coronavirus
Enteroviruses
Mycoplasma pneumoniae

(From Loda et al., 1972; Gwaltney, 1975; Kaye et al., 1971; and Monto and Ullman, 1974.)

persons, and (2) transmission of colds to experimental animals and human volunteers by viral inoculation.

Rhinoviruses differ from other viruses that may cause colds in having an optimal temperature for replication of 35° C. Hence, they do not grow well at body temperature and, possibly for this reason, do not cause disease of the lower respiratory tract. In contrast, cold viruses of other groups frequently cause more serious respiratory infections, such as croup, bronchiolitis, and pneumonia. *Mycoplasma pneumoniae* appears to be the only nonviral agent that is implicated in the cold syndrome, but this agent is rare as a cause of that disorder and is more commonly associated with atypical pneumonia. Although potentially pathogenic bacteria may be isolated from the nasal passages of children with colds (as they may be from normal children), they are not of etiologic significance.

Epidemiology. Colds occur year-round with their frequency being lowest in summer. The low environmental temperatures prevalent during winter do not appear to be a factor in this seasonal pattern of cold epidemiology; of greater importance is crowding of susceptible and infectious persons indoors. The major factor accounting for the frequency of colds and of recurrent episodes is the wide variety of serologically distinct viruses present in the community. Children are generally infected through contacts in schools and day-care centers, and young children represent the most important vectors of these viruses in the community. Rhinoviruses infect the nasal mucosa and appear to spread mainly by direct contact, for instance via hands that have been in contact with nasal secretions. Viruses that infect the pharynx and lower respiratory tract are more likely to be spread by the airborne route following aerosolization by coughing and sneezing.

Pathogenesis. Hyperemia and edema of the nasal mucosa with increased secretion of mucus by submucosal glands are the early pathologic findings in the noses of individuals infected by a "cold" virus. Ciliary activity is depressed during the period of acute infection, suggesting epithelial damage, but inflammatory infiltrates are not prominent.

The incubation period of a rhinovirus infection is two to four days. The infectious virus begins to spread late in the incubation period and may continue to spread throughout the period of acute illness.

Clinical Features. The characteristic features of the cold syndrome are rhinorrhea, nasal obstruction, sneezing, and coughing. Pharyngitis may be a complaint in children old enough to complain of a sore throat. Fever is not a prominent feature in adults but appears to be more common in uncomplicated colds in children. In young children the nasal obstruction and respiratory difficulty may interfere with feeding and sleeping. However, systemic symptoms such as a high fever, irritability, severe malaise, and myalgias are not part of the cold syndrome and should suggest the presence of complications or of other diseases.

Colds usually last four to seven days. Many patients have cold-like syndromes of much longer duration, often lasting several weeks, but because of the lack of specific diagnostic criteria the clinician is ordinarily unable to determine the etiology of such prolonged illnesses. However, such episodes must suggest the possibility of complications of the original cold or, especially when recurrences are unusually frequent, of a noninfectious basis for the symptoms, such as an allergic disorder.

Diagnosis. The identification of the cold syndrome is dependent on identification of the characteristic clinical symptoms. Facilities for the identification of etiologic viruses are not generally available, nor would the provision of such services be economically justifiable. An erythematous and inflamed nasal mucosa is said to be characteristic of infectious colds, whereas in allergic rhinitis the mucosa is pale and the exudate contains many eosinophilic leukocytes. However, the specific diagnostic value of these criteria has not been objectively established.

Therapy and Prevention. Relief of nasal obstruction is of greatest importance in infants since they are likely to be unable to mouth-breathe effectively. The secretions may be loosened by use of normal saline nose drops, and gentle suction with a bulb aspirator or a mechanical suction pump may be helpful in removing the secretions once so loosened. All aspects of the pharmacologic management of colds are at present controversial. Decongestants may be administered orally (phenylephrine or pseudoephedrine, either alone or in combination with an antihistamine) or as nose drops (saline solutions of ephedrine, epinephrine, or phenylephrine). Physiologic studies have documented that single doses of these drugs will diminish nasal airway resistance (Roth et al., 1977). However, it has not been shown that they do so during the natural course of the episode or that they are effective in reducing the incidence of complications. Additional concerns with respect to the use of decongestants are the possibility of local sensitization and of worsening of symptoms following cessation of administration.

Vitamin C given in pharmacologic doses (one gram or more per day administered orally) has been claimed to be effective both prophylactically in preventing episodes of colds and symptomatically in lessening the duration of symptoms. In controlled trials, both effects have been so small as to be of at best marginal value to the subjects. Furthermore, there is no good evidence that Vitamin C would not be toxic when administered in high doses for long periods of time and to large numbers of individuals. This is especially of concern when treating children, and the use of daily doses higher than those required nutritionally (approximately 50 mg per day) should be discouraged, especially in this age group (Chalmers, 1975).

Pharmacologic agents that stimulate host defenses or have antiviral activity have been effective in the prevention or treatment of a few viral respiratory infections. However, problems of potential toxicity and the necessity for widespread use of these agents to be effective would seem to make unlikely the possibility that they could make any substantial contribution to reducing the frequency of the common cold.

There is currently no evidence that any environmental measures can prevent colds in children who are living under normal conditions. Avoidance of contact with symptomatic individuals is not effective, since relatively asymptomatic children (i.e. those whose colds are in the incubation period) may be infective, and since the various viral agents are highly endemic in our society. The large number of viruses involved as etiologic agents for the common cold has greatly hampered efforts to develop a vaccine.

Complications. Colds appear clinically to be related to episodes of acute otitis media and sinusitis. It is generally assumed that obstruction of the eustachian tube and sinus ostia contribute to such an association. However, other mechanisms, such as alterations of host defense mechanisms during infection, have been proposed. In the absence of adequate studies using defined diagnostic criteria, it is impossible to assess these associations critically.

Although rhinoviruses do not seem to infect the lower respiratory tract, infections with these and other respiratory viruses are thought to be important precipitants of asthmatic attacks in children. The mechanism of this relationship is not known. Rhinovirus infections in volunteers have been shown to produce no lasting effects on pulmonary function. Therefore, such infections are not thought to contribute to the etiology of chronic lung disease.

Bacterial Rhinitis

General Considerations. The existence and potential importance of syndromes of bacterial rhinitis and nasopharyngitis have not been clearly documented. Such syndromes might be caused by such ubiquitous but potentially pathogenic bacteria as the pneumococcus, *Haemophilus influenzae* and Group A, beta-hemolytic streptococci. It is thought by many that such local mucosal infection might serve as a focus for infection of the middle ear, sinuses, meninges, or blood. These relationships cannot, however, be established without development of objective criteria for diagnosis of the local infection. In clinical practice, children often present with profuse purulent nasal discharge, which may be of prolonged duration. When gram-stained smears show large numbers of polymorphonuclear leukocytes and a predominance of a single bacterial species is confirmed by culture, it is reasonable to prescribe antimicrobial agents. The selection of drugs depends upon the organism identified; the general considerations are the same as those applied in selecting antimicrobial therapy for otitis media.

Several specific bacterial diseases may present with rhinitis. These are discussed briefly.

Congenital Syphilis. Nasal discharge is frequently the presenting feature of congenital syphilis and may occur in the absence of any of the other characteristic clinical signs (rash, mucosal lesions, hepatosplenomegaly, and skeletal changes). The infant is generally normal at birth, with rhinitis appearing at several weeks or months of age. The nasal mucosa is red and swollen and the discharge is thick and mucoid. Erosions and subsequent scarring affect both the nasal mucosa and the adjacent areas of skin on the face and lips. The discharge is laden with treponemes, and the diagnosis depends on dark-field examination or serologic tests. Infection of the mother may have occurred late in gestation, so that a negative serologic test obtained prenatally may not exclude this diagnosis. Early therapy is mandatory if late sequelae are to be avoided.

Pertussis. This disease is characterized by a prodromal catarrhal stage that precedes the more typical period of spasmodic whooping cough. The symptoms during the catarrhal period closely resemble those of the common cold although the nasal discharge is characteristically mucoid rather than watery. Older children and adults with pertussis may have a prolonged illness with upper respiratory symptoms and cough but without progression to classic whooping cough. Unfortunately, the specific diagnosis is often missed in such cases, and unnecessary spread of the disease may occur as a result; for instance, outbreaks have been reported in hospital personnel. Diagnosis of this infection can be made by isolation of *Bordetella pertussis* from nasopharyngeal swabs or by fluorescent antibody identification of the organism in smears made from the same source. Treatment with erythromycin (40 mg/kg/day) may prevent infection of contacts in epidemic situations and shorten the period of infectivity but is probably not effective in treating the clinical manifestations of the disease. Active immunization of infants with pertussis vaccine is required for control of the disease.

Diphtheria. Localized nasal diphtheria is less common than the pharyngeal and laryngotracheal forms of the disease. However, because nasal involvement, which may be either unilateral or bilateral, is localized, toxin absorption is limited and systemic signs are relatively mild. The suggestive features are prolonged, foul-smelling, and often serosanguinous nasal discharge. The presence of a membrane on the nasal septus should arouse immediate suspicion. The disease affects children and adults who have been inadequately immunized but is rare at present in the United States. The diagnosis depends upon culture of a toxigenic strain of *Corynebacterium diphtheriae*. Treatment should in general be administered when there is sufficient clinical suspicion of the disease, without waiting for a definitive diagnosis, and consists of administration of antitoxin of equine origin. Penicillin or eyrthromycin are usually given as well to limit further multiplication of the infective organism.

INFECTION OF THE PARANASAL SINUSES

General Considerations

Sinusitis is generally considered to occur frequently in children. However, objective diagnostic techniques to establish the presence or etiology of the disease have not been widely used. For instance, the validity of specific clinical findings in differentiating sinus infection from uncomplicated rhinitis has not been well established, and some of the radiographic findings that are thought to be indications of sinusitis are very frequently found in radiographs of normal children (Shopfner and Rossi, 1973). Because of these diagnostic difficulties, adequate information concerning the incidence of the disease and its optimal therapy is not yet available.

Pathogenesis

Sinusitis appears most frequently to be a complication of a viral upper respiratory infection. Suggested mechanisms for this relationship include (a) local vascular congestion, (b) narrowing and obstruction of the sinus ostia, (c) alterations in the local milieu for bacterial growth, and (d) reduction in the effectiveness of mucociliary action.

Disease entities that have been associated with sinusitis in children are listed in Table 32–2. Nasal allergy is thought to be a major cause of sinus disease in children. Sensitivity to environmental allergens (such as dusts, molds, or pollens), to foods, and to drugs such as aspirin have all been incriminated. The various malformations and traumatic defects presumably affect the sinuses by obstructing their ostia. Clouding of the sinuses

Table 32–2 DISORDERS ASSOCIATED WITH PARANASAL SINUSITIS

Anatomic
Nasal malformations
Nasal trauma
Tumors and polyps
Cleft palate
Foreign bodies
Dental infection
Cyanotic congenital heart disease

Physiologic
Barotrauma

Abnormalities of Local Defense Mechanisms
Allergy
Cystic fibrosis
Immotile-cilia syndrome and Kartagener syndrome

Abnormalities of Systemic Defense Mechanisms
Immunodeficiency, primary or secondary

and mucosal thickening have frequently been identified radiologically in children with cleft palate (Jaffe and DeBlanc, 1971), but the clinical significance of this is not clear. Radiologic signs of sinusitis have been reported to be seen especially frequently in children with cyanotic congenital heart disease (Rosenthal and Fellows, 1973). The sinus alterations may be due to vascular engorgement and proliferation of venous channels. Chronic sinus infection might contribute to the frequent occurrence of such complications as brain abscess in these children. Sinus disease in children with cystic fibrosis is generally identified in conjunction with the nasal polyps that are a frequent manifestation of the disease; the highly viscous mucous secretions may also play a role in sinus disease. The manifestations of Kartagener syndrome (situs inversus, bronchiectasis, and sinusitis) appear to result from a structural defect in cilia throughout the body (Eliasson, et al., 1977). The ciliary abnormality in Kartagener syndrome has recently been termed the "immotile cilia syndrome." Since approximately half the reported cases have not had situs inversus, this defect should be considered in the differential diagnosis of children with chronic or recurrent respiratory infections. The diagnosis can be suggested by physiologic tests of ciliary clearance and documented by ultrastructural examination of the respiratory epithelium. Sinus infection may occur in immunodeficiency disorders of all types. However, these disorders are uncommon in comparison to the frequency of sporadic cases of sinusitis; it is in general necessary to consider immune defects only when the sinusitis is unusually severe or persistent or when there has been significant infection of other organs as well.

Clinical Features

The clinical features of sinus infection are related to the age of the patient and to the sinus involved. In infants, only the maxillary and ethmoid sinuses are well developed and radiographically demonstrable. Thus, as early as the neonatal period, ethmoiditis is a prominent cause of chronic rhinorrhea. However, because the clinical signs are nonspecific, it is likely that most cases of ethmoiditis and maxillary sinusitis occurring in infancy are not distinguished clinically from cases of uncomplicated rhinitis. If pain occurs with sinus infection in infants, it would be manifested only as generalized irritability and would have limited localizing value.

In older children, the typical distribution of sinus pain may be elicited. The discomfort of maxillary sinusitis is felt below the eye or occasionally as toothache or temporal pain. Ethmoid involvement produces pain over the nose, in the temporal area, or, if the posterior ethmoid cells are involved, the mastoid region. The sphenoid sinus is rarely of clinical significance in children, being well developed only beyond three years of age, but when sphenoid sinusitis occurs, it may present with pain in the occipital, temporal, or postauricular areas. The frontal sinus does not generally produce clinical difficulty until age seven. In frontal sinusitis there may be localized tenderness and pain or discomfort in the supraorbital and frontal areas. There is considerable individual variation in the age limits of sinus development (Maresh, 1940). Furthermore, the diagnostic importance of local pain or discomfort is probably limited to cases in which there is complete obstruction of the sinus ostia. A similar range of symptoms has been found in adults with uncomplicated rhinitis who had normal sinus radiographs and in a group with evidence of acute or chronic sinusitis (Axelsson and Lunze, 1976).

Diagnosis

The diagnosis of sinusitis in infants and children is suggested by the presence of purulent rhinorrhea and nasal obstruction in conjunction with systemic signs such as fever and irritability. Other manifestations include headache or a sense of fullness, tenderness over the involved sinus, or a disturbed sense of smell. Because these signs are nonspecific, the diagnosis is often considered only when local or systemic spread of infection has occurred. The most common such presentation is with orbital or periorbital cellulitis. Maxillary sinusitis in older children may occasionally originate in apical infection of molars or premolars although this occurs much less commonly than in adults.

Clinical Evaluation. The presence of purulent rhinitis and local pain or tenderness should suggest the diagnosis of sinusitis. Rhinoscopy may be extremely helpful; the presence of a purulent sinus discharge or of obstruction of the sinus ostium confirms a diagnosis of sinusitis. Diminished maxillary or frontal transillumination is a relatively reliable sign of sinusitis of those areas in adults (Evans, et al, 1975), but this examination is probably not of value in children less than 12 years old (Chap. 25).

Radiologic examination may be of great value in supporting the clinical diagnosis of sinusitis or, when adequate views show well-aerated sinuses with normal mucosal thickness, in indicating the absence of sinus infection. The presence of an air–fluid level within a sinus should provide fairly conclusive evidence of sinusitis. However, the findings of mucosal thickening or opacity of developed sinuses are much more frequent in children with suspected sinusitis. The interpretation of these findings is open to considerable question, particularly in children less than six years of age. No studies have been reported of children in whom the radiologic diagnosis of sinusitis was confirmed by other objective means. However, mucosal thickening and sinus opacity have been found in radiographs of a large number of children having no clinical evidence of sinusitis (Shopfner and Rossi, 1973). The frequent finding of radiologically defined abnormalities of the sinus in normal children and in those with uncomplicated respiratory infections probably reflects the frequent involvement of the sinus mucosa in viral respiratory infections; the presence of such abnormalities, particularly in children less than six years old, does not by itself indicate the need for further diagnostic investigation or therapy. Radiographic examination of the sinuses thus is of greatest value in excluding the diagnosis of sinus disease where there is diagnostic difficulty and also in following the course of sinus involvement in patients who do not respond well to therapy or who have complications of sinus infection. A further difficulty in interpreting sinus radiography in children is the great variation in normal development and frequent failure of individual sinuses, most often the frontal, to develop at all. Such variants are also likely to be unilateral in individual subjects.

Etiologic Diagnosis. Specific identification of the causative organisms in sinusitis requires culture of aspirated sinus secretions by appropriate methods. Because potentially pathogenic bacteria are found in the nasal passages of most or all normal children, culture of nasal secretions is not helpful and may give misleading results (Evans et al., 1975). Sinus aspiration is indicated when accurate bacteriologic diagnosis is needed. Specific indications for sinus aspiration include (1) sinusitis in children who are seriously ill or who appear toxic, (2) the presence of a sinus infection that has not responded to initial antimicrobial drug therapy, (3) the onset of sinusitis in a patient who is receiving antibiotics, (4) the presence of suppurative complications, and (5) sinusitis in debilitated or immunologically deficient patients. In each of these instances, both specific identification of the causative organism or organisms and *in vitro* antibiotic susceptibility tests may be essential to proper patient management. The procedure may be performed by cannulation of the ostium of the affected sinus or by antral or frontal puncture. Care is required to avoid contamination of the secretions by nasal material. Examination of gram-stained smears is necessary to provide a rapid presumptive diagnosis and to help exclude consideration of bacteria that may later appear as contaminants in the cultures. Children who are ill enough to require these procedures should have cultures of blood and usually of such other potentially infected sites as the cerebrospinal fluid. Few systematic investigations of the bacterial etiology of sinusitis in children have been performed. Thus, much of the available information is derived from studies in which adequate cultures have been obtained from adults with acute maxillary sinusitis (Table 32–3) (Evans, et al., 1975; Urdal and Berdal, 1949; Axelsson and Unidekel, 1972; Rantanen, 1974; Chapnik and Bach, 1976). *Streptococcus pneumoniae* and *Haemophilus influenzae* are the predominant bacterial pathogens, one of these two organ-

Table 32–3   BACTERIAL SPECIES
IDENTIFIED IN SINUS EXUDATES IN
ACUTE MAXILLARY SINUSITIS

Bacterial Species	Per Cent of Cases
Streptococcus pneumoniae	25–45
Haemophilis influenzae	13–30
Group A beta-hemolytic streptococci	2–6
Neisseria sp.	0–1
Staphylococcus aureus	0–10
Enteric gram-negative bacilli	1–9
None (sterile exudates)	20–30

(From Evans et al., 1975; Urdal and Berdal, 1949;
Axelsson and Chidekel, 1972; Rantanen, 1974; and
Chapnick and Bach, 1976.)

isms having occurred in 50 to 75 per cent of
cases in various studies. It should be emphasized that infection due to *H. influenzae* occurs
frequently at all ages although it may be
commonest in young children. The majority
of *H. influenzae* strains isolated from infected
sinuses are nontypable and thus differ from
the strains causing such serious infections as
meningitis. Group A beta-hemolytic streptococci have been involved in a small proportion of cases. Many early investigations have
incriminated *Staphylococcus aureus* as an important pathogen in sinusitis. However, this
organism is rarely identified if care is used to
avoid contamination of the sinus specimens
with nasal material. A major problem in interpreting reports of the bacterial etiology of
acute sinusitis is the large number of additional bacterial species that have been incriminated in a small proportion of patients. Because of the difficulty of obtaining
satisfactory culture material, particularly
from young children, the importance of bacteria other than *S. pneumoniae* and *H. influenzae* as agents of acute sinus infection cannot
be evaluated at present. Unusual or drug-
resistant bacterial infection might be suspected when an acute infection does not respond
to antibacterial therapy. Further attempts at
obtaining a specific diagnosis would be indicated in such cases. Aspirated sinus exudates
have been bacteriologically sterile in approximately 25 per cent of cases; a few such cases
have yielded respiratory viruses when appropriate tissue culture techniques were used
(Evans et al., 1975); the relation of infectious
agents to most such cases is unknown.

Chronic sinusitis is unusual in children.
Recent studies of this disorder have shown
that anaerobic bacteria can frequently be isolated from sinus secretions obtained at the

time of surgery (Table 32–4) (Frederick and
Braude, 1974). This finding is of importance
in that such anaerobic infections may require
different antibacterial therapy from that
given for the common agents of acute sinusitis. Moreover, the potential clinical importance of anaerobic infection is shown by the
fact that the bacteria involved are the same as
those generally isolated in brain abscesses and
other intracranial complications of chronic
sinus infection. Thus, anaerobic cultures are
required to define the bacterial etiology of
cases of chronic sinusitis. Several bacterial
species are often present, and the organisms
are those that are part of the normal oral and
upper respiratory flora. Therefore, in suspected anaerobic infection, culture material
should be obtained surgically with strict attention to avoid contamination from nonsterile areas. Anaerobic infection is suggested
clinically by (a) the presence of a foul-
smelling discharge, (b) the occurrence of infection following surgical procedures or dental infection, (c) the presence of tissue destruction and abscess formation, and (d) a
mixed flora seen in gram stains or aerobic
cultures that are negative (Bartlett and Gorbach, 1976). Most reported cases of anaerobic
sinusitis have been of long duration. *Bacteroides* sp. and anaerobic streptococci are the
most common bacterial isolates in such cases,
but a variety of other organisms may be present.

Fungal sinusitis has rarely been reported in
children, and its occurrence must suggest a
disorder of local or systemic immunity. Rhinocerebral phycomycosis is an opportunistic
and highly invasive infection that generally
occurs in individuals who are diabetic or who
are receiving corticosteroid or other immunosuppressive therapy. Two cases have been

Table 32–4   ANAEROBIC BACTERIA
ISOLATED FROM SURGICAL SPECIMENS
OF PATIENTS WITH CHRONIC
MAXILLARY SINUSITIS

Bacterial Species	Per Cent of Patients
Anaerobic streptococci	57
Bacteroides funduliformis	14
B. fragilis	14
B. melaninogenicus	4
Veilonella	11
Corynebacteria sp.	4
Micrococcus	4

(From Frederick and Braude, 1974.)

reported in apparently healthy children (Blodi, et al., 1969). Aspergillosis of the maxillary sinus is a noninvasive infection that generally presents with unilateral proptosis. This disorder has not been reported to occur before adolescence.

Therapy

Attention to anatomic abnormalities and their surgical correction, investigation of allergies and removal of potentially significant allergens, and therapy of any underlying disorders are utilized when indicated. Local and systemic decongestants are widely used in the therapy of sinus disease; there is, however, no documentation that they provide more than transient, symptomatic relief (Roth et al., 1977; Lampert et al., 1975). If decongestants are to be used, 1 per cent ephedrine or 0.25 per cent phenylephrine can be administered intranasally as nose drops or as a spray. Drops should be instilled with the patient lying on his side with the head tilted downward. Sprays are given in the upright position. If Proetz displacement is utilized to promote sinus drainage, the same vasoactive decongestants can be added to the irrigating solution to increase exposure of the sinus ostia. Antihistamines may also be indicated when an allergic cause for the sinusitis is suspected.

Many investigations have shown that systemic, orally administered antibiotics provide symptomatic and objective improvement in acute sinus infections. In uncomplicated cases in which the causative organism is not known at the time of diagnosis, antibiotics active against both pneumococci and *H. influenzae* are required; the drugs and dosages used are the same as those employed for children with acute otitis media. Based upon the available evidence, these considerations are the same for all age groups beyond the neonatal period. In the first weeks of life sinus infection with group B streptococcus and enteric gram-negative bacilli has been reported. For such infections, broad-spectrum antibiotic therapy, usually including an aminoglycoside (gentamicin or kanamycin) plus a penicillin (ampicillin or penicillin G) is required initially; modifications may be made when culture results are available. At all ages, organisms other than *S. pneumoniae* and *H. influenzae* have been isolated from a consider-

able proportion of cases. Therefore, in unusually severe cases parenteral administration of broad-spectrum antibiotics in high doses is required until culture reports are available and a favorable clinical response has occurred. The therapy of sinus infection due to less common bacterial species is dependent upon identification of the organism and its antibiotic susceptibility. Surgical drainage is most important in chronic infection with anaerobic bacteria. For the majority of such infections, penicillin G or ampicillin provide effective antibacterial therapy and should be used in high doses. Alternative drugs for treatment of anaerobic infections include chloramphenicol and clindamycin, and these should be considered when penicillin-resistant bacteria have been identified or in the presence of such complications as intracranial abscess formation.

Most patients with acute sinusitis do well with medical management. Cases that do not show rapid improvement or that are particularly severe at the onset require drainage of the sinus cavity. Several techniques are available. The Proetz displacement method is the simplest of these and can be used where obstruction of the sinus ostium is not complete (Fig. 32–1). In this technique the nose and nasopharynx are filled with saline with the patient lying supine and the head hyperextended. Suction at the nostril is used to remove the irrigating solution and nasal secretions. With repetition of the irrigation, the sinus ostia are cleared and drainage of the sinus may be accomplished. A decongestant solution such as 0.25 per cent phenylephrine in saline may be used as the irrigating solution. When obstruction of the sinus ostium is complete, the infected sinus may be considered to be like an abscess cavity; the infection is likely to be clinically severe and surgical drainage is then required. Either cannulation of the natural ostium or trephination may be used for this purpose. Puncture of the maxillary antrum may be performed underneath the inferior turbinate or via the canine fossa. The procedure must be undertaken with great caution in children in whom eruption of the secondary dentition is not complete; prior radiologic visualization of the sinus is desirable to assess the depth of the sinus. The frontal sinus may be approached through the brow or supraorbital rim for irrigation, for which an isotonic saline solution is used. The reputed advantages of adding irrigation with

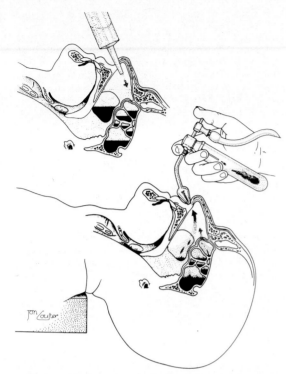

Figure 32–1 Sinus irrigation by the Proetz procedure. This technique may be considered in cases of chronic sinusitis that have not responded to antimicrobial therapy. *A*, The nose is first partially filled with normal saline. *B*, The saline is then removed by suction through one nostril while the other nostril is occluded. The intent of the procedure is to irrigate sinuses with partially patent ostia.

local antibiotics to the systemic therapy have not been documented.

Open surgical procedures for chronic infection are uncommonly required in young children and should be considered only when repeated irrigation has been unsuccessful in resolving the infection. Sublabial antrostomy is rarely indicated in children less than 10 years old; the risk of damage to the permanent dentition is a relative contraindication and anesthesia of teeth on the operated side has been reported (Paavolainen et al., 1977). Creation of a nasal antral window should accompany the sublabial antrostomy to assure goal drainage. Removal of nasal polyps, correction of septal deviation if it is sufficient to cause obstruction, or adenoidectomy may be required for some children with chronic sinusitis who do not improve with medical management.

SELECTED REFERENCES

Chapnik, J. S., and Bach, M. C. 1976. Bacterial and fungal infections of the maxillary sinus. Otolaryngol. Clin. North Am., *9*:43–54.
  This article presents a good review of the host defenses, microbiology, and antimicrobial therapy of sinusitis.

Evans, F. O., Syndor, J. B., and Moore, W. E. C., et al. 1975. Sinusitis of the maxillary antrum. N. Engl. J. Med. *293*:735–739.
  This article presents a critical study, in adults, of the diagnostic techniques used in, and the microbiology of, maxillary sinusitis.

Lampert, R. P., Robinson, D. S., and Soyka, L. F. 1975. A critical look at oral decongestants. Pediatrics, *55*:550–552.
  This article cites reasons for a cautious approach to the use of these drugs.

REFERENCES

Axelsson, A., and Chidekel, N. 1972. Symptomatology and bacteriology correlated to radiological findings in acute maxillary sinusitis. Acta Otolaryngol., *74*:118–122.
Axelsson, A., and Runze, U. 1976. Symptoms and signs of acute maxillary sinusitis. ORL, *32*:298–308.
Bartlett, J. G., and Gorbach, S. L. 1976. Anaerobic infections of the head and neck. Otolaryngol. Clin. North Am., *9*:655–678.
Blodi, F. C., Hannah, F. T., and Wadsworth, J. A. C. 1969. Lethal orbitocerebral phycomycosis in otherwise healthy children. Am. J. Ophthalmol., *67*:698–705.
Chalmers, T. C. 1975. Effects of ascorbic acid on the common cold: An evaluation of the evidence. Am. J. Med., *58*:532–536.
Chapnik, J. S., and Bach, M. C. 1976. Bacterial and fungal infections of the maxillary sinus. Otolaryngol. Clin. North Am., *9*:43–54.
Eliasson, R., Mossberg, B., Camner, P., et al. 1977. The immotile cilia syndrome. A congenital ciliary abnormality as an etiologic factor in chronic airway infections and male sterility. N. Engl. J. Med., *297*:1–6.
Evans, F. O., Syndor, J. B., Moore, W. E. C., et al. 1975. Sinusitis of the maxillary antrum. N. Engl. J. Med., *293*:735–739.
Frederick, J., and Braude, A. I. 1974. Anaerobic infection of the paranasal sinuses. N. Engl. J. Med., *290*:135–137.
Gwaltney, J. M., Jr. 1975. Medical reviews—rhinoviruses. Yale J. Biol. Med., *48*:17–45.
Jaffe, B. F., and DeBlanc, C. B. 1971. Sinusitis in children with cleft lip and palate. Arch. Otolaryngol., *93*:479–482.
Kaye, H. S., Marsh, H. B., and Dowdle, W. R. 1971. Seroepidemiologic survey of coronavirus (Strain OC34) related infections in a children's population. Am. J. Epidemiol., *94*:43–49.
Lampert, R. P., Robinson, D. S., and Soyka, L. F. 1975. A critical look at oral decongestants. Pediatrics, *55*:550–552.
Loda, F. A., Glezen, W. P., and Clyde, W. A., Jr. 1972. Respiratory disease in group day care. Pediatrics, *49*:428–437.

Maresh, M. M. 1940. Paranasal sinuses from birth to late adolescence. Am. J. Dis. Child., *60*:55–78.

Monto, A. S., and Ullman, B. M. 1974. Acute respiratory illness in an American community: The Tecumseh study. J.A.M.A., *227:164*–169.

Paavolainen, M., Paavolainen, R., and Tarkkanen, J. 1977. Influence of Caldwell-Luc operation on developing normal teeth. Laryngoscope, *87*:613–620.

Rantanen, T. 1974. Clinical function tests of the maxillary sinus ostium. Acta Otolaryngol., Suppl., *328*:1–38.

Rosenthal, A., and Fellows, K. E. 1973. Acute infectious sinusitis in cyanotic congenital heart disease. Pediatrics, *52*:692–696.

Roth, R. P., Cantekin, E. I., Bluestone, C. D., et al. 1977. Nasal decongestant activity of pseudoephedrine. Ann. Otol. Rhinol. Laryngol., *86*:235–242.

Shopfner, C. E., and Rossi, J. O. 1973. Roentgen evaluation of the paranasal sinuses in children. Am. J. Radiol., *118*:176–186.

Urdal, K., and Berdal, P. 1949. The microbial flora in 81 cases of maxillary sinusitis. Acta Otolaryngol., *37*:20–25.

Chapter 33

COMPLICATIONS OF NASAL AND SINUS INFECTIONS

Daniel D. Rabuzzi, M. D.
Arthur S. Hengerer, M. D.

The treatment of complications of nasal and paranasal sinus infections remains a significant portion of the practice of pediatric medicine. This is often true, despite the early and judicious use of antibiotic therapy, although with the advent of antibiotics the total number of these complications has been dramatically reduced over the years, and the average practitioner today may not be as well versed as older colleagues in the early recognition and therapy of these problems.

Table 33–1 COMPLICATIONS OF NASAL AND SINUS INFECTIONS

Local
    Synechiae
    Polyps
    Osteomyelitis
    Septal hematomas
    Septal abscesses
    Mucoceles
    Pyoceles

Orbital
    Cellulitis
    Abscesses

Intracranial
    Meningitis
    Brain abscesses
      Epidural
      Subdural
    Cavernous sinus thrombosis

Systemic
    Lower respiratory diseases
      Chronic bronchitis
      Bronchiectasis

The physician can only make the proper diagnosis if he or she knows the presenting characteristics of these complications and looks for them. It is the purpose of this chapter to provide an overview of such nasal and paranasal sinus infection complications so that the reader will be more attuned to their accurate diagnosis and treatment (Table 33–1).

NASAL INFECTION COMPLICATIONS

A child's nose is a prominent structure of facial anatomy, exposed to frequent blunt trauma. Coupling that fact with the known specific nasal diseases, it is then quickly appreciated why the fragile, pseudostratified, ciliated, columnar epithelium of the nasal mucosa is so frequently disturbed and prone to complications of infection.

Synechiae

Physiologic function of the normal nasal mucosa with its cyclical swelling allows opposing surfaces within the nasal cavity to contact one another. If, as a result of inflammatory, traumatic, or iatrogenic causes, a raw surface of granulating tissue exists, a fibroblastic matrix may be laid down along these opposing surfaces. Consequently, bands of scar tissue, so-called synechiae, will then be formed, stretching between any two anatomic structures within the nasal vault.

791

Once formed, the complications of mechanical blockage from these bands of scar tissue will occur with altered air currents and interference with the proper physiologic flow of the "mucous blanket." This may result in a chronic rhinorrhea and a change in the viscosity and the amount of postnasal drainage. Posterior pharyngeal irritation and possibly eustachian tube inflammation may be a result of this. Moreover, metaplastic changes in the nasal mucosa can occur with concomitant crusting, ulceration, and bleeding in the area anterior to the synechial formation. Synechiae located in the lateral aspects of the nose, between the turbinates and the floor of the nose, may alter normal sinus drainage from the hiatus semilunaris or from surgically created nasoantral windows. This occurrence could lead to an obstructive sinusitis.

Lysis of the synechial bands is usually corrective, providing the raw surfaces are allowed to heal unopposed. This is best accomplished by the use of Teflon sheets placed within the nasal vault between the lateral wall of the nose and the nasal septum. These sheets are sutured through-and-through to the nasal septum to allow them to stay in position for a 10 to 14 day period.

Septal Hematoma and Abscess

Septal hematoma, abscess, or both from nasal trauma or recurrent nasal and paranasal sinus infection is one of the most feared complications because of the significant cosmetic and functional sequelae that may result. Saddle nose deformity, nasal airway obstruction, nasal septal perforation, and extension of infection into paranasal or even intracranial structures are all problems that have occurred as complications of septal hematoma and abscesses. When the hematoma develops, the septal mucosa is erythematous and swollen, often touching the turbinates or lateral nasal wall. The swelling is doughy in consistency and may be quite tender. Depending on whether or not there is a communication within the cartilaginous septum, the hematoma or abscess cavity may be either unilateral or bilateral. This fact may be determined by direct visual examination and palpation. If only unilateral involvement exists, the likelihood of permanent complications is somewhat lessened because of the persistent nourishment to the cartilage through the opposite nasal mucoperichondrium.

Once recognized, a septal hematoma or abscess must be treated by adequate incision and drainage with wide opening of the tissue planes. This will require the use of general anesthesia in most children. The cavity should be packed lightly with one quarter inch iodoform gauze, and the patient should be placed on appropriate intravenous antibiotic therapy. High-dose penicillin is the initial drug of choice in these instances and should be given unless culture reports of the abscess drainage indicate the presence of resistant organisms. Recently there has been a trend toward the use of antibiotics such as nafcillin to protect against penicillinase-resistant organisms. When the treatment is not given early enough or when results are ineffective, additional significant complications can develop.

The interruption of the septal cartilage blood supply by the hematoma or abscess may result in eventual cartilage necrosis and resorption. An anterior septal perforation of varying size often develops in this necrotic area and will usually persist. The margins of these perforations often contain exposed cartilage edges and areas of granulation tissue, which maintain a superficial infection of saprophytic organisms. This, and the dryness caused by the irregular air currents passing through the perforation, will cause mucosal crusting and the subjective sensation of nasal obstruction. These crusts need to be removed frequently, a process often accompanied by bleeding, which at times may be quite significant. The child's annoyance with such crusting will often lead to habitual nose picking with resulting perforation enlargement. Depending on the size of the perforation, a "whistling" sound may also be created by nasal breathing, which is quite aggravating to child and parent alike. Repairs of such perforations by the use of various mucosal flaps or connective tissue grafts are only satisfactory if the perforation is less than 1 cm in diameter.

Further septal cartilage necrosis can cause collapse of all septal support with concomitant airway obstruction. Such collapse will alter the shape of the nasal vault, specifically in the so-called "valve" area between the septum and upper lateral cartilage, which is considered so important to the patient's awareness of nasal airflow. Similarly, the same collapse will also create the cosmetic deformity known as saddle nose. This external collapse may appear immediately if the cartilage loss is severe, or it may develop gradually with increasing age as a result of the loss or possibly from the alteration in the growth centers with maturity. Conservative repair of such a functional and cosmetic deformity need not wait until the child reaches maturity, but should be instituted 6 to 12 months after the active disease process has been controlled.

More serious complications secondary to septal cartilage infection are the effects of intracranial extension and abscesses. Since the angular veins between the nose and midportion of the face are without intraluminal valves, direct extension of infection into them may allow early development of septicemia and involvement of the cavernous sinus, meninges, and bony cranial vault. These complications will be surveyed later.

PARANASAL SINUS INFECTION COMPLICATIONS

Aside from those children suffering from generalized metabolic or inherited defects such as diabetes, cystic fibrosis, and aplastic anemias, chronic sinus infections are relatively rare in children under 16 years of age. This is in marked contrast to statistics for adults, in whom acute and chronic infections occur without associated systemic disease. In children, complications of acute sinus infections seem to occur more frequently than among the adult general population. These complications can be divided into those with local spread, those with intracranial involvement, and those with systemic symptoms.

Those complications that do ensue from acute and chronic sinus disease in children are linked directly to the anatomic relationship of the paranasal sinuses to other structures of the head, neck, and chest. These relationships are surprisingly constant (see Chapters. 23 and 31). Most commonly involved are the structures of the orbit, cranial vault, chest, and nares.

Orbital Complications

The discussion of this topic at this time in medical history has been radically changed by the advent of antibiotics. For this reason the previously defined classifications of the step-by-step development of the spread of sinus infections to other areas is no longer classical.

Table 33–2 CLASSIFICATION OF ORBITAL COMPLICATIONS

1 — Inflammatory Edema (Periorbital Cellulitis)
2 — Orbital Cellulitis
3 — Subperiosteal Abscess
4 — Orbital Abscess
5 — Cavernous Sinus Thrombosis or Intracranial Complications

The recent classification by Chandler et al. (1970) seems most practical (Table 33–2). The local, direct extension of disease causing the orbital complications is the result of several distinct factors limited to the facial structures of childhood. These influencing tendencies are the thinner bony septa of the sinus walls, larger vascular foramina, more porous bones, and open suture lines.

The paper-thin bony plates separating the ethmoid and maxillary sinuses from the orbit allow infection to spread to the orbit in this age group particularly (Bernstein, 1971). With ethmoid sinusitis the thickened, inflamed mucosa obstructs drainage into the nose, and when pus under pressure develops this leads to necrosis of the lamina papyracea by interrupting the periosteal blood supply. Contiguous and vascular spread of infection from the ethmoid labyrinth into the orbit will first produce edema and erythema of the eyelids, especially in their upper medial quadrants. Similarly, spread of infection from the maxillary antra will particularly cause lower lid swelling. From this stage, unless it is aggressively treated, it can rapidly progress to an orbital cellulitis. When that occurs, there is usually an increase in body temperature, tenderness over the lids increases markedly, and the globe itself may show some forward protrusion. Usually, extraocular mobility is present but limited, and some chemosis of the conjunctiva may be seen. Even at this stage, hospitalization and intravenous antibiotic therapy, along with topical nasal decongestants, will often abort any further progression of symptoms. Since the most virulent pathogens tend to be *Haemophilus influenza* and penicillinase-resistant staphylococcus, ampicillin and nafcillin would be the combined drugs of choice (Haynes and Cramblett, 1967; Watters et al., 1976). However, as this therapy is instituted, investigations must commence to rule out either a subperiosteal abscess or an intraorbital abscess. In days past, it would suffice to begin therapy and determine further treatment on whether or not there was a response to antibiotics over a 12 to 24 hour period. With the radiologic facilities of today, these diagnoses may be made much more rapidly and efficiently by the use of orbital tomography and computerized axial tomography (CAT) scanning.

The CAT scan gives an exquisite picture of an intraorbital lesion (Fig. 33–1). It can also define and differentiate both subperiosteal and intraorbital abscesses (Figs. 33–2 and 33–3). This allows for much more accurate and correctly timed operative intervention.

Should such radiologic innovations not be available to the clinician, the progressive symptoms that suggest purulent abscess formation are increasing edema and lid erythema with the inability to close the eye completely, marked orbital chemosis, proptosis of the eye either straight forward or in the down-and-out position (depending upon the site of abscess), further diminution of extraocular motion, and loss of visual acuity. These findings should, of course, be verified by a consulting ophthalmologist. Whatever the set of diagnostic circumstances, be they purely radiologic, purely clinical, or a combination of both, once the diagnosis of periorbital abscess is decided upon, surgical intervention must be carried out.

The proper method of draining a periorbital abscess is through an external ethmoidectomy skin incision midway between the inner canthus of the eye and the midnasal dorsum. The procedure is performed under general anesthesia with the use of a local anesthetic, with epinephrine (1:200,000) infiltrated into the skin for its vasoconstrictor effect. A layer

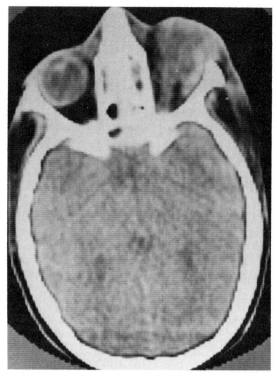

Figure 33–2 Intraorbital abscess. Note intact lamina papyracea.

dissection should be carried out down to and through the periosteum, as this will aid immeasurably in precluding inadvertent cutting of the angular vein and concomitant heavy bleeding. The elevation of the periosteum

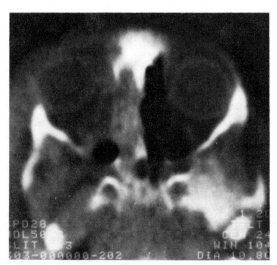

Figure 33–1 Magnified CAT scan showing ethmoiditis and subperiosteal orbital abscess.

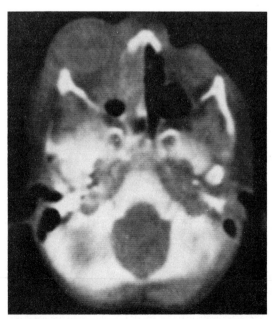

Figure 33–3 Subperiosteal abscess with lamina papyracea breakdown.

over the nasal projection of the maxillary bone and lamina papyracea of the medial wall of the orbit may expose the ethmoid sinus through a necrotic bony defect. If a subperiosteal abscess is present, it is rapidly drained. In addition to the abscess drainage, a partial ethmoidectomy should then be performed to remove diseased tissue, although without attempting a complete and meticulous dissection of all mucosa. Should a subperiosteal abscess not be found or should the CAT scan have shown an orbital abscess, then the periorbita must be incised and the intraorbital abscess found and drained. The wound is then closed in layers with one small drain from the incision line and another placed intranasally through the middle

meatus into the cleaned ethmoid sinus. If the maxillary sinus is the source of the orbital complication, then drainage should be done either through the inferior meatus or via the anterior maxillary bony wall with a spinal needle. This technique is discussed elsewhere in this chapter. Once the drainage has been accomplished and adequate chemotherapy is continued, resolution of the fever and associated symptoms is usually dramatic.

Unhalted infection and retrograde venous thrombophlebitis via the nasal and angular veins that surround the ethmoid labyrinth and orbital structures can ultimately spread to cause cavernous sinus thrombosis (Price et al., 1971) (Fig. 33–4). This devastating complication is diagnosed mainly by its orbital symp-

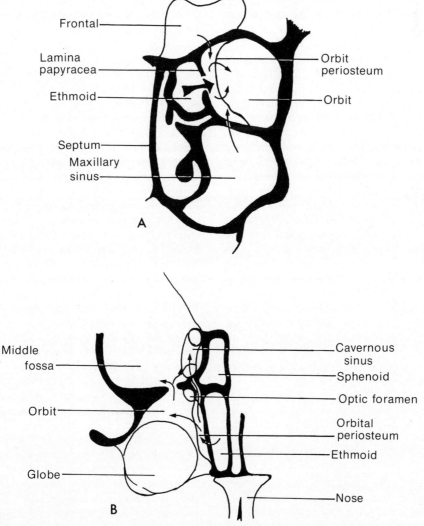

Figure 33–4 *A,* Spread of infection from sinuses to the orbit. *B,* Spread of infection from orbit to cavernous sinus.

tomatology, consisting of lid edema, erythema, and chemosis (which is most often present bilaterally). In addition, the paresis of the extraocular muscles innervated by the oculomotor, abducens, or trochlear nerves may be present, which eventually leads to a complete ophthalmoplegia. The body temperature is usually quite high from the marked toxicity and septic emboli, which cause the "picket fence" fever spikes. Massive antibiotic therapy, and more recently the adjunctive use of anticoagulants such as heparin, have improved the survival rates for these children.

A special comment should be made here regarding the sequelae of facial pain and headache that occur from the orbital complications and their further progression to intracranial areas. From the onset of sinus infection, some degree of discomfort is noted by all patients. Initially, it is the sense of congestion and pressure within the nasal region that can create the associated complaint of facial pressure and temporal region headache. As the step-by-step progression of the infection occurs, there is a shifting in location and intensity of pain. Once the orbital structures become involved, a severe, deep-seated pain behind the eyes develops, and with attempted eye movement aggravation of this pain occurs. If only the orbit is involved, the pain remains unilateral and is associated with headache, which may be localized or diffuse. The headache is due to the pus under pressure as well as to the localized vascular changes. With cavernous sinus involvement, the pain becomes more deeply placed in the center of the head. The headache is also severe as the sinus thrombosis and the venous pressure increase throughout the intracranial vessels.

Clinically, patients' response to this worsening pain is likely to be altered by the obtunded state that frequently accompanies the condition. Therefore, if the patient is severely toxic, there may be no real awareness of headache or facial pain.

Intracranial Complications

Intracranial spread of infection from the frontal, ethmoid, or sphenoid sinuses can produce further complications, such as meningeal irritation and infection, brain abscess, and peridural abscess. These problems should be managed by a multidisciplinary team composed of the pediatrician, neurologist or neurosurgeon, and the otolaryngologist.

The early and widespread use of antibiotics has caused osteomyelitis of the frontal or maxillary bones to become quite a rare entity, but it still may be seen in neglected patients or, more commonly, in undertreated patients. In infants and children, it is the spongy bone over the anterior wall of the maxilla that is usually infected, producing erythema, edema, and marked tenderness with swelling. Since the frontal sinus does not develop until the age of six years or older, complications of bony spread of sinus infection over the frontal area will not occur except in the older age group. The signs are similar in that swelling over the sinus, particularly with periosteal edema, is present. This often produces a "doughy" feeling to the skin over the affected area ("Pott's puffy tumor"). The patient should be treated with intravenous antibiotics and opening of the periosteum over the affected area to evacuate any collection of pus with insertion of drains. When surgery is performed, removal of only the obviously unhealthy and irreversibly diseased bone should be done. Long-term postoperative intravenous antibiotic therapy of two to three weeks' duration, followed by another six weeks of oral medication, has been found to allow resorption and regeneration of infected bone to the point that the surgeon can afford to be somewhat more conservative in his or her management than previously. The best possible surgical approach is through a noninfected area, so that a coronal incision and elevation of a scalp flap are ideal procedures for frontal sinus work. However, one is obliged to use a buccal incision for the maxilla, despite the obviously contaminated field. Fortunately, this has not seemed to have been a deterrent to rapid healing.

Meningeal inflammation secondary to the spread of infection from the nasal regions into the cranial vault will cause pain in the head and neck region, lethargy, fever, and nuchal rigidity. The pain in these patients is most often a diffuse, intense headache due to involvement of the meninges. The pain increases when the head is lowered to a dependent position or when the venous pressure is increased by coughing, crying, or straining. The same pathologic changes in the meninges are responsible for the pain created by head movement, especially neck flexion when done to demonstrate the rigidity. This occurs because of the stretching of the inflamed meninges and nerve roots, and is known as a positive Kernig's sign.

If this is suspected, a spinal tap for examination of cerebrospinal fluid must be done, and the patient must be hospitalized for administration of high doses of intravenous antibiotics. The response to this therapy is usually quite satisfactory once the offending organism has been identified and adequately treated. Brain and peridural abscesses tend to produce a somewhat more chronic and quiet symptom complex, which causes their diagnosis to be made relatively late in their course. This is especially true when the lesion is in the frontal lobe where clinical findings are minimal. Therefore, in anyone complaining of deep headaches, difficulty in concentrating, and general lethargy who also has an unresolved sinus problem, the clinician's responsibility is to rule out an intracranial problem (Blumenfeld and Skolnik, 1966). In these cases, the CAT scan has been an invaluable diagnostic tool, for it allows a noninvasive technique to be used for intracranial diagnostic purposes. If a brain abscess is discovered, it should be managed by a neurosurgeon. Later sinus surgery may be necessary for removal of residual intrasinus disease, but this is very rare in children.

Polyps and Mucoceles

The finding of nasal polyps in the prepubescent child is quite unusual and rarely secondary to chronic sinus disease. It is more likely that they would arise from a metabolic or immunologic problem, especially cystic fibrosis. For this reason, all these children deserve testing for immunoglobulin levels and low sweat chlorides. The treatment can then be directed to the basic underlying systemic problem.

Nasal polyps secondary to allergic–inflammatory causes are seen in the older pediatric age group about as frequently as in adults. This non-neoplastic polyp tissue consists of thickened edematous mucosal stroma, infiltrated with both eosinophils and polymorphonuclear leukocytes. Most often, the polyps project from the ethmoid sinuses via the middle meatus but may also be found in the superior meatus where they extend from both the posterior ethmoid air cells and the sphenoid sinus. The primary treatment of these polyps consists of strenuous antibiotic therapy and decongestants, with surgical excision being reserved only for those obstructive polyps that have become recalcitrant to this treatment. The smaller, nonobstructive polyps are usually not removed unless chronic sinus infection continues behind them. In many cases, the combination of a course of antibiotics and allergic desensitization will result in their complete resorption. In the event that surgery becomes necessary, a simple nasal polypectomy is the procedure of choice, since recurrence of these lesions without resolution of the basic medical problem is very common. In this age group, it is also obvious that any major intrasinus surgery must not be done until full facial growth has occurred.

In the discussion of nasal polyps, there is a distinct clinical entity known as the antrochoanal polyp. This polyp is almost always unilateral and tends to cause posterior choanal obstruction. It is a very pedunculated mass with a small stalk being present, extending from one of the maxillary sinus ostia through the nose into the posterior choana. The site of attachment of the stalk is in the sinus itself, most frequently on the lateral wall. These lesions do not respond to decongestants or antibiotic therapy and therefore must be removed surgically in every instance. The Caldwell-Luc approach with conservative removal of the bony anterior sinus wall and excision of only that mucosa around the site of the stalk is indicated. The polyp may then be removed through the nose or mouth. The important step is to remove the entire stalk; otherwise recurrence is frequent, especially if a simple avulsion technique is used.

Chronic sinus disease can on occasion produce complete obstruction of the ostia or ducts of the major paranasal sinuses. When this occurs, the mucous lining of the sinus continues to produce secretions, only now there is no effective egress available and a mucocele is formed. Over a period of years, the sinus walls may flatten and bow to accommodate the steadily increasing pressure created by the trapped mucus. When this process occurs from an obstructed nasofrontal duct, there will be a downward bulging of the orbital roof, producing an upper inner canthal swelling of the orbit with downward and outward deviation of the eye. On the other hand, mucoceles of the ethmoid and sphenoid sinuses are quite difficult to diagnose without radiographic evaluation because of the paucity of physical findings except for headache and a feeling of frontal pressure or impaired ocular muscle function. Therefore, diagnosis must be by radiograph, with both plane radiographs and tomography; or more recently the CAT scan has been used. By and large, since mucoceles or their infected equivalent, pyoceles, take years rather than months to develop to any significant size, it is very unusual to see these problems in the pediatric age group. However, if discovered, treatment must be by surgical intervention. A frontal sinus mucocele can be handled by use of an osteoplastic frontal sinusotomy with fat obliteration of the sinus and its nasofrontal duct. Ethmoid and sphenoid mucoceles are best treated by the external ethmoidectomy approach and drainage.

Lower Respiratory Tract Diseases

The spread of infection between the upper and lower respiratory tracts has been the subject of controversy and conjecture for many years (Farrell, 1936). In children with chronic nasal and paranasal sinus infection, there seems to be an increased incidence of cough and recurrent pneumonitis over and above that which would be expected on a purely incidental basis. This is most easily seen in the asthmatic child or the child with Kartagener syndrome in whom the immunologic and hereditary dysfunctions are readily apparent. However, there are many other children without any known metabolic or immunologic deficit who exhibit similar symptoms of malaise, low-grade fevers, chronic sinus mucosal disease, and recurrent tracheobronchitis or pneumonitis. It is in reference to these children that the term sinobronchial syndrome has been used.

The pathways of infection in this syndrome are probably twofold: first, by direct extension along the mucosa from the sinuses, via the pharynx with some laryngeal aspiration leading to intratracheal and bronchial disease; and second, by lymphatic spread from the sinuses via the mediastinum to the tracheobronchial tree. Studies have been done by several investigators to promote each concept (Sasaki and Kirchner, 1967). In the first instance, the mucosal spread could logically be seen to promote a chronic cough and recurrent tracheobronchial infection. On the other hand, it seems apparent that the repeated bouts of interstitial pneumonitis might be more readily explained when attributed to spread along known lymphatic pathways from the sinuses, through the mediastinum, and to the lungs themselves. The rare retropharyngeal or deep neck abscess seen without evidence of Waldeyer's ring infection may also be attributed to such spread.

Having discovered this systemic connection, when children have recurrent pulmonary disease the physician should search for associated chronic sinus infection via direct nasal examination and sinus radiographs. If the sinobronchial syndrome is diagnosed, then fairly aggressive antibiotic therapy and nasal decongestant therapy should be instituted. Cultures should be taken in the middle meati, even if no specific purulence is noted, to give some guidance as to the proper chemotherapeutic agent. Most commonly, either penicillin or one of its derivatives turns out to be the drug of choice in controlling the usual gram-positive infections. The maxillary sinuses seem to become secondarily infected. If good resolution of intrasinus disease does not occur after three weeks of therapy, then an antral irrigation should be done, and repeat cultures should be taken. This is classically performed by a puncture with a sharp, curved trocar or spinal needle through the inferior meatus. Recently, we have preferred to perform irrigation by direct puncture through the anterior sinus wall under local anesthesia in older children. This will hopefully resolve the sinusitis and eventually permit resolution of the pulmonary complications.

REFERENCES

Bernstein, L. 1971. Pediatric sinus problems. Otolaryngol. Clin. North Am., 4:127–142.

Blumenfeld, R. J., and Skolnik, E. M. 1966. Intracranial complications of sinus disease. Trans. Am. Acad. Ophthalmol. Otolaryngol., 70:899–908.

Chandler, J. R., Langenbrunner, D. J., and Stevens, E. R. 1970. The pathogenesis of orbital complications in acute sinusitis. Laryngoscope, 80:1414–1428.

Farrell, J. T. 1936. The connection of bronchiectasis and sinusitis. J.A.M.A., 106:92–96.

Haynes, R. E., and Cramblett, H. G. 1967. Acute ethmoiditis: Its relationship to orbital cellulitis. Am. J. Dis. Child., 114:261–267.

Price, D. D., Hameroff, S. B., and Richards, R. D. 1971. Cavernous sinus thrombosis and orbital cellulitis. South. Med. J., 64:1243–1247.

Sasaki, C. T., and Kirchner, J. A. 1967. A lymphatic pathway from the sinuses to the mediastinum. Arch. Otolaryngol., 85:432–445.

Watters, E. C., Waller, P. H., Hiles, D. A., et. al. 1976. Acute orbital cellulitis. Arch. Ophthalmol., 94:785–788.

Chapter 34

FOREIGN BODIES
OF THE NOSE

Robert S. Shapiro, M.D.

The otorhinolaryngologic, pediatric, radiologic, and general medical literature contains reports of unusual foreign bodies in the nose but few comprehensive discussions of this problem. This is understandable since nasal foreign bodies are commonly seen by the otolaryngologist and pediatrician and are usually removed quite easily. Frequently, however, there is a delay in referral to the otolaryngologist because a foreign body is not suspected to be present. Furthermore, certain foreign bodies can be quite difficult to remove and present a challenge in management. Removal of some of the animate foreign bodies (such as maggots) can prove to be quite difficult. A foreign body in the nasal cavity may accidentally be pushed backward and may be aspirated during an attempt at removal. This can result in acute respiratory obstruction. Nasal foreign bodies are more common in children than in adults, as children are more likely to put objects into the nose or to have objects placed there by other children.

ETIOLOGY

The foreign body may enter the nose by itself, or it may be placed there by the child or another person. Children are prone to making a game of placing objects into their nasal cavities and other body orifices. Children also tend to put objects into the noses of friends or younger siblings. This is especially common in retarded children. Some foreign bodies are iatrogenic, having accidentally been left in the nose following intranasal manipulation or surgery. Retrograde lodgement from cough-ing, regurgitation, and vomiting has been reported. Reports exist of teeth entering the nose during dental extractions.

Flies, insects, and fungi may enter the nose and may lead to an odorous discharge. This is more common in warmer climates. Predisposing factors include diabetes, syphilis, ozena, poor hygiene, and working with animals.

TYPES OF FOREIGN BODIES OF THE NOSE

Inanimate Foreign Bodies

The number of different objects that have been removed from the nose is virtually endless. Common foreign bodies include beans, nuts, peas, beads, chalk, eyelets, erasers, buttons, studs, pieces of sponge rubber, plasticine, pieces of wood, bones, sticks, paper, chewing gum, crayons, meat, pits (fruit stones), paper clips, jewelry, pieces of plastic, bread, small toys, and seeds. Essentially any object that can be placed in the nose has probably been found there (Fig. 34–1), and the literature contains numerous reports of unusual foreign bodies.

Marrone et al. (1968) reported on a patient with a tooth in the nose as the result of evulsion during endotracheal intubation for a surgical procedure. McAndrew (1976) reported the displacement of a lower wisdom tooth into the posterior nasal aperture during dental extractions. The tooth was located by radiograph. Wood and Case (1973) reported finding an apparent splinter of bone in the nasal cavity. This proved to be the fractured

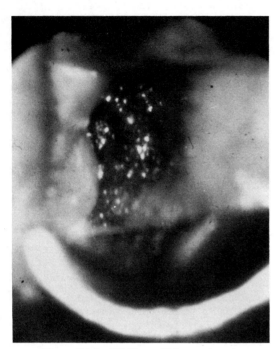

Figure 34–1 "Brillo pad" in nasal cavity.

end of a dental root tip fragment. Another foreign body of dental origin was described by Nazif (1971): a rubber dam clamp disappeared during a dental procedure; radiographs revealed the presence of the clamp in the nasal cavity.

Malhotra et al. (1970) described a very unusual foreign body in a man who was struck by the door of an Army vehicle. The patient subsequently noted inability to open his mouth, nasal obstruction, and pain and swelling on the side of his nose. Twenty four days later he presented for examination and was found to have a 3.5 inch long piece of a door handle from the vehicle in his nose. Dayal and Singh (1970) reported two cases of inanimate foreign bodies of the nasopharynx. One was a toy whistle, and the second was a large metallic foreign body that entered the nasopharynx through the ethmoid and frontal sinuses after an explosion. Awty (1972) described the removal of a large metal fragment lodged in the posterior nares and nasopharynx. This was a shell fragment from a gunshot injury. Tolhurst (1974) reported finding three foreign bodies in the nose at the time of repair of a cleft palate; there were two pieces of rolled paper and a small piece of wood. Utrata (1977) reported on a safety pin that had probably been present in the nose of a young child for two years. The object was

found perforated through the soft palate while the child was undergoing anesthesia for eye surgery. The child had been asymptomatic except for one episode of epistaxis six months before discovery of the foreign body. The safety pin had opened while in the nose, but it was removed under general anesthesia with an alligator forceps, and the palatal wound healed smoothly.

In a retrospective review of patients requiring admission to The Montreal Children's Hospital for removal of nasal foreign bodies under general anesthesia, the author found that 29 children were admitted for this reason between 1970 and 1977. The ages of the children ranged between 1.5 and 17 years. There were 16 girls and 13 boys. In one child the foreign body (a stone) passed into the stomach prior to the child going to the operating room, and surgery was cancelled. In four of the other children no foreign body was actually found. The foreign bodies found in the other 24 children are listed in Table 34–1. Three children had bilateral foreign bodies; two of these were sponges and the others were magnets. Eighteen children had foreign bodies or suspected foreign bodies in the right nasal cavity, and eight children had foreign bodies in the left nasal cavity (one passing spontaneously into the stomach). Of the children whose parents could be reached by telephone, 14 were right-handed and 2 were left-handed. No relation could be established between handedness and the particular nasal cavity in which the foreign body was placed. All foreign bodies were easily removed and there were no complications.

Table 34–1 FOREIGN BODIES OF THE NOSE REMOVED UNDER GENERAL ANESTHESIA AT THE MONTREAL CHILDREN'S HOSPITAL BETWEEN 1970 AND 1977

Type of Object	Number
Plastic objects	5
Buttons	4
Sponges	4 (2 bilateral)
Metal objects	2
Food	2
Paper clip	1
Magnet	1 (bilateral)
Eraser	1
Nut	1
Pit	1
Leather	1
Seed	1

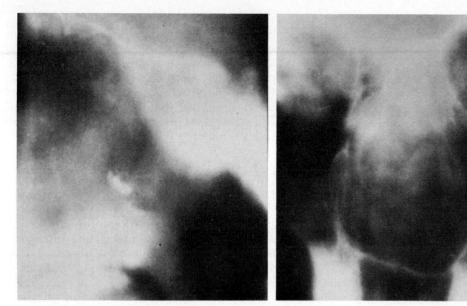

Figure 34–2 Lateral tomogram and anteroposterior tomogram showing large rhinolith filling the nasal cavity. This 15 year old girl had nasal obstruction for three years but no history of insertion of a foreign body into the nose. The rhinolith had displaced the septum. It was removed transnasally, and there was considerable bleeding, which was controlled with packing. The postoperative course was uneventful. (From Children's Hospital of Pittsburgh.)

These were only foreign bodies that required removal under general anesthesia. The majority of foreign bodies were removed in the outpatient department without general anesthesia.

Rhinoliths

Rhinoliths are formed from intranasal foreign bodies that become encrusted with mineral salts, usually calcium and magnesium (Fig. 34–2). The vast majority are thought to arise from exogenous foreign bodies. These are frequently fruit stones (pits). The theoretic possibility of endogenous nuclei such as blood clots and dried pus has been hypothesized, but most authors doubt this origin. Most reports show a preponderance of females among the patients with rhinoliths.

Animate Foreign Bodies

A wide variety of insects, maggots, intestinal worms, and leeches have been reported to be found in the nose. In hot climates flies may deposit their ova in the nose, with maggots resulting. This is rare in the healthy nose but is more common in patients with ozena or syphilis. Epistaxis, headache, lacrimation, and sneezing develop and are soon followed by a bloody discharge that becomes purulent. Ulceration and destruction of the nasal structures may occur. Death may result from meningitis (Smith, 1968). Maggots represent the larval stage of certain flies, such as the screw worm fly and the blow fly; a single screw worm fly may deposit as many as 300 eggs in five minutes (Hunter et al., 1976).

Rhinosporidium seeberi infestation is a fungal infection found mainly in India and Sri Lanka. Nasal polyps are formed and contain the spores in all stages of development. The masses appear as slender filiform or narrow leaf-like processes of a dull pink or reddish tint, with the surface studded with many minute, pale spots owing to the presence of the sporangia in the tissue (Smith, 1968). The growths are very friable and bleed easily when touched.

Ascaris lumbricoides, a nematode or intestinal round worm, is one of the most common helminthic parasites of man. Ascariasis has a world-wide distribution and is particularly common in regions with poor sanitation. Endemic regions exist in the United States, especially in southeastern parts of the Appalachian range. Humans are infected by ingestion of the mature eggs in fecally contaminated food or drink. These eggs hatch in the intestine, liberating minute larvae, which penetrate blood or lymph vessels in the intestinal wall. Some larvae reach the portal circulation and are carried to the liver, while others pass through the thoracic duct. By either route they finally reach the lungs, where they are filtered out of the blood stream, and in a few days many perforate the alveoli. After increasing in size, the larvae migrate up the respiratory passages to the epiglottis and then down the esophagus (Hunter et al., 1976). The parasite may lodge in the nose when regurgitated.

Leeches may cause epistaxis when present as foreign bodies in the nose. Alavi (1969) reported on 54 patients with leeches in the upper respiratory tract, 35 per cent of them presenting with epistaxis. Dayal and Singh (1970) reported on an 18 year old boy with a history of a leech entering the nose two months before examination. He complained of recurrent epistaxis. The leech was found hanging from the nasopharynx and was easily removed.

Aspergillus infections of the nose cause sneezing, rhinorrhea, headache, and the discharge of pieces of tough, greenish membrane, which may coexist with polyps and granulation tissue (Smith, 1968).

PATHOLOGY

The inanimate foreign bodies tend to cause edema and inflammation of the nasal mucous membrane. Ulceration and epistaxis may result. Granulation tissue may be produced. Sinusitis may also occur.

Baluyot (1973) reported that maggots in the nose cause varying degrees of inflammatory reaction, from a mild localized infection to massive destruction of the cartilaginous and bony nasal walls, with formation of deep, odorous, suppurating areas. The ascaris worms cause a varying degree of irritation by their presence and constant motion.

CLINICAL MANIFESTATIONS

The child with a foreign body in the nose may not bring this to the attention of his or her parents. It may remain asymptomatic and stay in the nose for a great length of time. Eventually a rhinolith may form around the foreign body. More frequently, however, a nasal discharge develops on the side of the nose with the foreign body. A unilateral rhinorrhea, particularly if purulent or odorous,

should alert one to the possibility of a foreign body. There may be pain, nasal obstruction, epistaxis, and sneezing. Examination usually shows edema with inflammation of the nasal mucosa. Ulceration may have occurred. The foreign body may also pass posteriorly and may be swallowed or aspirated. An ipsilateral serous otitis media may be present when the foreign material has been present for a long time.

A very common nasal foreign body that is particularly prone to causing infection is foam rubber. With foam rubber the nasal cavity very quickly develops a foul-smelling discharge. Seeds are common foreign bodies, and they may swell and become impacted. Stool and McConnel (1973) reported that special problems have arisen in recent years because of plastic toys. They cause little odor because of their low reactivity, and yet granulation tissue forms around them to give the gross appearance of a tumor.

With a rhinolith, nasal discharge is frequent, usually unilateral, and frequently foul-smelling. It may be purulent and tinged with blood. Epistaxis may occur, as may anosmia, headache, and sinusitis. The septum may be deviated. Bicknell (1970) reported perforation of the hard palate due to a rhinolith. Carder and Hill (1966) reported on an asymptomatic rhinolith. They found only two other asymptomatic rhinoliths in the literature. Smith (1968) reported that rhinoliths are more common in cases of cleft palate.

The diagnosis of the presence of a rhinolith can usually be made by visual inspection and palpation with a probe. The rhinoliths also show up well on radiographs. The films reveal a dense, irregular, but not necessarily homogeneous mass lying within the nasal passage. There may be local bone absorption or distortion due to pressure on the turbinates, with deflection of the septum. The medial wall of the antrum may be similarly indented (Harrison and Lamming, 1969).

Brown (1945) reported that nasal occlusion, headaches, and sneezing with serosanguineous discharge usually begin two or three days after parasitic infestation of the nose. The patient usually complains of intense pain and a sensation of "crawling." Delirium is not uncommon (Hunter et al., 1976). A septic temperature accompanies the reaction to the larvae, and the nose has a disagreeable fetid odor. Leukocytosis results from the accompanying secondary infection. Examination reveals marked swelling of the mucous membrane with obliteration of the cavity. The mucosa is fragile and bleeds easily. The worms are firmly attached and difficult to extract. The late stage of the infestation shows marked cartilaginous and bony destruction. Infestation with ascaris worms results in severe congestion and large amounts of mucopurulent discharge with absence of erosion of the cartilaginous and bony walls (Baluyot, 1973). The worms are easily recognized because of their size, measuring 6 to 10 inches.

Kecht (1969) reported a case of localized tetanus with facial paralysis, due to a wooden foreign body in the nasal cavity opposite the facial paralysis. Golding (1965) reported on an 18 month old child with a history of an unbearably foul odor emanating from his entire body for four weeks. No part of his body appeared to be free of the fetid odor. Bathing brought relief for only 15 minutes. His clothes had the same odor as his body. There was no evidence of illness otherwise, except for slight coryza. The child was found to have a piece of blanket in the right nasal cavity. One hour after removal of the foreign body the odor was gone. The odor did not recur. This was felt to be a case of bromidrosis or osmidrosis, which denotes a malodorous condition of human perspiration. Golding could find no other reports in the literature of a nasal foreign body being the cause of generalized bromidrosis. He did report that a colleague of his had a similar case, the etiology being a nasal foreign body.

DIAGNOSIS AND DIFFERENTIAL DIAGNOSIS

Diagnosis of the presence of an inanimate foreign body may be difficult. The first step is inspection of the nasal cavities with adequate illumination and a nasal speculum. An uncooperative child may require general anesthesia for proper examination. The diagnosis of a foreign body may be helped by vasoconstriction of the nasal mucosa with a nasal spray such as 1 per cent phenylephrine hydrochloride. Posterior rhinoscopy with a nasopharyngeal mirror is helpful in ruling out the presence of a foreign body in the nose far posteriorly. Radiographs may be of help in verifying the presence of a radiopaque foreign body (Fig. 34–3). Furthermore, sinus radiographs are useful in ruling out an ac-

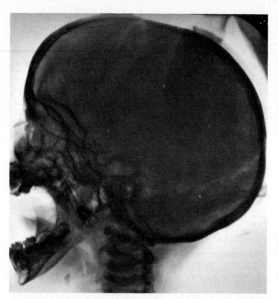

Figure 34–3 Lateral neck radiograph showing radiopaque foreign body (hair clip) in the nasopharynx of a two year old child. The presenting symptom had been bilateral nasal discharge. (From Children's Hospital of Pittsburgh.)

companying sinusitis. Radiopaque media studies are occasionally helpful with nonradiopaque foreign bodies. In any child with a nasal foreign body, both ear canals should be thoroughly checked, as the child who puts a foreign body into the nose is also likely to put things into the ears.

The diagnosis of parasitic and larval infestation of the nose is by anterior rhinoscopy with adequate illumination and a nasal speculum, as well as by posterior rhinoscopy with a nasopharyngeal mirror. The diagnosis of fungal infection is established by culture and microscopic demonstration of the hyphae and spores. However, *Rhinosporidium seeberi* cannot be cultured (Hunter et al., 1976).

In the differential diagnosis, such things as unilateral choanal atresia, polyps, sinusitis, and tumors should be considered. The radiologic differential diagnosis of a rhinolith includes calcified polyp, opaque foreign body of similar density (teeth or bone), osteoma, odontoma, and sequestration following local osteomyelitis (Harrison and Lamming, 1969).

MANAGEMENT

Stool and McConnel (1973) stated that "Any attempt at removal of a foreign body which does not succeed will make a bad situation worse. The child is usually apprehensive and the parents are aggravated. The physician, therefore, should be wary of falling into the trap of trying to do a removal without adequate instruments or good control of the patient." They also pointed out that removal of a foreign body is rarely an emergency. Time should be taken to obtain the proper instruments and illumination. If necessary, sedation or anesthesia can be provided.

The first step in attempting to remove a nasal foreign body without sedation or general anesthesia is to fully explain the situation and the procedure to the parents and the child. Adequate restraint is necessary in most young children. One very good method of restraint is for the child to sit on the parent's lap with the parent's arms around the child's arms and body. An assistant stabilizes the head. In the absence of an assistant, the parent can use one arm to hold the child's body and the other arm to stabilize the head by holding the forehead. The legs can be stabilized by an assistant or can be held between the parent's legs. Another method of restraint is to have the child lying on the back, immobilized by wrapping in a sheet or with a commercial restraint apparatus such as a Papoose Board.* An assistant is still required for stabilization of the head.

Adequate illumination should be provided with a head mirror or headlight. The use of

*Olympic Medical Corp., 4400 Seventh South, Seattle, Washington.

the headlight by the pediatrician allows both hands to be free. A nasal speculum should be used for visualization of the nasal cavity. Most objects can be grasped with a Hartman forceps (Fig. 34–4A). Another useful instrument is the alligator forceps. Some objects are best removed by passing a wire loop or a right-angled hook behind them before withdrawing (Fig. 34–4B). If necessary a topical nasal vasoconstrictor, such as 1 per cent phenylephrine hydrochloride, can be used prior to removing the foreign body. Topical anesthesia, such as with 4 per cent lidocaine hydrochloride or dilute cocaine, may also be of help.

Many techniques of foreign body removal have been described. Irvine (1973) recommended the use of a small curved oval ring. McMaster (1970) recommended the use of a fine wire loop ear curette. He bent the wire loop into an arc to form a shallow scoop. After using a topical vasoconstrictor, and a topical anesthetic if necessary, he passed the wire loop alongside the foreign body, following the curve of the scoop. Virnig (1972) recommended the use of a Fogarty biliary catheter for removal of foreign bodies. The catheter is passed along the floor of the nose, and the balloon is inflated when beyond the foreign body. The catheter and the foreign body are then withdrawn. Henry and Chamberlain (1972) recommended the use of a Foley catheter after spraying the nasal cavity with cocaine and epinephrine. They used a number 8 Foley catheter, passed into the nasopharynx along the inferior turbinate,

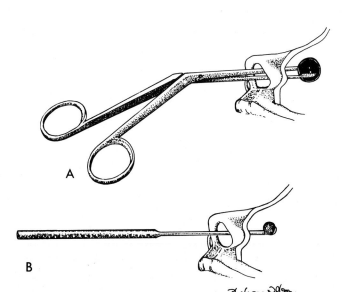

Figure 34–4 Removal of foreign body. A, Object grasped with a Hartman forceps. B, Wire loop passed behind foreign body prior to withdrawing.

passing beneath the foreign body. The balloon was inflated with 2 to 3 ml of saline, and the object was then removed as the catheter was withdrawn. Stool and McConnel (1973) reported on a method that does not require instrumentation. The child is placed in the supine position after the application of a nasal vasoconstrictor. The child's uninvolved nasal cavity is compressed with a finger, and the physician's mouth is placed over the child's as in applying mouth-to-mouth resuscitation. A sudden, strong blast of air is used to force the foreign body out through the anterior naris. Edmunds (1971) recommended spraying the involved nasal cavity with a vasoconstrictor and then immobilizing the child. A blower was then applied to the unobstructed naris. He timed the short, quick application of air blown into the unobstructed side with one of the child's cries. Messervy (1973) recommended that the child be placed in a sitting position, leaning slightly forward. The physician occludes the opening of the free nostril with a finger and the child takes a deep breath through the mouth and exhales forcibly through the nose. He recommended that this be tried at least 15 times before giving up. He also recommended that for children unwilling or unable to play this "game," sneezing while occluding the free nostril can be tried instead, pepper being utilized to initiate the reflex.

Stool and McConnel (1973) pointed out that pushing the object posteriorly into the nasopharynx should be avoided because of the possibility of the foreign body entering the trachea or esophagus. Occasionally general anesthesia is required for the removal of an inanimate foreign body, especially with an uncooperative child or with an impacted foreign body. Lowering the head during the procedure helps to prevent the foreign body from entering the larynx, trachea, or esophagus. An endotracheal tube is helpful. Lateral rhinotomy is occasionally necessary for the removal of severely impacted foreign bodies.

The treatment of rhinoliths consists of removal. If the rhinolith is too large to be removed in one piece, it can be broken with a strong forceps and removed in small pieces. If removal of the rhinolith requires displacing it posteriorly and recovering it from the nasopharynx, this should be done under a general anesthesia with the head lowered. Occasionally lateral rhinotomy is required for a massive rhinolith.

Hunter et al. (1976) recommended that larvae in the nose be anesthetized by applying benzol, ether, or chloroform, either on a cotton pledget or with an atomizer. An alternative method recommended by the same authors is irrigation with 20 per cent chloroform in sweet milk or 15 per cent chloroform in light mineral or vegetable oil. Following anesthesia of the larvae, they are removed with forceps and by having the patient blow the nose. If the patient is under general anesthesia, the larvae are removed by forceps or suction.

Ascaris worms are removed by forceps extraction. They need not be killed prior to removal. The intestinal infestation, however, must also be treated to prevent recurrence in the nose.

Rhinosporidium seeberi infestation is treated by surgical removal of the infected areas. Oral treatment with diaminodiphenylsulfone (DDS, dapsone) has recently been found to be effective in controlling nasal and nasopharyngeal rhinosporidiosis (Nair, 1979). Treatment of Aspergillus in the nose consists of thorough removal of all the fungus (Smith, 1968).

CONCLUSION

As a child may not admit to placing a foreign body in the nose, the physician must be alert to suspect a foreign body in the presence of a persistent unilateral nasal discharge, especially when the discharge is odorous, mucopurulent, or sanguineous. The removal of the foreign body should be done in a carefully planned manner with all appropriate instruments and illumination available. Precautions should be taken to prevent the foreign body from entering the larynx, trachea, or esophagus. General anesthesia should be utilized if necessary, rather than repeated, traumatic, unsuccessful attempts at removal in the uncooperative child. The ear canals should be checked for foreign bodies, as the child who is prone to placing things into the nose may very well have one in the ear canal as well.

SELECTED REFERENCES

Harrison, B. B., and Lamming, R. L. 1969. Case reports. Exogenous nasal rhinolith. Br. J. Radiol., *42*:838–840.

This article reviews the problem of rhinoliths in general and in particular has some detail concerning the radiologic aspects of rhinoliths.

Stool, S. E., and McConnel, C. S., Jr. 1973. Foreign bodies in pediatric otolaryngology. Some diagnostic and therapeutic pointers. Clin. Pediatr. (Phila.), *12*:113–116.
This article describes a practical approach to the diagnosis and management of foreign bodies in the ear, nose, and throat.

REFERENCES

Alavi, K. 1969. Epistaxis and hemoptysis due to Hirudo medicinalis (medical leech). Arch. Otolaryngol., *90*:178–179.

Awty, M. D. 1972. Removal of a large shell fragment from the nasopharynx. Oral Surg., *33*:513–519.

Baluyot, S. T., Jr. 1973. Foreign bodies in the nasal cavity. *In* Paparella, M. M., and Shumrick, D. A. (Eds.) Otolaryngology. Philadelphia, W. B. Saunders Co., pp. 62–68.

Bicknell, P. G. 1970. Rhinolith perforating the hard palate. J. Laryngol. Otol., *84*:1161–1162.

Brown, E. H. 1945. Screwworm infestation in the nasal passages and paranasal sinuses. Laryngoscope, *55*:371–374.

Carder, H. M., and Hill, J. J. 1966. Asymptomatic rhinolith: A brief review of the literature and case report. Laryngoscope, *76*:524–530.

Dayal, D., and Singh, A. P. 1970. Foreign body nasopharynx. J. Laryngol. Otol., *84*:1157–1160.

Edmunds, P. K. 1971. Removal of nasal foreign body. J.A.M.A., *217*:212.

Golding, I. M. 1965. An unusual cause of bromidrosis. Pediatrics, *36*:791–792.

Harrison, B. B., and Lamming, R. L. 1969. Case reports. Exogenous nasal rhinolith. Br. J. Radiol., *42*:838–840.

Henry, L. N., and Chamberlain, J. W. 1972. Removal of foreign bodies from esophagus and nose with the use of a Foley catheter. Surgery, *71*:918–921.

Hunter, G. W., Swartzwelder, J. C., and Clyde, D. F. 1976. Tropical Medicine, 5th ed. Philadelphia, W. B. Saunders Co.

Irvine, G. C. 1973. Foreign bodies in the ear and nose. A method of removal. East Afr. Med. J., *50*:116–117.

Kecht, B. 1969. Tetanus facialis durch Nasenfremdkörper. Monatsschr Ohrenheilkd Laryngorhinol., *103*:204–209.

Malhotra, C., Arora, M. M. L., and Mehra, Y. N. 1970. An unusual foreign body in the nose. J. Laryngol. Otol., *84*:539–540.

Marrone, M. P., Goodwin, M., and Genovese, M. 1968. A unique foreign body in the nose. Case report. Ann. Dent., *27*:156–158.

McAndrew, P. G. 1976. The lost tooth. J. Dent., *4*:144–146.

McMaster, W. C. 1970. Removal of foreign body from the nose. J.A.M.A., *213*:1905.

Messervy, M. 1973. Forced expiration in treatment of nasal foreign bodies. Practitioner, *210*:242.

Nair, K. K. 1979. Clinical trial of diaminodiphenyl-sulfone (DDS) in nasal and nasopharyngeal rhino-sporidiosis. Laryngoscope, *89*:291–295.

Nazif, M. 1971. A rubber dam clamp in the nasal cavity: report of case. J. Am. Dent. Assoc., *82*:1099–1100.

Smith, A. B. 1968. Epistaxis, foreign bodies, and parasites. *In* Stewart, J. P. (Ed.) Logan Turner's Diseases of the Nose, Throat and Ear, 7th ed. Bristol, John Wright & Sons, Ltd., pp. 60–62.

Stool, S. E., and McConnel, C. S., Jr. 1973. Foreign bodies in pediatric otolaryngology. Some diagnostic and therapeutic pointers. Clin. Pediatr. (Phila.), *12*:113–116.

Tolhurst, D. E. 1974. The ubiquitous foreign body. Cleft Palate J., *11*:237–239.

Utrata, J. 1977. Erosion of the soft palate by a foreign body in the nose. Ear Nose Throat J., *56*:403–404.

Virnig, R. P. 1972. Nontraumatic removal of foreign bodies from the nose and ears of infants and children. Minn. Med., *55*:1123.

Wood, G. L., and Case, J. H. 1973. A nasal splinter of dental origin. Dent. Surv., *49*:87–88.

Chapter 35

INJURIES OF THE NOSE, FACIAL BONES, AND PARANASAL SINUSES

Frank I. Marlowe, M.D.

GENERAL CONSIDERATIONS

Since entire textbooks have been written on the subject of facial injuries, it becomes obvious that the material to be presented in this chapter cannot be exhaustive or all-inclusive, but an attempt will be made to deal particularly with those aspects of each problem most peculiar to these injuries in children. In so doing, those basic principles that are of importance in children, as well as in adults, will be emphasized.

Children's exuberance, lack of fine physical control, and desire to explore their environments make them more susceptible to injuries involving the facial structures, especially during the early years. Offsetting this tendency to facial injury are the relative elasticity of the young child's facial bones and the somewhat lesser chance of exposure to the common causes of fractures in adults, such as high-velocity impacts and violent assault. In general, children suffer a surprisingly low incidence of severe facial fractures (Hall, 1972).

Despite the infrequency of facial fractures in children, the problem should not be construed as one of little magnitude. Of every ten deaths in children, four are the result of accidents; the highest incidence of these trauma-related deaths is in children between the ages of two and three years. In addition to these fatalities, 50,000 children are permanently crippled, and 2 million are temporarily incapacitated each year as a result of trauma.

Evaluation and treatment of the injured child present special challenges, and it cannot be reiterated too often that the child is not a small adult, but differs greatly from adults in terms of the type of injury sustained and his or her general physiologic response to the injury.

Attention to the ABCs of care of the adult trauma patient—airway, bleeding and shock, and cerebral and spinal cord injuries—is even more critical in caring for children who suffer trauma (Schultz, 1970).

Airway

The smaller anatomic dimensions and different tissue make-up of the child's airway predisposes the child to obstruction with very little mucosal edema or hematoma. These potential problems must thus be recognized early and managed rapidly. Blood, vomitus, or foreign bodies can fully or partially obstruct the airway, and in many cases these obstructions can be cleared quickly by sweeping a finger deep into the mouth and pharynx. Airway problems stemming from uncontrolled facial bleeding or grossly displaced facial tissues can often be alleviated rapidly and simply by moving the child to an upright position. Fractures of the mandible with severe posterior displacement may allow the tongue to drop posteriorly and occlude the airway. In such cases, the tongue may be pulled forward and sutured in this position, or an appropriate nasopharyngeal tube may be placed to maintain the airway. In all but very unusual and exceptional instances, immediate management of upper airway obstruction is most effectively handled by some form of intubation rather than by tracheostomy. Intubation is more rapidly accomplished, and usually personnel skilled in its use are more apt to be immediately available at the appropriate time. If the nature of the obstruction is temporary, endotracheal intubation may preclude the necessity for tracheostomy entirely. Even if the obstruction will probably require a long time to manage adequately, intermediate intubation will allow the physician time to perform the tracheostomy later under controlled conditions with good light, suction, and control of the patient's airway, making it a much safer procedure.

Since manipulation of the neck during intubation or tracheostomy may produce permanent neurologic damage, the possibility of a coexistent cervical spine injury must be kept in mind in the patient with airway obstruction.

Bleeding

The next important consideration is control of bleeding, which usually can be checked without too great difficulty in facial wounds by direct pressure. It must be borne in mind, however, that blood loss in cases of pediatric trauma is a critical factor, since the child has a much smaller circulating blood volume, and shock may follow the loss of as little as 100 to 200 cc of blood. Any readily apparent arterial bleeding should be clamped and ligated directly through the wound.

Shock is rarely the result of facial injury alone, but many factors predispose a child suffering from apparently minor facial trauma to shock. The critical nature of blood loss has already been mentioned. In addition, loss of body heat is an important consideration, as the child's relatively greater ratio of body surface to body volume makes him or her more prone to heat loss and to the development of hypothermia. Also, the child's ability to maintain homeostasis is much more endangered than the adult's by changes in blood volume, fluid volume, and blood pH. Because of this, children become ill faster than do adults, and there is much less time in which to recognize and treat these threats to homeostasis before they cause death.

The treatment for shock is dependent upon reestablishing an appropriate intravascular fluid volume (which may be done with crystalloids or blood products), controlling pain, conserving body heat, and controlling the patient's apprehension.

Central Nervous System

Once a clear airway has been assured and hemorrhage and shock have been controlled, consideration is given to the possible presence of associated injuries before definitive treatment of the facial trauma is undertaken. It has been said that patients do not die from facial injuries, but patients with facial injuries do die from associated injuries.

Injury to the central nervous system in instances of significant facial trauma is not uncommon; central nervous system injury may be intracranial or may involve an injury to the spinal cord. A careful evaluation of the child's level of consciousness, vital signs, and pupillary reactions is necessary to detect an intracranial injury, such as concussion, contusion, or hemorrhage. Nausea, vomiting, headache, or cerebrospinal fluid leakage from the nose or ear are also signs of cervical involvement. Localized pain or tenderness over the cervical spine, any alterations of mobility of the limbs, or changes in sensation in the limbs should also alert the physician to the possibility of an injury to the cervical spine. These symptoms and signs are particularly important to remember when manipulating the head and neck for placement of an endotracheal tube.

Radiographs of the cervical spine should be obtained, as should skull radiographs, in all instances of significant head trauma. If a neck injury is suspected, the head should be immobilized until radiographic evaluation can be carried out.

Attention may be drawn to thoracic injuries by the presence of pain, shortness of breath, or the presence of an obvious lag on one side of the chest, which may herald a pneumothorax. Localized tenderness or ecchymoses over the thoracic cage may indicate underlying rib fracture, a possible etiologic factor in pneumothorax.

Localized pain, tenderness, or obvious distention may call attention to an intra-abdominal injury. Changes in bowel sounds or the presence of "rebound" or of free blood in the abdominal cavity may also be noted in cases of severe abdominal injury.

Pain, swelling, or obvious deformity of any

of the extremities or joint areas is presumptive evidence of a musculoskeletal injury, and precautions must be taken so as not to aggravate the injury further.

Immediate consultation with the appropriate specialist, should any of the above findings be noted, is necessary to avoid serious consequences. Generally, the possible need for a thoracotomy or laparotomy takes priority over definitive care of the facial injury. In addition, evaluations of special organs, such as the eye and ear, must be made prior to institution of definitive care of a facial injury. For instance, a hematoma overlying the mastoid process, a hemotympanum, or frank bleeding or loss of cerebrospinal fluid from the ear canal indicate a basilar skull fracture. Although injuries to the eye may often seem "trivial" and swelling and discoloration of the eyelids, as well as subconjunctival hemorrhage, are commonly seen in association with other facial fractures, the possibility of ocular trauma must be borne in mind if disastrous results are to be avoided. Direct injury to the globe with leakage of fluid and possible iris prolapse is generally quite obvious, and the need for immediate ophthalmologic consultation is readily apparent. In some instances, however, the eye may appear to be normal, but a detached retina or hemorrhage into the vitreous may have occurred. In addition, a small intraocular foreign body may easily escape detection, even upon relatively close examination of the eyes. Assessment of visual acuity, even grossly, in each eye in turn, is absolutely essential.

Once the patient's general status is determined to be satisfactory and stable and the absence of any serious associated injury has been determined, evaluation of the facial injury may be undertaken.

Maxillofacial trauma in children differs from that seen in the adult in many ways. Good historical information is often more difficult to obtain in the child, and clinical and radiologic examinations are certainly more difficult, to the point where anesthesia may have to be utilized to allow adequate evaluation. In addition, the small size and poorly developed pneumatization of the sinus cavities make interpretation of radiographic studies more difficult, and false negative findings are not uncommon. Intracranial and cervical spine injuries appear to accompany maxillofacial trauma in children more frequently than they do in adults. This has been attributed in part to the fact that it takes a greater force to break the more elastic and stable bones of the child than it does to break an adult's bones. Thus, if the force is sufficient to break the bones of the face, it is usually sufficient to damage the child's central nervous system as well. These same developmental factors, plus the presence of unerupted teeth or mixed dentition in the mandible of the child, make internal fixation or fixation by interdental means more difficult. This problem is further compounded by the need for stabilization at an earlier time owing to the rapid healing of the facial bones in the child. Finally, unwarranted surgical treatment of the child may alter growth patterns and may lead to greater long-term functional losses and deformities than in the adult (Yarrington, 1977).

SOFT TISSUE INJURIES

The importance of early and proper wound care cannot be overemphasized, as it may eliminate totally or certainly minimize the need for future scar revision (McGregor, 1969).

Certain types of wounds deserve special consideration on the basis of the inflicting agent. For example, the treatment of dog bites is controversial. In general, if cleansing has been thorough these may be closed primarily within eight hours of the bite. Of course, proper attention must be given to tetanus and rabies preventive measures. Electrical burns usually involve the lips and oral tissues, and the extent of injury to the tissues is often difficult to evaluate. For this reason, one mode of acceptable treatment has been to allow spontaneous demarcation between living and dead tissue to occur with spontaneous separation of the necrotic tissue. The defect is than allowed to heal for 6 to 12 months before reconstruction is begun. One alternative is immediate excision of damaged tissues and reconstruction; another is using mucosal flaps to cover the injured tissues, possibly minimizing the tissue loss, with healing for 6 to 12 months followed by reconstruction as necessary.

Contusions of the soft tissues almost invariably heal spontaneously without a need for any more active treatment than cleansing and observation. A hematoma may accompany a contusion, but if the former is small it usually will resorb spontaneously without treatment.

On occasion, however, a hematoma may become encapsulated, producing a subcutaneous scar with a visible deformity. If this appears to be likely, the hematoma may be evacuated by incision when in the "gel" state, or by aspiration when liquefaction has occurred.

Abrasions require meticulous cleansing of the wound, which may necessitate anesthetizing the child in some way. All debris or foreign material must be removed by irrigation, mechanical debridement (sponge, brush, scalpel, dermabrader), or excision to preclude permanent "tatooing," which is difficult to treat secondarily (Fig. 35–1). Solvents, such as ether, may be necessary for the removal of oily or greasy, tarlike substances. Use of a nonadherent dressing allows good healing to take place.

With deeper wounds, such as lacerations and avulsions, in the absence of infection and with accurate approximation of the skin, healing of the epidermal wound occurs quite rapidly. Healing in the dermis takes considerably longer and may be more important from the standpoint of the ultimate appearance of the wound. The progression from a fibrin clot to a quiescent, avascular scar may take several months to several years, and clinically consists of a gradual change from a red, sometimes elevated scar with a surrounding area of induration to a pale, sometimes flat, soft scar. In unusual instances, this orderly progression is disrupted by the appearance of overabundant fibrous tissue in the dermis, which results clinically in a hypertrophic scar or keloid. The aphorism that "children heal well" may be entirely true, but a corollary is that the progression through the various phases of healing may be quite prolonged, and the likelihood of development of a hypertrophic scar and subsequent enlargement of this scar with future growth and development is greater. Wounds in the child can often retain signs of redness and elevation for several years after the initial wounding. Therefore, the physician must be particularly careful to avoid excessive skin tension in wound closure in children. Similarly, the surgeon must give more consideration to techniques such as Z-plasty that will reorder the lines of tension on the wound repair. In some instances, it is necessary to consider the effect of an extensive scar upon the future growth of the child. At times, the presence of a dense band of scar tissue over a growing bony prominence may acutally produce limitation of bone growth in that area. The factors of concern in wound care are (1 placement of the scar, (2) preparation of the wound, (3) stitch craft, and (4) postoperative care.

Scar Placement

In traumatic injuries, the scar has already been placed at the time of the wounding; however, an intimate knowledge of the tissue tension lines of the face, variously referred to as "relaxed skin tension lines" (RSTL), "lines of election," or erroneously as "Langer's lines," is still of great importance. This knowledge allows the surgeon to predict the quality of the ultimate healing and to choose the best incision for initial or later rearrangements of the wound or surrounding tissues. Scars placed in a "wrinkle line" or parallel to it tend to heal well, as do those placed in a line of election in nonwrinkled areas. Scars may also be "hidden" by placement in hair-bearing tissues, such as the scalp or eyebrow, or behind the ear in the postauricular sulcus. In addition, scars placed at natural junction zones of various facial features, such as the nasofacial sulcus or the nasolabial crease, tend to be less conspicuous to the casual observer.

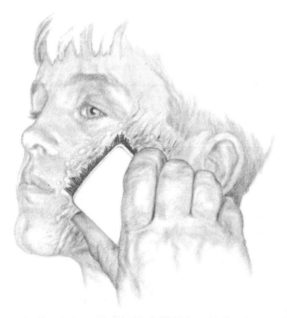

Figure 35–1   Accidental tattoo. (From Grabb, W. C., Kleinert, H. E., and Puckett, C. L. 1976. Technics in Surgery: Facial and Hand Injuries. Somerville, N.J., Ethicon, Inc.)

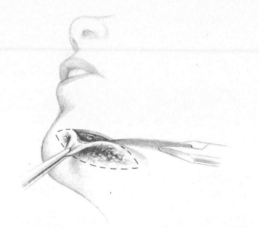

Figure 35–2   Trimming skin wounds with irregular edges. (From Grabb, W. C., Kleinert, H. E., and Puckett, C. L. 1976. Technics in Surgery: Facial and Hand Injuries. Somerville, N.J., Ethicon, Inc.)

Wound Preparation

Initial care of the wound is directed toward meticulous cleansing, as has been outlined in the care of abrasions. The excellent blood supply of the face allows excision of "damaged" tissue in the wound to be extremely conservative, and only obviously nonvital tissue should be sacrificed. This same excellent blood supply minimizes the problem of infection and allows primary closure of many facial wounds several hours after the injury. In the case of a clean wound, with little or no traumatized tissue, primary closure, or excision of the wound edges followed by primary closure, may be used, and the final result will be quite satisfactory (Fig. 35–2). In more extensive wounds, the more conservative approach dictates only thorough cleansing and removal of obviously nonviable tissue with salvage of all remaining tissue, which is replaced in its normal position and sutured. Since in extensive wounds it is seldom possible to achieve final reconstruction at the time of the primary treatment, the aim is to preserve as much tissue as possible for use in subsequent reconstruction. Irregular wounds are usually effectively closed by first approximating normal landmarks (eyebrow, eyelid, vermilion of the lip), distinctive portions of the wound itself that "mate" or "fit," or both landmarks and wound portions (Fig. 35–3). Where tissue has been lost, as in avulsion injuries, suturing of mucosa to skin or use of split skin grafts may be necessary.

The wound edges must be vertical, and the faces of these edges should be of the same thickness for the best scar. This usually requires undercutting or undermining of the skin edges. In wounds being sutured without tension, 3 to 5 mm of undermining will suffice to allow the proper amount of (slight) eversion of the wound edges. Where tension is a problem, undermining must be more extensive to allow for advancement of the skin to relieve the tension. The plane of undermining in the face is just deep to the dermis to avoid injury to the branches of the facial nerve, but this may be altered somewhat in the scalp and neck.

Finally, it is good to consider what is beneath the wound before embarking on closure. A beautifully executed wound closure over a nonrepaired transection of the parotid duct or a facial nerve branch is hardly a tribute to the surgeon's skills. In the same vein, it hardly seems worthwhile to use great care to close a soft tissue wound over multiple, severe bony injuries without first considering what subsequent treatment may be required: often the reduction and fixation of the bony injuries may best be done through the original wound, while at other times the manipulation of the bones takes place at just about the time of suture removal, and the wound is disrupted by traction and must be closed secondarily. If either of these situations appears likely to occur, it is often advisable to approximate the wound loosely with tape strips rather than to perform a suture closure.

Stitch Craft

Suture materials should be selected on the basis of the particular properties of the material and the specific application intended. In general, braided silk is easy to tie, and the knots hold well, but it has relatively low tensile strength. Synthetics, such as nylon, dacron, and polyethylene, are available as monofilaments or braided. They have good tensile strength and cause little tissue reaction but do not "handle" like silk and require a more meticulous knot-tying technique and more knot "throws." Catgut is the standard absorbable suture and may be chromicized to reduce tissue reaction and retard the rate of resorption; it is primarily employed as a buried suture to obliterate dead space and

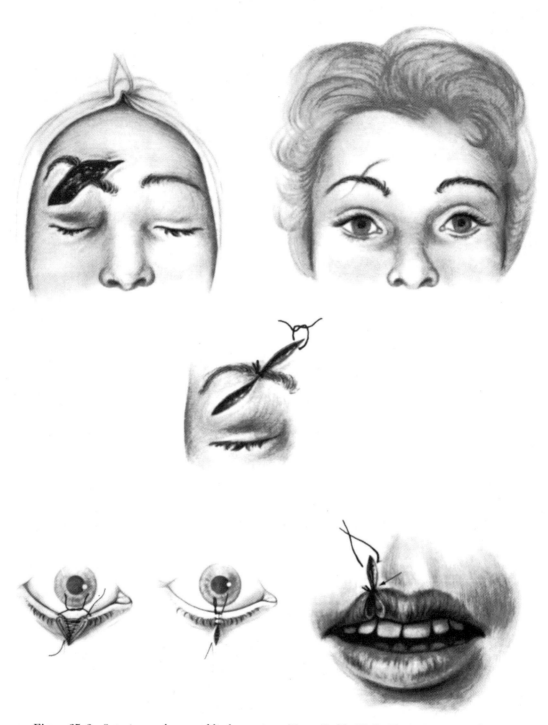

Figure 35-3 Suturing eyebrow and lip lacerations. (From Grabb, W. C., Kleinert, H. E., and Puckett, C. L. 1976. Technics in Surgery: Facial and Hand Injuries. Somerville, N.J., Ethicon, Inc.)

thus to help to prevent hematoma. Some of the newer synthetics, such as the polyglycolic acid derivatives, Dexon and Vicryl, combine the absorbable properties of catgut with the tissue tolerance qualities of the synthetic fibers.

Instruments should be selected carefully to minimize tissue trauma. Skin hooks and needle holders must be fine, tissue forceps atraumatic, and scissors sharp. Atraumatic needles with swaged-on sutures are generally best for plastic repairs.

Suture techniques vary widely and must be tailored to coaptation of the specific wound. Interrupted sutures provide accurate approximation with minimal chances of tissue strangulation. Continuous sutures are speedy to place and provide good hemostasis along the wound edge when interlocked. It should be remembered that the best scars result with the least tension on each suture; thus, for any given wound the more sutures that are made the less the tension on each suture. However, this concept must be balanced against the risk of tissue strangulation (Fig. 35–4).

Hematoma is the absolute nemesis of good wound healing as it (1) creates tension on the wound, (2) is a good culture medium for infecting organisms, and (3) contributes to failure of flaps and grafts by interfering with neovascularization. Careful suturing to obliterate dead space and the appropriate use of drains or suction will minimize this problem.

Postoperative Care

The aim of proper postoperative care is to preserve the status of the repair in such a manner as to insure optimal healing. This includes immobilization of the wound for healing, prevention of hematoma, and prevention of suture marks, and requires careful dressing, with pressure if appropriate, care in suture removal, and continued wound support.

Suture removal is a particularly significant consideration in children. When appropriate, the surgeon should select the subcuticular

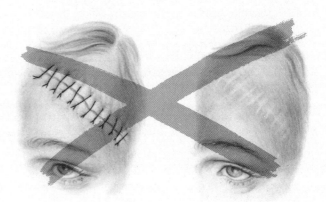

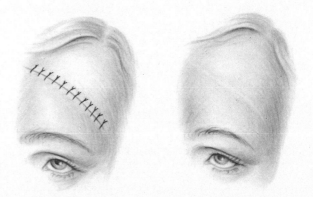

Figure 35–4 Preventing skin suture scars. (From Grabb, W. C., Kleinert, H. E., and Puckett, C. L. 1976. Technics in Surgery: Facial and Hand Injuries. Somerville, N.J., Ethicon, Inc.)

closure method or place adhesive paper strips over the wound closure.

Scar Revision

While it is often difficult to resist the demands of a concerned patient and anxious parents for immediate revisional surgery, such surgery is usually ill-advised before a year or longer has elapsed. This may be modified based on the appearance of the wound and estimates of its maturity (Chap. 30A).

Some scars may be highly visible because of differences in color or level from surrounding tissues and in the regularity of pattern of the scar, which tends to lead the eye along the entire length of the scar. Small discrepancies in level are often more significant than they might initially appear to be owing to the shadowing effect of light falling on the skin surface. While little can be done surgically to alter color differences, many procedures can be employed to minimize level differences.

Scar revision may take the form of local revision, limited to the scar itself, or revision requiring rearrangments of adjacent tissues. One local revision might be simple excision and resuturing of a scar that was the result of a technically poor primary closure. This may be done repeatedly, as in serial excision for burn scars or to replace split-skin grafts. Epithelial shaving for larger elevations and dermabrasion for smaller elevations may be used to correct disparities in level within a scar or between a scar and the surrounding

tissue. Running W-plasties and geometric broken-line closures are both attempts to fool the eye by changing the linear scar to an irregular or random scar, which is more difficult to follow and thus less noticeable.

Revisions involving adjacent tissue rearrangements include basic advancement, rotation, and transposition flaps, and variations of these flaps, such as the frequently mentioned but less frequently understood Z-plasty and the rhomboid flap. A detailed discussion of the construction and mechanics of transfer of these regional flaps is beyond the scope of this chapter, but some general remarks regarding their applicability is appropriate.

Z-plasty may be used for breaking a long, straight scar line; for lengthening a scar, such as to relieve a contracture or to revise a linear scar crossing a hollow (bridle deformity); or in a curvilinear scar that has produced a trap-door deformity (Fig. 35–5). In addition, it may be used to correct abnormal positioning of facial features, such as the outer canthus or oral commissure. It must be borne in mind, however, that the gains in length obtained by performing a Z-plasty are at the expense of losses in width and that the transpositions may result in tension changes in the surrounding tissues, which lead to areas of bunching and hollowing. The advantages of the revision must be balanced against these undesirable possibilities.

Rhomboid flaps are versatile variations of the transposition flap in which the transposition of the flap actually closes the donor defect. These flaps can also be modified or

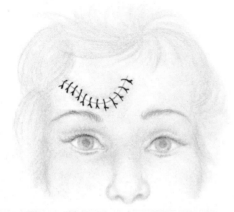
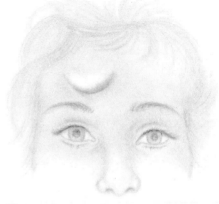

Figure 35–5 Trap-door deformity. (From Grabb, W. C., Kleinert, H. E., and Puckett, C. L. 1976. Technics in Surgery: Facial and Hand Injuries. Somerville, N.J., Ethicon, Inc.)

used in series to close larger defects, as in the flaps of Limberg and Dufourmentel (Fee, 1976).

Another useful variant of the transposition flap is the bilobed or Zimany flap, which is in essence a double transposition in a single step. This flap is used when the initial donor site does not lend itself to easy primary closure, so a further transposition is used to obliterate this site, and the second donor site is then repaired primarily (Tardy, 1972).

In the use of these and all other local or regional flaps, it is good to bear in mind that the closer the donor site is to the recipient site, the better will be the match as regards skin color and texture of the ultimate repair. This is also true of free grafts, with full or with partial thickness skin.

In spite of all the aforementioned recommendations, it must be realized that there is great, uncontrollable individual variation in healing characteristics, and this sets a limit to what can be achieved by pure surgical technique. It is impossible always to get a perfect scar, but to produce the best result in a given set of circumstances meticulous technique is essential, and failure in a single element is enough to give a poor result, however careful the attention may be to all other aspects of the repair.

EVALUATION OF FACIAL INJURY

The extent of facial injury may be assessed by three techniques: observation, palpation, and radiographic examination (Converse and Dingman, 1977).

Observation

Careful observation of all facial surfaces for indications of soft-tissue injury is the starting point. Any erythema or ecchymosis should be carefully noted. Any apparent facial asymmetry, either at rest or with movement of the face, should be noted carefully. It should be remembered that many people have some small degree of facial asymmetry on a developmental basis, so that the findings of the physical examination must be correlated with the patient's history. The eyelids should be opened to check for associated ocular injury, and examination of the muco-

sal surfaces of the oral cavity and pharynx must not be neglected.

Palpation

Palpation of the bony prominences of the face is next carried out, and this examination may be hampered somewhat by hematoma or edema, depending on the length of time that has elapsed since the injury. Tenderness at any site may indicate an underlying facial bone fracture, and comparison of the relative heights of the malar eminences (zygoma) is helpful in determining whether or not a fracture of the midfacial bones has occurred. A systematic and orderly palpation of the facial skeleton, even in the absence of obvious injury, may detect subtle deformities. A suggested plan of organization and the observations to be made as attention is focused on each of these areas appears in Table 35–1.

Radiographic Examination

Although radiographic examination of the facial bones is an important part of the overall evaluation of the facial injury, it cannot be relied upon exclusively. Often, gross facial bone displacements will not be readily apparent on radiographs and at other times apparent displacements of facial bones noted on radiography are not confirmed by clinical evaluation. The most informative radiographic views of the face are (1) Waters (occipitomental) views, (2) posteroanterior view, (3) lateral view, (4) lateral view of the nasal bones, (5) occlusive view of the nasal bones, (6) posteroanterior view of the mandible, (7) oblique view of the mandible, (8) occlusive view of the mandible, (9) Townes view (for ascending mandibular rami and condyles), and (10) tangential views of the zygomatic arch.

Additional and sometimes more precise information regarding a particular area may be obtained by the use of special radiographic techniques, including tomography, polytomography, and xeroradiography, which tend to give better delineation of the bony outlines. In addition, panoramic scanning radiographs are of particular value in visualizing fractures of the lower third of the face, including the lower portions of the maxilla and

Table 35–1 ORDERLY AND SYSTEMATIC EXAMINATION OF THE FACE

Areas to Examine:
Supraorbital and lateral orbital rims
Infraorbital rims
Malar eminences (zygoma)
Zygomatic arches
Nasal bones
Maxilla
Mandible
As attention is focused on each of these areas, certain observations should be noted.

Supraorbital and Lateral Orbital Rims
a) Bony depression or angulation
b) Tenderness
c) Eyebrow irregularity
d) Ocular proptosis or enophthalmos
e) Periorbital ecchymosis
f) Scleral ecchymosis
g) Swelling or ecchymosis of the upper eyelids
h) Limitation or lag in ocular movements
i) Diplopia (subjective)
j) Anesthesia of forehead
k) Muscular activity of forehead

Infraorbital Rims
a) Depression or angulation
b) Tenderness
c) Periorbital ecchymosis
d) Scleral ecchymosis
e) Limitation or lag in ocular movements
f) Diplopia in various directions of gaze (subjective)
g) Anesthesia of nasolabial fold and upper lip
h) Anesthesia of maxillary teeth

Malar Eminences
a) Comparison of height (unilateral depression)
b) Periorbital ecchymosis
c) Crepitus
d) Angulation

Zygomatic Arches
a) Depression or angulation
b) Periorbital ecchymosis
c) Tenderness
d) Limitation of mandibular excursion

Nasal Bones
a) Depression or angulation
b) Periorbital ecchymosis
c) Epistaxis
d) Tenderness
e) Crepitus
f) Loss of pyramidal support
g) Septal obstruction or deviation
h) Tenderness at base of columella

Maxilla
a) Dental malocclusion
b) Periorbital ecchymosis
c) Motion of maxilla
d) Asymmetry or collapse of dental arch form
e) Misplaced or damaged teeth
f) Tear of upper buccal sulcus or mucoperiosteum of palate

Mandible
a) Tenderness and pain (subjective)
b) Asymmetry of mandibular contour and lower lip
c) Asymmetry or collapse of dental arch
d) Dental malocclusion
e) Limitation of mandibular excursion
f) Abnormal motion
g) Misplaced or damaged teeth
h) Tear of lower buccal sulcus
i) Anesthesia of lower lip or teeth
j) Injury to tongue

(Reproduced with permission from Schultz, R. C. Facial Injuries, 2nd ed. Copyright 1977 by Year Book Medical Publishers, Inc., Chicago.)

the mandible. A further radiographic technique of value, often neglected, is the use of stereo views, particularly the stereo Waters view.

INJURIES OF SPECIFIC SITES

Nose

The primary difference between the child's nose and that of the adult, other than the obvious ones of size and configuration, consists of the proportionally smaller part of the nose of the child contributed by the bony nasal pyramid and the relatively greater elasticity of the bones and the immaturity of the suture lines. Because of these factors, injuries to the nasal bones of a child may not be as obvious as in an adult, and the overall elasticity and compliance of the structures may allow a significant cartilaginous injury with subsequent septal hematoma to coexist with unharmed bony structures. In addition, a relatively "minor" injury may result in arrested development and maturation of the nasal structures with a resultant infantile nasal configuration (Fig. 35–6). Soft tissue injuries of the nose are usually easily diagnosed by inspection, and repair, in the absence of tissue loss such as avulsion or amputation, is readily accomplished. Meticulous reapproximation of all tissue layers of the nose begins with the mucosa, including that of the nasal septum and turbinates. This is commonly accomplished with absorbable catgut sutures, and these may be placed to include the perichondrium and thus approximate the cartilagi-

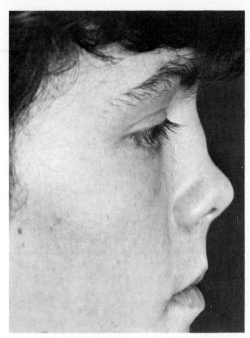

Figure 35–6 Saddle deformity resulting from injury to the nose. (Reproduced with permission from Schultz, R. C. Facial Injuries, 2nd ed. Copyright 1977 by Year Book Medical Publishers, Inc., Chicago.)

nous structures, such as the upper and lower lateral cartilages or the septal cartilage. Sutures may also be placed directly in the cartilage for accurate approximation as long as these are carefully placed to avoid strangulation or deformity of the cartilage. The superficial muscle tissues of the nose are generally adherent to the skin and they need not be repaired separately. Accurate approximation of the skin edges with appropriate regard to important anatomic features, such as the rim of the nasal ala, is the final stage in the soft tissue repair, although it is often advisable to splint the repair with an intranasal dressing of an appropriately lubricated packing material, such as adaptic gauze, and an external dressing of appropriate tape and a malleable or moldable splint.

In cases of tissue loss, avulsed segments of the lower nasal vault, if small, may be used as autografts and may be carefully sutured in place with a good chance of satisfactory survival. If the avulsed segments are not available, the use of composite grafts of skin and cartilage from the ear may be employed in the primary repair with a fair degree of success.

Cartilaginous and bony injuries to the nose are not diagnosed as easily as are soft tissue

injuries but are nonetheless important and may even occur in the newborn. A dislocated nasal septum as a result of trauma of delivery is readily reduced by gentle traction on the nose to effect realignment. Radiographs are generally of little value for demonstrating cartilaginous injuries, and in the case of children are often of little value in demonstrating bony injuries. This, coupled with the difficulties of satisfactorily examining the interior and exterior of the nasal structures in the child, contributes towards these injuries being considered "insignificant" and remaining untreated. Although displacement of these structures may not be great at the time of injury, gross deformity may result from continued growth and development of unaligned structures. For instance, hematomas of the septum must be evacuated immediately if a saddle deformity is to be prevented. This requires satisfactory incision and appropriate placement of dressings to prevent reaccumulation of blood, and this may require a general anesthetic. Infection of a hematoma, leading to a septal abscess, can cause rapid and disastrous loss of cartilage and requires immediate incision and drainage and vigorous antibiotic therapy. If the possibility of a septal hematoma or serious intranasal injury can be excluded, it is often better to wait several days to allow most of the edema and ecchymosis to resolve before attempting a definitive repair of the bony derangement. Bleeding from the nose of the child who has been struck suggests the presence of a fracture, and this is especially true if the bleeding is accompanied by edema and ecchymosis of the overlying tissues. Nasal bleeding may be the result of displaced nasal bones that have penetrated the nasal mucosa. In a recent study of nasal injury, seven signs suggestive of nasal fracture were noted to occur in this order of frequency: epistaxis, swelling of the nasal dorsum, ecchymosis of the eyes, tenderness of the nasal dorsum, radiographic evidence of fracture, nasal deformity, and crepitus of the nasal bones. This last finding is felt by some to be diagnostic of nasal fracture (Moran, 1977).

Immediate treatment of a nasal fracture is the same in children as in adults, and begins with control of any epistaxis, which usually ceases spontaneously. If epistaxis fails to stop spontaneously, the soft tissue portions of the nose may be grasped between the thumb and forefinger and pressure maintained for several minutes. Should no significant swelling

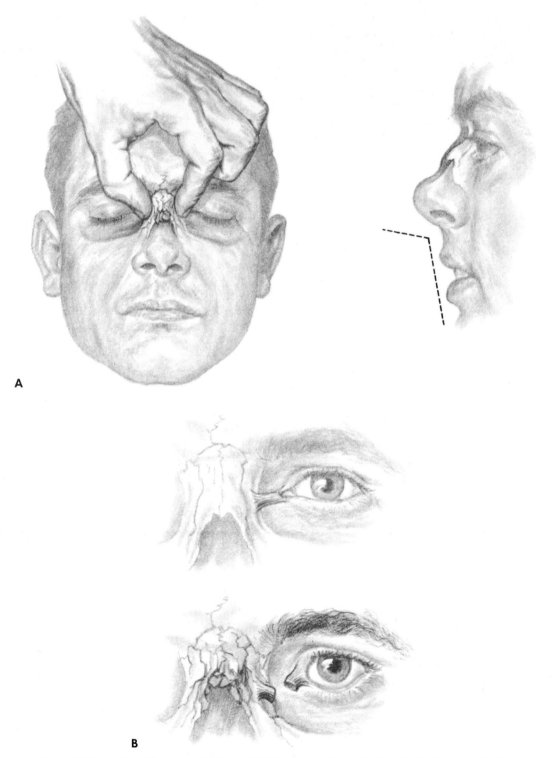

Figure 35–7   *A,* Nasal fractures. *B,* Naso-orbital fractures. (From Grabb, W. C., Kleinert, H. E., and Puckett, C. L. 1976. Technics in Surgery: Facial and Hand Injuries. Somerville, N.J., Ethicon, Inc.)

be noted at this point, evaluation of the external nose by inspection and palpation may be advisable. This applies also to examination of the intranasal structures, which requires satisfactory illumination, restraint, and vasoconstriction, along with a satisfactory source of suction. If there is doubt at this point as to the extent of the injury, one has the choice of carrying out further examination, including manipulation of the nasal cartilages and bones with appropriate instruments under general anesthesia, or of allowing time to pass in hopes that the tissue reaction will subside adequately enough to allow better clinical evaluation. It must be remembered, however, that the nasal tissues heal rapidly and that fixation with malposition may occur unless the fractures are properly reduced within a period of a few days.

Treatment of bony injuries in the young child revolves about satisfactory digital and instrument manipulation of the fractured fragments into appropriate positions, and then splinting to maintain the alignment. Comminuted nasal fractures are especially difficult to stabilize in children and may require splinting by means of external plates and fixation wires. Open reduction of nasal fractures in the young child is seldom justified although it may occasionally be helpful in treating older children.

It should be remembered that, in spite of apparently satisfactory reduction of nasal fractures and correction of cartilaginous or soft tissue injuries, there is no assurance that a deformity will not develop with progressive growth and development. The parents of these patients should be advised of the possible necessity for further treatment at some later date.

Some nasal fractures that require special consideration include the so-called "open-book" type of fracture, in which the fractured segments splay out to involve the frontal processes of the maxillae (Zaydon and Brown, 1964). This may be associated with fragmentation of the entire bony nasal bridge and its displacement into the ethmoid or frontal region (Fig. 35–7). These fractures of the nasofrontal and nasoethmoid regions may result in injuries to the nasofrontal ducts, the nasolacrimal apparatus, and the medial canthal ligaments with resultant later formation of a frontal mucocele, pseudohypertelorism and rounding of the medial canthus region, or epiphora and dacryocystitis. The treatment of these injuries is complex and largely surgical and may involve exploration of the frontal sinus or exploration of the medial portions of each orbit with direct wire fixation of the canthal ligaments to the repositioned bony structures of the lateral nasal wall and medial orbital wall (Weber and Cohn, 1977).

Midface

There are several special features to be considered in evaluating injuries to the midfacial region in the child (McCoy et al., 1966). In the very young, the size of the face relative to that of the cranial vault is quite small, so that injuries to this area are relatively infrequent. At approximately six years of age, the midfacial skeleton has achieved most of its ultimate growth, but there remain some anatomic differences between the midface skeleton of the six year old and that of an adult. The sinuses of the child are quite small and poorly pneumatized, and the bones are still quite resilient and tend to fracture in a greenstick manner. In addition, the mixed dentition of children is such that the decision to perform intermaxillary fixation must be considered carefully: at this age the roots of the deciduous teeth are gradually being resorbed, and there is frequent absence of teeth and a poor retentive shape to the crowns of some teeth. In addition, indiscriminate use of interdental wiring may damage the tooth buds and may result in losses or distortions of the permanent dentition.

Soft Tissue Injuries. These are particularly important in children, as injuries that damage a child's appearance inflict great damage on his or her self-esteem. This is a distinct possibility in the case of facial lacerations, and adequate attention must be paid to possible injuries to branches of the facial nerve. Proper management of such injuries must include careful preanesthetic evaluation of facial motion, and any injuries to a nerve must be repaired using microtechniques and the binocular operating microscope, possibly with the aid of a nerve stimulator, during the first 72 hours after injury if optimal results are to be obtained.

Soft tissue injuries to specific sites may require slightly different approaches (Bailey, 1977). Laceration of the cheek is probably the most commonly encountered soft tissue injury in children. While the superficial aspects of the repair are relatively simple, several structures deserve special consideration. Included among these are the branches of the facial nerve, the parotid gland and duct (Stensen duct), and the muscles of mastication and expression. A good guideline in the evaluation of these injuries is that those occupying an area posterior to a line dropped vertically from the lateral canthus and inferior to a line drawn from the external auditory canal to the nasal tip are most apt to involve significant injuries to the aforementioned structures (Fig. 35–8). Lacerations extending into the parotid gland may result in the development of a salivary fistula, which may be avoided by careful closure of the capsule of the gland and a meticulous, layered closure of the overlying soft tissue.

Injury to the parotid duct should be suspected when clear fluid is seen leaking from the wound surface. Patency of the duct is essential and may be obtained by suture closure over a fine polyethylene catheter. An alternative treatment is fistulization of the glandular segment of the duct into the oral cavity at some point other than the normal orifice. In very unusual circumstances, such as when extensive damage to the duct has occurred or it has been lost at its insertion into the gland, the identifiable portion may be ligated to produce atrophy of the gland. Injuries to facial nerve branches anterior to the region of the parotid duct do not usually result in significant loss of muscle function

because the superficial facial muscles are innervated in their posterior portions, and, therefore, repair of these small anterior branches, which have multiple anastomoses in most cases, is unnecessary. Clean divisions of the identifiable nerve branches require careful approximation of the nerve sheaths, with fine sutures and with the aid of magnification and appropriate microinstruments. In cases in which a significant portion of the nerve has been lost, the ends of the remaining portions can be marked for later use in free grafting or crossed anastomosis, as this type of sophisticated repair is rarely indicated at the time of primary treatment.

Wounds of the chin are somewhat unique in that the bulk of the subcutaneous tissue of the area is comprised of a somewhat avascular fat pad, and the tissues are therefore more prone to infection and subsequent resorption. Careful approximation of the injured tissues in layers, however, will usually insure satisfactory healing. Repair of lacerations of the lip requires careful attention to the alignment of the tissues, the most important landmark being the vermilion border. The vermilion–cutaneous junction should therefore be marked with an appropriate solution prior to the injection of any local anesthetic agent to avoid distortion of the tissue and to insure accurate reapproximation. In those lacerations that are through and through, the muscular closure of the orbicularis oris fibers is of

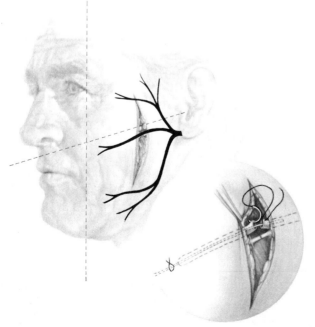

Figure 35–8 Suturing severed facial nerve and parotid duct. (From Grabb, W. C., Kleinert, H. E., and Puckett, C. L. 1976. Technics in Surgery: Facial and Hand Injuries. Somerville, N.J., Ethicon, Inc.)

great importance for insuring good physiologic function. When areas of tissue loss are less than 20 per cent, repair by direct closure is usually readily accomplished. In those losses involving greater amounts of tissue, the use of regional transposition flaps from the remaining uninvolved areas of the lip is in order.

Intraoral soft tissue wounds are often neglected under the erroneous assumption that these will always heal satisfactorily spontaneously. While this may be true of small punctate wounds, such as those inflicted by the other oral structures (teeth and alveolar fragments), it does not apply to more extensive injuries. On the other hand, however, too meticulous a closure without adequate consideration of drainage requirements for these injuries is equally undesirable and can result in the development of large hematomas of the buccal space or other undesirable sequelae. Intraoral wounds should be closed primarily whenever possible, avoiding distortion of natural landmarks and compromises of physiologic function just as is done in closures of cutaneous wounds. Suture closure can be carried out with permanent materials such as silk, although the use of absorbable materials such as chromic catgut is quite acceptable and may be preferred in areas in which suture removal presents a problem. Large, raw surfaces may require coverage by adjacent flaps (tongue flaps, regional mucosal flaps) or dermal grafts. In general, when patients have fractures that are compounded into the oral cavity and for which repair must be delayed, the intraoral soft tissue injury should be closed to reduce the incidence of infection and to convert the open to a closed fracture. Small or incomplete lacerations of the tongue may be left unsutured, especially in the uncooperative child who would have to be anesthetized to accomplish the suturing satisfactorily. In more extensive lacerations where the possibility of extensive scarring or the development of a permanent cleft of the tongue exists, careful suturing should be done. In addition, suturing of the tongue may be required as the method of choice for obtaining hemostasis in such a wound.

Lacerations involving the forehead and brow require careful attention to facial landmarks to reconstitute the hairline and eyebrow adequately. It should be realized that it is never necessary or advisable to shave the eyebrow in performing such repairs. In making secondary incisions or local tissue rearrangements, careful attention must be paid to the natural forehead lines. One of the more important anatomic structures of the midface from both a functional and aesthetic standpoint is the eyelids, and this dictates extremely meticulous attention to repair. Since this tissue is quite delicate and separates readily, it is not unusual to gain the false impression that tissue loss has occurred. The preferred repair of through-and-through lacerations involving the lid margin is careful approximation of conjunctiva, tarsus, and lid skin in layers, without using staggering methods or Z-plasty. While it is often recommended that the orbital septum be repaired with fine catgut sutures to prevent herniation of orbital fat, the septum is often left widely open following cosmetic blepharoplasty without any untoward result. Careful attention must be paid to appropriate repositioning of displaced lateral and medial canthal ligaments and to the integrity of the lacrimal duct system. Extensive injuries in this area warrant ophthalmologic consultation to evaluate the possibilities for restoration of function of the tear duct system and any associated intraocular injury. When tissue loss does occur in the lids, a graft may be obtained from the skin of an uninvolved upper lid in older children if some excess of this tissue exists, or thinned-out postauricular skin may be used.

In soft tissue injuries to the auricle, the presence of contusions and hematomas takes on more significance than it might in other specific anatomic sites. Contusions may predispose the underlying tissues to the development of perichondritis and possible loss of cartilage support. Hematomas must be drained adequately and conforming dressings applied so as to prevent any reaccumulation of the fluid if severe distortion from loss of cartilage or fibrous organization of the clot (cauliflower ear) is to be avoided. In the case of lacerations, initial efforts should be toward reconstruction of the external auditory canal and external meatus. The canal must be approximated meticulously or anastamosed and stented to maintain the patency of the canal and to prevent subsequent stenosis or obliteration. The next step in orderly repair of the auricle is accurate reapproximation of the helical rim. Following this, the remaining cartilage and skin areas are sutured. Tissue loss in cases of auricular trauma is of particular importance since there is no truly satisfactory donor site for secondary reconstruction except composite grafts from the opposite ear. Since the blood supply of the ear is abundant and the metabolic demands of the tissues are relatively low, the use of avulsed flaps of tissue with even extremely small pedicles carries a high rate of success. Even amputated composite tissue segments, if of a limited size (less than 25 per cent), often survive when relocated primarily. Case reports show that even when auricles have been totally avulsed replantation has been occasionally successful. On occasion, it is necessary to preserve the cartilaginous skeleton of the ear by removing damaged skin covering it and burying the segment beneath the postauricular skin. This may be done by making a small incision some distance superiorly or posteriorly in the scalp, so as not to interfere with the blood supply of the covering flap. The uniquely convoluted cartilage segment thus preserved becomes the keystone for subsequent reconstruction.

Bony injuries to the midface include those of the zygoma and orbital confines, those of the maxilla proper (including LeFort fractures), and those involving the alveolar process. Fractures of the bones of the face differ from fractures of bones of the remainder of the body in several respects. Because of their exposed position and minimal soft tissue cover, they may be fractured in spite of a relatively insignificant-appearing injury to the overlying tissues. In addition, injuries of a single isolated bone are the exception while combined injuries to several bones comprising a segment of the facial skeleton is the rule. When displacement occurs, it is invariably determined by the direction of the injuring force rather than by any effect of muscle pulls. This latter accounts for the tendency for reduced facial fractures to remain reduced and stable without unduly elaborate apparatus for traction and fixation. Fractures of the midfacial bones are usually readily apparent on physical examination, and attention is often drawn to the possibility of facial fracture by the presence of contused or abraded overlying soft tissues. In fractures of the maxilla, inspection may reveal flattening, shortening, or elongation of the face. The alignment of the teeth may be abnormal, with the upper teeth overlapping the lower or with the presence of an open bite. Abnormal mobility may be observed by grasping the anterior upper teeth or alveolus and attempting to move the maxilla up and down or in and out. In fractures of the zygoma or orbital rim, subconjunctival hemorrhage or ecchymosis

of the eyelids may be noted, and the patient may complain of numbness of the upper lip and gums. Careful palpation of the bony margins of the orbit may reveal separations or misalignments which may be confirmed by comparing both sides of the face. Placement of the index fingers on the high points of the cheeks or malar bones when viewed from above and behind the patient's head, helps the physician to detect fractures by measuring and comparing the levels of the fingers (and thus the bones). Variations in the level of the pupils or lateral canthi of the eyes may indicate depressions of the orbital rim (Fig. 35–9), another sign of fracture.

Emphysema of the cheek or periorbital tissues may result from a fracture that extends into the antrum or ethmoid complex and which allows air to pass into the soft tissues. Sneezing or blowing the nose may forcibly increase this emphysema.

The second commonest fracture of the facial bones is a fracture of the zygomatic complex. The signs of this fracture found upon examination include periorbital ecchymoses, flattening of the malar eminence, depression of the inferior rim of the orbit, and hypesthesia of the distribution of the infraorbital nerve. There may be tenderness at the infraorbital and lateral orbital rims and, on occasion, diplopia secondary to displacement of the lateral canthal tendon attached to the depressed bone. Displacement of the zygoma is most often associated with fracture separation at three points: along the infraorbital rim at the zygomaticomaxillary suture, along the lateral orbital rim at the zygomaticofrontal suture, and in the midportion of the zygomatic arch, at the junction of its temporal and zygomatic portions. Although isolated fractures of the zygoma do occur, they are much less frequent than are injuries associated with extension into the orbital floor along the orbital rim at the infraorbital foramen. Plane radiographs usually demonstrate these fractures well in the Waters view, and often show opacification of the maxillary antrum or the presence of an air/fluid level in the antrum on the side of the injury, which indicates bleeding into the antrum from torn mucosal lining. In cases of severe comminution of the orbital floor or dehiscence of orbital soft tissue through the floor, laminographic studies may be necessary to demonstrate the pathologic condition. In addition, stereoradiographic views and, more recently, xeroradiographic studies, have been found to

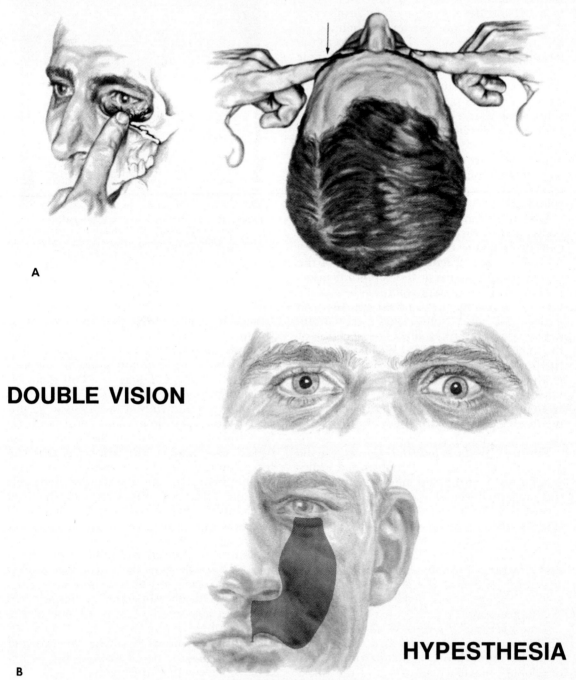

DOUBLE VISION

HYPESTHESIA

Figure 35–9 *A*, Zygomatic fracture. *B*, Diplopia and hypesthesia of the cheek often accompany a zygomatic fracture. (From Grabb, W. C., Kleinert, H. E., and Puckett, C. L. 1976. Technics in Surgery: Facial and Hand Injuries. Somerville, N.J., Ethicon, Inc.)

be extremely helpful in evaluating such injuries.

Displaced fractures of the zygoma usually require open reduction and internal fixation to avoid the development of deformities, a depression, and possible enophthalmos or diplopia. Multiple surgical approaches to the treatment of these fractures exist, and their application must be based on a careful consideration of the individual requirements of each patient (Lore, 1973). In general, the simplest and most direct approaches are preferred in children. Fractures of the zygoma may be reduced by direct traction or by approaches through the oral cavity or maxillary antrum or both. Fixation is then accomplished by direct wiring or internal splinting.

Fractures of the zygomatic arch proper are occasioned by direct, medially applied force, and the fracture most often consists of a central fracture, fracture at the origin of the zygoma and fracture at the temporal insertion accompanying depression of the middle segment. Swelling may be noted over the arch initially, but this is superseded by a definite depression or flatness following resorption of the edema and hematoma. Ecchymosis over the involved periorbital areas and associated tenderness with occasional depression may be noted. Mandibular excursions may be limited from impingement of the depressed fragments on the coronoid process of the mandible.

Fracture displacements of the zygomatic arch are usually readily demonstrated radiographically, and the best views are generally the tangential views, such as the submentovertex or the so-called "jug-handle views" (Fig. 35–10). A patient and skillful technician may be required to obtain these views in the anxious and frightened child. Reduction of these fractures is usually not difficult, and the structural nature of the arch and its cantilever-like arrangement make support or fixation unnecessary.

True *"blowout" fractures of the orbit* (Fig. 35–11) are probably quite rare in children owing to the lack of pneumatization of the developing maxillary antrum and the thickness of the bones of the inferior and medial walls of the orbit. The suggested mechanism of a blowout fracture is based on hydraulic pressures. Anterior pressure upon the globe forces the orbital contents posteriorly. This results in increased hydraulic pressure and increased pressure on the surrounding bony

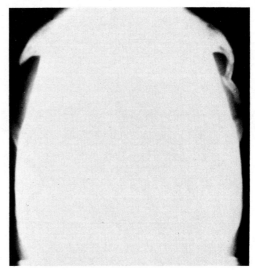

Figure 35–10 Radiograph of a zygomatic arch fracture. (From Dodd, G. D. 1977. Radiology of the nose, paranasal sinuses, and nasopharynx. *In* Golden, R., et al. (Eds.) Golden's Diagnostic Radiology, Sec. 2. Baltimore, Williams and Wilkins.)

frame. It is postulated that the thin areas fracture, and the orbital contents are forced through the opening into the surrounding sinus. The most common point of involvement is the floor and antrum. This theory is not without controversy, and a recent study has suggested a different mechanism. In this study, the orbital floor could consistently be fractured by pressure applied only to the orbital rim, and it was suspected that the forces on the rim alone caused a "buckling" of the floor. In this study, the hydraulic pressure effect was not part of the blowout mechanism. Orbital fractures are similar to fractures of the malar and zygomatic areas previously described and share many of the presenting symptoms and radiographic findings. Arbitrarily, they have been categorized as either "pure," in which no associated fracture of the orbital rim exists, or "impure," in which an associated fracture of one of the bony confines of the orbital rim does exist. Initially, ecchymoses involving the lids and periorbita may be noted without any significant displacement of the involved eye because of compensatory hematoma and edema within the orbit. This may be noted even though a significant amount of periorbital fat has herniated into the maxillary antrum. It has been stated that hypesthesia of the nasolabial area and upper lip is uncommon in blowout fractures and is more characteristic

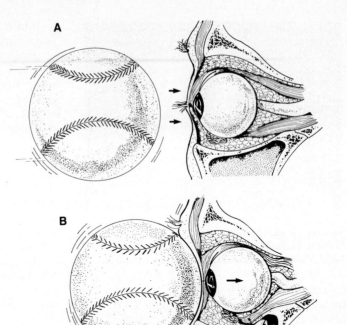

Figure 35–11 Blowout fracture of the orbit. (From Grabb, W. C., Kleinert, H. E., and Puckett, C. L. 1976. Technics in Surgery: Facial and Hand Injuries. Somerville, N.J., Ethicon, Inc.)

Torn inferior oblique and inferior rectus muscles

Fractured orbital floor

Periorbital fat   Maxillary sinus

of zygomatic fractures. This has been attributed to the fact that, in the former case, the infraorbital rim remains intact and tends to protect the infraorbital foramen. In the author's experience, hypesthesia of the infraorbital nerve may be *more* characteristic of a blowout fracture since the nerve is injured in its traverse through the infraorbital canal, contained in the thin bone of the orbital floor. This hypesthesia is usually of limited duration and probably represents contusion of the nerve rather than true disruption. Diplopia is an inconstant finding and has usually been attributed to actual muscle entrapment in the fracture site. This is probably most often *not* the case, as diplopia may be secondary to bleeding within the orbital soft tissues with consequent displacement of the globe, and/or hematoma within the muscle sheath itself, or the nerve sheath, with attendant limitation of range of motion on a neuromuscular basis. Ironically, the diplopia may be masked by the presence of edema and hematoma, which compensate for the depression of the orbital floor. Probably, the pathogenesis of most forms of persistent, and clinically significant, diplopia is atrophy and resorption of traumatized periorbital fat,

whether actually entrapped in a fracture site or merely contused. With the accompanying decrease in the volume of the orbital contents, the globe tends to settle into an enophthalmic position. Late enophthalmos and diplopia may occur even following apparently successful and technically excellent reductions of orbital fractures.

Orbital blowout fractures may be difficult to demonstrate radiographically, although an air/fluid level or partial opacification of the involved antrum on plane views are suggestive of this injury. Tomograms may reveal the so-called "teardrop" or "bomb-bay" signs (Fig. 35–12), which have been thought to be due to dehiscence of periorbital fat through the fracture site in the roof of the antrum. This can, however, be misleading, and when on occasion, these radiographic signs have been present, a small fracture of the orbital floor without dehiscence has been discovered at the time of surgery, and the radiographic finding was attributed to the presence of a submucoperiosteal hematoma of the antral roof. The decision as to whether or not these fractures should be treated is often a very difficult one, and must be an individual one based on the particular findings in, and re-

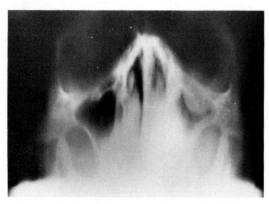

Figure 35–12 Radiograph of an orbital blowout fracture. (From Grabb, W. C., Kleinert, H. E., and Puckett, C. L. 1976. Technics in Surgery: Facial and Hand Injuries. Somerville, N.J., Ethicon, Inc.)

quirements of, each patient. Previously, the presence of diplopia, when associated with limitation of movement in a cardinal direction of gaze and infraorbital hypesthesia, and especially when accompanied by suggestive radiographic findings, was an absolute indication for surgical exploration. Recently, however, the trend has been away from exploration except in those cases in which true herniation of intraorbital contents or entrapment of muscles is clearly evident. Even in cases where true diplopia exists and limitation of range of motion of the eye can be demonstrated readily, it has become acceptable to observe the patient over a period of 7 to 14 days and to assess the resolution or progression of symptoms as the acute tissue reaction subsides. It has commonly been found that no intervention will be necessary after this period of time, and this concept of watchful waiting has partially been justified on the basis that surgical intervention immediately may not provide any assurance of normal function without diplopia or enophthalmos. The general criteria for surgical intervention are persistent diplopia and enopthalmos. Diplopia lasting longer than two weeks indicates a definite functional abnormality and a strong possibility of entrapment of muscle, while early enopthalmos suggests a significant loss of orbital tissues. Patients with these findings are considered candidates for surgical exploration and repair.

Fractures of the orbital rim with palpable step-offs must be corrected. Downward displacement of the globe may at first not be noticeable owing to the compensation by periorbital edema. Unlike the situation in the adult, after this type of fracture has healed in a child it is not as amenable to correction by refracturing or by bone grafting. Accurate reduction must therefore be done within the first five to seven days after injury. These same principles apply to the typical tripod fracture of the malar-zygomatic complex in which there is obvious asymmetry with a palpable step-off type of displacement and flattening of the malar eminence.

Approaches to the operative treatment of these fractures are largely similar to those used in fractures of the zygoma and consist of replacing herniated orbital tissues in their normal position and repositioning displaced bony fragments (Dingman and Natvig, 1964).

Maxillary fractures may occur in many forms, varying even between opposite sides of the same maxilla. An understanding of these fractures is possible if one considers them as LeFort originally described them: Type I (transverse), Type II (pyramidal), and Type III (craniofacial dysjunction) (Fig. 35–13). The most consistent symptom in these fractures is malocclusion, and the most common accompanying finding is elongation of the midface area. There is almost invariably periorbital swelling and ecchymosis, and palpation reveals mobility of the upper dental arch and surrounding maxilla. An anterior open bite is not an absolute indication of a maxillary fracture but is certainly presumptive evidence for one. The radiographic evaluation for suspected injury of the maxilla is similar to that for suspected injury to the zygomatic and malar complex.

Consideration of the LeFort classification system may be helpful in planning treatment, but variations of these fractures are so common as to demand even more individualized treatment than for other facial fractures (Mustarde, 1971). The need for access to the midfacial and dental arch areas means that techniques for maintaining the airway during anesthesia and postoperatively must be considered carefully. A tracheostomy is frequently performed in these cases, although its use should be predicated on firmer indications than the mere need for convenient access to the face. Nasotracheal intubation allows excellent access to the midface and teeth for application of arch bars, and even orotracheal intubation allows satisfactory access to these regions, although it requires that intermaxillary fixation be delayed until extubation has been accomplished. Commonly extubation occurs after 24 hours and is

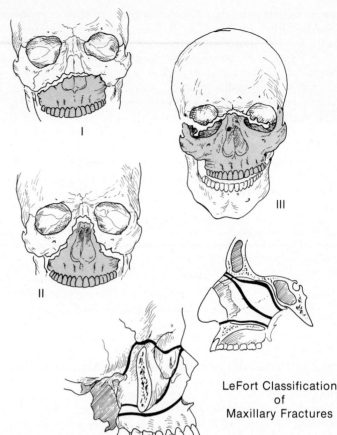

Figure 35–13 Maxillary fractures. (From Grabb, W. C., Kleinert, H. E., and Puckett, C. L. 1976. Technics in Surgery: Facial and Hand Injuries. Somerville, N.J., Ethicon, Inc.)

LeFort Classification of Maxillary Fractures

accomplished without anesthesia in adults. In children, however, this is a much less practical method, since although it does offer the benefit of leaving the mouth open in the immediate postoperative period, thereby reducing the danger of aspiration should the patient vomit while recovering from the anesthesia, extubation is more difficult.

In low transverse maxillary fractures (Guerin fracture or LeFort I fracture), when vertical displacement is minimal, interdental elastic fixation is usually sufficient and in children a firm, fibrous union is usually evident three to four weeks after fixation.

Pyramidal fractures (LeFort Type II) are central, midfacial fractures in the subzygomatic area and extend through the nasal bones and maxilla, usually at the zygomaticomaxillary suture areas. In common with fractures of the zygoma, they involve the maxillary antrum, inferior orbital rims, and the orbital floors, but in addition involve the central segment, which is displaced posteriorly with upward angulation to produce an open bite. The apex of this fracture commonly involves

the nasal bones and the bones of the medial aspect of the orbital floor. Surgical treatment is similar to that for open reduction of fractures of the zygoma and may require suspension of the maxilla from the intact frontal bone.

The LeFort Type III, or high-level, fracture is suprazygomatic and extends through the orbit and nasofrontal regions, constituting a separation of the midface from the cranium, as the term "craniofacial dysjunction" implies. The entire middle third of the face is fractured, with involvement of both zygomas, the nose, and the maxilla, presenting the characteristic appearance of a "bloated" edematous midface. Malocclusion, with an open, anterior open bite, is a characteristic of this type of fracture, and a "free-floating" maxilla is usually detectable by palpation. Once again, the cornerstone of surgical treatment is suspension of the fractured and displaced fragments from the adjacent stable cranial fragments by appropriate incisions and direct wiring through these incisions.

Various types of dental and alveolar injuries may be associated with fractures of the middle third of the face. A loosened tooth usually will solidify spontaneously; however, wire fixation to an adjacent tooth helps to assure its position and retention. A fractured segment of alveolus may be stabilized and alignment restored by wiring a tooth of the flail segment to an adjacent solid tooth or to an arch bar. Intermaxillary wire fixation will further secure the fracture and help to restore normal occlusion. Extensive alveolar fractures and avulsions, especially those having any periosteal or mucosal attachment, should be replaced and immobilized very securely. Most often, these segments will heal solidly in position.

Mandible

The management of fractures of the mandible in children is similar to their management in adults, with some notable exceptions (Freid and Baden, 1954). Initially, the deciduous teeth may not provide adequate support for intermaxillary fixation, and in children between the ages of 6 and 12 years the mixed dentition may prove to be inadequate for ligation of arch bars or intermaxillary fixation owing to the fact that the roots of the temporary teeth are undergoing resorption, and the teeth are exfoliating as the permanent teeth erupt to replace them. In addition, the rapid healing of fractures in children makes it mandatory that treatment be carried out within five to seven days if malunion is to be avoided. As in the case of other facial fractures, general anesthesia may more frequently be required for the management of fractures of the mandible in children, as fear and immaturity may limit the child's ability to cooperate. Finally, since many fractures of the body and ramus of the mandible are of the greenstick variety in children, early, but relatively short-term, fixation may provide for adequate and functional healing. Special consideration must be given to fractures of the condylar process, as possible interference with the growth center of this bone may result in developmental arrest and possible ankylosis of the joint.

As in fractures of the upper jaw, the most consistent physical finding in fractures of the mandible is malocclusion. While in fractures of the upper dental arch this is apt to be represented by an anterior open bite, a lateral crossbite is probably more common in fractures of the lower dental arch. Where the jaw is subluxed or dislocated there may be severe restriction of motion, with the jaw open and locked. Other common findings in fractures of the mandible are deformity, mobility of the fracture fragments, swelling, ecchymosis, and lingual deviation of the teeth, with associated tenderness to palpation of the involved area. The most useful radiographic views are the lateral or oblique, the posteroanterior, the Townes, and the occlusive. Recently, panoramic views (Panorex) have given a useful, wide view of the dental arches, which is often helpful. Finally, for diagnosing injuries to the temporomandibular joint area, tomograms may be useful.

In general, treatment of fractures of the mandible in the child should include early reduction and fixation for the shortest possible time consistent with good healing and stability, by the most conservative means available, but this must of necessity vary with the site of the injury. In young children, fractures usually occur in the anterior region of the mandible (mental or paramental) where the mandible is thin and contains many tooth buds. In addition, the cuspid region is particularly susceptible to trauma, as it is located at the anterior angle of the body of the mandible.

Following the diagnosis of a fracture, a treatment plan designed to be simple, effective, and to require the least amount of cooperation from the child must be formulated. It must also be practical, permit easy feeding, and cause no unusual discomfort. Reduction must correct the displacement, and immobilization must assure adequate surgical rest for the injured parts. In certain instances in which displacement is minimal and there is no significant discomfort or motion of the fracture line, simple rest and a soft diet, with perhaps the use of a Barton bandage, is adequate. For treatment of extensive fractures, interdental wiring in conjunction with acrylic splints may be required (Bernstein, 1969).

Special consideration must be given to fractures at special sites. Fractures at the precise midline of the mandible, the symphysis, are quite rare and when found are commonly associated with a fracture of one or both condyles. These fractures, both vertical and oblique, and often greenstick in nature, are exceedingly difficult to treat. The distracting forces acting on the fragments due to the attachment of multiple powerful muscles in this region compounds the problem.

Treatment of fractures of the body of the mandible spans the spectrum of simple immobilization with a Barton bandage for nondisplaced fractures, to reduction by either open or closed methods and fixation with splints or arch bars, with or without intermaxillary fixation. In general, prolonged fixation is not required in children (Kaban et al. 1977).

Fractures of the coronoid process are exceedingly uncommon and may require no treatment if malocclusion is not present or if there is no significant pain. Lateral crossbite may be seen in this injury initially, secondary to muscle spasm rather than to any fracture displacement.

Condylar fracture treatment is somewhat controversial but recently has tended towards a short period on a liquid diet or only very brief immobilization. Feared growth disturbances do not seem to materialize when normal temporomandibular joint function is maintained. Those few patients with residual deviation on opening the jaw may do special exercises to correct the deviation. While some authorities have suggested that "selected" fracture dislocations of the condyle be managed by open reduction of the fragments, the risks in this approach are significant, and possibly unwarranted, when one considers the extreme amount of remodeling that occurs in the condylar stump when jaw motion is constantly maintained. In addition, some recent evidence suggests that the condylar head, per se, is not as critical for growth as is normal function of the joint. Overzealous therapy for mandibular fractures in children, including prolonged intermaxillary fixation or interosseous wiring, may indeed be more apt to result in complications than would more conservative therapy.

Complications

Complications of facial injury in children are fortunately rare, but can be devastating. Facial deformity may result from soft tissue injuries or from bony injuries with malunion or interference with growth and development of the facial bones. Functional losses secondary to ankylosis of the mandible may occur with aseptic necrosis of the articular surface of the condyle as a consequence of complete separation of the condyle from the ramus. Permanent diplopia secondary to fracture of the zygoma and orbital floor may require corrections in the position of the orbital floor, eye muscle surgery, or both. A saddle nose deformity may result from unreduced nasal bone fractures or unrecognized septal hematoma or abscess. Fractures with displacement of the nasal and lacrimal bones and detachment of the palpebral ligaments may result in traumatic pseudohypertelorism. Cerebrospinal fluid rhinorrhea, with its ever-present risk of meningitis, may be a consequence of craniofacial disjunction.

Summary

In summary, the care of facial injuries in the child requires, in addition to the usual knowledge and understanding of these injuries in the adult, special consideration for the many significant differences between children and adults. One must also recognize that these special considerations are such that, occasionally, even with the most meticulously proper treatment, the results can be less than optimal. It is hoped that careful attention to the many details outlined in this section will minimize the number of such instances.

SELECTED REFERENCES

Converse, J. M., and Dingman, R. O. 1977. Facial injuries in children. *In* Reconstructive Plastic Surgery. Vol. 2, Chap. 26, Philadelphia, W. B. Saunders Co.
This excellent chapter is part of the new second edition of Dr. Converse's definitive multivolume text on reconstructive surgery and emphasizes child-adult differences in diagnosis and treatment. Other volumes in this series provide more detailed discussion and illustration of the numerous treatment methods available.

Dingman, R. O., and Natvig, P. 1964. Surgery of Facial Fractures. Philadelphia, W. B. Saunders Co.
Although this highly regarded standard text does contain a chapter on facial fractures in children (Chapter 11), its outstanding feature is the clear linedrawing depiction of the types of injuries and the beautifully illustrated operative techniques employed for their correction.

Lore, J. M., Jr. 1973. An Atlas of Head and Neck Surgery. Philadelphia, W. B. Saunders Co.
As indicated by the title, this work is an atlas of operative procedures, and as such contains a number of excellent plates dealing with facial fractures. Its organization is unusually clear and concise, and it points out indications for each procedure as well as pitfalls to avoid. The illustrations are particularly accurate and realistic.

McGregor, I. A. 1969. Fundamental Techniques of Plastic Surgery. Baltimore, Williams & Wilkins Co.

   A small, concise book with particular attention to basic soft tissue handling techniques in facial injuries.

Mustarde, J. C. 1971. Plastic Surgery in Infancy and Childhood, Chaps. V, VII, IX, XIV. Philadelphia, W. B. Saunders Co.

   The chapters noted, especially Chapter VII, Traumatic Injuries of the Jaws and Teeth by Drs. Rowe and Winter, provide excellently detailed accounts of the surgical management of various injuries in children of different ages.

REFERENCES

Bailey, B. J. 1977. Management of soft tissue trauma of the head and neck in children. Otolaryngol. Clin. North Am., *10*:193–204.

Bernstein, L. 1969. Maxillofacial injuries in children. Otolaryngol. Clin. North Am., *2*:397–401.

Converse, J. M., and Dingman, R. O. 1977. Facial injuries in children. *In* Reconstructive Plastic Surgery, Vol. 2, Chap. 26, Philadelphia, W. B. Saunders Co.

Dingman, R. O., and Natvig, P. 1964. Surgery of Facial Fractures. Philadelphia, W. B. Saunders Co.

Fee, W. E., Jr. 1976. Rhomboid flap principles and common variations. Laryngoscope, *86*:1706–1711.

Freid, M. G., and Baden, E. 1954. Management of fractures in children. J. Oral Surg. *12*:129–139.

Hall, R. K. 1972. Injuries of the face and jaws in children. J. Oral Surg., *1*:65–75.

Kaban, L. B., Mulliken, J. B., and Murray, J. E. 1977. Facial fractures in children. Plast. Reconstr. Surg. *59*:15–20.

Lore, J. M., Jr. 1973. An Atlas of Head and Neck Surgery. Philadelphia, W. B. Saunders Co.

McCoy, F. J., Chandler, R. A., and Crow, M. L. 1966. Facial fractures in children. Plast. Reconstr. Surg., *37*:209–215.

McGregor, I. A. 1969. Fundamental Techniques of Plastic Surgery. Baltimore, Williams & Wilkins Co.

Moran, W. B., Jr. 1977. Nasal trauma in children. Otolaryngol. Clin. North Am., *10*:95–101.

Mustarde, J. C. 1971. Plastic Surgery in Infancy and Childhood, Chaps. V, VII, IX, XIV. Philadelphia, W. B. Saunders Co.

Schultz, R. C. 1970. Facial Injuries. Chicago, Yearbook Medical Publishers.

Tardy, M. E., Jr. 1972. The bilobed flap in nasal repair. Arch. Otolaryngol., *95*:1–5.

Weber, S. C., and Cohn, A. M. 1977. Fracture of the frontal sinus in children. Arch. Otolaryngol.; *103*:241–244.

Yarrington, C. T., Jr. 1977. Maxillofacial trauma in children. Otolaryngol. Clin. North Am., *10*:25–32.

Zaydon, T. J., and Brown, J. B. 1964. Early Treatment of Facial Injuries. Philadelphia, Lea & Febiger.

Chapter 36

TUMORS OF THE NOSE, PARANASAL SINUSES, AND NASOPHARYNX

Victor L. Schramm, Jr., M.D.

Tumors of the nose, paranasal sinuses, and nasopharynx produce symptoms and signs that are common and nonspecific and, therefore, infrequently alarm either the patient or the patient's family. In addition, tumors in these areas occur much less frequently than do diseases related to upper respiratory tract infection, and hence may not be diagnosed early in their course. Fortunately, tumors of this region may be differentiated from infectious diseases by the chronology and severity of symptoms, by physical examination, and by simple noninvasive radiographic techniques. With proper identification and evaluation of masses in this region, nearly all tumors of the nose, nasopharynx, and paranasal sinuses may be managed successfully.

PRESENTING SYMPTOMS

Nasal obstruction, mouth breathing, slow eating, and rhinorrhea are symptoms common to most nasal and nasopharyngeal mass lesions. The rhinorrhea produced by benign diseases in these areas is usually serous or mucoid, with purulence developing as a result of secondary infections. Persistent, blood-tinged rhinorrhea is most frequently associated with a nasal hemangioma or granuloma but is also a consistent symptom of any malignancy in this area. Massive epistaxis in the young male is usually related to the presence of an angiofibroma. Tearing may be caused by a mass in the lateral nasal wall, particularly in the anterior floor of the nose.

Masses expanding beneath the skin of the nasal dorsum are most usually developmental anomalies, while masses protruding from the anterior nose are most commonly benign nasal polyps. Distortion of midfacial contour may be produced by tumors in the nose or maxillary sinus. A vague sensation of pressure in the region of the nose is suggestive of the presence of a benign lesion, but progressive facial pain, headache, facial numbness, otalgia, or diplopia are nearly always symptoms of malignancy. Hearing loss is frequently associated with nasal or nasopharyngeal disease, but its importance may be overlooked by the patient, family, or observer.

CLINICAL SIGNS

The physical signs produced by tumors in the midface and nasopharynx are readily observable. The characteristics of these masses usually will not only distinguish tumors from other conditions but also will allow the physician to make a distinction between benign and malignant disease in most instances. Nasal polyps may be unilateral or bilateral and are most commonly gray, glistening, and mobile. Ulceration of an unexposed polypoid mass may be noted in the case of a foreign body granuloma or hemangioma but is more common with malignancy. Any mass protruding from the nares will become ulcerated due to trauma and dehydration, and, therefore, observation of the intranasal portion is necessary to differentiate benign from malignant disease. Granular or friable polypoid masses in the nasal cavity are more frequently hemangiomas or foreign body granulomas than malignancies. The mass beneath the skin of the nasal dorsum with an overlying pit or a similar mass on the side of the nasal bone suggests a dermoid cyst. Masses without a skin pit, particularly those with a bluish or reddish hue and some intranasal component, will most frequently be gliomas.

Masses related to the maxilla or maxillary antrum are most commonly benign and may be distinguished as to their etiology by location and character. Masses of the low anterior maxilla producing distortion of the ala, gingivobuccal sulcus, or dentition are most frequently dentigerous or odontogenic cysts, globulomaxillary cysts, or benign giant cell tumors (Fig. 36–1). Sinus expansion in the premaxillary area is produced by fibro-osseous lesions, mucoceles, or inclusion cysts

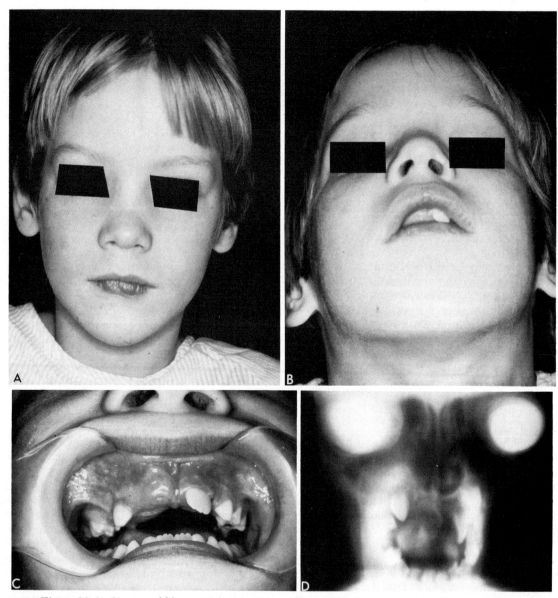

Figure 36–1 Six year old boy with benign giant cell tumor of the right maxilla. One year history of tearing and lacrimal infection (*A*) and gradual onset of a right maxillary mass and right nasal obstruction (*B*). Eruption of the right central incisor is delayed, and there is bone expansion in the right gingivobuccal sulcus (*C*). AP tomogram demonstrating mass expanding into maxillary sinus and inferior nasal cavity overlying unerupted lateral incisor (*D*).

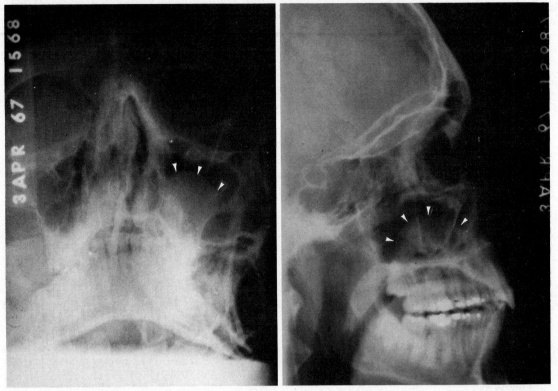

Figure 36–2 Globular water density mass representing an inclusion cyst arising from the anterior floor of the maxillary sinus (arrows). *Left,* Waters view; *right,* lateral view.

within the antrum. Lateral displacement of the orbital contents is common with disease in the ethmoid sinus; whereas upward displacement of the orbital contents occurs less frequently and is related to maxillary sinus disease. Infraorbital anesthesia, limitation of extraocular movement, proptosis, middle ear effusion, or trismus associated with a maxillary mass suggests malignancy.

The nasopharynx can usually be evaluated without general anesthesia by indirect mirror examination in older children or by palatal retraction or palpation at any age. Antral choanal polyps are the most commonly seen nonadenoid nasopharyngeal masses. They appear as gray or yellowish, smooth, mucosa-covered masses without nasopharyngeal connections. Polypoid masses that are not friable, are mucosa-covered, and that arise from the nasopharyngeal vault are usually retention cysts or less commonly dermoids, gliomas, or encephaloceles. A firm, globular nasopharyngeal mass in a male is most commonly an angiofibroma, while other ulcerated or firm submucosal lesions are epidermoid carcinomas, rhabdomyosarcomas, or occasionally lymphomas. When a nasopharyngeal mass is associated with trismus, middle ear effusion, blood-tinged rhinorrhea, or neurologic deficit in structures of the orbital apex or skull base, it is most likely a malignancy. Meningismus or meningitis is likely to be associated with rhabdomyosarcoma or carcinoma.

RADIOGRAPHIC EVALUATION

Radiographic examination of a patient provides important information on the location, extent, and effect of tumors of the nasal region on adjacent facial and cranial skeletal structures. The radiographic appearance of some tumors, such as the maxillary sinus inclusion cyst, may be diagnostic (Fig. 36–2). A polypoid nasopharyngeal mass of water density associated with unilateral maxillary sinus opacification is most likely an antral choanal polyp. The presence of a soft tissue mass of water density in the nose or paranasal sinuses may be difficult to evaluate, however, when the mass is adjacent to the thin, bony walls of the sinuses, pterygoid plates, or cribriform area. Expansion of bony structures, particularly with sclerotic margins, suggests a benign process, whereas indistinct bone erosion is more characteristic of malignancy.

The results of the tomographic examination may be particularly helpful in evaluating a tumor in a patient of any age. Computerized tomography partially overcomes the disadvantage of conventional radiographic evaluation in being able to distinguish between the density of bone and other densities. Computerized tomography is also helpful in determining intracranial extension of a mass. There are, however, two aspects of computerized tomography that should be taken into consideration: the prolonged immobilization necessary to complete the examination may require that children be given a general anesthetic, and a relatively higher radiation exposure is required for computerized tomography than for conventional radiographic examination.

A routine sinus series should be the initial radiographic evaluation. The most common finding for nasal tumors is that of a soft tissue mass. This in itself is not diagnostic, but the presence of such a mass when combined with other findings may suggest a specific diagnosis. A mass associated with nasal bone expansion is usually benign and most frequently is due to cystic fibrosis. If bone separation is noted, the presence of a dermoid cyst or encephalocele should be suspected. Computerized tomography is particularly helpful in evaluating the cribriform plate area. In addition, this technique may distinguish between bone erosion, which suggests the presence of malignancy, and simple bone expansion related to a benign process.

Routine sinus radiography may also be diagnostic of certain sinus tumors. A maxillary sinus inclusion cyst is seen as a globular, rounded density on the radiograph, and a mucocele may be distinguished by its expansile, sclerotic bony margin. Developmental incisural cysts and dental cysts can also frequently be delineated radiographically. Fibro-osseous lesions may be suggested by, but are not definitively diagnosed by, any radiographic technique. Computerized tomography may make it possible to distinguish between bone erosion and bone expansion when the results of routine radiographic evaluation are inconclusive. Computerized tomography with contrast enhancement can enable one to differentiate between vascular lesions, such as malignancies or vascular tumors, and fibro-osseous lesions and most other benign tumors.

A soft tissue mass in the nasopharynx may be any one of a number of different tumors, but when it is associated with a widened pterygopalatine fissure ("V" sign), it is likely to be an extension of a nasopharyngeal angiofibroma. Bowing of the posterior maxillary wall is frequently noted from expansion of a nasopharyngeal angiofibroma. Bone erosion, particularly in the sphenoid, is nearly always due to a rhabdomyosarcoma or carcinoma. Computerized tomography provides valuable information when a nasopharyngeal malignancy or angiofibroma is suspected; it can demonstrate central nervous system involvement or extranasopharyngeal extension of a mass (Fig. 36–3). The usefulness of angiography is limited to the diagnosis of an

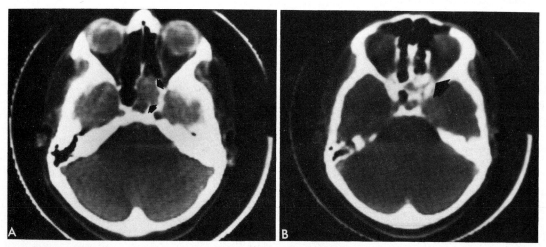

Figure 36–3 Computerized tomogram (CT) of 15 year old patient with nasopharyngeal carcinoma. Mass extending into posterior nasal cavity and sphenoid sinus (A) and involving the middle cranial fossa and posterior orbit (B).

angiofibroma and the preoperative embolization of this tumor.

MANAGEMENT APPROACH

The approach to management of tumors of the nose, sinuses, or nasopharynx depends on the certainty of the clinical diagnosis. A presumptive diagnosis based on the history, physical examination, and radiographic evaluation is confirmed pathologically in most instances. In a series of patients studied at the University of Pittsburgh (Schramm, 1979), the clinical impression agreed with the pathologic diagnosis in 88 per cent of the patients with nasal tumors and in 75 per cent of the patients with sinus or nasopharyngeal tumors. If a benign disease is determined to be the most likely cause of symptoms, the clinician should decide first if treatment is necessary and, if so, should plan an expedient excision.

In those situations in which the lesion is probably benign but the clinical evaluation is not diagnostic, an approach for excision should be planned so as not to compromise more radical excision if it proves necessary. An external facial approach in this situation is rarely necessary. If a malignancy is suspected, definitive treatment should be based on a histologic diagnosis. Specimens from nasal and nasopharyngeal lesions can be obtained directly. Biopsy specimens may be obtained from sinus tumors through a naso-antral window or by a transnasal route. Since the pathologic diagnosis of many of these tumors is difficult, the biopsy specimen must be representative and of adequate size to permit evaluation. Special stains of the biopsy material to demonstrate striations or mucin are helpful. Examination by electron microscopy is indicated in many of these tumors; this possibility should be discussed with the pathologist prior to obtaining the biopsy specimen. Because of the uncommon nature of many of these tumors, outside pathologic consultation is often beneficial. If the lesion is demonstrated microscopically to be benign, its excision can be completed.

Selected malignancies in the nose or the paranasal sinus areas may be removed by radical resection.

SURGICAL APPROACH

In general, the surgical approach to excision of neoplasms in this region need not be deforming. Nasal tumors can usually be approached intranasally. A lateral rhinotomy is cosmetically acceptable while exposing the anterior nasal cavity and the entire lateral wall of the nose to the nasopharynx (Schramm and Myers, 1978). Lesions in the posterior part of the nose may be approached transpalatally utilizing a palatal push-back technique. This gives exposure to the posterior nasal septum, nasopharynx, and sphenoid if necessary. Exposure of the nasal dorsum, nasal root, and glabella may be obtained through a bilateral alotomy "hood" approach in which an incision is made along the alar crease, transecting the columella at its base below the medial crura, and up the membranous septum. This incision, when connected to bilateral intracartilagenous incisions, allows elevation of the skin of the entire nose with little deformity resulting. A bilateral sublabial incision may be continued up the nasal dorsum in the same manner to give nearly the same exposure without any external incisions.

Maxillary sinus tumors may be removed through a gingivobuccal incision. This approach may be combined with a lateral rhinotomy for tumors of the ethmoid or maxilla. Biopsies of sphenoid sinus tissue may be obtained via an external ethmoid route, but surgery to remove lesions in the sphenoid is more appropriately performed from a transpalatal transseptal or a sublabial-transseptal approach. Nasopharyngeal surgery is accomplished by the transoral route, utilizing either the transpalatal push-back technique or direct nasopharyngeal exposure with palate retraction. Combinations of the craniofacial, transpalatal, and lateral rhinotomy approaches may be used to expose extensive lesions (Schramm et al., 1979) and to resect safely tumors located anywhere from above the glabella to the oral cavity, including the anterior and middle fossae of the skull. Plans for fitting the patient with a prosthesis should be completed prior to surgery whenever part of the facial structure or palate must be resected. Return of function following maxillectomy is excellent in children since there are almost always teeth to which an appliance may be fixed.

INCIDENCE OF TUMORS

The relative frequency of tumors recurring in this region has been difficult to assess because they are uncommon, and reports have focused primarily on individual tumors.

Table 36–1   DIFFERENTIAL DIAGNOSIS AND RELATIVE FREQUENCY OF
NASAL, NASOPHARYNGEAL, AND PARANASAL SINUS MASSES

Benign	Malignant
Nasal	
Polyp—antral choanal	Rhabdomyosarcoma
bilateral	Carcinoma
unilateral	squamous
cystic fibrosis	transitional
Hemangioma	undifferentiated
Squamous cell papilloma	adeno
Neural	Sarcoma
glioma	fibroma
neurofibroma	angio
neurilemoma	chondro
Dermoid/teratoma	osteo
Foreign body granuloma	Malignant (NFC)*
Fibroma (fibroepithelial polyp)	Esthesioneuroblastoma
Chondroma	Lymphoma
Nasopharyngeal	
Antral choanal polyp	Carcinoma
Angiofibroma	squamous cell
Teratoma/dermoid	transitional
Mucous cyst	undifferentiated
Hemangioma	Rhabdomyosarcoma
Glioma	Sarcoma (other)
Chondroma	Malignancy (NFC)*
Chordoma	Lymphoma
Rhabdomyoma	
Sinus	
Polyp—antral choanal	Rhabdomyosarcoma
Dental	Carcinoma
dentigerous cyst	transitional
odontogenic	squamous cell
Mucocele/mucous cyst	undifferentiated
Fibrous dysplasia	adeno
Ossifying fibroma	Sarcoma (other)
Giant cell tumor	Myxoma
Hemangioma	Lymphoma
Myxoma	
Melanotic neuroectodermal tumor	
Chondroma	
Mixed tumor	

*Not further classified

A perspective on the types and incidences of benign and malignant masses that arise in this area may be gained by a review of cases from the University of Pittsburgh and the Armed Forces Institute of Pathology (AFIP). Included in this study are 203 patients admitted to Eye and Ear Hospital or Children's Hospital of Pittsburgh between 1965 and 1975 and 349 benign and malignant tumor specimens acquired by the Otologic Pathology Registry of the AFIP between 1955 and 1975 (Schramm, 1979). Additional information has been obtained from a series of articles by Fu and Perzin (1974a, 1974b, 1974c, 1975, 1976a, 1976b, 1977a, 1977b) describing the clinicopathologic aspects of nonepithelial tumors in this region. Dehner (1973a, 1973b)

has also compiled a study that includes an excellent review of histologically benign and malignant lesions of the maxilla in children. The incidences of benign and malignant neoplasms reported from these divergent sources correlate well. The inclusion of patients with polyps and dentally related masses seen at the University of Pittsburgh makes the observations more clinically helpful.

Table 36–1 lists masses according to their differential diagnoses in the order of frequency with which they were noted in our study. The most common type of mass that occurs in the nasal cavities of children is the benign nasal polyp. Although benign nasal polyps are the result of an inflammatory rather than a neoplastic process, the relative frequency with which they occur in children makes consideration of this tumor important. A large majority of tumors in all three areas are nonepithelial. Carcinomas occur relatively more frequently in the nasopharynx than in the nose or sinuses.

MANAGEMENT OF NASAL TUMORS

Antral Choanal Polyps

Benign nasal polyps are the most frequently seen type of nasal tumor. Contrary to the usual belief, however, these polyps are relatively infrequently "allergic" in etiology. The most common type of polyp is the antral choanal polyp. The patient usually has a history of progressive unilateral nasal obstruction with mucoid or mucopurulent nasal drainage. Bilateral nasal obstruction eventually may occur as the polyp expands in the nasopharynx and obstructs the contralateral choana. A mass may also present in the oral cavity or may expand in dumbbell fashion to protrude from the anterior nares (Fig. 36–4). The appearances of all benign nasal polyps are remarkably similar. The mass is covered

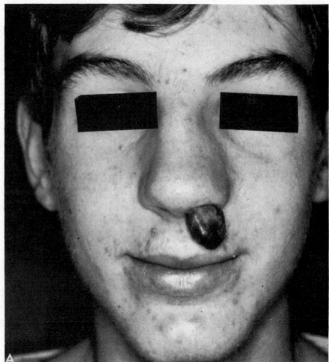

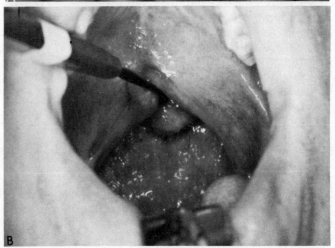

Figure 36–4 Bilobed antral choanal polyp. Exposure of protruding polyp has produced necrosis (A). Mass in nasopharynx visible with palatal retraction (B).

by glistening, smooth, grayish mucosa and is soft and mobile to palpation or manipulation. The antral choanal polyp will be seen most readily on indirect nasopharyngeal examination but may be visualized after topical nasal vasoconstriction as a mass protruding from the posterior aspect of the middle meatus. Unless the mass has been exposed as it protrudes from the nares, it is neither friable nor ulcerated. Radiographic evaluation will usually demonstrate unilateral maxillary and ethmoid opacification. Since the antral choanal polyp emanates from the mucosa of the maxillary sinus, it is not seen frequently prior to the age of four or five years. Surgical excision is indicated and should include Caldwell-Luc exposure of the maxillary antrum for removal of the antral attachment of the polyp. After antral mucosa has been dissected, the polyp is removed from the nasopharynx via the mouth. The temptation to simply avulse an antral choanal polyp with a snare should be avoided as the majority of polyps treated by avulsion may be expected to recur, requiring a second operative procedure and producing prolonged maxillary and ethmoid sinusitis. Because chronic infection due to obstruction of the maxillary sinus ostea is usually present, a nasoantral window should be considered at the time of primary surgery. When antral choanal polyps are removed by a Caldwell-Luc approach and a nasal antral window, the recurrence rate is nearly zero.

Nasal Polyps

The next most frequent type of nasal polyp disease is related to infection of the ethmoid sinuses. This produces unilateral multiple, or occasionally bilateral multiple, nasal polyps. The multiple polyps vary in size but have a grape-like appearance and are covered by glistening grayish mucosa. They may be seen protruding from the middle meatus and may fill the nose both anteriorly and posteriorly. Radiographically there is opacification of the ethmoid air cells as well as of the maxillary antrum due to middle meatus obstruction. It is not necessary to investigate the patient presenting with unilateral nasal polyps for the presence of an allergy, but any infection present must be treated and provision must be made for drainage of the ethmoid sinuses. Intranasal polypectomy with snare removal of the multiple polyps should precede an intranasal ethmoidectomy. Inflammatory

nasal polyps most frequently occur in patients over the age of five years. By this age, the ethmoid sinuses are well developed, and intranasal ethmoidectomy carries no unusual risk. Recurrent unilateral nasal polyps most frequently occur in patients who have not previously undergone intranasal ethmoidectomy. If an intranasal ethmoidectomy has been performed and the polyps recur, a Caldwell-Luc approach and a nasoantral window should be added to subsequent therapy. Such a procedure carries little risk, particularly in the patient over seven years of age in whom the anterior maxillary teeth have erupted.

Bilateral multiple nasal polyps may be seen either with infection alone or in conjunction with an allergic diathesis. Half of the patients with bilateral polyps not associated with cystic fibrosis will have an allergic component to their disease, while less than 10 per cent of patients with unilateral polyps will ultimately be demonstrated to have an allergy. Unfortunately, the histologic appearance of nasal polyps does not aid in establishing their etiology. The author reviewed 130 biopsy specimens of patients undergoing nasal polypectomy and found that the mucosa, interstitial tissue, and amount of inflammatory infiltrate were similar in all polyps. The polyps removed from patients with cystic fibrosis may be shown microscopically to have cystic spaces, but this finding is not limited to this group of patients. The patients with cystic fibrosis may also have a predominance of eosinophils in the inflammatory infiltrate of their polyps. Radiographic evaluation generally demonstrates opacification and mucosal thickening of all developed sinuses.

The treatment of bilateral multiple nasal polyps is the same as that outlined for unilateral polyps. If the polyps are recurrent or if physical examination or histologic evidence suggests that the patient has an allergy, the allergy should be identified and treated. Intrapolyp injections of steroids, a treatment that has been demonstrated to be effective in adults, is usually not necessary in children and should be avoided if possible. Allergic nasal polyps have shown a 50 per cent regression rate when treated with a topical steroid applied as an aerosal (Mygind et al., 1975). If the polyps are recurrent despite adequate medical, surgical, and allergic management, the possibility of cystic fibrosis should be evaluated by testing the level of sweat chlorides.

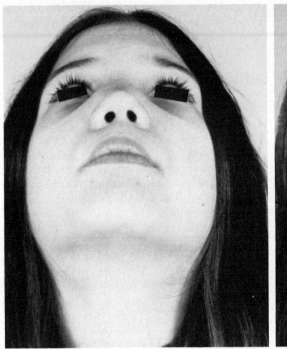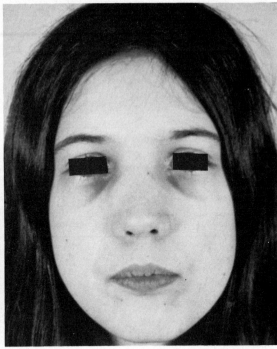

Figure 36–5 Expansion of nasal bones produced by polyps in a 14 year old girl with cystic fibrosis.

Nasal Polyps Associated with Cystic Fibrosis

About 20 per cent of patients with cystic fibrosis develop symptomatic nasal polyps. It is difficult to treat nasal polyps in this group of patients because the underlying disease cannot be alleviated. Even medical treatment with appropriate antibiotics and digestive enzymes does not alter the rate of occurrence of polyp disease in these individuals. The onset of nasal obstruction due to nasal polyps may occur in infancy or at any time thereafter. The polyps usually, although not invariably, occur bilaterally. Patients who develop polyps at an early age tend to have greater difficulty with more frequently recurring polyps than do those who develop polyps later. Patients with cystic fibrosis and nasal polyps may show expansion of the nasal dorsum and prominence of the anterior maxillary areas on physical examination (Fig. 36–5). Radiographically, all sinuses are usually opacified, with dense sclerotic margins about the maxillary antrum and loss of ethmoid trabeculation. Nasal bone expansion may also be noted radiographically (Fig. 36–6). The combination of chronic nasal obstruction, mouthbreathing, secondary nasal infection, and aspiration of purulent nasopharyngeal

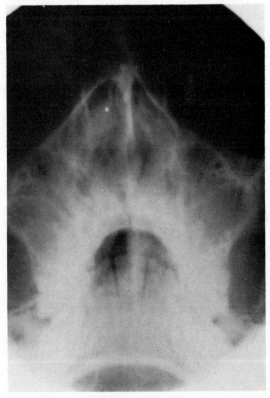

Figure 36–6 Expansion of nasal bones, nasal process of maxilla, and anterior maxillary wall demonstrated by Waters view radiograph.

secretions complicates the management of pulmonary problems in cystic fibrosis. For this reason, nasal polypectomy is usually indicated. In addition to snare removal of the nasal polyps, careful intranasal exenteration of all ethmoid sinus mucosa decreases the rate of recurrence of polyps in these patients. For older children, a Caldwell-Luc transantral ethmoidectomy and a nasoantral window is indicated. The mucosa that relines the sinuses after such a procedure is nearly devoid of glandular elements so that the tenacious sinus secretions produced in this disease are diminished. This, along with the improved sinus drainage obtained by this surgical approach to the intranasal and sinus disease, does result in decreased frequency of recurrence of nasal polyps and decreased intranasal and sinus infection (Jaffe et al., 1977; Schramm, 1979).

Benign Neoplasms

Intranasal hemangiomas form the next most common group of intranasal tumors. A hemangioma should be suspected in a patient with recurrent or persistent epistaxis. The lesion presents as a granular, friable mass, usually less than 1 cm in diameter, that may be located anywhere in the nasal cavity. Transnasal local excision of the hemangioma is necessary to prevent recurrent epistaxis. The intranasal hemangioma differs from the cutaneous group of hemangiomas in that it is usually not present at birth and does not regress with time. The nasal hemangioma occasionally may be difficult to distinguish clinically from an angiofibroma and pathologically from sarcoma.

Squamous cell papillomas also occur quite commonly in the nasal cavity and are usually recognized as warty-appearing masses in the nasal vestibule. Nasal bleeding and surrounding cellulitis frequently occur related to local trauma. Simple excision of the papilloma is adequate. Papillomas of the inverting type are quite uncommon in children, but when they do occur they present as polypoid, somewhat granular, reddish-tan intranasal masses. When inverting papillomas occur in children, they should be treated by wide local excision, usually utilizing a lateral rhinotomy approach. Foreign body or pyogenic granulomas may mimic hemangiomas in their appearance and clinical presentation as friable, inflamed masses. Local excision with electro-

cauterization of the granuloma base combined with antibiotic therapy usually effects a cure.

Benign nasal tumors of glandular origin increase in frequency with the patient's age and are most commonly mixed tumors in children. They may arise from the nasal septum or lateral nasal wall and may attain a relatively large size before being recognized. Although generally submucosal, when greater than 2 cm in diameter they may be ulcerated as a result of trauma or infection, and it is recommended that a biopsy specimen be obtained by incision for diagnosis prior to wide local excision of the mass.

Tumors of neural origin include gliomas, neurofibromas, and neurilemomas. They present as polypoid masses within the nose that may mimic benign polyps in their appearance. Usually they may be distinguished from benign polyps by their location, physical characteristics and appearance on radiographic examination. These polyps originate in locations away from the middle meatus. Opacification of the paranasal sinuses may be demonstrated radiographically but is due to secondary obstruction in the area of the middle meatus. Treatment for these lesions has been described in Chapter 31. Examination of a biopsy specimen is usually necessary to diagnose neurofibroma or neurilemoma. Depending on the size of the lesion, they may be locally excised through a transnasal route alone or with the addition of a lateral rhinotomy approach.

Fibromas or fibroepithelial polyps present with nasal obstruction caused by a firm mucosa-covered or squamous epithelium-covered mass. There is usually a history of intranasal trauma. Local excision biopsy confirms the diagnosis and is adequate therapy as well. Chondromas in children arise almost exclusively from the nasal septum. They are firm, mucosa-covered, less than 1 cm in diameter, and are cured by submucosal resection.

Nasal Malignancy

Nasal malignancy is uncommon and is frequently not suspected initially because its early symptoms are similar to those of benign diseases. A history of rapidly progressive nasal obstruction with serosanguineous nasal drainage suggests an intranasal malignancy. The clinical appearance of a nasal malignancy may vary, but usually a friable, reddish, ulcerating mass is present. The diagnosis is established by pathologic evaluation of biopsy material.

Rhabdomyosarcoma is the most common intranasal malignancy. The treatment for rhabdomyosarcoma of the nose is similar to that for rhabdomyosarcoma in other areas in the head and neck and includes wide local excision when possible, combined with radiation therapy and chemotherapy. Carcinomas, although they occur rarely in the nasal cavity, occur more frequently than do sarcomas of histologic types other than rhabdomyosarcoma. Treatment for carcinomas should be aggressive; in over 25 per cent of these patients, treatment can be successful if it is managed properly.

The diagnostic approach to all nasal, sinus, and nasopharyngeal malignancies is similar. In addition to biopsy confirmation of malignancy, tomography of the face in anterior, lateral, and basal projections will help to delineate the extent of disease. Computerized tomography for tumors in this area has become a very useful means of demonstrating both bone involvement and tumor extension.

The basic surgical approach to resectable disease in the nasal cavity is via a lateral rhinotomy. Tumors that involve the vault of the nasal cavity should not be considered unresectable, as the lateral rhinotomy may be combined with a frontal craniotomy to excise en bloc the roof of both ethmoid sinuses and cribriform plate, and may be extended posteriorly to include the anterior face of the sphenoid anterior to the optic chiasm. Tumors that arise in the posterior nasal septum may be excised by a transpalatal approach. Surgery for carcinoma should be combined with radiation therapy. Radiation therapy is less efficacious for sarcomas, but the addition of chemotherapy to the treatment regimen has now been demonstrated to be beneficial in the management of osteosarcomas and perhaps of chondrosarcomas as well.

TREATMENT OF SINUS NEOPLASMS

Benign and malignant neoplasms occur relatively less commonly in the sinuses than in the adjacent nasal and nasopharyngeal areas. Benign tumors most frequently involve the maxillary antrum and do so generally only after the age of six or eight when the maxillary sinus is fairly well developed. Special consideration must be given to developing teeth and bone growth centers in this area. When excising benign neoplasms, the developing tooth buds can usually be spared unless the tooth is involved in the neoplasm. Even if a developing tooth is exposed and bone is partially removed from around it, the tooth will usually develop and erupt. An anterior approach to the maxillary sinus avoids palatal growth centers as well as those located in the zygomatic process of the maxilla. Normal maxillary growth may be expected following Caldwell-Luc antrotomy at any age. More extensive surgery for aggressive benign disease or malignancy may necessarily interfere with growth centers. The most remarkable alteration in facial growth is noted following radiation therapy of 3000 R or more to the midface and skull base (Fig. 36–7). This may also affect the growth of the mandibular condyle so that late micrognathia may result.

Benign Tumors

The antral choanal polyp and dental-related benign diseases are the most frequently seen of the benign sinus masses. Treatment of antral choanal polyps has been previously discussed. The dentally related tumors may be either dentigerous or odontogenic in origin. They present as masses within or overlying the anterior maxilla. Sublabial removal of the bone and soft tissue cyst along with the involved tooth and local curettage of bone are usually curative. A detailed discussion of dental cysts is presented in Chapter 43.

The maxillary sinus retention cyst or mucocele may be discovered either as an expanding lesion in the area of the anterior maxilla (Fig. 36–8) or as an incidental finding on skull radiographs or sinus series taken for evaluation of headache or facial discomfort. Retention cysts that are asymptomatic and that do not obstruct the maxillary sinus ostia may not require treatment. They may, however, enlarge slowly to interfere with sinus physiology and should not be dismissed as invariably innocuous. The mucocele or large inclusion cyst may be evacuated either by a Caldwell-Luc antrotomy or through a nasoantral window. When a mucocele has been

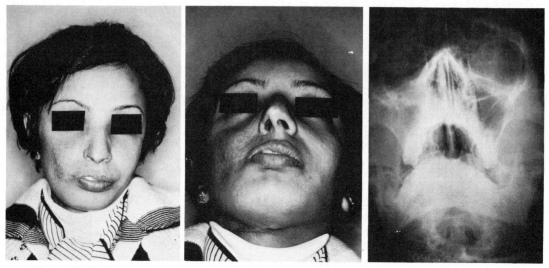

Figure 36–7 Facial asymmetry and malocclusion resulting as sequelae of radiation therapy for a maxillary sarcoma during childhood. Soft tissue atrophy of the irradiated midface and upper lip accentuate the flattening produced by lack of development of the lateral maxilla and zygomatic process. The chin appears to be rotated to the right and a cross bite is present because of incomplete growth of the right mandible.

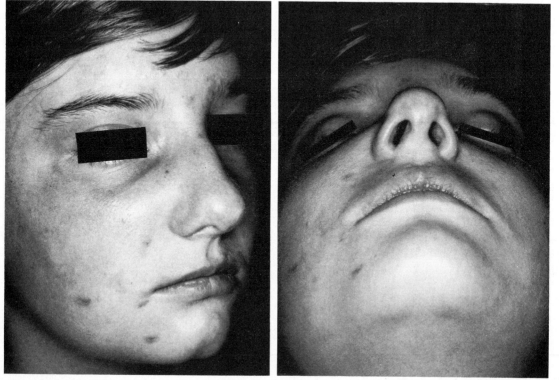

Figure 36–8 Expansion of the anterior maxilla produced by an inclusion cyst of the maxillary antrum simulating a fibro-osseous lesion.

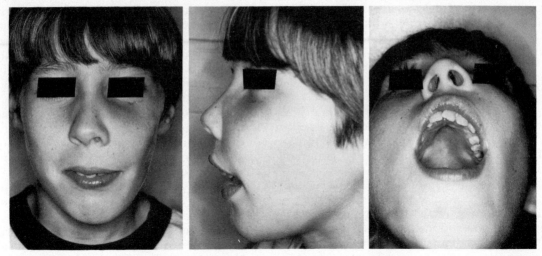

Figure 36–9 Fibrous dysplasia producing anterior, lateral, and palatal expansion of the maxilla.

removed, it is preferable to construct a permanent nasoantral window.

Fibro-osseous Lesions

The next most common and perhaps most important group of benign sinus neoplasms are the fibro-osseous lesions. Of these, fibrous dysplasia is relatively the most common. Patients with these lesions present with gradually progressive bony expansion of the anterior or lateral maxilla (Fig. 36–9). The ethmoid labyrinth may be primarily involved, and the antral cavity is frequently involved secondarily. The results of sinus radiography, polytomography (Fig. 36–10), and com-

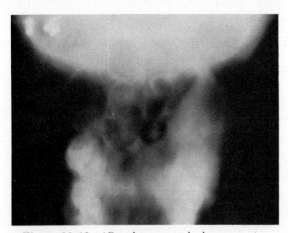

Figure 36–10 AP polytomograph demonstrating a radiodense mass of left maxilla ·enveloping erupted dentition and expanding with indistinct margins into the floor of the nose and palate. Fibrous dysplasia was confirmed histologically.

puterized tomography provide important information about the extent of the disease, which may be seen as a variably radiodense mass, but these examinations cannot distinguish one type of lesion from another. It is important to distinguish fibrous dysplasia, ossifying fibroma, cementifying fibroma, and giant cementoma pathologically, as the surgical treatment differs in each case.

Fibrous dysplasia is a clinically aggressive tumor that pathologically consists of fiber bone that persists as a maturation defect. The woven, immature bone pattern persists no matter how long the process has been present, and there is no maturation to lamellar bone. There is also no distinct junction between the pathologic process and surrounding bone, and the lesion thus cannot be treated by limited local excision, which would allow restoration of facial contour, and continued growth will require increasingly complicated excision. After pathologic confirmation of the diagnosis, patients with fibrous dysplasia should be managed by partial maxillectomy. This may be accomplished either through a sublabial incision or via a lateral rhinotomy.

The ossifying fibroma by contrast is a nonaggressive lesion that is well delineated microscopically, being made up of whirling masses of well-differentiated connective tissue with a variable amount of lamellar bone formation. When pathologic confirmation of the ossifying fibroma is obtained, local excision with a narrow margin of normal tissue is adequate treatment. The cementifying fibroma and giant cementoma are similar in clinical behavior to the ossifying fibroma and are treated in the same manner (Schmaman et al., 1970).

Giant Cell Granuloma

The giant cell reparative granuloma is a benign tumor that most frequently presents in the anterior maxillary area with symptoms of a gradually expanding mass and epiphora with secondary lacrimal infection. The lesion most frequently causes lacrimal obstruction initially and only later is identified as an expanding mass in the nose or premaxillary area. The lesion is contained within a bony capsule except in patients in whom cherubism, parathyroid osteopathy, and true giant cell tumors of long bones also exist. It is preferable to make a pathologic diagnosis prior to surgical excision of the mass.

Calcium and phosphorus levels should be obtained to rule out parathyroid disease, although hyperparathyroidism is rarely associated with this tumor in children. The surgical removal of this type of tumor generally includes sublabial local resection that avoids the developing dentition. Simultaneous cannulation of the superior and inferior lacrimal puncta with placement of Silastic tubes into the nasal lacrimal duct is suggested. Alternatively, for those patients who have had chronic lacrimal sac infections, a primary dacryocystorhinostomy may be performed. Deforming surgical excision need not be done, and the lesion usually becomes quiescent after an early, unpredictable clinical course.

Myxofibroma, Hemangioma

Myxofibromas and hemangiomas are the only other benign tumors that occur with any frequency in the paranasal sinus area. Both lesions must be confirmed pathologically and are best treated by wide local excision to reduce the incidence of the stubborn local recurrence that is otherwise noted (Canalis et al., 1976).

Sinus Malignancy

Primary sinus malignancy is quite uncommon in children. The sinuses may, however, be involved secondarily by tumors either in the nose or the nasopharynx. Of those lesions that do occur primarily in the sinuses, carcinomas and rhabdomyosarcomas occur with about equal frequency. Adenocarcinoma of minor salivary gland origin, osteogenic sarcoma, chondrosarcoma, fibrosarcoma, lymphoma, and undifferentiated malignancy may also be found.

Sinus malignancy in general has a characteristically rapid course. The initial symptoms of sinusitis are usually followed by expansion of facial contour, epiphora, epistaxis, and cranial nerve involvement, primarily of the trigeminal. Although the lesions are frequently not diagnosed until they are extensive, once a malignancy is suspected and is confirmed by the results of a biopsy, three general treatment approaches may be considered.

Some lesions of the sinus are resectable by a radical maxillectomy approach. Extension into the roof of the orbit and ethmoid should no longer preclude surgical excision, as combined craniofacial resection and radical maxillectomy may be possible. It should be noted that those patients who have had an epidermoid carcinoma or rhabdomyosarcoma removed with an adequate margin have a survival rate that is four to eight times as great as for those patients whose tumors' excision included a positive margin.

Radiation therapy and chemotherapy should be planned for nearly all patients with sinus malignancies. In the event that the disease is not locally resectable, drainage of the sinus through a Caldwell-Luc or nasoantral window approach is beneficial for evacuation of necrotic tumor and secondary infection. Even in those patients whose tumors are not locally resectable, a 10 per cent cure rate is possible through treatment that combines radiation therapy and chemotherapy.

TREATMENT OF NASOPHARYNGEAL TUMORS

Angiofibromas are the most commonly seen benign tumors occurring in the area of the nasopharynx. In fact, they are more common than the combined frequency of all other benign tumors of the nasopharynx. Excluding angiofibromas and nasopharyngeal malignancies, most tumors of the nasopharynx present as sessile or polypoid submucosal masses. Nasopharyngeal dermoid cysts and teratomas are the second most common benign tumors; they are usually recognized in infancy. Fibrous dysplasia, hemangiomas, gliomas, chondromas, and chordomas also may occur in the nasopharynx. Most of these lesions are treated by transoral or transpalatal local excision.

Nasopharyngeal Angiofibroma

The nasopharyngeal angiofibroma is a well-known tumor that occurs almost exclusively in males, most frequently during the pubescent or prepubescent years. The etiology of this benign tumor is unknown, although it nearly always arises in the area of the basisphenoid. Most patients present with a history of progressive nasal obstruction, and more than half have significant epistaxis. Clinically, the mass appears as a firm, grayish, mucosa-covered or friable, granular mass in the nasopharynx. Orbital involvement produces proptosis, and extension of the tumor through the pterygomaxillary fissure may produce swelling in the gingivobuccal sulcus or cheek.

Diagnosis of angiofibroma is most efficiently accomplished radiographically. Very few lesions in the nasopharynx produce the same radiographic pattern as the angiofibroma. Anterior bowing of the posterior maxillary wall and widening of the pterygomaxillary fissure when present suggest that the mass expanded slowly. Angiography demonstrates a vascular mass with a consistent pattern and feeding vessels, including the internal maxillary and ascending pharyngeal arteries (Fig. 36–11). Sessions and coworkers (1976) have compiled an excellent review of the radiographic characteristics of angiofibromas. It is desirable to obtain a biopsy specimen from an angiofibroma only if there is a question as to whether the lesion is benign or when a diagnosis is desired prior to referral of the patient for definitive therapy. Biopsy specimens, when obtained, should be removed in the operating room, where potentially brisk bleeding may be controlled.

Management of Angiofibromas

By far the most important step in the management of the angiofibroma is exact localization of the tumor. Retrograde carotid angiography with subtraction technique will usually define the extent of the lesion. It can be anticipated that many of the angiofibromas will involve the sphenoid sinus, the posterior nasal cavity, maxillary sinus, and pterygomaxillary space. Between 4 and 20 per cent of angiofibromas are reported to have extended intracranially (Ward et al., 1974); the patient must be evaluated with this in mind preoperatively. Embolization of the tumor via its main feeding arteries may be accomplished at the time of diagnostic angiography and can result in nearly complete obstruction of blood flow into the tumor (Fig. 36–11).

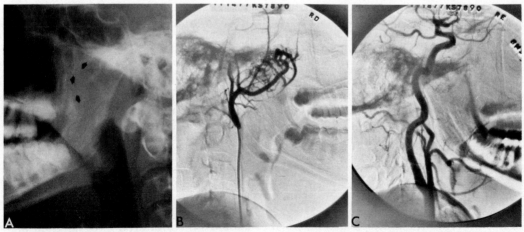

Figure 36–11 Nasopharyngeal angiofibroma. *A*, Soft tissue mass with distinct polypoid inferior margin producing anterior bowing of the posterior maxilla and pterygoid plates (arrows). *B*, External carotid angiogram with subtraction technique. Note the vascular mass without sphenoid sinus extension supplied primarily by the internal maxillary artery. *C*, Arteriogram following Gelfoam embolization and occlusion of the internal maxillary and ascending pharyngeal arteries (subtraction technique) with tumor stain no longer present.

When embolization is done with Gelfoam or blood clot emboli, bleeding at the time of surgical excision is minimized if surgery is carried out within a few days of angiography.

The extent and location of a nasopharyngeal angiofibroma can also be documented by computerized axial tomography (CAT). The routing CAT scan can demonstrate bone expansion or erosion and intracranial extension of the tumor. When intravenous contrast material is used to give vascular enhancement, the angiofibroma is noted to be highly vascular. A definitive diagnosis cannot be made at present by computerized tomography.

Treatment of Angiofibromas

Treatment of angiofibromas has been primarily surgical. With complete excision, recurrence of disease in up to 50 per cent of patients was common prior to the time when the full extent of the tumor could be defined preoperatively by radiographic examination. The treatment of choice at present is surgical excision, with radiation therapy or estrogen therapy reserved for those rare lesions that are unresectable. As yet, embolization alone has not been shown to be as reliable a treatment as excision. To provide the best chance for the patient's survival, excision should be performed only under conditions that will allow the use of angiography with embolization, evaluation by computerized tomography, management by experienced surgical and anesthesia teams, and, frequently, the support of neurosurgical consultation. Thus, it is suggested that most angiofibromas be treated in major surgical centers.

A plan for the surgical excision of an angiofibroma must be based on the knowledge of the exact extent of the tumor. There is presently no place for the snare and pack technique. Excision of the tumor must be done with an adequate margin of normal tissue to prevent local recurrence. The primary approach to the tumor is through a transoral, transpalatal route. The palatal push-back technique is preferred so that the posterior aspect of the bony palate and nasal septum may be removed. The vessels of the palatine foramen can be mobilized to gain wide exposure of the nasopharynx. If preoperative embolization has been utilized, temporary ligation of the external carotid system is generally unnecessary.

After adequate exposure of the lesion is accomplished, the anesthesiologist should prepare for rapid, large-volume blood replacement. Then, a circumferential excision should be completed, beginning over the clivus and extending along the preclivus and prevertebral fascia. If the tumor is not limited to the nasopharynx, as is commonly the case, then the transpalatal approach must be combined with a gingivobuccal incision with an extension around the maxillary tuberosity to provide access to the pterygomaxillary space, with a transpalatal, transseptal sphenoid approach for control of sphenoid sinus disease, or occasionally with a lateral rhinotomy or Caldwell-Luc approach for extension of the tumor into the posterior maxillary sinus or pterygomaxillary space. Massive pterygomaxillary or infratemporal fossa extension should be approached through a neck incision with elevation of the masseter muscle off of the mandible and removal of the coronoid process. Nasopharyngeal packing should be placed temporarily or for several days, depending on the amount of bleeding following excision.

Tumors that have extended intracranially should rarely be considered to be unresectable. Disease that extends superiorly through the sphenoid sinus is found in the anterior cranial fossa between the optic nerves. This area may be reached easily by a frontal craniotomy, although this approach may require division of the olfactory nerves. When the tumor mass has extended laterally into the cranial cavity, it has usually come from the nasopharynx through the superior orbital fissure lateral to the optic nerve, and this area can be visualized by frontolateral craniotomy. Vessels communicating with the tumor from the dura must be ligated; the tumor may thus be mobilized intracranially and removed as previously described by combined craniofacial resection.

With the advent of better techniques for surgical excision of such tumors, other methods of treatment will be less frequently utilized. Estrogen therapy has, at present, limited value, although it may decrease the symptomatic bleeding from these tumors. Radiation as a primary treatment modality should be considered experimental at present; relatively low-dose radiation therapy has been demonstrated to reduce the vascularity and size of angiofibromas (Briant et al, 1970; Fitzpatrick et al., 1980), but the potential for later development of osteoradionecrosis, delayed or abnormal bone growth, or late malignant transformation or malignant induction are contraindications to its use in the treatment of this benign disease (Batsakis et al., 1955). Further, the possible late development of malignancy of the thyroid or salivary glands from the low-dose radiation beyond the site of primary radiation has not been considered, though the association is known in patients who have had tonsil and adenoid radiation.

The relative frequency of occurrence of nasopharyngeal malignancy has been underestimated. In the series of 145 patients with nasopharyngeal tumors studied at the Armed Forces Institute of Pathology and the University of Pittsburgh, malignancy was found to occur slightly less commonly than benign disease in the nasopharynx even when angiofibromas were included among the benign diseases (67 malignant, 78 benign). Although the most common malignancy is the rhabdomyosarcoma, carcinomas occur almost as frequently. Lymphoma occurred in only 9 per cent of patients studied. Symptoms of nasal obstruction, hearing loss from middle ear effusion, and cervical lymphadenopathy appear as early symptoms of these lesions but are overlooked because of the common nature of these complaints. It is not until increasing pain, persistent bleeding, rapidly enlarging cervical masses, trismus, or central nervous system or cranial nerve complications occur that the malignant lesion is recognized (Fig. 36–12).

At this time the options for therapy are few and hope for survival is slight when a nasopharyngeal malignancy is diagnosed. Two factors may, however, improve this previously dismal outlook. It is presently possible to document quite exactly the extent of tumors in the nasopharynx by computerized tomography. With more precise definition of tumor location, radiation therapy may be more carefully planned and the frequency of incomplete destruction of tumor extensions may be minimized. In addition, chemotherapy, par-

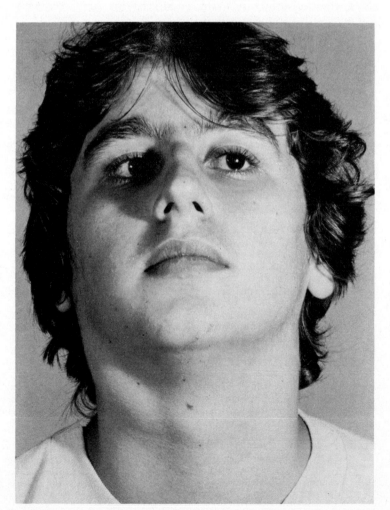

Figure 36–12 Right sixth cranial nerve paralysis and rapidly expanding right cervical mass resulting from undifferentiated nasopharyngeal carcinoma.

ticularly for rhabdomyosarcomas, is constantly improving.

The prognosis for the patient with a nasopharyngeal malignancy depends on the extent of the primary lesion and on the presence or possible presence of regional or distant metastasis. The tumor histology becomes important only when it becomes necessary to choose a chemotherapeutic agent or agents to be used in conjunction with radiation therapy. Virtually all these lesions may metastasize regionally or systemically. Radiation therapy for the primary site and the areas of lymphatic drainage in both sides of the neck is the standard treatment modality. Most patients who die of disease have systemic metastasis at the time of death, often without evidence of local disease (Straka and Bluestone, 1972; Fernandez et al., 1976). A treatment plan should be considered for all patients. Patients with rhabdomyosarcomas have shown improved survival rates when treated with radiation therapy and multiple-drug chemotherapy (Canalis et al., 1978). Patients with carcinomas that involve cranial nerves or the skull base or that extend into the pterygomaxillary fossa have a higher incidence of local recurrence and distant metastasis. Induction and postradiation maintenance chemotherapy is recommended at present for these advanced carcinomas.

REFERENCES

Batsakis, J. G., Klopp, C. T., and Newman, W. 1955. Fibrosarcoma arising in a "juvenile" nasopharyngeal angiofibroma following extensive radiation therapy. Am. Surg., 21:786–793.

Briant, T. D. R., Fitzpatrick, P. J., and Book, H. 1970. The radiological treatment of juvenile nasopharyngeal angiofibroma. Laryngoscope, 86(3):364–372.

Canalis, R. F., Smith, G. A., and Konrad, H. R. 1976. Myxomas of the head and neck. Arch. Otolaryngol., 102:300–305.

Canalis, R. F., Jenkins, H. A., Hemenway, W. G., et al. 1978. Nasopharyngeal and rhabdomyosarcoma. Arch. Otolaryngol., 104(3):122–126.

Dehner, L. P. 1973a. Tumors of the mandible and maxilla in children. Cancer, 31:364–384.

Dehner, L. P. 1973b. Tumors of the mandible and maxilla in children. II. A study of 141 primary and secondary malignant tumors. Cancer, 32:112–120.

Fernandez, C. H., Cangir, A., Samaan, N. A., and Rivera, R. 1976. Nasopharyngeal carcinoma in children. Cancer, 37:2787–2791.

Fitzpatrick, P. J., Briant, T. D. R., and Berman, J. M. 1980. The nasopharyngeal angiofibroma. Arch. Otolaryngol., 103(4):234–236.

Fu, Y. S., and Perzin, K. H. 1974a. Non-epithelial tumors of the nasal cavity, paranasal sinuses, and nasopharynx. A clinicopathologic study. I. General features and vascular tumors. Cancer, 33:1275–1288.

Fu, Y. S., and Perzin, K. H. 1974b. Non-epithelial tumors of the nasal cavity, paranasal sinuses, and nasopharynx. A clinicopathologic study. II. Osseous and fibro-osseous lesions, including osteoma, fibrous dysplasia, ossifying fibroma, osteoblastoma, giant cell tumor, and osteosarcoma. Cancer, 33:1289–1305.

Fu, Y. S., and Perzin, K. H. 1974c. Non-epithelial tumors of the nasal cavity, paranasal sinuses, and nasopharynx. A clinicopathologic study. III. Cartilaginous tumors (chondroma, chondrosarcoma). Cancer, 34:453–463.

Fu, Y. S., and Perzin, K. H. 1975. Non-epithelial tumors of the nasal cavity, paranasal sinuses, and nasopharynx. A clinicopathologic study. IV. Smooth muscle tumors (leiomyoma, leiomyosarcoma). Cancer, 35(5):1300–1308.

Fu, Y. S., and Perzin, K. H. 1976a. Non-epithelial tumors of the nasal cavity, paranasal sinuses, and nasopharynx. A clinicopathologic study. V. Skeletal muscle tumors (rhabdomyoma and rhabdomyosarcoma). Cancer, 37(1):364–376.

Fu, Y. S., and Perzin, K. H. 1976b. Non-epithelial tumors of the nasal cavity, paranasal sinuses, and nasopharynx. A clinicopathologic study. VI. Fibrous tissue tumors (fibroma, fibromatosis, fibrosarcoma). Cancer, 37(6):2912–2928.

Fu, Y. S., and Perzin, K. H. 1977a. Non-epithelial tumors of the nasal cavity, paranasal sinuses, and nasopharynx. A clinicopathologic study. VII. Myxomas. Cancer, 38(1):195–203.

Fu, Y. S., and Perzin, K. H. 1977b. Non-epithelial tumors of the nasal cavity, paranasal sinuses, and nasopharynx. A clinicopathologic study. VIII. Adipose tissue tumors (lipoma and liposarcoma). Cancer, 40(3):1314–1317.

Jaffe, B. F., Strome, M., Khaw, K. T., et al. 1977. Nasal polypectomy and sinus surgery for cystic fibrosis. A 10 year review. Symposium on Pediatric Otorhinolaryngology, Otolaryngol. Clin. North Am., 10(1):81–90.

Mygind, N., Pederson, C. B., Prytz, S., et al. 1975. Treatment of nasal polyps with intranasal beclomethasone dipropionate aerosol. Clin. Allergy, 5:159–164.

Schmaman, A., Smith, I., and Ackerman, L. V. 1970. Benign fibroosseous lesions of the mandible and maxilla. Cancer, 26:303–312.

Schramm, V. L., and Myers, E. N. 1978. Lateral rhinotomy. Laryngoscope, 88(6):1942–1045.

Schramm, V. L., Naroon, J., and Myers, E. N. 1979. Anterior skull base surgery for benign and malignant disease. Laryngoscope, 89(7):1077–1091.

Schramm, V. L. 1979. Inflammatory and neoplastic masses of the nose and paranasal sinuses in children. Laryngoscope, 89(12):1887–1897.

Sessions, R. B., Wills, P. I., Alford, B. R., et al. 1976. Juvenile nasopharyngeal angiofibroma: Radiographic aspects. Laryngoscope, 86:2–18.

Straka, J. A., and Bluestone, C. D. 1972. Nasopharyngeal malignancies in children. Laryngoscope, 82:807–816.

Ward, P. H., Thompson, R., Calcaterra, T., et al. 1974. Juvenile angiofibroma. A more rational therapeutic approach based upon clinical and experimental evidence. Laryngoscope, 84:2181–2194.

Chapter 37

ALLERGIC RHINITIS

Philip Fireman, M.D.

INTRODUCTION

Allergic rhinitis is the most common of all the allergic disorders, affecting over 20 million people in the United States. Because it is not a fatal disease and its symptoms may not be incapacitating, allergic rhinitis may at times be slighted or ignored by the surgical and medical community. Yet this frequent illness causes significant morbidity, which results in the expenditure of many millions of dollars in health care and the loss of millions of working and school days. Allergic rhinitis has a familial tendency and is induced by exposure to antigenic environmental factors, called allergens, with resultant sneezing, nasal pruritus, watery rhinorrhea, nasal mucosal edema, and subsequent nasal obstruction. The symptoms can be episodic or perennial; when symptoms recur annually during certain months, the syndrome is called seasonal allergic rhinitis. Typically, seasonal allergic rhinitis does not develop until after the patient has been sensitized by two or more pollen seasons. Seasonal allergic rhinitis is frequently referred to as "hay fever" or a "summer cold." These descriptive terms are misleading and should be discarded because fever is not a symptom associated with allergic rhinitis and neither hay nor the common cold virus is incriminated in the etiology of this syndrome.

The prevalence of allergic rhinitis in the general population is considered to be about 10 per cent, with the peak incidence in the postadolescent teenage child. Broder et al. (1974), in a study of a well-defined population in Tecumseh, Michigan, found the prevalence of allergic rhinitis to increase during childhood from less than one per cent during infancy, to a prevalence of 4 to 5 per cent from ages 5 to 9 years, to 9 per cent during adolescence, and 15 to 16 percent after adolescence. The prevalence of allergic rhinitis remains constant in the young adult but gradually declines during the middle years and in the elderly. Even though seasonal allergic rhinitis is infrequent in the very young child, perennial allergic rhinitis has been recognized in infancy and even in the neonate (Ingall et al., 1965). For reasons that are not clear, more male than female children are affected with allergic rhinitis prior to adolescence, whereas females are more often affected with nasal allergy after adolescence. Race and socioeconomic factors are not thought to be important factors in the expression of allergic rhinitis. The Tecumseh study also showed seasonal allergic rhinitis to be almost twice as common as perennial allergic rhinitis (Broder et al., 1974).

Even though syndromes identical to what we now classify as allergic rhinitis have been described for centuries, the concept of an immunologic pathogenesis dates to the beginning of the 20th century. At first, allergy diagnosis and therapy developed empirically, because the criteria for documentation of allergic disease and allergen–antibody interaction were difficult to quantify and were mostly subjective. The past 15 years have seen many advances in the elucidation of immunologic phenomena and have enabled the clinician to understand allergic diseases better. These discoveries have had considerable impact on the clinical practice of allergy and have provided a more scientific basis for many of the diagnostic and therapeutic procedures that developed without well-controlled documentation of efficacy over the past 50 years.

It is necessary to define the terms used by the allergist because the manner in which the words "immunology," "immunity," "allergy," "hypersensitivity," and "atopy" are used, and at times abused, indicates confusion as to their meaning. Medical dictionaries define *immunology* as the study of an antigen–antibody interaction which induces *immunity* and implies a beneficial protective response induced by the specific antigen. This definition of immunity is appropriate for the study of infectious diseases because the body will develop serum antibodies and sensitized lymphocytes to control the infectious agents upon reexposure; however, it is not appropriate to use this limited definition of immunity to describe the response to noninfectious environmental factors such as pollens, animal danders, and drugs. As used in this chapter, immunology will mean the study of antigens, antibodies, and their interaction, whether beneficial or not.

The term *allergy* was introduced by a pediatrician, Clemens von Pirquet, in 1906 to designate the host's altered reactivity to an antigen (allergen) that develops after previous experience with the same material; the end result could be helpful or harmful to the host (von Pirquet, 1906). This all-inclusive immunologic concept of allergy has been recently popularized by Coombs and Gell (1975) and may have merit in permitting an organized and systematic approach to understanding the pathogenesis of immune mechanisms. Nevertheless, the terms *allergy* or *allergic* as commonly used in clinical practice indicate an adverse reaction, and allergic rhinitis is best defined as that adverse pathophysiologic response of the nose and adjacent organs that results from the interaction of allergen with antibody in a host sensitized by prior exposure to that allergen. This immunologic definition of allergic rhinitis is accepted by most but not all clinical allergists and otolaryngologists because nonimmune processes can, on occasion, participate as additional contributory factors in the clinical expression of allergic diseases. *Hypersensitivity* indicates a heightened or exaggerated immune response that develops after more than one exposure to an allergen. Hypersensitivity will be considered synonymous with allergy. The terms *atopy* or *atopic* are also frequently used by allergists. These terms were introduced by Coca and Cooke in 1923 to classify those allergic diseases such as allergic rhinitis, asthma, and infantile eczema (atopic dermatitis) that had a familial predilection and implied genetic predisposition (Coca and Cooke, 1923). Other allergic diseases, such as contact dermatitis (poison ivy) or serum sickness, have no familial tendency and are referred to as nonatopic. It was also recognized that serum from these atopic individuals contained a factor identified as a reagin or skin-sensitizing antibody. This serum factor had the capacity to sensitize passively the skin of a nonsensitive individual, and after intradermal challenge of the passively sensitized skin site with specific allergen a wheal and flare reaction developed within 20 minutes. This passive transfer test, also known as the Prausnitz-Kustner test or PK test, had been described only several years earlier and was the first documentation of the specific serum and tissue antibody important in the pathogenesis of allergic diseases (Prausnitz and Kustner, 1921). As will be discussed later, more than 90 per cent of these reaginic antibodies are of the IgE immunoglobulin class (Yunginger and Gleich, 1975). Even though some allergists and clinical immunologists, including this author, frequently use the term *atopic* to identify these allergic patients and their families, the term *atopy* has never gained universal acceptance.

ETIOLOGY

The development of allergic rhinitis requires two conditions: the atopic familial predisposition to develop allergy and exposure of the sensitized patient to the allergen. Patients are not born with allergies but do have the capacity to develop symptoms spontaneously through repeated exposure to allergens in their environment. Inhalants are the principal allergens responsible for allergic rhinitis and may be present outdoors and indoors. These microscopic airborne particles include the pollens from weeds, grasses, and trees, mold spores, animal danders and environmental dusts, either house or occupational (Solomon and Mathews, 1978). Seasonal allergic rhinitis is primarily induced by pollens from the germination of "nonflowering" vegetation. In the temperate climates, the most important are tree pollens in the spring, grass pollens in the late spring and early summer, and ragweed in the late summer and early fall. Since there is variation from one geographic area to another, it is necessary for each clinician to become familiar with the pollination patterns in his or her region. "Flowering" vegetation, such as roses and fruit blossoms, rarely causes allergic rhinitis because these pollens are too heavy to be airborne and germination is facilitated by the action of bees. In warm climates, mold spores may be airborne year round, but in climates in which snow and freezing occur in the winter months, airborne mold spores are present intermittently during the spring, summer, and fall until there is significant frost. In patients with perennial allergic rhinitis, mold spores may be a significant inhalant allergen indoors along with epidermal animal danders and dust. The principal allergen in house dust has not been identified but a portion may be due to the house dust mite, dermatophagoides (Voorhorst et al., 1967). Most allergens, including the pollens, have not been chemically characterized, and each consists of multiple antigenic determinants. Food allergens are of lesser importance in the etiology of allergic rhinitis but cannot be ignored, especially in young children (Johnstone, 1967). Patients can be sensitive to one or multiple allergens. Although it is a well-established fact that exposure to an allergen is necessary to develop sensitivity and symptoms, it is not known why allergic individuals with the same exposure become sensitive to certain allergens but not to others. The threshold of reactivity to each allergen varies greatly from one patient to another; certain individuals react to small antigenic challenges and others tolerate a large allergen dose before developing symptoms. In addition to allergens, other factors can contribute to the development of nasal symptoms. These include aerosolized cosmetics, cigarette smoke, industrial fumes, and changes in temperature, humidity, and barometric pressure (Brown and Ipsen, 1968). Psychologic and social stresses and anxiety can also induce nasal congestion (Wolf et al., 1950). The importance of these additional contributory factors varies greatly from patient to .patient and should not be neglected in patient management.

Even though it is not possible to predict accurately the potentially atopic patient, the familial nature of allergic rhinitis has been recognized for years and a positive family history of atopy has been noted in 50 to 75 per cent of allergic patients (Cohen, 1974). Despite several extensive retrospective family and twin studies, there is no agreement as to the hereditary pattern in atopic diseases. Most investigators feel that several genetic loci are involved in the expression of allergic disease and inheritance is multifactorial. Recent immunologic studies have isolated some of these genetic influences. Elevated serum levels of IgE are sometimes associated with certain allergic diseases and a recessive genetic influence has been suggested (Marsh et al., 1974). Animal studies have shown that synthesis of specific antibodies to well-characterized antigens is controlled in part by immune response (Ir) genes, which are linked to the major tissue histocompatibility locus (HLA). The studies by Levine and coworkers (1972) have suggested that ragweed allergic rhinitis and immune responses to purified ragweed antigen E were linked to a particular HLA haplotype in successive generations of allergic families. Marsh et al. (1973) reported a significant correlation between haplotype HL–A7 and increased IgE antibodies to a low molecular weight purified ragweek antigen (Ra5) in a group of allergic rhinitis patients sensitive to this small portion of the ragweed allergen. Similar studies of other purified allergens are indicated in allergic rhinitis patients because the responses to the more complex allergens, such as are used in clinical practice, may or may not be controlled by similar or different genetic influences.

IMMUNOPATHOPHYSIOLOGY

Allergic rhinitis, along with allergic asthma and allergic urticaria, are described immunologically as immediate hypersensitivity syndromes and are mediated in large part by immunoglobulin E (IgE) antibodies (Ishizaka et al., 1966). The properties of IgE as compared to the other serum and secretory immunoglobulins are shown in Table 37–1. IgE is normally present in minute quantities as compared to the serum immunoglobulins IgG, IgA, and IgM. Because of their ability to fix to primate tissues, IgE antibodies are called homocytotropic. Specific IgE antibodies have been demonstrated both in secretions and in sera. Unlike IgG, IgE antibodies do not cross the placenta, and the fetus will not be passively sensitized by maternal IgE antibodies, yet the fetus is capable of synthesizing IgE (Miller et al., 1973). The IgE antibodies are synthesized after allergen challenge in large part by plasma cells located in lymphoid tissues adjacent to mucosal membranes. These IgE antibodies passively sensitize the membranes of tissue mast cells and circulating blood basophils. The exact nature

Table 37–1 PROPERTIES OF HUMAN SERUM AND SECRETORY IMMUNOGLOBULINS

	IgG	IgA	S-IgA°	IgM	IgD	IgE
Adult serum concentration (mg/ml)	10	2	—	1.5	0.03	0.0002
Antibody activity	+	+	+	+	?	+
Neutralization (antiviral, antitoxin)	+	±	+	+	−	−
Anaphylactic (histamine release)	±	−	−	−	−	+
Blocking antibody	+	±(?)	±(?)	−	−	−
Maternal–fetal transfer	+	−	−	−	−	−
Present in secretions	±	+	++	−	−	+
Fix to mast cell (homocytotropic)	±°°	−	−	−	−	+
Classic complement activation	+	−	−	+	−	−
Alternate complement pathway	−	+	+	−	−	+

°S-IgA is secretory IgA
°°Subclass 4 IgG antibodies may fix to mast cells

of the binding of IgE to mast cell and basophil cell membranes is not known, but it involves the Fc portion of the IgE molecule and an appropriate receptor in the cell surface (Ishizaka et al., 1973). During this sensitization phase there is no apparent deleterious host reaction. Upon subsequent challenge, the allergen combines with its specific IgE antibody at the cell membrane of the sensitized tissue mast cell and blood basophil (see Fig. 37–1). The interaction of IgE antibodies and allergen at the mast cell membrane does not appear to be capable of activating the complement sequence by the classical pathway, but studies have suggested that IgE antibodies may initiate complement activation by the alternate pathway (Ishizaka, 1976).

The combination of allergen and IgE antibody results in a sequence of energy-dependent enzyme reactions with alteration of the mast cell membrane, which initiates the release and synthesis of the specific pharmacologic mediators of the IgE immediate hypersensitivity reaction. These mediators include histamine, the slow-reacting substance of anaphylaxis (SRS-A), eosinophil chemotactic factor (ECF-A), platelet aggregation factor (PAF), and other kinins and vasoactive substances. These mediators are listed in Figure 37–1; they cause the increased vascular permeability, local edema, and increased eosinophil-laden secretions seen in allergic rhinitis. This reaction occurs in seconds or minutes after exposure to the allergens, and there is no extensive tissue destruction or

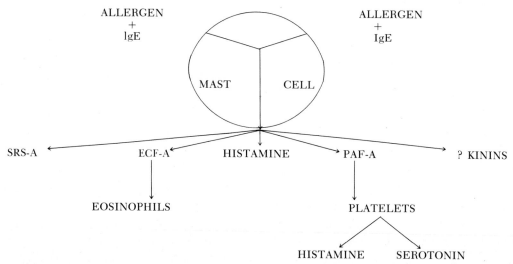

Figure 37–1 Diagrammatic representation of how allergen interaction with IgE antibody at mast cell surface initiates release of pharmacologic mediators of immediate hypersensitivity (allergic) reaction.

cytotoxicity. After mast cells go through a refractory period of several hours, the pharmacologic mediators of immediate hypersensitivity are resynthesized, and the mast cell will again be capable of responding to the specific allergen by release of its granules containing histamine and the other mediators. The tissue injury in this reaction can subside rapidly in minutes but may persist for hours or days depending upon the extent and duration of allergen exposure. Histamine from mast cells appears to be the principal chemical mediator in nasal allergy, and the mechanism by which it produces tissue edema is due to its ability to produce vasodilation and to increase capillary permeability (Riley and West, 1953). In addition, histamine and another vasoactive amino, serotonin, can be released from platelets that are aggregated by PAF from mast cells. The specific action of SRS-A in the pathophysiology of allergic rhinitis has yet to be demonstrated, even though SRS-A has been demonstrated in nasal polyp tissue (Kaliner et al., 1973). The function of the eosinophil that is attracted to nasal tissue by ECF-A has yet to be defined clearly. A regulatory or modulatory role for the eosinophil has been suggested because the enzymes histaminase and arylsulfatase, which effectively inactivate histamine and SRS-A, respectively, are more abundant in eosinophils than in other leukocytes (Wasserman et al., 1975). In addition, phospholipase, which inactivates PAF released from mast cells, is located primarily in the eosinophil. These mediators have a direct action on the vascular bed of the nose, and the edema and congestion of the nasal tissues can disturb the balance of autonomic nervous control of nasal functions. Since patients with allergic disease overreact to cholinergic stimuli, it may be that vascular dilatation and hypersecretion are aggravated by the disturbance and resulting imbalance of autonomic control. Other *in vitro* studies suggest that the inhibition of mediator release is promoted by those situations that will increase intracellular cyclic AMP (Orange et al., 1971). It has been noted that adrenergic agents, especially the more selective β-adrenergic agents, will increase intracellular cyclic AMP and thereby inhibit histamine release. This biochemical action may be the basis for the pharmacologic benefit of adrenergic agents. Cyclic AMP is normally catabolized by phosphodiesterase, and phosphodiesterase inhibitors may inhibit histamine release. Calcium and magnesium appear to be essential for the *in vitro* release of the histamine by the specific allergen from sensitized basophils (Lichtenstein and Osler, 1964). The immunologic effectors of the immediate hypersensitivity allergic reaction have been shown to be IgE antibodies in most situations; but it should be emphasized that it is the mediators, such as histamine, SRS-A, and ECF-A, that are responsible for the pathophysiology of the immediate hypersensitivity reaction.

Histologic examination of the nasal mucosa will demonstrate distended goblet cells in the presence of enlarged, congested mucous glands. The tissues are infiltrated with eosinophils and lymphoid cells with a paucity of neutrophils. The intracellular spaces are enlarged and the basement membrane is thickened. Mast cells are also present in the mucosal tissues, but the significance of their relative numbers has not been defined. Bryan and Bryan (1969) reported increased mast cells proportional to the severity of nasal allergy, but on the other hand, Connell (1969a) found increased mast cells in nonspecific and vasomotor rhinitis without any evidence of allergy. At the present time it appears that the number of mast cells cannot be utilized in discriminating the pathologic features of different types of rhinitis. The ground substance surrounding the cells and blood vessels changes during allergic rhinitis from its normal semisolid to a relatively fluid state (Rappaport et al., 1953). This change may account for the boggy appearance of the nasal mucosa frequently seen in allergic rhinitis.

Allergic rhinitis adversely affects nasal function which, besides the role as an airway, includes filtration of particulate matter from inspired air, humidification of air, olfaction, and phonation. Several investigators have developed methods for measuring nasal airway resistance in order to understand better the pathophysiology of allergic rhinitis. It has been shown that posture can affect airway resistance since the supine position was found to increase nasal resistance in allergic rhinitis threefold over that experienced in a sitting position (Rundcrantz, 1969). Exercise and increased activity can also temporarily reverse the nasal obstruction seen in allergic rhinitis (Richerson and Seebohn, 1968). These effects may contribute to the patient's interpretation of increased symptoms when in bed, due not only to allergenic contents of the furniture but also to the change in posture and activity. Using airway resistance studies and quantitative pollen challenges, Connell (1969b) has shown that a larger dose of allergen was required to increase resistance in the nasal mucosa that had remained unchallenged than was required to obtain the same effect after a week of daily exposures. He also demonstrated, in patients sensitized to several pollens, that repeated challenges with one allergen conditioned the nasal mucosa to react to a lower dose of the second allergen than would have been needed if given singly. This priming phenomenon could well account for the persistence of symptoms experienced in many patients towards the end of the pollen season in spite of decreased allergen exposure. It is also thought that this priming effect favors an increase in responsiveness to the nonspecific stimuli such as changes in humidity and temperature. It has been suggested that a defect exists in the nasal mucous membrane in patients with allergic rhinitis that permits inhaled allergen macromolecules an easier access to the immune recognition system than in nonatopic subjects. Salvaggio et al. (1964) found atopic subjects to have increased permeability to specific allergens instilled in the nose, but other more recent studies were unable to detect any differences in permeability between atopic and nonatopic subjects (Konton-Karakitsos et al., 1975).

SYMPTOMS AND SIGNS

Initial symptoms in seasonal allergic rhinitis progress from frequent sneezing and nasal pruritus to rhinorrhea and finally to nasal obstruction. Patients with perennial allergic rhinitis have more nasal stuffiness and obstruction than sneezing and pruritus. These symptoms not only vary considerably from season to season but also differ markedly at various times of night and day. Patients will complain of early morning and late evening symptoms, and sleep can frequently be interrupted because of nasal obstruction. Patients complain of not only nasal pruritus but also itching of the eyes, throat, and ears. Many children will constantly rub the nose with the hand or arm in an effort to relieve the nasal itch and perhaps to improve the nasal obstruction. Other children may press the palm of the hand upwards against the nose in an "allergic salute." Constant rubbing of the

nose often leads to the development of a transverse nasal crease, a horizontal groove across the lower third of the nose.

With nasal obstruction the patient will be a constant mouth breather and snoring will be a prominent nighttime symptom. It has been suggested that constant mouth breathing may contribute to the development of orofacial dental abnormalities requiring orthodontic procedures, but this has not been established definitively. Seasonal allergic rhinitis is frequently accompanied by allergic conjunctivitis with lacrimation, bilateral ocular pruritus, bilateral watery ocular secretions, and photophobia. Symptoms involving the adjacent sinuses may also be evident, especially maxillary discomfort or headaches when the symptoms of nasal obstruction are severe. In patients with eustachian tube dysfunction, allergic rhinitis may contribute to the development of serous otitis media. Loss of sense of smell and taste may also be described. Patients may also complain of generalized malaise, irritability, and fatigue; these symptoms are often difficult to differentiate from the side effects of the frequently used antihistamine therapy. Patients with seasonal pollinosis will describe a gradual increase in the severity of symptoms as the season progresses, especially on dry, windy days. At times, patients will relate a history of continuation of the symptoms beyond the pollen season, and many clinicians feel that repeated exposure to allergens increases the reactivity of the nasal mucosa so that ordinarily inocuous allergens and environmental factors can produce symptoms. The pattern of the patient's symptoms will frequently distinguish those with seasonal from those with perennial allergic rhinitis, especially in temperate climates with obvious seasonal climatic changes. In the warmer subtropical climates the seasonal pollen pattern may not be obvious, since the grass pollen season extends over many months and mold spores can remain in the air throughout the year. In much of the United States trees will pollinate in the spring, primarily in March and April; grasses in late spring and summer, especially May, June, and July; and ragweed during the last two weeks of August until the first frost. The southwest United States was traditionally pollen free, but the advent of irrigation and increased vegetation has changed that clinical impression. Ragweed tends to grow at the edges of cultivated fields and along highways and tends to cause increased symptoms during automobile trips. Even though airborne pollens spread for miles, increased concentrations of pollens are noted in areas of high plant density, and patients frequently complain of more symptoms in areas of high pollen density. If there is direct contact with a substantial quantity of pollen, patients may have very significant symptoms including angioedema, especially of the eyes, and on occasion, urticaria.

As mentioned earlier, ingested foods are rarely the cause of allergic rhinitis in the young child. It behooves the clinician to take a very careful environmental history and survey in all patients who complain of intermittent or year-round symptoms that do not fit the usual seasonal pattern outlined above. In general, these patients with year-round symptoms are much more of a diagnostic challenge than those with only intermittent complaints. The almost continuous exposure to house or industrial factors may induce perennial symptoms because congestion of the mucosal tissues may not have the opportunity to subside or return to normal during the few hours free of allergen exposure. It is also in these patients that the nonallergenic environmental factors tend to contribute to the symptomatology: these additional nonallergenic factors include changes in barometric pressure, temperature, and humidity and aerosolized irritants such as cigarette smoke, automobile fumes, industrial pollutants, and aerosolized cosmetics and drugs.

With development of the allergic reaction, clear nasal secretions will be evident, and the nasal mucous membranes will become edematous without much erythema. The mucosa appears boggy and blue-gray. With continued exposure to the allergen, the turbinates will appear to be not only congested but also swollen, and they will obstruct the nasal airway. If nasal obstruction is present, it may be necessary to shrink the mucosa with a vasoconstrictor to document the absence of nasal polyps, which are relatively uncommon in allergic rhinitis, occurring in less than 0.5 per cent of patients (Caplin et al., 1971). Conjunctival edema and hyperemia are frequent findings in patients with associated conjunctivitis. Allergic rhinitis patients with significant nasal obstruction and venous congestion, particularly children, may also demonstrate edema and darkening of the tissues beneath the eyes. These so-called "allergic shiners"

are not pathognomonic for allergic rhinitis; they also can be seen in patients with recurrent nasal congestion and venous stasis of any other cause. The conjunctiva may also demonstrate a lymphoid follicular pattern with a cobblestone appearance. Pallor of the palatine and pharyngeal tissues is also evident, and on occasion small follicular lymphoid hyperplasia is evident on the posterior pharyngeal surface without regional cervical lymphadenopathy or tonsillar hypertrophy. Purulent secretions are only seen in the presence of secondary infections.

LABORATORY STUDIES

The nasal secretions of patients with allergic rhinitis usually contain increased numbers of eosinophils. Eosinophilia may not be present in patients not recently exposed to specific allergens or in the presence of a superimposed infection. Steroids can significantly reduce eosinophilia, but antihistamine therapy has no significant effect on nasal eosinophils. The usefulness of nasal eosinophilia is, in large part, dependent upon the technique used to obtain the specimens and preparation of the slides for examination. It is difficult to quantify nasal eosinophilia accurately, and more than 3 per cent eosinophils seen on a nasal smear is considered an increase. Bryan and Bryan (1969) have noted that mast cells can also be observed in nasal secretions obtained by swabbing and abrading the posterior nasal mucosa, but this procedure is not practical in most pediatric patients. Infection is usually evidenced by a predominance of polymorphonuclear leukocytes on the nasal smear. Although several methods of measuring nasal airway resistance have been developed in the past few years, the diagnostic usefulness of quantifying this parameter in children is yet to be established and documented.

Laboratory confirmation of specific IgE antibody synthesis to specific allergens is not mandatory in every patient with seasonal allergic rhinitis. These laboratory tests should be reserved for those patients in which the presence of a seasonal pattern is not clear-cut. In certain patients it may be helpful to confirm the clinical impression with documentation of specific IgE antibodies by *in vivo* skin testing or *in vitro* serum radioimmunoassay (RAST) testing in order to reinforce the importance of environmental control. Skin testing with the suspected allergens is mandatory in all patients prior to initiation of immunotherapy with allergy extracts because the intensity of the local wheal and flare skin reaction will be utilized as a guide in determining the initial dose of allergen. Clinicians should be selective in the use of allergens for skin testing and should employ only *common* allergens of potential clinical importance in their patient. The most useful allergens in the study of allergic rhinitis are the pollens, molds, house dust, and epidermal danders. Allergens used for skin testing should be selected on the basis of prevalence in the patient's area of the country and the environment in which he or she lives and works.

There is no need to test for allergy to foods in patients with clear-cut seasonal allergic rhinitis; food testing should be reserved for those patients who are diagnostic problems, with intermittent or perennial symptomatology. The major problems with skin testing, especially for food allergens, have been the lack of potency, stability, and purity of the allergen solutions. The crude, undefined composition of allergens often produces false-positive reactions secondary to an irritating effect on the skin. It is well known that great care must be used in interpreting the results of food skin testing because there is often a discrepancy between the production of clinical symptoms and positive skin reactions to foods. If allergy testing is indicated, there is no need to test with a multitude of allergens. To avoid false-negative skin tests, antihistamine and adrenergic drugs should be withheld for 12 to 24 hours before skin tests are performed. Prick skin testing may be more reliable than intradermal skin testing; the specifics of such testing are outlined in standard allergy textbooks (Norman, 1978). As mentioned earlier, the *in vitro* allergosor-

bent radioimmunoassay (RAST) test for assessing the presence of serum IgE antibodies to various allergens has recently been employed as a diagnostic aid in allergic rhinitis. For certain allergens, this test has been shown to be as reliable as skin tests; however, its cost has been its major disadvantage. Table 37–2 compares the usefulness of skin testing as compared to RAST testing. On occasion, a nasal provocation test is useful in assessing a skin-test negative patient who is suspected of reacting to a particular allergen because of the recent observations that IgE antibodies may be present in nasal secretions but not evident by skin testing or the presence of serum IgE antibodies (Huggins and Brostoff, 1975). Provocation testing is performed by introducing the allergen into the nostril after its suspension or dilution in saline. A positive reaction is manifested by local pruritus, sneezing, and watery rhinorrhea and edema. It is always necessary to place a diluent control in the opposite nostril for comparison. The sublingual challenge with allergen is not a useful diagnostic tool for allergic rhinitis, in the opinion of this author. The *in vitro* cytotoxic leukocyte test with foods and other allergens has been advocated by some, but its usefulness as a laboratory test has not been confirmed in controlled studies by other investigators (Lieberman et al., 1974).

DIFFERENTIAL DIAGNOSIS

Children who present to the clinician with complaints of rhinorrhea and nasal obstruction may have symptoms not only of allergy but also of infections, foreign bodies, structural changes, drug reactions, or neoplasms. Nasal infections are usually characterized by burning and redness of the nasal mucosa and a purulent discharge. Without a doubt, the

Table 37–2 COMPARISON OF SKIN TESTING VS. RAST TESTING IN ALLERGIC DIAGNOSIS

Skin Test	RAST
Less expensive	No patient risk
Greater sensitivity	Patient convenience
Wide allergen selection	Not influenced by drugs
Results available immediately	Results are quantitative
Will detect non-IgE–mediated allergic reactions	Preferable to skin testing in certain patients: Patients with dermographism Patients with widespread dermatitis Uncooperative children

Table 37–3   COMPARISON OF ALLERGIC AND VASOMOTOR
(NONALLERGIC) RHINITIS

	Allergic	Vasomotor
Usual onset	Child	Adult
Family history of allergy	Usual	Coincidental
Collateral allergy	Common	Unusual
Symptoms		
Sneezing	Frequent	Occasional
Itching	Common	Unusual
Rhinorrhea	Profuse	Profuse
Congestion	Moderate	Moderate–marked
Physical examination		
Edema	Moderate–marked	Moderate
Secretions	Watery	Mucoid–watery
Nasal eosinophilia	Common	Occasional
Allergic evaluation		
Skin tests	Positive	Coincidental
IgE antibodies (RAST)	Positive	Coincidental
Therapeutic response		
Antihistamines	Good	Poor–fair
Decongestants	Fair	Poor–fair
Corticosteroids	Good	Poor–fair
Cromolyn	Fair	Poor
Immunotherapy	Good	None

common cold virus is the most frequent cause of upper respiratory infection, and at its outset a viral upper respiratory infection with its clear watery rhinorrhea and sneezing resembles allergic rhinitis. Redness of the nasal mucosa is characteristic of an upper respiratory infection and distinguishes it from allergic rhinitis. After several days the purulent nature of the nasal discharge clearly identifies the presence of infection or, in a confusing clinical situation, demonstration of the predominance of neutrophils on a smear of nasal secretions will confirm that impression. One must realize that nasal infections can be superimposed on allergic rhinitis.

Nasal obstruction and rhinorrhea, usually purulent, can also occur with foreign objects in the nares, but usually the symptoms are unilateral, and this differentiates the presence of foreign objects from allergic or infectious rhinitis. Nasal obstruction can also occur because of nasal polyps, which may not be associated with allergic disease but can be associated with cystic fibrosis or, rarely, with aspirin therapy. Polyps can usually be demonstrated by inspection and the use of a vasoconstrictor to reduce the local edema that may obscure the nasal polyps. Another cause for unilateral nasal obstruction may be deviation of the nasal septum or a neoplasm; both conditions are detectable upon visual examination of the nasal airway. Drugs administered systemically can simulate allergic rhini-

tis. Reserpine treatment of hypertension can produce nasal congestion, and a similar syndrome can be associated with the use of methantheline in the treatment of gastrointestinal disease and ulcers. The cessation of symptoms upon withdrawal of the drug will establish this diagnosis. The most common drug rhinopathy is rhinitis medicamentosa following topical administration of vasoconstrictors for more than three to five days. The mucosa becomes pale and edematous, quite similar to the situation seen in allergic rhinitis. It is important to question patients carefully to diagnose this condition, because some patients will consider the use of nose drops insignificant in their medical history. Frequently the seasonal allergic rhinitis or the upper respiratory infection for which the topical vasoconstrictor was initially applied has subsided by the time it is recognized that the problem is being perpetuated by the topical therapy. Another cause for nasal congestion is pregnancy, which may be considered in appropriate adolescent patients.

The above conditions can usually be differentiated from allergic rhinitis, but the separation of allergic from nonallergic perennial rhinitis and vasomotor rhinitis is often complicated. Nonallergic rhinitis may occur during childhood but more often is seen in adults. It simulates the perennial type of allergic rhinitis, but no immunologic etiology can be implicated. In nonallergic rhinitis, the edematous mucous membranes are often pale and eosinophilia may occasionally be present, but the usual methods of detecting a specific allergen and its mediating antibodies are unable to suggest a specific cause. Vasomotor rhinitis is a nonallergic form of persistent nasal disease also manifested by watery rhinorrhea and nasal obstruction. Vasomotor rhinitis is a vague category of chronic or intermittent nasal disease usually seen in older children and adults that does not lend itself to a specific definition. The patient complains of overresponsiveness of the nose to minimal changes of air temperature, obnoxious odors, and often change in position of the head. These patients seem to have unusual awareness of their symptoms and complain disproportionally to their magnitude. It is important to differentiate these patients with nonspecific, nonallergic rhinitis and vasomotor rhinitis from patients with allergic disease because of their different responses to therapy. Immunotherapy is not to be used in these diseases and drug therapy with antihistamine decongestants controls their symptoms inconsistently. As expected, these patients do not have historical or *in vivo* or *in vitro* tests to confirm allergic disease and eosinophilia is not as common a laboratory feature with this problem. A comparison of these different types of rhinitis is made in Table 37–3.

THERAPY

Successful therapy of allergic rhinitis involves three primary considerations: (1) identification and avoidance of the specific allergens and other contributory factors, (2) pharmacologic management, and (3) immunotherapy to alter the patient's immune response to the allergen.

Identification and Avoidance. Complete avoidance of the allergens is the best therapy for allergic disease because without exposure to allergens the allergic reaction will not take place. Once the specific allergens that are responsible for the symptoms are identified, each patient should make some effort to reduce the exposure to these allergens. Elimination of exposure to an animal dander by elimination of a feather pillow or removal of a pet from the house or elimination of a food allergen from the diet may provide complete or partial relief of symptoms. Avoidance of

more ubiquitous allergens such as pollens, dust, and molds may be more difficult. Patients who are sensitive to grass pollens should avoid increased exposure through gardening and grass cutting during the grass pollen season. Camping trips and picnics in the countryside should be postponed by ragweed-sensitive patients during the ragweed pollen seasons until another time of the year. Pollen rubbed into the nose and eyes can produce severe local edema, a point particularly important to remember in dealing with children, who often play outdoors in close contact with pollinating plants; patients should avoid direct contact with pollinating plants. House dust control measures, especially in the bedroom, can be a quite effective treatment for certain patients. These measures include providing rubberized or plastic airtight enclosures for mattresses and box springs; the use of synthetic bedding fabrics; and the removal of stuffed toys or stuffed furniture, heavy drapery, and dust catchers, such as book shelves and record cabinets, from the bedroom.

Environmental control measures should also include removal of hair carpet underpads and if feasible, sealing of the forced-air heating ducts and vents in the bedroom. Thorough weekly cleaning and vacuuming of the bedding and rugs in the bedroom effectively reduces the house dust allergen concentration. Electrostatic precipitrons can be installed in central forced-air heating and cooling systems, and these can substantially reduce not only house dust but also pollens and other airborne particles. Single-room air conditioners, which recirculate the air, can also effectively reduce pollen in the bedroom. Because single-room electrostatic precipitron units are less effective and may generate irritating ozone, they are not recommended. Mold-sensitive patients should be advised against raking leaves since the outdoor molds, especially Alternaria and Hormodendrum, thrive on dead leaves and cut vegetation. Damp basements and wallpaper, as well as glass-enclosed shower stalls, are often sources of molds in the home, and removal of the source of moisture will eliminate mold proliferation. If the moisture cannot be eliminated, mold retardants can be incorporated into the house paints or used in washing the walls. Molds in damp basements can be reduced by aerosolized paraformaldehyde or other antifungal agents. Unfortunately,

Table 37–4   REPRESENTATIVE ANTIHISTAMINES FOR
THERAPY OF ALLERGIC RHINITIS

Generic Name	Brand Name	Sedative Effect
Alkylamines		
Chlorpheniramine	Chlortrimeton	Mild
Dexchlorpheniramine	Polaramine	Mild
Brompheniramine	Dimetane	Mild
Triprolidine	Actidil	Mild
Ethylenediamines		
Tripelennamine	Pyribenzamine	Moderate
Methapyrilene	Histadyl	Moderate
Ethanolamines		
Diphenhydramine	Benadryl	Marked
Carbinoxamine	Clistin	Moderate
Doxylamine	Decapryn	Moderate

many patients do not have sufficient motivation to carry out adequate avoidance procedures in order to control their symptoms.

Pharmacologic Management. If the patient cannot completely avoid the allergen, the symptoms can be controlled with drugs in many cases. Antihistamines are preferred for treating mild to moderate allergic rhinitis. The antihistamines function by competing with histamine, the principal mediator of allergic rhinitis, for the H_1 cell receptor on endothelial and smooth muscle cells (Paton, 1973). There are several groups of antihistamines, which differ in chemical structure and in action (Table 37–4). Since the effectiveness of one group may diminish after several months or years of use, an antihistamine of another group may then be clinically efficacious. Therefore, the clinician should become familiar with the use of one or more antihistamines in each of the listed groupings. Chlorpheniramine or any of the several equivalents given early in the morning and at bedtime should provide good symptomatic control with the least number of side effects. Additional doses may be taken at four to six hour intervals. The effectiveness of antihistamines is sometimes interfered with by their side effects, which include drowsiness, headache, restlessness, nausea, and vomiting. These can sometimes be alleviated by switching to another group of antihistamines. Patients who become drowsy should be warned against driving an automobile or operating machinery after taking the medication and might be candidates for other modalities of therapy described below. When nasal obstruction by secretions is a prominent symptom, an alpha-adrenergic decongestant, such as phenylephrine, phenylpropanolamine, or cyclopentamine, should be used individually or in combination with an antihistamine to alleviate nasal mucosal engorgment, to decrease the nasal obstruction, and to improve the upper airway ventilation. Sometimes it is necessary to employ one or more trials of an antihistamine or antihistamine-decongestant combination in order to ascertain the most effective preparation for each patient. Topical nasal alpha-adrenergic vasoconstrictors usually provide prompt symptomatic relief but should not be used for more than several days. Many patients, after 7 to 10 days of using a topical decongestant, will develop so-called rebound vasodilatation and at times habituation. It is necessary to discontinue nose drops to relieve this "rhinitis medicamentosa."

If symptoms cannot be controlled with antihistamines, decongestants, and avoidance, several clinicians have suggested corticosteroid therapy. For pediatrics, the risk-to-benefit ratio of treating even severe allergic rhinitis with oral or parenteral corticosteroids is so high that we feel that they are usually contraindicated. However, aerosol topical corticosteroids, especially for short-term seasonal use, have proved useful in some patients. Beclomethasone, a poorly absorbed and rapidly metabolized topical corticosteroid, is currently enjoying considerable popularity in Europe for the treatment of allergic rhinitis without apparent systemic corticosteroid side effects (Mygind, 1973). This agent has been available in the United States for the treatment of bronchial asthma but is not yet released for the therapy of allergic rhinitis. The dose recommended by the European clinicians is 50 μg (one inhalation in each nostril) four times a day. Another topical aerosol pharmacologic agent available in Europe, but not yet available for the treatment of allergic rhinitis in the United States, is cromolyn sodium, which inhibits the release of mediators from mast cells. Although European investigators have found the drug to be effective in 75 per cent of patients treated, such high efficacy has not been reported in a recent study of allergic rhinitis patients in the United States (Handelman et al., 1977). If cromolyn does become available in the United States, its use will probably be limited to selected patients.

Immunotherapy. If symptomatic drug therapy and avoidance cannot adequately control symptoms or inadvertently provoke significant side effects, immunotherapy (hyposensitization) with allergen solutions may be indicated. Before proceeding with immunotherapy, the physician should institute a comprehensive investigation of the causative factors, and the patient's history of symptoms should be closely correlated with the presence of specific IgE antibodies, determined either by skin test results or by an *in vitro* radioimmunoassay (RAST). In several double-blind studies, immunotherapy or hyposensitization injections with solutions of pollen have been shown to be effective in reducing the symptoms of allergic rhinitis (Sadan et al., 1969). Studies of the clinical efficacy of nonpollen immunotherapy with house dust, molds, and animal dander allergens in perennial allergic rhinitis are not as conclusive as those reported for seasonal allergy (Norman, 1974). There is no place for immunotherapy with allergens that can be removed or avoided. This is especially true for food allergens. The use of animal danders for immunotherapy should be limited to those individuals, such as veterinarians and farmers, who cannot avoid exposure to animal products. Even though it is not known how immunotherapy promotes clinical improvement in allergic rhinitis, studies have shown a reasonable relationship between the higher doses of allergens administered, a decrease in specific IgE antibodies as measured by RAST over a period of months, an increase in IgG blocking antibodies, and a reduction in the release of leukocyte histamine *in vitro* (Patterson et al., 1978). After the decision is made to initiate immunotherapy, the clinician should carefully select the allergens to be employed. The

clinical history should be correlated with skin test results, and the magnitude of the local skin reaction should be a guide to the dose of allergen to initiate injection therapy. The clinician begins with relatively weak subcutaneous injections of aqueous- or alum-precipitated solutions of allergens. These are gradually increased in volume and concentration to the maximally tolerated dose as indicated by a moderate local reaction. It is imperative that the clinician does not induce systemic symptoms that provoke exacerbation of allergic rhinitis. After reaching the maximally tolerated dose, allergy injection therapy may be given on a perennial or year-round basis, during which the time interval between injections is increased from weekly to biweekly to monthly and given usually for several years. Another mode of immunotherapy is preseasonal weekly injections for several months prior to the season. Most patients with multiple seasonal sensitivities, certainly those with perennial allergic rhinitis, will more conveniently and practically be treated with a perennial schedule of injections approximately every four weeks. Immunotherapy may be expected to provide significant clinical improvement in 80 to 90 per cent of patients with pollen-induced allergic rhinitis. If improvement is not obtained after a two year trial with immunotherapy, the patient should be reevaluated, and discontinuation of immunotherapy should be considered. Duration of immunotherapy injections in patients who achieve clinical benefits is dependent upon the patient's overall clinical response. In the presence of clinical improvement, the patient should be given the opportunity to see if the clinical benefits are sustained after discontinuing the allergy immunotherapy. These patients should be given the opportunity to stop their immunotherapy after approximately five years of injections. Many children with allergic rhinitis tend to improve with time, but they are not "growing out" of the allergy because improvement is not related to physical growth but to an as yet undefined cause. It has been claimed that immunotherapy in children for seasonal allergic rhinitis may reduce their chances of developing pollen-induced asthma, but this report is open to many questions and has never been confirmed (Johnstone, 1957). In general, patients with seasonal allergic rhinitis are more responsive to immunotherapy than those with perennial allergic rhinitis.

The factors responsible for clinical improvement are multiple. Certain patients have exacerbations of symptoms after a spontaneous or induced remission for several seasons, and immunotherapy can be reinstituted without complication. Overall, the prognosis of allergic rhinitis, with or without therapy, is better than that for nonallergic and vasomotor rhinitis.

REFERENCES

Broder, I., Higgins, M. W., Mathews, K. P., et al. 1974. Epidemiology of asthma and allergic rhinitis in a total community, Tecumseh, Michigan. III. Second survey of community. J. Allergy Clin. Immunol., 53:127.

Brown, E. B., and Ipsen, J. 1968. Changes in severity of symptoms of asthma and allergic rhinitis due to air pollutants. J. Allergy, 41:254.

Bryan, M. P., and Bryan, W. T. K. 1969. Cytologic and cytochemical aspects of ciliated epithelium in the differentiation of nasal inflammatory disease. Acta Cytol., 13:515.

Caplin, I., Haynes, J. T., and Spohn, J. 1971. Are nasal polyps an allergic phenomenon? Ann. Allergy, 29:631.

Coca, A. F., and Cooke, R. A. 1923. On the classification of the phenomena of hypersensitiveness. J. Immunol., 8:163.

Cohen, C. 1974. Genetic aspects of allergy. Med. Clin. North Am., 58:25.

Connell, J. T. 1969a. Nasal mastocytosis. J. Allergy, 43:182.

Connell, J. T. 1969b. Quantitative intranasal pollen challenges. III. Priming effect in allergic rhinitis. J. Allergy, 43:33.

Coombs, R. R. A., and Gell, P. G. H. 1975. The classification of allergic reactions underlying disease. In Gell, P. G. H., Coombs, R. R. A., and Lachman, P. H. (Eds.). Clinical Aspects of Immunology, 3rd ed. Oxford, Blackwell Pub., p. 761.

Handelman, N. I., Friday, G. A., Schwartz, H. J., et al. 1977. Cromolyn sodium nasal solution in the prophylactic treatment of pollen induced seasonal allergic rhinitis. J. Allergy Clin. Immunol., 59:237.

Huggins, K. G., and Brostoff, J. 1975. Local production of specific IgE antibodies in allergic rhinitis patients with negative skin tests. Lancet, 2:148.

Ingall, M., Glaser, J., Meltzer, R. S., et al. 1965. Allergic rhinitis in early infancy: Review of the literature and report of a case in a newborn. Pediatrics, 35:108.

Ishizaka, K. 1976. Cellular events in the IgE antibody response. Adv. Immunol., 23:1.

Ishizaka, K., Ishizaka, T., and Hornbrook, M. M. 1966. Physicochemical properties of reaginic antibody. V. Correlation of reaginic activity with IgE globulin antibody. J. Immunol., 97:840.

Ishizaka, T., Sian, C. M., and Ishizaka, K. 1973. Mechanisms of passive sensitization. III. Number of IgE molecules and their receptor sites on human basophile granulocytes. J. Immunol., 111:500.

Johnstone, D. E. 1957. Study of the role of antigen dosage in the treatment of pollinosis and pollen asthma. Am. J. Dis. Child., 94:1.

Johnstone, D. E. 1969. Food allergy in children under two years of age. Pediatr. Clin. North Am., 16:211.

Kaliner, M. A., Wasserman, S. I., and Austen, K. F. 1973. Immunologic release of mediators from human nasal polyps. N. Engl. J. Med., 289:277.

Konton-Karakitsos, K., Salvaggio, J. E., and Mathews, K. P. 1975. Comparative nasal absorption of allergens in atopic and non-atopic subjects. J. Allergy Clin. Immunol., 55:241.

Levine, B. B., Strembas, R. H., and Fotino, M. 1972. Ragweed hayfever, genetic control and linkage to HL-A haplotypes. Science, 178:1201.

Lichtenstein, L. M., and Osler, A. G. 1964. Histamine release from human leucocytes by ragweed antigen. J. Exp. Med., 120:507.

Lieberman, P., Crawford, L., Bjelland, J., et al. 1974. Controlled study of the cytotoxic food test. J. Allergy Clin. Immunol., 53:89.

Marsh, D. G., Bias, W. B., and Hsu, S. H. 1973. Association of the HL-A7 cross reacting group with a specific reaginic antibody response in allergic man. Science, 179:691.

Marsh, D. G., Bias, W. B., and Ishizaka, K. 1974. Genetic control of basal immunoglobulin E level and its effect on specific reaginic sensitivity. Proc. Nat. Acad. Sci. USA, 71:3588.

Miller, D. L., Hirvonen, T., and Gitlin, D. 1973. Synthesis of IgE by the human conceptus. J. Allergy Clin. Immunol., 52:182.

Mygind, N. 1973. Local effect of intranasal beclomethasone aerosol in hay-fever. Br. Med. J., 4:464.

Norman, P. S. 1974. Specific therapy in allergy pro (with reservations). Med. Clin. North Am., 58:111.

Norman, P. S. 1978. In vivo methods of study of allergy: skin and mucosal tests, techniques and interpretation. In Middleton, E., Reed, C. E., and Ellis, E. F. (Eds.) Allergy: Principles and Practice, Vol. 1, St. Louis, The C. V. Mosby Co., p. 256.

Orange, R. P., Austen, W. G., and Austen, K. F. 1971. Immunologic release of histamine and SRS-A from human tissues. 1. Modulation by agents influencing cellular levels of cyclic 3-5-adenosine monophosphate. J. Exp. Med., 134:136.

Paton, W. D. M. 1973. Receptors for histamine. In Schacter, M. (Ed.) Histamine and antihistamines, Vol. 1, International Encyclopedia of Pharmacology and Therapeutics, Oxford, Pergamon Press.

Patterson, R., Lieberman, P., Irons, J. S., et al. 1978. Immunotherapy. In Middleton, E., Reed, C. E., and Ellis, E. F. (Eds.) Allergy, Principles and Practice, Vol. 2, St. Louis, The C. V. Mosby Co., p. 877.

Prausnitz, C., and Kustner, H. 1921. Studies uber Uberemphfindlichkeit, Centralbl. f. Baktinol. Abt. Orig., 86:160.

Rappaport, B. F., Sampter, M., Catchpole, H. R., et al. 1953. The mucoproteins of the nasal mucosa of allergic patients before and after treatment with corticotropin. J. Allergy, 24:35.

Richerson, H. B., and Seebohn, P. M. 1968. Nasal airway response to exercise. J. Allergy, 41:269.

Riley, J. F., and West, G. B. 1953. The presence of histamine in mast cells. J. Physiol. (London), 120:528.

Rundcrantz, A. 1969. Postural variations of nasal patency. Acta Otolaryngol., 68:1.

Sadan, N., Rhyne, M. B., Mellitis, E. D., et al. 1969. Immunotherapy of pollinosis in children. N. Engl. J. Med., 280:623.

Salvaggio, J. E., Cavanaugh, J. J. A., Lowell, F. C., et al. 1964. A comparison of immunologic responses of normal and atopic individuals to intranasally administered antigen. J. Allergy, 35:62.

Solomon, W. R., and Mathews, K. P. 1978. Aerobiology and inhalant allergens. In Middleton, E., Reed, C. E., and Ellis, E. F. (Eds.) Allergy, Principles and Practice, Vol. 2, St. Louis, The C. V. Mosby Co. p. 899.

von Pirquet, C. 1906. Allergie. Munch Med. Wochenschr., 53:1457.

Voorhorst, R., Spieksma, F. T. M., Varekamp, H., et al. 1967. The house dust mite (Dermatophagoides pteronyssinus) and the allergens it produces, identity with the house dust allergen. J. Allergy, 39:325.

Wasserman, S. I., Goetzl, E. J., and Austen, K. F. 1975. Inactivation of human SRS-A by intact human eosinophiles and by eosinophil arylsulfatase. J. Allergy Clin. Immunol., 55:72.

Wolf, S., Holmes, T. H., Treuting, T., et al. 1950. An experimental approach to psychosomatic phenomenon in rhinitis and asthma. J. Allergy, 21:1.

Yunginger, J. W., and Gleich, G. 1975. Impact and discovery of IgE in practice of allergy. Pediatr. Clin. North Am., 22:3.

INDEX

Page numbers in *italics* indicate illustrations. Page numbers followed by t indicate tables.

Branchial anomalies, 1393–1401
  of branchial arches, 1399
    cartilage, 1400, *1400*
  of branchial pouches, 1398
  of first branchial groove, 1393–1395, *1393*
    aplasia, 1393, *1393–1394*
    atresia, 1394
    duplication, 1394
    stenosis, 1394
  of second branchial groove, 1395–1398
    cyst, 1395, *1395*
    fistula, 1397
    sinus, 1396
Branchial apparatus, anomalies of. See *Branchial anomalies.*
Branchial arches
  in embryo, *6, 7*
  nerve supply of, 870t
Branhamella catarrhalis, otitis media and, 405
Breast-feeding, otitis media incidence and, 364, 365t
Brevicollis, 317
Bronchial congenital anomalies, 1237–1247
  abnormal bifurcation, 1242–1246
  agenesis, 1237, *1238*
  anomalous attachments, 1246
  atresia, 1237
  bronchial constriction, 1238
    bronchial hypoplasia, 1240
    bronchomalacia, 1240
    fibrous bronchostenosis, 1238, *1239*
    webs, 1238
  bronchial enlargement, 1240–1242
    bronchiectasis, 1240
    bronchogenic cysts, 1241–1242, *1242–1243*
    fistulas, 1242
    Kartagener syndrome, 1241, *1241*
  gastrointestinal tract attachments, 1247, *1246–1247*
  sequestered lung, *1245*, 1246
  tracheal, 1235
Bronchiectasis, 1258
  congenital, 1240
Bronchioles, development of, 1139
Bronchiolitis, 1255
Bronchitis, acute, 1254
Bronchomalacia, 1240
Bronchopneumonia, 1256
Bronchopulmonary dysplasia (BPD), 1213, 1273
  hyaline membrane disease and, 1208
Bronchoscope
  flexible, 1163, *1167*
  rigid, 1162
  size of, 1162t
  technique for introduction of, *1164*
Bronchoscopy, 1162–1168
  patient position for, *1163*
  preparation for, 1163
Bronchostenosis, fibrous, 1238, *1239*
Bronchus(i)
  anatomy and embryology of, 1138–1140, *1139, 1140*
  congenital anomalies of. See *Bronchial congenital anomalies.*
  foreign bodies of, 1302–1311
    incidence of, 1302–1304
    management of, 1306
      anesthesia in, 1307
      instruments for, 1307–1311

Bronchus(i) (*Continued*)
    pathophysiology of, 1304
    patient's history and clinical examination of, 1305
    radiographic assessment of, *1303*, 1305, *1305*
    symptoms and signs of, 1304t, 1306t
  obstruction of, dysphagia and, 909
  stridor and, 1194
  tumors of, 1318–1319
    adenoma, 1318
    fibroma, 1318
    lipoma, 1319
Brow, lacerations of, repair of, 821
Brucella, infection with, 1405
Brucellosis, 1404
Bullar furrows, 671, *672*
Burns
  electrical, 1115–1118, *1116–1117*
    facial, 809. See also *Facial injuries.*
  esophageal. See *Esophageal burns.*
  respiratory complications of, 1266–1267

Calculus, 941, *942*
Caldwell roentgenographic projection, *697*, 698
Caldwell-Luc antrotomy, 841
Calvarium, postnatal growth of, 23
Canal of Huguier, 104
Cancrum oris, 1016
Candida albicans
  oral candidiasis caused by, 977
  oropharyngeal manifestations of, 1007
Candidiasis
  mucocutaneous, oropharyngeal manifestations of, 1008
  oral, 977
Canker sores, recurrent, 976
Carcinoma. See also *Neoplasm* and *Tumor.*
  acinous cell, 1030
  epidermoid, of mouth, 1049
  mucoepidermoid, 1030
  nasal, 840
  squamous cell, of neck, 1435
Caries
  dental, 938, *939.* See also *Teeth, disorders of.*
  nursing bottle, 938
Carnegie system of classification, 1135
Carotid artery
  anomalies of, 333
  anomalous, in middle ear, 312
  injury of, 1422
  internal, aneurysm in, 312
Carotid artery systems, epistaxis and, 719, *720, 725*
Carotid body tumor, 318
Carotid sheath, 1365
Cartilage
  craniofacial
    basisphenoid, *10*
    prenatal, *9*
  cricoid, *1271–1272*
  skeletal growth and, 20, *21*
  tracheal, congenital deformity of, 1230
Cat-scratch disease, 1408
Catarrhal rhinitis, chronic, 716
Cauterization, epistaxis management and, 723

Equilibrium responses, 207, *208, 209*
Erythema multiforme, 1018
Eskimos
  otitis media incidence in, 361
  otorrhea incidence in, 360t
Esophageal burns, 1083–1092. See also *Esophagitis.*
  clinical categories of, 1086
  corrosives and, 1084–1092
    effect of on esophagus, 1084
    types of, 1084, 1085t
  diagnosis of, 1087
  history of, 1083
  incidence of, 1083, *1084*
  laws and, 1083
  management of, 1087–1092
    acute, 1087
    later, 1088–1091
      esophageal dilatation for, 1088, *1089–1090*
      gastrotomy for, 1089
      psychiatric consultation for, 1089
      retrograde bougienage for, 1090, *1090*
  pathology of, 1084–1086
    stages of, 1086
Esophageal strictures, acquired, 1092–1093
Esophagitis. See also *Esophageal burns.*
  complicated, management of, 1091
  diagnosis of, 1087
    esophagoscopy for, 1088
  types of, 1086
  uncomplicated, management of, 1087–1091
Esophagoscopes, removal of esophageal foreign bodies
    and, 1101, *1101–1102*
Esophagoscopy, 893–896
  complications of, 1106
  in esophagitis, 1088
  injuries from, 1114
  with flexible esophagoscope, *895*
  with rigid esophagoscope, *894–895*
Esophagram
  examination of neck and, 1374
  for dysphagia, 908
Esophagus
  anatomy and embryology of, 873
  atresia of, 874, *874*
  burns of. See *Esophageal burns.*
  congenital defect of, dysphagia and, 904
  congenital malformations of, 1053–1064
    esophageal atresia, 874, *874*
    esophageal duplication, 1061
    esophageal hiatal hernia, 1062
      diagnosis of, 1063
      treatment of, 1064
  disorders of, otalgia and, 221
  examination of, 891–896
    esophagoscopy in, 893–896, *894–895*
    radiographic, 891–893, *891–893*
  foreign bodies of, 1095–1108
    case histories of, 1106–1109
    duration of obstruction of, 1099
    endoscopic procedure and, 1099–1105
      selection of instruments for, 1101–1104,
        1101–1105
    esophageal status and, 1098, *1099*
    incidence of, 1095
    nature of, 1095–1098, *1096–1098*
    patient's history and, 1095
    radiography and, 1099

Esophagus (*Continued*)
    foreign bodies of, signs and symptoms of, 1095
      technique for removal of, 1105–1106
  functional abnormalities of, 1067–1081
    achalasia and, 1074–1076, *1075–1077*
    causes of, 1070t
    congenital esophageal stenosis and, 1078,
      1079–1080
    esophageal atresia and, 1071–1074, *1072–
      1073*
    esophageal spasm and, 1077
    gastroesophageal reflux and, *1080*, 1081
    manometry in, 1067–1069, *1068, 1072–1073*
    swallowing and, 1069–1071
    tracheoesophageal fistula and, 1071–1074,
      1072–1073
  injuries to, 1111–1119
    from accidents, 1111–1115
      animal bite, 1115
      endoscopic, 1114
      gunshot and knife, 1114
      vehicular, 1111–1112
    from chemicals, 1119
    from smoke and fire, 1118
  lesions of, dysphagia and, 910
  neurologic disorders of, 1128–1130, *1129*
  obstruction of, dysphagia and, 909
  physiology of, 877
  stricture of, 892, *893*
  vascular compression in, 874
Essential tinnitus, 274
  diagnostic criteria for, 274t
Ethmoidal sinuses. See *Sinus(es), ethmoid.*
Ethmoiditis
  acute, exophthalmos and, 742, *742*
  sinus infection and, 785
Eustachian tube
  abnormal function of, 369
  abnormal patency of, 397, *397*
  anatomy of, 366–369, *366, 367, 368, 369*
  anomalies of, 335
  catheterization, 377, *377*
  clearance function of, 370–375
  dysfunction of
    allergy and, 398, *399*
    cleft palate and, 399, *400*
    diagnosis of, 423
    hearing loss and, 58
    nasal obstruction and, 398
    related to abnormal conditions, 393–401,
      394
    symptoms of, 358
    vertigo and, 262
  embryology and development of, 90–91, *92*
  obstruction of, 393–397
    cholesteatoma and, 532
    functional, 394, *395*
    mechanical, 395, *396*
  pathogenesis of middle ear disease and, 369
  physiologic functions of, 370, *370*
  protective function of, 370–375
    model of, 373–375, *374, 375*
  testing of function of, 401–402
  ventilatory function of, 375–393
    assessment of, 375–377
    physiology of, 391–393, *392*, 392t
    tests of, 377–391

Hypopharynx (*Continued*)
  examination of, 890, *890*
    radiographic, *890*, 891
Hypoplasia
  of bronchial cartilage, 1240
  defined, 42
Hypoplastic anemia, congenital anomalies and, 323
Hyposalivation, 1026
Hypothalamus, acetylcholine production and, 685, 706
Hypoventilation, alveolar, surgical treatment of, 1001
Hypovolemia, salivation and, 1026

Iatrogenic ototoxicity, diseases of, 327
Ice cold caloric (ICC) irrigation, 210
Idiopathic diffuse interstitial fibrosis of lung, 1276
Idiopathic facial paralysis, 218
Idiopathic nasal disease, rhinorrhea and, 716
Idiopathic thrombocytopenia, oropharyngeal
    manifestations of, 1010
IgA, nasal production of, 686
    inflammatory nasal disease and, 711
IgE, nasal production of, 686
    allergic rhinitis and, 712
Immotile cilia syndrome, 785
  otitis media management and, 497
Immune response, acute otitis media with effusion
    and, 414–416
Immune system, defects in, otitis media and, 417
Immunity, defined, 850
Immunization, for diphtheria, 986
  Schick test for, 986
Immunoglobulin(s)
  allergic rhinitis and, 851, *852*
  nasal physiology and, 686
  properties of, 852t
  pulmonary production of, 1150
  role of in otitis media, 411
Immunoglobulin A (IgA), nasal production of, 686
    inflammatory nasal disease and, 711
Immunoglobulin E (IgE), nasal production of, 686
    allergic rhinitis and, 712
Immunology
  defined, 850
  of chronic otitis media with effusion, 416
  of otitis media, 410–413
    problems in study of, 410
  of pharynx, 411
Immunotherapy, in allergic rhinitis treatment, 860
Impedance, acoustic, 118–121, *119, 120*
    measurement of for hearing assessment, 162–164
Impedance bridge, *378*
  acoustic middle ear reflex and, 19
  tympanometry and, *164*, 165
Incisions, placement of in cosmetic surgery, 749–751,
    750
Incomplete morphogenesis, 41
Incudostapedial malunion, 325
Incus
  anomalies of, 330
  development of, 94
  dislocation of, traumatic, *630*
  folds of, 96
  surgical repair of, *342, 343*
Indians, American, otitis media incidence in, 361
Induction, genetic, 16

Infant(s)
  auditory responses of, 154
  hearing loss treatment plan for, 243, 248–251
  otitis media in, 361
Infant nutrition, middle ear disease and, 364t
Infection(s)
  lower respiratory. See *Lower respiratory infections.*
  prenatal, diseases associated with, 326
  upper respiratory. See *Upper respiratory infections.*
Infectious mononucleosis. See *Mononucleosis, infectious.*
Inflammatory nasal disease, 710–713
Inflation-deflation test of tympanic membrane,
    378–384, *378–383*
  eustachian tube dysfunction and, 400
  eustachian tube function and, 390, *390*
  instrumentation used in, *379*
Infundibulum, 670, 674
Injury. See also under specific site of injury.
  cosmetic surgery following, 747
    incision placement in, 751, *752*
Inner ear
  congenital problems of, 577–588
    acquired, 586
    genetic counseling for, 588
    pathoembryology of, 577–580, *578, 579*
  development of, *102–103*
  diseases of, 577–601. See also *Sensorineural deafness.*
    organ of Corti and, *578, 579*
  embryology and development of, 104–111
  sound transmission and, 121–123, *122*
Inspiration, physiology of, 1144
Internal carotid artery aneurysm, 312
Intracranial suppurative complications of otitis media
    and mastoiditis, 565–575, *566,* 567t
  brain abscess, 570, *571*
  extradural abscess, 568
  focal otitic encephalitis, 569
  lateral sinus thrombosis, 571
  meningitis, 567
  otitic hydrocephalus, 572
  subdural empyema, 569
Intramembranous ossification, 20, *21*
Intranasal cavity, 679
Intraoral soft tissue wounds, repair of, 821
Intratemporal complications and sequelae of otitis
    media, 513–561, *514.* See also under names of
    specific middle ear dysfunctions.
Intratympanic muscles, anomalies of, 333
Intrauterine infection, sensorineural hearing loss and,
    586
Isoniazid, 1407

Jackson, Chevalier,
  bronchoscopy and, 1302
  tracheotomy technique of, 1326
Jaw
  disorders of, otalgia and, 217
  tumors of
    benign, 1046
    malignant, 1049
Jervell and Lange-Nielsen syndrome, 584
Jugular bulb
  anomalies of, 33
  herniation of, 312
  high, 332

Neck (*Continued*)
  tumors of, fibrosarcoma, 1433
    hemangioendothelioma, 1436
    hemangiopericytoma, 1436
    incidence of, 1425t
      Hodgkin lymphoma, 1426–1428
      non-Hodgkin lymphoma, 1428–1430
    malignant melanoma, 1435
    neuroblastoma, 1433–1435
      clinical presentation of, 1433
      evaluation of, 1434
      pathology of, 1434
    rhabdomyosarcoma, 1431–1433, 1432t
      clinical presentation of, 1431
      evaluation of, 1432
      pathology of, 1431
    squamous cell carcinoma, 1435
    thyroid carcinoma, 1430–1431
      clinical presentation of, 1430
      evaluation of, 1431
      pathology of, 1430
Neck masses, 1379–1385
  congenital lesions and, 1379
    physical characteristics of, 1380t
  cystic hygroma and, 1380
  dermoid cyst and, 1381
  diagnosis of 1379–1383
    differential, 1384t–1385t
    by history, 1380t
    by location, 1382t–1383t, *1382*
    by physical characteristics, 1381t
  hemangioma and, 1381
  laryngocele and, 1381
  teratoma and, 1381
  thyroglossal duct cyst and, 1380
Neck reflex
  asymmetric tonic, 204, *204*
  symmetric tonic, 205, *205*
Neck righting reflex, 204, *204*
Necrotizing external otitis, 561
Necrotizing otitis media, 362
Needle aspiration
  examination of neck and, 1377
  suppurative adenitis and, 1403
Neisseria gonorrhoeae, pharyngitis caused by, 987
Neonatal respiratory diseases, 1205–1214
  acute, 1205–1213
    apnea, 1213
    atelectasis, 1210
    congenital diaphragmatic hernia, 1212
    diaphragmatic paralysis, 1213
    hyaline membrane disease, 1205–1208
      clinical presentation of, 1206
      complications of, 1207–1208
      pathophysiology of, 1205
      prevention of, 1208
      treatment of, 1206
    lobar emphysema, 1211
    meconium aspiration, 1209
    persistent fetal circulation, 1209
    pneumonia, 1209–1210
      Group B streptococcal, 1209
      nursery-acquired, 1210
    pneumothorax, 1212
    pulmonary cysts, 1211
    pulmonary hemorrhage, 1211
    transient tachypnea, 1208

Neonatal respiratory diseases (*Continued*)
  chronic, 1213–1214
    bronchopulmonary dysplasia (BPD), 1213
    Mikity-Wilson syndrome, 1214
  pathophysiology of, 1205
Neonate
  auditory responses of, 153
  complications from intubation of, 1271
  hearing loss treatment plan for, 241–243
  hoarseness in, 1183
  lip and palate of, development and anatomy of, 868
  nasal obstruction in, 708
  otitis media in, 361
  otitis media with effusion in, bacteriology of, 409
  respiration of, 684
  respiratory diseases of. See *Neonatal respiratory diseases.*
  swallowing mechanism in, 905
  tracheotomy on, *1330*
  vocal cord paralysis in, 1282
Neoplasia, hamartomas and, 41
Neoplasm. See also *Tumor* and *Carcinoma.*
  biopsy of, 643
  external ear. See *External ear, tumors of.*
  lymphoreticular, 640
  nasal cavity, rhinorrhea and, 715
  orbital, exophthalmos and, 743, *743, 744*
  salivary gland, 1029–1032
    benign, 1030
    in children, 1030t
    malignant
      high-grade, 1031
      low-grade, 1030
    metastatic, 1032
  temporal bone. See *Temporal bone, tumors of.*
Nerve. See under names of specific nerves.
Nerve supply, nasal, 682
Nerve tissue, tumors originating in, 640
Nervous system
  auditory. See *Auditory nervous system.*
  vocal cord paralysis and disorders of, 1279t
Neural crest cells, embryonic, *8, 9*
Neuralgia, aural, otalgia and, 222
Neuroblastoma
  of neck, 1433–1435
  olfactory, nasal obstruction and, 715
Neurocranium, prenatal, 9
Neurofibromatosis, 1125
  laryngeal, 1220, 1315
  oropharyngeal manifestations of, 1009
Neurologic examination, neurovestibular testing and, 202–204, 202t, 203t
Neuromas, acoustic, sensorineural hearing loss and, 591, *592*
Neuromusculature, facial, growth of, 29, *30*
Neuropathologic deficiencies, dysphagia and, 905, 909
Neuropore, anterior, in embryo, *6, 7*
Neurovestibular system
  embryology of, 200
  methods of examination of, 201–204
  patient's history for examination of, 199t
Neurovestibular testing, 199–211
Noma, 1016
Nonauditory tinnitus, 273
  myogenic causes of, 274
Nonchromaffin tympanojugular paraganglioma, 318
Nonselective immunologic degranulation, 687

Temporal bone (*Continued*)
  tumors of, epidermoid, 641
    metastatic, 639
    symptoms of, 642t
Temporal hypothesis of frequency discrimination, 130
Temporal lobe epilepsy, dizziness and, 267
Temporomandibular joint
  disease of, headache and, 734
  disorders of, otalgia and, 217
Tensor tympani, 93
  anomalies of, 333
  trauma to, 631, *631*
Tensor veli palatini muscle, 368, *369*
Teratogen, genetic induction and, 16, *16*
Teratoma, neck mass and, 1381
Tessier, Paul, 67
Tetanus, otogenous, otitis media and, 408
Tetanus immunization, neck injuries and, 1415
Thalidomide ototoxicity, 327
Therapy, auditory, 600
Third aortic arch, embryonic development of, 14
Thoracic duct, injuries of, 1422
Threshold of hearing, 112, *113*
  audiogram and, 159
Throat. See also under names of specific structures of
      throat.
  infections of, tonsillectomy and, 999
Throat cultures, pharyngitis and, 899
Thrombocytopenia, idiopathic, oropharyngeal
      manifestations of, 1010
Thrombosis, lateral sinus, 571
Thyroglossal duct cysts
  location of, 1400t
  neck mass and, 1380
Thyroid, lingual, 919
Thyroid carcinoma, 1430–1431
Thyroid function tests, hearing loss and, 239
Thyroid gland
  development of, 869
  disorders of, otalgia and, 221
  embryology of, 1359, *1359*
  injuries of, 1422
  palpation of, 1372, *1372*
Tinnitus, 271–276
  auditory system evaluation and, 273
  classification of, etiologic, 273–276
  ear disease diagnosis and, 139
  essential, 274
  Meniere disease and, 265
  objective, 271, 273–275
  ototoxic agents causing, 276t
  patient's history and, 272
  subjective, 272, 275
  vascular, 273
    causes of, 274t
Tissue
  embryonic craniofacial, 9
  mesenchymal, 20, *21*
    cellular migration in, 9
Tomographic sections
  coronal, 191–193, *192*
  parasagittal, 193–194, *193, 194*
Tomography, 190–195, *191*
  for exophthalmos, 739
  hoarseness and, 1188
Tongue
  anatomy and embryology of, 868–870, *869*

Tongue (*Continued*)
  burn injuries to, 1113
    electrical, 1115–1118, *1116–1117*
    smoke and fire, 1118
  congenital abnormalities of, 919–921, *919–922*
  examination of, 883
  geographic, 1017
  neurologic disorders of, 1126
Tongue-tie, 919
Tonsil(s)
  development and structure of, 872
  diseases of, otalgia and, 219
  lymphoma of, *884*
Tonsillectomy and adenoidectomy, 992–1004
  adverse effects of, 1003
  Children's Hospital of Pittsburgh study of, 997–1000
    criteria for entering, 998t
    criteria for exclusion from, 999t
    findings of, 999
  clinical indications for, 995
    currently acceptable, 1000
  clinical trials of, 995
  contraindications to, 1002, *1003*
  controversy regarding, 995
  cost vs. benefits of, 996, 997t
  frequency of, 994t
  history of, 992–994
  hospital care for, 1004
  otitis media management by, 486–494, *487*
    Children's Hospital of Pittsburgh study of, 490
    clinical trials of, 487–490, 487t, 488t, 489t
    effect of on eustachian tube function, 490–494,
        494–493
Tooth. See *Teeth.*
Tooth germ, deciduous, fetal, *11*
TORCH studies, hearing loss and, 239
Torticollis, paroxysmal, dizziness and, 268
Total communication, defined, 1576
Towne projection radiograph, 189, *189*
Toxoplasmosis, 1407
Toynbee phenomenon, 398, *398*
Toynbee test, 376, *376*
  eustachian tube function and, 387–389, *389*
Trachea
  anatomy and embryology of, 1138–1140, *1139, 1140*
  congenital defect of, dysphagia and, 904
  congenital malformations of. See *Tracheal congenital
      malformations.*
  examination of, neck palpation and, 1154
  foreign bodies of, 1302–1311
    incidence of, 1302–1304
    management of, 1306
      anesthesia in, 1307
      instruments for, 1307–1311
    pathophysiology of, 1304
    patient's history and clinical examination of, 1305
    radiographic assessment of, *1303*, 1305, *1305*
    symptoms and signs of, 1304t, 1306t
  obstruction of, dysphagia and, 909
  physiology of, 1146
  stridor and, 1194
  tumors of, 1316–1318, 1316t
    chondroma, osteochondroma and osteoma, 1317
    incidence of, 1317t
    papilloma, 1316
    tracheopathia osteoplastica, 1317
Tracheal congenital malformations, 1225–1237